The respiratory tract is commonly affected by infectious disease, and care of patients presenting with such illness ideally requires co-ordinated multidisciplinary teamwork. Such teams are managed by physicians with a breadth of knowledge spanning numerous specialities, which include infectious disease, tropical medicine, thoracic medicine, radiology, microbiology, surgery, paediatrics and intensive care. This volume collects together expertise from these fields and beyond, to provide a comprehensive reference source for all involved in the diagnosis and care of patients with respiratory infection.

Within three parts, the coverage includes both the upper and the lower respiratory tracts. A thorough overview of laboratory and radiological diagnostic methodology, pulmonary defence mechanisms and antimicrobial therapy provides the introduction. This is followed by coverage of major respiratory pathogens; each chapter forms a complete information dossier, detailing the full range from epidemiology and microbiology through to immunopathology and clinical management. Chapters in the third part serve to elaborate and emphasise key points by focusing on major respiratory syndromes and special situations such as paediatric problems, HIV, intensive care, cystic fibrosis and foreign travel.

This book is highly illustrated throughout, with clear, comprehensive and detailed coverage, and is sure to be a welcome and invaluable resource for all those concerned with appropriate and effective care of infectious disease within the respiratory tract.

Infectious diseases of the respiratory tract

To Belinda

Infectious diseases of the respiratory tract

EDITED BY MICHAEL E. ELLIS
KING FAISAL SPECIALIST HOSPITAL AND
RESEARCH CENTRE, RIYADH, SAUDI ARABIA

CAMBRIDGE
UNIVERSITY PRESS
1998

PUBLISHED BY THE PRESS SYNDICATE OF THE UNIVERSITY OF CAMBRIDGE
The Pitt Building, Trumpington Street, Cambridge CB2 1RP, United Kingdom

CAMBRIDGE UNIVERSITY PRESS
The Edinburgh Building, Cambridge CB2 2RU, United Kingdom
40 West 20th Street, New York, NY 10011-4211, USA
10 Stamford Road, Oakleigh, Melbourne 3166, Australia

First published 1998

Printed in the United Kingdom at the University Press, Cambridge

Typeset in Monotype Ehrhardt 9/12 [TAG]

A catalogue record for this book is available from the British Library

Library of Congress Cataloguing in Publication data

Infectious diseases of the respiratory tract / edited by Michael E.
Ellis.
p. cm.
Includes index.
ISBN 0 521 40554 8 (hardback)
1. Respiratory infections. I. Ellis, Michael E.
[DNLM: 1. Respiratory Tract Infections–diagnosis. 2. Respiratory
Tract Infections–therapy. WF 140 1427 1997]
RC740.I54 1997
616.2–dc21
DNLM/DLC
for Library of Congress 97–3051 CIP

Contents

Contributors

JONATHAN COURIEL
Department of Paediatrics, Booth Hall Children's Hospital, University of Manchester School of Medicine, Charlestown Road, Blackley, Manchester M9 7AA, UK

MARY DODD
Bradbury Cystic Fibrosis Unit, Wythenshawe Hospital, Southmoor Road, Manchester M23 9LT, UK

J. GRAHAM DOUGLAS
Department of Thoracic Medicine, Aberdeen Royal Infirmary, Foresterhill, Aberdeen AB9 2ZB, UK

MICHAEL E. ELLIS
Department of Medicine, King Faisal Specialist Hospital and Research Centre, Riyadh 11211, Saudi Arabia

JAMES A. R. FRIEND
Aberdeen Royal Infirmary, Foresterhill, Aberdeen AB9 2ZB, UK

RICHARD FROTHINGHAM
Division of Infectious Diseases and International Health, Department of Medicine, Duke University Medical Center, Durham VA Medical Center, 508 Fulton Street, Building 4, Durham, NC 27705-3875, USA

MONICA GRANDIEN
Department of Virology, Swedish Institute for Infectious Disease Control, 105 21 Stockholm, Sweden

A. D. HARRIES
Department of Medicine, Queen Elizabeth Central Hospital, PO Box 95, Blantyre, Malawi, Central Africa

JAVED KHAN
King Fahad National Guard Hospital, Riyadh, Saudi Arabia

MATS KALIN
Department of Infectious Diseases, Karolinska Hospital, S-171 76 Stockholm, Sweden

PETER McARTHUR
Department of Medicine, King Faisal Specialist Hospital and Research Centre, Riyadh, 11211, Saudi Arabia

J. T. MACFARLANE
Nottingham City Hospital, Hucknall Road, Nottingham NG5 1PB, UK

DAVID S. McKINSEY
Department of Epidemiology and Infectious Diseases, Research Medical Center, Kansas City, Missouri, USA

GARY MILLER
King Faisal Specialist Hospital and Research Centre, Riyadh 11211, Saudi Arabia

JAMES MOORECROFT
Bradbury Cystic Fibrosis Unit, Wythenshawe Hospital, Southmoor Road, Manchester M23 9LT, UK

EDMUND L. C. ONG
Infectious Diseases Unit, University of Newcastle Medical School, Newcastle General Hospital, Newcastle upon Tyne E4 6BE, UK

CHRISTOPHER M. PARRY
Wellcome Trust Clinical Research Unit, Centre for Tropical Diseases, Cho Quan Hospital, 190 Ben Ham Tu, Quan 5, Ho Chi Minh City, Vietnam, and Nuffield Department of Clinical Medicine, John Radcliffe Hospital, Headington, Oxford OX3 9DU, UK

BJORN PETRINI
Department of Microbiology, Karolinska Hospital, S–171 76 Stockholm, Sweden

HAROLD H. REA
King Faisal Specialist Hospital and Research Centre, Riyadh 11211, Saudi Arabia

HERBERT Y. REYNOLDS
Department of Medicine, The Milton S. Hershey Medical Center, The Pennsylvania State University, PO Box 850, Hershey, PA 17033, USA

P. VENKATESAN
Department of Infection and Tropical Medicine, Birmingham Heartlands Hospital, Birmingham B9 5ST, UK

NEIL V. L. WARAVDEKAR
Division of Pulmonary and Critical Care Medicine, Department of Medicine, The Milton S. Hershey Medical Center, The Pennsylvania State University, PO Box 850, Hershey, Pennsylvania 17033, USA

JOHN M. WATSON
Communicable Disease Surveillance Centre, Colindale, London NW9 5EQ, UK

ANTHONY K. WEBB
Bradbury Cystic Fibrosis Unit, Wythenshawe Hospital, Southmoor Road, Manchester M23 9LT, UK

JAMIE WEIR
Department of Radiology, Aberdeen Royal Infirmary, Foresterhill, Aberdeen AB9 2ZB, UK

ATHOL U. WELLS
Department of Respiratory Medicine, Green Lane Hospital, Auckland, New Zealand

M. J. WOOD
Department of Infection and Tropical Medicine, Birmingham Heartlands Hospital, Birmingham B9 5ST, UK

Preface

Infectious diseases of the respiratory tract are ubiquitous in all medical and surgical specialties, present a challenge in precise diagnosis and management, and are among the leading infectious causes worldwide of substantial morbidity and mortality both inside and outside hospital.

Patients who develop respiratory infection present various scenarios to a variety of physicians and specialties. For example, individuals with long-standing chronic lung disease such as chronic obstructive airways disease or cystic fibrosis may well be referred to a pulmonologist when they develop an infective exacerbation. A patient may develop pneumonia at home or in a residential institution – a generalist is often involved initially. At the other extreme, a hospitalised patient, on an intensive care unit for example, with nosocomial pneumonia will initially be managed by an intensivist. Non-infectious pulmonary disease may masquerade as pneumonia. These patients require a careful differential diagnostic approach, often under the direction of a general physician or pulmonologist. Returning foreign itinerants with fever and respiratory symptoms may have acquired a variety of travel-associated microbial illnesses – the expertise of the infectious disease specialist may then be called upon. However, the onus of diagnosis and management may be placed on any physician, depending upon the local medical care structure.

This text was therefore produced for a wide range of physicians who wish to equip themselves with a current comprehensive, clinically orientated source book on respiratory infections. Its primary objective is to provide a critically written reference source rather than a didactic step-by-step practical handbook, although practical aspects of clinical presentation and management are fully covered.

The first section contains overviews of four major areas. The initial chapter describes the current status of microbial diagnosis. This is followed by a comprehensive review of the application of radiological science and the major radiological features of pulmonary infections. These two chapters provide virtual self-contained summaries of these two areas. The third chapter overviews the current status of respiratory defence mechanisms. The major classes of antimicrobials are discussed in the concluding chapter of this first part. Part two expounds respiratory disease on a pathogen-by-pathogen or pathogen group basis. The third part describes the major respiratory syndromes and elaborates on differential disease settings such as intensive care and the challenge of the patient with chronic pulmonary infiltrates. Aspects of unusual or new agents and the changing characteristics of established pathogens are addressed.

Each chapter contains salient epidemiological and microbiological features, clinical presentation, radiological features, clinical and antimicrobial management, preventive and current status comments, as appropriate Most chapters are 'self-contained'. However, a degree of overlap does occur and is intentional, since this provides slightly different perspectives, serves to underscore important points or provides a succinct summary or overview, as in the case of the chapter on radiology.

In order to achieve an optimal balanced presentation and expert presentation of the field, contributors were chosen for their strong interest or acknowledged activity in their particular areas. All are currently actively involved in the clinical care of patients with respiratory infection They emanate from different parts of the globe as far afield as USA and New Zealand. Ten infectious diseases specialists and nine pulmonologists have contributed the majority of the chapters. Particular subspecialty expertise has been sought from the fields of immunology, surgery, intensive care, microbiology and radiology.

Considerable indebtedness is due to James Friend for his enthusiasm, helpful wisdom and comments, to Jocelyn Foster of Cambridge University Press, for her continued support throughout, and to Bernadette Martinez, Secretary of her Department of Medicine at the King Faisal Specialist Hospital and Research Centre who has laboured many hours with the manuscript preparation.

I would like to thank Belinda McBain for designing the cover logo which depicts *Aspergillus*.

Part 1: Diagnosis, host defence and antimicrobials

1 The laboratory diagnosis of respiratory infections

MATS KALIN*, MONICA GRANDIEN† and BJÖRN PETRINI*
Karolinska Hospital, Stockholm, Sweden; †Swedish Institute for Infectious Disease Control, Stockholm, Sweden

Introduction

Aetiological diagnoses in respiratory tract infections may be achieved by identifying the causative agent, antigenic subcellular products or specific nucleic acid sequences from that agent present in material from the infectious site. The aetiology may also be demonstrated by the finding of an antibody response to the infectious agent.

The process of diagnosing respiratory infections is complicated by the great diversity of microbial agents involved. Hence, a multitude of different methods for the identification of different types of bacteria, viruses, fungi, protozoa and helminths are available, and the problem of choosing the appropriate tests in the clinical setting at hand is often significant. Although diagnostic efforts may be limited because of the trivial nature of the infection or the availability of reasonably effective empirical therapy, an aetiological diagnosis is often indicated.

In addition to the great variety of microbial agents of potential importance in airway infections, a further problem is the existence of an abundant indigenous bacterial flora of the oral cavity, posing difficulties for obtaining uncontaminated specimens. It is often difficult to conclude whether identified microbial agents are the cause of an ongoing infectious process or merely colonisers of the oropharynx. For most viral agents as well as for *Legionella pneumophila*, *Mycobacterium tuberculosis*, *Pneumocystis carinii* and pathogenic dimorphic fungi the mere identification of the respective agent in respiratory tract secretions is considered to be a proof of ongoing disease with that agent. Atypical mycobacteria and opportunistic fungi as well as the common respiratory tract pathogens *Streptococcus pneumoniae*, *Haemophilus influenzae* and *Moraxella catarrhalis* often colonise the pharynx and a diagnosis cannot be based on their mere presence in airway secretions. The same is true for *Staphylococcus aureus* and Gram-negative rods, which are especially common in hospital-admitted patients. Even *Mycoplasma pneumoniae* and *Chlamydia pneumoniae* may be found in throat samples without relation to current disease, because they may be carried in asymptomatic individuals for many months after a clinical disease[1–3]. In the examples of *Candida* and cytomegalovirus even their presence in the distal airways is by no means invariably diagnostic of an ongoing infection, and a diagnosis must rest on other criteria, such as histopathology.

Considering the mentioned facts, it is evident that very sensitive methods such as the polymerase chain reaction (PCR) must be used judiciously when airway secretions are used to establish an aetiological diagnosis. Uncontaminated material may be obtained by aseptic aspiration of pleural, paranasal sinus, or middle ear effusions. Also, percutaneous fine-needle aspiration of a pneumonic process gives essentially uncontaminated material. Blood cultures are an important source for establishing the causative agent in severe respiratory tract infections, especially in severe cases of pneumonia, sinusitis and epiglottitis. In epiglottitis caused by *H. influenzae* type B the organism is almost always found in blood, and pneumococcal pneumonia is bacteraemic in about 25% of cases[4–8].

For lower respiratory tract infections numerous studies have shown that the number of disease-causing bacteria in pulmonary infections is at least 10^5, most often 10^6–10^8 cfu/ml of respiratory tract secretions[9–16]. Use of quantitative culture techniques with cut-off levels of10^5–10^6 cfu/ml will therefore contribute to an increased specificity if specimens are obtained in such a way that the presence of contaminating bacteria in concentrations exceeding this level is minimised. This can be achieved with transtracheal aspiration (TTA), percutaneous lung puncture, bronchoscopic protected specimen brush (PSB) and bronchoalveolar lavage (BAL). With sputum specimens, contamination is much more difficult to avoid, since the number of bacteria colonising the oropharynx may substantially exceed 10^6 cfu/ml. 'Routine' sputum cultures may therefore be very misleading and cannot be recommended. In contrast, the combined interpretation of Gram's stain and quantitative culture, preferably after washing of the specimen, makes sputum examination a reliable diagnostic method if the patient can deliver a purulent sample[9,17–20].

With all kinds of specimens the sensitivity of culture is seriously reduced if sampling is performed after the start of antibiotic therapy[6,10–12,21,22]. Blood and sputum cultures (as well as sputum Gram's stain) are almost meaningless, even after a few doses of antibiotics, and the yield of invasive methods such as TTA and bronchoscopy is also significantly reduced. Furthermore, false-positive cultures are more commonly encountered in patients on antibiotics, due to the frequent overgrowth of more resistant, potentially pathogenic bacteria[6,12,23].

This chapter is divided into four separate sections, each addressing a major group of aetiological agents, namely bacteria, fungi, viruses and mycobacteria. The reader should cross-refer to the relevant clinical chapters.

BACTERIAL INFECTION

Microbiological diagnosis of bacterial upper respiratory tract infections

Pharyngitis

Antigen detection methods
The most important objective with the aetiological diagnostic procedures for pharyngitis is to differentiate bacterial infection due to group

A streptococci from viral infection. Today several rapid immunological tests are available for the detection of the cell wall polysaccharide specific for group A streptococci from material collected by a throat swab. A result can be obtained while the patient is waiting in the clinic or the physician's office. The antigen detection tests that were first developed during the 1980s were based on an agglutination reaction, and were often difficult to interpret, especially for non-laboratory personnel. Modern tests are usually based on enzyme immunoassays and most often give very clear-cut results. The tests have become more simple and practical to use and the sensitivity has been increased.

The specificity of the antigen detection tests used today is usually close to 100%, but sensitivity has often been considerably lower[24,25] (Fig. 1.1). Compared to an optimised culture technique the sensitivity may be as low as 31–50%[25,26]. However, for patients with abundant growth it is over 80%, and it has been claimed that lower counts are usually seen in carriers. The test would then detect most clinical infections, but would not be useful for detection of asymptomatic carriage. Since a serological response is seen almost as frequently with a low as with a high bacterial count, the assumption that a negative antigen test in combination with a positive culture is characteristic of carriage rather than infection may not hold true.

From the above it is clear that if an antigen detection method is to be used, a positive test should usually be considered as diagnostic for group A streptococcal pharyngitis, whereas a negative one does not exclude a streptococcal aetiology. Therefore, patients with positive results should always be treated with antibiotics. For patients with negative tests different strategies may be used in different clinical settings, depending on the prevalence of streptococcal aetiology in the patient material seen, the performance of the used rapid test in the hands of the technician or nurse responsible for it and on the availability of culture facilities. It has been shown that the number of colonies isolated upon culture seems to be almost uniformly (87%) high during the first 36 hours after onset of the pharyngitis, and thereafter falls[26]. Antigen detection tests may then possibly be used for both diagnosing and excluding group A streptococcal infection if the patient is seen within two days after onset of the disease, whereas later

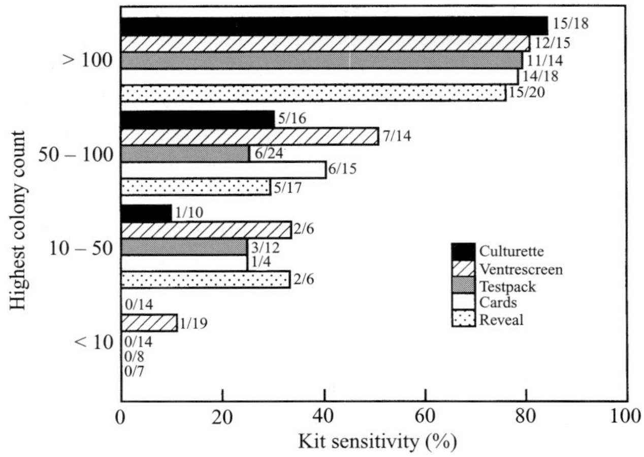

FIGURE 1.1 Streptococcal antigen detection kit sensitivity at different colony counts obtained by pharyngeal culture. Reproduced from Wegner *et al.* 1992 with permission.

in the course a negative antigen test must be interpreted cautiously. The co-operation with a clinical microbiological laboratory to check the specificity and sensitivity on a regular basis is recommended.

Culture

For definitive identification of group A streptococci in the pharynx, culture must be undertaken. Although rather conflicting results concerning the optimal culture technique have been obtained, several points are agreed[25–27]: (1) the specimen must be meticulously collected from tonsils, arches and the uvula in order to avoid false-negative results; (2) sheep blood agar incubated for 48 hours anaerobically or in a CO_2-containing atmosphere seems to give the best sensitivity. Incorporation of gentamicin, crystal violet or trimethoprim–sulphamethoxazole in the medium has been used to inhibit normal or colonising non-streptococcal flora, but the possible advantage of this remains unclear; (3) 48 hours of incubation is necessary; the plates should be read after both one and two days; and (4) training and quality control must be implemented. Even with these measures some 5% will probably be missed, but this figure may be much larger with, for example, one day aerobic blood agar.

A significant increase in the streptolysin-O titre can be measured in about a third of cases with light growth of *Streptococcus pyogenes* in throat culture and half of those with heavy growth[24,28]. It is assumed that those without antibody increase are colonised and not infected. However, the practical usefulness of antibody testing is limited by the fact that both acute- and convalescent-phase sera must be obtained and separated within 2–3 weeks. Antibody analyses are therefore helpful only in very special cases and for research purposes.

Streptococci other than group A may be more easily detected by the use of anaerobic culture conditions. Group C and G streptococci can definitely cause bacterial pharyngitis, but the risk of complications is minimal. The tendency today, therefore, is to optimise the diagnostic procedures used for detection of group A streptococci and give less attention to the identification of other streptococci.

More unusual causes of bacterial pharyngitis can be detected only by the use of special techniques and these agents must therefore be suspected on clinical grounds and their identification requested when the specimen is sent to the laboratory. The most important agent to suspect is *Corynebacterium diphtheriae*, which can be detected from an ordinary throat swab with the use of special media[29]. Also *Arcanobacterium hemolyticum*[30] and *Neisseria gonorrhea* may be found by culture on special media. Vincent's angina is diagnosed by microscopy of a direct smear. Diagnostic procedures for viruses, chlamydia and mycoplasma that can also cause pharyngitis are discussed below.

Acute otitis media

Because of the limited number of species involved and the good results achieved with empirical therapy, acute otitis media (AOM) is most often managed without attempts to obtain an aetiological diagnosis[31–33]. In cases of spontaneous perforation of the tympanic membrane a specimen for culture may be obtained from the external auditory canal, although contamination with skin flora may cause difficulties in interpretation. A definitive aetiological diagnosis can be obtained by culture of middle ear effusion after tympanocentesis. This procedure may be used in special cases such as patients with severe disease, infections in immunocompromised patients, therapeutic failure or rapidly recurrent infection. In the future PCR determinations on middle ear fluid may be an alternative method for diagnosis[34].

Sinusitis

A number of different agents may cause sinusitis. Acute community-acquired maxillary sinusitis is caused by *S. pneumoniae* or *H. influenzae* in about half of the cases, while a few per cent of the cases are caused by *M. catarrhalis*, *Streptococcus pyogenes*, *S. aureus* and Gram-negative enteric rods. Viral agents may be isolated simultaneously with bacteria or may occur in patients who have no bacterial growth. *C. pneumoniae* seems to be responsible for some cases of sinusitis. In chronic sinusitis and in sinusitis emanating from dental foci, anaerobic bacteria are relatively more important. Hospital-acquired sinusitis has been noted during recent years[35] and in these infections Gram-negative enteric bacteria and *Pseudomonas* spp. are often incriminated. Finally, several fungal species may cause sinusitis, both nosocomial and community-acquired. All these agents cannot be detected with the regular diagnostic set-ups commonly used. Instead, diagnostic efforts must be directed at identifying clinically relevant agents.

In most cases of acute community-acquired sinusitis no attempt to achieve an aetiological diagnosis is made, but the patient is treated empirically. Specimens for culture may be obtained in patients with severe disease, therapeutic failure or severe pain demanding relief. In patients with underlying or complicating conditions an aetiological diagnosis may be more urgently needed. Fungal infections cannot be adequately managed without an established aetiological diagnosis. Histopathology is often more sensitive than culture and provides vital information more rapidly.

Although the bacteria causing sinusitis probably originate from the nose and nasopharynx, these sites are also frequently colonised by several potentially pathogenic bacteria that cannot be excluded as aetiological agents. Therefore, there may be a dilemma in the interpretation of the significance of a culture. Also, specimens obtained by rinsing through the natural sinus ostium or by endoscopy generally give unreliable information, due to contamination. Only specimens obtained by sinus puncture are acceptable for obtaining an aetiological diagnosis based on culture. Aspirated material should be transported promptly to the microbiological laboratory for culture. Since anaerobic bacteria may be very sensitive to oxygen, the material should be cultured preferably within a few hours after sampling. Pending culture the material must be kept in an oxygen-free environment. This is best achieved by keeping the material in the syringe used during the aspiration with the needle closed by a rubber stopper.

Microbiological diagnosis of bacterial infections of the lower respiratory tract

Gram's stain and culture of sputum

In patients admitted with community-acquired pneumonia, examination of sputum is the basic procedure in the diagnostic work-up, but its usefulness has been seriously questioned[36]. It is evident that in many patients the disease-causing bacteria cannot be identified in sputum[6,36–8]. The reason for this is that many patients with pneumonia, especially elderly and seriously ill patients, fail to produce or expectorate any sputum, and others can produce only non-purulent specimens or have received antibiotics prior to sampling, in all of which circumstances Gram's stain and culture are considerably less informative[6,22].

Disease-causing bacteria identified by percutaneous lung aspiration are often found at the same frequency in simultaneously obtained sputum specimens, although a mixture of 3–5 bacterial species emanating from the oropharyngeal flora is a common finding[37]. Also, when results of blood culture and transtracheal aspirate culture are compared, it has been found that bacteria incriminated in a pneumonic process are usually present in concomitantly obtained sputum specimens, although within a mixture of pharyngeal flora[9,39–42].

The question then is whether pulmonary pathogens may be identified within the often abundant oropharyngeal flora. It has been shown that potentially pathogenic bacteria identified by TTA are more often found in purulent than in non-purulent sputum[39,43]. The extent of oropharyngeal contamination can easily be estimated in a Gram's stained smear of the specimen, from the proportions of leukocytes emanating from the infectious process and squamous epithelial cells emanating from the oropharynx (Fig. 1.2). Specimens containing only epithelial cells consist primarily of saliva. Such specimens should not be subjected to culture; the bacteria from the oropharyngeal flora outnumber any bacteria from the pneumonic process too extensively for any meaningful information to be available upon culture. Different criteria for assessing sputum purulence have been used, but there is general agreement that leukocytes should outnumber squamous epithelial cells, preferably by a factor of 2.5 or more[15,43].

In patients not treated with antibiotics and capable of producing a purulent sputum specimen, the Gram's stained smear should also be used to arrive at a presumptive diagnosis. The Gram's stain is rapid, simple, essentially specific (90%) and of a reasonable sensitivity (60–85%)[15,18,44,45]. Bacteria should be looked for with the oil immersion objective (× 1000) and only in purulent parts with no squamous epithelial cells, since the great number of oropharyngeal bacteria adjacent to such cells may interfere with the interpretation of the Gram's stain (Fig. 1.3). The use of Gram's stain is also important for increasing the yield by the cultural procedure: the sensitivity can be increased by directing the search for bacteria on the culture plates by the findings in the purulent parts of the Gram's stained smears[15,18,46] (Fig 1.4). Therefore, if Gram-positive lanceolate diplococci have been identified in the Gram's stain, one should look for colonies of *S. pneumoniae* when reading the culture plates; and if Gram-positive cocci in clusters or small Gram-negative coccobacilli have been identified, staphylococci and *H. influenzae*, respectively, should be looked for. The specificity of a cultural finding can be increased by support from a Gram's stained smear[17], which may be particularly important for diagnosing *M. catarrhalis* infections[47–49]. The use of Gram's stain as a basic procedure is important, since all potentially pathogenic bacteria may be presumptively identified and reported. Anaerobic bacteria may also be indicated by a Gram's stain finding, although their presence must be established by an invasive method rather than by sputum culture.

A further improvement of the accuracy of sputum Gram's stain and culture may be obtained by applying a washing procedure before processing the specimens[9,19]. By use of a quantitative culture technique it

Table 1.1. *Approximate numbers of bacteria in respiratory secretions and specimens (cfu/ml)*

	Before washing	After washing	Dilution factor	Threshold significant finding	Number in pneumonic process diagnosed
Aerobic bacteria in oropharynx	10^7	$<10^5$			
Pneumonic process	10^6				
Sputum	10^6	10^6			10^6
Protected specimen brush			10^3	10^3	10^6
Bronchoalveolar lavage			10–10^2	10^4–10^5	10^6

has been demonstrated that washing the sputum samples vigorously with tap water in an ordinary tea strainer (Fig. 1.5, Table 1.1) eliminates more than 99% of the total number of contaminating oropharyngeal bacteria, while the number of disease-causing micro-organisms is unaffected. Since the number of contaminating bacteria from the oropharynx is greatly reduced by the washing procedure, the identification of the disease-causing bacteria is facilitated both in the Gram's stains and on the culture plates. About 10^6 cfu/ml has been found of the disease-causing bacteria both in washed and in unwashed sputum as well as in parallel transtracheal aspirates[9]. Performing sputum cultures quantitatively with a cut-off limit of 10^5–10^6 cfu/ml therefore further increases the specificity and facilitates the reading of the culture plates.

By washing the sputum specimens and by using the Gram's stain information, both for preliminary identification and for the definitive identification of the bacteria by culture, the accuracy of both the rapid and the definitive aetiolgical diagnosis is optimised. The system facilitates the isolation of all disease-causing bacteria, which may then be subject to susceptibility-testing – important for almost all species. So-called 'routine' sputum cultures without any of these procedures can be very misleading, with a high percentage of both false-negative and false-positive results. They are, therefore, not helpful in the management of the patient and constitute laboratory work with a high cost: benefit ratio.

However, even with extensive laboratory efforts the diagnostic

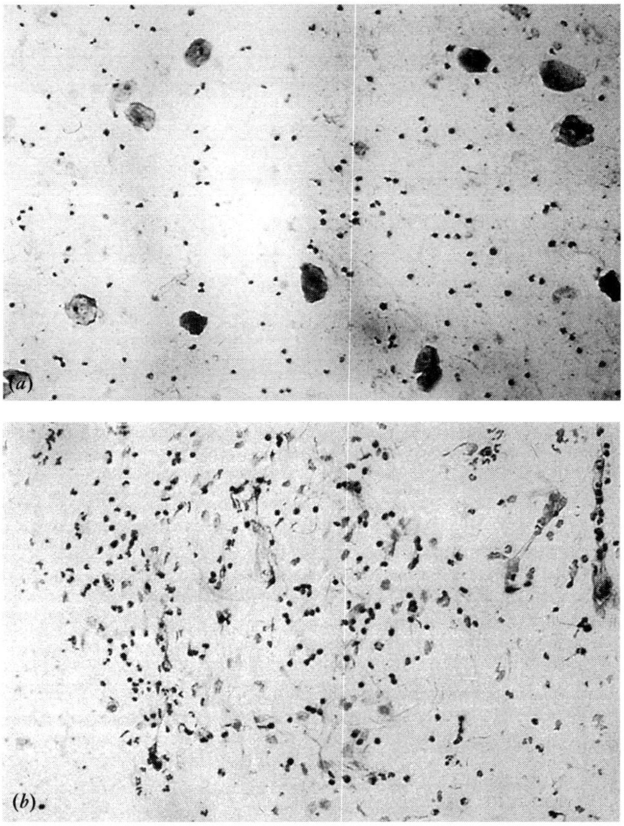

FIGURE 1.2 Sputum Gram's stain × 100 magnification. (*a*) Mixture of leukocytes emanating from the infectious process and squamous epithelial cells emanating from the oropharynx; and (*b*) only leukocytes; bacteria should be looked for in such areas.

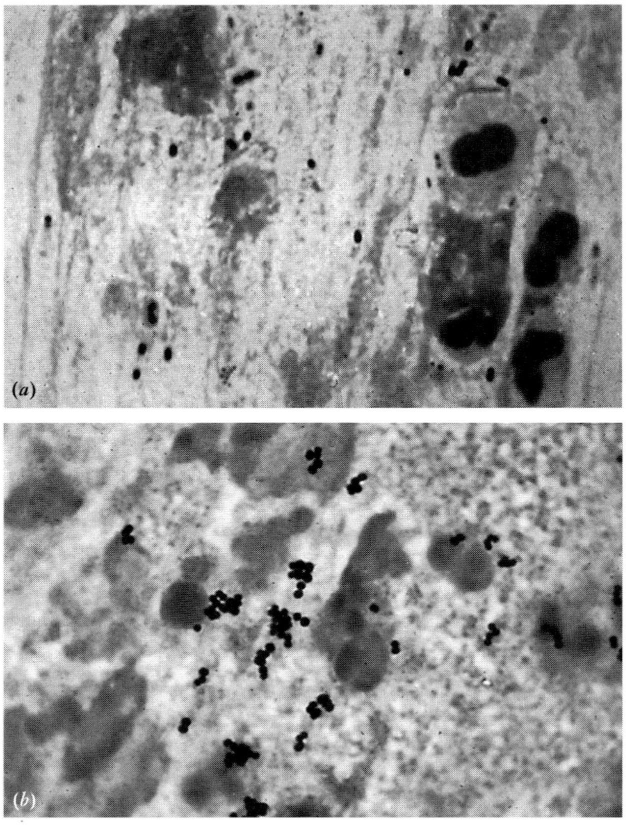

FIGURE 1.3 Sputum Gram's stain × 1000 magnification (*a*) Many Gram-positive lanceolate diplococci, i.e. *Streptococcus pneumoniae*, in purulent part of a Gram's stain. It is necessary to look for bacteria only in parts containing polymorphonuclear cells but no squamous epithelial cells. (*b*) *Staphylococcus aureus* in purulent part of sputum specimen.

yield from a sputum specimen is dependent on its quality. Good specimens can often be collected early in the morning. The patient must be instructed and helped to produce a sputum sample after deep cough. Specimens that consist of saliva alone or are heavily contaminated with saliva should be discarded and a new attempt to obtain a purulent sample made. Hypertonic saline inhalation and physiotherapist assistance may sometimes produce such a specimen. Saline injection through lamina cricothyroidea is a very effective way of producing a deep cough and hence adequate material, and seems to be free of complications[50]; this technique should probably be used more frequently. Patients with acute exacerbation of chronic bronchitis generally produce more purulent sputum samples than do non-bronchitic patients with pneumonia. A good, purulent specimen can be obtained from 50–75% of patients admitted with pneumonia[6].

When a purulent sample has been obtained, the jar must not be left with the patient, but transported to the microbiological laboratory as soon as possible. Two to five hours at room temperature may be enough to cause a reduction in the number of disease-causing bacteria and increase in the number of contaminants[51]. If the specimen cannot be transported promptly it should be kept at +4 °C. The use of culture media that are optimised for isolation and identification of the most important micro-organisms involved is essential, but details are discussed elsewhere[52].

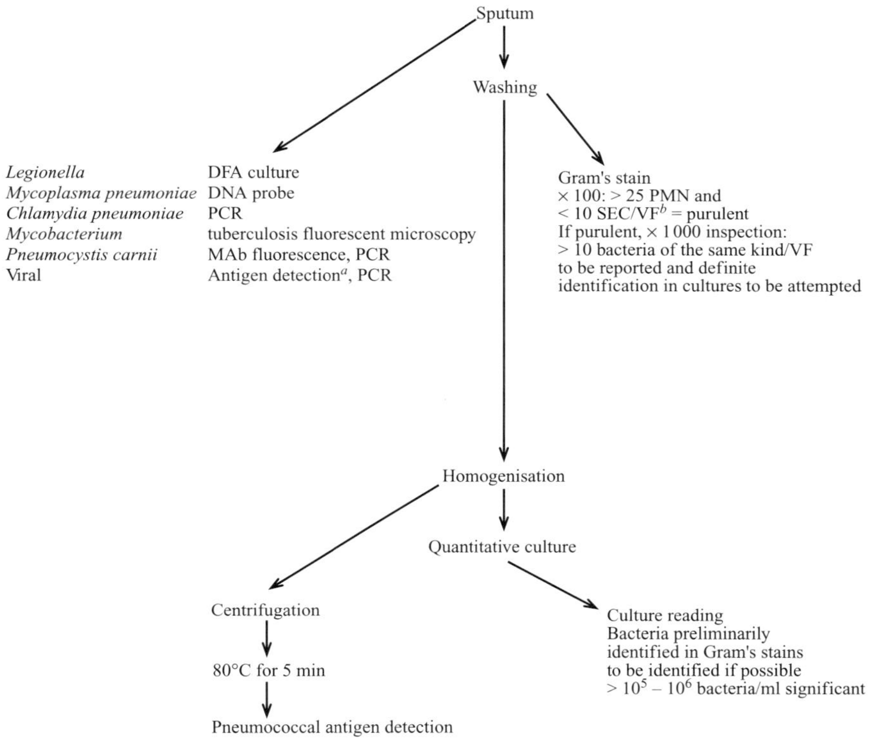

FIGURE 1.4 Algorithm for sputum processing. The different rapid methods can be used as needed, but the Gram's stain should be the basic procedure in all cases. DFA, direct fluorescence antibody; PCR, polymerase chain reaction; MAb, monoclonal antibody; [a]nasopharyngeal specimens preferred; [b] > 25 polymorphonuclear leukocytes and < 10 squamous epithelial cells per visual field.

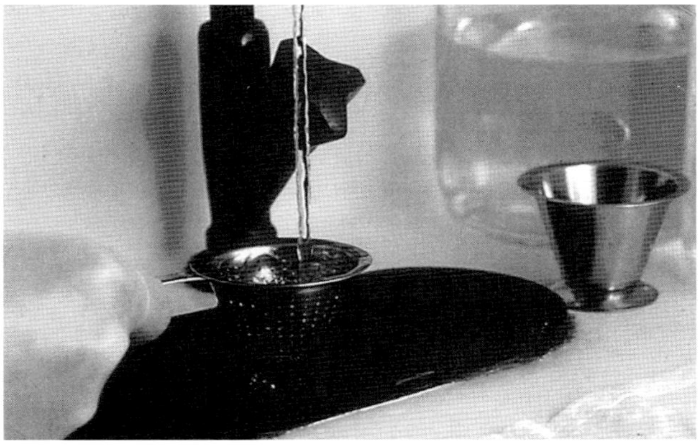

FIGURE 1.5 For washing, sputum is placed in an ordinary tea strainer and washed quite vigorously with tap water. With this procedure more than 99% of the oropharyngeal flora is eliminated, but the number of bacteria from the pneumonic process remains unchanged.

In patients with chronic bronchitis it is often difficult to determine the role of bacteria during exacerbations. Sputum culture results are notoriously difficult to interpret[53,54]. Quantitative bacterial cultures also have been found almost useless for establishing the diagnosis of a bacterial infection in patients with chronic obstructive pulmonary disease (COPD). However, Gram's stain of sputum, by revealing increased numbers of polymorphonuclear leukocytes and increased numbers of bacteria within purulent parts of the smear may be a better indicator of bacterial involvement[17,55]. The number of bacteria per oil immersion field should be more than ten, but most often many more bacteria are present.

For establishing the aetiology of nosocomial pneumonia, sputum culture and Gram's stain must be used with caution, since high numbers of potentially pathogenic bacteria are often found in the pharynx of hospitalized patients and it may be impossible to differentiate these from disease-causing bacteria. Gram's stain-directed quantitative culture from washed specimens may be usable in some settings, but has not been evaluated. Instead, invasive methods are advocated.

Antigen and DNA detection

As stated above, Gram's stain and culture are almost useless as diagnostic methods if the patient has already been started on antibiotics. Soluble pneumococcal polysaccharide antigen, on the other hand, may be detected for several days after initiation of antimicrobial therapy[8,15,45,50,56–60]. Polysaccharides are released in the airways from overproduction and from lysed pneumococci and are distributed widely in body fluids. The antigen concentration decreases only slowly after initiation of antibiotic treatment[57,61–63]. It has been known since the beginning of the century that capsular polysaccharides may be detected in serum and urine from many patients with pneumococcal disease. In the 1970s immunological methods that permitted more rapid and sensitive detection as well as detection of antigen in sputum specimens were developed[61,64–66].

Most pneumococcal antigen detection methods have been developed for the identification of the capsular polysaccharides, but examination for the species-specific cell wall C-polysaccharide is at least theoretically more attractive, with a lower risk of cross-reactions with contaminating bacteria[67–69]. Since there are 84 different capsular polysaccharides, the antisera to be used have to be directed against 84 different antigens for capsular polysaccharide detection. In contrast, for detection of the species-specific C-polysaccharide only one antibody specificity is needed in the reagent. In a few studies antibodies against only the most prevalent capsular types have been included in the antiserum used; thus the sensitivity and probably also the specificity has been increased[59, 70].

Several immunological methods have been used for pneumococcal antigen detection, including coagglutination, latex agglutination, counterimmunoelectrophoresis (CIE), or enzyme immunoassays (EIA)[8,45,50,56,60,61,65,66]. The agglutination tests are easy and rapid to perform, so a result can be reported within an hour after receipt of the specimen, i.e. at the same time as Gram's stain results. Since culture results are available only after 1–3 days, the rapid tests may give important preliminary information of value in the immediate management of the patient. If sputum is homogenised for quantitative culture as described above, a sputum antigen detection method can easily be included in the laboratory routines (Fig. 1.4). It is also important to note that the polysaccharide antigen concentration seems not to be affected by the sputum washing procedure described above[19, 58].

With sputum specimens from patients with pneumococcal pneumonia the sensitivity of the antigen detection methods has varied between 40 and almost 100%[6,8,50,56,58–60,69,71]. Reasons for the different sensitivities include the use of different methods, but also different criteria for diagnosing pneumococcal pneumonia. False-positive antigen findings occur, but in most studies of pneumonia the frequency has been low. In fact, contamination with saliva seems to be less important for the specificity of antigen-detection methods than for sputum Gram's stain and culture, and antigen detection has been found to produce reasonably accurate results also with non-purulent sputum specimens from pneumonia patients[6, 68, 69]. For the aetiological diagnosis of bacterial bronchitis, however, the results of antigen detection seem to be unreliable[61].

In most settings pneumococcal polysacharide antigen detection in serum and urine have contributed little to the diagnosis[6,57,60]. It has been shown by use of sensitive and quantitative EIA that the amount of antigen released into the circulation and the speed of clearance from the body is extremely variable for different types and in different patients, despite similar clinical presentations and courses[59]. With sensitive methods most bacteraemic and many non-bacteraemic patients may be diagnosed by examination of serum and urine[59,70]. Such methods are valuable for scientific purposes, but are most often considered to be too laborious for routine diagnostic purposes. Detection of antigen in serum or urine is most often considered to be specific, but children who are carriers and those who have otitis media had positive results in 4–16%[72]. In cases in which pleural fluid is present, it may be used for antigen detection with a higher sensitivity than culture[66].

For other species of classical bacteria, few usable antigens have been identified. The developement has been hampered by the lack of a gold standard for establishing the aetiology in pneumonia. *H. influenzae* type B capsular polysaccharide antigen is an exception and may be detected in serum, urine or sputum by use of simple immunological methods[73,74]. However, due to the low prevalence of *H. influenzae* type B as the cause of pneumonia in most clinical settings, it is not a cost-effective test.

Probes and PCR

Due to the frequent colonisation of the oropharynx with common respiratory bacterial pathogens, very sensitive methods such as PCR applied on sputum must be used cautiously. However, in a small study the results seemed promising[75]. Applied on serum, PCR may well be a useful method in the future, as is indicated by the recently described PCR method for identification of the pneumolysine and autolysine genes[76, 77]. Also, middle-ear fluid may be a useful material for PCR[34].

Serology

Diagnosis of infections with classical bacteria by demonstrating an antibody response has sometimes been accomplished for scientific purposes, but no method has been established as a routine. Usable antigens are less well defined and antibody responses are often late and irregular. In pneumococcal infections an antibody response is seen against both the capsular polysaccharide and the species-specific pneumolysin, but the sensitivity is rather low and paired sera separated by at least 10 days are needed[78–80]. Mixtures of outer membrane proteins have been used for serological diagnosis of *H. influenzae* infection, but their great diversity is a problem[81]. Whole bacterial cells have been used for demonstration of an antibody response in *Branhamella* infections[48,82]. None of these methods is close to being adopted as a routine method to be used in the clinical management of the patient.

Invasive methods for diagnosis of pulmonary infections: overview from a microbiology perspective

Invasive diagnostic techniques for the aetiological diagnosis of lung infections may be considered for three main groups of patients: (1) community-acquired pneumonia; (2) hospital-acquired, in particular ventilator-associated, pneumonia; and (3) immunocompromised patients with new or changing chest X-ray infiltrates.

Community-acquired pneumonia is most often managed outside hospital with no or minor diagnostic efforts. Also, in admitted patients empiric antimicrobial therapy is generally successful, and invasive diagnostic methods are too expensive and laborious as well as too uncomfortable and risky to the patient to be indicated for a majority of these patients. There is no question that the percentage of cases with a defined aetiology can be increased by the use of invasive diagnostic methods[10,83–85], but the cost-effectiveness and the risk:benefit ratios most often do not justify the use of them. Invasive methods may then be used in selected patients with severe disease or those not responding to therapy. The indications are increased if there are reasons to suspect tuberculosis, *P. carinii* or pathogenic fungi. In patients with AIDS and pulmonary disease, bronchoscopy is the established method to detect not only *P. carinii*, but also mycobacteria, *Cryptococcus*, *Histoplasma*, *Toxoplasma*, *Legionella*, cytomegalovirus and more common bacterial infections[86–90]. In cases in which a tumour or a foreign body is suspected bronchoscopy should be promptly performed.

For hospital-acquired pneumonia in non-ventilated, non-immunocompromised patients, the indications are similar to those in community-acquired pneumonia, although generally the patients are more seriously ill and the prognosis is worse. Colonisation with potentially pathogenic bacteria, especially Gram-negative rods, is also more common, and results from sputum culture are less reliable[91]. Invasive techniques may therefore be considered for many patients with hospital-acquired pneumonia. Today, the use of these methods is most often limited to patients who fail to respond to primary empirical antibiotic therapy, but widened indications may well be warranted[11,92–94]. In contrast, in ventilated patients a more aggressive diagnostic aproach has become a routine in many centres[11,93].

In immunocompromised patients with pulmonary infiltrates a wide variety of aetiological agents with different prognoses and treatments may be involved[11,95–100]. The choice of empirical therapy on clinical grounds is often difficult and because of the patient's abnormal host defences therapeutic failure may be life-threatening. Aggressive diagnostic efforts are therefore often warranted.

Therefore, invasive diagnostic methods for chest infections are most urgently needed in immunocompromised and in seriously ill, often ventilated, patients. These patients often have seriously abnormal laboratory parameters and therefore lung puncture or TTA may be dangerous. Serious bleeding diathesis, severe hypoxaemia, inability to co-operate and artificial ventilation preclude the use of these two methods. In contrast, none of the mentioned underlying conditions are absolute contraindications for fibreoptic bronchoscopy without biopsy, although all but mechanical ventilation make bronchoscopy more risky[95]. Although both TTA and especially lung puncture have been used in children[101], bronchoscopy during short anaesthesia is the preferred method. Further, bronchoscopy with, as needed, PSB, BAL and transbronchial biopsy (TBB), is the method of choice for several special pathogens such as *P. carinii*, *Mycobacterium tuberculosis*, pathogenic fungi, cytomegalovirus (CMV) and other herpesviruses. The procedure can be carried out during short anaesthesia and therefore also in patients who cannot co-operate. In ventilated patients bronchoscopy is simple to perform and is today being used with increasing frequency. There is an extensive literature on the indications and technical aspects of bronchoscopy in ventilator-associated pneumonia[11, 95, 102]. Generally, bronchoscopy has been found to contribute significantly to the aetiological diagnosis[103].

It should be noted in this context, however, that TTA is probably the most accurate method for diagnosing aerobic and especially anaerobic bacterial infections in non-ventilated, non-bronchitic patients with a sensitivity of almost 100% and a specificity of more than 95%[10, 12, 104].

Open lung biopsy remains the gold standard for establishing the aetiology in patients with lung diseases, especially for opportunistic pathogens and for non-infectious conditions. Because of its risks and more invasive nature, and due to the increasing accuracy obtained with other invasive methods, open lung biopsy is today used less often.

Specimens from patients with chest infections obtained by invasive methods represent exclusive diagnostic material that must always be utilised in an optimised way. It should be expediently transported to the microbiological laboratory and further processed immediately[11]. Even delay for a few hours may reduce the number of pathogenic organisms[105].

Transtracheal aspiration

TTA was used extensively during the 1970s and contributed significantly to an increased knowledge of aerobic and anaerobic bacterial aetiology in lower respiratory tract infections. In some centres great experience with this method was accumulated. In such places it may still be used today, because of its effectiveness in obtaining an aetiological diagnosis in patients with bacterial lung infection not treated with antibiotics. However, especially in inexperienced hands, TTA is associated with definite risks. In centres with no special expertise with this procedure, therefore, alternative methods, especially bronchoscopy, is preferred.

Under local anaesthesia, TTA involves inserting a needle through the cricoid membrane into the trachea, whereupon a sampling catheter is introduced through the needle[106]. If no material is obtained upon suction a small amount of sterile saline may be inserted before aspiration. However, undiluted material is preferred, since the insertion of saline interferes with the quantification of bacteria, which is crucial for the interpretation of the culture results (see below). Theoretically, contamination by the oropharyngeal flora should be completely avoided by this approach, if the trachea is sterile below the larynx. On the other hand, pulmonary pathogens should be easy to identify if they occur in the trachea in the same numbers as in the infectious process. It has been shown that this is most often the case and disease-causing bacteria can be identified in numbers most often of $\geq 10^6$/ml. A particular advantage with TTA is its accuracy in identifying anaerobic bacteria[101, 107].

In experienced hands the sensitivity of TTA in patients with bacterial pneumonia not treated with antibiotics approaches 99%[10,12,107]. In other words, a negative TTA in a patient not on antibiotics virtually excludes an infection with classical aerobic or anaerobic bacteria (*Mycoplasma*, *Legionella* and *Chlamydia* must be diagnosed by other means). By comparison with concurrent transthoracic aspiration and by performing TTA in patients without signs of infection it has been found that oropharyngeal contamination occurs in up to 75% of patients, but most often in low numbers[10,12,37,104]. With quantitative culture and a cut-off level of 10^5 bacteria/ml a specificity of 93–100% can be achieved. However, for patients with chronic bronchitis colonisation of the trachea with potentially pathogenic bacteria often exceeds this cut-off level, and the significance of bacterial infection is often difficult to assess with any method[17, 55, 108].

Complications of TTA include bleeding, puncture of the posterior tracheal wall, cutaneous and paratracheal abscesses, subcutaneous and mediastinal emphysema, pneumothorax, cardiac arrythmias and hypotension[106].

Bronchoscopy

Bronchoscopy is today used extensively for the identification of infectious agents in immunocompromised or seriously ill, often ventilated, patients[11,93,95,102,109]. In immunocompromised patients particularly a wide variety of micro-oganisms may be involved. For microbial agents that are always pathogenic, e.g. most viruses, *Legionella*, *M. tuberculosis*, *P. carinii* and pathogenic, dimorphic fungi, the mere identification of the respecive agent is diagnostic and oropharyngeal contamination is no problem. Bronchoalveolar lavage is then the preferred material because of its great volume for examination with several different methods and because material from the finest bronchi and alveoli is obtained. For *M. tuberculosis* or pathogenic fungi bronchial washing may also be used, whereas for *P. carinii* lavage of the alveoli is important for optimal sensitivity[11].

Detailed description of the bronchoscopic procedure and discussion of technical details may be found elsewhere[11, 95, 102, 109]. Briefly, the patient is premedicated with atropine to decrease the nasovagal response and oropharyngeal secretions. In non-ventilated patients the bronchoscope is usually inserted through the nose under topical anaesthesia and placed in the bronchus with suspected pathological changes or in case of a diffuse process in the lingular or right middle lobe bronchus. If both PSB and BAL are performed, PSB is the first sampling to be done. The bronchoscope is then wedged into a subsegment bronchus, whereupon BAL is performed by instilling sterile saline in 20-ml aliquots to a total volume of 120–240 ml.

In most settings, and especially in ventilator-associated pneumonia, classical bacteria are the most common aetiological agents. Typically community-acquired respiratory pathogens such as *S. pneumoniae*, *H. influenzae* and *M. catarrhalis* as well as *S. aureus* and Gram-negative enteric or non-enteric rods are most often incriminated. The problem is that all these bacteria may also colonise the oropharyngeal cavity and therefore infection and colonisation must be differentiated. This is especially difficult in ventilated patients, who often become colonised with *S. aureus* and Gram-negative rods.

Without special measures, specimens obtained through a flexible bronchoscope will become heavily contaminated by oropharyngeal flora[11,109–111]. Pharyngeal contamination occurs from aspiration during the procedure and from contamination of the brochoscope during its passage through the pharynx. Topical anaesthesia and suctioning through the working channel will increase contamination.

The most important means to reduce contamination and achieve an increased specificity with both the protected specimen brush (PSB) and bronchoalveolar lavage (BAL) is the use of quantitative cultures with appropriate cut-off levels[11,102,109] (Table 1.1). With PSB, contamination is further reduced by using a small brush within a double-lumen catheter sealed at the end with a Carbowax plug. This small brush collects 0.001–0.01 ml of material, so 10^3 bacteria on the brush correspond to 10^5–10^6 bacteria/ml in respiratory secretions, i.e. the lower concentration limit for bacteria in a chest infection. This threshold, 10^3 bacteria on the brush, has also been found to give an almost 100% specificity and still a good sensitivity[11, 16]. Since the brush is cut off into 1 ml of dilutent, this is often expressed as 10^3 cfu/ml, but it then actually corresponds to 100–1000 times that concentration in respiratory tract secretions.

For BAL, optimal fluid recovery and reduction of contamination is obtained by wedging the bronchoscope into a bronchus of the part of the lung to be examined, so that the bronchial lumen is completely occluded. The subsegment of the lung that is distal to the bronchoscope tip is then lavaged with 120–240 ml of fluid in 3–4 aliquots. About half is normally retrieved. The first aliquot is often used for non-bacterial diagnostics or is discarded. The great volume used will reduce the concentration of contaminating bacteria. Furthermore the respiratory secretions in the lung subsegment lavaged will also be diluted. It has been estimated that this dilution factor is 1/10–1/100, i.e. ten times less than that obtained with PSB. Therefore, 10^4 cfu/ml would be an appropriate threshold for a positive BAL. This level has in most studies been found to give the best balance between high sensitivity and high specificity[11, 112], although 10^5 cfu/ml has also been recommended[95]. Even 10^3 cfu/ml has been suggested as the best balance between sensitivity and specificity, providing only the last aliquot of 110 ml of lavage fluid is used for culture, and only non-respiratory normal flora is accepted as a positive finding[113]. The threshold used for PSB has been supported by comparison with quantitative cultures of open lung biopsy specimens[13], but the thresholds for BAL have been based predominantly on clinical correlations.

It must be remembered that the concentration of bacteria revealed on culture of a specimen may be influenced by a number of different factors: (1) as indicated above, there is a variation in the dilution obtained upon sampling both for PSB (1/100–1/1000) and for BAL (1/10–1/100). For PSB the amount of secretion on the brush may vary and for BAL the amount of respiratory secretion in the segment lavaged as well as the amount retrieved may vary; (2) the number of bacteria may be reduced during transportation[11, 105]; (3) the concentration of bacteria in a pneumonic process[114] may vary considerably, from 10^5 to 10^8 cfu/ml[9, 11,–16] with especially low numbers in the beginning of a pneumonic process[114]; (4) the start of antibiotic therapy will rapidly reduce the concentration of bacteria in the infectious process[6, 10, 21, 115]. The chances of getting bacterial concentrations by PSB or BAL above the accepted thresholds may therefore vary markedly.

In a review of 17 studies, including more than 1000 patients with the threshold of $\geq 10^3$ for PSB, a sensitivity of 79% and a specificity of 91% was found[11]. BAL with the threshold of $\geq 10^4$ had been used in eight studies with an aggregate sensitivity and specificity of 87% and 94%, respectively (Table 1.2). It can be seen from the resulting positive and negative predictive values that with both methods a pos-

Table 1.2. *Sensitivity, specificity and positive and negative predictive value of protected specimen brush (PSB) and bronchoalveolar lavage (BAL)*

	Threshold (cfu/ml)	Studies (*n*)	Total number of patients with pneumonia	Total number of patients without pneumonia	Sensitivity	Specificity	Positive predictive value	Negative predictive value
PSB	10^3	17	472	563	79	91	88	84
BAL	10^4	8	96	194	87	94	88	95

Modified after Baselski & Wunderink 1994[11].

itive finding speaks strongly for a bacterial pneumonia. A negative PSB does not exclude a bacterial infection, although this is almost always the case with a negative BAL. These conclusions are based on the means of the reviewed studies[11,116–121]. However, the risk of false-positive results with bacterial counts above the respective thresholds has varied considerably between different studies. A significant relationship has also been found between duration of mechanical ventilation and positive PSB in patients without pneumonia[119].

Though 10^3 cfu/ml on the PSB or 10^4 cfu/ml in the BAL fluid of one kind of bacteria must be interpreted as strong evidence for infection, and a completely negative culture before the start of antibiotics as clearly indicative of the absence of infection, borderline results must be interpreted with some caution and in the light of other laboratory and clinical information[11,114,122]. Withholding or withdrawing antibiotics from a patient with clinical signs of chest infection but negative bronchoscopy does not seem to be followed by any adverse consequences[11]. On the contrary, empirical antibiotic therapy may be connected with increased mortality[91]. Again, caution may be warranted, since low bacterial counts have been connected with the early phase of pneumonia[114]. Generally, however, a reliable negative diagnosis may be as important as a positive one, since other sites of infection or other conditions will then be identified more rapidly[122–124]. This is a very important point, since ventilator-associated pneumonia can be confirmed in less than half of the patients when the diagnosis is suspected on clinical and/or radiological grounds[11,14,103,124].

A further development of the BAL procedure has been achieved by Meduri *et al.*[122] by introducing the protected BAL (PBAL). A transbronchoscopic balloon-tipped catheter with a distal ejectable diaphragm is used in order to minimise the degree of contamination from the bronchoscope tip. After occlusion of the subsegmental bronchial lumen by inflation of the balloon, the distal diaphragm is expelled, whereupon the lavage is performed in the established way. With this technique a two-log difference in concentration was obtained between contaminants and true pathogens, which would create a clearer distinction between infected and non-infected patients. Moreover, a presumptive diagnosis was established by Gram's or Giemsa stains of BAL fluid in eight of eight patients with no false-positive results. The high cost of these special catheters is so far a significant drawback.

Some additional measures have been proposed to facilitate the interpretation of the microbiological results obtained with bronchoscopy. Calculation of 'bacterial indexes', i.e. the sum of the 10-log concentrations of the different or predominant bacterial species identified in BAL fluid, have been proposed by some authors to mirror the bacterial burden of the lung tissue more accurately than with ordinary quantitative BAL[125–127]. However, the procedure is not universally accepted as being superior to ordinary quantitation. A cytological marker of possible usefulness is the finding of elastin fibres[126]. These fibres originate from necrotising tissue, and may therefore indicate Gram-negative bacillary pneumonia. False-positive results due to adult respiratory distress syndrome may occur. The finding of antibody-coated bacteria seems to indicate the presence of pneumonia with a high specificity[128]. However, the sensitivity is not very high and Gram's stain seems to give approximately the same information. It has been shown that an increased amount of squamous epithelial cells (SEC) is correlated with contamination by oropharyngeal secretions, and it has been proposed, but not universally accepted, that specimens containing > 1% SEC be discarded[11,109,118]. Finally, the percentage of polymorphonuclear cells with intracellular bacteria seems to be correlated with the presence of pneumonia[116,112,129,130]. Although this method may provide a means of obtaining a rapid preliminary result of the BAL, it is far from settled what the optimal cut-off for intracellular organisms should be; from 2 to 25% has been proposed.

Direct microscopy of material obtained by bronchoscopy is of great importance for establishing a rapid definitive or presumptive diagnosis. For certain micro-organisms, such as *Legionella*, *Nocardia*, *Mycobacteria*, *P. carinii* and other fungi as well as for respiratory viruses, specific stains are available, with which the diagnosis can be established within a matter of hours (see the respective agent below). For these agents BAL fluid is usually preferred. For regular bacteria, Giemsa or Gram's stain may be used. Giemsa is the preferred method for visualising intracellular bacteria, whereas Gram's stain is used for morphological characterisation of bacteria. Since approximately 10^5 bacteria/ml is required for detection of bacteria in a direct smear, a positive direct Gram's stain from PSB or BAL is suggestive of active infection[11,95,109]. Indeed, the general experience is a high specificity, but a variable sensitivity with direct Gram's stain of both PSB and BAL[11,109,126]. The protected BAL seems to offer a kind of material giving a very high sensitivity as well as specificity by use of Gram's stain[112]. For preparation of smears from BAL for staining, cytocentrifugation of an adjusted cell suspension is the preferred method: by low-speed centrifugation of cells in suspension with simultaneous absorption of fluid onto a filter pad, a monolayer of cells with well-preserved morphology is obtained[131].

In a few reports quantitative culture of tracheal aspirates[132–134], blind bronchial sampling[135] or non-bronchoscopic BAL[136,137] have had a fairly high accuracy in mechanically ventilated patients, but generally these methods are considered to be inferior to PSB and BAL. Interestingly, in the study by Salata *et al.* the finding of elastin fibres in tracheal aspirates was a very specific finding, but only 52% of the patients with pneumonia were positive.

Complications

The use of bronchoscopy in order to arrive at an aetiological diagnosis is especially important in severely ill patients. However, in many of these patients, the risk of complications is also especially high. A decrease in oxygen saturation is always seen during bronchoscopy and patients may need extra oxygen during the procedure[11,102,112,138]. Bleeding may be a significant complication when transbronchial biopsy and to a lesser extent also bronchial brushings (more with the cytology brush than with the PSB) are used. Pneumothorax is uncommon, but may occur as a result of inadvertent distal sampling. Haemodynamic changes can occur as a result of sedative premedication or secondary to altered respiration during the procedure. Generally, with adequate precautions and in experienced hands, bronchoscopy can be considered to be a very safe method with few serious complications and a negligible risk of death as a result of the procedure[138]. The major risk factor is severe cardiovascular disease.

In ventilated and stable patients the procedure can usually be safely carried out if sampling is performed with consideration of the patient's condition. However, a complete BAL may not be possible in patients who are difficult to oxygenate, and transbronchial biopsy should be avoided in patients with bleeding abnormalities. In severely thrombocytopenic patients even PSB may be risky.

Non-intubated patients with severe hypoxaemia are at risk of respiratory failure and may require intubation before or after the bronchoscopy. Bleeding may be more difficult to control than in ventilated patients and transbronchial biopsy should be avoided in patients with thrombocytopenia or bleeding abnormality. Bronchoscopy with BAL seems to be a minor risk[138].

Lung aspiration

Percutaneous lung aspiration has been used in children, especially young children in developing countries, to obtain a specific diagnosis in cases of community-acquired pneumonia. The literature has been reviewed[139]. In one study *S. pneumoniae* was isolated in 165/211 (78%) patients with bacteraemic pneumococcal pneumonia. The reasons for obtaining false-negative results are missing the infection with the needle or failure to obtain a sample. False-positive results are very uncommon[140]. Complications have been few, but not negligible. Some cases of pneumothorax may need treatment.

For adults with community-acquired pneumonia this procedure is generally too risky, considering the low mortality and most often uncomplicated course of this disease. The diagnostic yield is, however, superior to that obtained with sputum and TTA[37,141]. In critically ill patients and in ventilated patients percutaneous lung aspiration could theoretically be considered. However, pneumothorax in this patient category is a significant complication and at the same time bronchoscopy is today a reliable and accurate method. Nevertheless, a few groups have published reports on the use of lung aspiration for the aetiological diagnosis in ventilated patients[142,143]. There seems to be no definitive advantage over bronchoscopy with BAL and PSB.

Open lung biopsy

Open lung biopsy has long been considered to be the gold standard for diagnosing the aetiology of lung infiltrates, especially diffuse infiltrates in immunosuppressed patients[100,144–147]. Though the introduction of the flexible bronchoscope with PSB and BAL has significantly facilitated the diagnostic procedure in patients with pulmonary infiltrates of unknown aetiology, these methods often fail to produce a definitive diagnosis, especially in cases with diffuse infiltrates and especially in immunocompromised hosts. For these patients open lung biopsy seems to be superior, although reports comparing methodologies directly are scarce[148]. A major advantage with open lung biopsy is that a tissue histology diagnosis is usually obtained; this is often necessary in fungal infections and the only definitive way to diagnose CMV pneumonia. Complications seem not to be a significantly greater problem with open lung biopsy than with TBB, but in patients with severe uncorrectable bleeding abnormalities biopsies must usually be avoided. Pneumothorax is a rather common complication, but seldom life threatening.

Atypical pneumonia agents

Accurate and rapid diagnostic methods for atypical agents such as *Legionella*, *Mycoplasma* and *Chlamydia* are important because there are only a limited number of effective antimicrobial agents. This is especially important for *Legionella* spp., since the prognosis may be significantly worse without adequate treatment. These bacteria are coloured either weakly or not at all by Gram's stain. Therefore, the finding of purulent sputum or mucoid sputum without contamination with squamous epithelial cells and without presence of visible bacteria may indicate an atypical aetiology.

Legionella

Serology

Documentation of a serum antibody response has been the most commonly used means for diagnosing *Legionella* infections (Table 1.3). This is usually accomplished by the use of the indirect immunofluorescent assay (IFA)[149,150]. A number of different antigens must be used for diagnosing all *Legionella* infections. However, 85% of cases of Legionnaire's disease, and almost all cases of severe disease, are caused by *L. pneumophila* serotype 1, which is therefore the most important organism to be represented in the antigen set-up. The experience with other antigens is more limited, and sensitivity and specificity are less well defined. About 75% of the patients with *L. pneumophila* serotype 1 infection will develop a significant (usually defined as four-fold) increase in specific antibody. Unfortunately, for some patients seroconversion may take up to nine weeks after onset of infection. High titres have often been used as a criterion for current disease, but such high titres may persist for more than a year after an acute infection. Presence of a high titre without a concomitant titre rise must, therefore, be interpreted with caution. The IFA test is essentially specific for *L. pneumophila* serotype 1, but cross-reactions and false-positive titre rises have been described. Since it will take from two to nine weeks before a titre rise can be seen, serology is useful only for scientific and epidemiological purposes and not for management of the individual case.

Table 1.3. *Methods for microbiological diagnosis of* Legionella *infection assuming that 85% of infections are caused by* L. pneumophila *serotype 1*

	Sensitivity[a] (%)	Specificity[a] (%)	Applicable for diagnosis
Sputum or bronchoalveolar lavage			
Culture	80–90	100	All *Legionella* spp.
DFA	20–70	95–99	*L. pneumophila*
DNA probe	60–90	95–99	All *Legionella* spp.
PCR	NA	NA	*L. pneumophila*
Urine			
Antigen	70	100	*L. pneumophila* serotype 1
Serum			
Antibody[b]	60	> 95	*L. pneumophila* serotype 1

DFA, direct fluorescent antibody; PCR, polymerase chain reaction; NA, not enough data available.

[a]Approximate numbers.

[b]Four-fold titre rise.

Culture

In contrast, the use of methods for the direct identification of *Legionella* in respiratory secretions should have an impact on therapy and outcome. The use and interpretation of such methods is facilitated by the fact that the presence of *Legionella* spp. in human material is considered to be a proof of active infection; i.e. if a particular method is specific for the identification of *Legionella* spp., detection of *Legionella* spp. in a clinical specimen with that method is 100% specific for the diagnosis of *Legionella* infection. *Legionella* bacteria may be detected in clinical specimens by culture, by direct fluorescent antibody, (DFA), by the identification of specific DNA, or by the detection of specific antigen in the urine.

Identification of *Legionella* spp. in respiratory secretions by culture is the most accurate method for diagnosis[149,151,152]. Moreover, with culture, all different *Legionella* spp. that cause human disease can be identified, although slightly different culture media to detect *Legionella* strains other than *L. pneumophilia* may be needed[153]. For all *Legionella* spp. buffered charcoal yeast extract (BCYE) is the base medium. Different antibiotic substances are usually added to this medium to prevent overgrowth of other more rapidly growing bacteria. Cephalosporins may be among the incorporated drugs, but may inhibit the growth of other Legionellaceae. Dyes that colour the *Legionella* organisms are often incorporated into the culture medium to facilitate detection of the minute colonies. Three to five days of incubation is usually needed for visible growth to occur. Media for culture of *Legionella* are today commercially available.

For patients with *Legionella* prosthetic valve endocarditis, other severe disease or immunosuppression, blood cultures may be positive if an appropriate technique is used.

Direct detection, antigen and DNA detection

Direct fluorescent antibody is the established rapid method for examining respiratory tract secretions[149,150,154]. In experienced hands this method is essentially specific. The sensitivity is variable and higher for BAL specimens than for sputum. A commercially available DNA probe seems to give results that are approximately equivalent to those of DFA if the threshold for a positive result is set to a level avoiding most false positives[155]. An advantage with the probe is that it is specific for the genus *Legionella* and can detect species other than *L. pneumophila*. A small study[156] has indicated that PCR may prove to be a sensitive tool to detect *L. pneumophila* from BAL specimens.

Specific antigen may also be detected in the urine by radioimmunoassay (RIA), EIA or latex agglutination, by which methods around 70% of the *Legionella* cases can be diagnosed[154,157]. These tests are specific for *L. pneumophila* serotype 1, and other serotypes or other *Legionella* species cannot be detected. *Legionella* antigen has also been detected in pleural fluid[158].

Mycoplasma pneumoniae

M. pneumoniae infections are very common and are seldom severe. Most infections are managed outside hospitals, probably without any contact with medical facilities at all. All established diagnostic measures are slow and can only occasionally contribute to an improved management of the patient. Such methods are of importance primarily for epidemiological and other research purposes.

During a *M. pneumoniae* infection the organism can usually be isolated from throat washings, nasopharyngeal specimens, sputum, or bronchial aspirate or lavage fluid[159–161]. However, even with a modified and improved medium[161], growth is slow and the culture method rather laborious; a diagnosis may be obtained only after 5–14 days of cultivation. Moreover, *M. pneumoniae* has been isolated several weeks after an acute mycoplasmal infection, and therefore, a positive result of culture is not 100% specific for active infection, but can represent infection in the several months prior to sampling[162].

An essentially specific diagnosis of *M. pneumoniae* infection can be obtained by identifying an antibody response to a glycolipid or surface protein antigen[159]. For a definitive diagnosis a fourfold or greater increase in titre is necessary; a single high titre may be suggestive of the aetiology. Several immunological methods have been used, the most common being the complement-fixing antibody assay. Today different forms of EIAs are increasingly being used[163,164]. The specificity of the serological assays has been questioned, but seems to be a problem primarily when whole cells are used as antigens. A positive serological result is not obtained until 1–3 weeks after the patient's first visit, so the value of these tests is primarily for scientific and epidemiological purposes. The demonstration of an IgM or IgA antibody response may be obtained somewhat earlier, but only occasionally in the first serum sample obtained from the patient[164–166].

The demonstration of cold haemagglutinin antibodies in the patient's serum may be suggestive of a *M. pneumoniae* infection[159,167]. These are IgM autoantibodies agglutinating human erythrocytes at 4 °C. Such antibodies are found in one-third to three-quarters of patients with *M. pneumoniae* infection[159,167]. Although these tests are not specific for *M. pneumoniae*, a positive test is highly suggestive in cases of pneumonia. Cold agglutinins appear at the end of the first week at a time when the patient often seeks medical advice. A rapid bedside test described by Garrow can be performed[168]; a positive rapid cold agglutinin test in cases of pneumonia is clearly suggestive of *M. pneumoniae* aetiology[159].

For the rapid detection of *M. pneumoniae* in pharyngeal or respiratory tract secretions, several methods have been developed, but although these are promising, none has become established in clinical practice. Direct antigen detection in clinical specimens has been accomplished with an antigen capture immunoassay[169] as well as a monoclonal antibody immunoblot assay[170]. Both methods show good sensitivity and specificity, but they are still rather laborious and have as yet not gained widespread use. Direct detection of *M. pneumoniae* in respiratory secretions has also recently been achieved by the use of an indirect immunofluorescence test, which shows promise for the future[171].

Direct identification of *M. pneumoniae* in clinical material has also been accomplished by detection of specific nucleotide sequences. The most commonly used method is the commercially available DNA–RNA probe. It is very specific, but sensitivity from pharyngeal specimens has varied between 22 and 100%[170,172,173]. Several recent studies have evaluated PCR for the detection of *M. pneumoniae* in clinical specimens[2,3,174]. Although the sensitivity has been found to be at least 100-fold greater than that of culture or the commercial DNA-probe, technical problems and lack of specificity have so far not permitted its use as a diagnostic tool. Not surprisingly, specimens from subjects with serological patterns suggesting infection in the more recent past have also been found to be positive, the reason probably being the rather frequent continued carriage of these bacteria after an infection.

Chlamydia species

For *Chlamydia* species the diagnosis is usually most often based on serology. Complement-fixing antibodies are only genus-specific, and this test does not provide optimal sensitivity either[175,176]. In cases of reinfection, the sensitivity may be low. However, by the use of a microimmunofluorescence (MIF) technique, a species-specific antibody response can be detected in most clinical cases[175–177]. The antigenic epitope seems to be a major outer membrane[175]. Both IgG and IgM antibodies may be diagnosed. In *C. pneumoniae* primary infections an early IgM and a later IgG response is the typical pattern, and in reinfections a further elevation of the IgG titre is typically seen. In infantile *C. trachomatis* pneumonitis, identification of an IgM response may be of value[175]. The complement-fixing test has been widely used for diagnosing *C. psittaci* infection. However, in the absence of exposure to contagious birds, a substantial part of the antibody increases seen with this method may be due to *C. pneumoniae* infection[176]. Therefore, the use of the MIF method is also necessary for diagnosing psittacosis.

C. trachomatis grows well in a variety of cell lines. *C. pneumoniae* can also be isolated from clinical specimens by use of appropriate cell lines[175,176]. For both species transportation is critical. The specimens must be properly frozen in special *Chlamydia* transport media. For *C. trachomatis,* culture may be part of the routine, whereas for *C. pneumoniae* culture is used only in a few specialised laboratories and mainly for research purposes. For *C. psittaci* isolation is not used.

Antigen detection of *C. trachomatis* by the use of direct immunofluorescence or EIA is established as a sensitive and specific means of diagnosis[175]. Direct demonstration of *C. pneumoniae* in respiratory secretions with fluorescent monoclonal antibody is more difficult, due to the limited number of organisms, and it is only 50% sensitive[176].

PCRs based on genetic coding for major outer membrane proteins (MOMP) have been developed for rapid identification or detection of all three major *Chlamydia* spp[178–180]. With this technique *C. pneumoniae* may be diagnosed in clinical specimens with a 25% higher sensitivity than with culture[176].

FUNGAL INFECTION

Microbiological diagnosis

Aspergillosis

The laboratory diagnosis of pulmonary aspergillosis is often difficult[181]. Serology may be helpful, but immunocompromised patients most often fail to develop an antibody response (Table 1.4). Culture may be difficult to interpret, because colonisation with this fungus is rather common. Antigen detection methods may be of some help, but the sensitivity is still low. PCR is as yet not a clinically useful method. In cases of *Aspergillus* sinusitis specimens for culture and histology can be more easily obtained, so once clinical suspicion has prompted a sampling procedure, the diagnosis can most often be settled if appropriate culture as well as histology are carried out.

The different forms of allergic reactions to *Aspergillus* spores may be diagnosed by clinical presentation, history of exposure and the presence of IgE and/or precipitating antibodies in serum.

In cases of aspergilloma, precipitating antibodies are always found, often in very high titres. Since the clinical and radiological presentation is usually typical, this diagnosis is seldom problematic. However, culture for *Aspergillus* is often falsely negative, and a laboratory diagnosis may be difficult in such cases. Occasionally, the aspergilloma may be caused by an unusual *Aspergillus* species that does not react with the commercial antigen used for the precipitin reaction[182]. Although the clinical diagnosis of chronic necrotising aspergillosis may be difficult, the laboratory confirmation is usually easy, with both serology and culture being positive.

The most difficult and important diagnosis is invasive aspergillosis. It seems clear that in cases in which *Aspergillus* is cultured from the respiratory tract of a neutropenic or otherwise severely immunocompromised patient, this should be considered diagnostic of invasive aspergillosis, especially in connection with a suggestive X-ray finding[181,183–186]. However, sputum is often absent in these patients and, if it is produced, cultures are seldom positive. Moreover, the growth of *Aspergillus* is slow and culture results are seldom obtained rapidly enough to contribute to the management of the patient[187]. Diagnostic antibody levels are generally not found in these immunosuppressed patients[188–190], but positive results have been reported with some serological methods[190,192].

The most promising method for obtaining an early and therefore clinically useful diagnosis of invasive aspergillosis is the detection of galactomannan antigen by use of any of several immunological techniques in serum, urine or bronchial secretions[188,193–197]. In one study 74% of leukemia patients with invasive aspergillosis were diagnosed

Table 1.4. *Microbiological diagnosis of different forms of pulmonary aspergillosis*

Disease	Culture	Antibodies	
		Precipitating	IgE
Allergic alveolitis	–	+	–
Eosinophilic pneumonia	–	–	+
Allergic bronchopulmonary aspergillosis	–	+	+
Aspergilloma	(+)	+	–
Chronic necrotising aspergillosis	+	+	–
Invasive aspergillosis	(+)	–	–

with antigen detection in serum; the specificity was 90% and by repeated sampling a diagnosis could be obtained at an early stage in several cases. The concentration of antigen was proportional to the severity of disease. However, in other studies the sensitivity has been around 50% and technical problems primarily with the most popular test, the latex agglutination kit, have occurred. In a small study a PCR test specific for *A. fumigatus* produced positive results with specimens from all four patients with invasive aspergillosis, but also with specimens from several colonised persons[198].

Pulmonary candidosis

Candida albicans is often found in sputum of patients receiving antibiotics for pneumonia, but is rarely a primary pulmonary pathogen. *C. albicans* predominates as a cause of both superficial and deep candida infections, although other species such as *Candida tropicalis*, *Candida krusei*, *Candida parapsilosis*, *Candida guillermondii*, *Candida parapsilosis* and *Candida* (*Torulopsis*) *glabrata* may also produce infection[199]. *Candida* isolated from airway secretions, however, nearly always reflects colonisation or contamination from the mouth or upper airways. Primary pulmonary candidosis is extremely rare[200,201]. Only a minority of patients with a compromised immune defence develop *Candida* infection in the trachea, bronchi or alveoli. Pulmonary candidosis was described in 3% of AIDS patients at autopsy[202]. However, pulmonary candidosis is very rare in the vast majority of AIDS patients. In sick newborns, aspiration of *Candida* from the mouth may cause deep-seated infection, and infants with cystic fibrosis have been reported to develop primary pulmonary candidosis more frequently than do normal siblings[203].

Predisposing factors for pulmonary candidosis are the same as for candidosis in general – namely, prolonged antibiotic therapy, diabetes, use of steroids and, in cases of disseminated infection, intravenous fluids, severe and longstanding granulocytopenia and gastrointestinal ulceration or operation. In disseminated candidosis, haematogenous *Candida* pneumonia can cause large infiltrates and severe disease as a part of the more generalised infection.

Clinical and radiological features of *Candida* pneumonia are nonspecific. Endobronchial inoculation may cause local or diffuse bronchopneumonia. In haematogenous dissemination nodular infiltrates appear in both lungs. Lung biopsy is the only way to diagnose invasive candidal infection in the alveoli.

For culture of *Candida* a routine bacteriological substrate such as a blood agar plate is sufficient. When yeast is suspected a Sabouraud agar plate is recommended, since it suppresses the bacterial flora. Incubation time should be seven days, although many *Candida* spp. grow within 2–3 days. The ideal incubation temperature is 30 °C, but the yeast grows as well at 37 °C at which temperature, however, the growth of bacterial contaminants is stronger.

Serological diagnosis of deep candidosis is enigmatic. Several test kits for candida antigen determination are commercially available, most of them with doubtful specificity or sensitivity. The Pastorex® latex test (Sanofi) for detection of mannan from *C. albicans* and several other *Candida* spp. detects 2.5 ng/ml of serum and has a specificity of over 95%. However, the presence of candidal mannan is variable in serum during disseminated candidosis, and a negative test does not exclude the diagnosis. The sensitivity of the test is approximately 50%[204]. Gas chromatographic determination of D-arabinitol/L-arabinitol ratios in urine is another more promising method for diagnosis of disseminated candidosis[205].

An alternative for blood or serum diagnosis of disseminated candidosis is the PCR. It is more sensitive than blood cultures for detecting disseminated candidosis verified at autopsy in transplanted patients[206]. Routine blood cultures are insensitive for fungal detection but the Isolator system (Dupont) may increase sensitivity of blood cultures in disseminated candidosis by up to 73%[207]. However, it is well known that fungal blood cultures may remain negative despite widespread candida dissemination to internal organs, and during antifungal therapy. Serum tests for precipitating antibodies against cytoplasmic antigens from *C. albicans* have a useful diagnostic value for deep candidosis[208], but they are produced slowly. Antibody tests against whole cell antigens are of less documented value.

Cryptococcal pulmonary infection

The respiratory tract is the classical portal of entry for cryptococcal infection. The pigeon harbours *Cryptococcus neoformans* var.*neoformans* in its intestine and spreads it by its faeces. Disease by this variant has worldwide distribution. *C. neoformans* var. *gattii*, on the other hand, is associated with the river red gum tree (*Eucalyptus camaldulensis*) and disease is restricted to areas where the tree grows, for example, Australia, California and some parts of Africa.

Pulmonary infection with *Cryptococcus* is usually indolent or asymptomatic in the normal host. In immunocompromised individuals, however, the pulmonary infection may give rise to dissemination with cryptococcaemia, meningitis or urogenital, skin, bone or visceral infection. Factors predisposing for cryptococcal infection are, for example, AIDS, cortisone or cytostatic treatment, sarcoidosis, organ transplantation, debilitation and neoplasia. Symptoms of pulmonary cryptococcosis may be cough, fever, mucoid sputum production and dyspnoea. Pleural effusion, chest pain or cavitation are rare.

C. neoformans capsular polysaccharide antigen can very specifically and sensitively be detected in cerebrospinal fluid (CSF), serum or urine by commercial latex agglutination tests in cases of cryptococcosis. However, there is a cross-reaction associated with disseminated infection with *Trichosporon beigelii*[209]. Moreover, cryptococci can be visualised by India ink in various secretions, but the sensitivity of this procedure is lower than that for antigen detection.

Cryptococci grow in routine bacteriological broths such as brain-heart infusion broth, and on blood–dextrose agar or Saubouraud agar plates usually after 2–3 days at 30 °C or 37 °C. The cultures should, however, be kept for three weeks, as delayed growth may occur in cases with low numbers of fungal organisms. Suspected cryptococci in broth or on agar can be verified by morphology with the use of wet smear and blancophor or India ink techniques. Thereafter, biochemical and other methods are applied for speciation. Specific antisera for serogroups A–D (var. *neoformans*) and B–C (var. *gattii*) are available. The fungus is readily recognised at histopathological examination on relevant biopsies, which can be helpful in the diagnosis of cryptococcosis. The capsule can be specifically stained by mucicarmine. It should be noted that the capsule is sometimes very thin or even absent, which has been described in a small number of patients with AIDS. Therefore, antigen detection and morphological investigation can be less reliable in these patients. In immunocompromised patients with suspected cryptococcal pulmonary infection, not only sputum but also CSF, blood, urine, prostatic fluid and other relevant specimens should be investigated for presence of cryptococci or cryptococcal antigen.

Pneumocystis carinii pneumonia

P. carinii was first idenitfied by Chagas in Brazil in 1909, and the organism was recognised as belonging to a distinct genus in 1912. Its current status is controversial; previously it was recognised as a protozoa, because of morphology and drug susceptibility, but nucleotide sequences of 16 S ribosomal RNA identifies it as a fungus[210].

The spread of infection is thought to be airborne, as supported by animal studies[211] and by local outbreaks, e.g. in leukaemic children and transplant recipients[212,213]. *P. carinii* thus seems to be able to spread from person to person. On the other hand, it has been found that 80% of four-year-old children have antibodies against *P. carinii*[214,215], suggesting that asymptomatic infection during childhood seems to be the rule. Reactivation of latent infection is probably common in immunosuppression, but reinfection and new infection are also possible.

Clinical disease is seen particularly in T cell deficient patients such as those with AIDS or those undergoing immunosuppressive therapy in malignant disease. *P. carinii* pneumonia (PCP) has been the AIDS-defining diagnosis in approximately 60% of HIV-infected patients in North America and Western Europe[216], but it is relatively uncommon in Africa[217].

A definitive diagnosis of PCP is possible by visualisation of the organism in airway specimens. This can be performed by methenamine silver staining, toluidine blue and modified Giemsa staining or by immunofluorescence employing monoclonal antibodies. The latter method is very sensitive[218]. The diagnostic yield depends largely on the specimen material: sputum gives a low diagnostic yield, induced sputum is variable – between 25 and 80%, BAL fluid is very sensitive at > 95% and transbronchial biopsy specimen is sensitive with an 85–95% yield[219].

The most sensitive laboratory method to diagnose *P. carinii* is the PCR, by which a specific DNA sequence from the organism is detected in sputum or bronchial lavage fluid[220,221]. It should be noted, however, that PCR can be positive also in the absence of present or past PCP, indicating possible colonisation[222].

Serology to detect antibodies to *P. carinii* has limited value in non-HIV infected patients and is of no practical use in HIV patients[215]. Most individuals are already seropositive in childhood, and titre rises are irregular. Detection of *P. carinii* antigens in serum was previously believed to be sensitive, but it was later proved to be of low sensitivity and specificity[223].

VIRAL INFECTION

Laboratory diagnosis

Most acute respiratory infections are caused by viruses (Table 1.5). They produce a variety of symptoms and cannot be differentiated from each other on clinical grounds. A precise (virus-specific) diagnosis is a prerequisite for the correct treatment of a viral infection in the lower respiratory tract and should always be attempted early in the course of a disease[224]. Likewise, the aetiology of viral lower respiratory infections in the immunosuppressed (Table 1.6) should be confirmed, since the use of antiviral, often life-saving, drugs must be based on knowledge of the causative virus.

There are two main approaches to diagnosis of viral infections:

(1) *Proving the presence of virus in the specimen*
  (a) by isolation of virus in tissue culture or in laboratory animals;
  (b) by detection of virus and viral antigens directly in the clinical specimen;
  (c) by detection of viral nucleic acids directly in the clinical specimen;

(2) *Demonstrating development of specific antibodies in the patient*
  (a) by proving a titre rise in a serum pair from the patient; or
  (b) by detecting virus-specific IgM in a single acute phase serum sample.

Proving the presence of virus in a specimen

In an acute viral respiratory infection, the virus is present in epithelial cells in the upper respiratory tract. Therefore, a virus causing a lower respiratory tract infection present in the nasopharynx. The quantity of virus shed is largest early in the course of the infection. Infectious virus may be found only during the first week of illness and specimens should be collected as early as possible. Immunologically normal individuals do not carry virus in their respiratory tract, with the exception of adeno- and enteroviruses, which can be found in low amounts for long periods after an infection. Isolation of one of these viruses is not a proof that they cause the infection.

High titres of virus are present in the nasopharynx in most acute respiratory infections and a single specimen from this location is enough for virus diagnosis. In immunocompromised patients, however, the presence of a virus must be proven in secretions collected from the lower respiratory tract (BAL or brush specimens) to obtain a specific aetiological virus diagnosis of a pneumonia.

Specimens can be collected either by aspiration of nasopharyngeal secretions (or washings) through a thin catheter attached to a mucus collector (tube) or – although this type of specimen yields less virus –

Table 1.5. *Viruses causing acute respiratory infections*

Respiratory syncytial virus
Influenza virus A and B
Parainfluenza virus types 1, 2, 3 and 4
Adenoviruses
Rhinovirus, enterovirus
Coronavirus

Table 1.6 *Viruses causing pneumonitis in immunosuppressed patients*

Cytomegalovirus
Herpes simplex virus
Varicella zoster virus
Adenoviruses

by use of swabs. Sterile saline can be used for washings. Specimens for detection of virus or viral antigens by immunoassays should not be unnecessarily diluted; swab specimens are not suitable for this type of test.

Diagnosis by isolation of virus in tissue culture or in laboratory animals
The specimen is mixed with an equal amount of virus transport medium immediately after collection. If a swab has been used, it is placed in a tube with virus transport medium (or a commercial transport tube). The specimen is immediately transported to the laboratory, preferably on ice.

In the laboratory the specimen is inoculated into a combination of cell cultures suitable for the viruses possibly occurring in the specimen. Occasionally, embryonated hen's egg is used, for influenza virus isolation, but in general, cell cultures are used for isolation of respiratory viruses.

The presence of virus in the cell culture is detected either by regular microscopic examination of the cell cultures, to monitor a cytopathic effect, or by testing for haemadsorbing capacity induced by influenza or parainfluenza viruses, which may not always cause a clear cytopathic effect. For final specific identification of the virus grown in cell cultures, immunofluorescence is generally used, although several other immunoassays are also used. Occasionally, a positive result may be obtained within three days (60% of the influenza virus strains). However, 7–10 days or more are often needed and a negative result will not be delivered until after 2–3 weeks, depending on the type of virus and on the laboratory routine. Cytomegalo- and parainfluenza viruses may replicate slowly, but respiratory syncytial virus positivity may also sometimes develop late. Centrifugation of a specimen onto a cell culture shortens the time for detection[225]. This is usually done in shell vial tissue cultures and has been described mainly for CMV[226], but has also been tried for other viruses infecting the respiratory tract[227–229]. In immunocompromised patients such short-term incubation is useful in clinical practice for detection of CMV in BAL; its sensitivity, however, is only 60% compared to conventional virus isolation[230].

Diagnosis by detection of virus or viral antigens directly in the clinical specimens
Immunofluorescence and solid phase immunoassays for detection of viral antigens have both proved to be efficient diagnostic methods for acute respiratory infections[231]. However, in the life-threatening CMV pneumonia in immunocompromised patients, antigen detection can not be used as the sole method for detecting CMV in alveolar cells in BAL because of its low sensitivity[230].

Immunofluorescence staining is performed on cells present in specimens collected from the respiratory tract, preferably nasopharyngeal aspirates[224]. A fair amount of intact cells must be present in the specimen. The cells are freed from mucus and laid down on several small areas on a microscope slide. After fixation in anhydrous acetone, the cell deposits are usually stained with mouse monoclonal antibodies, either directly labelled with fluoroisothiocyanate (FITC) or followed by antimouse-immunoglobulin FITC-labelled antibodies. One specimen may be investigated simultaneously for the presence of a variety of respiratory viruses, as the cell deposits are stained with different specific antiviral monoclonal antibodies. The method has been used successfully for a multitude of respiratory studies in the Western world[224,232] and in the developing world[233–235]. After acetone fixation the cell preparations can be stored frozen or sent by airmail for diagnosis or for quality control to a central laboratory[236].

The success of the method is dependent on the quality of the reagents[237]. After introduction of monoclonal antibodies for diagnosis, the specificity is usually high (Fig. 1.6). Compared to other diagnostic methods, such as virus isolation and solid phase immunoassays, the sensitivity varies with virus type and with quality of the specimen[234,238]. Immunofluorescence for respiratory syncytial virus diagnosis has a sensitivity equal to, or higher than, virus isolation. Likewise, the sensitivity by this method is high for diagnosis of parainfluenza type 3, but immunofluorescence diagnosis of other respiratory viruses is somewhat less sensitive than virus isolation.

Solid phase immunoassays can be used for the detection of viral antigens in respiratory tract specimens. Specimens should be collected from sites with very high virus concentrations and they should not be unnecessarily diluted. Also, for this type of investigation the specimen of choice is the nasopharyngeal secretion sampled by aspiration through a thin catheter introduced first through one nostril and then through the other. Among the assays, the enzyme-linked solid phase immunoassay (ELISA) is usually preferred, as it employs relatively stable reagents and is relatively inexpensive.

The assay is often performed in microtitre plates and a specimen can be investigated for a multitude of viruses in the same test run. Antibodies specific for the different viruses capture viral antigens from the specimens in different rows of wells in the plate. Bound antigens are indicated with enzyme-conjugated antibodies (often monoclonal antibodies), followed by a substrate that changes colour when reacting with the enzyme and results are obtained within a day. The results are reproducible, and read by a machine. Transportation and storage of specimens is facilitated, as infectious virus need not be present[239].

A variety of commercial test kits for diagnosis of respiratory syncytial virus or influenza virus by immunoassays have been developed. Usually, viral antigens from nasopharyngeal secretions are captured by

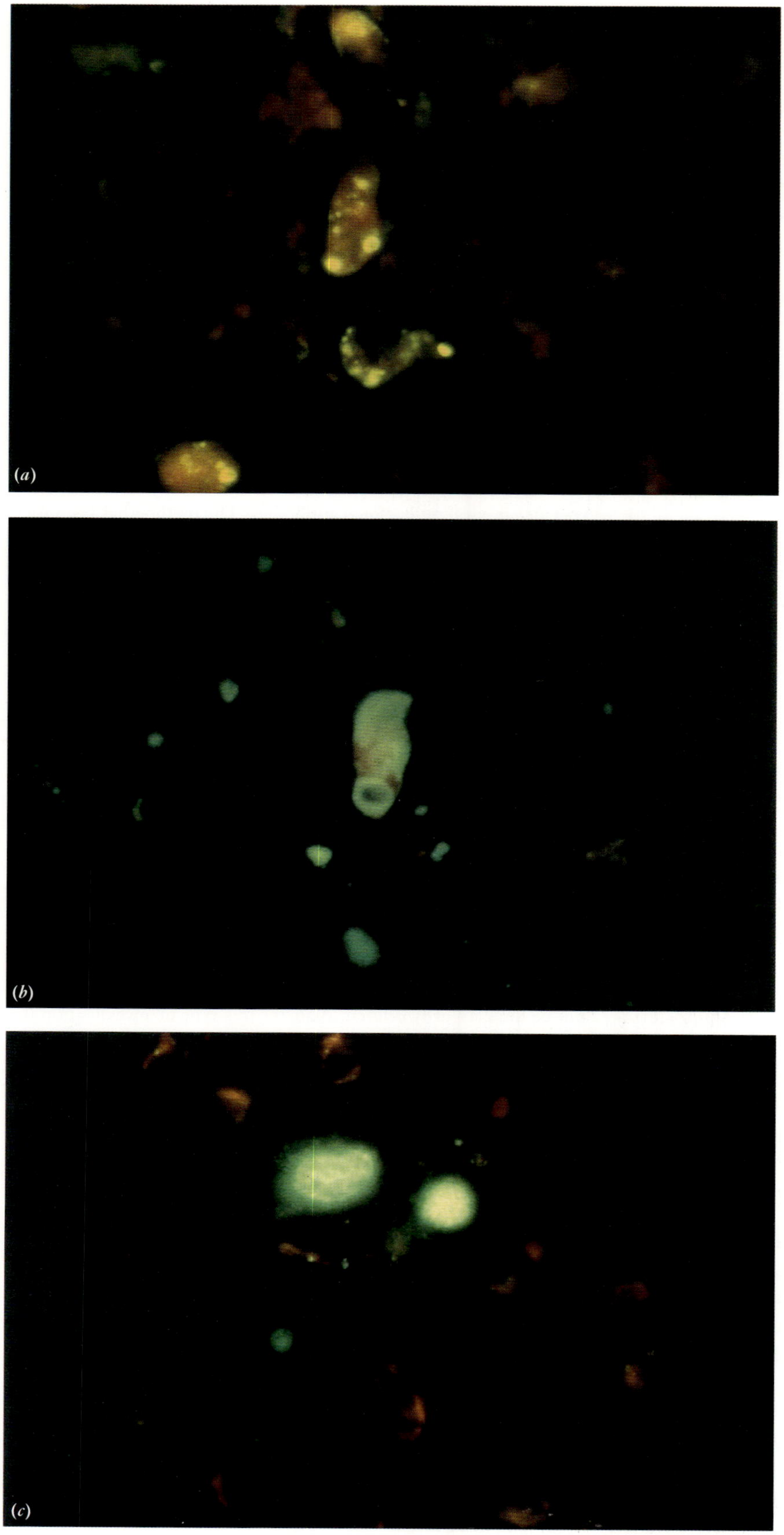

FIGURE 1.6 Detection by immunofluorescence of viral antigens in infected cells in clinical specimens. (*a*) Respiratory syncytial virus-infected cells showing typical cytoplasmic viral inclusions. (*b*) Influenza type B infected cells with cytoplasmic and perinuclear immunofluorescence. (*c*) Adenovirus-infected cells with accumulation of antigens in the nuclei.

specific antibodies[240] but a membrane enzyme immunofiltration assay has been described for influenza A[241]: viral antigens are trapped non-specifically in nylon membrane-bottomed microtitre wells. Other test kits employ a cellulose membrane for passive adsorption of viral antigens. The sensitivity of the commercial membrane test (85%) is somewhat lower than that of virus isolation[242]. Several reports have compared the accuracy for different kits and methods[243–247].

The time-resolved fluoroimmunoassay, TR-FIA, another immunoassay for detection of viral antigens, is used for large-scale diagnosis of viral respiratory infections in some parts of the world[248].

Detection of viral nucleic acids directly in clinical specimens

The gene hybridization technique has been evaluated for diagnosis of respiratory infections, but was not sensitive enough for reliable diagnosis. However, the polymerase chain reaction (PCR) has proved to be extremely sensitive for diagnosis directly from clinical specimens[249].

Most types of specimens in which virus or viral nucleic acids are expected to occur can be investigated by PCR. No infectious virus, and no intact cells from the respiratory tract are necessary for successful use of the technique. Amplification of genes by PCR is followed by detection of the gene product (amplimer) by gel electrophoresis and staining with ethidium bromide. Since respiratory infections are caused usually by RNA viruses (influenza, respiratory syncytial, parainfluenza- and rhinoviruses) a reversed transcription step producing complementary DNA is performed before the amplification by PCR. This step is not necessary for the DNA viruses (adenovirus and the herpes viruses).

A sensitive 'reversed transcription PCR – enzyme immunoassay' has been developed in which the amplified DNA in the solution is hybridised to a nested biotinylated RNA probe and quantitated in an enzyme immunoassay[250].

PCR also offers increased specificity. It has its place in diagnosis of, for example, the rhinoviruses, because of the existence of several distinct serotypes difficult to diagnose by immunological methods[251,252]. Although the technique is still demanding, expensive and vulnerable, PCR has shown its diagnostic superiority for demonstration of the presence of respiratory syncytial virus[253–256] and parainfluenza type 3[250] in clinical material.

Several papers have been published on the use of PCR for influenza diagnosis directly in clinical specimens[249,254,257,258]. The technique may also be used for nucleic acid sequencing of the H1 gene[259,260].

PCR has been shown to be the most sensitive method for detection of CMV in BAL from immunosuppressed patients with pneumonia[230,261] and the negative predictive value of the assay is high. At the same time, a pulmonary CMV infection should be seriously considered in patients with a positive CMV PCR in BAL[230]. The correlation is, however, less strong for HIV patients[262].

CMV viraemia in bone marrow transplant patients may predict development of a CMV pneumonia[263,264]. The presence of CMV matrix antigen, pp65, in peripheral blood leukocytes is a sensitive marker closely correlated with clinical symptoms[265–267] and the antigen can be repeatedly detected with immunoperoxidase or immunofluorescence stainings. The blood specimens need, however, to be processed within 3 hours after sampling, as they may otherwise give false-negative results. Likewise, PCR can be used for detection of CMV in peripheral blood leukocytes. Amplification of the major immediate early gene region by a nested PCR has a high sensitivity for detection of CMV. In renal transplanted patients a positive CMV PCR, however, is not as closely correlated with the appearance of clinical disease as is the CMV pp65 antigenaemia assay[268]. Despite the presumed latency of CMV in leukocytes, CMV leukocyte PCR can be standardised at a relevant level for screening of transplant patients[269,270].

By use of modern diagnostic tools and subsequent treatment with antiviral drugs, the mortality of CMV disease has been reduced to a minimum[264].

Diagnosis by serological investigation

Serodiagnosis has been widely used for diagnosis of respiratory infections. The first specimens should be taken within the first week of illness and the second serum sample (two weeks later for diagnosis of CMV and ornithosis, 2–4 weeks later). The demonstration of virus-specific IgM in a single serum sample also gives a virus-specific diagnosis. Serology, however, gives diagnosis late in the disease, as the investigation has to wait for the development of an antibody response in the patient. Furthermore, a lack of immunological response to the infection may be seen in immunocompromised patients.

Comparison of antibody titres in acute- and convalescent-phase sera

A significant titre rise can be demonstrated. While the complement fixation test has been widely used in the past, most laboratories now use the ELISA, which has the advantage of permitting separate measurement of the different immunoglobulin classes and subclasses. The ELISA technique is more sensitive than complement fixation and is superior for diagnosis in infants where an increase of the antibody level may be difficult to measure because of residual maternal antibodies.

Tests for specific antibodies of different immunoglobulin classes (IgG, IgM, IgA)

These are not routinely performed for respiratory viral infections, although the presence of IgM in a single serum specimen is diagnostic.

IgM detection for diagnosis has been reported for some respiratory viruses, but in most patients these antibodies are not detectable for several days of illness[271,272]. Combined testing for IgM and IgA is used in many diagnostic laboratories to increase the diagnostic sensitivity. For diagnosis of CMV, herpes simplex and varicella zoster virus infections in the lower respiratory tract, the detection of antibodies of IgG and IgM classes by ELISA supports a clinical diagnosis. However, in primary as well as in reactivated infections, anti-CMV antibodies may develop late in the disease. The fact that immunocompromised patients may fail to produce IgM even during symptomatic CMV infections should also be noted[273].

Table 1.7 summarises some major diagnostic techniques for viral respiratory pathogens.

Table 1.7. *Diagnosis of viral respiratory infection*

Virus	Antigen detection		Gene detection, PCR	Serology: two serum samples			IgM (single serum sample) ELISA
	IF	EIA		ELISA	CF	HI	
Respiratory syncytial virus	+ NPS	+ NPS	+(R)	+	+		(+)[a]
Influenza A	+ NPS	+ NPS	+	+	+	+	(+)[a]
Influenza B	+ NPS	+ NPS	+	+	+	+	(+)[a]
Parainfluenza 1	+ NPS	+ NPS	+(R)	+	+		
Parainfluenza 2	+ NPS	+ NPS	+(R)	+	+		
Parainfluenza 3	+ NPS	+ NPS	+(R)	+	+		(+)[a]
Adenovirus	+ NPS	+ NPS	+	+	+		(+)[a]
Rhinovirus			+[b]				
Measles[c]	+ NPS (4 days)		+(R)	+	+		+(from 2–3 days after rash)
Cytomegalovirus	(+)[d] L		+L	+			+
	pp65 in PBL		+PBL				
Herpes simplex virus	(+)[d] L		+L	+			+
Varicella zoster virus	(+)[d] L		+L	+			+

IF, immunofluorescence; EIA, enzyme immunoassay; PCR, polymerase chain reaction; CF, complement fixation; HI, haemagglutination; NPS, nasopharyngeal secretions; R, mainly research; PBL, peripheral blood leukocytes; L, bronchioalveolar lavage, BAL.

[a] Not suitable for routine diagnosis, because of late appearance (4–7 days after start of illness) and technical difficulties.

[b] Suitable for routine diagnosis because of the antigen diversity in the group.

[c] Measles is not mentioned in the text, but is included here for comparison.

[d] Sensitivity too low for antigen detection in bronchoalveolar lavage.

MYCOBACTERIAL INFECTION

Laboratory diagnosis of pulmonary tuberculosis or mycobacteriosis

Tuberculosis infection can be found in almost every body tissue, and mycobacterial investigation with culture, direct smear and, when appropriate, PCR and histopathological examination is advisable as soon as such an infection is suspected.

All respiratory specimens for mycobacterial cultures should be put in wide-mouthed, clean, sterile, tight containers as recommended by the laboratory. No additives should be used, neither saline, which dilutes the material, nor alcohol or formaldehyde, which kills the bacteria. If processing is delayed, refrigeration may prevent growth of contaminants in the specimen. Sputum is the simplest specimen material to obtain for diagnosis of pulmonary tuberculous infection, and if the patient produces sputum this is also the most relevant diagnostic material. A good specimen should contain 2–5 ml of sputum. The material should be free of saliva and be coughed up from the deep airways and collected early in the morning before any food is taken and after the mouth has been rinsed with sterile or chilled, boiled water. As the excretion of mycobacteria is intermittent, 2–3 or up to 6 specimens ideally from different days are advisable. It was reported that 95% of positive mycobacterial cultures and smears were found by examining three sputum samples[274]. The specimens should not be pooled because pooling may cause dilution of positive material and spread of contaminants. Patients unable to produce sputum spontaneously can produce good results with nebulised saline solution. The yield is not as good as that of expectorated sputum, but it is better than gastric aspirates[275].

Sputum specimens are well suited for diagnosis by direct smear examination but should always be homogenised and concentrated by centrifugation, (Fig. 1.7). Culture should be performed if the purpose is diagnosis of tuberculosis or mycobacteriosis. Direct smear without culture may be used only to judge the degree of contagiousness of the tuberculosis patient.

With the current PCR it is possible in sputum, as well as in other secretions, to obtain the diagnosis of *Mycobacterium tuberculosis* complex within 8 hours. Because of practical and economic restraints, only selected specimens are usually examined by PCR, as in the case of acid fast direct smear positive specimens when rapid confirmation of bacterium species is wanted. In critically ill patients with lung infiltrates and negative direct smear, or otherwise when a rapid diagnosis is necessary, PCR is very helpful, as the processing time is short. The sensitivity is equal to or even higher than that of culture (see below).

In the absence of sputum production, bronchoscopy with BAL is the preferred alternative method to provide specimens for the diagnosis of pulmonary tuberculosis. This method has been reported in some patient materials to yield even better results than sputum for both smear and culture[87]. Fiberoptic bronchoscopy was the exclusive means of diagnosing tuberculosis in 41% of sputum-producing patients and in 77% of those not producing sputum[276]. Specific lung segments may be probed by the bronchoscope and the yield of tubercle bacilli is usually higher than in gastric lavage. However, if bronchoscopy is preferred in a patient with sputum production; it is wise to have one or two sputa examined for acid fast bacteria before the

Table 1.8. *Approximate sensitivity of some common methods for bacteriological diagnosis of pulmonary tuberculosis*

	Sputum	Induced sputum	BAL	Gastric aspirate	Faeces	Pleural biopsy	Pleural fluid
Culture	High (bacteria/ml)	High	High	Medium	Medium	High	Low
Direct smear	Low (bacteria/ml)	Low	Low	Very low	Very low	Low	Very Low
PCR	High (bacteria/ml)	High	High	Medium	Medium	High	Low

bronchoscopy. This procedure may alert the bronchoscopist to the risk of inhaling tubercle bacilli from the patient.

If a gastric aspirate is chosen, it should be taken in the morning after overnight fasting. The patient is allowed to drink 200 ml of sterile water. Unboiled tap water may contaminate the culture with environmental mycobacteria. The patient has to swallow a thin tube, thereby emptying the content of the ventricle into a sterile bottle. The procedure should be repeated on two or three consecutive days for optimal diagnostic yield. Gastric wash is today largely replaced by BAL, which is more effective and almost as easy to perform.

When bronchoscopy is performed, biopsies may also be taken from suspected tuberculous lesions in the bronchial tree. Biopsy material should be put in a sterile tube without any additives. Thoracoscopy makes it possible to get tissue biopsies from the pleural cavity with a much higher isolation rate of tubercle bacilli than culture from pleural fluid[277]. Blind Abram's biopsies can also be performed from pleura with a good yield.

If thoracotomy is carried out in a patient with suspected tuberculosis, biopsies taken from lymph nodes, lung tissue and pleural tissue

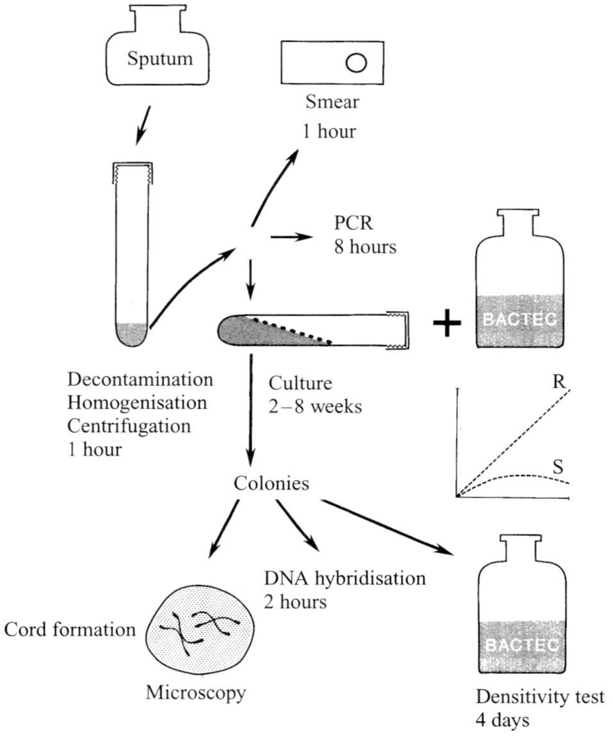

FIGURE 1.7 Laboratory diagnosis of pulmonary tuberculosis.

are advantageous. PCR can be performed on all these materials, but culture is still the basic diagnostic procedure.

Pleural fluid specimens may be mixed with heparin or citrate solution to avoid coagulation before they are sent to the laboratory for mycobacterial culture. At least 10 ml should be sent. As outlined above, culture of pleural fluid for tubercle bacteria is an insensitive examination that is suboptimal in the diagnosis of tuberculous pleuritis. Airway secretions often yield growth of tubercle bacteria in cases of tuberculous pleuritis even in the absence of lung infiltrates on X-ray.

In infants faecal culture is an alternative to airway specimens or gastric aspirate when pulmonary tuberculosis is suspected. However, the rate of contamination is higher than in airway specimens (Table 1.8).

In cases when tuberculosis is suspected, culture for mycobacteria should always be done. Direct smear is a valuable adjunct to culture, but its sensitivity is much lower, especially in patients excreting low numbers of mycobacteria. In unconcentrated sputum direct smear detects about 25% of culture-positive tuberculosis cases in our laboratory, whereas for homogenised and concentrated sputum the figure is approximately 50%. The latter figure accords well with other reports: Levy *et al.* found 53% sensitivity[274] and Gordin & Slutkin 46–55% sensitivity of smear in relation to culture[278]. However, Kim *et al.* found that 74% of culture-positive patients had positive smears[279]. The clinical stage of the disease, i.e. the quantity of mycobacteria excreted, as well as the technical procedures applied for both smears and cultures are important for the sensitivity of direct smears. If culture methods are suboptimal, for example, the sensitivity of smears will be higher than with the more sensitive culture techniques.

In extrapulmonary tuberculosis, whether associated with pulmonary tuberculosis or not, there may be a reason to perform mycobacterial cultures from urine, various secretions, abscesses or tissue biopsies. Fine-needle biopsy from lymph nodes with a syringe is often sufficient for a positive culture, but if concomitant histopathological examination is desired a surgical biopsy is better[280].

Blood cultures may be indicated when disseminated a-reactive tuberculosis or disseminated *M. avium* complex infection is suspected, as may be pertinent in patients with AIDS. In these cases the Bactec 13 A bottle (Becton Dickinson) with ^{14}C-labelled Middlebrook broth is recommended[281]. Obtaining specimens for blood culture is considerably easier and less troublesome for the patient than taking bone marrow specimens. The load of *M. avium* complex is very high in the disseminated form of infection in AIDS and the blood monocytes contain great numbers of mycobacteria. Therefore, the chance of diagnosing bloodstream infection is as good as that with bone marrow aspirate. In disseminated tuberculosis, on the other hand, there may be fewer circulating bacteria in the blood and a marrow specimen may be more likely to be positive for tubercle bacteria than a blood culture. Marrow specimens can be directly injected into 13 A Bactec bottles. It should be noted that histopathological examination of bone marrow and other tissues can often give comparatively rapid supplementary information on the aetiology of infection. For example, granuloma formation in the bone marrow may support a tentative diagnosis of mycobacterial infection.

In case of suspected tuberculous meningitis it is desirable that the specimen consists of 3–5 ml or more of CSF, as there are only a few mycobacteria per millilitre, making laboratory diagnosis slow and difficult. However, with PCR it is now possible to diagnose tuberculous meningitis swiftly[282].

PCR may in principle be applicable on any material for quick and specific tuberculosis diagnosis[283]. There are, however, some technical difficulties with the presence of certain inhibiting substances in tissues and blood which may cause falsely negative results. Each material must therefore be tested with the specific pretreatment technology applied at the local laboratory. Moreover, with this extremely sensitive method, amplifying DNA fragments a million times, there is a clear risk of cross contamination, unless rigorous measures are taken to avoid it. Therefore, PCR is a technique for the experienced laboratory. Kits for easier laboratory work with *M. tuberculosis* PCR are now appearing on the market[284].

Determination of tuberculostearic acid in sputum has been applied as a rapid method to diagnose pulmonary tuberculosis[285]. However, it requires expensive and complicated technical equipment[286].

Serological investigations in suspected tuberculosis have not been very rewarding, because of their lack of specificity and sensitivity. There are no currently used serological routine methods for diagnosing tuberculous infection. In the light of the promising results with the PCR technique it is less probable that any serodiagnostic method will become widespread[287].

Laboratory work

At the laboratory respiratory samples are homogenized and decontaminated from irrelevant bacteria, usually by 1–4% of NaOH, often combined with various mucolytic substances (Table 1.9). Suspensions are then neutralised by acid and centrifuged at 2500–4000 *g* before direct smears and cultures are made from the pellet. If PCR is to be done, an extra rinse of the pellet may be necessary.

The direct smear is the simplest and most rapid diagnostic procedure to detect mycobacteria in a specimen (Fig 1.7). Moreover, the specificity is very high in those laboratories experienced in the identification of positive smears. In conjunction with clinical data a positive direct smear can often give a preliminary diagnosis of tuberculosis. In some cases atypical mycobacteriosis is an alternative diagnosis, especially in immunosuppressed patients. However, it should be noted that the morphology of various species of mycobacteria is similar and therefore it is not possible to tell which species of mycobacteria is present in a direct smear. The specificity of direct smear is >99% in most laboratories, false positives mainly being found in cases with a low number of acid fast rods and in inexperienced laboratories. Direct smears should be stained by fluorescent dyes, e.g. auramin or auramin + rhodamin or by carbolfuchsin (Ziehl–Neelsen stain) (Table 1.10). The latter method gives a lower sensitivity and is more laborious to read than the fluorescent stains. Carbolfuchsin-stained slides must be read with 1000 × oil immersion in contrast to auramine-stained slides where 250 × air is sufficient. Approximately 10 000 mycobacteria/ml must be present for a 50% chance to detect a culture-positive specimen by direct microscopy using a 50 × magnification and reading 30 fields[288]. Moreover, culture is essential for definitive diagnosis including speciation and a drug susceptibility test. Culture detects as few as 10 bacteria/ml and is thus 1000-fold more sensitive than smear. A suggested model for reporting results of direct smears for mycobacteria is given in Table 1.11.

Table 1.9. *Common digestion procedures for specimens used to culture mycobacteria*

2–4% NaOH + *N*-acetyl-L-cysteine
17% benzalkonium chloride (Zephiran) + trisodium phosphate
2–4% NaOH + dithiothreitol (Sputolysin)
2–4% NaOH alone
1% NaOH + sodium lauryl sulphate

Table 1.10. *Common acid fast stains for mycobacteria*

Ziehl–Neelsen stain	Basic fuchsin in ethanol + phenol. Decolorise with HCl + ethanol. Counterstain with methylene blue
Auramine O fluorescent stain	Auramine ± rhodamine+ phenol + ethanol. Decolourise with HCl+ethanol. Counterstain with potassium permanganate

Classical culture of homogenized and centrifuged material is made on egg-based or agar-based solid media and read each week for eight weeks (Table 1.12). The time for *M. tuberculosis* to grow is usually 2–4 weeks, but certain strains grow much slower, and most atypical mycobacteria grow slowly.

Many laboratories use a sensitive and quick cultivation method for mycobacteria, employing a liquid medium, the Bactec system. Middlebrook 7H12 broth including ^{14}C-palmitic acid is used as a substrate and growth of mycobacteria is probed daily by detection of radioactive carbon dioxide (Fig. 1.7). Mycobacterial growth is verified by smear and subculture. Bottles are often positive within 2–3 weeks. The media for the Bactec system are comparatively expensive, but the versatility of the system makes it very attractive. Determination of chemotherapeutic sensitivity and DNA hybridisation for species diagnosis can be started immediately with material from the positive bottle without preceding subculture on solid media.

When growth has appeared on solid media or in Bactec bottles DNA hybridization by a commercial kit is applied for swift species diagnosis. If serpentine cords are formed, revealed by microscopy of smears, the probability for *M. tuberculosis* is high. Cord formation can often be seen also in material from Bactec bottles. *M. tuberculosis* complex and *M. avium* complex are the most common species in clinical materials. Among the pigmented organisms *Mycobacterium kansasii* and

Table 1.11. *Suggested reporting on acid fast bacteria found in sputum by the fluorochrome stain*

Number or rods	Report
0	Negative
1–2/30F	Equivocal – recommend new specimen
3–9/30F	Rare – positive
>10/30F	Positive
>1/F	Many – positive

F, microscopic field at 250–300 × magnification.

Table 1.12. *Some selective media for mycobacterial culture*

Löwenstein–Jensen	Coagulated eggs + defined salts + glycerol + potato flour
Antibacterial/antifungal supplement	Malachite green (0.25 g/l) Nalidixic acid + trimethoprim
Middlebrook 7H10–7H11	Agar base + defined salts + glycerol + albumin, vitamins, cofactors, oleic acid, catalase + dextrose or casein hydrolysate
Antibacterial/antifungal supplement	Malachite green (0.25 g/l) Azlocillin, nalidixic acid, polymyxin B, trimethoprim, amphotericin B

Table 1.13. *Examples of drugs suggested for sensitivity determinations in mycobacteria*

Mycobacterium tuberculosis complex	*Mycobacterium avium intracellulare* and other atypical mycobacteria
Isoniazid	Ethambutol
Rifampicin	Rifampicin, rifabutin
Pyrazinamide	Clarithromycin
Amikacin /streptomycin	Ciprofloxacin
Ethambutol	Amikacin
Ciprofloxacin	Clofazimin
Rifabutin	
Ethionamide	
Para-aminosalicylic acid	
Cycloserine	

Mycobacterium gordonae are the most prevalent. DNA probes exist for these four organisms. Other species of mycobacteria may be typed by biochemistry or gas chromatography. Within the *M. tuberculosis* complex the species *M. bovis* is identified by *in vitro* Tiophen-2-carboxylic acid hydrazide (TCH) sensitivity and pyrazinamide resistance, e.g. in the Bactec system, combined with lack of niacin production. *M. tuberculosis* is resistant against TCH and most often sensitive to pyrazinamide, and produces niacin[289]. Certain African strains are biochemically intermediate between *M. bovis* and *M. tuberculosis*.

Sensitivity tests should be performed on all new isolates of *M. tuberculosis* strains, and also when development of secondary resistance is suspected. Drug susceptibility tests for antimycobacterial substances are best done employing the liquid Bactec system and can be performed by inoculation of material directly from a positive broth culture, or from suspended colonies growing on solid media. The principle for determining *in vitro* sensitivity to antimycobacterial drugs using the Bactec system is the following: Bactec bottles are inoculated with the mycobacterial strain in appropriate dilution. There are two control bottles, one with this dilution and one diluted 100 times more. Also, a number of bottles contain antimycobacterial substances. Growth indices are compared daily from inoculated bottles with and without the presence of antimycobacterial drugs. If the growth index of mycobacteria in the presence of the tested drug is lower than in a drug-free control bottle with the mycobacteria diluted 1/100 the isolate is defined as sensitive to the drug. It is thus accepted that 1% of the bacteria in a sensitive isolate are resistant. In the case of pyrazinamide, which is active only at a low pH, a special Bactec bottle with pH 6.0 is used and a modifed calculation is applied according to the manufacturer's manual. It usually takes four days to perform a sensitivity test with the Bactec system. Suggested drugs for testing are presented in Table 1.13.

The PCR can be applied for the rapid direct diagnosis of *M. tuberculosis* from respiratory and other specimens (Fig. 1.7). It has been mostly applied on sputum specimens. Specificity and sensitivity of PCR for *M. tuberculosis* are similar to or better than those of culture[290,291]. Mycobacteria with reduced viability can also be detected by this technique. It is possible to detect *M. tuberculosis* in heavily contaminated specimens, for which culture may be impossible. The extraction of DNA is time consuming; the whole procedure to extract, amplify and detect the DNA takes approximately one day with today's kits. It is essential to avoid cross-contamination with DNA of the laboratory equipment, e.g. pipettes or solutions, which may otherwise cause false-positive results. Control systems should be employed to assure valid results and calibrate the level of sensitivity. Even in those cases of positive PCR tests, cultures should always be made for quality control, to obtain the strain for sensitivity determinations and to detect mixed infections.

Non-tuberculous mycobacteria

Specimen collection and laboratory methods are the same for non-tuberculous mycobacteria and *M. tuberculosis*. The laboratory techniques are designed to detect all sorts of mycobacteria, tuberculous as well as atypical. In the Western world *M. avium* complex dominates among non-tuberculous mycobacteria in most areas. Pulmonary infection with *M. avium* complex is more common in predisposed persons such as those with previous tuberculosis or with immunodeficiency. In persons with AIDS, *M. avium* complex may be detected in the airways, in the gastrointestinal tract and as a generalised infection with positive blood cultures. The spread of infection usually originates from the gastrointestinal tract rather than the airways. It is possible to obtain an ultimate diagnosis, e.g. in direct smear-positive sputum, by performing both *M. tuberculosis* PCR and *M. avium* complex PCR[292].

M. avium complex and other atypical mycobacteria do not form serpentine cords when grown on solid or liquid media, unlike *M. tuberculosis* complex. A preliminary classification can be made by microscopy of cultures by lack or presence of the characteristic cord formation. Definitive identification of *M. avium* complex or *M. kansasii* can be performed by commercial DNA hybridisation kit (GenProbe, California). Species other than *M. avium* complex and *M. kansasii* must be identified by such means as biochemistry or gas chromatography[293,294].

In vitro sensitivity determinations of atypical mycobacteria can be made much in the same way as for *M. tuberculosis* in the Bactec system. However, the inoculate should be about 1/100 of that for *M. tuberculosis* complex. Moreover, tests of synergistic activity of various drugs against *M. avium* complex can be performed for several two-drug combinations, especially combinations including ethambutol[295], which has effect on the cell wall permeability for other drugs[296]. The most relevant drug combinations are ethambutol plus rifampicin or rifabutin, ethambutol plus clarithromycin and ethambutol plus ciprofloxacin. Antimycobacterial regimens in patients with AIDS often contain these drugs in various combinations[297].

References

1. MARRIE TJ. *Chlamydia pneumoniae. Thorax* 1993; 48:1–4.
2. TJHIE JH, VAN KUPPEVELD FJM, ROOSENDAAL R. Direct PCR enables detection of *Mycoplasma pneumoniae* in patients with respiratory tract infections. *J Clin Microbiol* 1994; 32:11–16.
3. WILLIAMSON J, MARMION BP, WORSWICJ DA *et al.* Laboratory diagnosis of *Mycoplasma pneumoniae* infection 4. Antigen capture and PCR-gene amplification for detection of the mycoplasma: problems of clinical correlation. *Epidemiol Infect* 1992; 109:519–37.
4. AUSTRIAN R. Some observations on the pneumococcus and the current status of pneumococcal disease and its prevention. *Rev Infect Dis* 1981; 3 (Suppl):S1–S17.
5. AUSTRIAN R, GOLD J. Pneumococcal bacteremia with especial reference to bacteremic pneumococcal pneumonia. *Ann Intern Med* 1964; 60:759–76.
6. KALIN M, LINDBERG AA. Diagnosis of pneumococcal pneumonia: a comparison between microscopic examination of expectorate, antigen detection and cultural procedures. *Scand J Infect Dis* 1983; 15:247–55.
7. NORRBY SR, POPE KA. Pneumococcal pneumonia. *J Infect* 1979; 1:109–20.
8. REASERCH COMMITTEE OF BRITISH THORACIC SOCIETY AND PUBLIC HEALTH LABORATORY SERVICE. Community-acquired pneumonia in adults in British hospitals 1982–1983: a survey of aetiology, mortality, prognostic factors, and outcome. *Quart J Med* 1987; 239:195–220.
9. BARTLETT JG, FINEGOLD SM. Bacteriology of expectorated sputum with quantitative culture and wash technique compared to transtracheal aspirates. *Am Rev Resp Dis* 1978; 117:1019–27.
10. BARTLETT J. Diagnostic accuracy of transtracheal aspiration bacteriologic studies. *Am Rev Resp Dis* 1977; 115:777–82.
11. BASELSKI VS, WUNDERINK, RG. Bronchoscopic diagnosis of pneumonia. *Clin Microbiol Rev* 1994; 7:533–58.
12. BENNER EJ, MUNZINGER JP, CHAN R. Superinfection of the lungs: an evaluation by serial transtracheal aspiration. *West J Med* 1974; 121:173–8.
13. CHASTRE J, VIAU F, BRUN P, PIERRE J, DAUGE M-C, BOUCHAMA A, AKESBI A, GIBERT C. Prospective evaluation of the protective specimen brush for the diagnosis of pulmonary infections in ventilated patients. *Am Rev Resp Dis* 1984; 130:924–9.
14. FAGON JY, CHASTRE J, HANCE AJ *et al.* Detection of nosocomial lung infection in ventilated patients. Use of protected specimen brush and quantitative culture techniques in 147 patients. *Am Rev Resp Dis* 1988; 138:110–16.
15. KALIN M, LINDBERG AA, TUNEVALL G. Aetiological diagnosis of bacterial pneumonia by Gram stain and quantitative culture of expectorates. Leukocytes and alveolar macrophages as indicators of sample representativity. *Scand J Infect Dis* 1983; 125:153–60.
16. WIMBERLY N, FALING J, BARTLETT JG. A fiberoptic bronchoscopy technique to obtain uncontaminated lower airway secretions for bacterial culture. *Am Rev Resp Dis* 1979; 119:337–43.
17. BAIGELMAN W, CHODOSH S, PIZZUTO D, SADOW T. Quantitative sputum Gram stains in chronic bronchial disease. *Lung* 1979; 156:265–70.
18. HEINEMAN HS, CHAWLA JK, LOFTON WM. Misinformation from sputum cultures without microscopic examination. *J Clin Microbiol* 1977; 6:518–27.
19. KALIN M. Bacteremic pneumococcal pneumonia: value of nasopharynx culture and examination of washed sputum specimens. *Eur J Clin Microbiol* 1982; 1:394–6.
20. REIN MF, GWALTNEY JM JR, O´BRIEN WM, JENNINGS RH, MANDELL GL Accuracy of Gram´s stain in identifying pneumococci in sputum. *JAMA* 1978; 239:2671–3.
21. MONTRAVERS P, FAGON J-Y, CHASTRE J, LECSO M, DOMBRET MC, TROILLET J-L, GIBERT C. Follow-up protected specimen brushes to assess treatment in nosocomial pneumonia. *Am Rev Resp Dis* 1993; 147, 38–44.
22. SPENCER RC, PHILP JR. Effect of previous antimicrobial therapy on bacteriologic findings in patients with primary pneumonia. *Lancet* 1973; 2:349–51.
23. ÖRTQVIST Å, HAMMERS-BERGGREN S, KALIN M. Respiratory tract colonization, and occurrence of secondary infections, during hospital treatment of community-acquired pneumonia. *Eur J Clin Microbiol Infect Dis* 1990; 9:725–31.
24. GERBER MA, RANDOLPH MF, CHANATRY J, WRIGHT LL, DEMEO KK Antigen detection test for streptococcal pharyngitis: evaluation of sensitivity with respect to true infections. *J Pediatr* 1986; 108:654–7.
25. WEGNER DL, WITTE DL, SCHRANTZ RD. Insensitivity of rapid antigen detection methods and single blood agar plate culture for diagnosing streptococcal pharyngitis. *JAMA* 1992; 267:695–7.
26. KELLOGG JA, MANZELLA JP. Detection of Group A streptococci in the laboratory or physician´s office. Culture vs antibody methods. *JAMA* 1986; 255:2638–42.
27. KELLOG JA. Suitability of throat culture procedures for detection of group A streptococci and as reference standards for evaluation of streptococcal antigen detection kits. *J Clin Microbiol* 1990; 28:165–9.
28. KAPLAN EL, TOP FH JR, DUDDING BA, WANNAMAKER LW. Diagnosis of streptococcal pharyngitis: differentiation of active infection from the carrier state in the symptomatic child. *J Infect Dis* 1971; 123:490–5.
29. KRESH T, HOLLIS DG. *Corynebacterium* and related organisms. In: Balows A, Hausler WJ, Herrmann KL, Isenberg HD, Shadomy HJ, eds. *Manual of Clinical Microbiology*, 5th edn. Washington DC, American Society for Microbiology 1991:277–86.
30. CLARIDGE JE The recognition and significance of *Arcanobacterium hemolyticum. Clin Microbiol Newslett* 1989; 11:41–5.
31. BLUESTONE CD, STEPHENSON JS, MARTIN LM. Ten-year review of otitis media pathogens. *Pediatr Infect Dis J* 1992, 11:S7–S11.
32. KLEIN JO. Microbiologic efficacy of antibacterial drugs for acute otits media. *Pediatr Infect Dis J* 1993, 12:973–5.

33. ROSENFELD RM, VERTREES JE, CARR J *et al.* Clinical efficacy of antimicrobial drugs for acute otitis media: metaanalysis of 5400 children from thirty-three randomized trials. *J Pediatr* 1994; 124:355–67.

34. VIROLAINEN A, SALO P, JERO J, KARMA P, ESKOLA J, LEINONEN M. Comparison of PCR assay with bacterial culture for detecting *Streptococcus pneumoniae* in middle ear fluid of children with acute otitis media. *J Clin Microbiol* 1994, 32:2667–70.

35. UMBERTO G, MAULDIN GL, WUNDERINK RG *et al.* Cases of fever and pulmonary densities in patients with clinical manifestations of ventilator-associated pneumonia. *Chest* 1994; 106:221–35.

36. BARRETT-CONNOR E. The non-value of sputum culture in the diagnosis of pneumococcal pneumonia. *Am Rev Resp Dis* 1971; 103:845–8.

37. DAVIDSON M, TEMPEST B, PALMER DL. Bacteriologic diagnosis of acute pneumonia. Comparison of sputum, transtracheal aspirates, and lung aspirates. *JAMA* 1976; 235:158–63.

38. FOY HM, WENTWORTH B, KENNY GE, KLOECK JM, GRAYSTON JM. Pneumococcal isolations from patients with pneumonia and control subjects in a prepaid medical care group. *Am Rev Resp Dis* 1975; 111:595–603.

39. GECKLER RW, GREMILLION DH, MCALLISTER CK, ELLENBOGEN C. Microscopic and bacteriological comparison of paired sputa and transtracheal aspirates. *J Clin Microbiol* 1977; 6:396–9.

40. RATHBUN HK, GOVANI I. Mouse inoculation as a means of identifying pneumococci in sputum. *Johns Hopkins Med J* 1967; 120:46–8.

41. TEMPEST B, MORGAN R, DAVIDSON M, EBERLE B, OSEASOHN R. The value of respiratory tract bacteriology in pneumococcal pneumonia among Navajo indians. *Am Rev Resp Dis* 1974; 109:577–8.

42. THORSTEINSSON SB, MUSHER DM, FAGAN T. The diagnostic value of sputum culture in acute pneumonia. *JAMA* 1975; 233:894–5.

43. MURRAY PR, WASHINGTON JA. Microscopic and bacteriologic analysis of expectorated sputum. *Mayo Clin Proc* 1975; 50:339–44.

44. BELLIVEAU P, HICKINGBOTHAM N, MADERAZO EG, MAZENS-SULLIVAN M, ROBINSON A. Institution-specific patterns of infection and Gram´s stain as guide for empiric treatment of patients hospitalized with typical community-acquired pneumonia. *Pharmacotherapy* 1993; 13:396–401.

45. FARRINGTON M, RUBINSTEIN D. Antigen detection in pneumococcal pneumonia. *J Infect* 1991; 23:109–16.

46. LEVY M, DROMER F, BRION N, LETURDU F, CARBON C. Community-acquired pneumonia: importance of initial noninvasive bacteriologic and radiographic investigations. *Chest* 1988; 93:43–8.

47. AITKEN JM, THORNLEY PE. Isolation of *Branhamella catarrhalis* from sputum and tracheal aspirates. *J Clin Microbiol* 1983; 18:1262–3.

48. CATLIN BW. *Branhamella catarrhalis*: an organism gaining respect as a pathogen. *Clin Microbiol Rev* 1990; 3:293–320.

49. DAVIES BI, MAESEN FPV. Epidemiological and bacteriological findings on *Branhamella catarrhails* respiratory infections in the Netherlands. *Drugs* 1986; 31 (Suppl 3):28–33.

50. MACFARLANE JT, FINCH RG, WARD MJ, MACREA AD. Hospital study of adult community-acquired pneumonia. *Lancet* 1982; 2:255–8.

51. JEFFERSON H, DALTON HP, ESCOBAR MR, ALLISON MJ. Transportation delay and the microbiological quality of clinical specimens. *Am J Clin Pathol* 1975; 64:689–93.

52. WASHINGTON JA II (ed.). *Laboratory Procedures in Clinical Microbiology*. New York, Springer Verlag 1985.

53. AMERICAN THORACIC SOCIETY. Guidelines for the initial management of adults with community-acquired pneumonia: diagnosis, assessment of severity, and intial antimicrobial therapy. *Am Rev Resp Dis* 1993; 148:1418–26.

54. QUINONES CA, MEMON MA, SAROSI GA. Bacteremic *Haemophilus influenzae* pneumonia in the adult. *Sem Resp Infect* 1989; 4:12–18.

55. CHODOSH S. Treatment of acute exacerbations of chronic bronchitis: state of the art. *Am J Med* 1991; 91:6A-87S–6A-93S.

56. BOERSMA WG, LÖWENBERG A, HOLLOWAY Y, KUTTSCHRÜTTER H, SNIJDER JAM, KOETER GH. Pneumococcal capsular antigen detection and pneumococcal serology in patients with community acquired pneumonia. *Thorax* 1991; 46:902–6.

57. BOERSMA WG, LÖWENBERG A, HOLLOWAY Y, KUTTSCHRÜTTER H, SNIJDER JAM, KOETER GH. Pneumococcal antigen persistence in sputum from patients with community acquired pneumonia. *Chest* 1992; 102:422–7.

58. HOLLOWAY Y, BOERSMA WG, KUTTSCHRÜTTER H, SNIJDER JAM. Effect of washing sputum on detection of pneumococcal capsular antigen. *Eur J Clin Microbiol Infect Dis* 1991; 10:567–9.

59. SCHAFFNER A, MICHEL-HARDER C, YEGINSOY S. Detection of capsular polysaccharide in serum for diagnosis of pneumococcal pneumonia: clinical and experimental evaluation. *J Infect Dis* 1991; 163:1094–102.

60. VENKATESAN P, MACFARLLANE JT. Pneumococcal antigen in the diagnosis of pneumococcal pneumonia. *Thorax* 1992; 47:329–31.

61. EDWARDS EA, COONROD JD. Coagglutination and counterimmunoelectrophoresis for detection of pneumococcal antigens in sputum of pneumonia patients. *J Clin Microbiol* 1980; 11:488–91.

62. TELENTI A, SUAREZ LEIVA P. Persistence of pneumococcal antigens in sputum after pneumonia. *Scand J Infect Dis* 1984; 16:323–4.

63. BUKANTZ SC, GARA PF, BULLOWA JGM. Capsular polysaccharide in the blood of patients with pneumococcic pneumonia. Detection, incidence, prognostic significance and relation to therapies. *Arch Intern Med* 1942; 69:191.

64. DOCHEZ AR, AVERY OT. The elaboration of specific soluble substance by pneumococcus during growth. *J Exp Med* 1917; 26:477–93.

65. SPENCER RC, SAVAGE MA. Use of counter and rocket immunoelectrophoresis in acute respiratory infections due to *Streptococcus pneumoniae*. *J Clin Pathol* 1976; 29:187–90.

66. TUGWELL P, GREENWOOD BM. Pneumococcal antigen in lobar pneumonia. *J Clin Pathol* 1975; 28:118–23.

67. FARRINGTON M, RUBENSTEIN D. Antigen detection in pneumococcal pneumonia. *J Infect* 1991; 23:109–16.

68. HOLMBERG H, HOLME T, KROOK A, OLSSON T, SJÖBERG L, SJÖGREN A-M. Detection of C polysaccharide in *Streptococcus pneumoniae* in the sputa of pneumonia patients by an enzyme-linked immunosorbent assay. *J Clin Microbiol* 1985; 22:111–15.

69. ÖRTQVIST Å, JÖNSSON I, KALIN M, KROOK A. Comparison of three methods for detection of pneumococcal antigen in sputum of patients with community-acquired pneumonia. *Eur J Clin Microbiol Infect Dis* 1989; 9:725–31.

70. RUUSKANEN O, NOHYNEK H, ZIEGLER T, CAPEDING R, RIKALAINEN H, HOUVINEN P, LEINONEN M. Pneumonia in childhood: etiology and response to antimicrobial therapy. *Eur J Clin Microbiol Infect Dis* 1992; 11:217–23.

71. PARKINSON AJ, RABIEGO ME, SEPULVEDA C, DAVIDSON M, JOHNSON C. Quantitation of pneumococcal C polysaccharide in sputum samples from patients with presumptive pneumococcal pneumonia by enzyme immunoassay. *J Clin Microbiol* 1992; 30:318–22.

72. RAMSEY BW, MARCUSE E, FOY HM. Use of bacterial antigen detection in the diagnosis of pediatric lower respiratory tract infections. *Pediatrics* 1986; 78:1–9.

73. MARCON MJ, HAMOUDI AC, CANNON HJ.

Comparative laboratory evaluation of three antigen detection methods for diagnosis of *Haemophilus influenzae* type b disease. *J Clin Microbiol* 1984; 19:333–7.

74. WITT CS, MONTGOMERY JM, POMAT W, LEHMANN D, ALPERS MP. Detection of *Streptococcus pneumoniae* and *Haemophilus influenzae* type b antigens in the serum and urine of patients with pneumonia in Papua New Guinea: comparison of latex agglutination and counterimmunoelectrophoresis. *Rev Infect Dis* 1990;12 (Suppl 8):S1001–S1005.

75. GILLESPIE SH, ULLMAN C, SMITH MD, EMERY V. Detection of *Streptococcus pneumoniae* in sputum samples by PCR. *J Clin Microbiol* 1994; 32:1308–11.

76. RUDOLPH KM, PARKINSON AJ, BLACK CM, MAYER LW. Evaluation of polymerase chain reaction for diagnosis of pneumococcal pneumonia. *J Clin Microbiol* 1993; 31:2661–6.

77. SALO P, ÖRTQVIST Å, LEINONEN M. Diagnosis of bacteremic pneumococcal pneumonia by amplification of pneumolysin gene fragment in serum. *J Infect Dis* 1995; 171:479–82.

78. MUSHER DM, GROOVER JE, ROWLAND JM, *et al.* Antibody to capsular polysaccharides of *Streptococcus pneumoniae*: prevalence, persistence, and antibody response. *Clin Infect Dis* 1993; 17:66–73.

79. KONRADSEN HB, SØRENSEN UBS, HENRICHSEN J. A modified enzyme-linked immunosorbent assay for measuring type-specific anti-pneumococcal capsular polysaccharide antibodies. *J Immunol Methods* 1993; 164:13–20.

80. KALIN M, KANCLERSKI K, GRANSTRÖM M, MÖLLBY R. Diagnosis of pneumococcal pneumonia by enzyme linked immunosorbent assay of antibodies to pneumococcal hemolysin (pneumolysin). *J Clin Microbiol* 1987; 25:226–9.

81. MURPHY TF, APICELLA MA. Nontypable *Haemophilus influenzae*: review of clinical aspects, surface antigens, and the human immune response to infection. *Rev Infect Dis* 1987; 9:1–15.

82. HAGER H, VERGHESE A, ALVAREZ S, BERK SL. *Branhamella catarrhalis* respiratory infections. *Rev Infect Dis* 1987; 9:1140–9.

83. BATES JH, CAMPBELL GD, BARRON AL *et al.* Microbial aetiology of acute pneumonia in hospitalized patients. *Chest* 1992; 101:1005–12.

84. ÖRTQVIST Å, KALIN M, LEJDEBORN L, LUNDBERG L. Diagnostic fiberoptic bronchoscopy and protected brush culture in patients with community-acquired pneumonia. *Chest* 1990; 97:576–82.

85. TORRES, A., SERRA-BATLES, J., FERRER, A *et al.* Severe community-acquired pneumonia. *Am Rev Resp Dis* 1991; 144:312–18.

86. BAUGHMAN RP, DOHN MN, FRAME PT. The continuing utility of bronchoalveolar lavage to diagnose opportunistic infection in AIDS patients. *Am J Med* 1994; 97:515–20.

87. BAUGHMAN RP, DOHN MN, LOUDON RG, FRAME PT. Bronchoscopy with bronchoalveolar lavage in tuberculosis and fungal infections. *Chest* 1991; 99:92–7.

88. BAUGHMAN RP, RHODES JC, DOHN MN, HENDERSON H, FRAME PT. Detection of cryptococcal antigen in bronchoalveolar lavage fluid: a prospective study of diagnostic utility. *Am Rev Resp Dis* 1992; 145:1226–9.

89. JIMÉNEZ ML, ASPA J, PADILLA B, ANCOCHEA J, GONZÁLEZ A, FRAGA J, SANTOS I, MARTINEZ R, GÓMEZ HERRUZ P, LÓPEZ-BREA M. Fiberoptic bronchoscopic diagnosis of pulmonary disease in 151 HIV-infected patients with pneumonitis. *Eur J Clin Microbiol Infect Dis* 1991; 10:491–7.

90. WELDON-LINNE CM, RHONE DP, BOURASSA R Bronchoscopy specimens in adults with AIDS. Comparative yields of cytology, histology and culture for diagnosis of infectious agents. *Chest* 1990; 98:24–8.

91. FAGON JY, CHASTRE J, DOMART Y *et al.* Nosocomial pneumonia in patients receiving comtinuous mechanical ventilation. Prospective analysis of 52 episodes with use of a protected specimen brush and quantitative culture techniques. *Am Rev Resp Dis* 1989; 139:877–84.

92. FEINSILVER SH, FEIN AM, NIEDERMAN MS, SCHULTZ DE, FAEGENBURG GH. Utitily of fiberoptic bronchoscopy in non-resolving pneumonia. *Chest* 1990; 98:1322–6.

93. PINGLETON SK, CHASTRE J. Diagnosis of nosocomial pneumonia in mechanically ventilated patients. *Pulmonary Perspect* 1990; 7:1–4.

94. SCHELD WM, MANDELL GL. Nosocomial pneumonia: pathogenesis and recent advances in diagnosis and therapy. *Rev Infect Dis* 1991; 13 (Suppl 9):S743–S751.

95. GOLDSTEIN RA, ROHATGI PK, BERGOFSKY EH *et al.* American Thoracic Society. Clinical role of bronchoalveolar lavage in adults with pulmonary disease. *Am Rev Resp Dis* 1990; 142:481–6.

96. GENTILE G, MICOZZI A, GIRMENIA C, PAOLA A, DONATI PP, CAPRIA S. Pneumonia in allogeneic and autologous bone marrow recipients. A retrospective study. *Chest* 1993; 104:371–5.

97. MASCHMEYER G, LINK H, HIDDEMANN W *et al.* Pulmonary infiltrations in febrile patients with neutropenia. Risk factors and outcome under empirical antimicrobial therapy in a randomized multicenter study. *Cancer* 1994; 73:2296–304.

98. MERMEL LA, MAKI DG. Bacterial pneumonia in solid organ transplantation. *Semin Resp Infect* 1990, 5:10–29.

99. ROSENKOV EC III. Diffuse pulmonary infiltrates in the immunocompromised host. *Clin Chest Med* 1990; 11:55–64.

100. WILSON WR, COCKERILL FR, ROSENOW EC. Pulmonary disease in the immunocompromised host. *Mayo Clin Proc* 1985; 60:610–31.

101. BROOK I, FINEGOLD SM. Bacteriology of aspiration pneumonia. *Pediatrics* 1980; 54:1115–20.

102. MEDURI GU, BASELSKI V. The role of bronchoalveolar lavage in diagnosing nonopportunistic bacterial pneumonia. *Chest* 1991; 100:179–90.

103. FAGON JY, CHASTRE J, HANCE AJ, DOMART Y, TROILLET JL, GIBERT C. Evaluation of clinical judgement in the identification and treatment of nosocomial pneumonia in ventilated patients. *Chest* 1993; 103:547–53.

104. BERMAN SZ, MATHISON DA, STEVENSON DD *et al.* Transtracheal aspiration studies in asthmatic patients in relapse with infective asthma and in subjects without respiratory disease. *J Allergy Clin Immunol* 1975; 56:206–14.

105. REIN MF, MANDELL GL. Bacterial killing by bacteriostatic saline solotions – potential for diagnostic error. *N Engl J Med* 1973; 289:794–5.

106. BARTLETT, JG. The technique of transtracheal aspiration. *J Crit Illness* 1986; 1(1): 43–9.

107. RIES K, LEVISON ME, KAYE D. Transtracheal aspiration in pulmonary infection. *Arch Intern Med* 1974; 133:453–8.

108. BJERKESTRAND G, DIGRANES A, SCHREINER A. Bacteriological findings in transtracheal aspirates from patients with chronic bronchitis and bronchiectasis. *Scand J Infect Dis* 1975; 56:201–7.

109. BROUGHTON WA, MIDDLETON RM, KIRKPATRICK MB, BASS JB. Bronchoscopic protected specimen brush and bronchoalveolar lavage in the diagnosis of bacterial pneumonia. *Infect Dis Clin North Am* 1991; 5:437–52.

110. BARTLETT JG, ALEXANDER J, MAYHEW J, SULLIVAN-SIGLER N, GORBACH SL. Should fiberoptic bronchoscopy aspirates be cultured? *Am Rev Resp Dis* 1976; 1114:73–8.

111. FOSSIECK BE JR, PARKER RH, COHEN MH, KANE RC. Fiberoptic bronchoscopy and culture of bacteria from the lower respiratory tract. *Chest* 1977; 72:5–9.

112. MEDURI GU, CHASTRE J. The standardisation of bronchoscopic techniques for ventilator-associated pneumonia. *Chest* 1992; 102:557s–564s.

113. CANTRAL DE, TAPE TG, REED EC, SPURZEM JR, RENNARD SI, THOMPSON

AB. Quantitative culture of bronchoalveolar lavage fluid for the diagnosis of bacterial pneumonia. *Am J Med* 1993; 95:601–7.

114. DREYFUSS D, MIER L, LEBOURDELLES G *et al.* Clinical significance of borderline quantitative protected brush specimen culture results. *Am Rev Resp Dis* 1993; 147:946–51.

115. FOX RC, WILLIAMS CJ, WUNDERINK RG, LEEPER KV, JONES CA. Follow up bronchoscopy predicts therapeutic outcome in ventilated patients with nosocomial pneumonia. *Am Rev Resp Dis* 1991; 143:A109.

116. CHASTRE J, FAGON JY, SOLER P *et al.* Diagnosis of nosocomial bacterial pneumonia in intubated patients undergoing ventilation: comparison of the usefulness of bronchoalveolar lavage and the protected specimen brush. *Am J Med* 1988; 85:499–506.

117. FAGON JY, CHASTRE J, TROILLET JL *et al.* Characterization of distal bronchial microflora during acute exacerbation of chronic bronchitis. Use of the protected specimen brush technique in 54 mechanically ventilated patients. *Am Rev Resp Dis* 1990; 142:1004–8.

118. KAHN FW, JONES JM. Analysis of bronchoalveolar lavage specimens from immunocompromised patients with a protocol applicable in the microbiology laboratory. *J Clin Microbiol* 1988; 26:1150–5.

119. RODRIGUES DE CASTRO F, SOLÉ J, ELCUAZ R. Quantitative cultures of protected brush specimens and bronchoalveolar lavage in ventilated patients without suspected pneumonia. *Am J Resp Crit Care Med* 1994; 149:320–3.

120. TIMSIT J-F, MISSET B, FRANCOUAL S, GOLDSTEIN FW, VAURY P, CARLET J. Is protected specimen brush a reproducible method to diagnose ICU-acquired pneumonia? *Chest* 1993; 104:104–8.

121. POLLACK HM, HAWKINS EL, BONNER JR, SPARKMAN T, BASS JB. Diagnosis of bacterial pulmonary infection with quantitative protective catheter cultures obtained during bronchoscopy. *J Clin Microbiol* 1993; 17:255–9.

122. MEDURI GU, WUNDERINK RG, LEEPER KV, BEALS DH. Management of bacterial pneumonia in ventilated patients. Protected bronchoalveolar lavage as a diagnostic tool. *Chest* 1992; 101:500–8.

123. MEDURI GU. Ventilator-associated pneumonia in patients with respiratory failure. A diagnostic approach. *Chest* 1990; 97:1208–19.

124. MEDURI GU, MAULDIN GL, WUNDERINK RG *et al.* Causes of fever and pulmonary densities in patients with clinical manifestations of ventilator-associated pneumonia. *Chest* 1994; 106:221–35

125. JOHANSON WG, SEIDENFELD JJ, GOMEZ P, DE LOS SANTOS R, COALSON JJ Bacteriologic diagnosis of nosocomial pneumonia following prolonged mechanical ventilation. *Am Rev Resp Dis* 1988; 137:259–64.

126. PUGIN J, AUCKENTHALER R, MILI N, JANSSENS JP, LEW PD, SUTER PM. Diagnosis of ventilator-associated pneumonia by bacteriologic analysis of bronchoscopic and non-bronchoscopic blind bronchoalveolar lavage fluid. *Am Rev Resp Dis* 1991; 143:1121–9.

127. AUBAS S, AUBAS P, CAPDEVILA X, DARBAS H, ROUSTAN J-P, DU CAILAR J. Bronchoalveolar lavage for diagnosing bacterial pneumonia in mechanically ventilated patients. *Am J of Resp Crit Care Med* 1994; 149:860–6.

128. WUNDERINK RG, RUSSEL GB, MEZGER E, ADAMS D, POPOVICH J. The diagnostic utitity of the antibody-coated bacteria test in intubated patients. *Chest* 1991; 99:84–8.

129. CHASTRE J, FAGON JY, SOLER P *et al.* Quantification of BAL cells containing intracellular bacteria rapidly identifies ventilated patients with pneumonia. *Chest* 1989; 95:190S–192S.

130. SOLÉ-VIOLÁN J, RODRIGUEZ DE CASTRO F, REY A, MARTIN-GONZÁLEZ JC, CABRERA-NAVARRO P. Usefulness of microscopic examination of intracellular organisms in lavage fluid in ventilator-associated pneumonia. *Chest* 1994; 106:889–94.

131. KAHN FW, JONES JM. Diagnosing bacterial respiratory infection by bronchoalveolar lavage in the rapid diagnosis of lung disease. *Lab Menage* 1986; 24:31–5.

132. EL-EBIARY M, TORRES A, GONZALEZ J, DE LABELLACASA JP, GARCIA C, DE ANTA MTJ, FERRER M, RODRIGUEZ-ROISIN R. Quantitative cultures of endotracheal aspirates for the diagnosis of ventilator-associated pneumonia. *Am Rev Resp Dis* 1993; 148:1552–7.

133. MARQUETTE CH, GEORGES H, WALLET F *et al.* Diagnostic efficiency of endotracheal aspirates with quantitative bacterial cultures in intubated patients with suspected pneumonia. Comparison with the protected specimen brush. *Am Rev Resp Dis* 1993; 148:138–44.

134. SALATA RA, LEDERMAN MM, SHLAES DM *et al.* Diagnosis of nosocomial pneumonia in intubated, intensive care unit patients. *Am Rev Resp Dis* 1987; 135:426–32.

135. PAPAZIAN L, MARTIN C, MERIC B, DUMON J-F, GOUIN F. A reappraisal of blind bronchial sampling in the microbiologic diagnosis of nosocomial bronchopneumonia. A comparative study in ventilated patients. *Chest* 1993; 103:236–42.

136. GAUSSORGUES P, PIPERNO D, BACHMANN P, BOYER F, JEAN G, GERARD M. Comparison of nonbronchoscopic bronchoalveolar lavage to open lung biopsy for bacteriologic diagnosis of pulmonary infections in mechanically ventialted patients. *Intensive Care Med* 1989; 15:94–8.

137. ROUBY JJ, ROSSIGNON MD, NICOLAS MH, DE LASSALE EM, CRISITIN S, GROSSET J. A prospective study of protected bronchoalveolar lavage in the diagnosis of nosocomial pneumonia. *Anesthesiology* 1989; 71:679–85.

138. WEISS SM, HERT RC, GIANOLA FJ, CLARK JG, CRAWFORD SW. Complications of fiberoptic bronchoscopy in thrombocytopenic patients. *Chest* 1993; 104:1025–8.

139. SHANN F. Aetiology of severe pneumonia in children in developing countries. *Pediatr Infect Dis J* 1986; 5:247–52.

140. MIMICA I, DONOSO E, HOWARD JE *et al.* Lung puncture in the aetiological diagnosis of pneumonia. *Am J Dis Child* 1971 122:278–82.

141. MANRESA F, DORCA J. Needle aspiration techniques in the diagnosis of pneumonia. *Thorax* 1991, 46:601–3.

142. BEGER R, ARANGO L. Aetiologic diagnosis of bacterial nosocomial pneumonia in seriously ill patients. *Crit Care Med* 1985; 13:833–6.

143. TORRES A, JIMÉNEZ P, PUIG DE LA BELLACASA J, CELIS R, GONZÁLEZ J, GEA J. Diagnostic value of nonfluoroscopic percutaneous lung needle aspiration in patients with pneumonia. *Chest* 1990; 98:840–4.

144. COCKERILL II FR, WILSON WR, CARPENTER HA, SMITH TF, ROSENOW EC III. Open lung biopsy in immunocompromised patients. Arch Intern Med 1985; 145:1398–404.

145. GURURANGEN S, LWASON RAM, MORRIS JONES PH, STEVENS RF, CAMPBELL RHA. Evaluation of the usefulness of open lung biopsies. *Pediatr Hematol Oncol* 1992; 9:107–13

146. MCCABE RE, REMINGTON JS. Open lung biopsy. In: Shelhamer J, Pizzo PA, Parrillo JE, Masur H, ed. *Respiratory Disease in the Immunocompromized Host*. Philadelphia, Lipincott 1991: 105–17.

147. SNYDER CL, RAMSAY NK, MCGLAVE PB, FERRELL KL, LEONARD AS. Diagnostic open-lung biopsy after bone marrow transplantation. *J Pediatr Surg* 1990; 25:871–7.

148. ELLIS ME, SPENCE D, BOUCHAMA A *et al.* Open lung biopsy provides a higher and more specific diagnostic yield compared to broncho-alveolar lavage in immunocompromised patients. *Scand J Infect Dis* 1995; 27:157–62.

149. EDELSTEIN PH. The laboratory diagnosis of Legionnaires´disease. *Semin Resp Infect* 1987; 2:235–41.

150. WINN WC JR. Legionella and Legionnaires´disease: a review with emphasis on environmental studies and laboratory diagnosis. *Crit Rev Clin Lab Sci* 1985; 21:323–81.

151. VICKERS RM, STOUT JE, YU VL *et al.*

Culture methodology for the isolation of *Legionella pneumophila* and other Legionellacae from clinical and environmental specimens. *Semin Resp Infect* 1987; 2:274–9.

152. EDELSTEIN PH. Legionnaires´disease. State of the art clinical article. *Clin Infect Dis* 1993; 16:741–9.

153. LEE TC, VICKERS RM, YU VL *et al.* Growth of 28 *Legionella* species on selective culture media: a comparative study. *J Clin Microbiol* 1993; 31:2764–8

154. RUF B, SCHÜRMANN D, HORBACH I, FEHRENBACH FJ, POHLE HD. Prevalence and diagnosis of *Legionella* pneumonia: a 3-year prospective study with emphasis on application of urinary antigen detection. *J Infect Dis* 1990, 162:1341–8.

155. PASCULLE AW, VETO GE, KRYSTOFIAK S, MCKELVEY K, VRSALOVIC K. Laboratory and clinical evaluation of a commercial DNA probe for the detection of *Legionella* spp. *J Clin Microbiol* 1989, 27:2350–8.

156. JAULHAC B, NOWICKI M, BORNSTEIN M, MEUNIER O, PREVOST G, PIEMONT Y, FLEURETTE J, MONTEIL H. Detection of *Legionella* spp in bronchoalveolar lavage fluids by DNA amplification. *J Clin Microbiol* 1992, 30:920–4.

157. SATHAPATAYAVONGS B, KOHLER RB, WHEAT J, WHITE A, WINN WC. Rapid diagnosis of Legionnaires´ disease by latex agglutination. *Am Rev Resp Dis* 1983; 127:559–62.

158. OLIVERIO MJ, FISHER MA, VICKERS RM, YU VL, MENON A. Diagnosis of Legionnaires´ disease by radioimmunoassay of *Legionella* antigen in pleural fluid. *J Clin Microbiol* 1991; 29:2893–4.

159. BROUGHTON RA. Infections due to *Mycoplasma pneumoniae* in childhood. *Pediatr Infect Dis* 1986; 5:71–85.

160. CHANOCK RM, HAYFLICK L, BARILE MF. Growth on artificial medium of agent associated with atypical pneumonia and its identification as PPLO. *Proc Natl Acad Sci USA* 1962; 48:41–9.

161. TULLY JG, ROSE DL, WITCOMB RF *et al.* Enhanced isolation of *Mycoplasma pneumoniae* from throat washings with a newly modified culture medium. *J Infect Dis* 1979; 139:478–82.

162. BIBERFELD G, STERNER G. A study of *Mycoplasma pneumoniae* infections in families. *Scand J Infect Dis* 1969; 1:91–6.

163. DUSSAIX E, SLIM A, TOURNIER P. Comparison of enzyme-linked immunosorbent assay (ELISA) and complement fixation test for detection of *Mycoplasma pneumoniae* antibodies. *J Clin Pathol* 1983; 36:228–32.

164. UDUM SA, JENSEN JS, SØNDERGAARD-ANDERSEN J, LIND K. Enzyme immunoassay for detection of Immunglobulin M (IgM) and IgG antibodies to *Mycoplasma pneumoniae*. *J Clin Microbiol* 1992; 30:1198–204.

165. CIMOLAI N, CHEONG ACH. IgM antiP1 immunoblotting. A standard for the rapid serologic diagnosis of *Mycoplasma pneumoniae* infection in pediatric care. *Chest* 1992; 102:477–81.

166. GRANSTRÖM M, HOLME T, SJÖGREN AM, ÖRTQVIST Å, KALIN M. The role of IgA determination by ELISA in the early serodiagnosis of *Mycoplasma pneumoniae* infection in relation to IgG and μ-capture IgM methods. *J Med Microbiol* 1994; 40:288–92.

167. CHANOCK RM. *Mycoplasma* infections of man. *N Engl J Med* 1965; 273:1199–206.

168. GARROW DH. A rapid test for the presence of increased cold agglutinins. *Br Med J* 1958; 2:206–8.

169. KOK TW, VARKANIS G, MARMION BP, MARTIN J, ESTERMAN A. Laboratory diagnosis of *Mycoplasma pneumoniae* infection. 1. Direct detection of antigen in respiratory exudates by enzyme immuno assay. *Epidemiol Infect* 1988; 191:669–84.

170. MADSEN RD, WEINER LB, MCMILLAN JA, SAEED FA, NORTH JA, COATES SR. Direct detection of *Mycoplasma pneumoniae* antigen in clinical specimens by a monoclonal antibody immunoblot assay. *Am J Clin Pathol* 1988; 89:95–9.

171. HIRAI Y, SHIODE J, MASAYOSHI T, KANEMASA Y. Application of an indirect immunofluorescence test for detection of *Mycoplasma pneumoniae* in respiratory exudates. *J Clin Microbiol* 1991; 29:2007–12.

172. KLEEMOLA SR, KARJALAINEN JE, RATY RK. Rapid diagnosis of *Mycoplasma pneumoniae* infection: clinical evaluation of a commercial probe test. *J Infect Dis* 1990; 162:70–5.

173. KLEEMOLA M, JOKINEN C. Outbreak of *Mycoplasma pneumoniae* infection among hospital personnel studied by a nucleic acid hybridization test. *J Hosp Infect* 1992; 21:213–21

174. BERNET C, GARRET M, DE BARBEYRAC B, BEBEAR C, BONNET J. Detection of *Mycoplasma pneumoniae* by using the polymerase chain reaction. *J Clin Microbiol* 1989; 27:2492–6.

175. COOK PJ, HONEYBOURNE D. *Chlamydia pneumoniae J Antimicrob Chemother* 1994; 34:859–73.

176. GRAYSTONE JT. *Chlamydia pneumoniae* (TWAR) infections in children. *Pediatr Infect Dis J* 1994; 13:675–85.

177. WANG SP, GRAYSTONE JT. Immunologic relationship between genital TRIC, lymphogranuloma venereum, and related organisms in a new microtiter indirect immunofluorescence test. *Am J Ophthalmol* 1970; 70:367–74.

178. CAMPBELL LA, PEREZ MELGOSA M, HAMILTON DJ, KOU C-C, GRAYSTONE JT. Detection of *Chlamydia pneumoniae* by polymerase chain reaction. *J Clin Microbiol* 1992; 30:434–9.

179. GAYDOS CA, QUINN TC, EIDEN JJ. Identification of *Chlamydia pneumoniae* by DNA amplification of the 16S rRNA gene. *J Clin Microbiol* 1992; 30:796–800.

180. TONG CYW, SILLIS M. Detection of *Chlamydia pneumoniae* and *Chlamydia psittaci* in sputum samples by PCR. *J Clin Pathol* 1993; 46:313–17.

181. BODEY GP, VARTIVARIAN S. Aspergillosis. *Eur J Clin Microbiol Infect Dis* 1989; 8:413–37.

182. LAHAM MN, CARPENTER JL *Aspergillus terreus*, a pathogen capable of causing infective endocarditis, pulmonary mycetoma, and allergic bronchopulmonary aspergillosis. *Am Rev Resp Dis* 1982; 125:769–72.

183. KUSNE S, TORRE-CISNEROS J, MANEZ R, IRISH W, MARTIN M, FUNG J, SIMMONS RL, STARZL TE. Factors associated with invasive lung aspergillosis and the significance of positive *Aspergillus* culture after liver transplantation. *J Infect Dis* 1992; 166:1379–83.

184. REGER TR, VISSCHER DW, BARTLETT MS, SMITH JW. Diagnosis of pulmonary infection caused by *Aspergillus*: usefulness of respiratory cultures. *J Infect Dis* 1985; 152:572–6.

185. WEILAND D, FERGUSON RM, PETERSON PK, SNOVER DC, SIMMONS RL, NAJARIAN JS. Aspergillosis in 25 renal transplant patients. *Ann Surg* 1983; 198:622–9.

186. YU VL, MUDER RR, POORTSATTAR A. Significance of isolation of *Aspergillus* from respiratory tract in diagnosis of invasive pulmonary aspergillosis: results from a three-year prospective study. *Am J Med* 1986; 81:249–54.

187. BURCH PA, KARP JE, MERZ WG, KUHLMAN JE, FISHMAN EK. Favorable outcome of invasive aspergillosis in patients with acute leukemia. *J Clin Oncol* 1987; 5:1985–93.

188. KURUP VP, KUMAR A. Immunodiagnosis of aspergillosis. *Clin Microbiol Rev* 1991; 4:439–56.

189. DEREPENTIGNY L, REISS E. Current trends in immunodiagnosis of candidiasis and aspergillosis. *Rev Infect Dis* 1984; 6:301–12.

190. YOUNG RC, BENNET JE. Invasive aspergillosis: absence of detectable antibody response. *Ann Rev Respir Dis* 1971; 104:710–16.

191. MARIER R, SMITH W, JANSEN M, ANDRIOLE VT. A solid phase radioimmunoassay for the measurement of

antibody to *Aspergillus* in invasive aspergillosis. *J Infect Dis* 1979; 140:771–9.

192. TRULL A, PARKER J, WARREN RE. IgG enzyme linked immunosorbent assay for diagnosis of invasive aspergillosis: retrospective study over 15 years of transplant recipients. *J Clin Pathol* 1985; 38:1045–51.

193. ANSORG R, HEINEGG EH, RATH PM. *Aspergillus* antigenuria compared to antigenemia in bone marrow transplant recipients. *Eur J Clin Microbiol Infect Dis* 1994; 13:582–9.

194. ANDREWS CP, WEINER MH *Aspergillus* antigen detection in bronchoalveolar lavage fluid from patients with invasive aspergillosis and aspergillomas. *Am J Med* 1982; 73:372–80.

195. DUPONT B, HUBER M, KIM SJ, BENNET JE. Galactomannan antigenemia and antigenuria in aspergillosis: studies in patients and experimentally infected rabbits. *J Infect Dis* 1987; 155:1–11.

196. HAYNES KA, LATGE JP, ROGERS TR. Detection of *Aspergillus* antigens associated with invasive infection. *J Clin Microbiol* 1990; 28:2040–4.

197. TALBOT GH, WEINER MH, GERSON SL, PROVENCHER M, HURWITZ S. Serodiagnosis of invasive aspergillosis in patients with hematologic malignancy: validation of the *Aspergillus fumigatus* antigen radioimmunoassay. *J Infect Dis* 1987; 155:12–27.

198. TANG CM, HOLDEN DW, AUFAUVRE-BROWN A, COHEN J. The detection of *Aspergillus* spp by polymerase chain reaction and its evaluation in bronchoalveolar lavage fluid. *Am Rev Resp Dis* 1993; 148:1313–17.

199. AISNER J, SICKLES E, SCHIMPFF S *et al.* *Torulopsis glabrata* pneumonitis in patients with cancer. *JAMA* 1974; 230:584–5.

200. WENGROVER D, SEGAL E, KLEINMAN Y. Bronchopulmonary candidiasis is exacerbating asthma. Case report and review of the literature. *Respiration* 1985; 47:209–13.

201. MASUR H, ROSEN P, ARMSTRONG D. Pulmonary disease caused by *Candida* species. *Am J Med* 1977; 63:914–25.

202. SOBEL JD. Controversial aspects of candidiasis in the aquired immunodeficiency syndrome. In: Vanden Bossche H. *et al.* eds. *Mycoses in AIDS Patients*. New York, Plenum Press 1990.

203. JENNER BM, LANDAY LI *et al.* Pulmonary candidiasis in cystic fibrosis. *Arch Dis Child* 1979; 54:555–6.

204. HERENT P, STYNEN D, HERNANDO F, FRUIT J, POULAIN D. Retrospective evaluation of two latex agglutination tests for detection of circulating antigens during invasive candidosis. *J Clin Microbiol* 1992; 30:2158–64.

205. LARSSON L, PEHRSON C, WIEBE T, CHRISTENSSON B. Gas chromatographic determination of *C*-arabinitol/L-arabinitol ratios in urine: a potential method for diagnosis of disseminated candidiasis. *J Clin Microbiol* 1994; 32:1855–9.

206. CHRYSSANTOU E, ANDERSSON B, PETRINI B, LÖFDAHL S, TOLLEMAR J. Detection of *Candida albicans* DNA in serum by polymerase chain reaction. *Scand J Infect Dis* 1994; 26: 479–85.

207. TELENTI A, ROBERTS GD. Fungal blood cultures. *Eur J Clin Microbiol Infect Dis* 1989; 9:825–31.

208. VANMALI AN, LENTEK AL, FRANCO J, NGWENYA BZ Comparison of immunodiffusion and crossed-immunoelectrophoresis in the diagnosis of invasive candidiasis. *Eur J Clin Microbiol* 1983; 2:206–12.

209. MCMANUS EJ, JONES M Detection of a *Trichosporon beigelii* antigen cross-reactive with *Cryptococcus neoformans* capsular polysaccharide in serum from a patient with disseminated trichosporonon infection. *J Clin Microbiol* 1985; 21:681–5.

210. EDMAN JC, KOVACS JA, MASUR H. Ribosomal RNA sequence shows *Pneumocystis carinii* to be a member of the fungi. *Nature* 1988; 33:519–22.

211. HUGES WT. Natural mode of aquisition for *de novo* infection with *Pneumocystis carinii*. *J Infect Dis* 1982; 145:842–8.

212. BENSOUSAN T, GARO B, ISLAM S *et al.* Possible transfer of *Pneumocystis carinii* between kidney transplant recipients. *Lancet* 1990; 336:1066–7.

213. SINGER C, ARMSTRONG D, ROSEN PP *et al.* *Pneumocystis carinii* pneumonia: a cluster of eleven cases. *Ann Intern Med* 1975; 82:772–7.

214. MEUWISSEN JHET, TAUBER I, LEEWENBERG ADEM *et al.* Parasitologic and serologic observations of infection with *Pneumocystis* in humans. *J Infect Dis* 1977; 136:43–9.

215. PIFER LL, HUGHES WT, STAGNO S *et al.* *Pneumocystis carinii* infection: evidence for high prevalence in normal and immunosuppressed children. *Pediatrics* 1978; 61:35–41.

216. WALZER PD, PERL DP, KROGSTAD DJ *et al.* *Pneumocystis carinii* pneumonia in the United States. Epidemiologic, diagnostic, and clinical features. *Ann Intern Med* 1974; 80:83–93.

217. ELVIN KM, LUMBWE CM, MATHERON S *et al.* *Pneumocystis carinii* is not a major cause of pneumonia in HIV infected patients in Lusaka, Zambia. *Transact R Soc Trop Med Hyg* 1989; 83:553–5.

218. ELVIN K, BJÖRKMAN A, LINDER E, HEURLIN N, HJERPE A. *Pneumocystis carinii* pneumonia: detection of the organism in sputum and bronchoalveolar lavage fluid. *Br Med J* 1988; 297:381–4.

219. LIDMAN C. Clinical aspects of *Pneumocystis carinii* pneumonia in HIV infection with a special emphasis on prophylaxis. Thesis, Karolinska Institute, Stockholm 1993.

220. OLSSON M, ELVIN K, LÖFDAHL S, LINDER E. Detection of *Pneumocystis carinii* DNA in sputum and bronchoalveolar lavage by polymerase chain reaction. *J Clin Microbiol* 1993; 32:221–6.

221. KITADA K, OKA S, KIMURA S, SHIMADA K, SERIKAWA T, YAMADA J, TSUNOO H, EGAWA K, NAKAMURA Y. Detection of *Pneumocystis carinii* sequences by polymerase chain reaction: animal models and clinical application to noninvasive specimens. *J Clin Microbiol* 1991; 29:1985–90.

222. ELVIN K. Laboratory diagnosis and occurrence of *Pneumocystis carinii*. Thesis, Karolinska Institute, Stockholm 1993.

223. MADDISON SE, WALLS KW, HAVERKOS HW *et al.* Evaluation of serologic tests for *Pneumocystis carinii* antibody and antigenemia in patients with acquired immunodeficiency syndrome. *Diagn Microbiol Infect Dis* 1984; 2:69–73.

224. GARDNER PS, MCQUILLIN J. *Rapid Viral Diagnosis, Application of Immunofluorescence*. London, Butterworths 1980.

225. ENGLER HD, SELEPAK ST. Effect of centrifuging shell vials at 3,500 x g on detection of viruses in clinical specimens. *J Clin Microbiol* 1994; 32:1580–2.

226. GLEAVES CA, SMITH TF, SHUSTER EA, PEARSON GR. Comparison of standard tube and shell vial cell culture techniques for the detection of cytomegalovirus in clinical specimens. *J Clin Microbiol* 1985; 21:217–21.

227. LEE SHS, BOUTILIER JE, MACDONALD MA, FORWARD KR. Enhanced detection of respiratory viruses using the shell vial technique and monoclonal antibodies. *J Virol Methods* 1992; 39:39–46.

228. MATLEY N, NICHOLSON D, RUHS S, ALDEN B, KNOCK M, SCHULZ K, SCHMUECKER A. Rapid detection of respiratory viruses by shell vial culture and direct staining by using pooled and individual monoclonal antibodies. *J Clin Microbiol* 1992; 30:540–4.

229. SCHIRM J, LUIJ DS, PASTOOR GW, MANDEMA JM, SCHRÖDER FP. Rapid detection of respiratory viruses using mixtures of monoclonal antibodies on shell vial cultures. *J Med Virol* 1992; 38:147–51.

230. ERIKSSON B-M, BRYTTING M, ZWEYGBERG-WIRGART B, HILLERDAL G, OLDING-STENKVIST E, LINDE A. Diagnosis of cytomegalvirus in bronchoalveolar lavage by polymerase chain reaction, in comparison with virus isolation and detection of viral antigen. *Scand J Infect Dis* 1993; 25:421–7.

231. GRANDIEN M. Viral diagnosis by antigen detection techniques *Clin Diagnostic Viral* 1996; 5: 81–90.

232. ØRSTAVIK I, GRANDIEN M, HALONEN, P *et al.* Viral diagnosis using the rapid immunofluorescence technique and epidemiological implications among children in different European countries. *Bull World Health Org* 1984; 62:307–13.

233. BALE JR. Creation of a research program to determine the aetiology and epidemiology of acute respiratory tract infection among children in developing countries. *Rev Infect Dis* 1990; 12 (Suppl 8):S861–S866

234. KALIN M, GRANDIEN M. Rapid diagnostic methods in respiratory infections. *Curr Opin Infect Dis* 1993; 6:150–7.

235. SALIH M, HERRMANN B, GRANDIEN M *et al.* Viral pathogens and clinical manifestations associated with acute lower respiratory tract infections in children of the Sudan. *Clin Diagn Virol* 1994; 2:201–9.

236. GARDNER PS, GRANDIEN M, MCQUILLIN J. Comparison of immuno-fluorescence and immunoperoxidase methods for viral diagnosis at a distance: a WHO collaborative study. *Bull WHO* 1978; 56:105–10.

237. SHEN K, ZHAORI G, SWEYGBERG-WIRGART B, YING M, GRANDIEN M, WAHREN B, LINDE A. Detection of respiratory viruses in nasopharyngeal secretions with immunofluorescence technique for multiplex screening – an evaluation of the Chemicon assay. *Clin Diagnostic Virol* 1996; 6: 147–54

238. WORLD HEALTH ORGANIZATION. Use of monoclonal antibodies for rapid diagnosis of respiratory viruses. *Bull WHO* 1992; 70: 699–703.

239. GRANDIEN M, PETTERSSON C-A, GARDNER PS, LINDE A, STANTON A. Rapid viral diagnosis of acute respiratory infections: comparison of enzyme-linked immunosorbent assay and the immunofluorescence technique for detection of viral antigens in nasopharyngeal secretions. *J Clin Microbiol* 1985; 22:757–60.

240. DÖLLER G, SCHUY W, TJHEN KY, STEKELER B, GERTH HJ. Direct detection of influenza virus antigen in nasopharyngeal specimens by direct enzyme immunoassay in comparison with quantitating virus shedding. *J Clin Microbiol* 1992; 30:866–9.

241. DUVERLIE G, HOUBART L, VISSE H, CHOMEL JJ, MANUGUERRA JC, HANNOUN C, ORFILA J. A nylon membrane enzyme immunoassay for rapid diagnosis of influenza A infection. *J Virol Methods* 1992; 40:77–84.

242. CHOMEL JJ, REMILLEUX MF, MARCHAND P, AYMARD M. Rapid diagnosis of influenza A: comparison with ELISA immuno-capture and culture. *J Virol Methods* 1992; 37:337–44.

243. DOMINGUEZ EA, TABER LH, COUCH RB. Comparison of rapid diagnostic techniques for respiratory syncytial and influenza A virus respiratory infections in young children. *J Clin Microbiol* 1993; 31:2286–90.

244. JOHNSTON SLG, BLOY H. Evaluation of a rapid enzyme immunoassay for detection of influenza A virus. *J Clin Microbiol* 1993; 31:142–3.

245. LEONARDI GP, LEIB H, BIRKHEAD GS. Comparison of rapid detection methods for influenza A virus and their value in health-care management of institutionalized geriatric patients. *J Clin Microbiol* 1994; 32:70–4.

246. MILLER H, MILK R, DIAZ-MITOMA F. Comparison of the VIDAS RSV assay and the Abbott testpack RSV with direct immunofluorescence for detection of respiratory syncytial virus in nasopharyngeal aspirates. *J Clin Microbiol* 1993; 31:1336–8.

247. TAKIMOTO S, GRANDIEN M, ISHIDA MA *et al.* Comparison of enzyme-linked immunosorbent assay, indirect immunofluorescence assay, and virus isolation for detection of respiratory viruses in nasopharyngeal secretions. *J Clin Microbiol* 1991; 29:470–4.

248. HALONEN P, MEURMAN O, LÖVGREN T, HEMMILÄ I, SOINI E. Detection of viral antigens by time-resolved fluoroimmunoassay. *Curr Topics Microbiol Immunol* 1983; 104:133–45.

249. CHERIAN T, BOBO L, STEINHOFF MC, KARRON RA, YOLKEN RH. Use of PCR–enzyme immunoassay for identification of influenza A virus matrix RNA in clinical samples negative for cultivable virus. *J Clin Microbiol* 1994; 32:623–8.

250. KARRON RA, FROEHLICH JL, BOBO L, BELSHE RB, YOLKEN RH. Rapid detection of parainfluenza virus type 3 RNA in respiratory specimens: use of reverse transcription–PCR–enzyme immunoassay. *J Clin Microbiol* 1994; 32:484–8.

251. BALFOUR-LYNN IM, VALMAN HB, STANWAY G, KHAN M. Use of the polymerase chain reaction to detect rhinovirus in wheezy infants. *Arch Dis Child* 1990; 67:760.

252. IRELAND DC, KENT J, NICHOLSON KG. Improved detection of rhinoviruses in nasal and throat swabs by seminested RT-PCR. *J Med Virol* 1993; 40:96–101.

253. PATON AW, PATON JC, LAWRENCE AJ, GOLDWATER PN, HARRIS RJ. Rapid detection of respiratory syncytial virus in nasopharyngeal aspirates by reverse transcription and polymerase chain reaction amplification. *J Clin Microbiol* 1992; 30:901–4.

254. CLAAS EC, VAN MILAAN AJ, SPRENGER MJ, RUITEN-STUIVER M, ARON GI, ROTHBARTH PH, MASUREL N. Prospective application of reverse transcriptase polymerase chain reaction for diagnosing influenza infections in respiratory samples from a children's hospital. *J Clin Microbiol* 1993; 31:2218–21.

255. CUBIE HA, INGLIS JM, LESLIE EE, EDMUNDS AT, TOTAPALLY B. Detection of respiratory syncytial virus in acute bronchiolitis in infants. *J Med Virol* 1992; 38:283–7.

256. FREYMUTH F, EUGENE G, VABRET A, PETITJEAN J, GENNETAY E, BROUARD J, DUHAMEL JF, GUILLOIS B. Detection of respiratory syncytial virus by reverse transcription-PCR and hybridization with a DNA enzyme immunoassay. *Clin Microbiol* 1995; 33: 3352–355

257. DONOFRIO JC, COONROD JD, DAVIDSON JN, BETTS RF. Detection of influenza A and B in respiratory secretions with the polymerase chain reaction. *PCR Methods Appl* 1992; 1:263–8.

258. ZHANG W, EVANS DH. Detection and identification of human influenza viruses by the polymerase chain reaction. *J Virol Methods* 1991; 33:165–89.

259. BRESSOUD A, WHITCOMB J, POURZAND C, HALLER O, CERUTTI P. Rapid detection of influenza virus H1 by the polymerase chain reaction. *Biochem Biophys Res Commun* 1990; 167:425–30.

260. ZUCKERMAN MA, LEVANTIS P, OXFORD JS. Direct sequence determination of the influenza B HA-1 gene after PCR amplification of clinical specimens from an infected volunteer. *J Virol Methods* 1993; 44:35–44.

261. MYERSON D, LINGENFELTER PA, GLEAVES CA, MEYERS JD, BOWDEN RA. Diagnosis of cytomegalovirus pneumonia by the polymerase chain reaction with archived frozen lung tissue and bronchoalveolar lavage fluid. *Am J Clin Pathol* 1993; 100:407–13.

262. HEURLIN N, ELVIN K, LIDMAN C, LIDMAN K, LUNDBERGH P. Fiberoptic bronchoscopy and sputum examination for diagnosis of pulmonary disease in AIDS patients in Stockholm. *Scand J Infect Dis* 1990; 22:659–64.

263. MEYERS JD, LJUNGMAN P, FISHER LD. Cytomegalovirus as a predictor of cytomegalovirus disease after marrow transplantation: importance of cytomegalovirus viremia. *J Infect Dis* 1992; 162:373–80.

264. LJUNGMAN P. Cytomegalovirus infections in transplant patients. *Scand Infect Dis* Suppl 1996; 100: 59–63.

265. VAN DER BIJ W, SCHIRM J, TORENSMA R, VAN SON WJ, TEGZESS AM. The TH. Comparison between viremia and antigenemia for detection of cytomegalovirus in blood. *J Clin Microbiol* 1988; 26:2531–5.

266. VAN DER BIJ W, TORENSMA R, VAN SON WJ *et al.* Rapid immunodiagnosis of active

cytomegalovirus infection by monoclonal antibody staining of blood leucocytes. *J Med Virol* 1988; 25:179–88.

267. REVELLO MG, PERCIVALLE E, DI MATTEO A, MORINI F, GERNA G. Nuclear expression of the lower matrix protein of human cytomegalovirus in peripheral blood leukocytes of immunocompromised viraemic patients. *J Gen Virol* 1992; 73:437–42.

268. MEYER-KÖNIG U, SERR A, HUFERT FT, STRIK M, KIRSTE G, HALLER O, NEUMANN-HAEFELIN D. Laboratory diagnosis of HCMV-related disease in renal transplant patients – pp65 antigen detection versus nested PCR. *Clin Diagn Virol* 1995; 3:49–59.

269. EHRNST A, BARKHOLT L, LEWENSOHN-FUCHS I *et al.* CMV PCR monitoring in leucocytes of transplant patients. *Clin Diagn Virol* 1995; 3:139–53.

270. EHRNST A. The clinical relevance of different laboratory tests in CMV diagnosis. *Scand J Infect Dis* Suppl 1996; 100: 64–71.

271. VIKERFORS T, GRANDIEN M, JOHANSSON M, PETTERSSON C-A. Detection of an immunoglobulin M response in the elderly for early diagnosis of respiratory syncytial virus infection. *J Clin Microbiol* 1988; 26:808–11.

272. VIKERFORS T, LINDEGREN G, GRANDIEN M, VAN DER LOGT J. Diagnosis of influenza A virus infections by detection of specific immunoglobulins M, A, and G in serum. *J Clin Microbiol* 1989; 27:453–8.

273. WEBER B, PROSSER F, MUNKWITZ A, DOERR HW. Serological diagnosis of cytomegalovirus infection: comparison of 8 enzyme immunoassays for the detection of HCMV-specific IgM antibody. *Clin Diagn Virol* 1994; 2:245–59.

274. LEVY H, FELDMAN C, SACHO H, VAN DER MEULEN H, KALLENBACH J, KOORNHOF H. A reevaluation of sputum microscopy and culture in the diagnosis of pulmonary tuberculosis. *Chest* 1989; 95:1193–7.

275. ROBERTS GD. Bacteriology and bacteriologic diagnosis of tuberculosis. In: Schlossberg D ed. *Tuberculosis*. New York, Springer-Verlag 1983:23–31.

276. AL-KASSIMI FA, AZHAR M, ALI-MAJED S, AL-WASSAN AD, AL-HAJJAJ MS, MALIBARY T. Diagnostic role of fibreoptic bronchoscopy in tuberculosis in the presence of typical X-ray pictures and adequate sputum. *Tubercle* 1991; 72:145–8.

277. DEPARTMENT OF HEALTH AND PUBLIC POLICY, American College of Physicians. Diagnostic thoracocentesis and pleural biopsy in pleural effusions. *Ann Intern Med* 1985; 103:799–802.

278. GORDIN F, SLUTKIN G. The validity of acid-fast smears in the diagnosis of pulmonary tuberculosis. *Arch Pathol Lab Med* 1990; 114:1025–7.

279. KIM TC, BLACKMAN RS, HEATWOLE AM. Acid fast bacilli in sputum smears of patients with tubeculosis: prevalence and significance of negative smears pretreatment and positive smears post-treatment. *Am Rev Resp Dis* 1984; 129:264–70.

280. RADHIKA S, GUPTA SK, CHAKRABARTI A, RAJWANSHI A, JOSHI K. Role of culture for mycobacteria in fine-needle aspiration. Diagnosis of tuberculous lymphadenitis. *Diagn Cytopathol* 1989; 5:260–2.

281. MIDDLEBROOK G, REGGIARDO Z, TIGERTT WD. Automatable radiometric detection of growth of *Mycobacterium tuberculosis* in selective media. *Am Rev Resp Dis* 1977; 115:1066–71.

282. SHANKAR P, MANJUNATH N, MOHAN KK, PRASAD K, BEHARI SHRINIWAS M, AHUGA GK. Rapid diagnosis of tuberculous meningitis by polymerase chain reaction. *Lancet* 1991; 339:5–7.

283. CLARRIDGE JE III, SHAWAR RM, SHINNICK TM, PLIKAYTIS BB. Large-scale use of polymerase chain reaction for detection of *Mycobacterium tuberculosis* in a routine mycobacteriology laboratory. *J Clin Microbiol* 1993; 31:2049–56.

284. BENNESDEN J, THOMSEN VO, PFYFFER GE *et al.* Utility of PCR in diagnosing pulmonary tuberculosis. *J Clin Microbiol* 1996; 34:1407–11.

285. LARSSON L, ODHAM G, WESTERDAHL G, OLSSON B. Diagnosis of pulmonary tuberculosis by selected-ion monitoring: improved analysis of tuberculostearate in sputum using negative-ion mass spectometry. *J Clin Microbiol* 1987; 25:893–6.

286. BROOKS J, DANESHVAR M, FAST D, GOOD R. Selective procedures for detecting femtomolar quantities of tuberculostearic acid in serum and cerebrospinal fluid by frequency-pulsed electron capture gas–liquid chromatography. *J Clin Microbiol* 1987; 25:1201–6.

287. CHAN SL, REGGIARDO Z, DANIEL TM, GIRLING DJ, MITCHINSON DA. Serodiagnosis of tuberculosis using an ELISA with antigen 5 and a hemagglutination assay with glycolipid antigens: results in patients with newly diagnosed pulmonary tuberculosis ranging in extent of disease from minimal to extensive. *Am Rev Resp Dis* 1990; 142:385–9.

288. SMITHWICK RW. *Laboratory Manual for Acid-fast Microscopy*. Atlanta, Centers for Disease Control, 1976.

289. ROBERTS GD, KONEMAN EW, KIM YK. Mycobacterium. In: Balows A, Hansler Jr WJ, Herrman KL, Isenberg HD, Shadomy HJ, eds. *Manual of Clinical Microbiology American Society for Microbiology*, Washington DC, American Society for Microbiology 304–339.

290. BÖDDINGHAUS B, ROGALL T, FLOHR T, BLÖCKER H, BÖTTGER EC. Detection and identification of mycobacteria by amplification of rRNA. *J Clin Microbiol* 1990; 28:1751–9.

291. SAVIC B, SJÖBRING U, ALUGUPALLI S, LARSSON L, MIÖRNER H. Evaluation of polymerase chain reaction, tuberculostearic acid analysis, and direct microscopy for the detection of *Mycobacterium tuberculosis* in sputum. *J Infect Dis* 1992; 166:1177–80.

292. VAN DER GIESSEN JWB, EGER A, HAAGSMA J, VAN DER ZEIJST BAM. Rapid detection and identification of *Mycobacterium avium* by amplification of 16S rRNA sequences. *J Clin Microbiol* 1993; 31:2509–12.

293. BUTLER WR, AHEARN DG, KILBURN JO. High-performance liquid chromatography of mycolic acids as a tool in the identification of *Corynebacterium*, *Nocardia*, *Rhodococcus*, and *Mycobacterium* species. *J Clin Microbiol* 1986; 23:182–5.

294. TISDALL PA, ROBERTS GD, ANHALT JP. Identification of clinical isolates of mycobacteria with gas–liquid chromatography alone. *J Clin Microbiol* 1979; 10:506–14.

295. HOFFNER SE, SVENSON SB, KÄLLENIUS G. Synergistic effects of antimycobacterial drugs on *Mycobacterium avium* complex determined radiometrically in liquid medium. *Eur J Microbiol* 1987; 6:530–5.

296. HOFFNER SE, KÄLLENIUS G, BEEZER AE, SVENSON SB. Studies on the mechanisms of the synergistic effects of ethambutol and other antibacterial drugs on *Mycobacterium avium* complex. *Acta Leprolog* 1989; 7 (Suppl 1):195–9.

297. HORSBURGH CR JR. *Mycobacterium avium* complex infection in the acquired immunodeficiency syndrome. *N Engl J Med* 1991; 324:1332–8.

2 Radiological aspects of lung infection

JAMIE WEIR

Aberdeen Royal Infirmary, Scotland, UK

Introduction

The imaging of patients who have, or who are suspected of, having a lung infection should be based on two important and widely differing concepts. The first is the analysis of the chest radiograph, a basic investigation of unparalleled use to any clinician. This radiograph should be used as the start of any investigative chain leading to other more complicated diagnostic tests and occasionally to radiological therapeutic intervention. The second concept is based on the understanding of disease as related to the individual patient under investigation. To make full use of any imaging modality, the following fundamental points have to be considered.

(a) Does the patient have a pre-existing lung and/or a systemic condition? and,

(b) Does the patient have an altered immunity state for whatever reason?

It is also important to ascertain the ethnic origin of the patient, whether the patient comes from the tropics or has recently travelled to a known site of infection. The radiographical and clinical picture may also be atypical if the patient has either been given inappropriate therapy particularly antibiotics or has only taken a partial course of the correct drugs. A chest radiograph or indeed any imaging investigation, can rarely be specific in identifying the causal organism unless the answers to the above are known. Classical infections such as *Mycobacterium tuberculosis* and *Pneumocystis carinii* may give pathognomonic changes on a chest radiograph providing the patient was 'normal' beforehand, but both conditions can present very different radiological signs in other patients, for example, those with HIV disease.

These two above concepts do therefore closely link the radiologist and the clinician if successful patient management is to be forthcoming. The radiologist is required to analyse individual imaging investigations together with forming flow chart protocols for various abnormalities. The clinician needs to combine these imaging results with the patient's overall status for proper understanding of a specific disease.

This may seem so obvious that it does not need stating but close clinico-radiological co-operation is essential in order to avoid unnecessary, inappropriate and misleading investigations which result in a delayed diagnosis and poor patient care.

The chest radiograph

Despite the chest radiograph almost reaching its centenary, it still remains the fundamental tool for the radiological diagnosis of chest infection. It is also highly unlikely that it will be superseded for some considerable time despite the rapid advances in non-ionising techniques. Table 2.1 outlines the abnormalities that may exist in patients with lung disease, whether seen on a standard radiograph or on computed tomography (CT).

Table 2.1. *Features on a chest radiograph that may indicate infection*

1.	Presence of underlying lung disease	
2.	Consolidation (increased lung opacity)	
3.	Nodules and nodular shadowing	
4.	Reticular shadowing	
5.	Linear shadowing	
6.	Atelectasis	
7.	Cavitation	
8.	Calcification	
9.	Lymphadenopathy	
10.	Abnormality of the	pleura
		mediastinum
		diaphragm
		chest wall

The pathological basis of the ten points requires further analysis in order to understand the radiological changes that may be present in patients with infection.

Pre-existing lung disease

If the patient has an abnormality in the lung, secondary infection is common. Patients with cavity formation, for example, from previous tuberculosis, have a predilection for fungus growth. Patients with bronchiectasis have an increased instance of air space infection close to affected bronchi. Fibrosis, emphysema, atelectasis and cavities all may be present before an acute infective episode, or alternatively, may be its result. The documentation of pre-existing lung disease is therefore important as the longevity of any abnormality defines its significance in relation to acute or chronic infection.

Increased lung opacity (consolidation)

Pathologically, consolidation is replacement of alveolar air by fluid or debris. The fluid is either a transudate or an exudate. Debris can include live or dead cells, tumour or in rare cases other materials such as that found in alveolar proteinosis. Radiologically, it is better to use the term 'alveolar air replacement' to describe an area of opacity on a chest radiograph that is due to alveolar obliteration. Alveolar air replacement in its pure form exists without any loss of volume, but with loss of vascular markings and occasionally with an air bronchogram. It may be heterogenous or homogenous, unilateral or bilateral, local or diffuse. Its pattern may also aid in the diagnosis of the infective agent.

Nodules and nodular shadowing

A nodule is defined as any well-circumscribed mass lesion up to 3 cm in diameter. Nodular shadowing implies multiple nodules, usually less than 1 cm in diameter. Both types of lesion may be present in infection and suggest various infective agents. *Nocardia* may present as a discrete focal lesion, and multiple nodules are characteristic of cytomegalovirus.

Reticular shadowing

Small linear opacities that resemble a fishnet are described as reticular. The term implies an interstitial abnormality, the best example being seen in patients with Langerhans cell granulomatosis (Histiocytosis X). It is occasionally seen in patients with AIDS who have opportunistic infections particularly *P. carinii* pneumonia (see below).

Linear shadows

Linear or band like shadows are caused by a wide variety of pathology including scars, atelectasis, pleural tags, septal lines and any cause of bronchial wall thickening and mucoid impaction. Bronchial wall thickening occurs in bronchiectasis, bronchiolitis, asthma, cystic fibrosis, lymphangitis carcinomatosa and in cases of pulmonary oedema. Bronchial wall thickening has to be considerable before line shadows appear visible on a chest radiograph, extending from the hila in defined anatomical patterns. The presence of dilatation associated with the thickening is also important in distinguishing bronchiectasis from the other causes.

Atelectasis (loss of volume or collapse)

Pneumonia is the commonest cause for collapse in the paediatric age group due to the small airways being blocked by mucus. This does occur in the adult but tumour is more likely, particularly in the lung carcinoma age group. Atelectasis may also result from lung retraction and/or compression by an intrathoracic space occupying lesion, for example mass or fluid. Scarring and adhesive conditions such as hyaline membrane disease also result in collapse. Linear or discoid atelectasis is due to hypoventilation with alveolar collapse[1] and is not associated with bronchial occlusion. It is therefore widely seen in postoperative patients and in any condition resulting in poor respiratory and diaphragmatic movement. It may be sufficient to cause hypoxaemia and its severity is frequently underestimated on the chest radiograph. Round atelectasis is a specific term resulting from a chronic area of collapse adjacent to pleural disease and hence often found in asbestosis. It was first described by Blesovsky and its mechanism is still not fully understood[2]. It is usually oval in shape, and contains either an air bronchogram or air shadows within it. The adjacent bronchi and vessels are curved around the mass which has often been present for many years (Fig. 2.1 (*a*) and (*b*)). A specific diagnosis may be possible with CT[3].

Cavitation

A cavity is defined as a mass within the lung parenchyma which has undergone necrosis and communicates with the bronchial tree. An abscess is slightly different as it may, or may not, communicate with a bronchus. Numerous conditions have cavitation as a feature and it is not particularly helpful in differentiating types of infection. However, fungal infections commonly cavitate as do necrotising

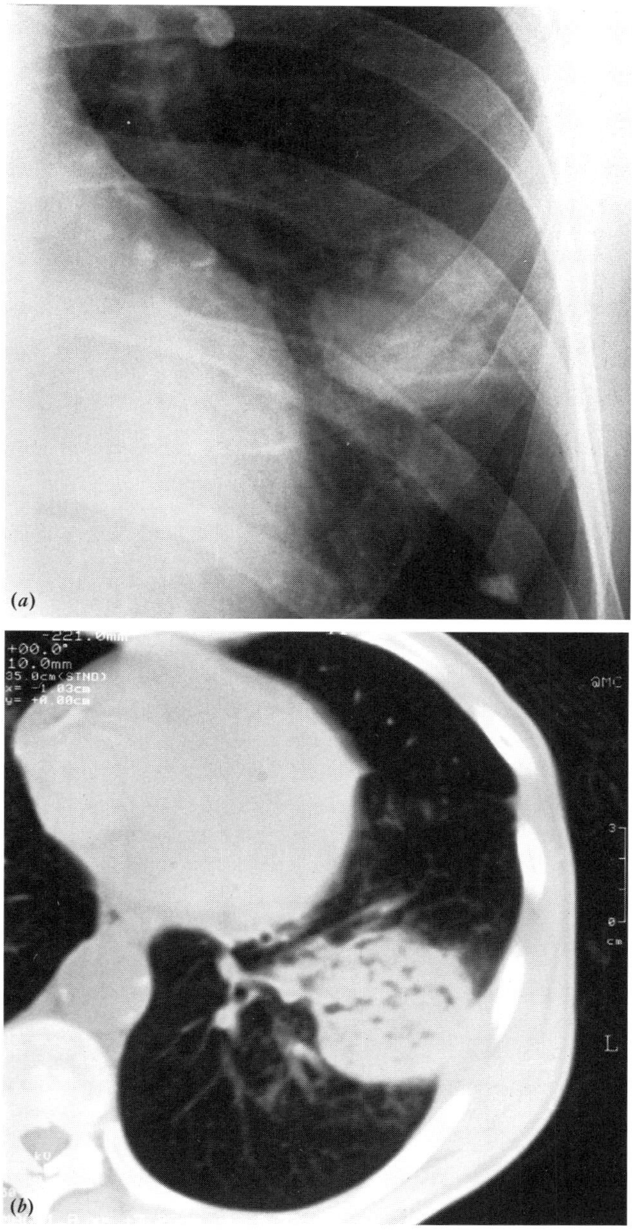

FIGURE 2.1 (*a*), (*b*) Round atelectasis. (*a*) PA chest radiograph showing an area of dense consolidation in the lateral aspect of the left lower lobe, that had remained unchanged for 2 years in a patient with recurrent but intermittent fever. (*b*) CT scan showing well-defined consolidation with pockets of gas within it. The vessels are curved around the lesion and there is close relationship to the pleura. Percutaneous needle biopsy specimen grew anaerobic bacteria.

pneumonias such as *Klebsiella*. The thickness of the cavity wall does help in differentiating benign from malignant lesions, a figure of 4 mm or less being usual in the former and over 4 mm in the latter. It is not, however, a golden rule as some infective cavities are thick walled for example *Aspergillus* and mucormycosis and some carcinomas, particularly squamous, are thin walled.

Calcification

Concentric laminated calcification is only seen in infective causes such as tuberculosis and histoplasmosis. Ring calcification is seen in hamartomas or other cartilage tumours and punctate calcification in granulomas. The presence of calcification in old tuberculosis results from the healing of caseation and may be quite widespread.

Lymphadenopathy

Hilar and mediastinal lymphadenopathy in infection may be due to either reactive hyperplasia or direct spread of infection. The distribution of the lymphadenopathy is often useful in determining the infective agent, for example, in primary tuberculosis, lymphadenopathy may be the only manifestation of the disease. The chest radiograph is poor at discriminating the mediastinum and CT is essential if it is important to document nodal enlargement. Nodal sampling via mediastinoscopy or mediastinotomy is made more accurate by CT mapping of the affected areas.

Abnormalities of the pleura, mediastinum, diaphragm and chest wall

Lung infection may spread directly to any of these adjacent structures causing abscess formation or continued spread of the disease. Pneumonia is often accompanied by a small pleural effusion, usually sterile, but this may become infected and progress to an empyema. The differentiation of a simple effusion from an empyema may be difficult if not impossible on a simple chest radiograph and needle sampling should be undertaken more frequently than at present if the condition is suspected clinically. Infections that do not respect tissue barriers, such as actinomycosis, may begin in the lung, pass through the pleural space, cause rib periostitis and present clinically as a chest wall abscess subpleural and subdiaphragmatic infected fluid collections may also be caused by an initial pneumonic process. Direct mediastinal spread of infection results in acute mediastinitis and often carries a poor prognosis. Infections may also spread into the pericardium resulting in pericarditis and pericardial fluid, for example tuberculosis.

It is also important to note that: (a) patients with proven lung infection may have a 'normal' chest radiograph;[4] (b) there may be considerable disparity between the severity of the infection and the severity of the changes on the radiograph; and (c) radiological changes may pre-date or post-date clinical signs and symptoms.

The standard P–A (postero-anterior) chest radiograph may be taken at a low kV (e.g. 70) which gives good contrast and bony detail but poor penetration and mediastinal outline or high kV (e.g. above 120) which gives the opposite. The lung parenchyma is therefore better shown at high kV, the radiation dosage is lower but the presence of calcium is harder to detect. The use of the lateral chest radiograph has become markedly restricted recently, and it is now out of vogue, a sad state for it can be extremely useful when the P–A film may need help for interpretation. The lateral film may also show abnormalities not visible on the P–A film, particularly in the posterior basal segments of the lower lobes, the areas around the hila and for the detection of small pleural effusions.

Computed tomography

In the late 1970s and the early 1980s, chest computed tomography (CT) was mainly confined to staging for malignancy, and the resolution of lung parenchyma was relatively poor. However, with the advent of high resolution CT (HRCT) over the last few years, it is now possible to obtain exquisite views of the pulmonary lobules, interstitial and alveolar spaces and detect subtle changes in structure[5–7] (Fig. 2.2(*a*) and (*b*)). Sections 1 mm thick are now standard, and various protocols exist for the assessment of bronchiectasis[8], diffuse and focal lung disease[9] and in guiding open (and closed) lung biopsy.

Structures down to 0.3 mm (300 microns) may now be resolved, and variations in diffuse lung disease, not discernible before, are now well recognised.

The ability to detect parenchymal abnormality in the presence of a normal chest radiograph has also marked advantages.

HRCT findings in lung disease are broadly based on four patterns: nodular, reticular, increased lung opacity and 'spaces'. Lung infection may involve one, or all, of these patterns depending on the nature of the infection, its severity, its stage and its rate of progression or healing. Nodular opacities can result from both air space consolidation and interstitial abnormalities. Interstitial nodules are classically present in sarcoidosis and other granulomata, whereas air space consolidation is seen early in lobar pneumonia, pulmonary oedema and bronchiolitis obliterans. Reticular shadowing is multifocal in causation with peribronchial thickening, interlobular septal and interstitial thickening, subpleural infiltration and honeycombing all contributing to the production of 'lines' on HRCT.

Increased lung opacity may be of two main subdivisions: 'ground glass' opacification and air space consolidation. 'Ground glass' opacification is a non-specific term referring to loss of the normal air filled alveoli but with retention of the vascular markings. Its presence usually indicates active disease and is seen in diseases such as pulmonary oedema, idiopathic pulmonary fibrosis and *P. carinii* pneumonia. Air space consolidation can be detected early on HRCT. 'Spaces' or cystic lung disease may be due to any cause of honeycomb lung, dilated bronchi in bronchiectasis, cysts, bullae or cavitating solid lung lesions. Most of these conditions are readily distinguishable on HRCT.

CT has a useful role to play in providing additional information of the distribution of parenchymal lung disease in immunosuppressed non-AIDS patients prior to bronchoscopic biopsy[10,11]. The results of bronchoscopic procedures are more likely to be successful if the disease is central rather than peripheral, a pattern that cannot be reliably demonstrated on a plain chest radiograph.

There is always a downside to any investigation and with CT, standard or HRCT, it is the radiation dosage. For comparison, a routine CT chest is equivalent in patient dosage to approximately 200 chest radiographs. Nevertheless, HRCT in limited amounts is undoubtedly the best available method at the present time for directly imaging the lung parenchyma.

Magnetic resonance imaging

This is a non-ionising technique dependent on magnetic fields and has no known biological hazard at the strengths used in diagnostic apparatus. The resolution is relatively poor when it comes to visualisation of the lung parenchyma but its spectacular demonstration of mediastinal structures in any plane, and its ability to show tissue interfaces has made the technique invaluable to certain patients. (Fig. 2.3).

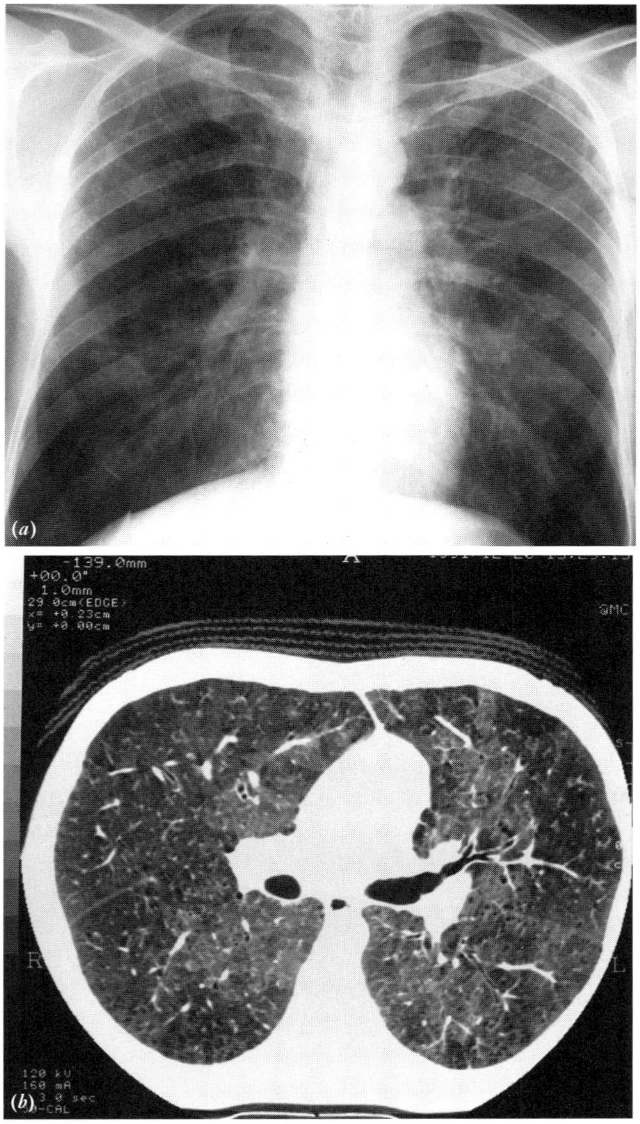

FIGURE 2.2 (*a*), (*b*) Extrinsic allergic alveolitis. (*a*) 32-year-old with extrinsic asthma showing upper lobe interstitial shadowing with an ill-defined alveolar component. (*b*) HRCT of 1 mm thickness through the upper lobes demonstrating individual pulmonary lobules with alveolar air replacement, ground glass consolidation and some localised air trapping.

Recently, improved resolution due to coil technology, software upgrades and rapid scan times, has made it possible to visualise the lung parenchyma[12] but it is at the moment less valuable in lung infection than HRCT. This will probably change with the ever-increasing sophistication of the technique.

Nuclear medicine

Two radionuclides are currently in use for detecting areas of infection in the thorax, ^{111}In (Indium) and ^{67}Ga (Gallium). Lung abscess is well shown by ^{111}In labelled white cells due to the uptake of the labelled granulocytes into the area of infection. ^{111}In can also be used in assessing the infection associated with bronchiectasis.

Accumulation of ^{67}Ga in the lungs occurs in infection but is also seen in pneumoconiosis, sarcoidosis and fibrosing alveolitis. It is therefore, rather non-specific. ^{67}Ga can also be used in the assessment of patients with AIDS as discussed by Bekerman *et al.*[13]. They demonstrated various patterns of uptake depending upon the state of disease. One of their groups showed abnormal radionuclide uptake with normal chest radiography and no pulmonary symptoms indicating a worse stage of the disease than was originally apparent. Thallium and gallium have been used in combination in immunodeficiency AIDS in patients with mycobacterial infections, to assess differential uptake[14]. The results, as yet unconfirmed, suggest that thallium and gallium mismatching is specific in AIDS-related *Mycobacterium* infection and that the accuracy of early diagnosis is enhanced by this technique.

Lung biopsy

Percutaneous lung biopsy using a cutting needle for histology or a fine needle for cytology is a well-established technique for the diagnosis of mass lesions and occasionally focal or diffuse inflammatory abnormalities. The use of fine needle aspiration (FNA) in the diagnosis of lung infection has a limited application and tends only to be used as a last resort[15,16]. Its use in the immunocompromised patient is

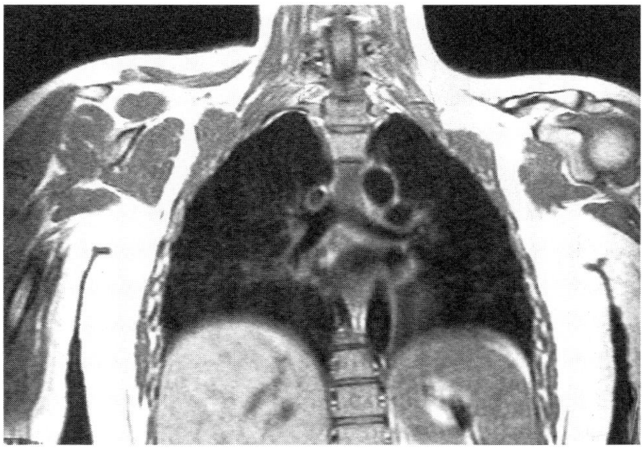

FIGURE 2.3 Normal coronal MRI demonstrating mediastinal and pulmonary anatomy.

associated with an increased incidence of complications, usually pneumothorax, which may persist and be difficult to treat[17,18]. However, those centres that have good bacteriological facilities find the technique useful in difficult cases, and its use will certainly increase.

Specific organisms and their radiological appearances

Although a considerable number of lung infections may have no specific radiological appearances, there may be indicators that point to a particular organism or group of organisms. Hence, the following categorisation of pneumonias reflects the radiological interpretation and will act as a guideline to physicians faced with certain radiological appearances and a pneumonia of unknown aetiology. Full descriptions of particular organisms with further radiographical examples will be found elsewhere in this book.

Community acquired pneumonia may be radiologically similar to a variety of non-infective consolidated lung diseases such as hypersensitivity pneumonias, bronchiolitis obliterans organising pneumonia (BOOP), drug reactions, vasculitides and alveolar haemorrhage[19]. Serological and histological studies may be necessary to determine such aetiologies.

Gram-positive bacteria

Staphylococcus aureus

This pneumonia seldom presents outside hospital, is unusual in healthy people and is now a common cause of bronchopneumonia. Radiologically, the pattern of staphylococcal pneumonia differs between children and adults. In children, there is a rapid bronchopneumonia, with over 50% of cases developing pneumatoceles (Fig. 2.4). They appear during the first week of illness and usually disappear completely. In adults, the pneumonia is often bilateral and may lead to single or multiple cavities or abscesses. If the infection is blood borne, multiple small nodules develop throughout the lung fields which may cavitate.

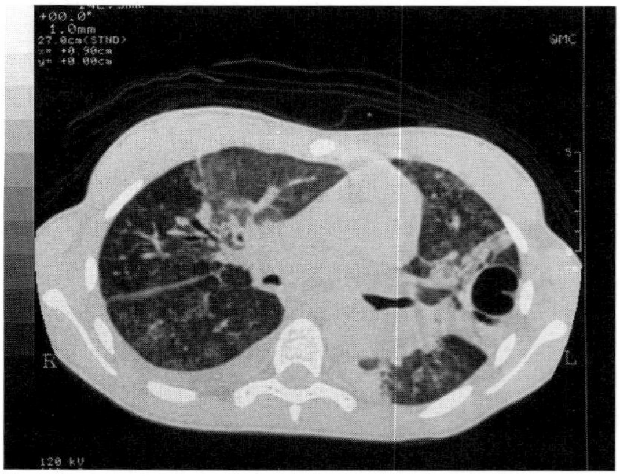

FIGURE 2.4 Staphylococcal pneumonia and pneumatocele. CT scan. 13 year-old girl with bilateral lung consolidation and multiple pneumatoceles.

Streptococcus pneumoniae

The radiological changes of streptococcal pneumonia mirror the four classical pathological changes of congestion, red hepatisation, grey hepatisation, and resolution, but the clinical course of the disease rarely follows this path due to early antibiotic therapy, pre-existing lung disease or altered immunity. The consolidation begins in the peripheral air spaces, frequently the lower lobes and spreads to other bronchopulmonary segments, often with an air bronchogram. Cavitation is rare, with resolution usually taking about 2 weeks but this may be delayed to up to 10 weeks particularly in older patients.

Gram-negative bacteria

Enterobacteriaceae

Klebsiella

Klebsiella pneumonia tends to be a disease of men, associated with chronic lung disease, diabetes mellitus and particularly chronic alcoholism. Radiologically, the pneumonia initially develops similar to pneumococcal pneumonia but the features that distinguish it are (a) bulging of the fissures due to an increase in lung volume by fluid secretion, (b) cavity formation (Fig. 2.5 (*a*) and (*b*) rare in pneumococcal pneumonia and (c) increased incidence of empyema.

Escherichia coli, Proteus, Yersinia and Salmonella

These can all be found as causes of pneumonia, but the radiological changes are varied and rather non-specific.

Haemophilus influenzae

In adults, pneumonia caused by *H. influenzae* tends to occur in patients with either pre-existing lung disease, diabetes mellitus or asplenia for whatever cause. In children, the organism causes an upper respiratory tract infection that may spread down the bronchial tree, and in both adults and children can cause severe epiglottitis with airway obstruction. Radiologically, the pneumonia is often basal, bilateral and indistinguishable from *S. pneumoniae.* It rarely cavitates but pleural effusions are common.

Pseudomonas aeruginosa

Patients with a tracheostomy, debilitating disease, steroid therapy, bronchiectasis or cystic fibrosis are prone to *Pseudomonas* lung infection. The radiological pattern is similar to staphylococcal infection with extensive lower lobe involvement, abscess formation and widespread nodular shadowing (Fig. 2.6).

Legionnaire's disease

Legionella pneumophila pneumonia is almost always accompanied by an abnormal chest radiograph with unilateral peripheral air space consolidation that progresses rapidly over a few days (Fig. 2.7). Cavitation, bilateral infection and lower lobe enlargement are all rare[20–22].

Anaerobic bacteria

This type of infection usually results from aspiration but may occasionally be blood borne. Consequently, the pneumonia often develops in the dependent parts of the lung with the right lung being more commonly involved than the left. The consolidation often persists for weeks and frequently cavitates to produce a lung abscess with accompanying pleural effusion and empyema[23,24]. Resolution is slow and may take months.

Blood borne anaerobic infections such as that caused by *Fusobacterium necrophorum* (Fig. 2.8) produce multiple cavitating areas scattered throughout both lung fields, similar to those seen in haematogenous staphylococcal infection.

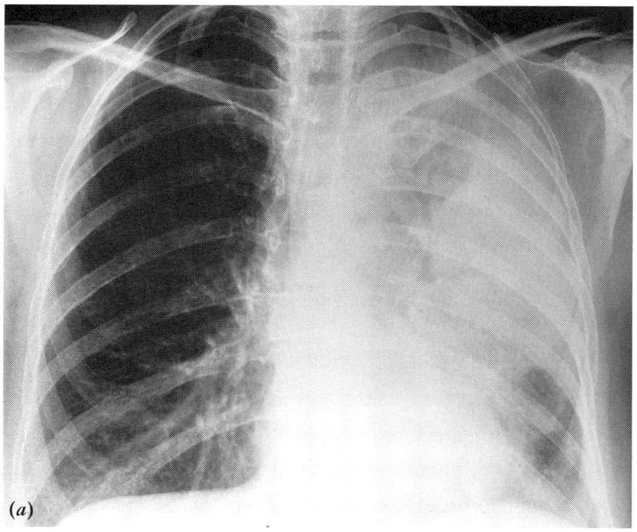

(*a*)

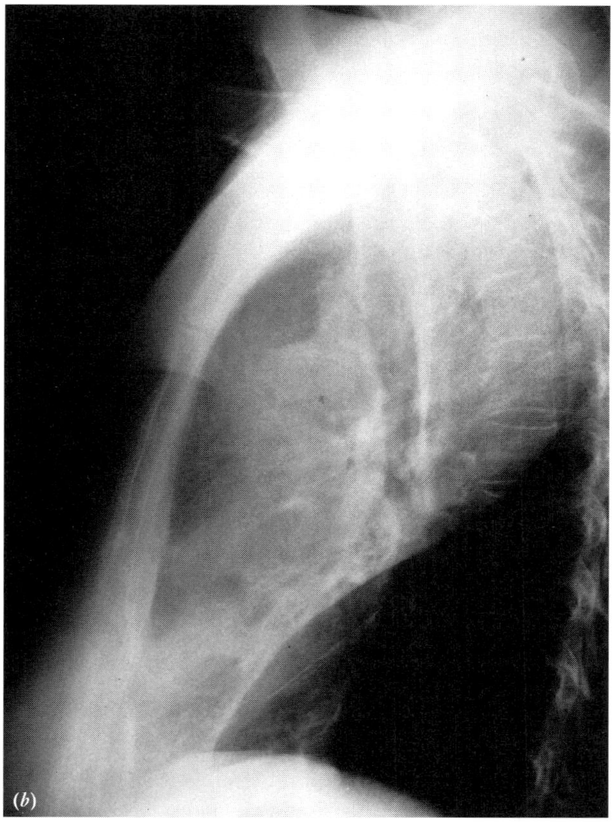

(*b*)

FIGURE 2.5 (*a*), (*b*) *Klebsiella* pneumonia. PA film demonstrates dense left upper lobe consolidation, which on the lateral film bulges the oblique tissue downwards due to lobar enlargement with retained secretions.

Mycobacterium tuberculosis

Primary TB

Primary tuberculous infection can involve one or all of the following: lung parenchyma, hilar/mediastinal nodes, bronchial tree and pleura.

In the lung parenchyma, the classical lesion is the Ghon focus, an area of consolidation that caseates and heals by fibrosis and calcification. It may occur in any part of the lung, with cavitation being rare.

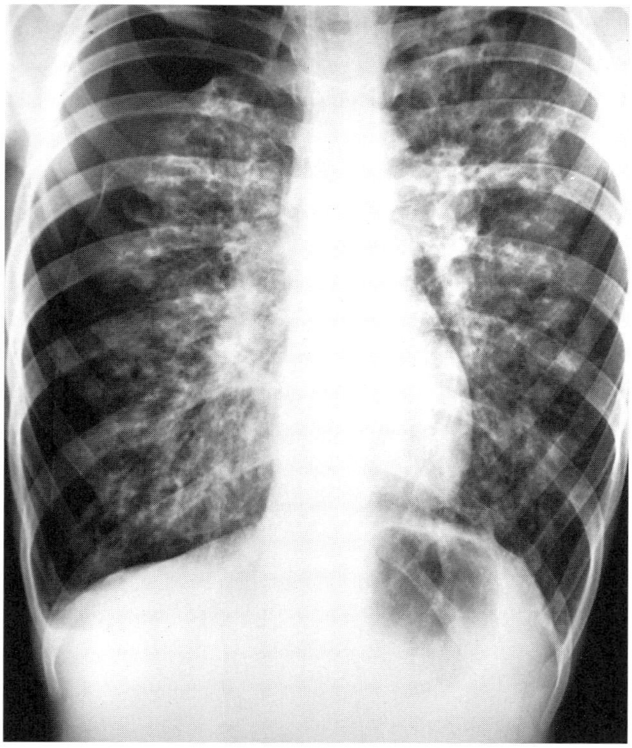

FIGURE 2.6 *Pseudomonas* infection. 19-year-old boy with cystic fibrosis showing widespread bronchiectasis, a right pneumothorax and patchy infective consolidation due to *Pseudomonas* throughout both lungs.

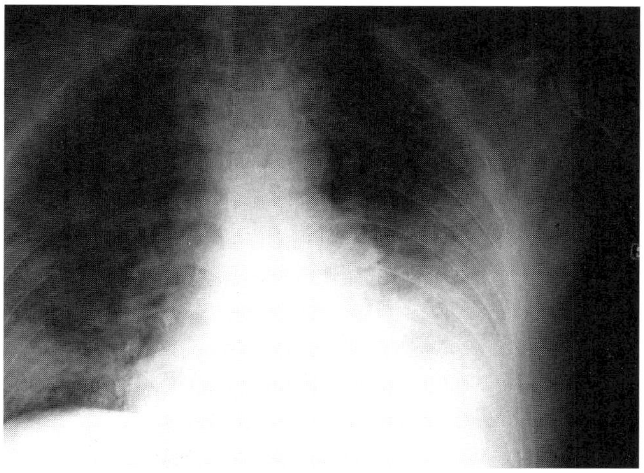

FIGURE 2.7 *Legionella* infection. Peripheral consolidation which, in this case, is bilateral but without specific features to indicate the causal organism.

Hilar and mediastinal lymphadenopathy which may be considerable (Fig. 2.9) differentiates primary from secondary TB as it does not occur in the latter. It is more common in children than adults and may, or may not, be accompanied by any visible parenchymal lesion (Fig. 2.10).

Tuberculous involvement of the airways may cause areas of collapse or occasionally obstructive emphysema. The radiological appearances may be minimal.

Pleural disease usually manifests itself by a pleural effusion that persists and is predominately lymphocytic. It may be the only sign of tuberculous infection and in adults with an undiagnosed pleural effusion, this disease should be high on the list of differential diagnoses.

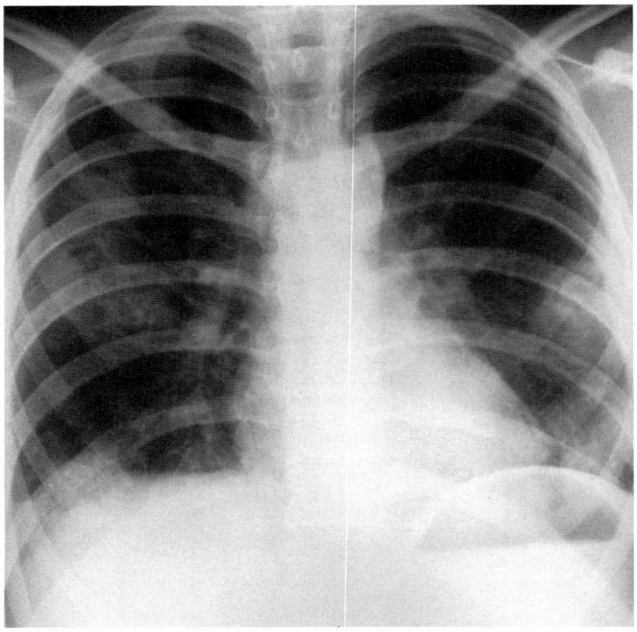

FIGURE 2.8 *Fusobacterium necrophorum.* Multiple cavitating areas of consolidation due to blood-borne anaerobic infection.

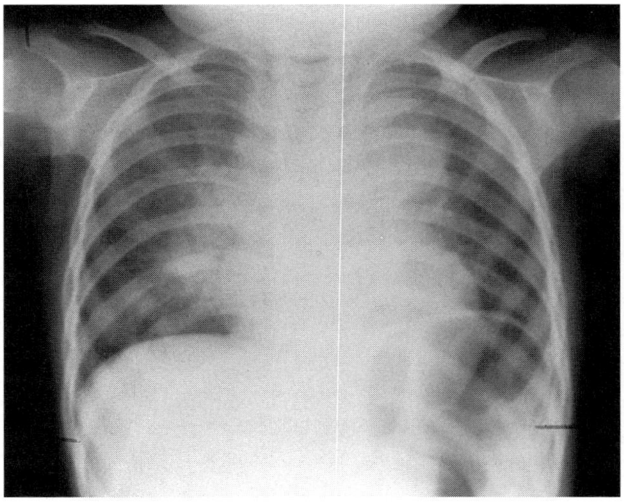

FIGURE 2.9 Pulmonary *Mycobacterium tuberculosis.* Widespread mediastinal and hilar lymphadenopathy in an Asian child born and domiciled in Scotland.

Secondary TB

Lung re-infection

The classical post primary lung infection develops in the posterior apical aspect of the upper lobes, or occasionally in the apical segments of the lower lobes[25]. Consolidation which may be widespread soon cavitates with progressive loss of volume (Fig. 2.11). The consolidation which is initially patchy, tends to coalesce and may spread rapidly, while other areas show healing with fibrosis. Cavitating areas of caseation may spread to the bronchial tree and cause bronchopneumonia.

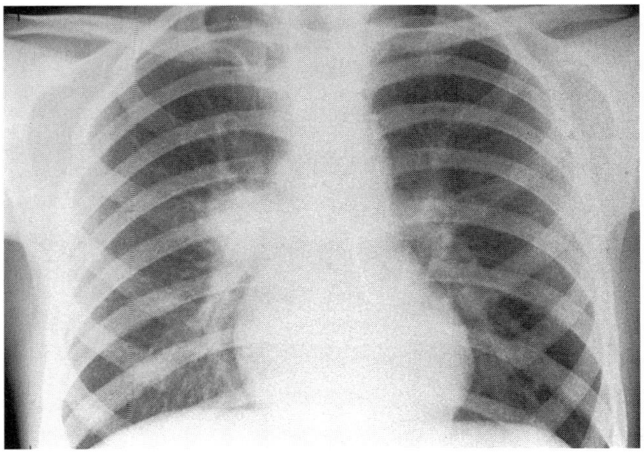

FIGURE 2.10 Primary *Mycobacterium tuberculosis* 22-year-old white Caucasian with unilateral hilar lymphadenopathy as the sole presentation of primary TB.

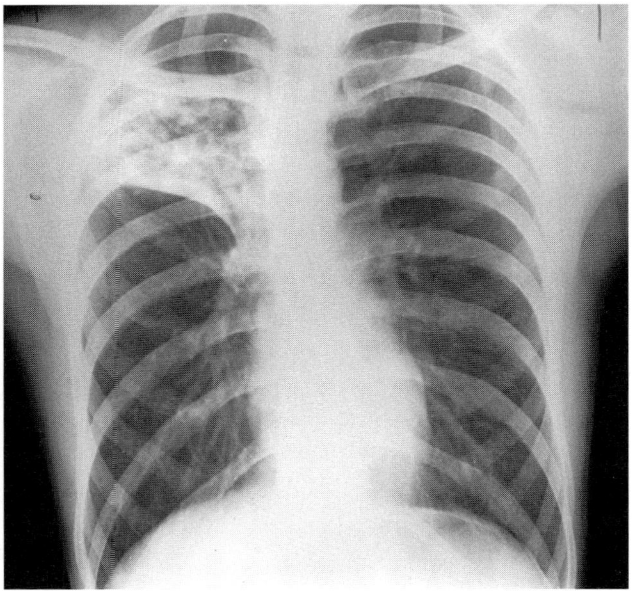

FIGURE 2.11 *Mycobacterium tuberculosis.* Typical changes of consolidation, cavitation and loss of volume in the right upper lobe.

Miliary TB

Multiple small discrete nodules throughout both lung fields, often 1 mm or less in size, that slowly progress to 3–5 mm if untreated, before the patient succumbs (Fig. 2.12). With appropriate treatment, the nodules disappear quite rapidly in comparison to other tuberculous lung disease leaving a normal lung parenchyma.

Localised bronchiectasis

Localised thickening and dilatation of bronchii to the apico-posterior aspects of the upper lobes may cause haemoptysis and this bronchiectasis can be seen on HRCT.

Tuberculoma

One or more solid lesions often containing calcium may result from primary or secondary infection, are often found incidentally, and may have been present for many years (Fig. 2.13). The larger they are, the more likely they are to contain active bacilli, which can reactivate and spread at any time.

Non-tuberculous (atypical) mycobacteria (NTM)

Their importance both clinically and radiologically has been increasing over the last two decades, particularly with the spread of the infections worldwide. Radiologically there are no specific features to differentiate atypical mycobacteria from *M. tuberculosis* (see Fig. 2.14). However, NTM diseases tend to have thinner walled cavities, a high incidence of endobronchial spread, are found with pre-existing lung disease and rarely show haematogenous dissemination[26,27].

Patients with AIDS who have mycobacterial infection[28,29] more frequently have *Mycobacterium avium–intracellulare* than *M. tuberculosis.* They may show the characteristic changes of tuberculous infection, but a significant proportion either show non-specific changes or may have a normal chest radiograph[30].

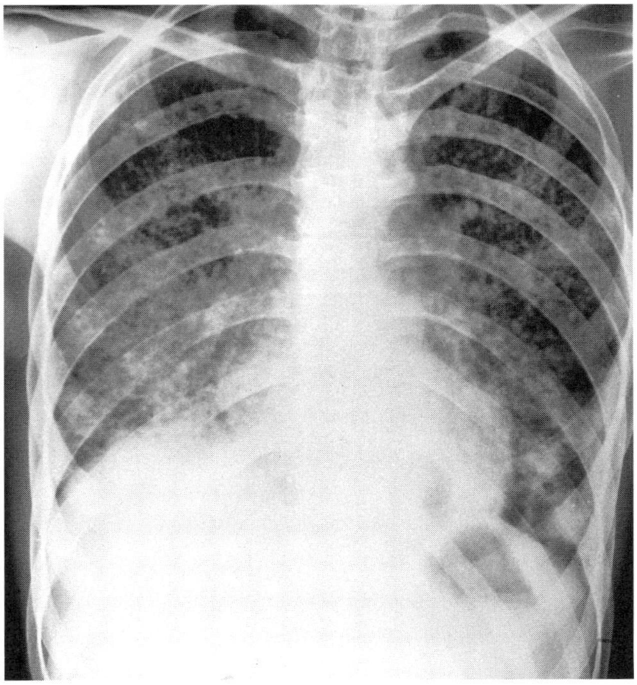

FIGURE 2.12 Miliary tuberculosis. Widespread miliary nodules throughout both lung fields in a patient who recently had cardiac surgery.

Rickettsia, Chlamydia and *Mycoplasma* pneumonia

Rickettsia

Coxiella burnetii is a rickettsial organism causing 'Q' fever, with a variable incidence of pneumonia. In a recent series by Pickworth[31], 21 cases of proven 'Q' fever with pneumonia were analysed. The most common findings were segmental opacities, with loss of volume and lobar consolidation, with slow resolution. Multiple opacities are occasionally seen, which may progress to areas of round pneumonia, and may alert the clinician to this infective agent. In most cases, however, there are no specific findings on the chest radiograph.

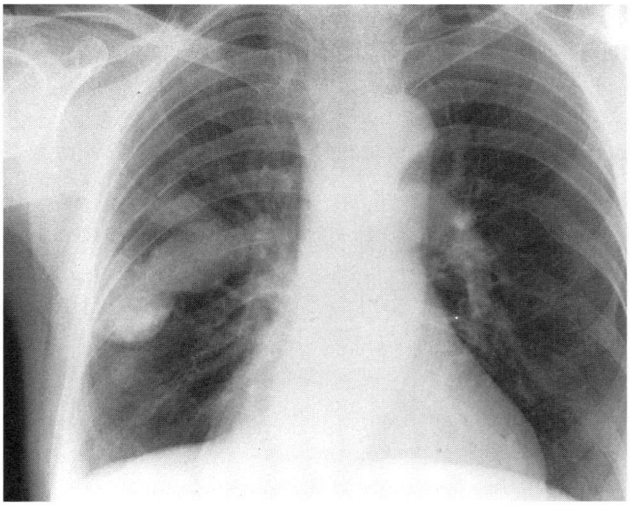

FIGURE 2.13 Tuberculoma. Multiple but localised well-defined nodules with calcification, that were unchanged for 9 years.

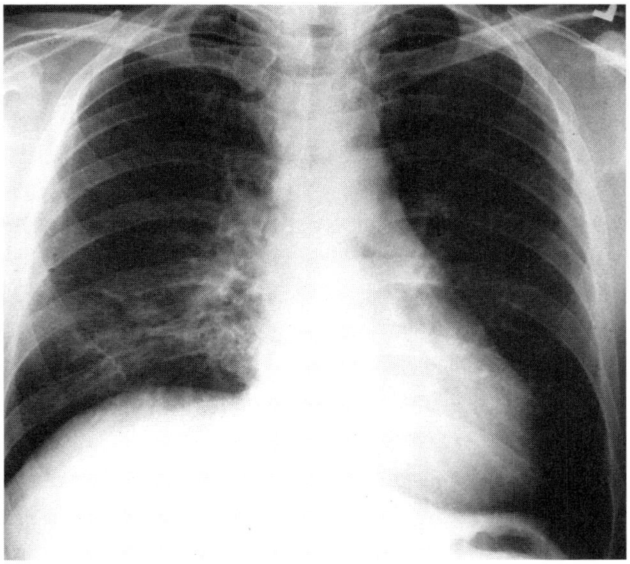

FIGURE 2.14 *Mycobacterium kansasii.* Non-specific pneumonic consolidation in the right middle lobe.

Chlamydia

Chlamydia trachomatis

This may cause pneumonia in infants under 6 months of age following transmission of infection from their mother's vagina. There is interstitial shadowing with infiltration and over-expansion[32,33]. In adults, the pneumonia can be seen in AIDS patients, other immunocompromised persons and occasionally in normal individuals. Again, diffuse interstitial pneumonia is the usual radiographical findings.

Chlamydia psittaci

Psittacosis is usually caused by transmission from infected parakeets or parrots. There is patchy reticulo-nodular shadowing extending from the hila with lobar consolidation and often subsegmental collapse. Hilar lymphadenopathy also commonly occurs. The changes may progress over several months and fatal end stage lung disease can develop if the source of infection is not removed. Comparison of the radiographic features of Legionnaire's disease, pneumococcal pneumonia, mycoplasma infection and psittacosis has been well described[34].

M. pneumoniae

This is a common pneumonia in the community and radiologically looks similar to many viral infections. Peri-bronchial and peri-vascular intestinal infiltrates, patchy consolidation (usually in the lower lobes) and homogenous acinar ground glass consolidation, combined with hilar lymphadenopathy are the main radiological features of this pneumonia[35]. Pleural effusion is rare.

Viral pneumonias

The diagnosis of viral pneumonias is often made on an exclusion basis, as the majority of viral infections cause a non-specific bronchopneumonia or localised interstitial disease, combined with other clinical indicators including failure to respond to antibodies and lack of sputum production. The accuracy of distinguishing bacterial from non-bacterial pneumonia on a chest radiograph is often poor[36], and imaging in whatever form may only give a guideline to possible infective agents unless pathognomic (rare) signs are present.

The two main groups of viruses are classified depending on their nucleic acid form; RNA based or DNA based.

RNA viruses

Measles

The majority of patients with measles who develop a pneumonia have secondary bacterial infection, with only a small proportion having true viral lung infection. Measles pneumonia causes an interstitial shadowing frequently accompanied by hilar lymphadenopathy[37].

Respiratory syncytial virus (RSV)

The RSV causes severe bronchiolitis and bronchopneumonia in infants and young children with radiological evidence of patchy areas of consolidation, localised air trapping and bronchial wall thickening. The RSV also occurs in adults who may be immunocompromised.

Influenza and parainfluenza viruses

Both viruses cause non-specific areas of consolidation, often in the lower lobes, which may then progress to large areas of confluent consolidation. They may also present with widespread interstitial and alveolar shadowing which has a similar appearance to acute pulmonary oedema.

DNA viruses

Cytomegalovirus

This infection causes pneumonia predominately in patients with altered immunity, particularly after transplant surgery, or in those with haematological disorders. There are no specific features to the chest radiograph but a mixture of parenchymal and interstitial shadowing, with pleural effusion are the commonest features with definitive nodules being present in around 30% of patients (Fig. 2.15). Spontaneous pneumothorax and pneumomediastinum occurred in a significant (28% and 17% respectively) proportion of the 35 patients reviewed by Olliff & Williams[38]. Cytomegalovirus (CMV) pneumonitis in AIDS patients should be suspected in patients with extrathoracic CMV or Kaposi's sarcoma, and should, if possible be differentiated from PCP infection. The radiographic appearances of CMV pneumonitis in AIDS include reticular shadowing, ground glass opacification, bronchial wall thickening and dense consolidation[39].

Chickenpox pneumonia

The varicella zoster virus manifests itself as two clinical entities, chickenpox and shingles, both of which can cause pneumonia. Most cases are those related to chickenpox infection, which radiologically shows changes of widespread nodular shadowing that may become confluent near the hila. The nodules may develop rapidly over 24 hours and take any time between a week to many months to resolve. The pneumonia can be severe and fulminant and can be associated with immunocompromised individuals particularly those with leukaemia (Fig. 2.16). A characteristic pattern in adults, of multiple small calcified opacities throughout both lungs is occasionally seen following resolution of the viral pneumonia. (Fig. 2.17).

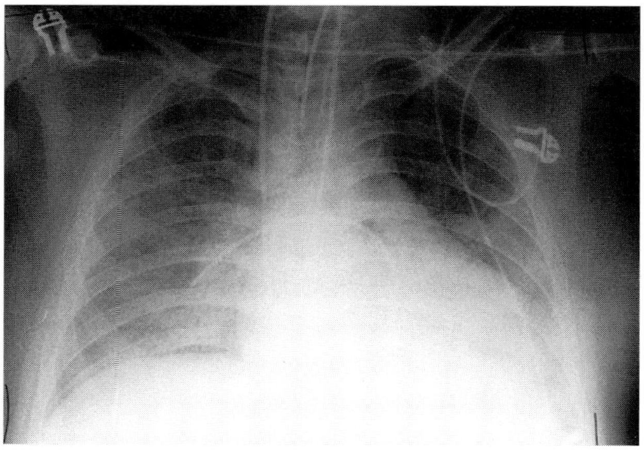

FIGURE 2.15 Cytomegalovirus. CMV infection post renal transplant. Widespread interstitial shadowing with nodules. The patient was in intensive care with endotracheal intubation, a pulmonary arterial line and respiratory failure.

Herpes simplex

Herpes simplex (HSV) infection (types 1 and 2) causes a non-specific pneumonia with alveolar shadowing progressing to confluence and exudate formation. It is seen in immunocompromised patients and also in those with severe burns. The virus has been isolated in a significant percentage of patients with the adult respiratory distress syndrome (ARDS), who have an increased morbidity and mortality as a result.

Adenoviruses

The adenoviruses cause upper and lower respiratory tract infections in infants and children. The chest radiograph shows bronchopneumonia with air trapping and over-inflation. Lobar collapse may also occur. About half the cases progress to chronic lung disease including bronchiectasis, fibrosis and obliterative bronchiolitis. It may also cause a hypertranslucent lung (Macleod's syndrome) if the disease is contracted during infancy.

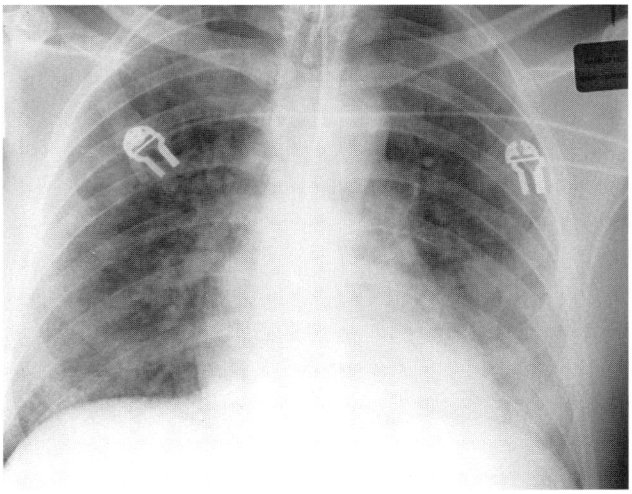

FIGURE 2.16 Acute chickenpox pneumonia. Widespread nodular shadowing throughout both lung fields in a patient with disseminated varicella.

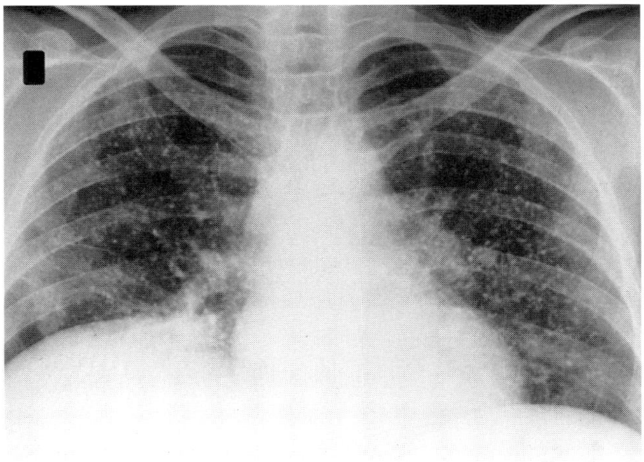

FIGURE 2.17 Previous chickenpox pneumonia. Previous bilateral infection resulting in widespread minute calcified nodules. The patient had no previous knowledge of an infective episode.

Actinomycosis and nocardiosis

Both these organisms have several features that are similar to fungi but they are separately classified. They both may present on a chest radiograph as a solid peripheral mass, indistinguishable from a primary bronchial carcinoma.

Actinomycosis

From a radiological aspect, the pneumonia of actinomycosis is similar to that of any other cause of consolidation with one important exception. The disease does not respect tissue boundaries and can produce pleural infection, rib periostitis and present as a chest wall abscess (Fig. 2.18(*a*) and (*b*)). This rarely happens in any other infection. Complete resolution occurs following appropriate antibiotic therapy but the development of lung abscess, chronic fibrosis and sinus formation may occur if the disease is unrecognised or only partially treated[40].

Nocardiosis

A similar radiographic pattern to actinomycosis is caused by infection with *Nocardia*. A dense area of consolidation, frequently with cavitation and pleural disease is common but nocardia can also be widespread and patchy with interstitial shadowing[41–43]. *Nocardia* is relatively rare and is confined mainly to immunosuppressed patients, or to those with chronic disease.

Fungus diseases

Aspergillosis

The main species causing human infection is *Aspergillus fumigatus*. Radiologically, this fungus disease has a wide spectrum of appearances depending on the three main types of disease present[44–46].

Hypersensitivity abnormalities

Allergic bronchopulmonary aspergillosis (ABPA) is one form of hypersensitivity resulting in asthma, eosinophilia and mucoid impaction of the airways. Lobar or whole lung collapse may occur with casts of the bronchial tree being expectorated or removed at bronchoscopy. Proximal bronchiectasis with normal distal branching is characteristic of this disease, and can be seen on bronchography or more beautifully on HRCT (Fig. 2.19). Marked dilatation of segmental bronchi can show as a 'gloved finger' opacity on the chest radiograph. The other types of hypersensitivity include extrinsic allergic alveolitis, where there is a background pattern of ground glass consolidation, again best seen on HRCT (Fig. 2.2(*a*) and (*b*)) or the asthma associated with Loefler's syndrome.

Mycetoma

Mycelial growth of the fungus can occur in any lung cavity, often post tuberculous, but also in a wide variety of other conditions including bronchiectasis, cavitating tumours and pulmonary sequestration. Although most mycetomata are caused by *A. fumigatus*, any fungus can be involved in producing an intracavity foreign body. On a chest radiograph, mycetomas often occupy a thin walled cavity and produce a halo of air on computed tomography[47] (Fig. 2.20). They can grow quite quickly or remain stable for many years (Fig 2.21).

Calcification of the fungus ball may also occur (Fig 2.22). For those patients not suitable for surgery, a new form of therapy has recently been documented[48,49], comprising intracavity injection of amphotericin B in either gelatine or glycerin paste under CT guidance. The solidification of the material within the cavity allows for slow specific release of the amphotericin B and the initial results are encouraging.

Invasive aspergillosis

Frank invasion of the lung parenchyma by *Aspergillus* occurs in patients with immunosuppression either due to AIDS or following cancer therapy, organ transplantation or leukaemia. One or more areas of dense consolidation, often with cavitation and an air crescent are the main signs of the disease, with progression to involve the whole lobe[50,51]. Recovery usually only occurs if the disease is diagnosed early.

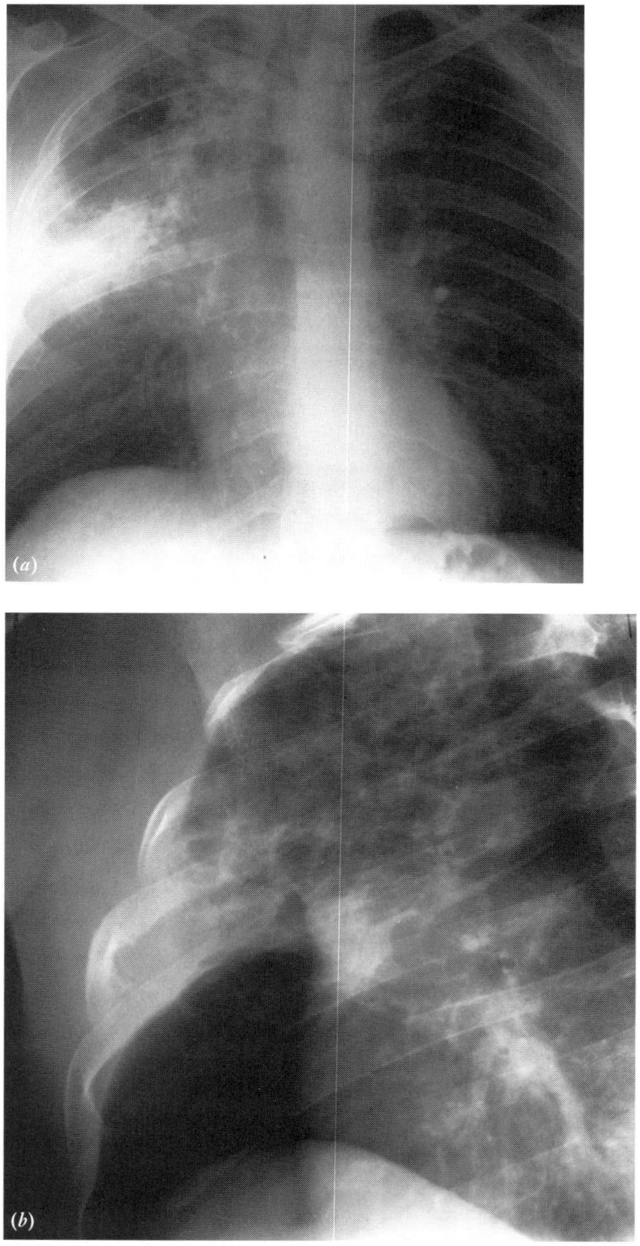

FIGURE 2.18 (*a*), (*b*) Actinomycosis. Dense upper lobe consolidation with pleural thickening and rib periostitis.

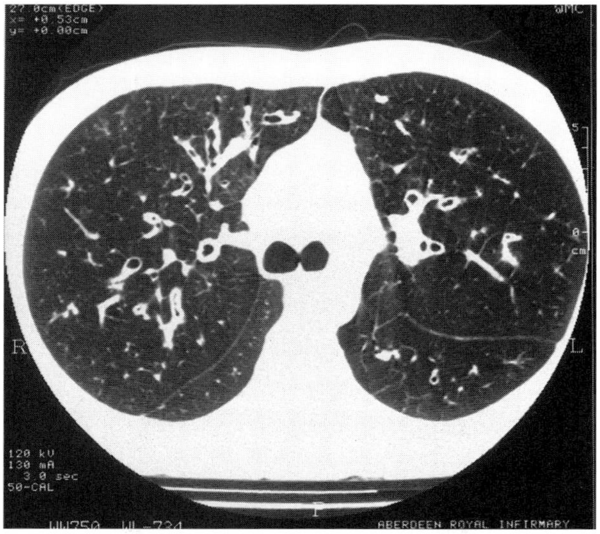

FIGURE 2.19 Allergic bronchopulmonary aspergillosis. HRCT shows typical beaded appearances of bronchiectasis in the anterior segment of the right upper lobe.

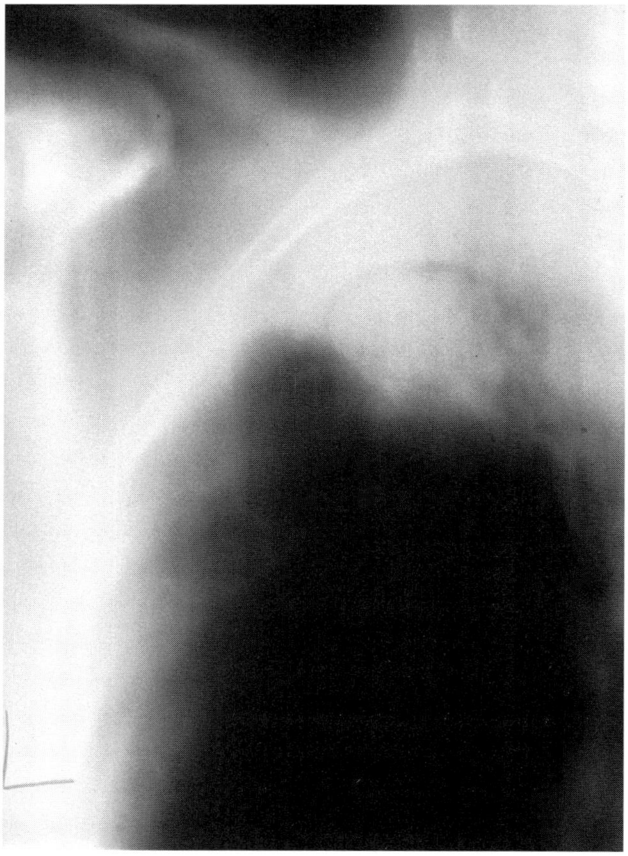

FIGURE 2.20 Mycetoma. Quickly growing mycetoma in an old tuberculous cavity. The cavity was empty 6 months previously.

Invasive aspergillosis on HRCT shows the consolidation to be peribronchial and the nodules to be centrilobular[52]. Invasion of blood vessels is a prominent pathological feature, and direct involvement of the aorta has also been reported[53].

Mucormycosis

Patients with mucormycosis have underlying haematological disorders such as leukaemia or lymphoma or other immunocompromising disorders. There is a rapid invasion of lung tissue, including blood vessels with early cavitation and a poor prognosis[46,54]. A dense area of consolidation with prominent cavitation and sometimes associated with a localised pneumothorax are the main radiological features (Fig. 2.23).

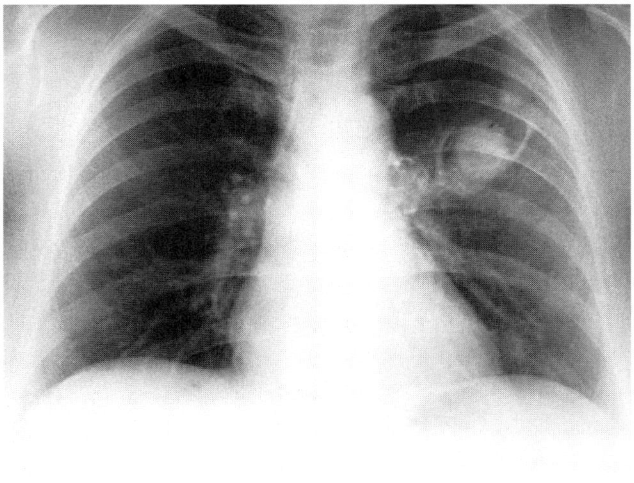

FIGURE 2.21 Mycetoma. Left mid zone mycetoma in an asymptomatic patient that has remained unchanged for 25 years!

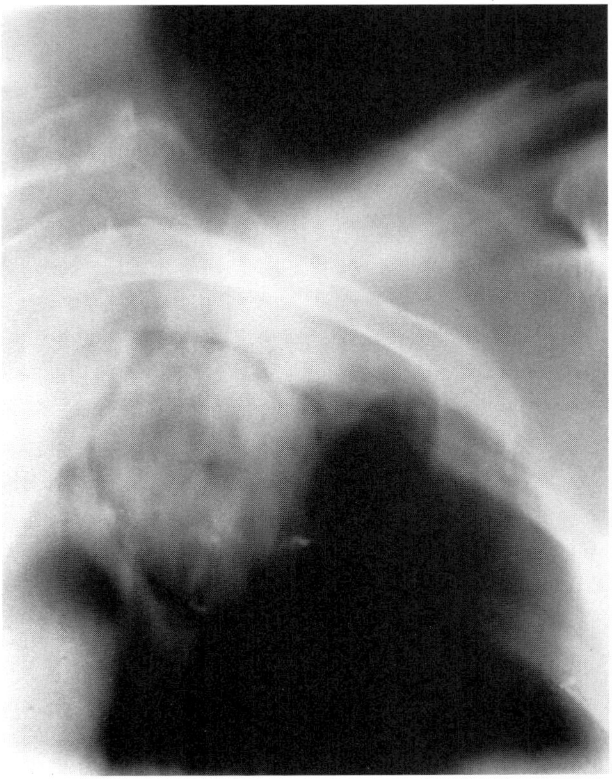

FIGURE 2.22 Mycetoma. Flecks of calcification in a mycetoma.

Histoplasmosis

Although the organism is spread worldwide, most cases are seen from endemic areas of North America. Acute infection causes non-specific air space pneumonia, but often with hilar lymphadenopathy, which tends to distinguish it from other bacterial or viral pneumonias. Persons who are heavily exposed to the organism may develop either an acute fatal illness or show very little in the way of symptoms or signs yet later have the characteristic calcified nodules on the chest radiograph (Fig 2.24). Occasionally, a solid nodule can occur often with calcification, a histoplasmoma, and it is usually accompanied by tell-tale hilar node calcification. Chronic histoplasmosis can have radiological features that include loss of lung volume, bullae with fluid levels, and interstitial and peribronchial thickening[55].

The radiographical findings of disseminated histoplasmosis in AIDS patients are varied and non-specific[56]. They range from diffuse nodularity, through linear opacities to normal chest radiographs.

Candidiasis

Candida may cause an opportunistic infection in immunocompromised hosts, usually those with leukaemia or lymphoma. Rather non-specific findings include diffuse bilateral, often lower lobe, patchy consolidation, which may be accompanied by a pleural effusion[57].

Cryptococcosis

Of increasing importance in patients with AIDS, *Cryptococcus* causes either a localised peripheral area of consolidation that resembles a

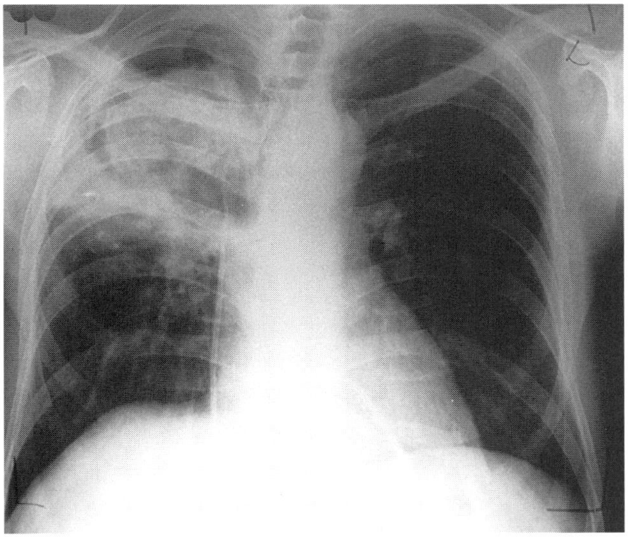

FIGURE 2.23 Mucormycosis. Rapidly cavitating pneumonic consolidation in the right upper lobe with a localised pneumothorax in an immunocompromised patient. The diagnosis of mucormycosis was made at postmortem 2 days later.

mass, or may be diffuse with multiple, ill-defined, nodules[58,59]. Feigin described three types of cryptococcosis: air space collection of fungus with a well-defined mass, granulomatous infection with infiltration, consolidation and lymphadenopathy and lastly airway colonisation which has no specific radiological features[60].

Law *et al.* have described a case of pulmonary cryptococcosis mimicking methotrexate pneumonitis[61] and suggest that this infection should be added to the list of differential diagnoses of the latter condition.

Coccidioidomycosis and blastomycosis

Coccidioidomycosis and blastomycosis are virtually confined to the Americas and unless travellers have acquired the infection, will not be seen outwith certain areas. Radiologically, coccidioidomycosis either causes localised cavitating disease similar to tuberculosis or may be disseminated with widespread nodulation. The radiological patterns in blastomycosis are varied and non-specific ranging from peripheral pneumonic consolidation to single and multiple nodules[62].

Protozoan infections

Pneumocystis carinii pneumonia (PCP)

Significant lung infection with *P. carinii* only occurs if the host has severe underlying immunological deficiency as found, for example, in patients with AIDS or on steroid therapy for haemopoietic or malignant conditions. The radiological appearances are varied, ranging from a normal chest radiograph through to bullous cystic lung disease. The usefulness of CT in the 10% of patients with suspected or proven PCP infection who have a normal chest radiograph has been highlighted by several authors[63–65]. The ground glass opacification of alveolar consolidation is seen earlier and with more clarity on HRCT[66] and its progression can be accurately followed by this technique. The alveolar consolidation is usually bilateral, with bronchial wall thickening (Fig. 2.25). Linear opacities as a feature of PCP infection have been described[67]. Localised unilateral pneumonic consolidation particularly in AIDS patients may be seen together with cystic spaces and bronchial dilatation[68,69]. The bullous or cystic spaces have a wall thickness of 1 mm or less with smooth margins and may be caused by localised air trapping secondary to bronchiolitis. While most resolve on long-term follow-up, they can persist and remain although usually smaller than on initial presentation.

Tumefactive *P. carinii* infection in AIDS has recently been reported to occur in hilar lymph nodes, the pleural apex and the psoas muscle[70], with fatality occurring rapidly in two of the three cases. The spread of the infective organism is likely to be haematogenous and the inhalation of pentamidine has been implicated as a predisposing factor in the dissemination of the extra pulmonary disease.

Amoebiasis

Pleuropulmonary infestation usually results from rupture of a liver abscess with involvement through the diaphragm, hence the predominance of the right base as the commonest site for any abnormality. Consolidation with pleural effusion are the main findings with occasional progression to lung abscess, mediastinal and or pericardial involvement. A large series of 501 patients from Mexico with thoracic disease as a consequence of amoebic liver abscesses has been described by Ibarra-Perez[71] with rupture of the abscess through the diaphragm occurring in 326 patients, into either the pleura, the lung or rarely the pericardium.

Helminth infestation

Hydatid disease

The lung is the second commonest site for infestation by *Echinococcus*, after the liver. Both organs have a capillary bed that acts as a filter allowing the larvae to become static and grow. Classically the hydatid cyst is a peripheral oval or spherical density with normal

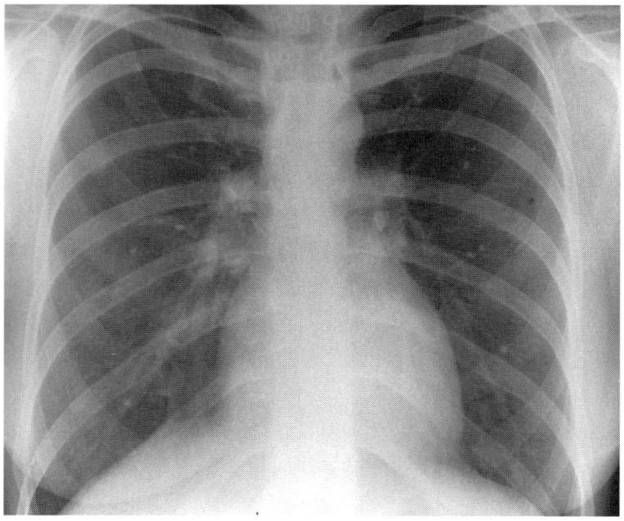

FIGURE 2.24 Histoplasmosis. Small well-defined calcifications in a patient from an endemic area.

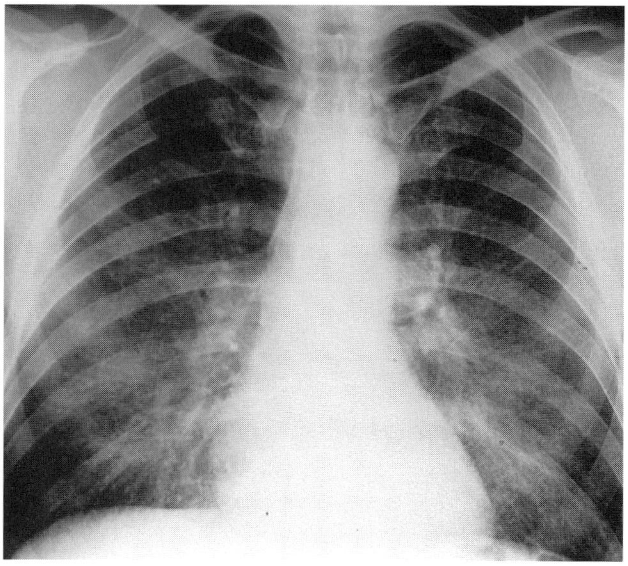

FIGURE 2.25 *Pneumocystis carinii* pneumonia. Bilateral ground glass consolidation with some interstitial shadowing at the left base.

lung surrounding it (Figs. 2.26(*a*) and (*b*), Fig. 2.27). Multiple cysts suggest multiple infestations. If the cyst ruptures, air can become trapped between the host and the parasite, forming a 'perivesicular pneumocyst'. Membranes may also float on the air-fluid level within the cyst producing the 'water lily' sign, on the erect chest film or on CT. Both these specific and classic signs are, however, quite rare, occurring in less than 5% of patients. Cyst rupture is often accompanied by increasing surrounding lung consolidation with secondary infection. The cysts may cause distortion of the normal landmarks, compression of mediastinal, diaphragmatic or chest wall structures and can rupture into either the lung parenchyma, the airways, the mediastinum or the pleural space with a pleural effusion and often a pneumothorax[72].

Tropical infections

The majority of tropical infections and infestations are localised to specific geographical areas of contamination, and only become a problem when seen outside their normal range, mainly in travellers. The possibility of a 'peculiar' infection must always be considered when dealing with such a patient. A full radiological description of tropical diseases affecting the lungs is outwith the scope of this chapter and is well covered by other texts[73–79]. See also Chapter 26.

Miscellaneous conditions

Bronchiectasis

Bronchiectasis is frequently accompanied by chronic airway infection or by surrounding parenchymal lung infection particularly in an acute exacerbation. The organisms are bacterial and often antibiotic resistant. The reason for including the disease in this 'imaging' chapter is to show the change in radiological diagnosis from bronchography to HRCT[8]. Sections of 1 mm with 10 mm increments through the lung fields show exquisite lung and airway pathology with accurate demonstration of localised or widespread bronchiectasis of whatever variety (Figs 2.28, 2.29 and 2.30). Selective bronchography with fibreoptic bronchoscopy is now reserved for those patients who may require clarification or further assessment of their disease prior to surgery. The demise of bronchography is accompanied by the removal from the market of the previously used specific contrast agent, dionosil. HRCT is now used exclusively for the diagnosis and follow-up of patients with bronchiectasis and has become the gold standard with the proviso that high quality images are obtainable when correct protocols are followed. Normal CT sections of 8 to 10 mm in thickness are of little value because of partial volume effects and they should not be used for either confirming or excluding this disease.

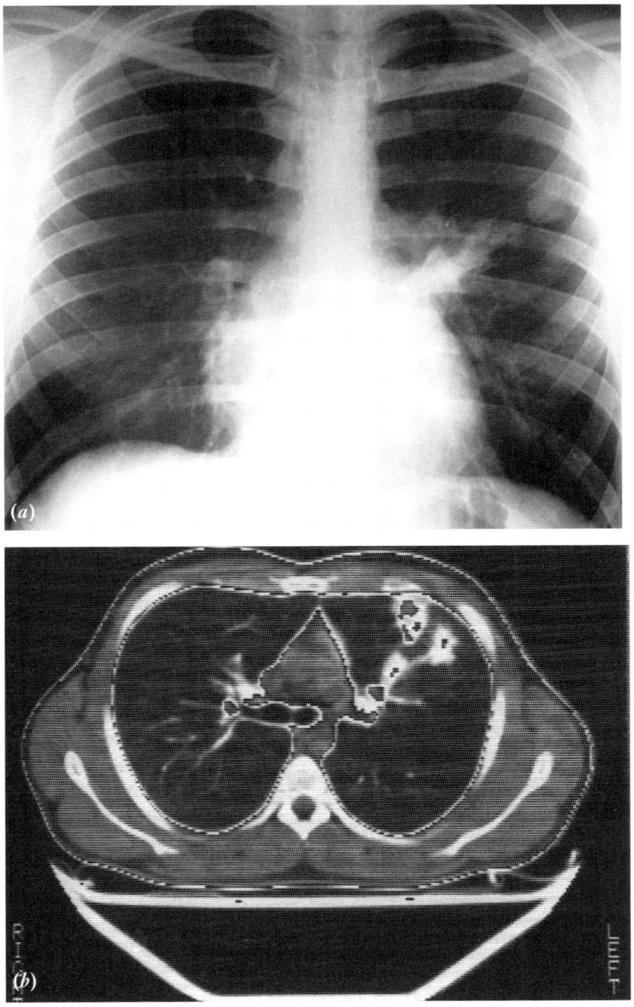

FIGURE 2.26 (*a*) Hydatid disease. (*b*) Multiple well-defined oval lesions in the left upper lobe in a sheep farmer.

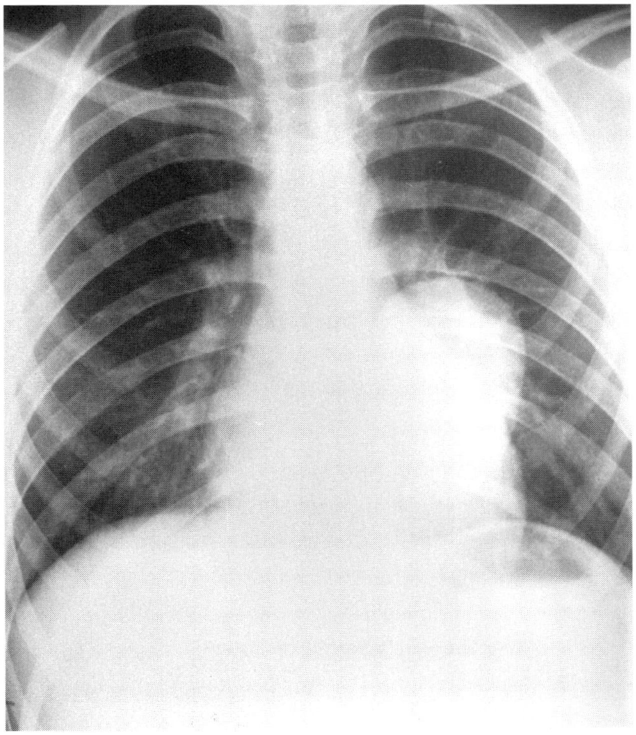

FIGURE 2.27 Hydatid disease. Well-defined single mass in the posterior aspect of the left lower lobe in a boy of 14 from the Western Isles of Scotland.

Septic pulmonary emboli

Radiologically, the majority of patients with septic pulmonary emboli will have multiple peripheral nodules, often with an obvious feeding vessel (Fig. 2.31(*a*) and (*b*). Wedge-shaped sub-pleural densities, cavitation, nodules with an air bronchogram and pleural fluid are other features[80]. CT has been shown to be of value in this diagnosis, if performed early in the disease, by showing the characteristics of the nodules and their feeding vessels[81].

The AIDS patient with lung infection

Acute infection is an important cause of morbidity and mortality in patients with AIDS and has to be differentiated from drug induced lung disease, lymphoma, Kaposi's sarcoma and other unrelated

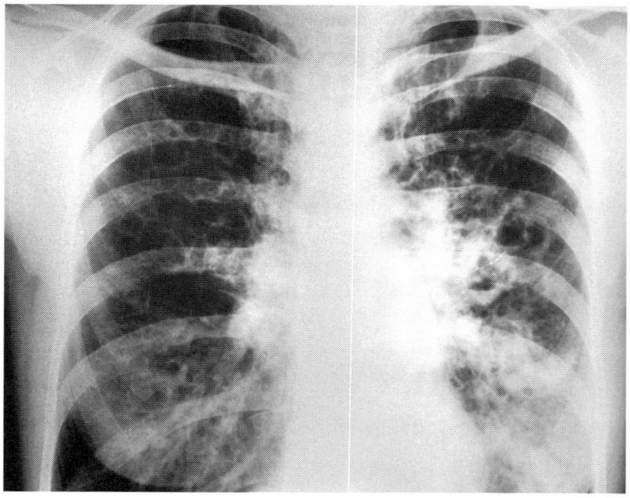

FIGURE 2.28 Bronchiectasis. Widespread bilateral bronchiectasis with multiple fluid levels in the saccular dilatations.

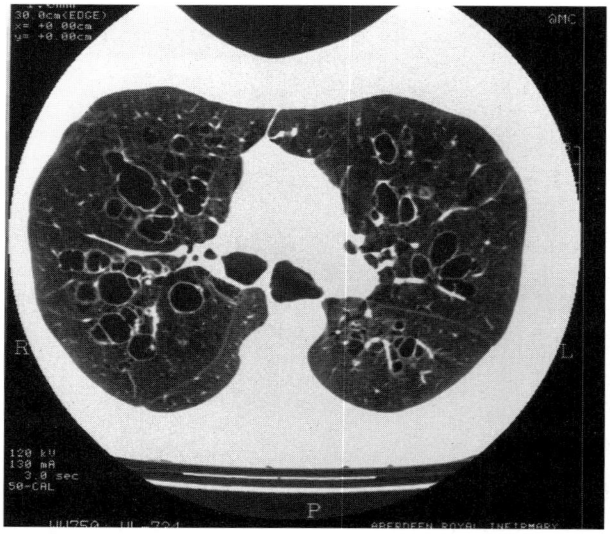

FIGURE 2.29 Bronchiectasis. Dilatation of the bronchi associated with irregularity and enlargement of the main bronchi seen in the Munier Kuhn syndrome.

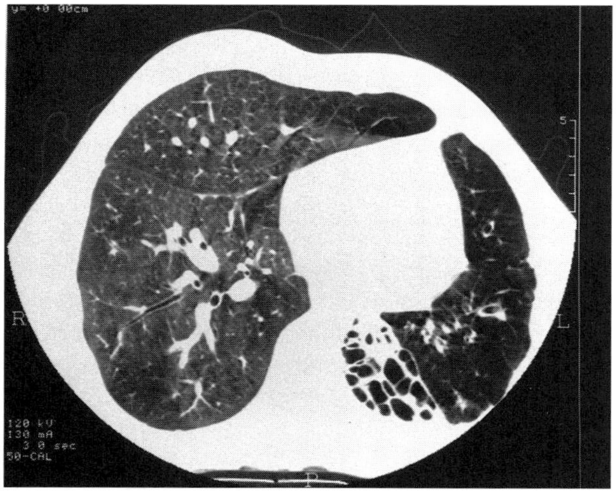

FIGURE 2.30 Bronchiectasis. Left lower lobe bronchiectasis of severe degree.

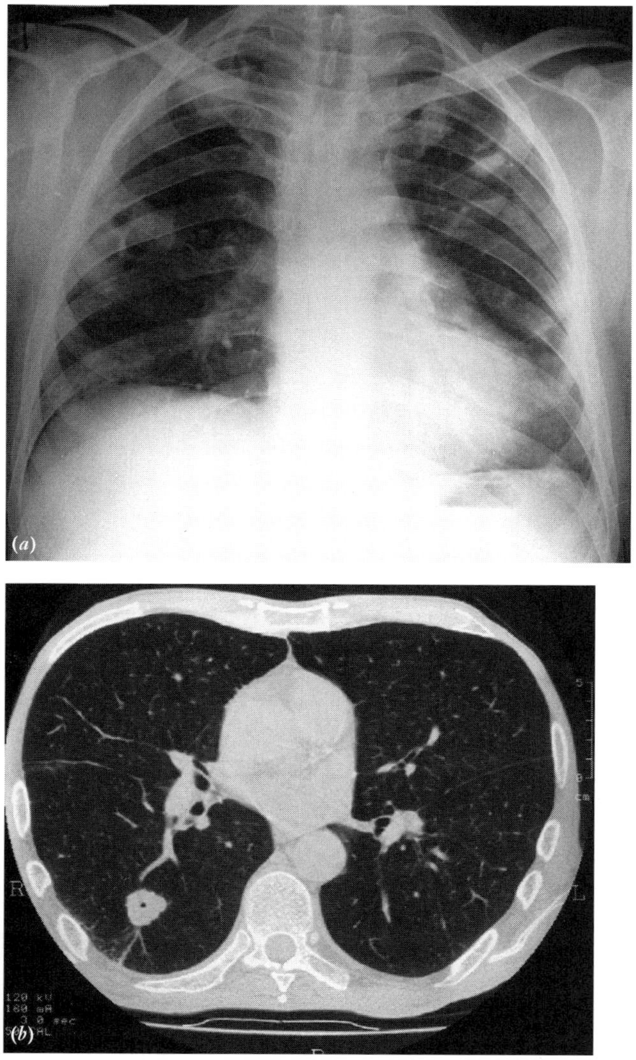

FIGURE 2.31 (*a*) Septic pulmonary emboli. (*b*) Widespread cavitating septic emboli with feeding vessels on CT.

conditions such as pulmonary embolism[82]. The commonest acute infection is *P. carinii*[83] (Fig 2.32). The classical appearances of PCP and mycobacterial diseases may be present in AIDS but many atypical patterns exist (Figs. 2.33 and 2.34) and appreciation of the numerous diverse appearances of these diseases is necessary for correct management[84,85]. PCP occurs in about 70% of AIDS patients at some point in their illness, with 10% initially having a normal chest radiograph. The use of prophylactic pentamidine nebulisers has reduced the incidence of acute infection but has allowed extrathoracic manifestations of the disease to occur in a more chronic form[70]. Bacterial infections with common organisms such as *Haemophilus* have an increased incidence in AIDS patients. They usually present as a focal area of lobar consolidation, different from the picture of PCP described above.

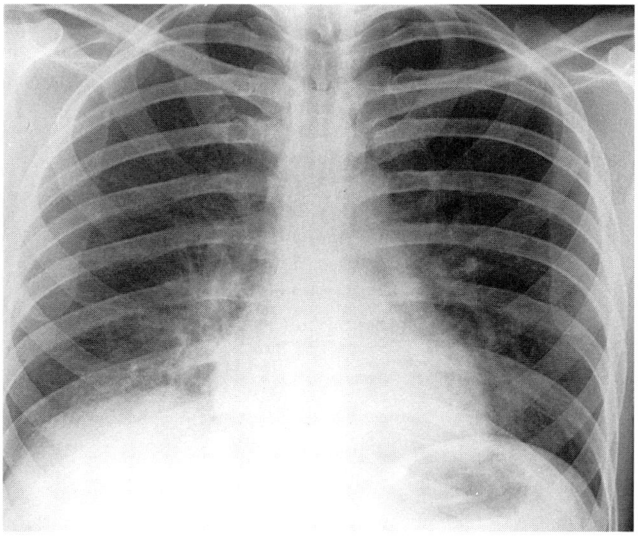

FIGURE 2.32 *Pneumocystis carinii* pneumonia. PCP infection, mainly in the right lower lobe, in a patient with AIDS.

M. tuberculosis occurs in around 10% of AIDS patients, often showing characteristic appearances of upper lobe consolidation and cavitation.

The disease may progress to include hilar and mediastinal lymphadenopathy similar to primary infection and pneumonic consolidation in a variety of sites in any lobe. Greenberg *et al.* recently reported findings in 133 AIDS patients with proven pulmonary TB. Their findings showed approximately one third of patients had a primary TB pattern, another third a post-primary pattern, and the remaining third was made up of atypical infiltrates (13%) minimal radiographic changes (5%) normal radiograph (14%) and a miliary pattern (3%). The results also showed that, as the CD4 count lowered, the percentage of patients showing the typical post primary pattern also reduced and that with counts of less than 200/mm^3, the chances of a normal radiograph with proven TB increased to 20%[86]. The implication is that the chest radiograph, long regarded as a good indicator of TB, lacks both sensitivity and specificity in patients with AIDS, particularly those with low CD4 counts. The contrast CT appearance of lymphadenopathy is said to be characteristic with necrotic central areas surrounded by enhancing rims of lymphoid tissue. The appearance is not seen in lymphoma or Kaposi's tumour but is recognised in fungal infections such as cryptococcosis.

M. avium-intracellulare is also commonly found in these patients, with pulmonary and non-pulmonary involvement, and poor response to standard antituberculous drugs.

The fungal diseases of candidiasis, aspergillosis (Fig 2.35) and cryptococcosis occur relatively infrequently in AIDS patients and show a variation in radiographic abnormalities including nodules, areas of consolidation both of which may cavitate, and lymphadenopathy. A few patients may have insolated pleural effusions.

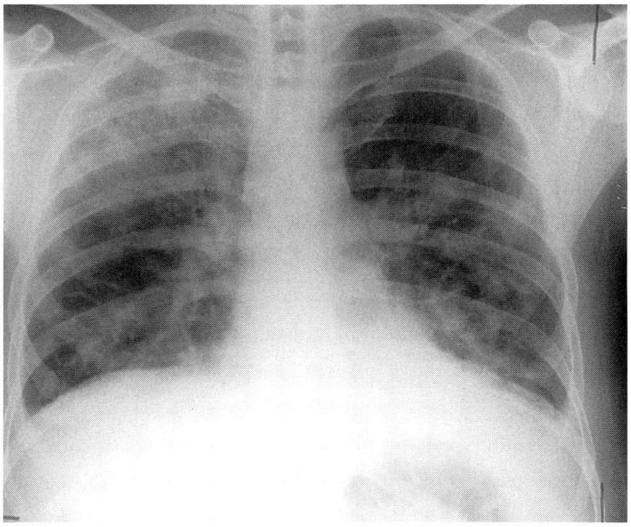

FIGURE 2.33 AIDS. *Mycobacterium avium intracellulare* in the left lower lobe and Kaposi's sarcoma in the right upper lobe.

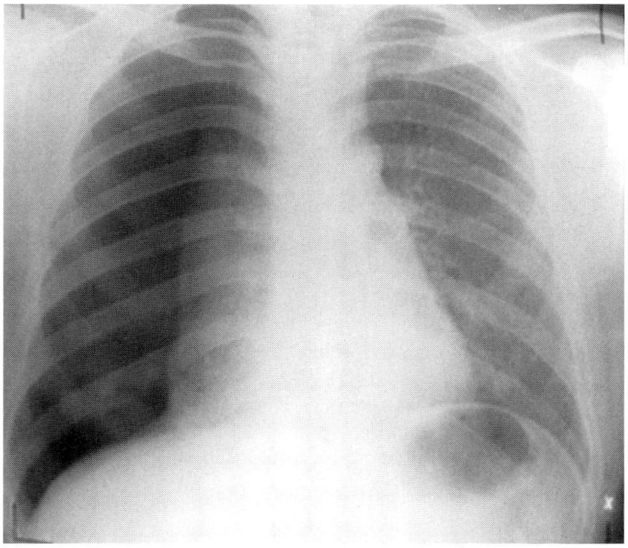

FIGURE 2.34 AIDS. Miliary TB in an African patient with AIDS. There is a large right pneumothorax due to the tuberculosis.

Table 2.2. *Common HIV-associated infections*

Pattern	Diseases	CT correlations
Normal	PCP	Air-space modules; patchy, diffuse ground-glass infiltrates
	Disseminated tuberculosis; disseminated fungal infection	Occult infiltrates; cavities; miliary disease
	Non-specific interstitial pneumonitis, LIP (uncommon); KS (uncommon)	
Diffuse infiltrates	PCP	Diffuse ground-glass infiltrates; +/– cystic changes
	PCP plus other infections (CMV, MAI, MTB; fungi)	
	Disseminated tuberculosis; disseminated fungal infection	Low-density lymphadenopathy
	Non-specific interstitial pneumonitis, LIP (uncommon)	
	KS	Peribronchial/perivascular infiltrates and/or nodules; occult pleural nodules +/– effusions
Focal infiltrates	Pyogenic bacteria	Occult cavitation; parapneumonic effusions
	PCP (apical distribution related to aerosolized pentamidine)	
	Tuberculosis; fungal infections	
Nodules	Non-Hodgkin's lymphoma	
	KS	Peribronchial/perivascular subpleural nodules
	Septic emboli	Cavitary/perivascular nodules
	Tuberculosis; fungal infections	May be low-density following IV contrast administration
Adenopathy	*M. tuberculosis, C. neoformans; H. capsulatum*	Low density; nodes; rim enhancement
	KS; non-Hodgkin's lymphoma	
	P. carinii (uncommon)	Calcified nodes (aerosolized pentamidine)
Pleural effusions	KS	Pleural nodules
	Tuberculosis; non-Hodgkin's lymphoma; pyogenic empyema; *P. carinii* (uncommon)	

Abbreviations: LP = lymphocytic interstitial pneumonitis. KS = Kaposi's sarcoma, CMV = cytomegalovirus, MAI = *Mycobacterium avium-intracellulare*, MTB = *Mycobacterium tuberculosis*.
Reproduced with permission from Drs Naidich & McGuinness, *Radiologic Clinics of North America*, 1991, 29 (5); 1014[83].

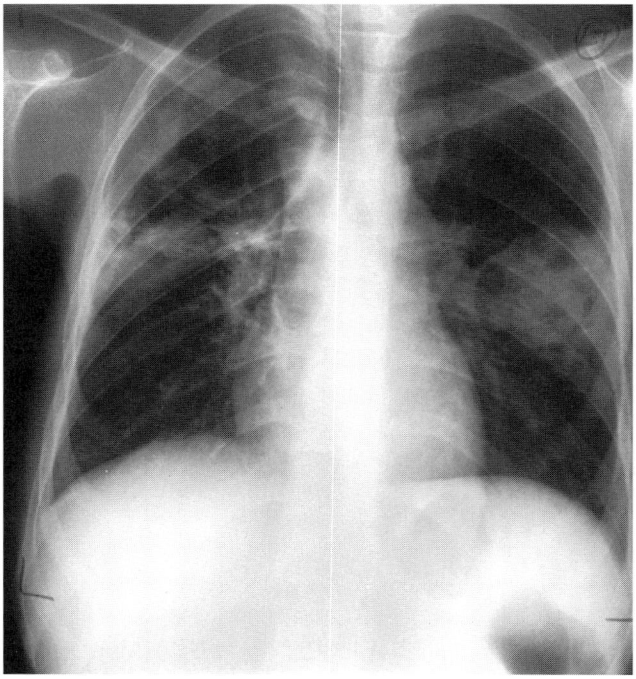

FIGURE 2.35 AIDS. An immunocompromised African patient with AIDS who has an aspergillosis mycetoma in the left mid zone and active tuberculosis in the right upper lobe.

Table 2.2 shows the common infections and the possible appearances on either plain chest radiography or HRCT.

Lung infections in immunocompromised (non-AIDS) patients

The opportunistic infections involved may be local or diffuse as in the AIDS patients above, and the type of infecting organism depends to some extent on the type of immune problem[87]. Patients with T-cell function abnormalities, for example, are prone to mycobacterial disease. Gram-positive and negative bacteria are commonly found, often with cavitation (Fig. 2.36). Fungi also present either as a solid, often cavitating peripheral lesion or as diffuse nodules due to haematogenous dissemination with both appearances being similar to those produced by bacterial and viral agents. Viral disease, often CMV, produces diffuse interstitial or reticulonodular disease and may be indistinguishable from bacterial pneumonias in the latter stages. Protozoan infection with PCP is very common, with early ground glass consolidation leading to widespread alveolar shadowing with an air bronchogram. PCP may also cause nodules, localised

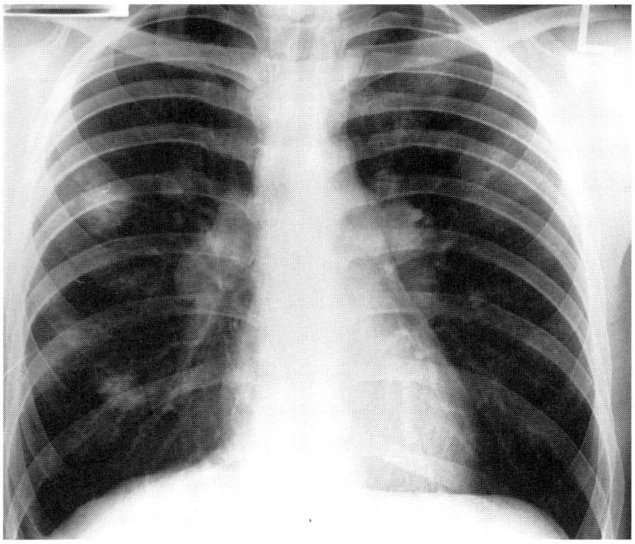

FIGURE 2.36 Agammaglobulinaemia. Multiple blood-borne areas of bacterial pneumonia in a patient with congenital agammaglobulinaemia.

dense areas of consolidation and a pleural effusion. It has recently been shown that HRCT[11] is better than a chest radiograph in the differential diagnosis of lung infection in the non-AIDS immunocompromised patient.

Conclusions

For imaging patients with lung infection, the requirements are good quality chest radiographs, preferably high kV, a CT scanner capable of thin section scans with high resolution and a skilled interventional radiologist for diagnostic and therapeutic procedures. The presence of a nuclear medicine department and an MRI facility are also becoming more important. Lastly, by the very nature of lung infection, the results of imaging will only be as good as the clinico-radiological co-operation.

Acknowledgements

I would like to thank Dr John Calder, Consultant Radiologist, Royal Victoria Infirmary, Glasgow for the use of Figs. 2.34 and 2.35.

Table 2.2 is printed by kind permission of Dr Naidich, New York.

References

1. WESTCOFF JL, COLE S. Plate atelectasis. *Radiology* 1985; 155:1–9.
2. BLESOVSKY A. The folded lung. *Br J Dis Chest* 1966, 60:19–22.
3. MCHUGH K, BLAQUIERE RM. CT features of rounded atelectasis. *AJR* 1989; 153(2), 257–60.
4. EPLER GR, MCLOUD TC, GAENSLER EA, MIKUS JP, CARRINGTON CB. Normal chest roentgenograms in chronic diffuse infiltrative lung disease. *N Engl J Med* 1978; 298:801–9.
5. GRENIER P, VALEGE D, CLUZEL P, BRAUMER MW, LENOIR S, CHASTANG C. Chronic diffuse interstitial lung disease: diagnostic value of chest radiography and high resolution CT. *Radiology* 1991; 179:123–32.
6. MATHIESON JR, MAYO JR, STAPLES CA, MULLER NL. Chronic diffuse interstitial lung disease: comparison of diagnostic accuracy of CT and chest radiography. *Radiology* 1989; 171:111–16.
7. WEBB WR. High resolution CT of the lung parenchyma. *Radiol Clin North Am* 1989; 27:1085–97.
8. GRENIER P, MAURICE F, MUSSET D, NAHUM H. Bronchiectasis: assessment by thin-section CT. *Radiology* 1986; 161:95–9.
9. BEIGIN CJ, COBLENTZ CL, CHILES C, BELL DY, CASTELLINO RA. Chronic lung diseases: specific diagnosis using CT. *AJR* 1989; 152:1183–8.
10. JANZEN DL, ADLER BD, PADLEY SPG, MÜLLER NL. Diagnostic success of bronchoscopic biopsy in immunocompromised patients with acute pulmonary disease: predictive value of disease distribution as shown on CT. *AJR* 1993; 160:21–4.
11. JANZEN DL, PADLEY SPG, ADLER BD, MULLER NL. Acute pulmonary complications in immunocompromised non-AIDS patients: comparison of diagnostic accuracy of CT and chest radiography. *Clin Radiol* 1993; 47:159–65.
12. MAYO JR, MACKAY A, MULLER NL. MR imaging of the lungs: value of short TE spin-echo pulse sequences. *AJR* 1992; 159:951–6.
13. BEKERMAN C, BITRAN J, WEINSTEM R, BENNETT C, RYO V, PINSKY S. Abstract. *J Nucl Med* 1987; 29:648.
14. LEE VW, COOLEY TP, FULLER JD, WARD RJ, FARBER HW. Pulmonary mycobacterial infections in AIDS: characteristic pattern of thallium and gallium scan mismatch. *Radiology* 1994; 193:389–92.
15. CONCES DJ JR, CLARK SA, TARVER RD, SCHWENK GR. Transthoracic aspiration needle biopsy: value in the diagnosis of pulmonary infections. *AJR* 1989; 152:31–4.
16. TORRES A, JIMENEZ P, PUIG DE LA BELLACASA J, CELIS R, GONZALEZ J, GEA J. Diagnostic value of nonfluoroscopic percutaneous lung needle aspiration in patients with pneumonia. *Chest* 1990; 98:840–4.
17. SCOTT WWJ, KUHLMAN JE. Focal pulmonary lesions in patients with AIDS: percutaneous transthoracic needle biopsy. *Radiology* 1991; 180:419–21.
18. WALLACE JM, BATRA P, GONG H, OVENFOS CO. Percutaneous needle lung aspiration for diagnosing pneumonitis in the patient with AIDS. *Am Rev Resp Dis* 1985; 131:389–92.
19. LYNCH JB, SITRIN RG. Noninfectious mimics of community-acquired pneumonia (Review). *Semin Resp Infec* 1993; 8:14–45.
20. EVANS AF, OAKLEY RH, WHITEHOUSE GH. Analysis of the chest radiograph in Legionnaire's disease. *Clin Radiol* 1981; 32:361–5.
21. DEITRICH PA, JOHNSON RD, FAIRBANK JT, WALKE JS. The chest radiograph in Legionnaire's disease. *Radiology* 1978; 127: 577–82.
22. WUNDERINK RG, WOLDENBERG LS, ZEISS J, DAY CM, CIEMINS J, LACHER DA. Radiologic diagnosis of autopsy-proven ventilator associated pneumonia. *Chest* 1992; 101:458–63.
23. BARTLETT JG. Anaerobic bacterial infections of the lung. *Chest* 1987; 91:901–9.
24. LANDAY MJ, CHRISTENSEN EE, BYNUM LJ, GOODMAN C. Anaerobic pleural and pulmonary infections. *AJR* 1980; 134:233–40.
25. WOODRING JH, VANDIVIERE JH, FRIED AM, DILLON ML, WILLIAMS TD, MELVIN IG. Update: the radiographic features of pulmonary tuberculosis. *AJR* 1986; 146:497–506.
26. ALBELDA SM, KERN JA, MARIHELLI DL. Expanding spectrum of pulmonary disease

caused by non-tuberculous *Mycobacteria*. *Radiology* 1985; 157:289–96.

27. WOODRING JH, VANDIVIERE HM. Pulmonary disease caused by nontuberculous *Mycobacteria*. *J Thorac Imag* 1990; 5:64.
28. MARINELLI DL. Non-TB infection in AIDS. *Radiology* 1986; 160:77–82.
29. LEVINE B, CHAISSON RE. *Myobacterium kansasii*: a cause of treatable pulmonary disease associated with advanced human immunodeficiency virus (HIV) infection. *Ann Intern Med* 1991; 114:861–8.
30. PITCHENIK AE, RUBINSON HA. The radiographic appearance of tuberculosis in patients with the acquired immune deficiency syndrome (AIDS) and pre-AIDS. *Am Rev Resp Dis* 1985; 131:393–6.
31. PICKWORTH FE, EL-SOUSSI M, WELLS IP, MCGAVIN CR, REILLY S. Radiological appearances of 'Q' fever pneumonia. *Clin Radiol* 1991; 44:150–3.
32. EDELMAN RR, HANN LE, SIMON M. *Chlamydia trachomatosis* pneumonia in adults: radiographic appearance. *Radiology* 1984; 152:279–82.
33. RADKOWSKI MA, KRANZLER JK, BEEM OM, TIPPLE MA. *Chlamydia* pneumonia in infants: Radiography in. *AJR* 1981; 137:703–6.
34. MACFARLANE JT, MILLER AC, SMITH WHR, MORRIS AH, ROSE DH. Comparative radiographic features of community acquired legionnaires' disease, pneumococcal pneumonia, *Mycoplasma* pneumonia, and psittacosis. *Thorax* 1984; 39:28–33.
35. GUCKEL C, BENZ-BOHM G, WIDEMANN B. Mycoplasmal pneumonias in childhood: roentgen features, differential diagnosis and review of literature. *Paediatr Radiol* 1989; 19: 499–503.
36. TEW J, CALENOFF L, BERLIN BS. Bacterial or non-bacterial pneumonia : accuracy of radiographic diagnosis. *Radiology* 1977; 124:607–12.
37. FAWCITT J, PARRY HE. Lung changes in pertussis and measles in childhood: a review of 1894 cases with a follow up study of the pulmonary complications. *BJR* 1957; 30: 76–82.
38. OLLIFF JFC, WILLIAMS MP. Radiological appearances of cytomegalovirus infections. *Clin Radiol* 1989; 40:463–7.
39. MCGUINNESS G, SCHOLES JV, GARAY SM, LEITMAN BS, MCCAULEY DI, NAIDICH DP. Cytomegalovirus pneumonitis: spectrum of parenchymal CT findings with pathologic correlation in 21 AIDS patients. *Radiology* 1994; 192:451–9.
40. FRANK P, STRICKLAND B. Pulmonary actinomycosis. *Br J Radiol* 1974; 47:373.
41. FEIGIN DS. Nocardiosis of the lung: chest radiographic findings in 21 cases. *Radiology* 1986; 159:9–14.
42. HENKLE JQ, NAIR SV. Endobronchial pulmonary nocardosis. *JAMA* 1986; 256:1331–2.
43. RABY N, FORBES G, WILLIAMS R. Nocardia infection in patients with liver transplants or chronic liver disease: radiologic findings. *Radiology* 1990; 174:713.
44. GEFTER WB, WEINGRAD TR, EPSTEIN DM, OCHS RH, MILLER WT. 'Semi-invasive' pulmonary aspergillosis: a new look at the spectrum of *Aspergillus* infections of the lung. *Radiology* 1981; 140:313–21.
45. GREENE R. Pulmonary aspergillosis: three distinct entities or a spectrum of disease. *Radiology* 1981; 140: 527–30.
46. LIBSHITZ HI, PAGANI JJ. Aspergillosis and mucormycosis: two types of opportunistic fungal pneumonia. *Radiology* 1981; 140:301–6.
47. ROBERTS CM, CITRON KM, STRICKLAND B. Intrathoracic aspergilloma: role of CT in diagnosis and treatment. *Radiology* 1987; 165:123–8.
48. MUNK PL, VELLET AD, RANKIN RN, MÜLLER NL, AHMAD D. Intercavity aspergilloma: transthoracic percutaneous injection of amphotericin gelatin solution. *Radiology* 1993; 188:821–3.
49. GIRON JM, POEY CG, FAJADET PP, BALAGNER GR, ASSOUN JA, RICHARDI GR, HADDAD JH, CACERES JC, SENAC JP, RAILHAC JJ. Inoperable pulmonary aspergilloma: percutaneous CT guided injection with glycerin and Amphotericin B pase in 15 cases. *Radiology* 1993; 188: 825–7.
50. HEROLD CJ, KRAMER J, SERTL K, KALHS P, MALLEK R, IMHOF H, TSCHOLAKOFF D. Invasive pulmonary aspergillosis: evaluation with MR imaging. *Radiology* 1989; 173:717–21.
51. KUHLMAN, JE, FISHMAN EK, SIEGELMAN SS. Invasive pulmonary aspergillosis in acute leukemia: characteristic findings on CT, the CT halo sign and the role of CT in early diagnosis. *Radiology* 1985; 157:611–14.
52. LOGAN PM, PRIMACK SL, MILLER RR, MÜLLER NL. Invasive aspergillosis of the airways: radiographic, CT, and pathologic findings. *Radiology* 1994; 193:383–8.
53. KATZ JF, YASSA NA, BHAN I, BANKOFF MS. Invasive aspergillosis involving the thoracic aorta: CT appearance. *AJR* 1994; 163:817–19.
54. ZAGORIA RJ, CHOPLIN RH, KARSTAEDT N. Pulmonary gangrene as a complication of mucormycosis. *AJR* 1985; 144:1195–6.
55. GOODWIN RA JR, DES PREZ RM. Histoplasmosis. *Am Rev Resp Dis* 1978; 117:929–56.
56. CONCES DJ JR, STOCKBERGER SM, TARVER RD, WHEAT LJ. Disseminated histoplasmosis in AIDS: findings on chest radiographs. *AJR* 1993; 160:15–19.
57. PAGANI JJ, LIBSHITZ HI. Opportunistic fungal pneumonias in cancer patients. *AJR* 1981; 137:1033–1039.
58. MILLER WTJ, EDELMAN JM, MILLER WT. Cryptococcal pulmonary infection in patients with AIDS: radiographic appearance. *Radiology* 1990; 175:725–8.
59. KHOURY MB, GODWIN JD, RAVIN CE, GALLIS HA, HALVORSEN RA, PUTMAN CE. Thoracic cryptococcosis: immunologic competence and radiological appearance. *AJR* 1984; 142:893–6.
60. FEIGIN DS. Pulmonary cryptococcosis: radiologic–pathologic correlates of its three forms. *AJR* 1983; 141:1263–72.
61. LAW KF, ARANDA CP, SMITH RL, BERKOWITZ KA, ITTMAN MM, LEWIS ML. Pulmonary cryptococcosis mimicking methotrexate pneumonitis. *J Rheumat* 1993; 20:872–3.
62. SHEFLIN JR, CAMPBELL JA, THOMPSON GP. Pulmonary blastomycosis: findings on chest radiographs in 63 patients. *AJR* 1990; 154:1177–80.
63. MOSKOVIC E, MILLER R, PEARSON M. High resolution computed tomography of *Pneumocystis carinii* pneumonia in AIDS. *Clin Radiol* 1990; 42:239.
64. MCLOUD TC. Pulmonary infections in the immunocompromised host. *Radiol Clin North Am* 1989; 27:1059.
65. MCLOUD TC, NAIDICH DP. Thoracic disease in the immunocompromised patient. *Radiol Clin North Am* 1992; 30: 525.
66. BERGIN CJ, WIRTH RL, BERRY GJ, CASTELLINO RA. *Pneumocystis carinii* pneumonia: CT and HRCT observations. *J Comput Assist Tomogr* 1990; 14:756–759.
67. PAGE JE, WILSON AG. Linear opacities as a feature of pneumocystis pneumonia. *Br J Radiol* 1990; 63:597–601.
68. KUHLMAN JE, KAVURA M, FISHMAN EK, SIEGELMAN SS. *Pneumocystis carinii* pneumonia: spectrum of parenchymal CT findings. *Radiology* 1990; 175:711–14.
69. PANICEK DM. Cystic pulmonary lesions in patients with AIDS. *Radiology* 1989; 173:12.
70. EAGAR GM, FRIENDLAND JA, SAGEL SS. Tumefactive *Pneumocystis carinii* infection in AIDS: report of three cases. *AJR* 1993; 160:1197–8.
71. IBARRA-PEREZ C. Thoracic complications of amoebic abscess of the liver: report of 501 cases. *Chest* 1981; 79: 672–7.
72. BEGGS I. The radiology of hydatid disease: a review. *AJR* 1985; 145:639–8.
73. AWE RJ, MATTOX KL, ALVEREZ BA, STORK WJ, ESTRADA R, GREENBERG DS. Solitary and bilateral pulmonary nodules due to

Dirofilaria immitis. *Am Rev Resp Dis* 1975; 112:445–9.

74. COCKSHOTT WP, LUCAS AV. Radiological findings in *Histoplasma duboisii* infections. *Br J Rad* 1964; 37:653–660.
75. COCKSHOTT WP, PALMER PES. Exotic diseases in travellers. *Curr. Imaging* 1990; 2:142–52.
76. HERLINGER H. Pulmonary changes in tropical eosinophilia. *Br J Rad* 1963; 36:880–901.
77. PETTERSON T, STEUSTROM R, KYRONSEPPA H. Disseminated lung opacities and cavitation associated with strongyloides stercoralis and *S mansoni* infections. *Am J Trop Med and Hyg* 1974; 23:158–62.
78. PALMER PES. Diagnostic imaging in parasitic infections. *Pediat Clin North Am* 1985; 32:1019–39.
79. PRYYANANDA B, PRADATSUNDARASAR A, VIRANUVATTI V. Pulmonary gnathostomiasis. *Ann Trop Med and Parasit* 1985; 49:121–2.
80. KUHLMAN JE, FISHMAN EK, TEIGEN C. Pulmonary septic emboli: diagnosis with CT. *Radiology* 1990; 174:211–13.
81. HUANG RM, NAIDICH DP, LUBAT E, SCHINELLA R, GARAY SM, MCCAULEY DI. Septic pulmonary emboli: CT radiographic correlation. *AJR* 1989; 153:41–5.
82. BROWN MJ, MILLER RR, MÜLLER NL. Acute lung disease in the immunocompromised host: CT and pathologic examination findings. *Radiology* 1994; 190:247–54.
83. NAIDICH DP, MCGUINNESS G. Pulmonary manifestations of AIDS – CT and radiographic correlations. *Radiol Clin North Am* 1991; 29:999–1017.
84. AMOROSA JK, NAHASS RG, NOSHER JL, GOCKE, DJ. Radiologic distinction of pyrogenic pulmonary infection from *Pneumocystis carinii* pneumonia in AIDS patients. *Radiology* 1990; 175:721.
85. KUHLMAN JE, KNOWLES MC, FISHMAN EK, SIEGLEMAN MD. Premature bullous pulmonary damage in AIDS: CT diagnosis. *Radiology* 1989; 173:23–6.
86. GREENBERG SD, FRAGER D, SUSTER B, WALKER S, STRAVROPOULOS C, ROTHPEARL A. Active pulmonary tuberulosis in patients with AIDS: spectrum of radiographic findings (including a normal appearance). *Radiology* 1994; 193:115–19.
87. MOORE EH. Diffuse lung disease in the current spectrum of immunocompromised hosts (non-AIDS). *Radiol Clin North Am* 1991; 29:983–97.

3 Respiratory defences against infection

NEIL V. L. WARAVDEKAR and HERBERT Y. REYNOLDS
Milton S. Hershey Medical Center, Pennsylvania State University, USA

Introduction

Despite the deceiving appearance of being clean, the air we breathe contains a variety of smokes, pollens, hazardous chemicals, debris and microorganisms. Airway contact with microbes is continuous. Although minor infections are frequent, it is surprising that serious infections such as pneumonia are relatively rare in the immunocompetent host. With an elaborate array of host defence mechanisms, the respiratory system is able to remain largely free from infection. A specific inciting event, either acquired or inherited, is needed to overcome this competent defence. Disruption of anatomic barriers, decreased clearance of secretions, depressed cough reflex and derangements or alterations in immune status are but a few of the mechanisms whereby this intricate system can be compromised (Table 3.1). The respiratory defence system acts differently from a usual surveillance mechanism in that it becomes active on a periodic basis when the need arises. Although the respiratory defence system is co-ordinated from the nose and mouth to level of the alveolar unit, it will be considered separately as the airways and the alveoli. Each has unique adaptations to resist and combat infection which are integrated to maintain a disease-free state.

Airway structure

The airways of the respiratory system are covered by a mucosa which varies in cell type throughout the system. The airway surface is composed of three distinct layers: an epithelium, the basement membrane and the submucosa. The naso- oropharynx with the exception of the nasal turbinates is lined by a stratified squamous epithelium. Pseudostratified columnar epithelium with cilia and mucus secreting apparatus covers the turbinates and the endobronchial surface from the trachea down to the respiratory bronchioles. Regeneration of these cells occurs about every 7 days. Cilia, up to 200 per cell, are grouped in tufts which beat at a speed of approximately 600 times per minute[1] with the net effect of propelling mucus and debris toward the upper airways where it can be removed. In the peripheral airways the cells tend to be more cuboidal and cilia are shorter. In the submucosa bronchial glands are found which produce mucus that is extruded onto the mucosa and plasma cells are present which synthesise IgA and other immunoglobulins. Tissue mast cells as well as afferent and efferent fibres from autonomic nerves are also located in the submucosa. The epithelial cells are ciliated and possess tight junctions between cells which limit bacterial penetrance[2]. Several cell types of the epithelium can produce secretions[3] and these include goblet cells, Clara cells, serous cells and dendritic cells. Goblet cells are mucus-producing cells which are interspersed between ciliated cells throughout the airways with a ratio of one goblet cell for every five ciliated cells. Clara cells are non-ciliated secretory cells found predominantly in the terminal bronchioles where there are few goblet cells. Serous cells possess numerous absorptive microvilli. Although found in the airways of rodents and foetuses, they have not been identified in the adult human. Dendritic cells can have several cytoplasmic processes projecting toward the mucosal surface. Fig. 3.1 provides a schematic representation of the above structures.

Bronchus associate lymphoid tissue (BALT) can be found at points of airway bifurcation and will be discussed in a subsequent section. Bathing the surface of the epithelium is a gel-like substance which is composed of mucus, immunoglobulins, cells, local mediators,

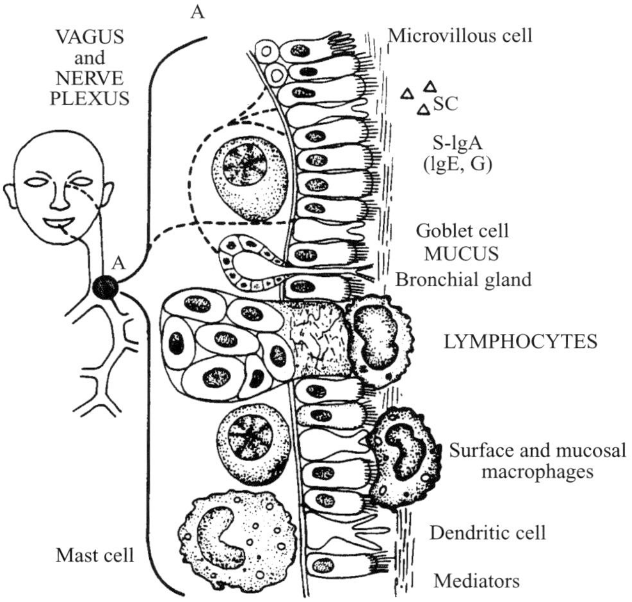

FIGURE 3.1 Schematic of conducting airway (A) with expanded view of mucosa and submucosa. Mucus and fluid containing immunoglobulin and secretory component (SC) cover the ciliated pseudostratified epithelium. Brush cells with microvilli and dendritic cells with processes which do not reach the mucosal surface can be noted. A plexus of autonomic nerves exerts control over cellular and glandular secretion. Lymphocytes can be extruded to the surface. Plasma cells which produce secretory immunoglobulin A (S-IgA) and mast cells which release histamine are found in the submucosa. (Ref. 65, with permission.)

Table 3.1. *Host defence mechanisms to airway challenge*

Host defences	Defect	Potential infection problem
Surveillance mechanisms		
Ciliated and squamous epithelium in naso-oropharynx	Poor nutrition	Colonisation with pathogenic gram-negative bacteria
Conducting airways		
Mechanical barriers (larynx) and airway angulation	Bypassing barriers with an endotracheal tube or tracheostomy	Aspiration, direct entry of microorganisms into airway
Mucociliary clearance	Structural defects in cilia	Stagnant secretions, bronchiectasis
Cough	Depressed cough reflex	Poor removal of secretions
Bronchoconstriction	Hyperactive airways, intrinsic asthma	*Aspergillus*, use of corticosteroids
Local immunoglobulin coating-secretory IgA	(a) IgA deficiency	Sinopulmonary infections
	(b) Functional deficiency from breakdown by bacterial IgA, proteases	Abnormal colonisation with certain bacteria (bronchitis)
Alveolar milieu		
Other immunoglobulin classes (opsonic IgG)	Acquired hypogammaglobulinemia, IgC_4, IgG_2 deficiency	Pneumonia with encapsulated bacteria
Iron-containing proteins (transferrin, lactoferrin)	Iron deficiency	May not inhibit certain bacteria (*Pseudomonas, Escherichia coli*)
Alternate complement pathway activation	C_3 and C_5 deficiency	Trouble with infection but not life threatening
Surfactant	Decreased synthesis, acute lung injury	Loss of opsonisation activity Alveolar collapse (atelectasis)
Alveolar macrophages	Subtle effects from immunosuppression, cannot kill intracellular microbes	Propensity for *Pneumocystis carinii* and *Legionella sp.* infections; poor inactivation of *Mycobacterium*
Polymorphonuclear granulocytes	Absent because of immunosuppression; intrinsic defect in motility or lack of chemotactic stimulus	Poor inflammatory response, propensity for gram-negative bacillary infection and fungus (*Aspergillus*)
Augmenting mechanisms		
Initiation of immune responses (humoral antibody and cellular)	Not described except as part of deficiency syndrome	Inadequate S-IgA or IgG antibody (?viral or mycoplasma infection and with encapsulated bacteria)
Generation of an inflammatory response (influx of polymorphonuclear granulocytes, eosinophils, lymphocytes and fluid components)	Generally reflects status and supply of PMNs	Same as for PMNs C_5 deficiency might decrease inflammatory response

From Ref. 64.

microbial antigens and debris. While it is apparent that there is adequate secretory function, opposing this is absorption of the fluid from the airways[4] such that an equilibrium is established balancing secretion and absorption such that the net change in volume is minimised. Brush cells are located at all airway levels[5] and through numerous microvilli which are submerged in the mucous blanket absorption may occur.

The physical barriers to infection

Anatomic factors

Inspired air usually enters the nose in its course down the respiratory tree; the nose presents one of the first barriers to infection. The nasal hairs act to filter larger particles, particularly those greater than ten millimicrons which become impacted on them because of airflow.

Due to the construction of the nasal passages, there is turbulent flow as air passes the septum and nasal turbinates whereby particulate matter becomes deposited on the mucosal surface. Particles of similar size to those filtered by the nasal hairs are subsequently washed out of the nose by an increase in secretions (rhinorrhea) or expelled by sneezing. Particulate matter may move further down the pharynx and be swallowed or expectorated as phlegm. Air passing over the turbinates, and mucosa acquires the correct humidity such that the lower airways do not become desiccated. As the nasal airflow makes a gentle 90 degree turn downward, particles impact on the posterior pharynx due to inertial forces and are subsequently removed. With mouth breathing, particularly during times of exertion, this inertial impaction in the posterior pharynx is the primary means of air filtration as the nasal barriers are bypassed. Likewise, the efficient humification process that occurs over the turbinates is also bypassed and air may have to travel well into the trachea before it attains proper humidification and warmth appropriate for the alveolar surface[6]. In the posterior pharynx where the bulk of particulate matter is deposited is a collection of lymphoid tissue comprising the tonsils and adenoids (Waldeyer's ring) and this allows easy access of lymphocytes and phagocytic cells to antigenic materials.

As the air moves further down passing through the vocal cords and entering the trachea, there is a decrease in the rate of flow and laminar air flow ensues. Particles of less than ten millimicrons are carried with the airstream. Due to the dichotomous branching of the bronchial tree (through about 16 generations), these particles are deposited on the airway mucosa where ciliated cells and the mucociliary escalator clear them from the lungs. Particulate matter of one millimicron in diameter or less can enter the alveoli but due to its small mass and slow sedimentation velocity it may not settle in the terminal airway[7]. In the distal airspaces the airflow is decreased and particles are deposited as a result of diffusion. Here the alveolar macrophages act as the principle scavengers to maintain a clean environment. Fig. 3.2 is a schematic representation of the above process. It can be seen that pollens and dusts which are much larger than 10 μm are removed in the upper airways or may produce symptoms of rhinorrhea, sneezing, hay fever, etc., while aerosolised microbes which are much smaller can gain access to the alveoli and perhaps produce infection.

Reflex mechanisms in the airways

It is an assumption that coughing, sneezing and wheezing (bronchoconstriction) are signs which require treatment; however, their importance in maintaining the integrity of the airways is becoming appreciated[8]. These reflexes are important in protecting the airways against aspirated secretions and particulates as well as removing mucus. The cough reflex is an excellent way for secretions in the larger airways to be expelled and is far superior to therapeutic interventions such as inhaled positive pressure breathing, chest physiotherapy and incentive spirometry in accomplishing this. This reflex occurs with a deep inspiration followed by glottic closure which is mediated by the cricopharyngeal muscles. Subsequently, there is elevation of the intrapleural pressure by contraction of the diaphragm, chest wall and abdominal muscles. The glottis is suddenly opened and the pressure which has been generated in the trachea and bronchi is quickly expelled resulting in peak flow rates greater than 12 l/s. This force propels mucus upward and out of the respiratory tract. The reflex works exceedingly well in the normal person and

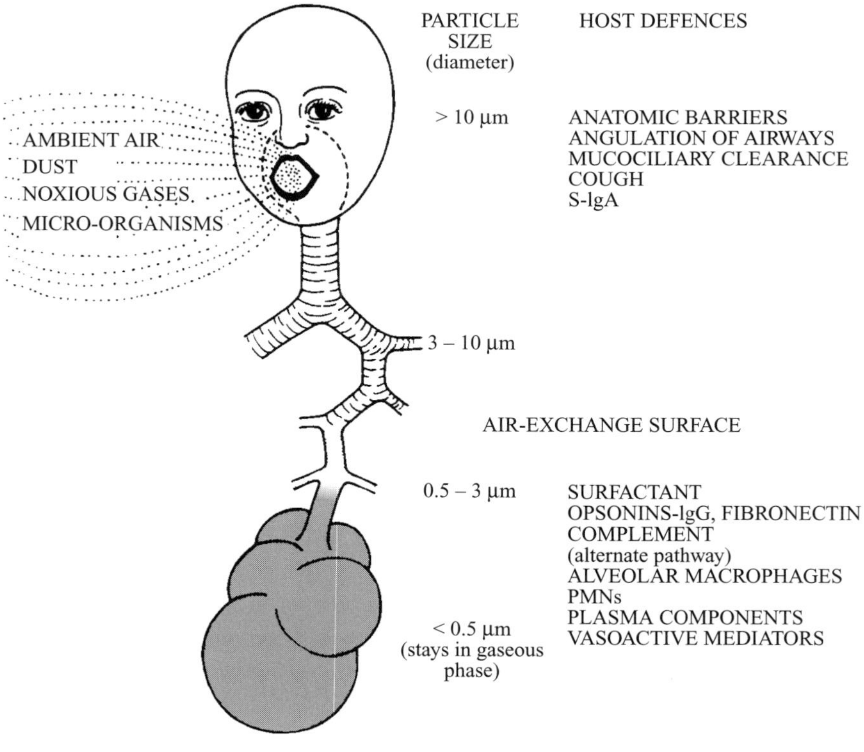

FIGURE 3.2 Host defences: naso-oral pharynx, conducting airways and alveoli. Air is inhaled through the mouth or nose and travels to the alveoli where gas exchange occurs. Large particulate matter is filtered in the naso-oral pharynx and conducting airways while smaller particles and microbes may reach the alveolar space. Host defences in the upper airways are predominantly mechanical barriers and mucociliary clearance. In the distal airspace, phagocytic cells and soluble factors (opsonins) maintain the integrity of the system. (From Ref. 63, with permission.)

aspirated objects and mucus are removed with relative ease, but with disease states such as bronchitis, bronchiectasis and cystic fibrosis, coughing may be less effective. Suppression of cough by medications or central nervous system insult has a similar effect. In patients with Kartagener's syndrome, coughing acts as the primary means for clearance of secretions as the cilia are dysfunctional. The sneeze is similar to the cough and clears materials from the upper respiratory tract.

Bronchoconstriction is a way of limiting the permeation of substances from the airways into the lungs. Irritant receptors which are located in the nose, pharynx, larynx and airways send input to the medulla of the brain where it is integrated and relayed via efferents in the vagus nerve[9] to produce constriction of smooth muscle surrounding the airway lumen and reduction in bronchial diameter.

Colonisation of the airways

The naso-oropharynx is replete with microorganisms, both aerobic and anaerobic, which comprise the normal flora[10]; these exist in apparent symbiosis with the normal host. There are no obvious deleterious effects from this relationship, but the exact role of this union is unknown. Microorganisms commonly found in nasal and throat cultures from normal individuals can include *Neisseria* spp., *Staphylococcus* spp., *Streptococcus* spp. and *Moraxella catarrhalis*. Patients with chronic obstructive pulmonary disease (COPD) have an increased incidence of colonisation with *Streptococcus pneumoniae*, *Haemophilus* spp. and fungi. Anaerobic bacteria are plentiful in the mouth, particularly around the teeth and gums and are readily cultured from oral secretions in great quantity. Aerobic Gram-negative organisms are found relatively infrequently in the naso-oropharynx with only 15% of normals showing organisms such as *Escherichia coli* or *Pseudomonas* spp. in culture[11]. Viruses are rarely cultured and their presence may imply that an infection exists. Traditionally, the bronchi and lower airways have been considered to be sterile[12,13]; however, more recent data lead one to suspect that normals may have a low level of colonisation in these 'sterile' regions[14]. With diseases such as cystic fibrosis or bronchiectasis where there are large amounts of retained mucus or airway abnormalities, there can be areas of localised microbial infection.

Microbes are very efficient in gaining a foothold once introduced to the mucosa of the respiratory tree (Fig. 3.3). Viruses tend to invade the cell directly and integrate themselves into the host cell genome such that they direct the cellular replication; however, the cell is usually destroyed as a result of this process. The ciliated and microvillous cells in the respiratory epithelium serve as major points of attack by the microbes. *Mycoplasma pneumoniae* can shear off cilia by binding to receptors and *Bordetella pertussis* has a similar action, but attaches to the proximal rather than to the distal cilium. Microvillous cells which can be found interspersed between ciliated cells are the point of attachment for organisms such as *Neisseria*. The proper milieu must exist for attachment of bacteria to ciliated structures and this may include metabolic changes in the mucosal cells which are found in the debilitated host[15]. Bacterial proteases can play a role in allowing attachment to the mucosa. *S. pneumoniae* elaborates a protease which degrades secretory immunoglobulin A (S-IgA) and may thereby neutralise this defence mechanism. Similar proteolytic enzymes are produced by *H. influenzae*, *Neisseria meningitidis*, *Pseudomonas aeruginosa* and other Gram-negative bacteria. In addition ciliastatic factors which are paralytic to cilia can be produced by organisms such as *Pseudomonas aeruginosa*[16]. Structures on bacteria such as pili on *Neisseria* sp. can aid in the adhesion of organisms. From this it is easy to recognise that the interaction between microorganisms and respiratory defences is a dynamic process[17] with microbes using various means to overcome barriers the host has imposed against them.

Ciliary defects

Microbes can produce toxic or lytic effects on the cilia which can be a way of entering the cell and permeating the respiratory epithelial barrier. Cilia are essential for the clearance of mucus and secretions from the airways as witnessed in many respiratory infections when the ciliary apparatus is disrupted and secretions must be removed by vigorous coughing. Bronchiectasis and bronchitis represent two forms of disease where there is chronic inflammation of the airways and altered ciliary function occurs. The end result is ineffective clearance of mucus and secretions and creation of an ideal culture medium for bacteria. Ultrastructural defects of the cilia can alter their motility and have dramatic effects on the host defence system. Individuals with such abnormalities have a proclivity for developing respiratory tract infections.

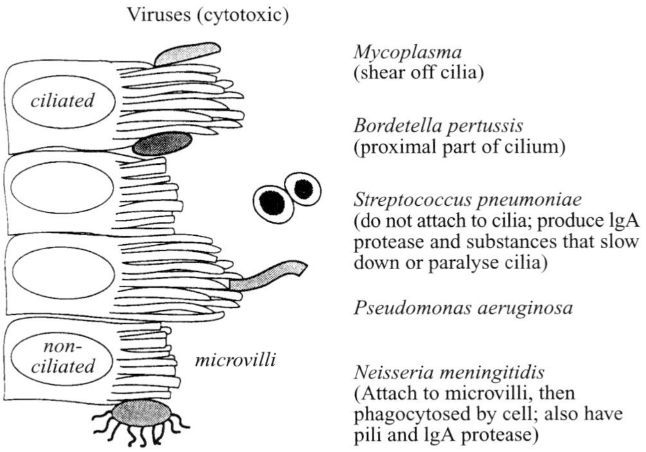

FIGURE 3.3 Schematic showing respiratory epithelium and interaction with microbes. Cells with microvilli or cilia are primarily affected. *Mycoplasma pneumoniae* attaches to receptors on the cilia and shears them from the cell. *Bordetella pertussis* acts in a similar fashion but attaches to a more proximal portion of the cilium. *Streptococus pneumoniae* does not attach to the cilia, but produces substances that slow or stop ciliary beating. *Pseudomonas aeruginosa* can attach to cilia but appears to require metabolic derangements in a chronically ill host. *Neisseria meningitidis* attaches directly to microvilli. Numerous microorganisms are capable of producing IgA proteases which degrade secretory IgA which has been produced. Viruses tend to directly invade cells. (From Ref. 66, with permission.)

Cilia on epithelial cells in the respiratory tract are similar to flagella found on bacteria and the tail structure of the sperm. Absence of dynein arms results in unco-ordinated ciliary movement and has been found to be the cause of Kartagener's syndrome[18,19]. A second defect which results in repeated respiratory tract infections but is not associated with situs inversus is the absence of the radial spoke structures[20]. Subsequently, deletion of the central microtubules with transposition of one of the pairs of peripheral microtubules to the center of the structure has been described[21]. These defects were first proposed as 'immotile cilia syndromes'; however, it has been recognised that these defects produce dyskinesis rather than immotility and result in defective mucociliary transport.

Attack by various pathogens or the presence of congenital abnormalities are not the only factors which cause decreased ciliary function. It has long been known that tobacco smoke impairs the function of cilia[22]. Hypoxia, hypercapnia and acidosis have all been shown to decrease ciliary motion as have metabolic derangements such as hypocalcaemia and hypokalaemia. The influence of drugs on ciliary function should not be overlooked[23]. Digitalis, acetylcholine and catecholamines are stimulatory whereas atropine slows movement. Thus, it appears that there are many endogenous and exogenous influences that affect ciliary motility which in the proper circumstances may lead to disease states.

Secretory products of the airway mucosa

Immunoglobulins

Secretions from the naso-oropharynx and conducting airways contain a variety of products from the parotid and salivary glands, the nasal mucosa, the lacrimal glands, goblet cell and bronchial gland secretions. Among the protein content, up to 10% can be due to immunoglobulins[24]. The predominant form of immunoglobulin varies in different portions of the respiratory tract (Fig. 3.4). Although concentrations of immunoglobulin are measured in the mucosal secretions, they are synthesised by plasma cells which reside in the submucosa. Immunoglobulin A (IgA) is found in largest proportion in the conducting airways; only small amounts of immunoglobulin G (IgG) and scant amounts of immunoglobulin E (IgE) are measured in the normal host[25]. The relative concentrations of IgA and IgG persist as one moves from the upper airway to the trachea and bronchi; it is only in the smaller bronchi and alveolar space that the concentration of IgG exceeds that of IgA[26]. Thus IgG may play a more predominant role in the defence of this portion of the respiratory system.

Most secretory IgA (S-IgA) is in a dimeric form and has a secretory component and J chain attached which are two non-immunoglobulin polypeptide chains[27]. The secretory component and J chain are produced by cells of the epithelium whereas the lymphoid cells of the submucosa synthesise the IgA monomers. S-IgA can only be extruded into the airway secretions after these components have been complexed together. The heavy chain structure defines two subclasses of IgA–IgA_1 and IgA_2 which possess the $alpha_1$ and $alpha_2$ chains respectively[28]. Delaroix *et al.* have reported that bronchial secretions contain approximately twice the amount of IgA_1 as compared to IgA_2[29]; however, the concentration of IgA_2 in these secretions is significantly higher than that in serum.

Since IgA predominates in the upper airway secretions it would appear that its role is important in the initial host defences; however, its exact function remains to be elucidated. As it is difficult to define the specific functions of IgA, Reynolds and Merrill reviewed several concepts about S-IgA in the respiratory tract[30] and summarised:

(i) The concentration of S-IgA is quite high in the naso-oropharynx and upper airways but decreases in the distal portions of the lung reflecting its importance in providing a barrier against microbial adherence and absorption through the epithelial surface. As S-IgA has poor opsonin activity and questionable complement activation, it may have a much lesser role in protecting the distal airways and alveoli.

(ii) S-IgA may contain antibody activity against allergens, bacteria and viruses for humoral immunity can be established after respiratory immunisation, natural infection or exposure. Once immunity is established, it confers some protection against challenge with homologous microbes. Thus, the antibody activity of S-IgA in the naso-oropharynx appears to be one of its most convincing protective roles.

(iii) As the period of immunity is relatively short, a booster or amnestic response from later challenge is needed but this response can be variable at best.

(iv) Although S-IgA does have some innate resistance to proteolytic degradation which may be related to its secretory component, some microbes produce IgA proteases which are capable of rendering S-IgA ineffective and may partially explain the colonisation of airways in patients with diseases such as chronic bronchitis. Thus it appears that S-IgA does have an important role in host defence in the upper respiratory tract.

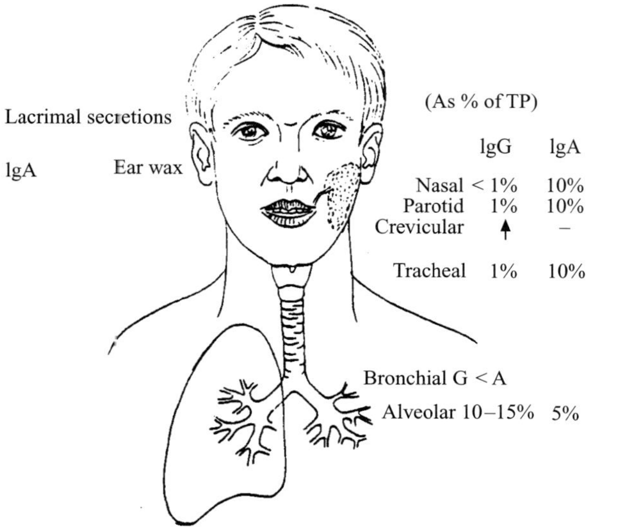

FIGURE 3.4 The predominant immunoglobulin type varies in airway fluids. IgA exceeds IgG in upper airways secretions while in the alveolar fluid the relationship is reversed. The relative proportions of IgA and IgG are given as a percentage of the total fluid protein (TP). (From Ref. 64, with permission.)

Immunoglobulin G is much smaller than S-IgA and does not require a secretory component for transport. IgG is found in lower quantity than IgA down to the level of the terminal airways and alveoli where it occurs in higher amounts. IgG will be considered in a later section.

Complement

The complement system consists of inactive proteins. When stimulated by antibody (classic pathway) or by substances such as endotoxin (alternate pathway), the cascade is activated. When activated, this system efficiently causes lysis of micro-organisms, release of lysosomal enzymes, chemotaxis and opsonisation in addition to regulating immune reactions. Complement has been isolated from airway secretions and may play an important role in resistance to respiratory infection. Mice which have had complement levels depleted show decreased clearance of tracheal inoculates of *S. pneumoniae*[31].

Iron binding proteins

Iron is an essential ingredient for life of some micro-organisms and to survive within a host's cells they must have a readily available source of this element[32]. In plasma, transferrin binds up iron which is being transported and in mucosal secretions lactoferrin performs a similar function. Siderophores are chelating mechanisms which bacteria have developed to compete for iron. From bronchoalveolar lavage data, it appears that lactoferrin, produced by epithelial cells and polymorphonuclear cells, predominates in the airways and that transferrin is found in the alveoli possibly secreted by lymphocytes or macrophages[33]. The net effect of these iron transport proteins is to complex free iron in mucosal or alveolar secretions, sequester it from bacteria and suppress their growth. In addition, Arnold, Brewer and Gauthier have shown iron binding proteins possess bacteriocidal activity against *Streptococcus mutans, S. pneumoniae* and *E. coli*[34]. More recently *Legionella pneumophila* has been added to this list[35]. Iron binding proteins appear to play a role in the non-immune host defences of the respiratory system.

Lysozyme

Lysozyme is released by granulocytes and has been found in sizeable quantity in mucosal secretions. It is itself bacteriocidal, but in the presence of complement it may be bacteriolytic[36]. This activity with regard to common respiratory pathogens remains somewhat controversial.

Cellular defence mechanisms in the airways

Within the conducting airways numerous opportunities exist for host defences to combat antigens and microbiological agents which have not been eliminated. There is a misconception that the lung is not a significant lympho-reticuloendothelial organ. However, the respiratory tract with its lymph nodes and lymphatic system is part of this network. Within the mediastinum, lymph nodes surround the trachea and carina and the hila of the lungs. In the upper respiratory tract is Waldeyer's ring. Diffusely distributed throughout the airways is bronchus-associated lymphoid tissue. Our focus will be on the bronchus associated lymphoid tissue (BALT) and the phagocytic cells found in the airways.

Bronchus associated lymphoid tissue

We have already mentioned that in portions of the airway where deposition of particulate matter occurs, lymphoid tissue can be found. The close relationship of the tonsils and adenoids to the posterior pharynx is an excellent example. BALT is small aggregates of submucosal lymphoid tissue clustered at points of airway bifurcation. Its location suggests that it plays a role in immunity by intercepting antigens when they impact on the airways, although its function in humans is not fully appreciated[37]. BALT is very species dependent and may not be present in normal humans. BALT consists of a few follicles of cells covered by an epithelium of flattened irregularly shaped cells with an absence of cilia or secretory structures above the follicle, while below the BALT in the basement membrane lymphoid cells infiltrate through the collagen fibres and muscle. The possibility that these structures participate in immune reactions is supported by the work of Racz *et al.* where BALT in immunised rabbits was shown to trap antigen[38].

The BALT follicles consist of clusters of lymphocytes, reticulum cells and macrophages with the lymphocytes being the predominate cell type. The lymphocytes are of small and medium size and are not arranged with any structural orientation which may resemble a lymph node. B cells have been shown to predominate over T cells with ratios of approximately 4:1, respectively, and this is nearly a complete reversal of the lymphocyte ratios found in blood or lymph nodes. While surface immunofluorescence staining has shown that IgA and IgM are more prevalent than IgG, cytoplasmic staining has not shown intracellular immunoglobulin; thus, these cells are not considered to be plasma cells. The macrophages are similar to the dendritic and interdigitating types and appear to be involved in antigen presentation to lymphocytes.

Within the distal airways there exist other less-defined collections of lymphoid tissue which are distinct from lymph nodes or parenchymal lymphoid aggregates. These lymphoepithelial cells can be found at the bronchoalveolar junctions situated where they can encounter macrophages migrating between the airways and interstitial tissue and may play a vital role in the immune regulation of the distal lung.

Antigen-presenting cells

When an antigen enters the airways it must be cleared via removal or inactivation or an immune response may possibly be initiated. If the antigenic material is not cleared, it will be initially phagocytosed, processed and subsequently presented to the T-lymphocyte where it is recognised as foreign and an immune response ensues, thus the concept of antigen presenting cells. Within the airways are numerous cells which are capable of initiating this process and include macrophages and dendritic cells. Langerhans cells, endothelial cells, B-lymphocytes and fibroblasts can serve in similar function[39]. Although macrophages may be found on the mucosal surface of the airways their numbers are few and these most probably represent alveolar macrophages which are being removed from the lungs. It is the dendritic cells which are found in relatively high numbers (up to 1% of all epithelial cells) throughout the airways that appear to have a greater role in antigen presentation[40]. It is notable that the cytoplasmic processes of these cells do not extend into the bronchial lumen so that airway antigen must adhere to or penetrate the mucosa for processing to begin. While different from macrophages, dendritic cells remain capable of phagocytosis. Dendritic cells have been found in vascular walls, visceral pleura and alveolar septa and are increased in number by cigarette smoke[41]. In the mouse, these cells function well in antigen presentation to T-cells. A scheme for various immune circuits within the respiratory tract is offered (Fig. 3.5).

The alveolar space

Within the upper respiratory tract and conducting airways anatomic barriers, branching of the tracheobronchial tree, mucociliary clearance and cough provide mechanisms whereby particulate matter is excluded or removed from the airways. As the pseudostratified columnar epithelial thins to give way to the delicate alveolar sacs, host defence mechanisms are dramatically altered. Past the respiratory bronchioles there are no goblet cells or mucus secreting glands; hence there is no mucus production or mucociliary clearance. Cough is extremely ineffective in clearing particles of 0.5 to 3 µm which have evaded removal. Specialised interactions exist within the alveoli for coping with antigenic material, microbes or particulates (Fig. 3.6). Four distinct mechanisms have been discussed for this process[42].

(i) Particulate matter becomes coated with opsonins from the epithelial lining fluid and this enhances phagocytosis by the alveolar macrophage.
(ii) The alveolar macrophage through physical contact with lymphocytes or with cytokines produced by them can be activated such that its bacteriostatic or bacteriocidal function is enhanced.
(iii) The alveolar macrophage can process antigenic substances and present the antigen to an appropriate lymphocyte that will begin an immune response possibly culminating in antibody production.
(iv) An inflammatory reaction can be initiated through chemotaxis which attracts polymorphonuclear neutrophils into the alveolar space.

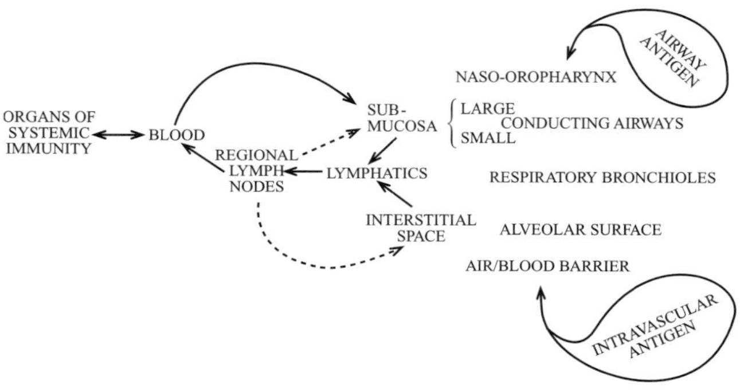

FIGURE 3.5 A representation of immune circuits within the respiratory tract. Antigens arriving in the airways can be deposited on the naso-oral pharynx or conducting airways. Antigens in the pulmonary artery blood can reach the capillaries and breach the air–blood barrier. Airway antigens may stick to bronchus associated lymphoid tissue or the mucosa and be processed by macrophages or dendritic cells. Alveolar macrophages ingest antigens in the alveolar space. Antigens and the 'carrying' cells (macrophages and dendritic cells) are transported to hilar or mediastinal lymph nodes by the lymphatics where, with T-lymphocytes, an immune response is initiated. After reaching these lymph nodes, immune cells or antigens require access to systemic immune circuits to maximise the response and to induce B-lymphocytes or plasma cells to return home or to the orginal site. Local circuits (dashed lines) from regional nodes could lead back to the submucosa and interstitial areas without requiring a systemic loop, but these are uncertain. (From Ref. 30.)

Fig. 3.6 is a schematic representation of this process. The alveolar macrophage is considered to have a prominent role in these interactions.

Cells within the alveolar space

Millions of cells may be retrieved by bronchoalveolar lavage (BAL) of the distal airspaces with a few hundred milliliters of fluid in the normal individual. Reynolds and Newball noted that such lavage

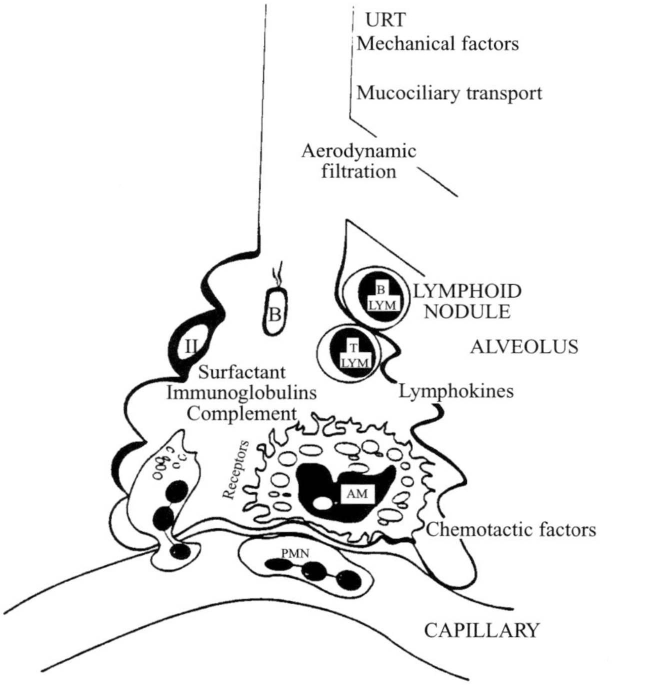

FIGURE 3.6 A representation of host defences in the alveolar space. A bacterium (B) of critical size that escapes removal in the upper respiratory tract (URT) by mechanical factors and mucociliary transport is deposited in the alveolus. Here, it may encounter surfactant which is produced by the Type II alveolar cells and/or immunoglobulins produced by B-lymphocytes (B LYM) or plasma cells. The alveolar macrophage (AM) may phagocytose the mmicrobe when it has been conditioned by complement components. Opsonic antibody can also facilitate attachment of the bacterium to the AM through specialised surface receptors. Alternative mechanisms to enhance clearance and killing of the microbes exist. The AM can produce chemotactic factors that will attract polymorphonuclear neutrophils (PMN) which have marginated in the lung capillary adjacent to the alvolus and initiate an immune response or the bacterium may trigger T-lymphocytes (T LYM) to release lymphokines which may activate AM phagocytic or bacteriocidal activity. (From Ref. 24.)

fluid contains many alveolar macrophages (85%), about 10% lymphocytes, 5% red blood cells, 1–3% PMNs and only scant numbers of ciliated epithelial cells, eosinophils and mast cells[26].

Alveolar macrophages

It appears that the alveolar macrophages (AM) develop from monocyte precursor cells and within the interstitium of the lung undergo further maturation and differentiation before they are mature. In fact, in the normal host only a small proportion of the AM are found within the alveoli as has been reported by the BAL Co-operative Group[43]. AM have also been recovered in small numbers from the conducting airways during bronchial lavage[44,45] and may represent those being transported out of the body via mucociliary clearance, although some of these may be participating in the defence of the distal airways. AM demonstrate remarkable phagocytic activity and are responsible for ingesting not only particulate material but also microbes and host cells which have evaded defence mechanisms and made their way down to the alveoli, and must be cleared[46]. Although quite avid as phagocytes, it appears that ingested materials are degraded and destroyed in a slower process than occurs with phagocytic cells in the bloodstream. Also these are not the only phagocytic cells present in the alveoli as neutrophils can be recruited if they should be necessary and lymphocytes can be if a cell-mediated response is needed. The AM are able to perform their tasks by virtue of numerous bio-active products including cytokines, enzymes, bio-active lipids, proteins and various others[47].

Lymphocytes

Of the lymphocytes present in the alveolar space, T-lymphocytes represent the largest number constituting about 70%. The majority of the T-cells are of the T-helper (T_H) subtype (CD_4) and about 30% represent T-suppressor cells (T_S or CD_8)[48]. A T_H/T_S ratio of 1:5 is found which is comparable to that in peripheral blood. T-cells produce many lymphokines including interleukin 2 and are of the HLA-DR antigen type[49]. Plasma cells and B cells make up the remainder of the lymphocytes found within the alveolar space. Fig. 3.7 depicts some of the interactions possible between macrophages and lymphocytes.

Cellular interactions in the alveolar space

Numerous interactions between alveolar macrophages and other cells in the alveolar space can occur with secretory cell products being used as mediators (cytokines). Under influence of Vitamin D and other unrecognised factors, cells of the monocyte line differentiate into AM. These phagocytes have the important pulmonary function to keep the alveolar space free of debris, antigenic material, and microbes. If 'activated', the AM can produce and secrete many cellular products and enzymes (cytokines) which can affect other cells. Chemotactic factors can serve to attract PMNs when they are needed, similarly, interleukin-1 can recruit T-lymphocytes. Activated T-cells produce various lymphokines which also modulate the function of other cells. Interleukin-2 in addition to stimulating the proliferation of other T-cells can activate killer T-cells and stimulate B-cells which can lead to production of antibody. T-cells through interferon and migratory inhibition factor can act to activate AM and thus regulate their function. T-suppressor cells may down-regulate AM function.

Non-cellular components in the alveolar space

Opsonins

BAL fluid contains some acellular constituents which are capable of acting as nonimmune opsonins. Surfactant has been shown to coat strains of staphylococci and *E. coli*[50,51]. *In vitro* bacterial uptake by macrophages has been stimulated by large fragments of fibronectin[52]. It can be inferred that, since alveolar macrophages have been shown themselves to secrete fibronectin and it is recovered from the epithelial lining fluid, it should have some role as a pulmonary opsonin. Although not a component of BAL fluid, the acute phase proteins such as C-reactive protein may have a similar role[53].

Immunoglobulins

Antibodies directed against a specific antigen represent the principal immune opsonins. Fig. 3.4 has shown a quantitative representation of the major immunoglobulins in the respiratory tract. IgA probably

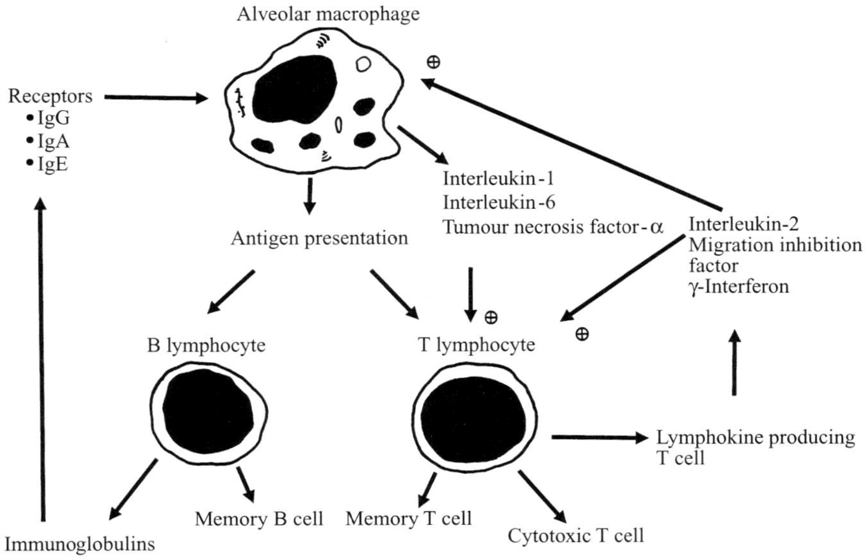

FIGURE 3.7 Interactions between the alveolar macrophage and lymphocytes. Numerous potential cellular interactions exist between the alveolar macrophage (AM) and B- or T-lymphocytes. The AM can present antigen to the lymphocytes resulting in immunoglobulin production in B-cell lines or further differentiation in T-cell lines. Cytokines can be produced by the AM which will stimulate T-cells (ex. Interleukin 1, Interleukin 6, Tumour Necrosis Factor α). Lymphokines produced by T-cells (ex. Interleukin 2, Migration Inhibition Factor, γ-Interferon) can have positive feedback on the AM.

does not have potent opsonic activity. Immunoglobulin M (IgM) is found in only trace amounts in the epithelial lining fluid (ELF).

The antibody which is principally responsible for immune mediated opsonisation is IgG. It is found in sizeable quantity in the ELF and represents about 5% of the protein content. Its proportion of the four heavy chain classes closely approximates those in serum. In the non-smoker, IgG1 and IgG2 predominate (65% and 28%, respectively) with the remainder being IgG3 (1.8%) and IgG4 (5.2%)[54]; these values are roughly those found as serum concentrations. Cigarettes smokers tend to have less IgG2 (decreased from 28% to 13%). IgG1 and IgG3 have the ability to fix complement and thus are regarded as the most important of the four subclasses. IgG2 has been shown to contain type specific antibodies against polysaccharide antigens such as those found on *S. pneumoniae* and *H. influenzae*[55]. It is also the subclass responsible for anti-teichoic acid antibody against *S. aureus* and antibody against lipopolysaccharide of *P. aeruginosa*[56]. IgG4 although present in low concentrations in ELF can act as a reaginic antibody. It may be increased in hypersensitivity pneumonitis[57]. An absence of IgG4 can lead to bronchiectasis or recurrent respiratory tract infection[58].

The development to polysaccharide vaccines against such agents as *S. pneumoniae, H. influenzae*, and *N. meningitidis* which are administered by parenteral route demonstrate that humoral immunity confers protection in respiratory tract because systemic antibody diffuses into an infected, inflamed alveolar space.

Complement

Complement components are found in the ELF. In the human, properdin factor B is present[59] and C4 and C6 are present in lower proportions than in the serum. Clq has not been identified[26]. Although it is not perfectly clear whether this system is operational in the alveoli, activation of the cascade sequence could result in lysis and destruction of microbial agents. The C3b component can act as an opsonin and promote phagocytosis by macrophages and PMNs or it can generate C5a which can serve as a PMN chemoattractant. By experimental removal of the complement system, a predisposition to infection with encapsulated organisms has been found[31].

Integrated defences in the alveolar space

Once a microbe has successfully evaded defence mechanisms and gained entrance into the alveolar space, it will be bathed in the epithelial lining fluid which covers the alveolus as it expands and contracts with breathing. Opsonins may coat the microbe and render it more readily ingested by a phagocyte. When coated with immunoglobulin, especially IgG, even encapsulated bacteria are phagocytosed in a more efficient process as is seen with *S. pneumoniae, H. influenzae* and *Klebsiella pneumoniae*[60]. Activation of complement may play a role in destroying infective agents in the alveoli. The flagship of the host defences is the alveolar macrophage which acts as the primary phagocyte in the alveoli. Once inside the AM, the organism may be destroyed directly or if the microbe is too potent to be killed, the macrophage can become activated and complete this process by interaction with various cells including the T-lymphocyte[61]. Antigen which is presented to the T-cell causes its stimulation which brings into action the immune function of this group of cells which can involve the production of cytokines and monokines or the production of antibodies. Various other cell lines including the polymorphonuclear neutrophil which produces an inflammatory response can be recruited to aid in the defence process[62].

Certain microbes have the potential to be difficult to handle for tissue macrophages and thus AM also. These include: *Mycobacterium tuberculosis, Listeria monocytogenes, Toxoplasma gondii, L. pneumophila*, cytomegalovirus, herpes simplex virus, human immunodeficiency virus (HIV-1) and others[63]. Control of the intracellular replication of such microbes is attained by macrophage activation or antigen presentation such that cellular immunity is acquired. Thus, within the alveolar space, various defences exist to attack and destroy invading organisms with additional mechanisms which can be brought into action should there be a failure or inadequacy of the system.

References

1. RUTLAND W, GRIFFIN M, COLE PJ. Human ciliary beat frequency in epithelium from thoracic and extrathoracic airways. *Am Rev Resp Dis* 1982;125:100–5.
2. MARADA JL. Loosening tight junctions – lessons from the intestine. *J Clin Invest* 1989;83:1089–94.
3. GAIL DB, LENFANT CJM. Cells of the lung: biology and clinical implications. *Am Rev Resp Dis* 1983;127:366-87.
4. KILBURN KH. A hypothesis for pulmonary clearance and its implications. *Am Rev Resp Dis* 1968;98:449–63.
5. REID L, JONES R. Bronchial mucosal cells. *Fed Proc* 1979;38:191–6.
6. MCFADDEN ER JR, DENISON DM, WALLER JF *et al.* Direct recording of the temperatures in the tracheobronchial tree in normal man. *J Clin Invest* 1982;69:700-5.
7. MARTIN TR. Defense mechanisms and immune reactions in the respiratory system. In Peirson DJ & Kacmarek RM, eds *Foundations of Respiratory Care*, New York: Churchill Livingstone; 147–62.
8. FULLER RW, JACKSON DM. The physiology and treatment of cough. *Thorax* 1990;45:425–30.
9. BARNES PJ. Neural control of the human airways in health and disease. *Am Rev Resp Dis* 1986;134:1289–314.
10. MACKOWIAK PA. The normal microbial flora. *N Engl J Med* 1982;307:83–93.
11. ROSENTHAL S, TAGER I. Prevalence of gram negative rods in the normal pharyngeal flora. *Ann Intern Med* 1975;83:355–7.
12. LAURENZI GA, POTTER RT, KASS EH. Bacterial flora of the lower respiratory tract. *N Engl J Med* 1961;265:1273–8.
13. POTTER RT, POTMAN F, FERNANDEZ J *et al.* The bacteriology of the lower respiratory tract: bronchoscopic study of 100 clinical cases. *Am Rev Resp Dis* 1968;97:1051.
14. HALPERIN SA, SURATT PM, GWALTNEY JM, GROSCHEL DHM, HENDLEY JO, EGGLESTON PA. Bacterial cultures from the lower respiratory tract in normal volunteers with and without experimental rhinovirus infection using a plugged double lumen catheter system. *Am Rev Resp Dis* 1982;125:678–80.
15. NEIDERMAN MS, MERILL WW, FERRANTI RD, PAGANO KM, PALMER LB,

REYNOLDS HY. Nutritional status and bacterial binding in the lower respiratory tract in patients with chronic tracheostomy. *Ann Intern Med* 1984;100:795–800.

16. WILSON R, MUNRO N, HASTIE A *et al.* *Pseudomonas aeruginosa* produces low molecular weight molecules which damage human respiratory epithelium *in vitro* and slow mucociliary transport on the guinea pig trachea *in vivo. Chest* 1989;95:S214.
17. REYNOLDS HY. Bacterial adherence to respiratory tract mucosa – a dynamic interaction leading to colonization. *Sem Resp Med* 1987;2:8–19.
18. ELIASSON R, MOSSBERG B, CAMNER P, AFZELIUS BA. The immotile cilia syndrome: A congenital ciliary abnormality as an etiologic factor in chronic airway infections and male sterility. *N Engl J Med* 1977;297:1–6.
19. PEDERSON H, MYGIND N. Absence of azonemal arms in nasal mucosa cilia in Kartagener's syndrome. *Nature* 1976;262:494–5.
20. STURGESS J, CHAO J, WONG J, ASPIN N, TURNER JAP. Cilia with defective radial spokes. *N Engl J Med* 1979;300:53–6.
21. STURGESS J, CHAO J, TURNER JAP. Transposition of ciliary microtubules – another cause of impaired ciliary motility. *N Engl J Med* 1980;303:318–22.
22. DALHAMN T. The effect of cigarette smoke on ciliary activity in the upper respiratory tract. *Arch Otolaryngol* 1959;70:166–8.
23. KENSLER CJ, BATTISTA SP. Chemical and physical factors affecting mammalian ciliary activities. *Am Rev Resp Dis* 1966;93 (No.3, Part 2):93–102.
24. REYNOLDS HY. Respiratory infections may reflect deficiencies in host defence mechanisms. *Disease-a-Month* 1985;31:1–98.
25. MERRILL WW, HYUN H, STROBER W, RANKIN J, FICK BB, REYNOLDS HY. Correlations between respiratory tract proteins from upper (nasal) and lower (bronchial lavage) sites. *Am Rev Resp Dis* 1982;125:268A.
26. REYNOLDS HY, NEWBALL HH. Analysis of proteins and respiratory cells obtained from human lungs by bronchial lavage. *J Laborat Clin Med* 1974;84:559–73.
27. THOMPSON RE, REYNOLDS HY, WAXDAL MJ. Structural composition of canine secretory component and immunoglobulin A. *Biochemistry* 1975;142:2853–60.
28. MESTECKY J, MCGHEE JR. Immunoglobulin A: molecular and cellular interactions involved in IgA biosynthesis and immune response. *Adv Immunol* 1987;40:153–245.
29. DELAROIX DL, DIVE C, RAMBAUD JA, VAERMAN JP. IgA subclass in various secretions and serum. *Immunology* 1982;47:383–5.
30. REYNOLDS HY, MERRILL WW. Lung immunology: humoral and cellular immune responsiveness of the respiratory tract. *Curr Pulmonol* 1981;3:381–422.
31. GROSS GN, REHN SR, PIERCE AK. The effect of complement depletion on lung clearance of bacteria. *J Clin Invest* 1978;62:373–8.
32. FINKELSTEIN RA, SCIORTINO CV, MCINTOSH MA. Role of iron in microbe–host interactions. *Rev Infect Dis* 1983;5:S759–S77.
33. REYNOLDS HY, CHRETIEN J. Respiratory tract fluids: analysis of content and contemporary use in understanding lung diseases. *Disease-a-Month*, 1984;30:1–103.
34. ARNOLD RR, BREWER M, GAUTHIER JJ. Bactericidal activity of human lactoferrin: sensitivity of a variety of microorganisms. *Infect Immunol* 1980;28:893–8.
35. BORTNER CA, MILLER RD, ARNOLD RR. Bactericidal effect of lactoferrin on *Legionella pneumophila*. *Infect Immunol* 1986;51:373–7.
36. KLEBANOFF SJ. Antimicrobial mechanisms in neutrophilic polymorphonuclear leukocytes. *Sem Hematol* 1975;112:117–42.
37. BIENENSTOCK J, BEFUS D. Gut and bronchus associated lymphoid tissue. *Am J Anat* 1984;170:437–45.
38. RACZ P, TENNER-RACZ K, MYRVIK QN, FAINTER LK. Functional architecture of bronchus associated lymphoid tissue and lymphoepithelium in pulmonary cell-mediated reactions in the rabbit. *J Reticuloendo Soc* 1977;22:59–83.
39. SERTL K, TAKEMURA T, TSCHACHLER E, FERRANS VJ, KALIMER MA, SHEVACH EM. Dendritic cells with antigen-presenting capability reside in airway epithelium, lung parenchyma and visceral pleura. *J Exp Med* 1986;163:436–51.
40. HOLT PG, SCHON-HEGRAD MA, OLIVER J. MHC class II antigen-bearing dendritic cells in pulmonary tissues of the rat. *J Exp Med* 1988;167:262–74.
41. SOLER P, MOREAU A, BASSET F, HANCE AJ. Cigarette smoking-induced changes in the number and differential state of pulmonary dendritic cells/Langerhans cells. *Am Rev Resp Dis* 1989;139:1112–17.
42. REYNOLDS HY. Immunologic system in the respiratory tract. *Physiol Rev* 1991;71:1117–33.
43. THE BAL COOPERATIVE GROUP STEERING COMMITTEE. Bronchoalveolar lavage constituents in healthy individuals, idiopathic pulmonary fibrosis and selected comparison groups. *Am Rev Resp Dis* 1990;141:S169–S202.
44. FICK RB, RICHARDSON HB, ZAVALA DC, HUNNINGHAKE GW. Bronchoalveolar lavage in allergic asthmatics. *Am Rev Resp Dis* 1987;135:1204–9.
45. RANKIN JA, MARCY T, ROCHESTER, CL, SUSSMAN, J, SMITH, S, BUCKLEY, P, LEE D. Human airway macrophages – a technique for their retrieval and a descriptive comparison with alveolar macrophages. *Am Rev Respir Dis* 1992; 145: 928–33.
46. FELS AOS, COHN ZA. The alveolar macrophage. *J Appl Physiol* 1986;60:353–69.
47. SIBILLE Y, REYNOLDS HY. Macrophages and polymorphonuclear neutrophils in lung defence and injury – State of the art. *Am Rev Resp Dis* 1990;141:471–501.
48. HUNNINGHAKE GW, CRYSTAL RG. Pulmonary sarcoidosis: a disorder mediated by excess helper T lymphocyte activity at sites of disease. *N Engl J Med* 1981;305:429–34.
49. SALTINI C, SPURZEM JR, LEE JJ, PINKSTON P, CRYSTAL RG. Spontaneous release of interleukin-2 by lung T-lymphocytes in active pulmonary sarcoidosis is primarily from the Leu+DR+T cell subset. *J Clin Invest* 1988;77:1962–70.
50. O'NEILL SJ, LESPERANCE E, KLASS DJ. Human lung lavage surfactant enhances staphylococcal phagocytosis by alveolar macrophages. *Am Rev Resp Dis* 1984;130:1177–9.
51. CONROD JD. The role of extracellular bactericidal factors in pulmonary host defences. *Sem Resp Infect* 1986;1:118–29.
52. CZOP JK, MCGOWAN SW, CENTER DM. Opsonin-independent phagocytosis by human alveolar macrophage: augmentation by human plasma fibronectin. *Am Rev Resp Dis* 1982;125:607–9.
53. MOLD C, ROGERS CP, KAPLAN RL, GEWURZ H. Binding of human C-reactive protein to bacteria. *Infect Immunol* 1982;38:392–5.
54. MERRILL WW, NAEGEL GP, OLCHOWSKI JJ, REYNOLDS HY. Immunoglobulin G subclasses: Quantitation and comparison with immunoglobulins A and E. *Am Rev Resp Dis* 1985;131:584–91.
55. SIBER GR, SCHUR PH, AISENBERG AC, WEITMAN SA, SCHIFFMAN G. Correlation between serum IgG_2 concentrations and the antibody response to bacterial polysaccharide antigens. *N Engl J Med* 1980;303:178–82.
56. FICK RB, OLCHOWSKI J, SQUIER SU, MERRILL WW, REYNOLDS HY. Immunoglobulin-G subclasses in cystic fibrosis: IgG_2 response to *Pseudomonas* lipopolysaccharide. *Am Rev Resp Dis* 1986;133:418–20.
57. CALVANICO NJ, AMBEGAONKAR SP, SCHLUETER DP, FINK JN. Immunoglobulin

levels in bronchoalveolar lavage fluid from pigeon breeders lung. *J Laborat Clin Med* 1980;96:129–40.

58. BECK CS, HEINER DC. Selective immunoglobulin G_4 deficiency and recurrent infections of the respiratory tract. *Am Rev Resp Dis* 1981;124:94–6.

59. ROBERTSON J, CALDWELL JR, CASTLE JR, WALDMAN RH. Evidence for the presence of components of the alternate (properdin) pathway of complement activation in respiratory secretions. *J Immunol* 1976;117:900–3.

60. REYNOLDS HY. Immunoglobulin G and its function in the human respiratory tract. *Mayo Clin Proc* 1988;63:161–74.

61. MURRAY HW. Interferon-gamma, the activated macrophage and host defence against microbial challenge. *Ann Intern Med* 1988;108:595–608.

62. REYNOLDS HY. Lung inflammation: normal host defence or a complication of some diseases. *Ann Rev Med* 1987;38:295–323.

63. REYNOLDS HY. Host defence impairments that may lead to respiratory infections. *Clin Chest Med* 1987;8:339–58.

64. REYNOLDS HY. Normal and defective respiratory host defences. In Pennington, JE, ed. *Respiratory Infections: Diagnosis and Management*, 2nd ed. New York: Raven Press; 1989: 1–33.

65. REYNOLDS HY. Pumonary host defences: state of the art. *Chest* 1989;95:S223–30.

66. REYNOLDS HY. Integrated host defence against infection. In Crystal RG, West JB, eds. *The Lung: Scientific Foundation*. New York: Raven Press; Year: 1899–911

4 General principles of antimicrobial therapy

P. VENKATESAN and M.J. WOOD
Bimingham Heartlands Hospital, UK

Introduction

The respiratory tract represents a varied and complex tissue into which antimicrobial agents need to penetrate. The rational selection of antimicrobial agents for the treatment of respiratory tract infections demands an understanding of their spectra of activity, their time-dependent interactions with micro-organisms and their pharmacokinetic properties. In recent years our knowledge of the interaction between antibiotics and pathogens and of the pharmacokinetics of antimicrobials in the respiratory tract has blossomed, with particular interest in the β-lactams, macrolides and quinolones (the antibiotics most frequently used for the treatment of respiratory infections). The emergence of antibiotic resistance in many respiratory pathogens has now reduced the utility of many previously commonly used antibiotics and has challenged the standard choices in the empirical treatment of infections.

Pharmacokinetics in the respiratory tract

The different pathogens that infect the respiratory tract multiply in different tissue compartments. Some, such as *Legionella pneumophila* and *Chlamydia pneumoniae*, are intracellular organisms, whereas others, such as *Streptococcus pneumoniae* and *Haemophilus influenzae* multiply extracellularly. It is also possible to distinguish between infection in the air spaces, such as the lumen of the bronchi, bronchioles and alveoli, and infection in the tissues of the bronchial mucosa and alveolar interstitium. For an antimicrobial to be effective in treating respiratory tract infections, an adequate concentration of the antimicrobial agent must be delivered to the particular tissue compartment (if necessary, into the cells themselves) which is the site of bacterial replication. This usually means that the local concentration of the antimicrobial agent at the site of infection should be higher than the concentration needed to inhibit replication of the pathogenic organism *in vitro* (usually termed the minimum inhibitory concentration or MIC). It may not, however, always be necessary to achieve this ideal since studies have shown that sub-inhibitory concentrations of antibiotics can alter bacterial morphology, enhance phagocytosis or intracellular killing of bacteria or produce other effects that aid host defences against infection[1].

For the treatment of acute exacerbations of chronic bronchitis, the antibiotic needs to achieve therapeutic concentrations within the bronchial mucosa and the lumen of the airways, while in classical lobar pneumonia the antibiotic must reach the alveolar lining fluid and the parenchymal interstitium: for intracellular pathogens, the agent needs to concentrate within the phagocytic cells of the lung.

Antibiotics may reach infected respiratory tissue by one of two routes. In most situations orally or parenterally administered antibiotics are absorbed into, and delivered, via the bloodstream. In a few situations, such as prophylaxis, the treatment of cystic fibrosis, fungal infections, respiratory syncytial virus (RSV) and *Pneumocystis carinii* pneumonia (PCP), the agents can be administered by inhalation and therefore reach the bronchial mucosa and other tissues from the bronchial lumen[2]. With either route, certain factors and barriers determine the eventual distribution of antimicrobial into the infected tissue compartments[3] (Fig. 4.1).

The general pharmacokinetic properties of an antibiotic (its absorption, metabolism and excretion) will determine the total concentration of the agent that is found in the plasma but the degree to which it penetrates into respiratory tissue compartments depends upon a number of other factors. The endothelium lining the capillaries represents the first major barrier to antibiotic penetration. This may be overcome by antibiotics either passing through the membranes of endothelial cells, a process of non-ionic diffusion called permeation, or by passive diffusion through pores between cells in so-called fenestrated capillary beds. Such pores permit the

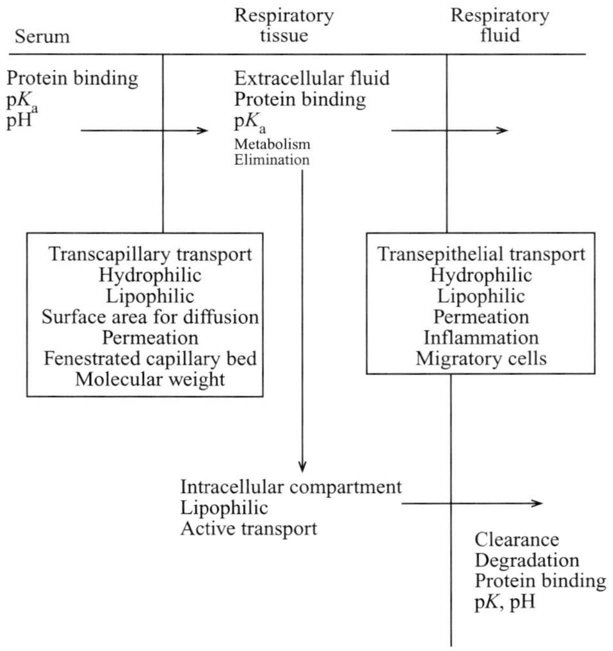

FIGURE 4.1 Factors influencing the penetration of antibiotics into respiratory tissues and fluids.

movement of molecules with a molecular weight of less than 1 kDa and favour hydrophilic molecules that are dissolved in the aqueous phase. Passive diffusion along a concentration gradient is the major mechanism of transfer of low molecular weight antibiotics from blood into tissues. Not all blood-borne antibiotic is available for passive diffusion into tissue. The amount of an antibiotic that is available is dependent on two parameters: its degree of protein binding, with only the unbound portion of an antibiotic able to penetrate into tissues; and the p*K*a. The latter determines the degree to which the antibiotic is ionised at serum pH and is important when the physicochemical nature of the antibiotic determines its ability to cross the capillary wall. Fenestrated capillary beds are not, however, present throughout the entire respiratory tract. They are absent in the pulmonary circulation but present in the bronchial circulation[4,5]. This is a major hindrance to hydrophilic antibiotics. None the less, hydrophilic antibiotics can achieve bactericidal concentrations in respiratory tissues, principally because of the combination of a considerable pulmonary blood flow and a very large surface area across which diffusion can occur.

Un-ionised, lipophilic antibiotics are not dependent on intercellular pores for their penetration. Thus, lipid soluble agents such as trimethoprim, rifampicin, chloramphenicol, macrolides and isoniazid (but not β-lactam antibiotics which are poorly lipid soluble) are capable of readily passing through the lipid-protein cell membranes along the concentration gradient by non-ionic diffusion.

Active transport is an energy dependent mechanism which has been shown to be important for antibiotic penetration into certain tissues. Some pharmacokinetic data do suggest the existence of saturable transport mechanisms for antibiotics within the respiratory tract but these are of unproven relevance. In a study of ceftazidime in ventilated intensive care patients, for instance, increasing the serum concentrations of antibiotic beyond a certain point was not matched by proportional increases in concentrations in the bronchial secretions[6].

Once in tissues, antimicrobials may partition between the extracellular and intracellular compartments. About 20% by weight of most tissues is composed of extracellular fluid (ECF). Entry of antibiotic into cells is mainly dependent on lipid solubility: drugs that are lipid soluble readily penetrate cells and are distributed throughout the ECF and cellular compartments. Such antibiotics have a large 'apparent' volume of distribution. Non-lipophilic drugs such as β-lactams do not penetrate cells and are confined to the ECF, where their concentration parallels that in the serum. The availability of antibiotic for cell penetration is also a function of extracellular protein binding, p*K*a and tissue pH. Active transport mechanisms are also involved in antibiotic uptake by cells: studies have suggested active transportation of macrolides, clindamycin and quinolones into alveolar macrophages[4,5,7]. After intracellular penetration, antibiotics may be eliminated by reabsorption into the venous circulation or by degradation. Certain cells of the blood-bronchoalveolar barrier, termed Clara cells, have a metabolic function, and may be responsible for the local degradation of antibiotic[8].

From the tissues, antibiotics may pass across the respiratory epithelium to the lumen of the respiratory tract. The factors affecting this transfer are similar to those affecting the transit of antibiotics from serum to tissue. The epithelial cells of alveoli and bronchi are bound together by many tight junctions limiting permeability[9]. Although these inter-cellular junctions may be loosened by inflammation, thus aiding the transfer of hydrophilic antibiotics, lipophilic antibiotics are at an advantage in passing through the epithelial cells. An additional mechanism of drug transfer is the carriage of antibiotics within inflammatory cells as they cross the epithelium to reach sites of infection and inflammation within the bronchial and alveolar lumen[10,11].

The alveolar macrophages probably contribute to this transfer and release antibiotic into the alveolar space. The epithelial lining fluid (ELF) bathes the terminal bronchioles and alveoli and contains the alveolar macrophages. Once an antibiotic has reached either the ELF or the bronchial mucus, its ability to deal with pathogens is affected by the rate at which it is cleared, its protein binding and the pH. The acidic pH found in abscesses (and to a lesser extent in ELF and sputum) tends to reduce the activity of certain antibiotics, particularly the aminoglycosides. Clearance occurs as the ELF or mucus is cleared by cilial action and removed from the respiratory tract. Degradation of antibiotic occurs in the presence of local enzymes, particularly bacterially derived ones, and aminoglycosides and polymyxins are bound to and inactivated by purulent material.

An alternative approach to obtain therapeutic concentrations of antibiotics in bronchial secretions and ELF is to administer them via the respiratory tract. This can be achieved either by instilling antibiotics intra-tracheally in ventilated patients or by inhalation of nebulised solutions. For widespread distribution throughout the lung, nebulisers must generate very small particles[12]. Even when this is achieved, the inhalation of antibiotic will be limited by the pulmonary function of the patient[13]. Furthermore, inhaled drugs are not distributed equally throughout the lungs and certain parts of the lung will receive less antibiotic than others, with the apices receiving more than the bases.

In general, the pharmacokinetics of antibiotics in the upper respiratory tract parallels their behaviour in the bronchial tree and lungs. In the pharynx, the appearance of an antibiotic in saliva depends on serum protein binding, serum and saliva pH, and the p*K*a and lipid/water partition of the antibiotic.

Given the complexity of the pharmacokinetics of antibiotics in the respiratory tract, it will be apparent that the serum antibiotic concentration alone is not a reliable indicator of antibiotic efficacy in respiratory tract infections. Therefore experimental animal and human models have been developed to study antibiotic concentrations in various tissue compartments and to correlate these with efficacy against different pathogens. Such models utilise tissue biopsies and sampling of ELF, sputum and (for infections of the upper respiratory tract) saliva or middle ear fluid. Bronchoscopy and bronchoalveolar lavage have made an important contribution in human studies[4,14]. These studies have facilitated the development and testing of antibiotics used in respiratory tract infections.

Antibiotic–bacterial interactions

There are now sufficient scientific data to establish the optimal means of antibiotic administration to maximise the antimicrobial activity and to minimise drug-related toxicity. Bacterial death as a result of antibiotic exposure may be either concentration dependent or concentration independent. Aminoglycosides, for instance, have concentration-dependent antibacterial activity and yet their toxicity is related to high trough concentrations. There are now several studies suggesting that the total daily dose of an aminoglycoside is best given as one single injection. On the other hand, β-lactam agents kill bacteria best when the antibiotic concentration remains constantly approximately four times greater than the MIC of the organism. Hence these antibiotics have time-dependent (but concentration-independent) killing and the goal of therapy is to maintain concentrations above the MIC of the pathogen for as long as possible. Although it has not been directly tested in respiratory tract infections, theory would suggest that maximising the time above MIC by use of continuous infusion or choice of agents with longer half-lives would result in improved efficacy of β-lactam antibiotics.

Classes of antibiotics

β-Lactams

β-lactams bind to various bacterial penicillin binding proteins (PBPs), which also function as transpeptidase enzymes. These enzymes mediate the final cross-linking stage in the synthesis of peptidoglycan. By inhibiting the action of transpeptidases β-lactams interfere with cell wall synthesis and cause bacterial lysis. A peptidoglycan cell wall is common to all Gram-positive and Gram-negative bacteria and is also present in spirochaetes and actinomycetes. Therefore, all these bacteria are potentially susceptible to the β-lactams but, in practice, some resist the action of certain members of this class. Resistance arises through the possession of inactivating β-lactamase enzymes, alteration in PBPs or decreased permeability of the outer bacterial cell wall.

In general, β-lactams are hydrophilic molecules and require high serum concentrations to achieve significant bactericidal concentrations in respiratory tissue. Within respiratory tissue they are mainly confined to the ECF and only a fraction reaches bronchial secretions and alveolar lining fluid. Provided that adequate doses are used, bactericidal concentrations can still be achieved at sites of infection. Plasma half-lives tend to be short and therefore repeated dosing is required to maintain therapeutic levels of antibiotic.

Penicillins

Benzylpenicillin

Benzylpenicillin is bactericidal against many Gram-positive bacteria, most Gram-negative cocci and some Gram-negative anaerobes. It is the agent of choice in treating susceptible *S. pneumoniae*. Amongst Gram-positive organisms, it is not active against *Enterococcus faecalis*. Furthermore, it is not active against Gram-negative bacilli or staphylococci which possess β-lactamase activity.

As benzylpenicillin is acid labile it does not survive passage through the stomach and has to be administered parenterally. Plasma protein binding is 50% and the plasma half-life is about 1 hour. It rapidly penetrates into tissues, particularly sites of inflammation. It has an established record in the treatment of pneumococcal pneumonia. However, most *Staphylococcus aureus* strains now produce β-lactamases and antibiotic resistance among *S. pneumoniae* is also of increasing concern.

Alteration in PBPs is the main resistance mechanism in *S. pneumoniae*. Since the first clinical isolation of penicillin resistant *S. pneumoniae* in 1965, resistance has been reported in all countries in which it has been sought[15]. In certain countries and regions, such as Spain, parts of Eastern Europe, South Africa, Mexico, Alaska and Papua New Guinea, prevalence of resistant pneumococci exceeds 10% and in some cities within these countries prevalence rates as high as 40% have been reported[16]. Although the MICs for various cephalosporins are higher in penicillin-resistant isolates compared with penicillin-sensitive isolates[17], respiratory infections caused by penicillin-resistant pneumococci can usually be treated successfully with a suitable cephalosporin. Linares *et al.*[18] systematically studied the susceptibility of penicillin-resistant pneumococci to 24 different β-lactam antibiotics and found that some, but not all, cephalosporins were more active than benzylpenicillin. The more active ones included cefotaxime, ceftriaxone and cefpirome. Other cephalosporins were less active than penicillin and are therefore not recommended for empirical use in areas with a high prevalence of penicillin resistance.

Anti-staphylococcal penicillins

The anti-staphylococcal penicillins are relatively stable to staphylococcal β-lactamase. Those currently used are chiefly the isoxazolyl penicillins inclusive of cloxacillin and flucloxacillin, which are also active against other aerobic Gram-positive cocci, with the exception of *E. faecalis*. Oral absorption is excellent, exceeding 80%, the protein binding is high (>90%) and the plasma half-life is about 1 hour. Tissue penetration is rapid and pharmacokinetics resemble benzylpenicillin[19]. Efficacy in the treatment of staphylococcal pneumonia is well established but of concern for the future is the emergence and spread of methicillin-resistant *S. aureus*.

Ampicillin/amoxycillin

Compared with benzylpenicillin, ampicillin is less active against Gram-positive organisms, with the exception of *E. faecalis*, and more active against Gram-negative organisms. Its spectrum against respiratory tract pathogens includes *H. influenzae* and some *Escherichia coli* but does not extend to *Moraxella catarrhalis* or *Klebsiella, Enterobacter* and *Serratia* spp.

Oral absorption of ampicillin is limited by acid lability and amounts to about 30%. The acid stability of ampicillin has been improved by the development of prodrugs, such as pivampicillin, talampicillin and bacampicillin and serum levels of ampicillin attained after the oral administration of such a prodrug are considerably higher than those attained after administration of ampicillin itself[20]. Chemical modification to amoxycillin increases acid stability and absorption to 90%. Plasma protein binding is relatively low at 20% and the plasma half-life is about 1 hour. The concentration of ampicillin in bronchial secretions and ELF is less than 20% of serum concentrations[21,22]. Despite this poor penetration, the dose of antibiotic used ensures that bactericidal concentrations are achieved in tissue. As with the lower respiratory tract there is adequate penetration of ampicillin into middle ear fluid[23]. After oral dosing with amoxycillin, 500 mg 8-hourly, a serum concentration of 4.13 mg/l and a lung tissue concentration of 2.68 mg/kg are obtained[24].

β-Lactamase inhibitors

There are three clinically utilised β-lactamase inhibitors: clavulanic acid, sulbactam and tazobactam. They possess limited intrinsic antibacterial activity but are potent inhibitors of many of the plasmid-mediated β-lactamases found in *E.coli*, *M. catarrhalis*, *Bacteroides fragilis* and *H. influenzae*. They are used in combination with other β-lactam antibiotics: clavulanic acid with amoxycillin or ticarcillin, sulbactam with ampicillin, and tazobactam with piperacillin. *In vitro* clavulanic acid and tazobactam were equally potent in inhibiting 35 β-lactamases and were significantly more potent than sulbactam[25]. In the respiratory tract β-lactamase production is most relevant in *H. influenzae* and *M. catarrhalis*. In North America about 20% of *H. influenzae* isolates are β-lactamase producers[26]. In Europe the figure is closer to 10%[27] while, in some African countries, β-lactamase is produced by 80% of isolates[28]. The principle β-lactamase produced is TEM-1. In *M. catarrhalis* the principal β-lactamases are designated BRO-1 and BRO-2 and are present in 90% of isolates[29]. *M. catarrhalis* may cause co-infections with non-β-lactamase producing pathogens and β-lactamases produced by the former may affect the ability to treat the latter, a phenomenon termed 'indirect pathogenicity'.

Clavulanic acid is used in conjunction with amoxycillin (in a 1:2 ratio in the oral preparation and 1:5 in the intravenous preparation) as co-amoxiclav and with ticarcillin in a 1:15 ratio. Sulbactam is combined with ampicillin in a 1:1 ratio and tazobactam with piperacillin in a 1:8 ratio. Both clavulanic acid and sulbactam can be detected in lung tissue[30,31] and in comparable ratios to amoxycillin or ampicillin[32]. Tazobactam penetrates well into bronchial secretions and concentrations persist for a good period[33].

Although, in one study, β-lactamase activity in sputum was not inhibited by clavulanic acid, good clinical responses occurred with co-amoxiclav therapy[34] and β-lactamase/β-lactam combinations have been used with particular success in the therapy of respiratory infections when anaerobic organisms were likely pathogens, e.g. lung abscesses or chronic otitis media.

Anti-pseudomonal penicillins

Carbenicillin, mezlocillin, ticarcillin, azlocillin and pipericillin have a spectrum of activity similar to ampicillin, but with less Gram-positive activity and poor stability against most enterobacterial β-lactamases but with additional activity against *Pseudomonas* species. Azlocillin and piperacillin also have activity against *Klebsiella* species. These penicillins are particularly used to treat pseudomonal infections in patients with cystic fibrosis, even though their penetration into bronchial secretions is poor[35]: concentrations in sputum are less than 20% of serum concentrations. β-lactamase production can be induced by some of these penicillins and, together with the relatively poor tissue concentrations, suggests that, for severe infections such as pseudomonal pneumonia, adjunctive therapy with an aminoglycoside or a quinolone should be used.

Cephalosporins

All cephalosporins are derivatives of 7-aminocephalosporanic acid but they have widely differing spectra of activity. Cephalosporins tend to have broader spectrums of activity and resistance is less of a problem than their penicillin relatives. None have activity against *Legionella* spp. or *E. faecalis*. The most widely used classification of the group is into three 'generations'. The first generation are agents stable to staphylococcal β-lactamase, and are active against most Gram-positive bacteria, but are broken down by most enterobacterial β-lactamases. This generation has largely been superseded by the subsequent two generations, both of which are resistant to a range of Gram-negative β-lactamases. In the second generation, this extends the spectrum to include *H. influenzae* and various Enterobacteriaciae. Cefoxitin, which is really a cephamycin rather than a cephalosporin, has the advantage of being active against *Bacteroides* species. Cefuroxime is more β-lactamase stable than its second generation relatives, cefaclor, cefamandole and cefoxitin.

The third generation cephalosporins are even more β-lactamase stable and this results in exceptional potency against most enterobacteria, except some *Citrobacter*, *Enterobacter*, and *Serratia* species. Some third-generation agents have good antipseudomonal activity and some do not. Third-generation agents which lack activity against *P. aeruginosa* include cefotaxime, ceftriaxone and ceftizoxime: those with anti-pseudomonal activity include cefoperazone, ceftazidime, cefpirome and cefepime. In some instances the wider Gram-negative activity is accompanied by less anti-staphylococcal activity.

Pharmacokinetics are similar to the penicillins. There are a number of orally administered cephalosporins, such as cefaclor, cephalexin, cefuroxime, cefixime and ceftibuten but most cephalosporins must be administered parenterally. They are hydrophilic and tissue penetration is limited but adequate. The concentration of antibiotic in bronchial secretions and ELF is typical for a β-lactam antibiotic, being usually less than 20% of serum concentrations, in general higher concentrations being obtained with the second and third generation agents than the first generation compounds[14,36–39].

Cefuroxime

Cefuroxime can be administered orally in the form of an ester, cefuroxime axetil, which has an oral bioavailability of about 40% when taken with food. The plasma half-life is about one hour and protein binding is 30%. Tissue penetration is rapid and adequate. After a 500 mg oral dose of cefuroxime axetil the concentration of drug in bronchial tissue is 1.8 mg/kg and in ELF is 0.7 mg/l compared with a serum concentration of 3.5 mg/l[38]. Cefuroxime and cefuroxime axetil have proved comparable to aminopenicillins in the treatment of pneumonia and bronchitis[40]. Parenteral cefuroxime, in common with all other second and third generation cephalosporins has been successfully used in the treatment of Gram-negative hospital-acquired pneumonia.

Cefotaxime

The plasma half-life of cefotaxime is about 1 hour and protein binding is 40%. Penetration into bronchial secretions is considerably improved at high doses. After a dose of 1 g intravenously the ratio of serum to sputum concentrations is 24:1 while after a 2 g dose it is 6:1[41]. Sputum concentrations with a 2 g dose reach 3 mg/l. Cefotaxime is clinically effective in treating respiratory tract infections due to susceptible bacteria[42].

Ceftriaxone

Ceftriaxone is highly protein bound and has a half-life considerably longer than other cephalosporins, being 6 to 9 hours. Sustained levels in serum maintain concentrations in tissues. Thus, even with once daily dosing, adequate levels are maintained in both serum, lung parenchymal tissue and sputum[43].

Ceftazidime

Ceftazidime has very low protein binding and a plasma half-life of about 2 hours. Penetration into the lung may be limited by a saturable transport mechanism: in a study on ceftazidime in ventilated intensive care patients, increasing serum concentrations of antibiotic were not matched by a proportionate increase in bronchial secretions above a certain dose of antibiotic[6]. While ceftazidime has a particular role in treating pseudomonal infection, it also has proven efficacy in treating various community-acquired respiratory tract infections[44].

Cefpirome

In vitro cefpirome is more active than cefotaxime and ceftazidime against several Gram-positive and Gram-negative bacteria but less active than ceftazidime against *P. aeruginosa*. It has a plasma half-life of 2.3 hours[45] and its sputum penetration is similar to other cephalosporins[46]. In treating lower respiratory tract infections, it is as effective as ceftazidime and ceftriaxone[47].

Cefepime

Cefepime has a very broad spectrum of activity extending to *P. aeruginosa*. The plasma half-life is about 2 hours. Tissue penetration is similar to other cephalosporins. Concentrations achieved in bronchial mucosa are 60% of the concentration in serum[36]. In clinical trials it has proved equi-effective with other cephalosporins in treating lower respiratory tract infections[42,44].

Table 4.1 summarises the antimicrobial spectrum of cephalosporins.

Other β-lactams

Carbapenems

Carbapenems, including imipenem and meropenem, are a new class of β-lactam antibiotic. They have a very broad spectrum of activity and are stable to almost all β-lactamases. Their spectrum includes anaerobes and organisms resistant to other antibiotics such as *Serratia, Enterobacter* and many *Pseudomonas* species. Imipenem, but not meropenem, is rapidly degraded by a renal dehydropeptidase and is administered in a 1:1 ratio with a dehydropeptidase inhibitor cilastatin. Carbapenems penetrate bronchial secretions to concentrations about 20% of those in serum[48,49]. In patients receiving 1 g six-hourly of imipenem-cilastatin the mean sputum concentration of imipenem was 4.4 mg/l compared with a peak serum concentration of 34.9 mg/l[48]. For imipenem, protein binding is low at 25% and plasma half-life is about 1 hour. Studies have proven the clinical efficacy of imipenem-cilastatin in treating nosocomial respiratory tract infections, especially those caused by *Pseudomonas* or *Acinetobacter* species[50,51] but caution must be exercised in patients with neurological disorders, since convulsions have been precipitated: meropenem does not seem to have this drawback.

Aztreonam

Aztreonam is a mono-cyclic β-lactam active against aerobic, Gram-negative bacteria including *P. aeruginosa*. It is not effective against Gram-positive organisms and anaerobes. It penetrates into bronchial secretions, with concentrations of 4.8 to 18.7 mg/l after a 2 g dose[52] and has been shown to be efficacious in treating Gram-negative pneumonia[53].

Macrolides

Macrolides consist of a macrocyclic lactam ring with two sugars attached. The most important compounds contain 14, 15 or 16 carbons. Macrolides bind to the 50 *S* subunit of the ribosome of bacteria and thereby inhibit protein synthesis. They have a very broad spectrum of activity which importantly includes pathogens responsible for atypical pneumonia – *Legionella* spp., *Mycoplasma pneumoniae* and *Chlamydia* spp. Resistance is not a problem in the atypical pathogens. In experimental conditions resistance to erythromycin has been selected in *L. pneumophila*[54], but in a retrospective survey of clinical isolates, collected in the USA between 1981 and 1990, no resistance was encountered to erythromycin, clarithromycin, roxithromycin or dirithromycin[55].

Macrolides are lipophilic and cross cell membranes. This results in high tissue concentrations and entry into the intracellular compartment, especially within lysosomes. Plasma and tissue half-lives are longer than β-lactams.

The 14-carbon macrolides induce hepatic microsomal enzymes and interfere with theophylline clearance, resulting in increased blood levels (and potential toxicity).

Macrolides are useful as treatment for patients who are allergic to penicillins and are effective in most pneumococcal, streptococcal and mycoplasmal infections. They are the drugs of choice for *Legionella* and *Chlamydia* infections.

Erythromycin

Erythromycin is a 14-carbon macrolide with good activity against Gram-positive bacteria and many Gram-negative anaerobes but not against the Enterobacteriaciae. Its activity is also unreliable against *H. influenzae*, with MICs ranging from 0.25 to 20 mg/l. It is also active against some atypical mycobacteria and many strains of *Nocardia* and *Actinomyces*. Resistance is well documented in *S. pneumoniae*, and occurs particularly in penicillin-resistant strains. In a survey of *S. pneumoniae* isolates in a Parisian hospital Buu-Hoi *et al.* found that resistance to erythromycin rose from 1% to 19% from 1976 to 1986[56]. This increase in resistance paralleled the increase in erythromycin prescriptions over that period. In other countries the prevalence of resistance to erythromycin is not as high, for instance, in the United Kingdom 6.5% of *S pneumoniae* isolates are resistant[57].

Oral absorption of commonly used erythromycin salts is poor, being less than 30% and the poor absorption contributes to a high frequency of upper gastrointestinal toxicity. Ester prodrugs, such as erythromycin acistrate and stearate, are better absorbed. Intravenous erythromycin is very irritant and thrombophlebitis is common. Protein binding is high at 80% and the plasma half-life is 1.5 hours. Tissue penetration is good and the tissue:serum concentration ratio ranges from 0.5 to 5.0. High tissue concentrations are achieved in the

Table 4.1. *A comparison of cephalosporins*

Generation	Spectrum	Cephalosporin	Route of administration	Serum half-life (h)
I	Staphylococci (++)	Cephazolin	Parenteral	1–2
	Enterobacteria (+)	Cephalothin	Parenteral	0.5–1
	H. influenzae (+)	Cephalexin	Oral	1
		Cephradine	Oral/parenteral	1
		Cefaclor	Oral	0.5–1
		Cefadroxil	Oral	1.5–2
II	Staphylococci (++)	Cefuroxime	Oral/parenteral	0.5–1
	H. influenzae (+++)	Cephamandole	Parenteral	0.75–1
	Enterobacteria (++)			
II	As above plus some Anaerobes	Cefoxitin	Parenteral	0.75–1
III	Enterobacteria (+++)	Cefotaxime	Parenteral	1–1.5
	H. influenzae (++)	Ceftriaxone	Parenteral	8
	Staphylococci (+)			
III	Enterobacteria (+++)	Ceftazidime	Parenteral	2
	P. aeruginosa (++)	Cefoperazone	Parenteral	2
	Staphylococci (+)			
III	Enterobacteria (+++)	Cefixime	Oral	4
	H. influenzae (+++)			
	Staphylococci (–)			
	P. aeruginosa (–)			
III/IV	Enterobacteria (+++)	Cefepime	Parenteral	2
	P. aeruginosa (++)	Cefpirome	Parenteral	2
	Staphylococci (++)			

lung. Within tissue, erythromycin is mainly found in the intracellular compartment[7,58]. Less erythromycin appears in the extracellular fraction and therefore lower concentrations are found in bronchial secretions[58,59].

Clarithromycin

Clarithromycin is another 14-carbon macrolide with a similar spectrum of activity to erythromycin. MICs are very low for *M. pneumoniae* (<0.008 mg/l)[60] and *Chlamydia pneumoniae* (0.007 mg/l)[61] and clarithromycin is about twice as active as erythromycin against *H. influenzae* (MICs can still be 2–4 mg/l)[62].

The advantage of clarithromycin is good acid stability and, hence, predictable serum concentrations after oral administration. Less frequent dosing is required and the frequency of gastrointestinal side-effects is lower than for erythromycin[63]. Tissue penetration is very good owing to the lipophilic nature of clarithromycin. Following a 500 mg oral dose, a serum concentration of 2.51 mg/l and a lung tissue concentration of 17.47 mg/kg were recorded[64]. Intracellular penetration is good and this compartmentalisation acts as a reservoir and extends the plasma half-life to about 4 hours.

In trials involving unselected upper and lower respiratory tract infections clarithromycin has proved as effective as erythromycin[63] and β-lactams[65,66].

Azithromycin

Azithromycin is a 15-carbon macrolide (azalide), less potent than erythromycin against Gram-positive organisms[67] but four times as active against *H. influenzae*[62] and with good activity against the atypical respiratory pathogens[61].

It is very acid stable and 37% of an oral dose is absorbed[68] but plasma concentrations remain very low, a 500 mg dose giving mean peak concentrations in plasma of only 0.4 mg/l. Tissue penetration, however, is extremely good and the ratio of tissue:plasma concentrations ranges from 10 to 100 for various non-respiratory sites[68]. In one study, a single oral dose of 500 mg resulted in a serum concentration of 0.13 mg/l and a peak bronchial mucosal concentration of 3.89 mg/l[69]. Such low serum concentrations might be a disadvantage when bacteraemia is a strong possibility (in *S. pneumoniae* pneumonia, for example). Azithromycin penetrates well into cells, and inflammatory cells can transport antibiotic into ELF and sputum[11]. After a single 500 mg, oral dose of azithromycin antibiotic is still detectable in serum and tissue 96 hours later and peak concentrations are reached 48 hours after the dose[69]. Antibiotic persistence reduces the frequency of dosing and has also enabled very short courses, such as three days of treatment for exacerbations of chronic bronchitis[70].

Azithromycin has proved as effective as β-lactams[71] and erythromycin[72] in the treatment of respiratory tract infections (chiefly exacerbations of chronic bronchitis) and is associated with fewer side-effects.

Roxithromycin

Roxithromycin is an oxime derivative of erythromycin and has a similar spectrum of activity. Compared with other macrolides it has high protein binding and this results in higher serum levels but lower tissue diffusion[73]. None the less, therapeutic concentrations are obtained in nasal mucosa, tonsillar tissue and lung[64] and, within tissues, it is concentrated intracellularly[7]. It has comparable activity to erythromycin in the treatment of lower respiratory tract infections and similar effects upon theophylline concentrations[74].

Aminoglycosides

Aminoglycosides bind to the 30 *S* subunit of the bacterial ribosome, inhibit protein synthesis and also perturb cell membrane permeability. They are bactericidal. Their spectrum covers some Gram-positive organisms (staphylococci but not streptococci), the Enterobacteriaciae and Gram-negative aerobes, but not anaerobes. Some aminoglycosides are active against mycobacteria. Acquired resistance is now widespread and there is usually cross-resistance between aminoglycosides.

Aminoglycosides are not absorbed after oral administration. They are hydrophilic, have low protein binding and poor tissue penetration. The most important toxic effects are those on the eighth nerve, both vestibular and cochlear branches, and the kidney. The different degrees of toxicity of the various aminoglycosides are summarised in Table 4.2[75]. Toxicity limits the attainment of the high serum levels needed in order to achieve therapeutic concentrations in bronchial secretions. Even when therapeutic concentrations are reached in such secretions the activity of aminoglycosides is reduced by the acid pH of sputum[76] and binding to chromatin and DNA released from dead inflammatory cells[77]. They thus have several drawbacks in the treatment of suppurative respiratory infections. Gentamicin, netilmicin, tobramycin and amikacin are very similar in toxicity (Table 4.2). Given similarity in toxicity, spectrum of activity and pharmacokinetics the cheapest agent, gentamicin, is usually to be preferred and there is rarely a therapeutic advantage in choosing a considerably more expensive aminoglycoside such as amikacin.

Gentamicin

Gentamicin is active against staphylococci, Enterobacteriaciae and Gram-negative aerobes. Activity against *Pseudomonas* species is variable and it does not have significant activity against mycobacteria. Acquired resistance is reported in several species.

Gentamicin is administered parenterally. Protein binding is less than 25% and the plasma half-life is 1 to 4 hours. Concentrations in bronchial secretions are less than 30% of serum levels[78] and are higher, but more transient, after intravenous compared with intramuscular administration. Gentamicin has also been administered by aerosol inhalation[13]. By this route, higher concentrations of antibiotic can be reached in bronchial secretions compared with parenteral administration and these concentrations can be maintained for a longer period. A small quantity of the aerosolised gentamicin is absorbed systemically but this is only of concern in patients with renal impairment[79].

Gentamicin is chiefly used for severe Gram-negative nosocomial infections, but for Gram-negative pneumonia should probably be used in combination with a β-lactam. It is also useful as part of combination therapy for severe *S. aureus* pulmonary infections.

Table 4.2. *Relative toxicity of aminoglycosides (adapted from Reference[75])*

	Vestibular	Cochlear	Renal
Streptomycin	4	1	<1
Neomycin	1	4	4
Kanamycin	1	3	1
Amikacin	1	3	1
Gentamicin	3	2	2
Tobramycin	2	2	2
Netilmicin	2	2	1

Amikacin

The spectrum of activity of amikacin is similar to gentamicin except that it is significantly bactericidal against mycobacteria and retains activity against many organisms with acquired resistance to the aminoglycosides. As for any aminoglycoside, tissue penetration is poor with bronchial secretion concentrations being less than 30% of serum concentrations[80]. None the less it has proved clinically effective in the treatment of serious Gram-negative pneumonia in combination with other antibiotics[53]. In clinical studies aerosolised amikacin has also proved useful in both prophylaxis and treatment of infections in patients with cystic fibrosis[81].

Tobramycin

The spectrum of tobramycin is similar to gentamicin, as are the pharmacokinetics and tissue penetration[82]. Tobramycin can be administered by the aerosolised route with little systemic absorption and is as effective as other aminoglycosides in clinical trials[79].

Streptomycin

Streptomycin has the usual aminoglycoside spectrum of activity but is particularly active against mycobacteria, being effective against *M. tuberculosis* and some atypical mycobacteria, such as *M. kansasii* and *M. ulcerans*. Resistance may be caused by either decreased permeability to streptomycin (when it can be overcome with penicillin) or due to changes in the bacterial ribosomes.

Streptomycin is administered by the intramuscular route. Protein binding is about 30% and the plasma half-life is about 3 hours. It is rapidly distributed in the extracellular compartment but does not penetrate into thick-walled abscesses. The most serious toxicity is vestibular. Streptomycin is no longer part of first-line treatment for tuberculosis, but has a useful reserve role and is still used in countries with limited access to other agents.

Fluoroquinolones

Quinolones inhibit bacterial DNA gyrase which is involved in the supercoiling and packaging of bacterial DNA. The earlier compounds, such as nalidixic acid were of no use in respiratory infections but the newer fluoroquinolones have a broad spectrum of activity and much improved pharmacokinetics (Table 4.3). Their spectrum includes most Enterobacteriaceae, *H. influenzae, M. catarrhalis* and

Table 4.3. *A comparison of quinolones*

	Nalidixic	Norfloxacin	Ofloxacin	Ciprofloxacin	Sparfloxacin
Spectrum	Enterobacteria *H. influenzae*	Enterobacteria *H. influenzae* *Neisseria* spp.	Enterobacteria *H. influenzae* *Neisseria* spp. *S. aureus*	Enterobacteria *H. influenzae* *Ps. aeruginosa* *Neisseria* spp. *S. aureus*	Enterobacteria *H. influenzae* *Ps. aeruginosa* *Neisseria* spp. *S. aureus* *S. pneumoniae*
Oral absorption	>90%	50–80%	100%	50–84%	40%
Lung penetration	poor	poor	good	good	good
Theophylline interaction	–	++	+	++	–
Clinical use	Urinary tract infection	Urinary tract infection gonorrhoea	Urinary tract respiratory tract infections gonorrhoea	Urinary tract respiratory tract, gastro- intestinal infections gonorrhoea	Respiratory tract infection

the atypical pathogens. They are less active against *S. aureus*, *P. aeruginosa* and *S. pneumoniae*. Naturally resistant organisms include *E. faecalis*, *Acinetobacter* and non-*aeruginosa* species of *Pseudomonas*. Acquired resistance is non-transferable but is increasingly seen in staphylococci, *P. aeruginosa* and some Enterobacteriaceae. There is cross resistance between the various fluoroquinolones.

The fluoroquinolones have very favourable pharmacokinetic attributes[83]. Oral absorption is good, protein binding is low and tissue penetration is excellent. The latter is facilitated by small molecular size and the occurrence of antibiotic in an un-ionised state, given that pI values are very close to serum pH of 7.4. Once in tissues, active transport mechanisms concentrate antibiotic in the intracellular compartment[84]. Tissue concentrations in the lung tend to be twice those in serum[85,86]. Antibiotic readily reaches ELF and sputum: concentrations are similar to serum concentrations but ELF levels are more than twice as high[87,88]. The latter may be because of the contribution of antibiotic release from alveolar macrophages. Salivary concentrations of fluoroquinolones are also very good. Many fluoroquinolones can be administered intravenously when their pharmacokinetic properties are similar to those after oral use.

Some fluoroquinolones, e.g. pefloxacin and, to a lesser extent, ciprofloxacin, are excreted by hepatic metabolism and such compounds may depress the cytochrome P450 enzyme pathway and reduce the elimination of theophylline[89]. Fluoroquinolones are not recommended in children, or pregnant or lactating women since, in some animal species, cartilage damage in developing joints has been produced.

Ciprofloxacin

Ciprofloxacin is reliably active against many respiratory pathogens. *In vitro* it is more active against *L. pneumophila* than macrolides, although less active than rifampicin. Macrolides and tetracyclines are more active against *M. pneumoniae* and *Chlamydia* spp. Activity against *S. pneumoniae* is variable with MIC_{90}s between 0.5 and 4 mg/l. Resistance has been induced *in vitro* to both *S. pneumoniae* and *H. influenzae*, but the frequency of such induction is less than with other antibiotics[90]. Ciprofloxacin has good activity against most Gram-negative pathogens but the MIC_{90}s for *Pseudomonas* spp. can vary from 0.5 – >2.0 mg/l and more resistant organisms can emerge during the course of treatment.

Ciprofloxacin is water soluble. After an oral dose, 50 – 84% of the drug is absorbed, plasma protein binding is relatively low at 30% and the plasma half-life is about 4 hours. Tissue penetration is good and rapid. In one study, after an oral dose of 500 mg the concentration of ciprofloxacin in bronchial mucosa was 4.4 mg/kg, compared with 3.0 mg/l in serum[24]. Concentrations in respiratory secretions are twice as high as serum[87]. The penetration of ciprofloxacin into saliva and upper respiratory tract secretions explains its efficacy in clearing oropharyngeal carriage of *Neisseria meningitidis*[91].

In clinical trials ciprofloxacin has proved comparable or better than β-lactams in the treatment of exacerbations of chronic bronchitis or pneumonia[92,93], but, compared with β-lactams it is seems less effective at achieving bacteriological cure, particularly for pneumococci[93]. Clinical failures have also been reported in the treatment of pneumococcal pneumonia[94] and, given its variable activity against *S. pneumoniae* and the pre-eminence of this pathogen, ciprofloxacin cannot yet be recommended as first-line treatment for community-acquired pneumonia. For nosocomial, primarily Gram-negative, pneumonia ciprofloxacin has proved a useful agent[95]. In treating sensitive *P. aeruginosa* infections in patients with cystic fibrosis ciprofloxacin is as effective as combination therapy with a β-lactam plus an aminoglycoside with the advantage that it can be given orally[85]: the spread of resistance after repetitive use of ciprofloxacin in this patient population has now limited the use of quinolones in this setting. In experimental animal models, ciprofloxacin has proved effective in treating infections caused by atypical pathogens but experience in the treatment of atypical pneumonia in humans is still limited[54,96].

Ofloxacin

Ofloxacin has a similar spectrum of antimicrobial activity to ciprofloxacin but the optical isomer of ofloxacin, levofloxacin, which is undergoing clinical trials, is twice as potent *in vitro*[97]. Oral absorption of ofloxacin is virtually 100%, the plasma half-life is about 6 hours and plasma protein binding is 25%. Tissue penetration is comparable to ciprofloxacin. After an oral dose of 600 mg the concentration of ofloxacin in lung tissue was 17.7 mg/kg compared with a serum concentration of 8.7 mg/l[98].

In clinical trials of both community-acquired respiratory tract infections and nosocomial pneumonia, ofloxacin has achieved similar results to ciprofloxacin and is clinically and bacteriologically as effective as β-lactams[93] Ofloxacin is not metabolised before excretion and does not raise theophylline levels[89].

Sparfloxacin

Sparfloxacin also has a similar spectrum of activity against Gram-negative pathogens as ciprofloxacin, but has improved activity against Gram-positive pathogens. The MIC_{90}s against *S. pneumoniae* range from 0.2 to 1.0 mg/l, which are considerably better than those of ciprofloxacin, and which may overcome one of the drawbacks of earlier fluoroquinolones in the treatment of respiratory infections. Sparfloxacin also has good activity against mycobacteria.

Sparfloxacin is lipophilic. In animal studies 40% of an oral dose is absorbed. The plasma half-life is prolonged at 20 hours and protein binding is about 40%. Tissue penetration is excellent and intracellular penetration is good. The concentration of sparfloxacin achieved in bronchial mucosa is twice the serum concentration but in bronchial secretions it is only half of the serum concentration[83]. There does not appear to be an interaction with theophylline.

Trimethoprim

Trimethoprim is a synthetic antimicrobial that inhibits bacterial folate metabolism by interfering with bacterial dihydrofolate reductase (DHFR). Its selective toxicity is based on its greater affinity for the bacterial DHFR enzyme compared with its human counterpart. Trimethoprim has a wide range of activity including Gram-positive bacteria, most aerobic Gram-negative bacteria and *H. influenzae*. Anaerobes, and the atypical respiratory pathogens (except for *Legionella* spp.) are generally resistant. *M. catarrhalis* isolates are invariably resistant[29]. Acquired high-level resistance to trimethoprim (by production of a mutant DHFR) has been reported in many species, including *S. pneumoniae* and *H. influenzae*. In a recent survey of 2212 isolates of *H. influenzae* in England and Scotland 6.8% were resistant to trimethoprim[99].

Over 95% of an oral dose of trimethoprim is absorbed. Plasma protein binding is moderate and tissue penetration is good (the apparent volume of distribution exceeds that of the total body water). The concentration of trimethoprim in bronchial secretions is greater than that in serum, with a mean sputum concentration of 4.5 mg/l compared with a serum concentration of 2.6 mg/l[100]. A new trimethoprim derivative, bromidoprim, has a longer half-life and can be given once, instead of twice, a day[101].

Trimethoprim combined with sulphamethoxazole has an important role in the treatment and prophylaxis of *Pneumocystis carinii* pneumonia (PCP). Otherwise, the use of trimethoprim in combination with sulphamethoxazole is no longer generally warranted. The arguments regarding synergy and control of the emergence of resistance by use of the combination have been discredited and most of the side effects were attributable to the sulphonamide component[102]. Furthermore, there are conflicting data whether or not sulphamethoxazole can be detected in bronchial secretions[100,102]: its poor tissue penetration is thought to be due to its high protein binding[102]. Certainly, clinically, trimethoprim alone is as effective as co-trimoxazole in treating respiratory tract infections[102].

Lincosamines

Clindamycin is a lincosamine antibiotic which binds to the 50 S ribosomal subunit of bacteria and interferes with protein synthesis. It has very good activity against anaerobic organisms and Gram-positive aerobes but it is not active against Gram-negative aerobes. Its spectrum extends to include protozoa such as *Pneumocystis carinii*.

Resistance to clindamycin is linked with resistance to erythromycin, which also binds to the 50 *S* subunit. Acquired resistance has been described in *S. pneumoniae* and *Bacteroides* spp.

Clindamycin has excellent oral absorption. It is highly protein bound but, because it is lipophilic, tissue penetration is very good. Active transport mechanisms result in uptake into neutrophils and, probably, other phagocytic cells[103]. Adequate levels appear in sputum[104] and clindamycin has an established role in the treatment of lung abscesses and other anaerobic respiratory infections[105].

Metronidazole

Metronidazole is thought to act via a reduced form of the drug causing damage to the DNA of micro-organisms. This reduction can only be achieved in anaerobic conditions and therefore the spectrum of activity of metronidazole is limited to anaerobic bacteria and anaerobic protozoa. Acquired resistance is rare.

Oral absorption exceeds 90% but the rate of absorption is very variable. It may also be administered by rectal suppositories or by intravenous infusion. Plasma protein binding is low and tissue penetration is good with serum, saliva and sputum concentrations after dosages of 400 mg three times a day being roughly the same at steady state[106].

Tetracyclines

Tetracyclines interfere with bacterial protein synthesis and are predominantly bacteriostatic against a broad range of respiratory pathogens, including many Gram-positive and Gram-negative bacteria, *Chlamydia, Mycoplasma, Rickettsia, Coxiella* spp. and spirochaetes and *Actinomyces israelii*. They are not active against *P. aeruginosa*. In a survey in the UK, acquired tetracycline resistance was found in 8.1% of *S. pneumoniae* isolates, 4.5% of *H. influenzae* and 3% of *M. catarrhalis*[57]. Resistance is yet to be reported in the atypical respiratory pathogens but has been found in genital *Mycoplasma* species[107]. Cross-resistance among the members of the group is the general rule.

Oral absorption varies amongst the various tetracyclines. Doxycycline and minocycline are lipophilic and the most readily absorbed. Their protein binding is high but tissue penetration is excellent. They thus penetrate most effectively into bronchial secretions and concentrations in sputum are about half those in serum[108–110].

Tetracyclines are deposited in bone and developing teeth and should not be used in children under the age of 8 years or in pregnant women.

The usefulness of tetracyclines in respiratory tract infections has been considerably compromised by the spread of resistance, but they are still drugs of choice for *Chlamydia psittaci, Coxiella burnetii,* mycoplasma and rickettsial infections.

Glycopeptides

The two glycopeptides, vancomycin and teicoplanin, prevent formation of peptidoglycan by inhibiting the transfer of the sub-units across the cell wall. They are only active against Gram-positive organisms and have a particular role in the treatment of infections caused by enterococci and methicillin-resistant staphylococci. They are equally active against *S. aureus* but vancomycin is more active against coagulase-negative staphylococci (CNS) and teicoplanin is more active against enterococci and streptococci. Acquired resistance is still rare but has occurred in CNS and *E. faecalis*.

Neither drug is absorbed by mouth but, unlike vancomycin, teicoplanin can be administered intramuscularly. They are widely distributed. Teicoplanin has a much longer terminal half-life and need only be given once daily. Either vancomycin or teicoplanin is clinically effective in treating lower respiratory tract infections due to *S. aureus*[111], but either is only indicated in situations where there is methicillin-resistance or β-lactam allergy.

Anti-mycrobacterial drugs

Some of the drugs (such as streptomycin, rifampicin and cycloserine) used to treat mycobacterial infections have activity against other pathogenic bacteria, whereas others, such as isoniazid and ethambutol are specific for mycobacteria. Acquired drug-resistance tuberculosis is becoming increasingly prevalent and resistance to individual and multiple drugs is described. The genetic basis for resistance has not been elucidated in all instances[112]. Drugs used in the treatment of *M. tuberculosis* infections are not necessarily active against the atypical mycobacteria. Drugs used to treat the latter include clarithromycin, azithromycin, ethambutol, rifabutin and clofazimine.

Isoniazid

Isoniazid is the most bactericidal of the anti-tuberculous drugs and is a necessary component of all short-course regimens for tuberculosis. Oral absorption is virtually complete, plasma protein binding is very low and tissue penetration is excellent[113]. It penetrates into macrophages and is cidal for intracellular mycobacteria. Its toxicity is well recognised: hepatitis (about 2% during standard regimes), peripheral or optic neuritis and hypersensitivity reactions.

Rifampicin

In addition to being bactericidal against *M. tuberculosis* rifampicin is active against Gram-positive cocci, meningococci, *H. influenzae* and *Legionella* spp. It is an important adjunct to macrolides in the treatment of severe Legionnaire's disease and is useful in treating severe staphylococcal infections. In the latter situation, however, resistance develops rapidly if rifampicin is used as a single agent and therefore it must be used in combination with another anti-staphylococcal agent. Unlike some other agents it retains activity against slowly multiplying and dormant *M. tuberculosis*. It is active against some non-tuberculous mycobacteria, such as *Mycobacterium kansasii* and *Mycobacterium marinum* but not the *M. avium–intracellalare* complex. Oral absorption is virtually complete and protein binding is high. As rifampicin is lipophilic, tissue and cellular penetration is good and levels reached in tissues exceed serum levels[114,115].

Pyrazinamide

Pyrazinamide is bactericidal and acts at acidic pH. It is therefore thought to act within the acidic phagolysosomes in which mycobacteria reside, but some dispute this[116]. Like rifampicin it retains activity against slowly multiplying and dormant mycobacteria. Oral absorption exceeds 80% and tissue penetration is good.

Ethambutol

Ethambutol is only bacteriostatic against mycobacteria and does not possess activity against other bacteria. Primary resistance is unusual but resistance emerges rapidly when mycobacteria are exposed to the drug alone. Oral absorption is about 80% and tissue penetration is good with entry into the phagolysosomes within alveolar macrophages[117].

Anti-fungals

Amphotericin B

Amphotericin B binds to sterols, which are found in fungal but not in bacterial membranes: thus amphotericin B is principally active against fungi, including *Aspergillus fumigatus, Blastomyces dermatitidis, Candida* spp., *Coccidioides immitis, Cryptococcus neoformans, Histoplasma capsulatum* and *Paracoccidioides brasiliensis.* Resistance is reported in various *Candida* spp., especially *Candida lusitaniae*.

Amphotericin B must be administered intravenously but is insoluble in water: it is prepared as a micellar suspension with sodium desoxycholate or as liposomal or lipid-complexed preparations. Over 90% is bound to plasma proteins[118], and hence, only a small proportion is left to penetrate into tissues. The highest tissue concentrations are reached in the liver, spleen, kidneys and lungs[119]. Amphotericin B has significant toxicity: immediate effects are fever, rigors and vomiting but, of more significance are hypokalaemia, anaemia and renal damage, necessitating frequent monitoring. With the traditional formulation, doses of 0.6–1.0 mg/kg/day may be used but administration in lipid-complexed formulations allow doses of amphotericin B of 3–5 mg/kg/day to be administered with less toxicity.

Sufficient concentrations of amphotericin B are reached in the lungs for amphotericin B to be effectively used to treat invasive respiratory fungal infections. Although the liposomal formulation has fewer side-effects, lung concentrations are more unpredictable[120]. Amphotericin B is not detectable in bronchial secretions in experimental dogs[121] and this explains its failure in controlling aspergillomas and endobronchial infection. To overcome this problem amphotericin B has been instilled directly into cavities containing aspergillomas, with variable success[122] and aerosolised amphotericin B has also been used for pulmonary infection.

5-Flucytosine

5-Flucytosine (5-FC) is a synthetic pyrimidine that is converted to 5-fluorouracil (5-FU) by cytosine deaminase within fungal cells. 5-FU is then incorporated into RNA to interfere with protein synthesis: it also has effects on fungal DNA synthesis. The activity of 5-FC is restricted to yeasts which possess cytosine deaminase, such as *Candida* spp and cryptococci. Acquired resistance develops rapidly during therapy and 5-FC should always be used in combination with another effective antifungal agent.

5-FC is administered orally and is well absorbed and widely distributed into tissue and bronchial secretions[121]. Its major toxicity is bone marrow depression, probably related to small amounts of 5-FU release, and hepatotoxicity and monitoring of serum levels should be undertaken to minimise the risk of this, particularly in patients with existing myelosuppression.

The combination of 5-FC and amphotericin B has been successfully used for pulmonary candidiasis and some success has been reported in treating severe aspergillosis[123].

Azoles

The azole anti-fungals inhibit the synthesis of ergosterol and thereby prevent its incorporation into the fungal cell membrane. Many have a broad spectrum of antifungal activity but laboratory sensitivity testing is very difficult to perform and method dependent. Resistance occurs in some *Candida* spp. Little pharmacokinetic data are available specifically for the respiratory tract for the systemic azoles, ketoconazole, miconazole, fluconazole and itraconazole.

Fluconazole

Fluconazole has a broad spectrum of activity including *B. dermatitidis*, most *Candida* spp., *C. immitis*, *C. neoformans* and *H. capsulatum*. *Aspergillus* spp. *Candida glabrata* and *Candida krusei* are resistant to fluconazole. Oral absorption is excellent. Plasma protein binding is low and very little is metabolised resulting in a long half-life. It is widely distributed into most body sites. It has been used with success for therapy and secondary prophylaxis of cryptococcosis in AIDS patients but experience with isolated pulmonary cryptococcosis is anecdotal. There are few data regarding its use in other deep fungal infections.

Itraconazole

Itraconazole has a similar antifungal spectrum to that of fluconazole but, in addition, is active against *Aspergillus* spp. It is lipophilic and oral absorption is variable (and better with food). Plasma protein binding is high but, nevertheless, therapeutic concentrations are achieved in lungs, liver and bone tissue. There are reports of successful treatment of pulmonary aspergillosis[124] and it has become the drug of choice for pulmonary histoplasmosis, blastomycosis[125] and coccidioidomycosis[126].

Anti-virals

Amantadine/rimantadine

These two tricyclic amines inhibit replication of all strains of influenza A but not influenza B. Oral absorption is excellent and tissue penetration is good with concentrations in respiratory secretions at least equivalent to serum levels[127]. Both amantadine[128] and rimantadine[129] have been used in the prevention and treatment of influenza A during known outbreaks.

Ribavirin

Ribavirin is a nucleoside analogue that interferes with viral synthesis of guanosine triphosphate. It can be administered orally or intravenously but is rapidly degraded. It can also be given via a small particle aerosol generator[12] and aerosolised ribavirin has proved beneficial in the treatment of severe respiratory syncytial virus (RSV) bronchiolitis in infants and for influenza infections in adults: infection caused by RSV is its main indication since the benefits in influenza are modest[12,130]. There have also been case reports of its effective use in measles pneumonitis[131] and systemically administered ribavirin reduces the mortality in other viral infections such as Lassa fever[132] and haemorrhagic fever with renal syndrome[133].

Acyclovir

Acyclovir is a nucleoside analogue which is phosphorylated by viral thymidine kinase and subsequent to further phosphorylation specifically inhibits herpes viral DNA polymerase. It is mainly active against herpes simplex and varicella zoster virus. Less than 30% is absorbed after oral administration and in situations of severe illness the intravenous route is preferred. Plasma protein binding is low and tissue penetration is good. A short half-life of 3 hours necessitates frequent dosing. Acyclovir has been shown to be of benefit in varicella pneumonia[134] and there are case reports of successful use in herpes simplex pneumonitis[135].

The valine ester of acyclovir, valaciclovir, enables significantly higher plasma concentrations of acyclovir to be achieved after oral administration. This may be of advantage in prophylaxis against herpes infections, but in most respiratory infections caused by herpes simplex or varicella zoster virus, acyclovir should be administered intravenously and improved oral absorption does not represent an advantage.

Ganciclovir

Phosphorylated ganciclovir competes with guanosine triphosphate for incorporation into viral DNA. Ganciclovir is active against herpesviruses, including human cytomegalovirus (CMV). It is usually administered intravenously and oral bioavailability is only 4%: despite this an oral preparation is now available for use in CMV retinitis in AIDS patients. Protein binding is very low (only 1–2%) and tissue penetration is thought to be good. Results with ganciclovir in the treatment of established CMV pneumonia in immunocompromised individuals have been improved by adjunctive therapy with specific immunoglobulin[136].

Pentamidine

The mode of action of this antiprotozoal compound is uncertain but pentamidine is a second-line agent (after co-trimoxazole) in the treatment and prophylaxis of *P. carinii* pneumonia in immunocompromised patients. It also has some activity against aerobic Gram-positive cocci and *C. albicans*.

Pentamidine is poorly absorbed by mouth but can be delivered by the inhaled or intravenous routes. To reach alveolar spaces very small aerosol particles of $< 2\ \mu$ must be generated by suitable nebulisers. Penetration of aerosolised pentamidine is relatively poor into the apices of the lung, consolidated lung and generally in patients with obstructive airways disease. In non-apical lung, alveolar concentrations achieved after inhalation are almost 100 times those produced by the same dose given intravenously[137]. In studies in autopsy patients it has been found that the lung concentration of pentamidine is very low in those patients who had only received one or two intravenous doses but in patients who have died after several doses the lung concentration is considerably higher[138]. Thus it appears that pentamidine accumulates in the lung gradually. For this reason inhaled pentamidine is advocated as an adjunct to intravenous pentamidine for the first few days of treatment until tissue concentrations reach therapeutic levels.

References

1. DAIKOS GK. Continuous *versus* discontinuous antibiotic therapy: the role of the post-antibiotic effect and other factors. *J Antimicrob Chemother* 1991;27:157–60.
2. THYS J-P, AOUN M, KLASTERSKY J. Local antibiotic therapy for bronchopulmonary infections. In Pennington JE, ed. *Respiratory Infections: Diagnosis and Management*. 3rd ed. New York: Raven Press; 1994:741–66.
3. BARZA M, CUCHURAL G. General principles of antibiotic tissue penetration. *J Antimicrob Chemother* 1985;15, Suppl A:59–75.
4. BALDWIN DR, HONEYBOURNE D, WISE R. Pulmonary disposition of antimicrobial agents: *in vivo* observations and clinical relevance. *Antimicrob Agents Chemother* 1992;36:1176–80.
5. HONEYBOURNE D, BALDWIN DR. The site concentrations of antimicrobial agents in the lung. *J Antimicrob Chemother* 1992;30:249–60.
6. LANGER M, CANTONI P, BELLOSTA C, BOCCAZZI A. Penetration of ceftazidime into bronchial secretions in critically ill patients. *J Antimicrob Chemother* 1991;28:925–32.
7. CARLIER MB, ZENEBERGH A, TULKENS PM. Cellular uptake and subcellular distribution of roxithromycin and erythromycin in phagocytic cells. *J Antimicrob Chemother* 1987;30, Suppl B:47–56.
8. GAIL DB, LENFANT CJ. Cells of the lung: biology and clinical implications. *Am Rev Resp Dis* 1983;127:366–87.
9. EFFROS RM, MASON GR, SIETSEMA K, HUKKANEN J, SILVERMAN P. Pulmonary epithelial sieving of small solutes in rat lungs. *J Appl Physiol* 1988;65:640–8.
10. GIRARD AE, GIRARD D, RETSEMA JA. Correlation of the extravascular pharmacokinetics of azithromycin with in-vivo efficacy in models of localized infection. *J Antimicrob Chemother* 1990;25, Suppl A:61–71.
11. VALLEE E, AZOULAY-DUPUIS E, POCIDALO JJ, BERGOGNE-BEREZIN E. Activity and local delivery of azithromycin in a mouse model of *Haemophilus influenzae* lung infection. *Antimicrob Agents Chemother* 1992;36:1412–17.
12. KNIGHT V, GILBERT BE. Aerosol treatment of respiratory viral disease. *Lung* 1990;168, Suppl:406–13.
13. ILOWITE JS, GORVOY JD, SMALDONE GC. Quantitative deposition of aerosolised gentamicin in cystic fibrosis. *Am Rev Resp Dis* 1987;136:1445–9.
14. BALDWIN DR, ANDREWS JM, ASHBY JP, WISE R, HONEYBOURNE D. Concentrations of cefixime in bronchial mucosa and sputum after three oral multiple dose regimens. *Thorax* 1990;45:401–2.
15. APPELBAUM PC. Antimicrobial resistance in *Streptococcus pneumoniae*: an overview. *Clin Infect Dis* 1992;15:77–83.
16. LINARES J, PALLARES R, ALONSO T *et al.* Trends in antimicrobial resistance of clinical isolates of *Streptococcus pneumoniae* in Bellvitge Hospital, Barcelona, Spain (1979–1990). *Clin Infect Dis* 1992;15:99–105.
17. SPANGLER SK, JACOBS MR, PANKUCH GA, APPELBAUM PC. Susceptibility of 170 penicillin-susceptible and penicillin-resistant pneumococci to six oral cephalosporins, four quinolones, desacetylcefotaxime, Ro 23-9424 and RP 67829. *J Antimicrob Chemother* 1993;31:273–80.
18. LINARES J, ALONSO T, PEREZ JL *et al.* Decreased susceptibility of penicillin-resistant pneumococci to twenty-four beta-lactam antibiotics. *J Antimicrob Chemother* 1992;30:279–88.
19. KISS UJ, FARAGO E, GOMORY A, SZAMARANSZKY J. Investigations on the flucloxacillin levels in human serum, lung tissue, pericardial fluid and heart tissue. *Int J Clin Pharmacol Ther Tox* 1980;18:405–11.
20. MAESEN FPV, BEEUWKES H, DAVIES BI, BUYTENDIJK HJ, BROMBACHER PJ, WESSMAN J. Bacampicillin in acute exacerbations of chronic bronchitis – a dose range study. *J Antimicrob Chemother* 1976;2:279–85.
21. STEWART SM, ANDERSON IME, JONES GR, CALDER MA. Amoxycillin levels in sputum, serum and saliva. *Thorax* 1974;29:110–14.
22. INGOLD A. Sputum and serum levels of amoxycillin in chronic bronchial infections. *Br J Dis Chest* 1975;69:211–16.
23. KRAUSE PJ, OWENS NJ, NIGHTINGALE CH, KLIMEK JJ, LEHMANN WB, QUINTILIANI R. Penetration of amoxicillin, cefaclor, erythromycin-sulfisoxazole, and trimethoprim-sulfamethoxazole into the middle ear fluid of patients with chronic serous otitis media. *J Infect Dis* 1982;145:815–21.
24. HONEYBOURNE D, ANDREWS JM, ASHBY JP, LODWICK R, WISE R. Evaluation of the penetration of ciprofloxacin and amoxycillin into the bronchial mucosa. *Thorax* 1988;43:715–19.
25. PAYNE DJ, CRAMP R, WINSTANLEY DJ & KNOWLES DJ. Comparative activities of clavulanic acid, sulbactam, and tazobactam against clinically important beta-lactamases. *Antimicrob Agents Chemother.* 1994;38:767–72.
26. JORGENSEN JH. Update on mechanisms and prevalence of antimicrobial resistance in *Haemophilus influenzae. Clin Infect Dis* 1992;14:1119–23.
27. KAYSER FH, MORENZONI G, SANTANAM P. The Second European Collaborative Study on the frequency of anti-microbial resistance in *Haemophilus influenzae. Eur J Clin Microbiol Infect Dis* 1990;9:810–17.
28. CULLMANN W. Importance of beta-lactamase stability in treating today's respiratory tract infections. *Respiration* 1993;60, Suppl 1:10–15.
29. FUNG CP, POWELL M, SEYMOUR A, YUAN M, WILLIAMS JD. The antimicrobial susceptibility of *Moraxella catarrhalis* isolated in England and Scotland in 1991. *J Antimicrob Chemother* 1992;30:47–55.
30. COX AL, MEEWIS JMJM, HORTON R. Penetration into lung tissue after intravenous administration of amoxycillin/clavulanate. *J Antimicrob Chemother* 1989;24, Suppl B:87–91.
31. FRANK U, SCHMIDT-EISENLOHR E, JOOS-WURTTEMBERGER A, HASSE J, DASCHNER F. Concentrations of sulbactam/ampicillin in serum and lung tissue. *Infection* 1990;18:307–9.
32. VALCKE YJ, ROSSEEL MT, PAUWELS RA, BOGAERT MG, VAN DER STRAETEN ME. Penetration of ampicillin and sulbactam in the lower airways during respiratory infections. *Antimicrob Agents Chemother* 1990;34:958–62.
33. JEHL F, MULLER-SERIEYS C, DE LARMINAT V, MONTEIL H, BERGOGNE-BEREZIN E. Penetration of pipericillin-tazobactam into bronchial secretions after multiple doses to intensive care patients. *Antimicrob Agents Chemother* 1994;38:2780–84.
34. STOCKLEY RA, DRAGICEVIC P,

BURNETT D, HILL SL. Role of beta-lactamases in the response of pulmonary infections to amoxycillin/clavulanate. *J Antimicrob Chemother* 1989;24, Suppl B:73–81.

35. MARLIN GE, BURGESS KR, BURGOYNE J, FUNNELL GR, GUINESS MDG. Penetration of pipericillin into bronchial mucosa and sputum. *Thorax* 1981;36:774–80.

36. CHADA D, WISE R, BALDWIN DR, ANDREWS JM, ASHBY JP, HONEYBOURNE D. Cefipime concentrations in bronchial mucosa and serum following a single 2 gram intravenous dose. *J Antimicrob Chemother* 1990;25:959–63.

37. BALDWIN DR, MAXWELL SRJ, HONEYBOURNE D, ANDREWS JM, ASHBY JP, WISE R. The penetration of cefpirome into the potential sites of pulmonary infection. *J Antimicrob Chemother* 1991;28:79–86.

38. BALDWIN DR, ANDREWS JM, WISE R, HONEYBOURNE D. Bronchoalveolar distribution of cefuroxime axetil and *in-vitro* efficacy of observed concentrations against respiratory pathogens. *J Antimicrob Chemother* 1992;30:377–85.

39. FRAMPTON JE, BROGDEN RN, LANGTREY HD, BUCKLEY MM. Cefpodoxime proxetil. A review of its antibacterial activity, pharmacokinetic properties and therapeutic potential. *Drugs* 1992;44:889–917.

40. BRAMBILLA C, KASTANAKIS S, KNIGHT S, CUNNINGHAM K. Cefuroxime and cefuroxime axetil versus amoxycillin plus clavulanic acid in the treatment of lower respiratory tract infections. *Eur J Clin Microbiol Infect Dis* 1992;11:118–24.

41. LODE H, KEMMERICH B, GRUHLKE G, DZWILLO G, KOEPPE P, WAGNER I. Cefotaxime in bronchopulmonary infections – a clinical and pharmacological study. *J Antimicrob Chemother* 1980;6, Suppl A:193–8.

42. BARCKOW D, SCHWIGON CD. Cefipime versus cefotaxime in the treatment of lower respiratory tract infections. *J Antimicrob Chemother* 1993;32, Suppl B:187–93.

43. FRASCHINI F, BRAGA PC, SCARPAZZA G *et al.* Human pharmacokinetics and distribution in various tissues of ceftriaxone. *Chemotherapy* 1986;32:192–9.

44. LEOPHONTE P, BERTRAND A, NOUVET G *et al.* A comparative study of cefepime and ceftazidime in the treatment of community-acquired lower respiratory tract infections. *J Antimicrob Chemother* 1993;31, Suppl B:165–73.

45. KAVI J, ANDREWS JM, ASHBY JP, HILLMAN & WISE R. Pharmacokinetics and tissue penetration of cefpirome, a new cephalosporin. *J Antimicrob Chemother* 1988;22:911–16.

46. SHISHIDO H, NAGAI H, MIYAKE S, KABURAGI T, SATOH K, DEGUCHI K. Penetration of cefpirome into sputum in chronic respiratory infections: comparison of administration of 0.5 g and 1.0 g in the same patient. *Int J Clin Pharmacol* Research 1993;13:225–9.

47. NORRBY SR. Cefpirome: efficacy in the treatment of urinary and respiratory tract infections and safety profile. *Scand J Infect Dis* Suppl 1993;91:41–50.

48. MACGREGOR RR, GIBSON GA, BLAND JA. Imipenem pharmacokinetics and body fluid concentrations in patients receiving high-dose treatment for serious infections. *Antimicrob Agents Chemother* 1986;29:188–92.

49. MULLER-SERIEYS C, BERGOGNE-BEREZIN E, ROWAN C, DOMBERT MC. Imipenem penetration into bronchial secretions. *J Antimicrob Chemother* 1987;20:618–19.

50. ACAR JF. Therapy of lower respiratory tract infections with imipenem/cilastatin: a review of worldwide experience. *Rev Infect Dis* 1985;7, Suppl 3:S513–17.

51. WATHEN CG, CARBARNS NJ, JONES PA *et al.* Imipenem-cilastatin in the treatment of respiratory infections in patients with chronic airways obstruction. *J Antimicrob Chemother* 1988;21:107–12.

52. BOCAZZI A, LANGER M, MANDELLI M, RANZI AM, URSO R. The pharmacokinetics of aztreonam and penetration into the bronchial secretions of critically ill patients. *J Antimicrob Chemother* 1989;23:401–7.

53. BJORNSON HS, RAMIREZ-RONDA C, SAAVEDRA S, RIVERA-VAZQUEZ CR, LIU C, HINTHORN DR. Comparison of empiric aztreonam and aminoglycoside regimens in the treatment of serious gram-negative lower respiratory infections. *Clin Therap* 1993;15:65–78.

54. MEYER RD. Role of the quinolones in the treatment of legionellosis. *J Antimicrob Chemother* 1991;28:623–5.

55. JOHNSON DM, ERWIN ME, BARRETT MS, GOODING BB, JONES RN. Antimicrobial activity of ten macrolide, lincosamine and streptogramin drugs tested against *Legionella* species. *Eur J Clin Microbiol Infect Dis* 1992;11:751–5.

56. BUU-HOI AY, GOLDSTEIN FW, ACAR JF. A seventeen-year epidemiological survey of antimicrobial resistance in pneumococci in two hospitals. *J Antimicrob Chemother* 1988;22, Suppl B:41–52.

57. POWELL M, MCVEY D, KASSIM MH, CHEN HY, WILLIAMS JD. Antimicrobial susceptibility of *Streptococcus pneumoniae, Haemophilus influenzae* and *Moraxella (Branhamella) catarrhalis* isolated in the UK from sputa. *J Antimicrob Chemother* 1991;28:249–59.

58. BRUN Y, FOREY F, GAMONDES JP, TEBIB A, BRUNE J, FLEURETTE J. Levels of erythromycin in pulmonary tissue and bronchial mucus compared to those of amoxycillin. *J Antimicrob Chemother* 1981;8:459–66.

59. MARLIN GE, DAVIES PR, RUTLAND J, BEREND N. Plasma and sputum erythromycin concentrations in chronic bronchitis. *Thorax* 1980;35:441–5.

60. CASSELL GH, DRNEC J, WAITES KB *et al.* Efficacy of clarithromycin against *Mycoplasma pneumoniae*. *J Antimicrob Chemother* 1991;27, Suppl A:47–59.

61. RIDGWAY GL, MUMTAZ G, FENELON L. The in-vitro activity of clarithromycin and other macrolides against the type strain of *Chlamydia pneumoniae* (TWAR). *J Antimicrob Chemother* 1991;27, Suppl A:43–5.

62. MASKELL JP, SEFTON AM, WILLIAMS JD. Comparative *in-vitro* activity of azithromycin and erythromycin against Gram-positive cocci, *Haemophilus influenzae* and anaerobes. *J Antimicrob Chemother* 1990;25, Suppl A:19–24.

63. ANDERSON G, ESMONDE TS, COLES S, MACKLIN J, CARNEGIE C. A comparative safety and efficacy study of clarithromycin and erythromycin stearate in community-acquired pneumonia. *J Antimicrob Chemother* 1991;27, Suppl A:117–24.

64. FRASCHINI F, SCAGLIONE F, PINTUCCI G, MACCARINELLI G, DUGNANI S, DEMARTINI G. The diffusion of clarithromycin and roxithromycin into nasal mucosa, tonsil and lung in humans. *J Antimicrob Chemother* 1991;27, Suppl A:61–5.

65. BACHAND RT. Comparative study of clarithromycin and ampicillin in the treatment of patients with acute bacterial exacerbations of chronic bronchitis. *J Antimicrob Chemother* 1991;27, Suppl A:91–100.

66. NEU HC, CHICK TW. Efficacy and safety of clarithromycin compared to cefixime as outpatient treatment of lower respiratory tract infections. *Chest* 1993;104:1393–9.

67. BARRY AL, JONES RN, THORNSBERRY C. *In vitro* activities of azithromycin (CP 62,993), clarithromycin (A-56268; TE-031), erythromycin, roxithromycin, and clindamycin. *Antimicrob Agents Chemother* 1988;32:752–4.

68. FOULDS G, SHEPARD RM, JOHNSON RB. The pharmacokinetics of azithromycin in human serum and tissues. *J Antimicrob Chemother* 1990;25, Suppl A:73–82.

69. BALDWIN DR, WISE R, ANDREWS JM, ASHBY JP, HONEYBOURNE D. Azithromycin concentrations at sites of

pulmonary infection. *Eur Resp J* 1990;3:886–90.

70. BRADBURY F. Comparison of azithromycin versus clarithromycin in the treatment of patients with lower respiratory tract infection. *J Antimicrob Chemother* 1993;31, Suppl E:153–62.

71. HOEPELMAN AIM, SIPS AP, VAN HELMOND JLM *et al.* A single-blind comparison of three-day azithromycin and ten-day co-amoxiclav treatment of acute lower respiratory tract infections. *J Antimicrob Chemother* 1993;31, Suppl E:147–52.

72. MANFREDI R, JANNUZZI C, MANTERO E *et al.* Clinical comparative study of azithromycin versus erythromycin in the treatment of acute respiratory tract infections in children. *J Chemother* 1992;4:364–70.

73. NILSEN OG. Comparative pharmacokinetics of macrolides. *J Antimicrob Chemother* 1987;20, Suppl B:81–8.

74. PAULSEN O, CHRISTENSSON BA, HEBELKA M *et al.* Efficacy and tolerance of roxithromycin in comparison with erythromycin stearate in patients with lower respiratory tract infections. *Scand J Infect Dis* 1992;24:219–25.

75. PRICE KE, GODFREY JC, KAWAGUCHI H. *Adv Appl Microbiol* 1974;18:191–307.

76. BODEM CR, LAMPTON LM, MILLER DP, TARKA EF, EVERETT ED. Endobronchial pH: relevance to aminoglycoside activity in gram-negative bacillary pneumonia. *Am Rev Resp Dis* 1983;127:39–41.

77. MENDELMAN PM, SMITH AL, LEVY J, WEBER A, RAMSEY B, DAVIS RL. Aminoglycoside penetration, inactivation, and efficacy in cystic fibrosis sputum. *Am Rev Resp Dis* 1985;132:761–5.

78. PENNINGTON JE, REYNOLDS HY. Concentrations of gentamicin and carbenicillin in bronchial secretions. *J Infect Dis* 1973;128:423–34.

79. CROSBY SS, EDWARDS WAD, BRENNAN C, DELLINGER EP, BAUER LA. Systemic absorption of endotracheally administered aminoglycosides in seriously ill patients with pneumonia. *Antimicrob Agents Chemother* 1987;31:850–3.

80. DULL WL, ALEXANDER MR, KASIK JE. Bronchial secretion levels of amikacin. *Antimicrob Agents Chemother* 1979;16:767–71.

81. SCHAAD UB, WEDGWOOD-KRUCKO J, SUTER S, KRAEMER R. Efficacy of inhaled amikacin as adjunct to intravenous combination therapy (ceftazidime and amikacin) in cystic fibrosis. *J Pediatr* 1987;111:599–605.

82. ALEXANDER MR, SCHOELLS J, HICKLIN G, KASIK JE, COLEMAN D. Bronchial secretion concentrations of tobramycin. *Am Rev Resp Dis* 1982;125:208–9.

83. DECRE D, BERGOGNE-BEREZIN E. Pharmacokinetics of quinolones with special reference to the respiratory tree. *J Antimicrob Chemother* 1993;31:331–43.

84. CARLIER MB, SCORNEAUX B, ZENEBURGH A, DESNOTTES JF, TULKENS PM. Cellular uptake, localisation and activity of fluoroquinolones in uninfected and infected macrophages. *J Antimicrob Chemother* 1990;26, Suppl B:27–39.

85. PEDERSEN SS. Clinical efficacy of ciprofloxacin in lower respiratory tract infections. *Scand J Infect Dis* 1989;Suppl 60:89–97.

86. RITROVATO CA, DEETER RG. Respiratory tract penetration of quinolone antimicrobials: a case in study. *Pharmacother* 1991;11:38–49.

87. BERGOGNE-BEREZIN E, BETHELOT G, EVEN P, STERN M, REYNAUD P. Penetration of ciprofloxacin into bronchial secretions. *Eur J Clin Microbiol* 1986;5:197–200.

88. BALDWIN DR, WISE R, ANDREWS JM, ASHBY JP, HONEYBOURNE D. The distribution of temafloxacin in bronchial epithelial lining fluid, alveolar macrophages and bronchial mucosa. *Eur Resp J* 1992;5:471–6.

89. WIJNANDS WJA, VREE TB, VAN HERWAARDEN CLA. The influence of quinolone derivatives on theophylline clearance. *Br J Clin Pharm* 1986;22:677–83.

90. PIDDOCK LJV, JIN YF. Selection of quinolone-resistant mutants of *Haemophilus influenzae* and *Streptococcus pneumoniae*. *J Antimicrob Chemother* 1992;30:109–10.

91. GAUNT PN, LAMBERT BE. Single dose ciprofloxacin for the eradication of pharyngeal carriage of *Neisseria meningiditis*. *J Antimicrob Chemother* 1988;21:489–96.

92. BASRAN GS, JOSEPH J, ABBAS AMA, HUGHES C, TILLOTSON GS. Treatment of acute exacerbations of chronic obstructive airways disease – a comparison of amoxycillin and ciprofloxacin. *J Antimicrob Chemother* 1990;26, Suppl F:19–24.

93. THYS JP, JACOBS F, BYL B. Role of quinolones in the treatment of bronchopulmonary infections, particularly pneumococcal and community-acquired pneumonia. *Eur J Clin Microbiol Infect Dis* 1991;10:304–15.

94. KORNER RJ, REEVES DS, MACGOWAN AP. Dangers of oral fluoroquinolone treatment in community acquired upper respiratory tract infections. *Br Med J* 1994;308:191–2.

95. PELOQUIN CA, CUMBO TJ, NIX DE, SANDS MF, SCHENTAG JJ. Evaluation of intravenous ciprofloxacin in patients with nosocomial lower respiratory tract infections. Impact of plasma concentrations, organism, minimum inhibitory concentration, and clinical condition on bacterial eradication. *Arch Intern Med* 1989;149:2269–73.

96. HAVLICHEK D, POHLOD D, SARAVOLATZ C. Comparison of ciprofloxacin and rifampicin in experimental *Legionella pneumophila* pneumonia. *J Antimicrob Chemother* 1987;20:875–81.

97. DAVIS R, BRYSON HM. Levofloxacin. A review of its antibacterial activity, pharmacokinetics and therapeutic efficacy. *Drugs* 1994;47:677–700.

98. WIJNANDS WJA, VREE TB, BAARS AM, HAFKENSHEID JCM, KOBLER BEM, VAN HERWAARDEN CLA. The penetration of ofloxacin into lung tissue. *J Antimicrob Chemother* 1988;22, Suppl C:85–9.

99. POWELL M, FAH YS, SEYMOUR A, YUAN M, WILLIAMS JD. Antimicrobial resistance in *Haemophilus influenzae* from England and Scotland in 1991. *J Antimicrob Chemother* 1992;29:547–54.

100. HUGHES DTD. The use of combinations of trimethoprim and sulphonamides in the treatment of chest infections. *J Antimicrob Chemother* 1983;12:423–34.

101. SALMI HA. Bromidoprim in acute respiratory tract infections. *J Chemother* 1993;5:532–6.

102. BRUMFITT W, HAMILTON-MILLER JMT, HAVARD CW, TANSLEY H. Trimethoprim alone compared to co-trimoxazole in lower respiratory infections: pharmacokinetics and clinical effectiveness. *Scand J Infect Dis* 1985;17:99–105.

103. KLEMPNER MS, STYRT B. Clindamycin uptake by human neutrophils. *J Infect Dis* 1981;144:472–9.

104. SMITH BR, LEFROCK JL. Bronchial tree penetration of antibiotics. *Chest* 1983;6:904–08.

105. BARTLETT JG. Anaerobic bacterial infections of the lung and pleural space. *Clin Infect Dis* 1993;16, Suppl 4:S248–55.

106. SIEGLER D, KAYE CM, REILLY S, WILLIS AT, SANKEY MG. Serum, saliva and sputum levels of metronidazole in acute exacerbations of chronic bronchitis. *Thorax* 1981;36:781–3.

107. MCCORMACK WM. Susceptibility of Mycoplasmas to antimicrobial agents: clinical implications. *Clin Infect Dis* 1993;17, Suppl 1:S200–1.

108. GARTMANN J. Doxycycline concentrations in lung tissue, bronchial wall, bronchial secretions. *Chemotherapy* 1975;21:19–26.

109. HARNETT BJS, MARTIN GE. Doxycycline in serum and in bronchial secretions. *Thorax* 1976;34:144–8.

110. MAESEN FPV, DAVIES BI, VAN NOORD JA. Doxycycline in respiratory infections: a re-assessment after 17 years. *J Antimicrob Chemother* 1986;18:531–6.

111. LEWIS P, GARAUD JJ, PARENTI F. A multicentre open clinical trial of teicoplanin in infections caused by Gram-positive bacteria. *J Antimicrob Chemother* 1988;21, Suppl A:61–7.

112. WALLACE RJ. Current therapy of mycobacterial infections. *Curr Opin Infect Dis* 1993;6:758–63.

113. WEBER WW, HEIN DW. Clinical pharmacokinetics of isoniazid. *Clin Pharmacokinetics* 1979;4:401–22.

114. ACOCELLA G, NICOLIS FB, LAMARINA A. A study of the kinetics of rifampicin in man. *Chemotherapia* 1967;5:87.

115. TULKENS PM. Intracellular pharmacokinetics and localization of antibiotics as predictors of their efficacy against intraphagocytic infections. *Scand J Infect Dis* 1991;Suppl 74:209–17.

116. RASTOGI N, POTAR MC, DAVID HL. Pyrazinamide is not effective against intracellularly growing *Mycobacterium tuberculosis*. *Antimicrob Agents Chemother* 1988;32:287.

117. BIRNBERGER A, STELTER WJ. Ethambutol concentrations in lung tissue and serum. *Praxis der Pneumologie* 1981;35:1054–5.

118. POLAK A. Pharmacokinetics of amphotericin B and flucytosine. *Postgrad Med J* 1979;55:667–70.

119. ATKINSON AJ, BENNETT JE. Amphotericin B pharmacokinetics in humans. *Antimicrob Agents Chemother* 1978;13:271–6.

120. JANGNEGT R, DE MARIE S, BAKKER-WOUDENBERG IAJM, CROMMELIN DJA. Liposomal and lipid formulations of amphotericin B. *Clin Pharmacokinetics* 1992;23:279–91.

121. PENNINGTON JE, BLOCK ER, REYNOLDS HY. 5-fluorocytosine and amphotericin B in bronchial secretions. *Antimicrob Agents Chemother* 1973;61:324–6.

122. HARGIS L, BONE RC, STEWART J, RECTOR N, HILLER FC. Intracavitary amphotericin B in the treatment of symptomatic pulmonary aspergillosis. *Am J Med* 1980;68:389–94.

123. ATKINSON GW, ISRAEL HL. 5-Fluorocytosine treatment of meningeal and pulmonary aspergillosis. *Am J Med* 1977;55:496–504.

124. DENNING DW, STEVENS DA. Antifungal and surgical treatment of invasive aspergillosis: a review of 2,121 published cases. *Rev Infect Dis* 1990;12:1147–201.

125. DISMUKES WE, BRADSHER RW,JR., CLOUD GC *et al.* Itraconazole therapy for blastomycosis and histoplasmosis. *Am J Med* 1992;93:489–97.

126. GRAYBILL JR, STEVENS DA, GALGIANI JN, DISMUKES WE, CLOUD GA. The NAIAD-Mycoses Study Group. Itraconazole treatment of coccidioidomycosis. *Am J Med* 1990;89:282–90.

127. AOKI FY, SITAR DS. Amantadine kinetics in healthy elderly men: implications for influenza prevention. *Clin Pharmacol Ther* 1985;37:137–44.

128. NICHOLSON K, WISELKA MJ. Amantadine for influenza A. *Br Med J* 1991;302:425–6.

129. TOMINACK RL, HAYDEN FG. Rimantadine hydrochloride and amantadine hydrochloride use in influenza A virus infections. *Infect Dis Clin N Am* 1987;1:459–78.

130. HALL CB, MCBRIDE JT, WALSH EE *et al.* Aerosolised ribavirin treatment of infants with respiratory syncytial virus infection. *N Engl J Med* 1983;315:1443–7.

131. FORNI AL, SCHLUGER NW, ROBERTS RB. Severe measles pneumonitis in adults: evaluation of clinical characteristics and therapy with intravenous ribavirin. *Clin Infect Dis* 1994;19:454–62.

132. MCCORMICK JB, KING IJ, WEBB PA *et al.* Lassa fever: effective therapy with ribavirin. *N Engl J Med* 1986;314:20–6.

133. HUGGINS JW, HSIANG CM, COSGRIFF TM *et al.* Prospective, double-blind, concurrent, placebo-controlled clinical trial of intravenous ribavirin therapy of haemorrhagic fever with renal syndrome. *J Infect Dis* 1991;164:1119–27.

134. HAAKE DA, ZAKOWSKI PC, HAAKE DL, BRYSON Y. Early treatment with acyclovir for varicella pneumonia in otherwise healthy adults: retrospective controlled study and review. *Rev Infect Dis* 1990;12:788–98.

135. GEORGES JC, MAHASSEN P, MATTEI MF, DOPFF C, DE FAUP-ROCHETON B. Herpes simplex virus pneumonia following transplantation. *Aggressologie* 1992;33, Suppl 3:151–3.

136. REED EC, BOWDEN RA, DANDLIKER PS, LILLEBY KE, MEYERS JD. Treatment of cytomegalovirus pneumonia with ganciclovir and intravenous cytomegalovirus immunoglobulin in patients with bone marrow transplants. *Ann Intern Med* 1988;109:783–8.

137. MONTGOMERY AB, DEBS RJ, LUCE JM *et al.* Selective delivery of pentamidine to the lung by aerosol. *Am Rev Resp Dis* 1988;137:477–8.

138. DONNELLY H, BERNARD EM, ROTHKOTTER H, GOLD JWM, ARMSTRONG D. Distribution of pentamidine in patients with AIDS. *J Infect Dis* 1988;157:985–9.

Part 2: Respiratory infections due to major respiratory pathogens

5 Pneumococcal pneumonia

MATS KALIN
Karolinska Hospital, Sweden

Introduction

Streptococcus pneumoniae is the most common cause of pneumonia and is an infectious agent posing a most serious threat to human health. Though mortality in developed countries has decreased significantly since the preantibiotic era, it is still considerable and morbidity has not changed substantially. Mortality in children in developing countries is still alarmingly high.

During the last few decades, a rapid emergence of resistance against most of the commonly used antimicrobial drugs and the identification of the seriousness of pneumococcal infections in asplenic individuals and in those with advanced HIV have added to the burden of pneumococcal disease. However, the introduction of a vaccine has provided some hope.

Though the clinical presentation of pneumonia has been known for at least 2500 years, the pathology for 170 years, and the importance of the pneumococcus in pneumonia for more than 100 years, major deficiencies still exist in our understanding of pathogenesis[1–5].

Microbiology

S. pneumoniae (pneumococcus) is a Gram-positive, often lanceolate-shaped diplococcus with a polysaccharide capsule. Though the classification as streptococci has not always been accepted, the pneumococcus has several characteristics in common with other streptococci. The cell wall composition is similar, and like other streptococci it is catalase-negative and ferments glucose by the hexose monophosphate pathway to form lactic acid. Also, by nucleic acid homology it has been found to be closely related to many other streptococci and genetic material can be transferred to, and from, other streptococcal species by natural transformation.

On culture growth pneumococci are alpha-haemolytic but are distinguished from other alpha-haemolytic streptococci by optochin sensitivity and by sensitivity to surface-active agents such as ox bile or sodium desoxycholate. Such agents seem to remove or inactivate the inhibitors of the very active pneumococcal cell wall autolysins. Pneumococci are facultatively anaerobic and have rather specific growth requirements including 5–10% carbon dioxide in approximately 10% of the strains.

Cell structure

As in other Gram-positive bacteria, the pneumococcal cell wall is composed of peptidoglycan (murein) and teichoic acid. The predominant component apart from peptidoglycan is the C-polysaccharide, a ribitol teichoic acid containing phosphorylcholine and galactosamine[6,7], which is covalently bound to the peptidoglycan layer (Fig. 5.1). The C-polysaccharide is distributed on both the outer and inner sides of the peptidoglycan layer, and its thickness varies considerably between different strains[8]. The C-polysaccharide is analogous to the group (i.e. in most cases species)-specific polysaccharides of other streptococci, and is specific for the species *S. pneumoniae*. The exact chemical structure of the C-polysaccharide has been established (glucose, 2-acetamido-2-,4-,6-trideoxygalactose, galactoseamine, ribitolphosphate, and choline phosphate). Interestingly, each of these components has been identified as a constituent of different capsular polysaccharides, possibly pointing to an evolutionary origin of the capsular substances from the C-polysaccharide.

The cell wall also contains several proteins[2,9]. The M-protein is equivalent to the M-protein of *Streptococcus pyogenes* (group A), and is similarly type-specific. However, the pneumococcal M-protein is unrelated to capsular types and not known to be related to virulence or immunity to the extent found in Group A streptococci. Other proteins present in the cell wall are the surface protein A, the important autolysin, its powerful inhibitor, the Forsman (F) antigen, as well as two enzymes that are released during autolysis, neuramidase and pneumolysin. The F antigen apparently consists of C-polysaccharide covalently bound to a lipid moiety, i.e. a lipoteichoic acid, with the C-polysaccharide component being exposed on the surface and the lipid part anchored in the lipid bilayers of the plasma membranes[8,10]. The phosphorylcholine residue of the cell wall participates in the action of autolysin; when it is replaced by another amino alcohol such as ethanolamine, the autolytic capability is lost[7].

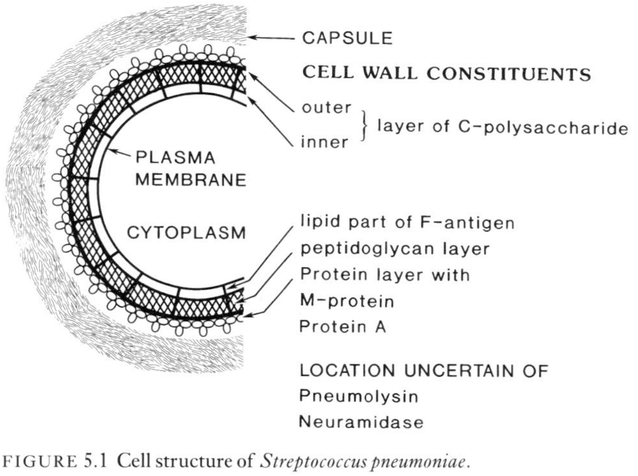

FIGURE 5.1 Cell structure of *Streptococcus pneumoniae*.

In all wild strains of *S. pneumoniae* the cell wall is surrounded by a polysaccharide capsule, which seems to be covalently linked to the cell wall peptidoglycan[11] (Fig. 5.2). Ninety different serotypes have been identified. Normally, the capsule is the only exposed antigen with all the cell wall antigens being concealed by the capsular material[8].

Epidemiology and pathogenesis

S. pneumoniae has, for more than 100 years, been known as the most common cause of pneumonia[1,3]. In the beginning of the twentieth century, young, mostly male, adults in Western countries were frequently prone to pneumococcal pneumonia in whom a case fatality rate approaching 30% was recorded. Sir William Osler named pneumococcal pneumonia 'the captain of the men of death'[3,12,13]. In the developed world today severe pneumococcal pneumonia is primarily a disease of the elderly[14–20], while in developing countries it continues to be a very significant threat to young people also. It is estimated that at least one million children below the age of 5 each year die from pneumococcal pneumonia[21,22].

The total incidence of pneumococcal pneumonia in Western populations is around 1–5/1000 person–years, being several times higher in the very young and in the elderly (Table 5.1). Of all cases of community-acquired pneumonia, at least 40–50% are caused by *S. pneumoniae*[1,3,12,15,23–34]. *S. pneumoniae* also seems to be the most frequent cause of severe community-acquired pneumonia[35,36]. The annual incidence of pneumococcal bacteraemia in North America and Europe is at least 10–20 per 100 000 individuals (Fig. 5.3). This is probably underestimated, since not all individuals falling ill with a clinical presentation consistent with pneumococcal bacteraemia will have blood cultures taken. Of the diagnosed cases of bacteraemia, at least half are associated with pneumonia. Though the case fatality rate in pneumococcal pneumonia decreased significantly with the advent of antibiotics in the 1940s, the incidence has remained almost unchanged[1,13]; the shift towards being a severe disease only in the elderly and in those with underlying diseases is, however, evident. Interestingly, the frequency of pharyngeal carriage has fallen dramatically[26], but the incidence of pneumococcal infection remains unchanged. Two recent studies have shown that the risk of invasive disease may be more than 20-fold greater for small children if they are attending day care centres than if they are taken care of at home or at family day care[37,38].

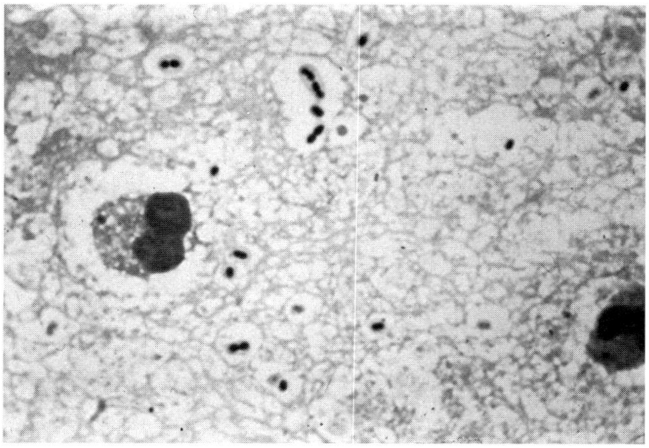

FIGURE 5.2 Gram's stain with visible polysaccharide capsule.

Table 5.1. *Diseases caused by* Streptococcus pneumoniae *in Europe and North America, approximate numbers*

Category of Disease	% of all cases Caused by *S. pneumoniae*	Cases caused by *S. pneumoniae*	
		Annual attack rate per 100 000 individuals	Case fatality rate %
Sinusitis	35		
Otitis media	30	1000	
Bacterial bronchitis	20		
Pneumonia	40	200	5
Bacteraemia	5–15	20	20
Meningitis	20	2	30
Endocarditis	1	0.4	
Arthritis		0.2	
Cellulitis		0.1	
Osteomyelitis		0.1	

In the pre-antibiotic era, the case fatality rate was almost 80% in bacteraemic and 13% in non-bacteraemic cases[3,12–14]. Pneumococcal bacteraemia developing from a pneumonic process via the lymphatic system, from a paranasal sinus via the subarachnoid space, or directly via the nasal mucosa[1], is still associated with a considerably higher case fatality rate (11%–41%, in most studies round 20%), compared to non-bacteraemic pneumococcal disease (around 5%)[14,15,17–20,28,31,39–42]. The mortality is particularly high in cases with extrapulmonary foci,

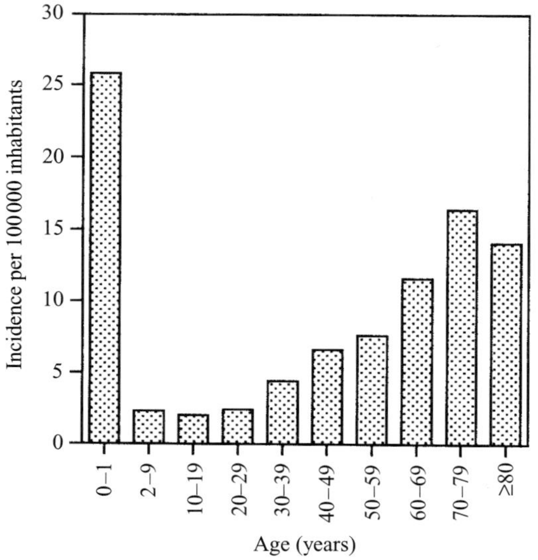

FIGURE 5.3 Age-specific incidence of invasive pneumonoccal disease in Sweden. (Adapted after Burman, Norrby and Trollfors.)

in the elderly and in patients with underlying diseases such as hypogammaglobulinaemia, splenic dysfunction, alcoholism, liver cirrhosis, chronic heart, lung and kidney diseases, myeloma, lymphoma and some other malignancies.

Pneumococcal disease is globally endemic. Epidemics may occur in settings such as the South African gold mines, where the arrival of new susceptible men caused rapid spread[1]. Several other epidemics have been described, also recently, most often in closed institutional settings like schools and military units[43–46], but account for only a minority of the cases.

Capsular types

Ninety different serotypes of *S. pneumoniae* have been identified. The typing system is based on the differences in the chemical and antigenic structure of the polysaccharide capsule[47]. Thus, 90 chemically distinct capsular types have been described. The last six types have recently been identified. Still more types may be added in the future. Some of the types are antigenically related to each other, and such related types are together included in groups. Antisera raised against one of the types in a group cross-react to some extent with the other types in the same group. Between the groups, and between types not included in groups, there is no, or very limited, cross-reactivity. The Danish nomenclature is generally used, designating types that are antigenically related a group number and a type letter (such as 9A, 9L, 9N and 9V), while types without close relationship to other types are given numbers only (such as 1, 2, 3, 4, 5).

Most of the capsular types have been infrequently isolated during the time period that different types have been recognised, i.e. since the beginning of the century, indicating that these capsular polysaccharides are conferring less virulence to the pneumococcus than are the more commonly encountered polysaccharides[1–4,13,24,31,33,48–54]. Among the more prevalent types significant differences in type distribution have been noted. Certain types, notably 6A, 19F and 23F since the beginning of the century have consistently predominated in young carriers of pneumococci, and together with types 14, 18 and 7F have been responsible for most of the pneumococcal diseases in children (Fig 5.4). The age-specific pathogenicity of these types is probably dependent on the poor immunogenicity of their polysaccharides in children less than 5 years of age[53,55]. Type 3, on the other hand, has been among the most common types as long as typing has been carried out and is a predominating type among the elderly in most geographical areas, probably reflecting an especially high virulence. Finally, types 1 and 2, contrary to most other types, are infrequently isolated from carriers, may be spread epidemically, and most often cause lobar rather than bronchopneumonic infection[2,3,12,13].

In many areas of the world, the pneumococcal type distribution pattern has changed dramatically during the twentieth century: in the beginning of the century types 1 and 2 accounted for up to 65% of the cases of lobar pneumonia, and during the pre-antibiotic era types 1, 2, and 3 together accounted for up to 75% of the bacteraemic cases[2,3,12,13,52,56,57] (Fig. 5.5). Today, type 2 is almost never isolated in Western countries, and type 1 is most often seen in less than 10%[27,49,51,53,54]. Type 5 was common several decades ago, but is today infrequent in North America and Europe. Interestingly, the type distribution pattern has changed over time in a very similar way in all Western countries, while in some developing countries it is today remarkably similar to that seen in North America and Europe during the first decades of the twentieth century[2,58], indicating a different susceptibility to different pneumococcal types in hosts living under different socioeconomic circumstances.

Pathogenesis

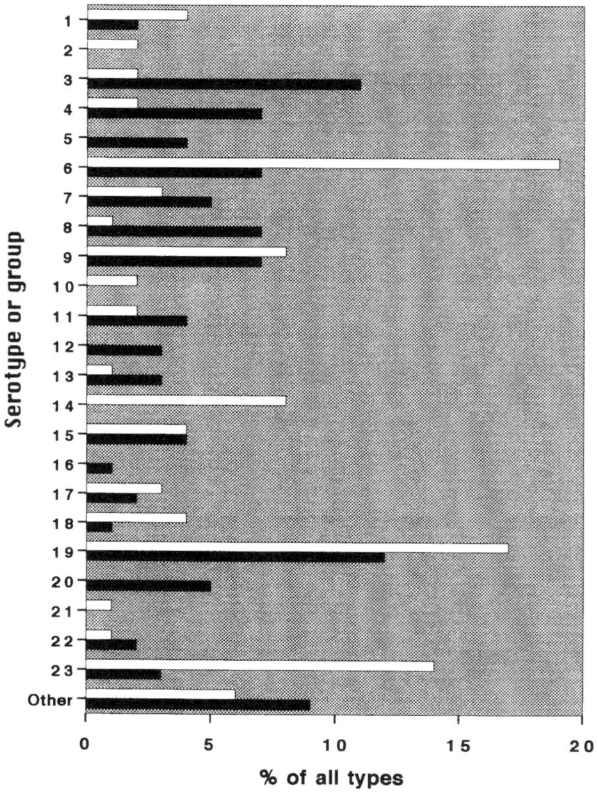

FIGURE 5.4 Serotype distribution in pneumococcal pneumonia in children and adults. Black indicates ≥ 15 years of age, white ≤ 15 years of age. (Adapted after Ref. 33.)

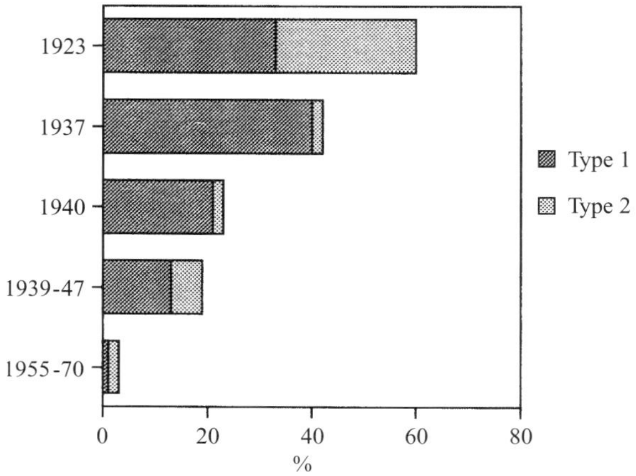

FIGURE 5.5 The frequencies of isolation of types 1 and 2 in Denmark in different years.

Despite the fact that an impressive amount of knowledge had been accumulated already in 1938, when White wrote his famous review of *The Biology of the Pneumococcus*[5], major deficiencies still exist in our understanding of pathogenesis in pneumococcal infection almost six decades later[2,4]. The mechanisms by which the pneumococci damage the human host are still obscure. Despite an often vigorous inflammatory reaction in the lung, structure is most often completely restored if a patient survives a pneumococcal pulmonary infection. Overwhelming growth within the pulmonary air space seems to be the primary mechanism by which the pneumococcus affects its host, but the aetiology of the (often severe) toxic symptoms remains obscure.

Mechanism of development of pneumonia

Pneumonia may occur by inhalation or aspiration of microorganisms, from bacteraemia, or by contagious spread. It is generally accepted that aspiration is the predominant way by which pneumococci reach the lung[1,59–61]. Aspiration of small amounts of pharyngeal material occurs regularly during sleep also in healthy individuals[62], but the bacteria which thereby reach the normally sterile subglottical space are usually effectively eliminated by cough, mucociliary transport, or if they reach the alveoli, by ingestion by macrophages or polymorphonuclear leukocytes[60]. Pneumonia may thus arise when the amount and virulence of aspirated bacteria overwhelm the defence mechanisms.

Pharyngeal carriage of *S. pneumoniae*, is a prerequisite for a pneumococcal pneumonia to develop, and may be very common in small children[59,63] and in patients with chronic obstructive pulmonary disease (COPD)[64], while in healthy adults rates of 3–18% are most often found today, the higher figure being more representative for parents of small children[26,65]. However, by using more sensitive methods for isolation, significantly higher carrier rates may be found. Several serotypes may be carried concomitantly[3,59,66]. Pneumococci seem to adhere to specific receptors on pharyngeal cells and a particular strain may be carried for several months[67]. During carriage there is a systemic type-specific antibody response, more regularly in older hosts. Pneumococcal disease usually develops early in the course of acquisition of the carrier state[66,68]. Viral respiratory tract infections are associated with an increase of the number of *S. pneumoniae* bacteria in carriers as well as with increases in carriage rates and pneumococcal infections. Carriage may also continue several weeks after a pneumococcal infection, and most antibiotics are ineffective in eliminating the bacteria from the nasopharynx.

The defence mechanisms normally preventing a pneumonic lesion from developing can be impaired by a number of chronic and acute conditions[1–3,60]. The amount of aspirated material may be increased in conditions with reduced consciousness, such as alcohol intoxication or CNS disease. The mucociliary transport system is constantly impaired in COPD, pulmonary oedema and during some viral infections; severe viral infections may also impair the function of alveolar macrophages and leukocytes[60,69–73] and bacteria seem to adhere preferentially to cells damaged by virus infections[64,74].

The pneumococcus is a prototypic extracellular pathogen, capable of causing disease only as long as it remains outside the phagocytes. It is unable to degrade its own hydrogen peroxide, which is released to the outside of the cell. Once inside a phagocytic vacuole, the pneumococci die.

The capsule

It has been known since the beginning of the century that the polysaccharide capsule is crucial for the virulence of the pneumococcus[1,2,4]. Rough strains without capsules are virtually avirulent, the number of pneumococci that are required to establish a lethal infection in laboratory animals being increased by a factor of 10^5. Though necessary for virulence, the capsular polysaccharides are non-toxic when injected into laboratory animals as pure substances. The mechanisms by which they promote virulence is by protecting the bacteria against immediate ingestion by animal phagocytes. However, there is a considerable difference in virulence among the 90 known capsular types; some of the capsular structures are connected with significant invasiveness, while most of them seem to confer only minor virulence. Another important factor is the thickness of the capsule – a substantially thicker capsule giving more protection against phagocytosis[2]. The binding of type-specific anti-capsular antibodies to the capsule, changes the structure of the cellular surface so that phagocytosis is facilitated. However, as described above, the capacity of raising antibodies against the capsular polysaccharides is remarkably different for different types in different age groups.

The cell wall

Toxic products produced during growth or degradation have been thought to be responsible for the often dramatic clinical presentation of a pneumococcal infection, but no single toxin or other cell product has been definitively identified as responsible. However, cell wall constituents seem to be largely responsible for the inflammatory reaction[1,2,9,75] (see Fig. 5.1). The phosphorylcholine residue of the C-polysaccharide is highly immunogenic, eliciting antibody response, complement activation and binding of an acute phase reactant beta-globulin of human serum, the C reactive protein (CRP). Furthermore, the latter reaction results in opsonisation and activation of complement. Two enzymes, neuramidase and pneumolysin, released primarily during autolysis may also be of importance in the pathogenesis[2,9,76]. The mechanism of release may be the reason for autolysin-deficient strains being less virulent than autolysin-producing variants. Also, the surface protein A may be involved in the pathogenetic events during pneumococcal infection[2,9] and both pneumolysin- and protein A-deficient strains show reduced virulence in experimental animals with prolonged survival of the animals after pneumococcal challenge. The same effect can also be achieved by active or passive immunisation of the animals against either of these two antigens. Pneumolysin also seems to be directly injurious both to the respiratory epithelium and to the pulmonary vascular endothelium[77,78]. However, although several new pathogenic facets have emerged in recent years, the importance of different mechanisms by which pneumococcal cell wall or other constituents, alone or in concert with each other and with host factors, damage the host are still largely obscure.

Antibody response and complement activation

Antibodies are crucial in the defence against infections caused by *S. pneumoniae*. In individuals lacking a normal B-cell defence, it is therefore one of the principal pathogens. Though an antibody response is elicited against several structures of the pneumococcus, such as the C-polysaccharide, the phosphorylcholine residue, and the pneumolysin, the only antibodies that are known to be of importance for mammalian defence against pneumococci are those directed against the type specific polysaccharide[1,2,9,68,79]. For example, in the constantly prevailing epidemic situation among South African gold mines, newcomers have often been struck by pneumococcal disease during the first six months, while thereafter the risk has been dramatically reduced due to the development of antibodies against the prevalent types[1,80]. It has now been shown that the risk of developing pneumonia with a certain serotype is very small in the presence of type-specific antibody, which normally develops in response to pharyngeal carriage[68]. The capsular polysaccharides are pure polysaccharides and as such elicit only a T-cell-independent antibody response. This implies that there most often will be an antibody response after antigenic stimulation by a particular polysaccharide, but no immunogenic memory and hence no booster response upon new contact with the same polysaccharide[2]. T-cell-independent antigens also elicit a poor antibody response in small children with their immature immune system; the weak or absent IgG2 response seems to be of particular importance. An adult or almost adult type of antibody response is acquired against most of the capsular types after 2 years of age. However, against some of the capsular polysaccharides, notably 6A, 14, 19F, and 23F, an adult type of antibody response is noted considerably later, so that a particular susceptibility to these types is seen until at least 5 years of age[55].

Complement activation seem to be an important part of the defence of mammalian hosts against pneumococcal infections, and congenital complement deficiencies may be associated with increased susceptibility to pneumococcal disease[1,2,4,60,61]. Complement is activated in several ways: by the reaction between C-polysaccharide and CRP, as well as by the hosts immunogenic reaction to the C-polysaccharide and to the type-specific polysaccharide. Activation of both the classic and the alternative pathways occurs.

Underlying conditions

Many underlying conditions are important for susceptibility to pneumococcal infection. Invasive disease is seen mainly in people with one of several such factors[12,15,16,51,18–20,42,81] (Table 5.2).

Table 5.2. *Conditions associated with increased susceptibility to pneumococcal disease*

Immunoglobulin deficiency
Congenital complement deficiency
Asplenia
Sickle cell disease
Nephrotic syndrome
Multiple myeloma
Malignant lymphoma
Bone marrow transplant
HIV disease
Alcoholism
Cirrhosis of the liver
Chronic renal failure
Chronic obstructive pulmonary disease
Chronic heart failure
Diabetes mellitus
Increased aspiration tendency
Cerebrospinal fluid leak
Age below 2–5 years
High age

Patients with anatomical (after trauma or surgery for medical reasons) or functional (as in sickle cell disease or after radiation) asplenia are at an 30–600 times increased risk of acquiring fulminant disease with encapsulated bacteria[1,82–84]. The risk is greatest in malignant disease and least marked after surgery for trauma. Patients splenectomised for non-malignant haematological disorders are at intermediate risk level. The risk is particularly high in small children and during the early years following splenectomy. Children with sickle cell disease are at a particularly high risk before 2 years of age because of their immature immune system. *S.pneumoniae* is responsible for at least half of the cases of infection with encapsulated bacteria in asplenic individuals and for most of the fatal ones. The reason for splenectomised individuals being more susceptibile to infection with encapsulated bacteria is probably the spleen's unique role in the clearance of non-opsonised organisms[2,85,86]. The spleen and the liver are the major organs involved in clearance of intravascular microorganisms, and the liver is, due to its size, the more important organ for opsonised agents, which are effectively bound to receptors on liver macrophages. The macrophages of the spleen, however, are unique in their ability to adhere and engulf non-opsonised encapsulated bacteria as well. In the absence of type-specific antibody or complement activation, a functioning spleen is therefore crucial. In asplenic individuals the number of intravascular bacteria may increase exponentially, and a clinical picture of overwhelming septicaemia with septic shock may develop. Since children have been exposed to fewer capsular types compared with adults, they are more prone to post-splenectomy septicaemia. In the abscence of other immunological defects, the capacity to mount an IgG response to pneumococcal polysaccharides, including the pneumococcal vaccine, seems to be essentially normal in asplenic individuals, and vaccination is an important prophylactic measure in these individuals. However, since the IgM response to polysaccharides is reduced in asplenic individuals, vaccination is generally recommended to be carried out two weeks before splenectomy if this can be arranged. In patients with Hodgkin's disease and other lymphomas, vaccination should be undertaken before both splenectomy and the start of chemotherapy. In patients who do not respond to the vaccine, especially in children with sickle cell disease, penicillin prophylaxis may be indicated. In recent years a reduction of the incidence of *S. pneumonia* infections has been noted in asplenic individuals older than two years of age. An increased awareness as well as the introduction of the 14-valent pneumococcal polysaccharide vaccine in 1978 may have been of importance[84,87].

Cirrhosis of the liver is also known to be associated with an increased susceptibility to serious pneumococcal infection, probably because of a reduced number of phagocytic cells. Many other chronic diseases, such as chronic heart failure, chronic obstructive pulmonary disease, diabetes mellitus and alcoholism have also been associated with increased susceptibility to pneumococcal disease.

Several other host defence deficiencies are also of importance[2,4,12]. Patients with a- or hypo-gammaglubulinaemia are prone to respiratory tract infections in early life, with the pneumococcus being the principal pathogen. IgG2 and IgG4 deficiencies are particularly important. Patients with secondary Ig deficiency, as in myeloma, may also develop severe pneumococcal infections. Although most individuals with IgA deficiency are symptom-free, some may have an increased incidence of respiratory infections due to extracellular organisms such as *S. pneumoniae* and *Haemophilus influenzae*. As indicated, complement is also important for the normal host defence against pneumococci. Hence, congenital or secondary C3 deficiency is connected with an increased frequency of pneumococcal infections. Some individuals with C2 deficiency in addition seem to be at increased risk.

The incidence of pneumococcal disease is greatly increased in the very young and in the elderly[3,12,15,23]. In small children the reason for the increased susceptibility is low antibody levels due to lack of exposure and an immature immune system with a particular deficient response to IgG2. In addition, children are more exposed to pneumococci because of their close contacts with other children, who may be carriers of pneumococci and who may be ill with viral respiratory infections (thus increasing the pneumococcal carriage rates and the numbers of bacteria in the carriers)[59,63,66]. In elderly individuals important factors seem to be a decline in T-cell numbers and function related to atrophy of the thymus, an inability of T-helper cells to secrete interleukin 2, a decreased humural response, and an impaired chemotaxis[88].

Pneumococcal disease and HIV

Individuals with human immunodeficiency virus (HIV) infection develop progressive dysfunction of both the cell-mediated and the humoral immune system[89]. The former is generally the more important for progressive HIV disease. Infections developing in individuals with a defective cellular response are the typical ones seen in advanced HIV disease. However, despite the defence against pneumococcal infection being virtually exclusively dependent on the normal function of B-cells, it is clear that the risk of such infections is greatly increased in HIV[89–96]. One factor of importance may be that a blunted B-cell response seem to be more prominent for T-cell independent antigens, like the pneumococcal polysaccharides, than for T-cell dependent antigens like proteins[97]. The incidence of pneumococcal bacteraemia appears to be 50–100-fold increased in patients with acquired immunodeficiency syndrome (AIDS) compared with the population in general. Approximately 5% of all admissions of AIDS patients are due to bacterial pneumonia. Pneumococcal pneumonia may be the first manifestation of HIV-infection in a substantial number of patients[90]. Symptomless also, HIV seems to be associated with a significantly increased risk of pneumococcal infection. The course of pneumococcal pneumonia may be more serious in HIV-infected individuals, and 30–60% of the cases may be associated with bacteraemia[89,92,93,95]. In general, clinical presentation is similar to that in non-HIV-infected individuals, but uncommon presentations have been described[89,95]. The case fatality rate for patients with pneumococcal pneumonia in asymptomatic HIV-infected individuals approximates that for non-HIV-infected patients. In AIDS patients it may be significantly higher in certain settings[92].

Clinical presentation

Few diseases have been so thoroughly described in the literature as pneumococcal pneumonia. The epidemiology and natural history, unaffected by antibiotic treatment, have been outstandingly described by Heffron in his excellent and comprehensive review of the accumulated knowledge of pneumococcal pneumonia until 1938[3].

The onset of pneumococcal pneumonia is often preceded by symptoms from a foregoing viral disease like coryza, mild upper respiratory tract illness and general malaise. The typical onset of the pneumococcal infection is a single sudden rigor with rapidly increasing fever and corresponding tachypnea and tachycardia[12,30,61]. This is followed by pleuritic chest pain and cough productive of sputum which is typically pinkish ('rusty') and may become greenish. Such a typical onset is often seen in young and middle-aged people, though all symptoms may not be present in each case. In elderly patients the onset may be insidious with few symptoms suggesting a pneumococcal pneumonia[12,30,98]. Respiratory symptoms may be minor or absent and the patient may even be afebrile. Occasionally toxic symptoms including general malaise, nausea, vomiting, diarrhoea, and headache predominate. In the elderly, confusion may be a salient symptom.

Repeated chills are not typical for pneumococcal pneumonia and may indicate an alternative aetiology. Chest pain may be severe and sometimes may be suggestive of pulmonary embolus. Lower lobe pneumonia can elicit diaphragmatic irritation, and abdominal pain or referred shoulder pain may dominate the presentation. Onset with abdominal pain as the most marked symptom is particularly common in children.

Without antimicrobial chemotherapy the patient continues to be toxic with sustained high fever and pleuritic chest pain for 7 to 10 days, whereupon defervescence and general improvement suddenly emerges (the 'crisis')[12].

Death may occur at any point in the course from respiratory or circulatory failure, from septic complications including meningitis or endocarditis, from non-infectious complications or from secondary hospital-acquired infections. In the antibiotic era, almost half of the deaths have occurred during the first 24 hours after admission when antibiotic therapy could have done little to change the course[14,20,39,98] (Fig. 5.6).

Physical examination

On examination, the patient with pneumococcal pneumonia is typically feverish, ill-looking with tachycardia and tachypnoea and sometimes cyanosis. The motion of the affected hemithorax is restricted, there is dullness on percussion with inspiratory rales and bronchial breath sounds. A pleuritic rub is occasionally noted. Upper abdominal tenderness resulting from diaphragmatic irritation may occur. Later in the course, abdominal distension due to paralytic ileus may be seen.

In elderly and severely toxic patients, who often have difficulties in co-operating fully, the findings may be few and non-characteristic. It is therefore not possible to exclude pneumococcal pneumonia without further investigations, most importantly the chest X-ray. If the patient is admitted during the first 24 hours after the initial rigor, physical findings may also be minor.

Laboratory findings

The chest X-ray may be normal if performed during the first 24 hours. After this time it typically reveals a homogeneous density which may be lobar or segmental[14,81,98,99] (Fig 5.7). The involvement of more than one lobe is common and has, in some studies, been connected with a more serious prognosis. A limited amount of pleural effusion is seen in a third of cases on lateral decubitus X-rays.

A marked polymorphonuclear leukocytosis is typically present[30,61]. In patients with severe infection, leukopenia may instead be found and is a poor prognosis indicator. The ESR is often not significantly raised when the patient presents, but then usually rises and stays high several weeks after clinical improvement. C-reactive protein (CRP) probably more accurately mirrors the clinical course because of its rapid increase at the start of the disease and its short half-life time[98]. CRP is most often raised to 20 to 100 times the normal value in pneumococcal pneumonia, also in elderly patients with atypical presentation, and it may be useful in the differentiation from atypical and viral pneumonia. In cases with rapid clinical improvement, CRP will be normalised within days, while in cases with suppurative complications the value remains elevated.

Aetiological diagnosis

A pneumococcal aetiology can be definitively established only by isolating the organism from a normally sterile site. Blood cultures are positive in only about 25% of admitted patients who can be sampled before initiation of antibiotic treatment and infrequently in those already receiving an antibiotic[1,14,27,31,100]. In a few more cases a definitive aetiology may be obtained by culture of pleural fluid. Invasive methods may be useful in certain situations or settings. Percutaneous lung aspiration culture is almost 100% specific and very sensitive[22]. Likewise, transtracheal aspiration generally gives accurate results, but false positive results occur. Given the high success rate with empiric antibiotic therapy in community-acquired pneumonia these two methods are not acceptable to the patient in ordinary settings[101]. Bronchoscopy with protected specimen brush and bronchoalveolar lavage, on the other hand, is time-consuming, but accurate and safe and is today probably the most accurate and feasible diagnostic approach in cases where an aetiologic diagnosis is crucial for the management of the patient and in cases when the patient does not respond to empiric antimicrobial chemotherapy[101–104].

In most cases of pneumonia today no aetiological diagnosis is obtained. The reason is that many patients have received antibiotic therapy before they are subjected to sampling for culture and obtaining adequate specimens, i.e. purulent sputum, is often difficult or impossible. However, by use of several different diagnostic methods a presumptive diagnosis can be arrived at in the majority of cases[27,28,100,101] (Table 5.3). In patients not treated with antibiotics and capable of producing a purulent sputum specimen, a Gram's-stained smear is a simple, specific (90%) and reasonably sensitive (60–85%) method to arrive at a presumptive diagnosis of a pneumococcal aetiology[27,101,105,106] (Fig. 5.8). With such specimens, culture is also most often positive, especially if done quantitatively after homogenisation of the specimen[65,107]. The accuracy of the sputum culture can be further improved if the bacteria preliminary identified within purulent parts of the Gram's stain smear are attempted to be identified on the culture plates[27,105]. Moreover, by applying a washing procedure before processing the sputum specimens, more than 99% of the contaminating oropharyngeal flora may be eliminated, improving specificity and easiness of interpretation of both Gram's-stains and cultures[65,107].

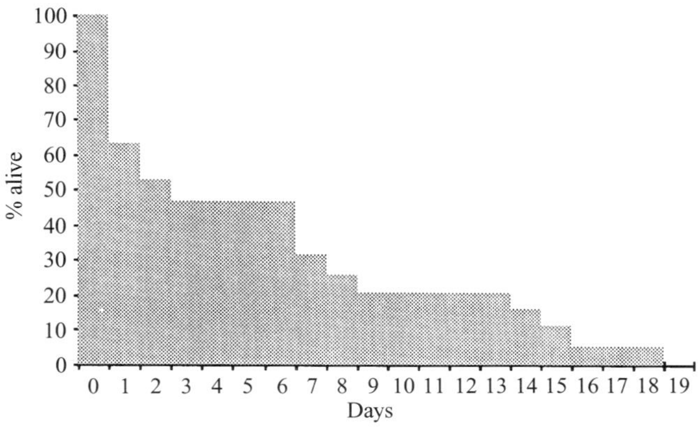

FIGURE 5.6 Interval between admission and death in bacteremic pneumococcal pneumonia in Sweden 1977–84. (Reproduced with permission from Örtqvist *et al.*, 1988[98].)

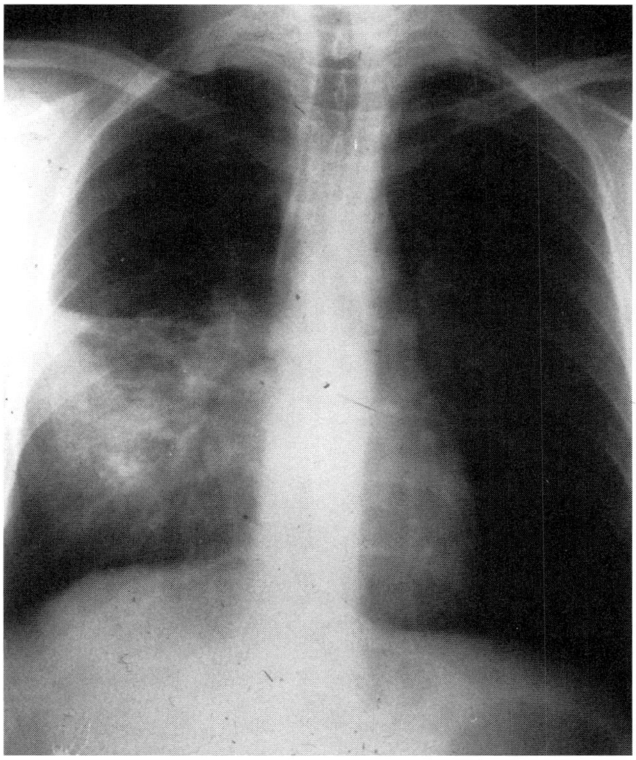

FIGURE 5.7 *Streptococcus pneumoniae* lobar pneumonia.

Table 5.3. *Frequency of positive results obtained with seven different methods for identification of pneumococci in pre- and post-treatment specimens from 93 patients with acute community-acquired pneumonia of probable pneumococcal origin*

	Pre-treatment samples		Post-treatment samples	
	Patients examined *n*	Patients positive %	Patients examined *n*	Patients positive %
Blood culture	64	25	17	6
Antigen detection in				
serum	34	3	77	9
urine	40	8	74	18
urine concentrated	40	18	74	24
sputum	50	56	66	56
Sputum culture	51	80	67	13
Sputum Gram's stain	49	65	65	17

Adapted after Kalin & Lindberg, 1983[27].

For patients on antibiotics, sputum Gram's stain and culture are almost useless[27,31,101]. However, soluble polysaccharide antigen may be detected in sputum by immunological methods such as coagglutination, latex agglutination, counterimmunoelectrophoresis (CIE), or enzyme immunoassays (EIA) with almost unchanged sensitivity for several days after start of antibiotic treatment[27,28,100,101,108–110]. Most antigen detection methods have been developed for detection of capsular polysaccharides, but examination for the species-specific C-polysaccharide is at least theoretically more attractive with lower risk of cross-reactions with contaminating bacteria[101,111]. Different methods for antigen detection and different criteria for diagnosing pneumococcal pneumonia produce a variable sensitivity range of between 50% and 100%. False positive reactions occur, but in most studies of pneumonia the frequency has been low. Antigen detection methods seem to give fairly accurate results also with non-purulent sputum specimens. However, when applied to serum or urine they contribute little to the diagnosis. The polysaccharide antigen concentration is not affected by the washing procedure[65,109].

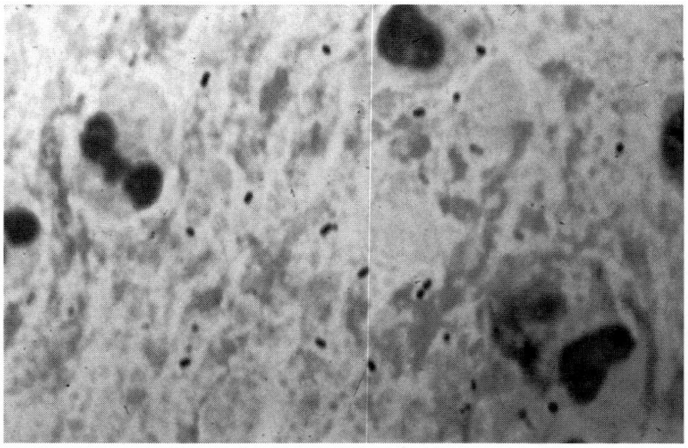

FIGURE 5.8 Sputum Gram's stain with many polymorphonuclear leukocytes and lanceolate-shaped Gram-positive diplococci. This finding is diagnostic for a pneumococcal aetiology.

Nasopharyngeal colonisation with pneumococci has been found to be strongly indicative of pneumococcal aetiology in adults with pneumonia. Given the low carriage rate in most populations today, the specificity will be acceptable for obtaining a presumptive diagnosis when other methods are failing (80–97%)[65,112,113].

Complications

There are several complications of pneumococcal pneumonia and these are summarised in Table 5.4. Atelectasis may occur before, or after, antibiotic therapy has been instituted. It may be prevented or managed by physiotherapy, or may resolve with or without minor scarring. Bronchoscopic aspiration may be indicated on rare occasions. More extensive pleural effusions, though most often sterile, may delay recovery and cause discomfort and impaired breathing. In such cases thoracocentesis is indicated. In most cases, however, the effusion is resorbed with minor or no scarring[99]. In the pre-antibiotic era, frank empyema (Fig. 5.9) was seen in 5% of the cases[3,12,95], but with adequate antibiotic therapy this complication is today noted in less than 2%[30,99,114]. Sustained fever and pleuritic pain, together with signs of pleural effusion, are seen. Without drainage, empyema leads to pleural scarring and impaired pulmonary function. With partially organised empyemas, ultrasound may be used to facilitate adequate drainage. Pyopneumothorax and bronchopleural fistulas were rare complications in the preantibiotic era also[3,12,95]. In most cases today with adequate antibiotic therapy, complete normalisation of the affected lung parenchyma and pleural space occurs within 8–18 weeks as indicated by follow-up chest X-rays[99]. Necrosis and cavitation are rare complications with a pure pneumococcal aetiology[115–117].

Pneumococcal pericarditis has become exceedingly rare, and the diagnosis therefore may be very difficult[118]; most patients also have pneumonia and empyema. Prompt adequate management with

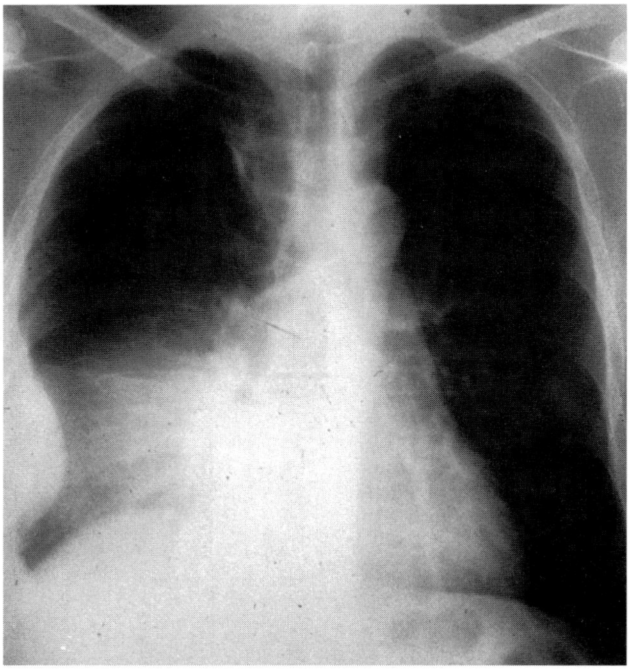

FIGURE 5.9 Chest X-ray showing empyema.

Table 5.4. *Complications of pneumococcal pneumonia*

Bacteraemia
Septic shock
Atelectasis
Pleural effusion
Empyema
Pyopneumothorax
Bronchopleural fistulas
Lung abscess
Pericarditis
Arthritis
Meningitis
Endocarditis
Peritonitis
Cellulitis
Brain abscess
Herpes labialis

surgical drainage is crucial. Both arthritis and meningitis occur more often without concomitant pneumonia as a result of bacteraemia probably emanating from the airways. Patients with impaired resistance to pneumococcal infection (see above) are more prone to develop meningitis during a pneumonia than are patients without significant underlying health problems. In conjunction with pneumonia it is more often seen in alcoholics, and before the advent of antibiotics the triad of pneumonia, meningitis and endocarditis was a classical presentation with 100% mortality in this patient group[3]. Pneumococcal meningitis may also develop as a result of contiguous spread in patients with CSF leakage following skull trauma. Pneumococcal endocarditis is today uncommon both as a primary disease and as a complication to pneumonia[119,120]. The proportion of infectious endocarditis due to *S. pneumoniae* has decreased significantly since the pre-antibiotic era, and is today most often little more than 1%. In some populations, for example, the Alaskan natives, the incidence of pneumococcal endocarditis is still significant, due to a more than 10-fold higher incidence of pneumococcal bacteraemia[119]. *S. pneumoniae* endocarditis is often aggressive, and heart valve replacement is frequently necessary[119,120].

Pneumococcal peritonitis is an extremely rare complication of pneumonia today. It was, however, previously a rather frequent complication of nephrotic syndrome and cirrhosis of the liver. Occasional cases of pneumococcal appendicitis have been described[121]. Cellulitis due to *S. pneumoniae* as a primary infection or as a consequence of bacteraemia was an infrequent occurrence also in the pre-antibiotic era. In one series it was reported to occur in 2% of cases of lobar pneumonia[3]. Facial cellulitis in children with hypogammaglobulinaemia is, however, well recognised[122], but in adults only some 15 cases have been described[95,123,124], two of which were due to direct extension from an underlying pulmonary focus. A few cases of epiglottitis with bacteraemia have been described[125]. Muscle abscesses and rhabdomyolysis have been described as caused by *S. pneumoniae* in a few instances[126, 127]. In 1943 *S. pneumoniae* was reported to be the aetiological agent in brain abscesses in 12.5% of the cases[128], while in more recent series 0–5% of the cases have been caused by this agent[95].

In patients with anatomical or functional (as in sickle cell disease) asplenia focal infections are the exception rather than the rule. The presentation is most often one of overwhelming septicaemia, with septic shock and sometimes purpura fulminans[82,83,129]. The mortality is high even with prompt antibiotic therapy and intensive care.

The frequency of secondary, hospital-acquired infection in community-acquired pneumonia has been found to be significant in a few previous American studies[130], but has recently been found to be below 1%[131].

Herpes labialis is a common complication in pneumococcal disease and occasionally may help suggest the aetiology when diagnostic methods have failed.

Management

Before the rapid emergence of resistance seen during the last two decades (see below) most antibiotics except aminoglycosides were shown to be effective in the treatment of pneumococcal pneumonia[1,30,132]. Among more recent antibiotics, the fluorinated quinolones are effective in most cases. However, bacteriological eradication is less effective than with other antibiotics, and many therapeutic failures have been reported[133,134]. The treatment of choice in uncomplicated cases of pneumococcal infection has been penicillin G or oral penicillin V 1–3 G daily in at least four divided doses. With the development of resistance against penicillin, the situation is today more complex. In patients with empyema, endocarditis or meningitis, and in critically ill patients, significantly higher doses, up to 12 G daily, are recommended. True penicillin allergy is uncommon and when it does occur cross-allergy with cephalosporins is unusual[135]; a cephalosporin is therefore in most cases the primary alternative both for oral and parenteral treatment. In patients with a history of anaphylactic reaction to any one of the betalactam agents, vancomycin, erythromycin or clindamycin are preferred.

The response to adequate antibiotic treatment in pneumococcal pneumonia is most often prompt, and a significant improvement is usually seen within 24–48 hours. In patients not improving within two to three days, another aetiology or a mixed aetiology[12,101] or a complication like empyema, meningitis or endocarditis should be suspected and ruled out by adequate diagnostic procedures. However, in many patients, no particular explanation is found and it can only be concluded that some patients respond slowly to therapy.

Antibiotic resistance in *S. pneumoniae*

Pneumococci were among the first organisms to acquire resistance to antimicrobials; both against optochin in 1912 and sulphapyridine in the 1930s. Resistant mutants soon developed after introduction of these drugs[1,132]. With the introduction of penicillin in the 1940s, the situation was dramatically changed: all strains were found to be very sensitive (MIC $\leq$ 0.01 μg/ml) – most patients responded rapidly and development of resistance was not a problem. However, by 1943 mutants resistant to penicillin were selected experimentally, so the emergence of strains with reduced susceptibility (MIC 0.12–1.0 μg/ml) in 1967 and of penicillin-resistance (MIC $\geq$ 2.0 μg/ml) and multiresistance involving most of the commonly used drugs 10 years later, is no surprise given the constantly increased consumption of antibiotics[59,132,136,137]. Today, strains with reduced susceptibility and resistance to penicillin and several other drugs can be found in most geographical areas, with different prevalences[132,136,137]. However, the great majority of strains are still fully susceptible. In some areas, however, notably South Africa, Spain, Hungary and Pakistan, the percentage of strains resistant to betalactam drugs now approaches 50%[80,136,138–146] (Table 5.5; Table 5.6; Fig. 5.10). The emergence of penicillin-insensitive pneumococci has, in several areas, been found to be preceded by an increased consumption of antibiotics[59,80,138,140,144,145].

Table 5.5. *Resistance to different antibiotics in* S. pneumoniae *in some countries, 1995, percentage of examined strains*

	Penicillin 0.12–1.0	Penicillin ≤ 2.0	Erythromycin ≤ 1.0	Tetracycline ≤ 8.0	Chloramphenicol ≤ 8.0
Spain	20	20	13	38	29
France	12	12	35	20	9
Hungary	20	26	45	59	28
USA	14	10	10	8	4
UK	2	2	9	5	1
Sweden	3	0.5	4	5	2

Table 5.6. *MIC for other betalactam-agents in pneumococci resistant to penicillin*

	Susceptible	Intermediate	Resistant
PcG	0.01	1	8
Ampicillin	0.01	1	8
Cefaclor	0.5	32	64
Cefalothin	0.1	4	16
Cefuroxime	0.06	2	16
Cefotaxime	0.01	0.5	2
Ceftriaxone	0.01	0.5	1
Imipenem	0.01	0.5	1

The mechanism by which pneumococci acquire resistance to penicillin is by alteration of the structure of one or more of the five high molecular weight penicillin binding proteins (PBP), so that their affinity for penicillin is reduced[132,146–150]. Stepwise changes of the PBPs have occurred, resulting in the emergence of strains with successively decreased binding of penicillin, corresponding to successively increased penicillin MICs. The PBPs, which are enzymes responsible for cell wall peptidoglycan synthesis, are the common targets for all β-lactam drugs, so reduced susceptibility to penicillin is always accompanied by reduced sensitivity to all other β-lactam drugs as well[137,132,151,152]. However, some β-lactam drugs, notably cefotaxim, ceftriaxone and meropenem, have thus far been less affected and in certain clinical settings have therefore, been effective for the treatment of infections caused by Penicillin-insensitive pneumococci (Table 5.7).

For the treatment of respiratory tract infections caused by intermediately resistant pneumococci, an increased dose of penicillin may be used in most cases, while for resistant strains cefotaxime, ceftriaxone, imipenem or non-β-lactam drugs may be preferred[80,137,140,151,153]. Pneumococcal meningitis poses special problems because of the limited penetration of antibiotics into the cerebrospinal fluid in combination with the need for bactericidal antibiotic concentrations; a bactericidal titre of at least ≥ 1:8 has been found necessary for effective bacterial killing to be achieved[137,152,154]. This can most often be reached with cefotaxime, ceftriaxone or meropenem against intermediately resistant strains, but only occasionally against resistant strains whose MICs are > 2–4 μg/ml. Strains with particularly high MICs to third generation cephalosporins leading to therapeutic failures have been identified and may increase in frequency in the future[145,146,155,156]. A further factor of importance in this context is the defective autolysis seen in the majority of penicillin-resistant pneumococci[132]. Exposure to a β-lactam drug in concentrations exceeding the MIC, results in inhibition of these strains, but very high concentrations may be required to achieve bacterial killing. Other drugs such as chloramphenicol which exhibit bacterial killing have been unsatisfactory for penicillin-insensitive strains[80,157].

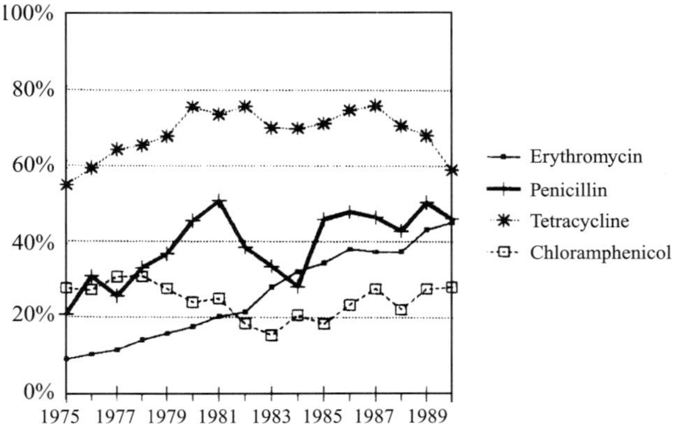

FIGURE 5.10 Antibiotic resistance in Hungary 1975–90. (Reproduced with permission from Marton *et al.*[145].)

The clinical experience achieved thus far indicates that treatment of meningitis with penicillin or ampicillin has been associated with increased rates of therapeutic failures both with resistant strains and with those with reduced susceptibility[80,137,140,151,155,158,159]. For intermediately resistant strains, cefotaxime, ceftriaxone or imipenem have most often been effective, while for strains with higher MIC-values there is no clearly effective alternative; combinations including two or more of these three β-lactam drugs, vancomycin and rifampicin have been used with variable success.

The molecular mechanisms involved in the emergence of β-lactam resistance in *S. pneumoniae* have been elucidated in recent years (Fig 5.11). By meticulous analysis of a large number of pneumococcal strains with different susceptibility patterns from several different geographic areas, evidence has accumulated pointing to emergence of resistance mediated through altered PBPs. Intra-species recombinational events have occurred, in which segments of native pneumococcal PBP genes have been replaced with the corresponding segments from related streptococcal species[147,148,150]. Such

Table 5.7. *Resistance patterns in strains of* S. pneumoniae *isolated in Spain and in South Africa*

Percentage of the total number of strains with any kind of resistance

	Spain	South Africa
Tetracycline	14	51
Tetracycline Chloroamphenicol	20	3
Tetracycline Chloramphenicol Penicillin	15	73
Penicillin	6	7
Tetracycline Chloramphenicol Penicillin Erythromycin	3	1
Tetracycline Penicillin	2	
Chloramphenicol	2	
Tetracycline Chloramphenicol Erythromycin	1	2
Tetracycline Penicillin	0.5	

Data from Fenoll *et al.*[138] and from Friedman & Klugman 1992*a*[139].

events have given rise to mosaic genes, coding for hybrid PBP-enzymes with decreased affinity for penicillin. Strains with such enzymes have had an increased chance of survival in an environment of substantial antibiotic pressure. In a few areas, probably because of particularly high antibiotic pressure, some strains have acquired several different gene fragments in a stepwise fashion, thus giving rise to complicated mosaic genes coding for grossly altered PBPs with low affinity for penicillin, thus implying high MICs. A few such evolved penicillin-resistant clones have been particularly successful and have spread between countries and even continents[136,146,149,150,160,161].

The prevalence of resistance to non-β-lactam drugs including tetracycline, erythromycin, clindamycin, chloramphenicol, and co-trimoxazole has also been reported to be alarmingly high and continually increasing in several countries[132,138–140,142,162]. Of particular concern is the great number of strains which are multi-resistant. Penicillin-resistant strains seem to be more prone to be resistant to non-β-lactam drugs as well. The most worrying current trends in Western countries, apart from Spain, are the rapid spread of β-lactam-resistant clones in some areas and the rapid increase of macrolide resistance[132,146,161].

Prophylaxis and control

Vaccination against pneumococcal disease was employed at the beginning of the twentieth century in South African gold miners, among whom the disease was widespread and carried a high mortality[1]. However, it was not until 1945, that it was clearly shown that a protective antibody response could be elicited by vaccination with purified capsular polysaccharides and that this protection was strictly type specific[163]. Due to the waning interest in pneumococcal infections after the introduction of penicillin, pneumococcal vaccine was not licensed until 1978 after the 'rediscovery' of the seriousness and impact of pneumococcal infections[14]. In the first commerciably available vaccine, the 14 most prevalent capsular polysaccharides were included, but in 1983 the number of polysaccharides included in the

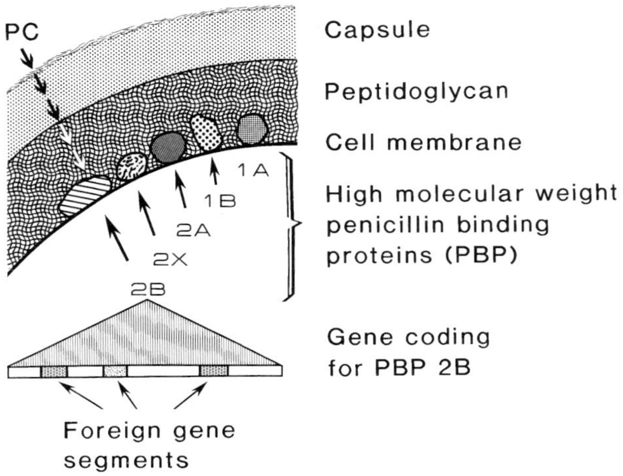

FIGURE 5.11 Schematic of the molecular basis for penicillin resistance in *S. pneumoniae*.

vaccine, based on worldwide prevalence studies as well as on immunological considerations was increased to 23[53]. The 23-valent vaccine covers at least 90% of the prevalent pneumococcal types in children as well as in adults in most parts of the world.

The pneumococcal polysaccharide vaccines have been shown to be about 80% protective in young male Africans and North Americans against invasive infection with the types included in the vaccine[1,164,165,166]. Unfortunately, in many patient groups with severe defects in the defence against pneumococcal infections, for example, those with immunoglobulin deficiency, myeloma, patients receiving immunosuppressive or cytotoxic therapy for transplant or malignant diseases, and those with advanced HIV disease, the vaccine response is severely impaired, in contrast to normal hosts[164–169]. Poor immunogenicity of the vaccine is also seen in children below 2 years of age and is due to their immature response to the T-cell independent polysaccharide antigens. Moreover, the antibody response to some types, notably the most prevalent children types, 6A, 14, 19F and 23F remains poor until at least 5 years of age[55, 164].

In developed countries, the most important target groups for the pneumococcal vaccine are individuals with underlying conditions predisposing to pneumococcal disease and elderly people in general with, or without, underlying diseases[164–169] (Table 5.8). As stated above, patients with some important underlying diseases respond poorly, while in those with asplenia, lymphoma before chemotherapy, nephrotic syndrome, chronic renal failure, liver cirrhosis, alcoholism, COPD, chronic heart disease, diabetes mellitus and HIV without AIDS, the response may be impaired but not absent. Since the incidence and/or the seriousness of pneumococcal disease in patients with these diseases is increased compared with the population in general, they are important target groups for an effective vaccine. In elderly individuals in general, both the incidence and severity of pneumococcal infections are high, while antibody response to the vaccine is only slightly impaired with increasing age[53,68,164, 170]. The pneumococcal vaccine has been shown to be protective in asplenic individuals, though to a limited degree in the very young – who unfortunately are at the highest risk[84,87,167,171]. For other risk groups who are able to mount an antibody response, for example, patients with diabetes mellitus, chronic heart or lung disease, an estimated protective efficacy of 60–80% against invasive disease with types included in the vaccine has been indicated by case control studies and by the indirect cohort studies[164,167,169]. For those with more profound immunosuppressive underlying diseases, including immunoglobulin deficiencies, malignant lymphomas and multiple myeloma, there is no clinical indication of protective efficacy, though patients with lymphomas may be able to respond to the vaccine prior to start of chemotherapy.

For the elderly, the results of several performed studies have been conflicting: there is only one published, prospective, randomised, controlled study[172] indicating an efficacy (77% decrease in pneumonia incidence), while there are several studies indicating lack of efficacy[164–166,173]. However, there are also three retrospective case-control studies showing about 70% protection against type-specific bacteraemic pneumococcal pneumonia[164]. Moreover, the data from the national pneumococcal surveillance study maintained by the Centers for Disease Control and Prevention, USA, has produced several reports on the protective efficacy of the vaccine by use of an indirect cohort method comparing the frequency of vaccine- and non-vaccine-types in vaccinated and unvaccinated individuals falling ill with invasive pneumococcal disease; the latest report indicates a protective efficacy of 75% in the immunocopetent elderly[167]. Finally, in a prospective case control study published in 1991, there was protective efficacy of 61%, against the types represented in the vaccine for immunocompetent individuals[169] (Table 5.9). No protection was found for immunocompromised patients. The protection declined with advancing age of the patient as well as with time after vaccination. No protection was found against non-vaccine types.

The lack of efficacy in most of the placebo-controlled prospective studies is probably due primarily to two facts: (i) the patient recruitment has been too small with the anticipated number of invasive pneumococcal events (non-invasive disease has not been included due to the uncertainty of the available diagnostic procedures), (ii) and patients with moderately immunosuppressive disease or therapy have been included. The vaccine response in such patients may be limited and irregular, thus reducing the possibilities of showing an efficacy for individuals responding.

Thus, the licensed pneumococcal polysaccharide vaccine is highly efficacious in preventing invasive pneumococcal disease in young immunocompetent persons. The vaccine also seems to be effective for preventing invasive disease in elderly immunocompetent individuals.

Table 5.8. *Recommendations for use of the 23-valent pneumococcal polysaccharide vaccine according to the Immunisation Practices Advisory Committee at the Center for Disease Control, USA*

1. Immunocompetent adults with chromic illnesses at an increased risk of pneumococcal disease or its complications
Chronic heart disease
Chronic pulmonory disease
Diabetes mellitus
Alcoholism
Liver cirrhosis
Cerebrospinal fluid leak
Individuals ≤ 65 years old
2. Immunocompromised adults at an increased risk of pneumococcal disease or its complications
Splenic dysfunction or asplenia
Hodgkins disease or other malignant lymphoma
Multiple myeloma
Chronic renal failure
Nephrotic syndrome
Organ transplant with immunosuppressive therapy
3. Children ≥ 2 years old with chronic illnesses specifically associated with increased risk of pneumococcal disease or its complications
Splenic dysfunction or asplenia, including sickle cell disease
Nephrotic syndrome
Cerebrospinal fluid leaks
Conditions associated with immunosuppression
4. Asymptomatic or symptomatic HIV infection in individuals > 2 years of age

Table 5.9. *Protective efficacy of pneumococcal polysaccharide vaccine against invasive infection with types included in the vaccine in immunocompetent patients*

Age (years)		Protective efficacy, % (95% CI) in relation to time since vaccination		
	n	< 3 years	3–5 years	> 5 years
< 55	125	93	89	85
		82/97	74/96	62/94
55–64	149	88	82	75
		70/95	57/93	38/90
65–74	213	80	71	58
		51/92	30/88	–2/83
75–84	188	67	53	32
		20/87	–15/81	–67/72
≥ 85	133	46	22	–13
		–31/78	–90/68	–174/54

Adapted after Shapiro *et al.*, 1991, *NEJM* 325: 1453[169].

Efficacy declines in the extreme elderly, but seems to be reasonable until 75–80 years of age. In immunocompromised individuals, not able to mount an antibody response, no efficacy is seen, while in those with moderately immunosuppressive diseases the efficacy is probably related to the immune responsiveness. There is a waning protection with time after vaccination related to decline in anticapsular antibody concentrations. Revaccination may therefore, be performed 3–10 years after the first vaccination if there is a continued risk of serious disease, especially if a rapid decline in pneumococcal antibody levels is diagnosed or anticipated[68,167,168,174]. It is still uncertain whether the vaccine conveys any protective efficacy against non-bacteraemic pneumococcal pneumonia[165,166]. Serious side-effects are virtually absent after primary vaccination and side-effects are similar in type and frequency if revaccination is performed at least 4 years later. Pneumococcal vaccination of patients at discharge from hospital with conditions constituting an indication for pneumococcal vaccination, has been recommended as efficient and cost effective[175,176].

In view of the high incidence and serious prognosis of pneumococcal infections pneumococcal vaccination should be considered in HIV-infected individuals[89,91,92,95,168]. The vaccine should probably be given as early as possible, since also asymptomatic HIV infection is associated with an increased susceptibility to pneumococcal disease and since the vaccine response is better the earlier in the course of an HIV infection it is given. The decreasing B-cell response seen during the course of HIV leads to progressively impaired antibody response to pneumococcal polysaccharide vaccine with decreased CD4 counts[96]. In asymptomatic individuals, the antibody response is essentially normal, while in patients with lymphadenopathy and AIDS-related complex (ARC) it is significantly decreased, and in AIDS patients the response to both T-cell dependent and independent antigens is partially or completely lost. In ARC/AIDS patients with CD4 cells below 400, the antibody response can be significantly improved with 4–54 weeks of zidovudine therapy prior to vaccination[176]. Revaccination should probably be offered 5–6 years after the first vaccination.

Major problems with vaccination against pneumococcal disease by use of the capsular polysaccharide vaccine are the poor response in many important target populations including children below 2 years of age, and the lack of immunogenic memory and booster effect upon revaccination. Immunogenic memory, as well as improved responsiveness in small children, has recently been shown to be achieved with pneumococcal capsular polysaccharides conjugated to a protein carrier[48,177–181]. However, at present only a limited number of polysaccharide–protein conjugates can be included in a vaccine, and since the distribution of prevalent capsular types is quite different in different population ages and in different geographical areas, there is a significant problem in determining which serotypes to include. However, the success of the *H. influenzae* conjugate vaccines for prevention of invasive *H. influenzae* type B disease holds promise for the future[182]. Different vaccines, appropriate for different target groups, may be necessary.

Areas for research

The structure and function of the pneumococcal cell has not been fully elucidated. Pneumolysin seems to be an important product, but its potency and importance as a toxin, as well as the possible implications for management and prophylaxis, have not been fully clarified. Other soluble or cell wall proteins may also be of importance in this context. The epidemiology of *S. pneumoniae* needs further study. The spread of strains in the community and the relation between carriage, pneumococcal disease, antibody development and underlying conditions should be areas for research, particularly now that typing methods other than serotyping are available. Pathogenesis of pneumococcal pneumonia, including the primary events before the pneumococci reach the alveoli, the causes of the sudden onset and the severe toxic symptoms as well as the factors behind development of bacteraemia are further factors which require elucidation.

Immunity against different capsular polysaccharides and other cell constituents requires clarification if vaccines are to be improved. Development of conjugate vaccines with much heightened immunogenicity is well on its way, but will need further intensive efforts. The protective efficacy, as well as the effectiveness of the pure polysaccharide vaccines and of different conjugate vaccine preparations in different population groups, will be very important areas for research in the near future. The prevalence of different pneumococcal types in different populations will need continued surveillance in order for the vaccines to be modified to give maximal protection.

The spectrum of clinical presentations of disease caused by *S. pneumoniae* and the prognosis in various settings need continued study in light of the changes noted during the twentieth century. Methods for aetiological diagnosis clearly need improvement, both for case management and for evaluation of protective efficacy in vaccine programmes. Management with antibiotics has to be continuously evaluated as new antibiotics become available and, more importantly, given the rapid emergence of antibiotic resistance of *S. pneumoniae*. Measures directed towards avoiding or reducing the emergence of antibiotic resistance are important to evaluate. The frequency and rate of resistance development in different areas is very different, hence antibiotic policies and other factors will not be uniform.

Summary

S. pneumoniae is the most common cause of pneumonia and is one of the infectious agents posing the most serious threats to human health. The incidence of pneumococcal pneumonia is at least 2 per 1000 person–years and is higher in small children and elderly. The precise incidence is impossible to establish due to lack of reliable diagnostic methods. The case fatality rate is round 5% in non-bacteraemic cases, 20% in bacteraemic pneumonia, and 30% in meningitis. Susceptibility to pneumococcal disease is especially high in small children in developing countries and in patients in the developed world with a number of underlying disorders, including functional asplenia, immunoglobulin and complement deficiencies, multiple myeloma, malignant lymphomas, chronic heart, lung and kidney diseases, alcoholism and HIV-infection.

Though major deficiencies still exist in our understanding of the pathogenesis of pneumococcal disease, it is clear that the function of B-lymphocytes is crucial, particularly in the production of IgG2. Antibody response is developed during pharyngeal colonisation, which is common in early childhood, and during infection. An antibody response is seen against several of the pneumococcal cell structures, but only antibodies directed against the capsular polysaccharide substances are protective. Thus, a certain specificity of antibody confers protection against only 1 of 90 known serotypes. Fortunately, only some 10–20 serotypes are prevalent at a given time in a given population, and most of the serotypes are not seen.

During the last few decades, a rapid emergence of resistance against penicillin and most of the other commonly used antimicrobial drugs has taken place, and in several geographic areas an alarmingly high prevalence of resistant strain has been noted. Resistance seem to have developed globally. In a few areas high level resistance clones have developed, which are constantly spreading between countries and even continents. The emergence of antibiotic resistance has created serious problems in the management of pneumococcal infections, especially meningitis.

Due to the seriousness of pneumococcal disease much effort has been put into the development of a vaccine. The presently available vaccine is a mixture of 23 capsular polysaccharides and provides 70% protection against invasive disease with the included types (covering about 90% of prevalent types in most areas) in hosts able to mount an antibody response against the polysaccharides. Unfortunately, many of the vaccine target groups, including children below the age of 2 and many immunosuppressed patients, are unable to respond to the vaccine. Moreover, immunogenic memory and booster effect upon revaccination are not acquired with vaccines consisting of pure polysaccharides. Therefore, vaccines with the polysaccharides conjugated to protein carriers are now being developed and these hold promise for the future, although the great number of prevalent serotypes poses special problems.

References

1. AUSTRIAN R. Some observations on the *Pneumococcus* and the current status of pneumococcal disease and its prevention. *Rev Infect Dis* 1981; 3 (Suppl):S1–S17.
2. BRUYN GAW, ZEGERS BJM, V.FURTH R. Mechanism of host defense against infection with *Streptococcus pneumoniae*. *Clin Infect Dis* 1992; 14:251–62.
3. HEFFRON R. Pneumonia: With Special Reference to *Pneumococcus* Lobar Pneumonia. A Commonwealth Fund book. Cambridge, MA: The Commonwealth Fund 1939 (Reprinted by Harvard Univeristy Press 1979).
4. JOHNSTON RB. Pathogenesis of pneumococcal pneumonia. *Rev Infect Dis* 1991; 13 (Suppl 6):S509–17.
5. WHITE, B. *The Biology of the Pneumococcus*. New York: The Commonwealth Fund; 1938 (Reprinted by Harvard Press 1979).
6. JENNINGS HJ, LUGOWSKI C, YOUNG NM. Structure of the complex polysaccharide C-substance from *Streptococcus pneumoniae* type 1. *Biochemistry* 1980; 19:4712–19.
7. TOMASZ A. Surface components of *Streptococcus pneumoniae*. *Rev Infect Dis* 1981; 3:190–211.
8. SØRENSEN UBS, BLOM J, BIRCH-ANDERSEN A, HENRICHSEN J. Ultrastructural localization of capsular, cell wall polysaccharide, cell wall proteins and F antigen in the *Pneumococci*. *Infect Immun* 1988; 56:1890–6.
9. BOULNOIS GJ. Pneumococcal proteins and the pathogenseis of disease caused by *Streptococcus pneumoniae*. *J Gen Microbiol* 1992; 138:249–59.
10. FISCHER W, BEHR T, HARTMANN R, PETER-KATALINIC J, EGGE H. Teichoic acid and lipoteichoic acid of *Streptococcus pneumoniae* possess identical chain structures. A reinvestigation of teichoic acid (C polysaccharide). *Eur J Biochem* 1993; 215:851–7.
11. SØRENSEN UBS, HENRICHSEN J, CHEN HC, SZU SC. Covalent linkage between the capsular *polysaccharide* and the cell wall peptidoglycan of *Streptococcus pneumoniae* revealed by immunochemical methods. *Microb Pathog* 1990; 8:325–34.
12. CECIL RL, BALDWIN HS, LARSEN NP. Clinical and bacteriologic study of 2000 typed cases of lobar pneumonia. *Arch Intern Med* 1927; 40:253–80.
13. FINLAND, M. Pneumonia and pneumococcal infections, with special reference to pneumococcal pneumonia. *Am Rev Resp Dis* 1979; 120:481–502.
14. AUSTRIAN R, GOLD J. Pneumococcal bacteraemia with especial reference to bacteraemic pneumococcal pneumonia. *Ann Intern Med* 1964; 60:759–76.
15. BURMAN LÅ, NORRBY R, TROLLFORS B. Invasive pneumococcal infections: Incidence, predisposing factors and prognosis. *Rev Infect Dis*, 1985; 7:133–42.
16. FILICE GA, DARBY CP, FRASER DW. Pneumococcal bacteraemia in Charleston County, South Carolina. *Am J Epidemiol* 1980; 112:828–35.
17. MARRIE TJ. Bacteremic pneumococcal pneumonia: a continuously evolving disease. *J Infect* 1992; 24:247–56.
18. MUFSON MA, KRUSS DM, WASIL RE, METZGER WI. Capsular types and outcome of bacteraemic pneumococcal disease in the antibiotic era. *Arch Intern Med* 1974; 134:505–10.
19. MUFSON MA, OLEY G, HUGHEY D. Pneumococcal disease in a medium-sized community in the United States. *JAMA* 1982; 248:1486–9.
20. ÖRTQVIST Å, KALIN M, JULANDER I, MUFSON MA. Deaths in pneumococcal

pneumonia. A comparison of two populations – Huntington WVa, and Stockholm, Sweden. *Chest* 1993; 103:710–16.

21. MONTO AS. Acute respiratory infection in children of developing countries: challenge of the 1990s. *Rev Infect Dis* 1989; 11:498–505.
22. SHANN F. Etiology of severe pneumonia in children in developing countries. *Pediatr Infect Dis J* 1986; 5:247–252.
23. BREIMAN RF, SPIKA JS, NAVARRO VJ, DARDEN PM, DARBY CP. Pneumococcal bacteraemia in Charleston County, South Carolina. A decade later. *Arch Intern Med* 1990; 150:1401–5.
24. FACKLAM RR BREIMAN RF. Current trends in bacterial respiratory pathogens. *Am J Med* 1991; 91 (Suppl 6A):3S–11S.
25. FANG G-D, FINE M, ORLOFF J, ARISUMI D, KAPOOR W. New and emerging etiologies for community-acquired pneumonia with implications for therapy. A prospective multicenter study of 359 cases. *Medicine (Baltimore)* 1990; 69:307–16.
26. FOY HM, WENTWORTH B, KENNY GE, KLOECK JM, GRAYSTON JM. Pneumococcal isolations from patients with pneumonia and control subjects in a prepaid medical care group. *Am Rev Respir Dis* 1975; 111:595–603.
27. KALIN M LINDBERG AA. Diagnosis of pneumococcal pneumonia: a comparison between microscopic examination of expectorate, antigen detection and cultural procedures. *Scand J Infect* Dis 1983; 15:247–55.
28. MACFARLANE JT, FINCH RG, WARD MJ, MACREA AD Hospital study of adult community-acquired pneumonia. *Lancet* 1982; 2:255–8.
29. MACFARLANE J. An overview of community acquired pneumonia with lessons learned from the British Thoracic Society study. *Sem Resp Infect* 1994; 9:153–65.
30. MUSHER DM. State-of-the-art clinical article. Infections caused by *Streptococcus pneumoniae*: clinical spectrum, pathogenesis, immunity, and treatment. *Clin Infect Dis* 1992; 14:801–9.
31. NORRBY SR, POPE KA. Pneumococcal pneumonia. *J Infect* 1979; 1:109–20.
32. ÖRTQVIST Å, HEDLUND J, GRILLNER L *et al.* Etiology, outcome and prognostic factors in patients with community-acquired pneumonia requiring hospitalization. *Eur Respir J* 1990; 3:1105–13.
33. OSEASOHN R, SKIPPER BE, TEMPEST B. Pneumonia in a Navajo community. A two-year experience. *Am Rev Respir Dis* 1978; 117;1003–9.
34. PECHÈRE JC. Epidemiology of microorganisms causing community-acquired pneumonia. *JAMA* 1990; Suppl vol 6 (3):10–13.
35. MOINE P, VERCKEN J-B, CHEVRET S, CHASTANG C, GAJDOS P. Severe community-acquired pneumonia. Etiology, epidemiology, and prognosis factors. *Chest* 1994; 105:1487–95.
36. TORRES A, SERRA-BATLLES J, FERRER A *et al.* Severe community-acquired pneumonia. Epidemiology and prognostic factors. *Am Rev Resp Dis* 1991; 144:312–18.
37. GESSNER BD, USSERY XT, PARKINSON AJ, BREIMAN RF. Risk factors for invasive disease caused by *Streptococcus pneumoniae* among Alaska native children younger than two years of age. *Pediatr Infect Dis J* 1995; 14:123–8.
38. TAKALA AK, JERO J, KELA E, RÖNNBERG, P-R, KOSKENNIEMI E, ESKOLA J. Risk factors for primary invasive pneumococcal disease among children in Finland. *JAMA* 1995; 273:859–64.
39. GRANSDEN WR, EYKYN SJ, PHILLIPS I. Pneumococcal bacteraemia: 325 episodes at St Thomas's Hospital. *Br Med J* 1985; 290:505–8.
40. KUIKKA A, SYRJÄNEN J, RENKONEN O-V, VALTONEN VV. Pneumococcal bacteraemia during a recent decade. *J Infect* 1992; 24:157–68.
41. SIEGMAN-IGRA Y, SCHWARTZ D, ALPERIN H, KONFORTI N. Invasive pneumococcal infection in Israel. *Scand J Infect Dis* 1986; 18:511–17.
42. WATANAKUNAKORN, C., GREIFENSTEIN, A., STROH, K *et al.* Pneumococcal bacteraemia in three community teaching hospitals from 1980 to 1989. *Chest* 1993; 103:1152–6.
43. DEMARIA A, BROWNE K, BERK SL, SHERWOOD E, MCCABE WR. An outbreak of type 1 pneumococcal pneumonia in a men's shelter. *JAMA* 1980; 244:1446–9.
44. HODGES, R.G. & MACLEOD, C.M. Epidemic pneumococcal pneumonia V. Final consideration of the factors underlying the epidemic. *Am J Hyg* 1946; 44:237–43.
45. MERCAT A, NGUYEN J, DAUTZENBERG N. An outbreak of pneumococcal pneumonia in two men's shelters. *Chest* 1991; 99:147–51.
46. QUICK RE, HOGE CW, HAMILTON DJ, WHITNEY CJ, BORGES M, KOBAYASHI JM. Underutilization of pneumococcal vaccine in nursing homes in Washington state: report of a serotype-specific outbreak and a survey. *Am J Med* 1993; 94:149–52.
47. HENRICHSEN J. The pneumococcal typing system and pneumococcal surveillance. *J Infect* 1979; 1(suppl 2):31–7.
48. BALTIMORE RS. New challenges in the development of a conjugate pneumococcal vaccine. *JAMA* 1992; 268:3366–7.
49. GRAY BM, DILLON HC. Clinical and epidemiologic studies of pneumococcal infection in children. *Pediatr Infect Dis J* 1986; 5:201–7.
50. KALIN M, LINDBERG AA. Distribution of pneumococcal types in the Stockholm region 1976–78. *Scand J Infect* Dis 1980; 12:91–5.
51. KLEIN JO The epidemiology of pneumococcal disease in infants and children. *Rev Infect Dis* 1981; 3:246–53.
52. LUND E. Distribution of *Pneumococcus* types at different times in different areas. *Bayer-Symposium III*, 1971:49–56.
53. ROBBINS JB, AUSTRIAN R, LEE CJ *et al.* Considerations for formulating the second generation pneumococcal capsular polysaccharide vaccine with emphasis on the cross-reactive types within groups. *J Infect Dis* 1983; 148:1136–59.
54. SMART LE, PLATT DJ, TIMBURY MC. A comparison of the distribution of pneumococcal types in systemic disease and the upper respiratory tract in adults and children. *Epidemiol Infect* 1987; 98:203–9.
55. DOUGLAS RM, PATON JC, DUNCAN SJ, HANSMAN DJ. Antibody response to pneumococcal vaccination in children younger than five years of age. *J Infect Dis* 1983; 148:131–7.
56. FINLAND M, BARNES MW. Changes in occurrence of capsular serotypes of *Streptococcus pneumoniae* at Boston City Hospital during selected years between 1935 and 1974. *J Clin Microbiol* 1977; 5:154–66.
57. TILGHMAN RC, FINLAND M. Clinical significance of bacteraemia in pneumococcal pneumonia. *Arch Intern Med* 1937; 59:602–19.
58. GREENWOOD BM, HASSAN-KING M, ONYEMELUKWE G. Pneumococcal serotypes in West Africa. *Lancet* 1980; 1:360.
59. AUSTRIAN R. Some aspects on the pneumococcal carrier state. *J Antimicrob Chemother* 1986; 18 (Suppl A):35–45.
60. BUSSE WW. Pathogenesis and sequelae of respiratory infections. *Rev Infect Dis* 1991; 13(Suppl 6):S477–85.
61. COONROD JD. Pneumococcal pneumonia. *Sem Respir Infect* 1989; 4:4–11.
62. HUXLEY EJ, VIROSLAV J, GRAY WR, PIERCE AK. Pharyngeal aspiration in normal adults and patients with depressed consciousness. *Am J Med* 1978; 64:564–8.
63. HENDLEY JO, SANDE MA, STEWART PM, GWALTNEY JM. Spread of *Streptococcus pneumoniae* in families. I. Carriage rates and distribution of types. *J Infect Dis* 1975; 132:55–61.
64. MURPHY TF, SETHI S. Bacterial infection in chronic obstructive pulmonary disease. *Am Rev Resp Dis* 1992; 146:1067–83.

65. KALIN M. Bacteremic pneumococcal pneumonia: value of nasopharynx culture and examination of washed sputum specimens. *Eur J Clin Microbiol* 1982; 1:394–6.

66. GWALTNEY JM, SANDE MA, AUSTRIAN R, HENDLEY JO. Spread of *Streptococcus pneumoniae* in families. II. Relation of transfer of *S.pneumoniae* to incidence of colds and serum antibody. *J Infect Dis* 1975; 132:62–8.

67. LODA FA, COLLIER AM, GLEZEN WP, STRANGERT K, CLYDE WA, DENNY FW. Occurence of *Diplococcus pneumoniae* in the upper respiratory tract of children. *J Pediatrics* 1975; 87:1087–93.

68. MUSHER DM, GROOVER JE, ROWLAND JM *et al.* Antibody to capsular polysaccharides of *Streptococcus pneumoniae*: prevalence, persistence, and antibody response. *Clin Infect Dis* 1993; 17:66–73.

69. ANONYMOUS. How does influenza pave the way for bacteria [Editorial]. *Lancet* 1982; 1:485–6.

70. JAKAB GJ. Mechanisms of virus-induced bacterial superinfections of the lung. *Clin Chest Med* 1981; 89:53–67.

71. LARSON HE, PARRY RP, TYRELL DAJ. Impaired polymorphonuclear leukocyte chemotaxis after influenza virus infection. *Br J Dis Chest* 1980; 74:56–62.

72. MCINTOSH K. Pathogenesis of severe acute respiratory infections in the developing world: respiratory syncytial virus and parainfluenza viruses. *Rev Infect Dis* 1991; 13(Suppl 6):S492–500.

73. VERHOEF J, MILLS EL, DEBETS-OSSENKOPP Y, VERBRUGH HA. The effect of influenza virus on oxygen-dependent metabolism of human neutrophils. *Adv Exp Med Biol* 1982; 41:647–54.

74. PLOTKOWSKI M-C, PUCHELLE E, BECK G, JACQOUOT J, HANNOUN C. Adherence of type 1 *Streptococcus pneumoniae* to tracheal epithelium of mice infected with influenza A/PR8 virus. *Am Rev Resp Dis* 1986; 134:1040–4.

75. TUOMANEN E, TOMASZ A, HENGSTLER B, ZAK O. The relative role of bacterial cell wall and capsule in the induction of inflammation in pneumococcal meningitis. *J Infect Dis* 1985; 151:535–40.

76. BERRY AM, YOTHER J, BRILES DE, HANSMAN D, PATON JC. Reduced virulence of a defined pneumolysin-negative mutant of *Streptococcus pneumoniae. Infect Immunun* 1989; 57:2037–42.

77. RUBINS JB, DUANE PG, CHARBONEAU D, JANOFF EN. Toxicity of pneumolysin to pulmonary endothelial cells *in vitro. Infect Immun* 1992; 60:1740–6.

78. STEINFORT C, WILSON R, MITCHELL T. Effect of *Streptococcus pneumoniae* on human respiratory epithelium *in vitro. Infect Immun* 1989; 57:2006–13.

79. KALIN M, KANCLERSKI K, GRANSTRÖM M, MÖLLBY R. Diagnosis of pneumococcal pneumonia by enzyme linked immunosorbent assay of antibodies to pneumococcal hemolysin (Pneumolysin). *J Clin Microbiol* 1987; 25:226–229.

80. KOORNHOF HJ, WASAS A, KLUGMAN K. Antimicrobial resistance in *Streptococcus pneumoniae*: a South African perspective. *Clin Infect Dis* 1992; 15:84–94.

81. ORT S, RYAN JL, BARDEN G, DÉSOPO N. Pneumococcal pneumonia in hospitalized patients: clinical and radiological presentations. *JAMA* 1983; 249:214–18.

82. KINGSTON ME, MCKENZIE CR. The syndrome of pneumococcemia, disseminated intravascular coagulation and asplenia. *Can Med Assoc* J 1979; 121:57–61.

83. SINGER DB. Postsplenectomy sepsis. *Persp Pediatr Pathol* 1973; 1:285–311.

84. WONG W-Y, OVERTURF GD, POWARS DR. Infection caused by *Streptococcus pneumoniae* in children with sickle cell disease: epidemiology, immunologic mechanisms, prophylaxis, and vaccination. *Clin Infect Dis* 1992; 14:1124–36.

85. BROWN EJ, HOSEA SW, FRANK MM. The role of the spleen in experimental pneumococcal bacteraemia. *J Clin Invest* 1981; 67:975–82.

86. HOSEA SW, BROWN EJ, HAMBURGER MI, FRANK MM. Opsonic requirements for intravascular clearance after splenectomy. *N Engl J Med* 1981; 304:245–50.

87. KONRADSEN HB, HENRICHSEN J. Pneumococcal infections in splenectomized children are preventable. *Acta Paediatr Scand* 1991; 80:423–7.

88. SIMONS RJ, REYNOLDS HY. Altered immune status in the elderly. *Sem Respir Infect* 1990; 5:251–9.

89. JANOFF EN, BREIMAN RF, DALEY CL, HOPEWELL PC. Pneumococcal disease during HIV infection. Epidemiologic, clinical, and immunologic perspectives. *Ann Intern Med* 1992; 117:314–24.

90. GARCIA-LEONI ME, MORENO S, RODENO P, CERCENADO E, VICENTE T, BOUZA E. Pneumococcal pneumonia in adult hospitalized patients infected with the human immunodeficiency virus. *Arch Intern Med* 1992, 152:1808–12.

91. JANOFF EN, O´BRIEN J, THOMPSON P *et al. Streptococcus pneumoniae* colonization, bacteraemia, and immune response among persons with human immunodeficiency virus infection. *J Infect Dis* 1993; 167:49–56.

92. PESOLA GR, CHARLES A. Pneumococcal bacteraemia with pneumonia. Mortality in acquired immunodeficiency syndrome. *Chest* 1992; 101:150–5.

93. POLSKY B, GOLD, JWM, WHIMBERLEY E *et al.* Bacterial pneumonia in patients with the acquired immune deficiency syndrome. *Arch Intern Med* 1986; 104:38–41.

94. REDD SC, RUTHERFORD GW, SANDE MA, LIFSON AR, HADLEY WK, FACKLAM RR. The role of human immunodeficiency virus infection in pneumococcal bacteraemia in San Francisco residents. *J Infect Dis* 1990; 162:1012–17.

95. RODRIGUEZ-BARRADAS MC, MUSHER DM, HAMILL RJ, DOWELL M, BAGWELL JT, SANDERS CV. Unusual manifestations of pneumococcal infection in human immunodeficiency virus-infected individuals: the past revisited. *Clin Infect Dis* 1992; 14:192–9.

96. RODRIGUEZ-BARRADAS MC, MUSHER DM, LAHART C *et al.* Antibody to capsular polysaccharides of *Streptococcus pneumoniae* after vaccination of HIV-infected subjects with 23-valent pneumococcal vaccine. *J Infect Dis* 1992; 165:553–6.

97. BALLET JJ, SULCEBE G, COUDERC LJ, DANON F, RABIAN C, LATHROP M. Impaired antipneumococcal antibody response in patients with AIDS-related persistent generalized lymphadenopathy. *Clin Exp Immunol* 1987; 68:479–87.

98. ÖRTQVIST Å, GREPE A, JULANDER I, KALIN M. Bacteremic pneumococcal pneumonia in Sweden: clinical course and outcome and comparison of the clinical picture with non-bacteraemic pneumococcal pneumonia and *Mycoplasma* pneumonia. *Scand J Infect Dis* 1988; 20:163–171.

99. JAY SJ, JOHANSON WG, PIERCE AK. The radigraphic resolution of *Streptococcus pneumoniae* pneumonia. *N Engl J Med* 1975; 293:798–801.

100. RESEARCH COMMITTEE OF BRITISH THORACIC SOCIETY AND PUBLIC HEALTH LABORATORY SERVICE Community-acquired pneumonia in adults in British hospitals 1982–1983: a survey of aetiology, mortality, prognostic factors, and outcome. *Quart J Med* 1987; 239:195–220.

101. FARRINGTON M, RUBINSTEIN D. Antigen detection in pneumococcal pneumonia. *J Infect* 1991; 23:109–16.

102. BROUGHTON WA, MIDDLETON RM, KIRKPATRICK MB, BASS JB. Bronchoscopic protected specimen brush and bronchoalveolar lavage in the diagnosis of bacterial pneumonia. *Infect Dis Clin North Am* 1991; 5:437–452.

103. MEDURI GU, BASELSKI V. The role of bronchoalveolar lavage in diagnosing nonopportunistic bacterial pneumonia. *Chest* 1991; 100:179–90.

104. ÖRTQVIST Å, KALIN M, LEJDEBORN L, LUNDBERG L. Diagnostic fiberoptic bronchoscopy and protected brush culture in patients with community-acquired pneumonia. *Chest*, 1990; 97:576–82.

105. HEINEMAN HS, CHAWLA JK, LOFTON WM. Misinformation from sputum cultures without microscopic examination. *J Clin Microbiol* 1977; 6:518–27.

106. REIN MF, GWALTNEY JM JR, O´BRIEN WM, JENNINGS RH, MANDELL GL. Accuracy of Gram´s stain in identifying *Pneumococci* in sputum. *JAMA* 1978; 239:2671–3.

107. BARTLETT JG, FINEGOLD SM. Bacteriology of expectorated sputum with quantitative culture and wash technique compared to transtracheal aspirates. *Am Rev Resp Dis* 1978; 117:1019–27.

108. BOERSMA WG, LÖWENBERG A, HOLLOWAY Y, KUTTSCHRÜTTER H, SNIJDER JAM, KOETER GH. Pneumococcal antigen persistence in sputum from patients with community acquired pneumonia. *Chest* 1992; 102:422–7.

109. HOLLOWAY Y, BOERSMA WG, KUTTSCHRÜTTER H, SNIJDER JAM. Effect of washing sputum on detection of pneumococcal capsular antigen. *Eur J Clin Microbiol Infect Dis* 1991; 10:567–569.

110. VENKATESAN P, MACFARLANE JT Pneumococcal antigen in the diagnosis of pneumococcal pneumonia. *Thorax*, 1992; 47:329–331.

111. ÖRTQVIST Å, JÖNSSON I, KALIN M, KROOK A. Comparison of three methods for detection of pneumococcal antigen in sputum of patients with community-acquired pneumonia. *Eur J Clin Microbiol Infect Dis* 1989; 9:725–31.

112. HEDLUND J, KALIN M, ÖRTQVIST Å. Nasopharyngeal culture in the pneumonia diagnosis. *Infection* 1990; 18:283–5.

113. BURMAN LÅ, TROLLFORS B, ANDERSSON B *et al.* Diagnosis of pneumonia by cultures, bacterial and viral antigen detection tests, and serology with special reference to antibodies against pneumococcal antigens. *J Infect Dis* 1991; 163:1087–93.

114. LIGHT RW, GIRARD WM, JENKONSON SG, GEORGE RB. Parapneumonic effusion. *Am J Med* 1980; 69:507–12.

115. HAMMOND JMJ, LYDDELL C, POTGIETER PD, ODELL J. Severe pneumococcal pneumonia complicated by massive pulmonary gangrene. *Chest* 1993, 104:1610–12.

116. KEREM E, ZIV YB, RUDENSKI B, KATZ S, KLEID D, BRANSKI D. Bacteremic necrotizing pneumococcal pneumonia in children. *Am J Respir Crit Care Med* 1994; 149:242–4.

117. YANGCO BG, DERESINSKI SC. Necrotizing or cavitating pneumonia due to *Streptococcus pneumoniae*: report of four cases and review of the literature. *Medicine* 1980; 59:449–57.

118. BERK SL, RICE PA, REYNHOLDS CA, FINLAND M. Pneumococcal pericarditis: a persisting problem in contemporary diagnosis. *Am J Med* 1981;70:247–51.

119. FINLEY JC, DAVIDSON M, PARKINSON AJ, SULLIVAN RW. Pneumococcal endocarditis in Alaska natives. A population-based experience, 1978 through 1990. *Arch Intern Med* 1992; 152:1641–5.

120. POWDERLY WG, STANLEY SL JR, MEDOFF G. Pneumococcal endocarditis: report of a series and review of the literature. *Rev Infect Dis* 1986; 8:786–91.

121. HELTBERG O, KORNER B, SCHOUENBORG P. Six cases of acute appendicitis with secondary peritonitis caused by *Streptococcus pneumoniae*. *Eur J Clin Microbiol* 1984; 3:141–3.

122. POWELL KR, KAPLAN SB, HALL CB, NASELLA MA, ROGHMANN KR. Periorbital cellulitis: clinical and laboratory findings in 146 episodes, including tear countercurrent immunoelectrophoresis in 89 episodes. *Am J Dis Child* 1988; 142:853–7.

123. HAUBRICH RH, KEROACK MA Pneumococcal crepitant cellulitis caused by a bronchocutaneous fistula. *Chest* 1992; 101:566–7.

124. LAWLOR MT, CROWE HM, QUINTILIANI R. Cellulitis due to *Streptococcus pneumoniae*: case report and review. *Clin Infect Dis* 1992; 14:247–50.

125. DAUM RS, NACHMAN JP, LEITCH CD, TENOVER FC. Nosocomial epiglottitis associated with penicillin- and cephalosporin-resistant *Streptococcus pneumoniae* bacteraemia. *J Clin Microbiol* 1994; 32:246–8.

126. PEETERMANS WE, BUYSE B, VANHOOF J. Pyogenic abscess of the gluteal muscle due to *Streptococcus pneumoniae*. *Clin Infect Dis* 1993; 17:939.

127. SPATARO V, MARONE C. Rhabdomyolysis associated with bacteraemia due to *Streptococcus pneumoniae*: case report and review. *Clin Infect Dis* 1993; 17:1063–4

128. MCFARLAN AM. The bacteriology of brain abscess. *BMJ*, 1943; 2:643–4.

129. WARA DW. Host defence against *Streptococcus pneumoniae*. The role of the spleen. *Rev Infect Dis* 1981; 3:299–309.

130. TILLOTSON JR, FINLAND M. Bacterial colonization and clinical superinfection of the respiratory tract complicating antibiotic treatment of pneumonia. *J Infect Dis* 1969; 119:597–624.

131. ÖRTQVIST Å, HAMMERS-BERGGREN S, KALIN M. Respiratory tract colonization, and occurrence of secondary infections, during hospital treatment of community-acquired pneumonia. *Eur J Clin Microbiol Infect Dis* 1990; 9:725–31.

132. KLUGMAN K. Pneumococcal resistance to antibiotics. *Clin Microbiol Rev* 1990; 3:171–96.

133. SULLIVAN MC, COOPER BW, NIGHTGALE CH, QUINTILIANI R, LAWLOR MT Evaluation of the efficacy of ciprofloxacin against *Streptococcus pneumoniae* by using a mouse protection model. *Antimicr Agent Chemother* 1993; 37:234–9.

134. THYS JP, JACOBS F, BYL B. Role of quinolones in the treatment of bronchopulmonary infections, particularly pneumococcal and community-acquired pneumonia. *Eur J Clin Microbiol Infect Dis* 1991; 10:304–15.

135. BEELEY L. Allergy to penicillin. *Brit Med J* 1984; 288:511–12.

136. APPELBAUM PC. Antimicrobial resistance in *Streptococcus pneumoniae*: an overview. *Clin Infect Dis* 1992;15:77–83.

137. JACOBS MR. Treatment and diagnosis of infections caused by drug-resistant *Streptococcus pneumoniae. Clin Infect Dis* 1992; 15:119–27.

138. FENOLL A, BOURGON MC, MUNOZ R, VICIOSO D, CASAL J. Serotype distribution and antimicrobial resistance of *Streptococcus pneumoniae* isolates causing systemic infections in Spain, 1979–1989. *Rev Infect Dis* 1991; 13:56–60.

139. FRIEDLAND IR, KLUGMAN KP. Antibiotic-resistant pneumococcal disease in South African children. *Am J Dis Child* 1992; 146:920–3.

140. LINARES J, PALLARES R, ALONSO T *et al.* Trends in antimicrobial resistance of clinical isolates of *Streptococcus pneumoniae* in Bellvitge Hospital, Barcelona, Spain (1979–1990). *Clin Infect Dis* 1992; 15:99–105.

141. JACOBS MR, KOORNHOF HJ, ROBINS-BROWNE RM *et al.* Emergence of multiply resistant *Pneumococci*. *N Engl J Med* 1978; 299:735–40.

142. MARTON A. Pneumococcal antimicrobial resistance: the problem in Hungary. *Clin Infect Dis* 1992; 15:106–11.

143. MASTRO TD, GHAFOOR A, NORMANI N. Antimicrobial resistance of *Pneumococci* in children with acute lower respiratory tract disease. *Lancet* 1991; 337:156–9.

144. JOHNSON AP, SPELLER DCE, GEORGE RC, WARNER M, DOMINGUE G, EFSTRATIOU A. Prevalence of antibiotic

resistance and serotypes in pneumococci in England and Wales: results of observational surveys in 1990 and 1995. *Br Med J* 1996; 312:1454–6.
145. MARTON A, GULYAS M, MUNOZ, R TOMASZ A Extremely high incidence of antibiotic resistance in clinical isolates of *Streptococcus pneumoniae* in Hungary. *J Infect Dis* 163:542–8.
146. DOERN GV, BRUEGGEMAN A, HOLLEY HP, RAUCH AM. Antimicrobial resistance of Streptococcus pneumoniae recovered from outpatients in the United States during the winter months of 1994 to 1995: results of a 30-center national surveillance study. *Antimicrob Agent Chemother* 1996; 40:1208–13.
147. COFFEY TJ, DOWSON CG, DANIELS M *et al.* Horizontal transfer of multiple penicillin-binding protein genes, and capsular biosynthetic genes, in natural populations of *Streptococcus pneumoniae*. *Mol Biol* 1991; 5:2255–60.
148. JABES D, NACHMAN S, TOMASZ A. Penicillin-binding protein families: evidence for the clonal nature of penicillin resistance in clinical isolates of *Pneumococci*. *J Infect Dis* 1989; 159:16–25.
149. HAKENBECK R, BRIESE T, CHALKLEY L *et al.* Antigenic variation of penicillin-binding proteins from penicillin-resistant clinical strains of *Streptococcus pneumoniae*. *J Infect Dis* 1991; 164:313–19.
150. MUNOZ R, MUSSER, JM, CRAIN M *et al.* Geographic distribution of penicillin-resistant clones of *Streptococcus pneumoniae*: characterization by penicillin-binding protein profile, surface protein A typing, and multilocus enzyme analysis. *Clin Infect Dis* 1992; 15:112–18.
151. LINARES J, ALONSO T, PERZ JL, AYATS J, DOMINGUEZ MA, PALLARES R, MARTIN R. Decreased susceptibility of penicillin-resistant *Pneumococci* to twenty-four beta-lactam antibiotics. *J Antimicrob Chemother* 1992; 30:279–88.
152. NEAL TJ, O´DONOGHUE MAT, RIDGEWAY EJ, ALLEN KD. *In-vitro* activity of ten antimicrobial agents against penicillin-resistant *Streptococcus pneumoniae J Antimicr Chemother* 1992; 30:39–46.
153. MOINE P, VALLEÉ E, AZOULAY-DUPUIS E *et al. In vivo* efficacy of a broad-spectrum cephalosporin, ceftriaxone, against penicillin-susceptible and -resistant strains of *Streptococcus pneumoniae* in a mouse pneumonia model. *Antimicrob Agents Chemother* 1994; 38:1953–8.
154. MCCRACKEN GH JR, SAKATA Y. Antimicrobial therapy of experimental meningitis caused by *Streptococcus pneumoniae* strains with different susceptibilities to penicillin. *Antimicrob Agent Chemother* 1985; 27:141–5.
155. FRIEDLAND IR, SHELTON S, PARIS M *et al.* Dilemmas in diagnosis and management of cephalosporin-resistant *Streptococcus pneumoniae* meningitis. *Pediatr Infect Dis J* 1993; 12:196–200.
156. SLOAS MM, BARETT FF, CHESNEY PJ, ENGLISH BK, HILL BC, TENOVE FC, LEGGIADRO RJ. Cephalosporin treatment failure in penicillin- and cephalosporin-resistant *Streptococcus pneumoniae* meningitis. *Pediatr Infect Dis J* 1992; 11:662–6.
157. FRIEDLAND IR, KLUGMAN KP. Failure of chloramphenicol therapy in penicillin-resistant pneumococcal meningitis. *Lancet* 1992; 339:405–8.
158. FRIEDLAND IR, PARIS M, EHRETT S, HICKEY S, OLSEN K, MCCRACKEN GH. Evaluation of antimicrobial regimens for treatment of experimental penicillin- and cephalosporin-resistant pneumococcal meningitis. *Antimicrob Agents Chemother* 1993; 37:1630–6.
159. VILADRICH PF, GUDIOL F, LINARES J *et al.* Evaluation of vancomycin for therapy of adult pneumococcal meningitis. *Antimicrob Agents Chemother* 1991; 35:2467–72
160. MCDOUGAL LK, FACKLAM R, REEVES M *et al.* Analysis of multiply antimicrobial-resistant isolates of *Streptococcus pneumoniae* from the United States. *Antimicrob Agents Chemother* 1992; 36:2176–84.
161. SOARES S, KRISTINSSON KG, MUSSER JM, TOMASZ A. Evidence for the introduction of a multiresistant clone of serotype 6B *Streptococcus pneumoniae* from Spain to Iceland in the late 1980s. *J Infect Dis* 1993; 168:158–63.
162. GESLIN P, BUU-HOI A, FRÉMAUX A, ACAR FJ. Antimicrobial resistance in *Streptococcus pneumoniae*: an epidemiological survey in France, 1970–1990. *Clin Infect Dis* 1992, 15:95–8.
163. MACLEOD CM, HODGES RG, HEIDELBERGER M, BERNHARD WG Prevention of pneumococcal pneumonia by immunisation with specific capsular polysaccharides. *J Exp Med* 1945; 82:445–65.
164. BRUYN GAW, V.FURTH R. Pneumococcal polysaccharide vaccines: indications, efficacy and recommendations. *Eur J Clin Microbiol Infect Dis* 1991; 10:897–910.
165. FEDSON DS Pneumococcal vaccination in the prevention of community-acquired pneumonia: an optimistic view of cost-effectiveness. *Sem Resp Infect* 1993; 8:285–93.
166. FINE MJ, SMITH MA, CARSON CA *et al.* Efficacy of pneumococcal vaccination in adults. A meta-analysis of randomized controlled trials. *Arch Intern Med* 1994. 154:2666–77.
167. BUTLER JC, BREIMAN RF, CAMPBELL JF, LIPMAN HB, BROOME CV, FACKLAM RR. Pneumococcal polysaccharide vaccine efficacy. An evaluation of current recommendations. *JAMA* 1993; 270:1826–31.
168. IMMUNIZATION PRACTICES ADVISORY COMMITTEE. Pneumococcal polysaccharide vaccine. *Morb Mort Wkl Rep* 1989; 38:64–76.
169. SHAPIRO ED, BERG AT, AUSTRIAN R *et al.* The protective efficacy of polyvalent pneumococcal polysaccharide vaccine. *N Engl J Med* 1991; 325.1453–60.
170. MUSHER DM, LUCHI JM, WATSON DA, HAMILTON R, BAUGHN RE. Pneumococcal polysaccharide vaccine in young adults and older bronchitics: determination of IgG responses by ELISA and the effect of adsorbtion of serum with non-type-specific cell wall polysaccharide. *J Infect Dis* 1990; 161:728–35.
171. AMMAN AJ, ADDIEGO J, WARA DW, LUBIN B, SMITH WB, MENTZER WB. Polyvalent pneumococcal polysaccharide immunization of patients with sickle cell anemia and patients with splenectomy. *N Engl J Med* 1977; 297:897–900.
172. GAILLAT J, ZMIROU D, MALLARET *et al.* Essai clinique du vaccin antipneumococcique chez des personnes agees vivant en institution. Revue dépidemiologie et de sante Publique, 1985; 33:437–44.
173. LAFORCE FM, EIKOFF TC. Pneumococcal vaccine: an emerging consensus. *Ann Intern Med* 1988; 108:757–9.
174. MUFSON MA, HUGHEY DF, TURNER CE, SCHIFFMAN G. Revaccination with pneumococcal vaccine of elderly persons 6 years after primary vaccination. *Vaccine* 1991; 9:403–7.
175. FEDSON DS, CHIARELLO LA. Previous hospital care and pneumococcal bacteraemia. *Arch Intern Med* 1983; 143:885–9.
176. GLASER JB, VOLPE S, AGUIRRE A, SIMPKINS H, SCHIFFMAN G. Zidovudine improves response to pneumococcal vaccine among persons with AIDS and AIDS-related complex. *J Infect Dis* 1991; 164:761–4.
177. FATTOM A, LUE C, SZU C *et al.* Serum antibody response in adult volunteers elicited by injection of *Streptococcus pneumoniae* type 12F polysaccharide alone or conjugated to diphtheria toxoid. *Infect Immun* 1990; 58:2309–12.
178. GIEBINK GS, KOSKELA M, VELLA PP, HARRIS M, LE CT. Pneumococcal capsular polysaccharide-meningococcal outer membrane protein complex conjugate vaccines: immunogenicity and efficacy in experimental pneumococcal otitis media. *J Infect Dis* 1993; 167:347–55.

179. PATON JC, LOCK RA, LEE C-J *et al.* Purification and immunogenicity of genetically obtained pneumolysin toxoids and their conjugation to *Streptococcus pneumoniae* type 19F polysaccharide. *Infect Immun* 1991; 59:2297–304.

180. SARNIAK S, KAPLAN J, SCHIFFMAN G, BRYLA D, ROBBINS JB, SCHNEERSON R. Studies on pneumococcus vaccine alone or mixed with DTP and on pneumococcus type 6B and *Haemophilus influenzae* type b capsular polysaccharide-tetanus toxoid conjugates in two- to five-year-old children with sickle cell anemia. *Pediatr Infect Dis J* 1990;9:181–6.

181. STEINHOFF MC. Developing and deploying pneumococcal and *Haemophilus* vaccines. *Lancet* 1993; 342: 630–1.

182. SHAPIRO ED. Infections caused by *Haemophilus influenzae* type b. The beginning of the end? *JAMA* 1993; 269:264–6.

6 Staphylococcal pneumonia

MICHAEL E. ELLIS
King Faisal Specialist Hospital and Research Centre, Riyadh, Saudi Arabia

Introduction

Staphylococcal pneumonia is a cause of substantial morbidity and mortality. Previously, *Staphylococcus aureus* was thought to be an uncommon aetiological agent in both community and hospital-acquired pneumonia, possibly because relatively little attention had been focused on it relative to other causes of pneumonia, for example, nosocomial Gram-negative pneumonia. Evidence is accruing, however, that places a greater emphasis on this pathogen. Recent literature suggests its contribution to pneumonia is increasingly recognised, emergence of methicillin resistant *S. aureus* in both the community and hospital is presenting therapeutic and management challenges, it may be under-diagnosed in HIV positive patients and there are significant shifts from previously perceived epidemiological-clinical features. *S. aureus* is the organism responsible for staphylococcal pneumonia and there is no definitive evidence that *Staphylococcus epidermidis* causes pneumonia.

Table 6.1. *Important cellular components*

Peptidoglycan	Fixed
Teichoic acid	
Protein A	
Microcapsule	
Specific surface adhesions	
Clumping factor	
Coagulase	Soluble
Catalase	
Hyaluronidase	
Lipase	
α, β, γ, δ, TSST-1 toxins	
Toxic oxygen radicals	

Microbiology, pathology and immunology

S. aureus is a 0.9 mμ coccus, and member of the family micrococcacae whose triple axes division leads to a clustered appearance; occasionally five-membered chains occur. It is a Gram-positive organism but may appear Gram-negative within phagocytes or if aged. Facultatively anaerobic and growing on non-selective media/blood agar *S. aureus* prefers aerobic conditions under which well-demarcated, smooth, convexed colonies have enhanced production of golden carotenoid pigment. Characteristics permitting differentiation from *S. epidermidis* and *Staphylococcus saprophyticus* include plasma coagulation (coagulase positivity), mannitol fermentation and positive deoxyribonuclease reactivity.

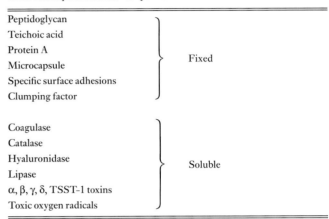

The important ultrastructural antigenic components (Table 6.1) are cell wall surface polysaccharide and protein binding peptidoglycan, teichoic acid and protein A. Although peptidoglycan confers stability, opsonic IgG antibodies are stimulated, which are only partly host protective and, in addition, may induce toxic antigen–antibody complex mediated reactions. Interleukin-1 is also produced from monocytes. Peptidoglycan and teichoic acid can activate the alternative pathway of complement, whilst the classical pathway is activated through C1q binding and antibody/cell wall constituent interactions. Phagocytic attraction is then mediated via C5a and phagocytic attachment occurs. Peptidoglycan is also known to generate tumour necrosis factor which further activates polymorphs. Protein A, linked to peptidoglycan is of the utmost importance in biological and immunopathological reactions. For example, each molecule attaches to two molecules of immunoglobulin via the Fc portion, resulting in inhibition of phagocytosis of antibody-coated bacteria. There are 80 000 binding sites per bacterium. The gene coding for protein A has been cloned and sequenced. Protein A can also directly lead to platelet injury.

Ribitol-phosphate teichoic acid appears necessary for phage receptor function, for maintaining the normal physiological milieu of the cell, and extracellular teichoic acid may be protective to the bacterium by diverting complement components away from the bacteria by consuming human IgG and complement. Raised teichoic acid antibodies may be a good indicator of invasive staphylococcal disease, for example, in endocarditis and in cystic fibrosis patients.

Some strains of *S. aureus* possess a capsule. Only a few strains have morphologically distinct large capsules and these are associated with mucoid colonies. They are called Smith strains and are of serotypes 1 and 2. These are not common human pathogens. Many more strains possess capsules visible only by electronmicroscopy (microcapsules). Most *S. aureus* strains isolated from clinical material are microencapsulated. The microcapsule surface antigens are, to some degree, antiphagocytic as evidenced by the enhanced polymorph ingestion that occurs in the presence of anticapsular antibody. This permits colonisation with the organism and permits spread within the host.

Surface protein receptor/binding sites also favour colonisation and further spread via attachment to the many proteins found in the host cell, for example, wound fibronectin, fibrinogen, vitronectin, thrombospondin, collagen and laminin of basement membranes.

Elaboration of these host cell proteins on damaged endothelial cells and on foreign bodies such as intravascular devices, prostheses and osseus implants, permits adhesion of *S. aureus* via staphylococcal surface adhesins. Adhesion is irreversible due to covalent binding forces. The binding domain for *S. aureus* has been identified in some of the host proteins, for example, fibrinogen, which lies within the terminal part of the gamma chain[1]. Similarly, the specific fibronectin adhesion site on *S. aureus* and the corresponding genes have been identified recently[2]. This phenomenon impedes phagocytosis, establishing a substantial infection focus which can act as a source for bacteraemia, metastatic staphylococci foci, and poor therapeutic outcome unless the foreign body is removed. Following adhesion, there is rapid formation of a glycocalyx around the organisms which presents a physical barrier to antibiotic penetration[3]. However, antibiotics have been known to penetrate into this biofilm[4]. Adaptive antibiotic resistance as a result of the foreign body has also been suggested[5].

Clumping of staphylococci is a phenomenon due to the presence of cell wall fibrinogen binding clumping factor. This clumping factor is found in coagulase-producing organisms but differs from free coagulase enzyme production. In capsulated strains, however, the capsule surrounds the clumping factor.

It is clear that, after intact skin/mucus membrane and other mechanical barriers, the polymorph is the principal host defence mechanism. Thus patients with impaired polymorph phagocytic function are at high risk for *S. aureus* infection. These include such predisposing conditions as alcoholism, diabetes mellitus, chronic liver disease, renal dysfunction and malnutrition. Antibody integrity is thought not so clinically important, despite *in vitro* evidence of increased phagocytic uptake in the presence of antibody, including complement defective situations[6].

A number of soluble enzymes and toxins, which are important in pathogenesis, are secreted by *S. aureus*. Among these, coagulase, catalase, hyaluronidase, lipase and toxins are the most understood. Coagulase precipitates fibrin in the immediate vicinity of the bacteria. This impedes phagocytic access. By self-coating with host fibrin, *S. aureus* avoids phagocytosis. Catalase is an important bacterial defence mechanism, which can destroy the bactericidal toxic oxygen radicals produced by host neutrophils. Lipase ensures survival and dissemination of *S. aureus* and hyaluronidase hydrolyses the matrix of connective tissue ensuring dissemination.

Four haemolytic toxins are produced, α, β, γ, δ, which are all broad spectrum cell membrane poisons particularly to erythrocytes, platelets and leukocytes to a variable degree. In addition, α toxin is dermatonecrotic and δ toxin stimulates cyclic AMP production leading to inhibition of ileal water absorption and to diarrhoea, features which characterise disseminated *S. aureus* infection. Leucocidin is another membrane poison but is non-haemolytic. It consists of two different antigen components which act synergistically on leukocyte membranes resulting in permeability access to cations and discharge of lysosomal granules. Staphylococcal enterotoxins A–E are associated with food poisoning, whilst enterotoxin F and toxic shock syndrome-associated toxins (TSST-1) have been indicated in staphylococcal toxic shock syndrome. TSST-1 behaves as a superantigen producing a strong clonal lymphoproliferative driven release of interleukin-1/tumour necrosis factor and other cytokines resulting in severe clinical sepsis[7]. Two types of exfoliative toxins have been identified, which can split the cementing intracellular matrix to produce the staphylococcal scalded skin syndrome.

Table 6.2. *Antibiotic resistance*

β-lactamase
PBP2[1]
Tolerance
Altered normally present PBP

PBP = penicillin binding protein.

Resistance to antimicrobials (Table 6.2) particularly β-lactams, including methicillin, is also an adaptive genetically versatile property of *S. aureus*[8–11] and may be due to: (i) plasmid-mediated β-lactamase production. These bacteria will usually be susceptible to β-lactam stable antibiotics such as cloxacillin. Approximately 75% of staphylococci are penicillinase producers and resistant to penicillin G/V; (ii) chromosomally mediated alteration of penicillin binding protein (PBP) with a reduced affinity for binding methicillin (intrinsic resistance). PBP are cell membrane enzymes responsible for cell wall synthesis but are capable of binding β-lactam antibiotics which then prevent the antimicrobial activity of the β-lactam. In the case of methicillin resistant *S. aureus* (MRSA), these are PBP2[1]. Only a minority of MRSA cells express methicillin resistance and therefore resistance may not be detected by regular laboratory methods, a phenomenon called heteroresistance. Intrinsic resistance can be detected by a high MIC (> 20 μm/ml) for methicillin; (iii) tolerance as defined by disproportionate MBC/MIC (conventionally taken as a 32-fold increase in MBC/MIC), and possibly due to autolytic enzyme failure; (iv) another mechanism relates to the presence of altered penicillin binding capacity of normally present PBPs and the absence of PBP2[1] binding proteins. MRSA strains frequently associated with multiple resistance to other antibiotics have emerged in recent years and is a worrying trend, often associated with nosocomial disease and outbreaks in many hospitals. The MRSA may reach epidemic proportions and proves difficult to eradicate from the environment. Some strains are even resistant to glycopeptide antibiotics such as teicoplanin, and treatment failures have been reported.

In summary, the first barrier of host defence is provided by intact skin and mucosa, where breach of these barriers, which include traumatised skin allows access of *S. aureus* to fibronectin and other proteins, which permits adhesion and initial bacterial invasion. An effective polymorphonuclear mobilisation and ingestion response is then essential, together with an intact opsonisation system involving complement, immunoglobulins and other facets of the immune system to contain the bacteria. Intracellular killing of *S. aureus* is achieved by the production of toxic oxygen radicals. The role of the cell-mediated immune system remains unclear.

Following seeding of the lung via bronchogenous or haematogenous routes, there is an intense pathological reaction as a result of the potent toxins and enzymes previously described. The effect of lipase and hyaluronidase and α toxin particularly facilitate dissemination through the tissue to produce a suppurative pathology with necrosis and abscess formation. This may later communicate with the pleural space or lead to pneumatoceles. Involvement of arterial walls leads to septic lung infarction.

Epidemiology and predisposing factors

S. aureus infections are commonly implicated in a wide range of both hospital and community acquired infections. These encompass involvement of skin and soft tissue, bone and joint, renal, cardiovascular including endocarditis, and intravascular access devices, central nervous, muscle and respiratory systems. Currently, *S. aureus* accounts for approximately 15% of bacteraemias in the UK[12] and is the second most common cause of bacteraemias seen in some hospitals[13]. *S. aureus* is generally acknowledged as being an uncommon, if not rare, cause of pneumonia in adults. For example, over a 12-year period in the Trent region in the UK, only 61 cases among adults were identified[14]. There are no precise statistics, but it is felt that *S. aureus* infections in general, and including pneumonia, may be increasing[14,15]. This is not surprising, given the rise in prevalence of predisposing conditions for *S. aureus* sepsis, for example, rising population of the elderly, use of immunosuppressive therapeutics, HIV disease, institutionalised care, antimicrobial resistance and invasive device usage. Over a 3-year period in a US tertiary care hospital, between 1989 and 1992, 162 *S. aureus* infections were seen, compared to 139 in a preceding 5-year period[16]. Of *S. aureus* infections seen between 1989 and 1992, 22/162 (13.6%) were pneumonic/pleural space infections. Most of these were required nosocomially. MRSA accounted for just over half of all strains[16].

In a 2500 bed hospital in Taipei, 138 cases of non-intravenous drug abusing patients with *S. aureus* septicaemia were seen in a 2-year period, 1985–1986, of which 34 (24%) had pulmonary involvement[17]. As a cause of pulmonary infections overall, data from large studies suggest that up to 10% of all community-acquired pneumonias are due to *S. aureus*[18,19]. However, some series report higher rates. For example, among 96 adult patients with community-acquired pneumonia seen at the National University Hospital, Singapore, *S. aureus* was found almost as commonly as *Haemophilus influenzae* and *Mycoplasma pneumoniae*, (4.2% of patients compared to 5.2% and 5.2%, respectively)[20]. As a cause of nosocomial pneumonia, in general, this is approximately 10%[21]. Again, this lower figure has been challenged, for example, among 500 intensive care patients from five hospitals in Kentucky, the most common isolates from sputum was *S. aureus* (26.6%), whereas *Pseudomonas* species were second most frequent at 24.8%[22]. Other centres have reported the increasing importance of *S. aureus* among critically ill patients, particularly in the genesis of ventilator-associated pneumonia[23]. In a recent study from Spain, one-quarter of all episodes of *S. aureus* ventilator-associated pneumonia, was caused by methicillin-resistant strains[24].

S. aureus has been thought to be an uncommon cause of community-acquired pneumonia in HIV positive patients, accounting for less than 2% of all such pneumonias diagnosed in life[25]. Autopsy studies, however, specifically reporting bacterial infections, have given an incidence of over 40%[25]. Although a substantial proportion of such findings may have been in the setting of a terminal event, they nevertheless do suggest that many cases are under- diagnosed in life.

The tremendous variation in the incidence of *S. aureus* pneumonia is partly a reflection of patient population studied. The diagnostic methodology used is also important since the organism can be carried in the oropharynx in up to 50% of adults. The significance of the organism in regular sputum samples may therefore be difficult. Protected specimens from the lower airways as well as tissue biopsy is therefore necessary for solid diagnosis. These aspects have been discussed at length in Chapters 1 and 27.

An increasing frequency of MRSA strains has been detected since the 1960s. Currently, up to between 9–40% of *S. aureus* isolates from hospitalised/institutionalised patients are MRSA[26,27]. In a recent study of ventilator-associated pneumonia, MRSA was found in 11/49 of patients (22%)[24]. However, the frequency of MRSA appears to vary from hospital to hospital and country to country. It can be lower than 0.5% in some Scandinavian hospitals, for example[28]. The elderly, patients in tertiary-care facilities and patients with severe underlying disease or who are critically ill, seem to be at particular risk. The upsurge of MRSA poses problems for treatment, further nosocomial spread including outbreaks, and possible impact on morbidity and mortality.

There appears to be a close association of cases of *S. aureus* pneumonia and influenza epidemics. Thus in Woodhead's series, most cases of *S. aureus* community-acquired pneumonia occurred between December and May[14]. This has not always been found. For example, there was no seasonal variation detected among bacteraemic *S. aureus* pneumonic patients in a large community teaching hospital in Sweden. However, 66% of those patients acquired their infection from hospital[29].

Nasopharyngeal colonisation by *S. aureus* in the general population of healthy adults is approximately 30%, rising to between 50 and 90% in certain populations which include health care workers, intravenous drug abusers, diabetics and patients on dialysis. There has also been a suggestion that the mainstem bronchi of hospitalised patients become increasingly colonised in time with *S. aureus*, and act as a source for pneumonia[30]. Person-to-person transmission occurs mainly via hand-to-hand contact. Staphylococcal respiratory infection then occurs as a result of dissemination of the organism from the skin via a haematogenous route or inhalation/aspiration from an upper respiratory tract reservoir. It is therefore not surprising that *S. aureus* respiratory infections are particularly common in settings providing overcrowding or reduction in standards of personal care such as certain institutionalised organisations, for example, nursing homes, psychiatric care facilities and paediatric nurseries. Ventilated or tracheostomised ICU patients and those on dermatological wards are also at risk.

There are several risk situations for staphylococcal pneumonia (Table 6.3). The first is a failure of the host mechanical defence barrier, for example, in patients with endotracheal intubation. In Musher's review, endotracheal/tracheal tube/laryngectomy/laryngeal dysfunction/predispositions to aspiration were identified in the cases of aerogenous pneumonia[16]. These situations allow for bypass of the normal mechanical defence system, thereby allowing *S. aureus*, usually present in the nasopharynx and bronchi, to gain access to the

Table 6.3. *Host risk factors*

Wounds, abrasions, catheters
Upper respiratory tract anatomical abnormality, endotracheal tubes
Overcrowding/break in personal hygiene
Institutionalisation/hospitalisation
Prolonged antibiotics
Previous viral, mycoplasma infection
Indwelling vascular devices
Endocarditis, other suppurative foci
Chronic pulmonary disease
The elderly, the very young
Liver disease
Renal impairment
Diabetes mellitus
Malignancy
Immunosuppressive therapy
HIV
Chronic granulomatous disease

distal lower respiratory tract. Insertion of intercostal chest drains has also been associated with the subsequent development of empyema. A breach in the skin can also act as a portal of entry for *S. aureus* and subsequent bacteraemia with a potential for a haematogenous spread to the lungs. This occurs in patients with intravenous drug abuse, patients with long-term intravenous catheters, those with AV shunts receiving regular haemodialysis, patients with burns, or in patients with focal localised infections of the skin or heart. The latter includes those with endocarditis, particularly tricuspid valve endocarditis and patients with suppurative thrombophlebitis from which sources haematogenous dissemination to the lungs is a real possibility. Persons with soft tissue cellulitis and abscesses are also at risk from haematogenous spread. Staphylococcal pyomyositis is common in some tropical countries and such patients pose a risk for staphylococcal pneumonia[31]. Unhygienic treatment of wounds with herbal packing for example, may be the portal of entry in some community-acquired, non-intravenous drug abuse associated cases of bacteremic *S. aureus* pneumonia[17].

An association between staphylococcal pneumonia and cranioencephalic trauma has been described[32,24], and may be due to lack of antibiotic exposure prior to the trauma, aspiration during initial resuscitative procedures and following colonisation after pulmonary/tracheal trauma.

Individuals with lower respiratory tract abnormalities are particularly predisposed to bronchogenous staphylococcal lung infection. Thus, *S. aureus* pneumonia may occur secondary to, and distal to, an obstructive bronchial carcinoma, in patients with chronic respiratory disease such as bronchiectasis, or cystic fibrosis. Chronic pulmonary disease features in approximately 50% of patients with *S. aureus* pneumonia[14,33].

The occurrence of staphylococcal pneumonia after viral and other infections, particularly influenza A, is well documented. The classic study of Chickering and Park in which post- mortem lung cultures were obtained from most of the 5% of 8000 soldiers with influenza who had died, showed *S. aureus* in 50% and strongly suggested an association with the fatal pneumonia[34]. During the 1968–1969 Hong Kong influenza epidemic, there was a three-fold increase in the incidence of staphylococcal pneumonia in patients admitted to hospital with pneumonia in Atlanta. This was thought to account for the excess pneumonia mortality[35]. Patients with staphylococcal pneumonia during an influenza epidemic tend to be younger and have less underlying chronic disease[35]. Influenza A has been found to depress mucociliary clearance, possibly through an associated severe tracheitis, is associated with leukopaenia, and adherence of *S. aureus* to respiratory epithelium is enhanced. Though less common, severe staphylococcal pneumonia has been described in children and adults in association with influenza B which *per se* is usually less virulent than A[36]. The interaction between influenza and bacterial infection is discussed in Chapter 9. Influenza A appears to produce severe lung injury with persistent alveolitis and patchy consolidation associated with collagen deposition. These changes may be cumulative with sequential viral infections[37]. Subsequent aerosol inhalation of staphylococci in animal models in various damaged lungs, has been found to be associated with a severely depressed inflammatory response and defective intrapulmonary killing[37].

Mycoplasma pneumoniae infection may be complicated by severe staphylococcal suprainfection, possibly related to transient depression of T-lymphocyte function[38].

Staphylococcal pneumonia may occur after measles infection, thought to be due to direct respiratory tract damage by the virus or via alterations in immune defence or vitamin A deficiency.

The systemic humoral and cellular immune integrity of the host, particularly the polymorphonuclear function, is a key factor in response to infection once the organism has breached the mechanical defence barriers. Thus, *S. aureus* pulmonary infections usually occur in adults > 60 years of age or in very young children. In adults, there is usually a substantial number of patients who have underlying conditions associated with polymorph dysfunction. In a recent series, 50% of patients had severe liver dysfunction, diabetes mellitus, renal dysfunction, haematological/solid organ malignancy or were on immunosuppressive therapy such as steroids[33]. The frequency of association with such predisposing conditions appears to be less in individuals developing secondary staphylococcal pneumonia during the course of influenza[35].

Individuals with defective polymorph function linked to chronic granulomatous disease are at high risk of recurrent staphylococcal infections. This appears to be related to defective bactericidal oxygen radical formation.

Although the classical T-lymphocyte defect in HIV positive individuals should not predispose patients to staphylococcal infection, *S. aureus* nevertheless appears to be the most common bacterial pathogen in HIV persons. However, *S. aureus* pneumonia accounts for 5–10% of such cases[39,40]. In one study, 23% of 129 consecutive episodes of respiratory tract disease were associated with recovery of the organism from the respiratory tract, and in eight cases of pneumonia it was thought to be the causative agent[39]. Post-mortem studies have suggested that *S. aureus* pneumonia in such patients may be under-estimated[25]. Although many AIDS patients may have primary risk factors *per se* for *S. aureus* infection, e.g. intravenous drug abuse and indwelling IV catheters, specific defects in *S. aureus* killing by neutrophils have also been identified[41]. Prior involvement of the respiratory tract by Kaposi's sarcoma or *Pneumocystis carinii* to produce mucosal destruction, may be a further factor[42,39].

Clinical features

Presentation of staphylococcal pneumonia is variable depending on the age, predisposing factors and the setting[14,15,33]. Many cases of staphylococcal pneumonia occur in young children, although the incidence in recent years has been falling (Chapter 23). In children aged < 2 years and particularly in the newborn, the presentation may be non-specific with irritability, anorexia and signs of respiratory distress which may be due to pneumothorax rather than consolidation.

In adults, any age-group can be affected but, in general, older adults are more frequently involved. Thus, in Kaye's series, the median age was 61 years (range 26–83)[33], in Woodhead's series 50% were aged < 45 years with two peaks at 16–35 years and at 56–65 years of age[14]. An average age of 52 years was seen in Fisher's series[15]. Features of concomitant medical illness are usually apparent. A recent or ongoing history of viral or other non-staphylococcal respiratory tract infection, may be present. There may be an extra pulmonary primary focus such as cellulitis, intravenous drug abusing marks or indwelling devices (in particular in patients whose disease has a haematogenous pathogenesis).

The onset of disease can be abrupt, within 2–3 days, in about 20% of cases and a fulminant course is occasionally seen in these, particularly in patients with a bronchogenic mode of acquisition. In others, patients may be moderately ill, whilst some have a subacute relatively mild mode of presentation.

Fever, cough productive of purulent sputum, pleuritic chest pain and haemoptysis are common. Tachypnoea and cyanosis may be marked. Systemic toxicity, particularly with high fever, chills, and accompanied by confusion and systolic hypotension, may be present in as many as one-fifth of patients admitted with community acquired *S. aureus* pneumonia[14].

Approximately one-sixth of cases referred to hospital have non-pulmonary features predominating, such as shock, vomiting, congestive cardiac failure or acidosis, which may overshadow the pulmonary focus and lead to misdiagnosis[14].

Specific respiratory examination findings include those of consolidation, with or without pleural effusion.

The possibility of a co-existing staphylococcal endocarditis should be borne in mind, particularly in community, younger or intravenous drug abusing patients without a recognisable primary focus or underlying predisposition, associated with repeated positive blood cultures. There may be various accompanying cutaneous manifestations such as Osler's nodes or Janeway's patches (Fig. 6.1). The presence of urinary red cells, white cell casts, a positive rheumatoid factor or a positive teichoic antibody test is supporting evidence for endocarditis. Echocardiography should be performed if the diagnosis of endocarditis is entertained.

A recent study of ventilator-associated pneumonia due to *S. aureus* has suggested that patients were 3.5 times more likely to have MRSA rather than methicillin sensitive *S. aureus* (MSSA). Patients with MRSA were much more likely to have received steroids, have been ventilated, to be older and to have chronic obstructive airways disease, received previous antibiotics, to be bacteraemic or to develop shock and to die[24].

A number of complications may arise (Table 6.4). The occurrence of pneumatoceles is uncommon but can be life threatening. It is more likely to occur in children. The presence may be suggested by a sudden change in the patient's condition. Thus the occurrence of sudden breathlessness, circulatory failure and surgical emphysema should alert the physician to this possibility. Pneumatoceles may occur as a result of initial obstruction to the site of draining microabscesses in some individuals and in children, also due to the absence of collateral ventilatory pores of Kohn[43].

Lung abscess may also complicate *S. aureus* pneumonia, particularly in patients with impaired expectoration, i.e. the young, the old and those receiving endotracheal intubation. This complication should be suspected if the pneumonic course is punctuated by the production of excessive amounts of putrid sputum, persistent fever, persistent malaise, anaemia and leucocytosis. Finger clubbing may develop rapidly.

Pleural effusions are not infrequently found. Empyema usually occurs as a result of direct extension from a lung abscess or following placement of an intercostal drain for removal of non-sterile pleural effusions[44]. There may be signs of pleural effusion with dullness, diminished breath sounds and perhaps bronchial breathing at the

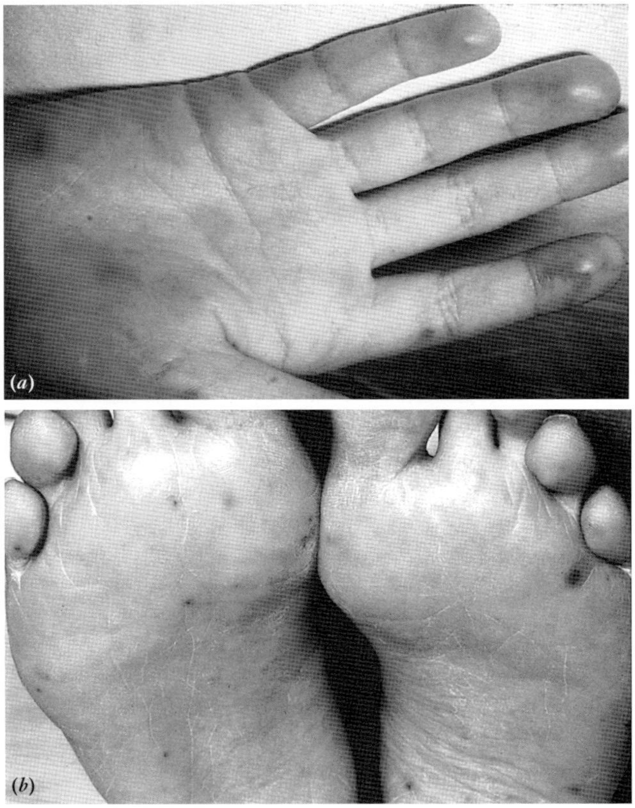

FIGURE 6.1 (*a*) Cutaneous manifestations including Janeway's patch in patient with endocarditis. (*b*) Emboli due to *S. aureus*.

Table 6.4. *Complications of* S. aureus *pneumonia*

Abscess
Empyema
Pneumatocele
Pneumothorax
Bronchopleural fistula
Pancoast syndrome
Haematogenous spread
TSS
Rash
Sepsis syndrome

upper limit. Chest pain may recur and fever persist. A bronchopleural fistula may develop with an air-fluid on chest radiography.

Haematogenous dissemination may also result in distant organ septic metastases, usually to the brain via vertebral veins, where the presentation may be silent, or the patient may develop signs of a space occupying lesion which include focal headaches, convulsion or partial paresis.

The toxic shock syndrome has been described in association with staphylococcal pneumonia[43] in which the characteristic erythematous rash progressing to desquamation, particularly on the hands and feet, is present. In addition, a primary desquamating peripheral erythematous rash, unassociated with other features of the toxic shock syndrome, such as hypotension, hyperaemic mucosa or multi-system involvement, has also been described[45].

Pancoast syndrome due to staphylococcal pneumonia is a rare association[46].

Laboratory features

There is usually a peripheral polymorph leukocytosis with a total white count raised to between 15×10^9–25×10^9/l with an accompanying mild anaemia. However the white count can be low as a result of an underlying immune suppression or secondary to overwhelming sepsis. The presence of thrombocytopaenia would suggest DIC. Positive blood cultures are found in up to one third of all primary staphylococcal pneumonias[14,33,44]. However, patients with MRSA pneumonia are more likely to be bacteraemic compared to those with MSSA[24].

Microbiological diagnosis is solid if a positive culture for *S. aureus* is obtained from the blood, pleural fluid or abscess. Since *S. aureus* is carried in the nasopharynx of many healthy persons, its finding *per se* is not indicative of lung pathology. However, the presence of many Gram-positive cocci in clusters and within polymorph laden white cells in a good sputum sample, would strongly suggest the diagnosis. Sheathed bronchoscopical brush specimens, coupled with quantitative culture counts, would provide a higher degree of diagnostic specificity (Chapter 1). It is vital, in view of the increasing problem with MRSA to identify MRSA isolates by disc diffusion, microdilution MIC or oxacillin agar screening tests and to obtain full sensitivity profiles.

Radiological appearances

No chest radiographical feature is diagnostic of *S. aureus* pneumonia and a variety of presentations have been described. In Fisher's series, bilateral lung involvement was more common and cyst/abscess formation occurred in 15/21 patients (71%). Pleural effusions were reported in eight of 21 patients (38%) of which four were empyema[15], similar to other reports[33]. Diffuse parenchymal infiltrates (bilateral as common as unilateral) have been the commonest presentation. Occasionally the infiltrates are lobar in distribution. There have been very few instances (0–16%) of abscess or cavity formation (Fig. 6.2 (*a*), (*b*)) in more recent reports[33,44]. However, post-mortem examinations reveal pulmonary abscess formation in 90% of patients who died from *S. aureus* pneumonia[15]. The reduced incidence of abscess and cavity formation in the more recent series may reflect earlier recognition and institution of appropriate antimicrobial therapy. Early, well-demarcated, multiple/bilateral rounded lesions suggestive of a haematogenous origin (Fig. 6.3 (*a*), (*b*), (*c*))[16] may progress to cavitation within a week. More diffuse lesions are said to be a feature of bronchogenic causation. Lobar consolidation is more a feature in young children. Other radiographical lesions include bronchopleural fistulae with air fluid levels, pneumothorax (Fig. 6.4 (*a*)) and pneumatocele (Fig. 6.5). The air crescent sign commonly seen in invasive aspergillosis or pulmonary haematoma may occasionally be seen in *S. aureus* lung infection[47].

Outcome and management

The mortality of staphylococcal pneumonia is in general high and of the order of 30–40% for both community-acquired and hospital-acquired infections[14,24,33,44]. Factors which have been associated with a fatal outcome include older age, confusion, reduced conscious level, renal dysfunction, acidosis, bacteraemia, admission to ICU and significant underlying medical conditions[14,15,16,44]. Bacteremia particularly, carries a high mortality rate[29]. It is however difficult to be sure of the precise contribution of the pneumonia to the mortality, particularly in patients with a complex milieu of other medical and surgical problems. However, excess deaths in an influenza epidemic were primarily due to staphylococcal pneumonia and some of these occurred in adults < 50 years of age who did not have underlying diseases[35]. A recent study of *S. aureus* ventilator-associated pneumonia indicated that direct pneumonia-related mortality was 20-fold higher in individuals who had MRSA compared to those with MSSA[24]. The reason for this does not appear to be related to increased virulence of MRSA or to a higher patient risk profile in those with MRSA but may be due to poor vancomycin delivery to the airways for those with MRSA, and delay in instituting appropriate antibiotics with activity against MRSA. The finding of a difference in mortality in patients with MRSA compared to those with MSSA has, however, not been uniformly reported[48].

Prompt institution of an intravenous penicillin is the mainstay of effective treatment for MSSA pneumonia (Table 6.5). Since most hospital and community strains of MSSA are resistant to β-lactam antibiotics, initial therapy should be with a stable β-lactam antimicrobial such as cloxacillin, nafcillin or methicillin. For cloxacillin, the adult dosage is 4–12 g/day in 4–6 equal doses. Benzyl penicillin may be substituted at a dose of 8–16 mega units/day if the strain proves to be susceptible. Duration of treatment is for a minimum of 2 weeks intravenously, extending to 6 weeks if a haematogenous source or metastatic complication is diagnosed. If endocarditis is proven or suspected, concomitant management with cardiologists and cardiothoracic surgeons is essential. Alternatives in true penicillin allergy include clindamycin 600 mg Q6 hourly or vancomycin 500 mg Q6 hourly. Since the mechanism of action of vancomycin is by inhibition of cell wall peptidoglycan synthesis, RNA synthesis and alteration of permeability of intracellular membranes, this antimicrobial may also

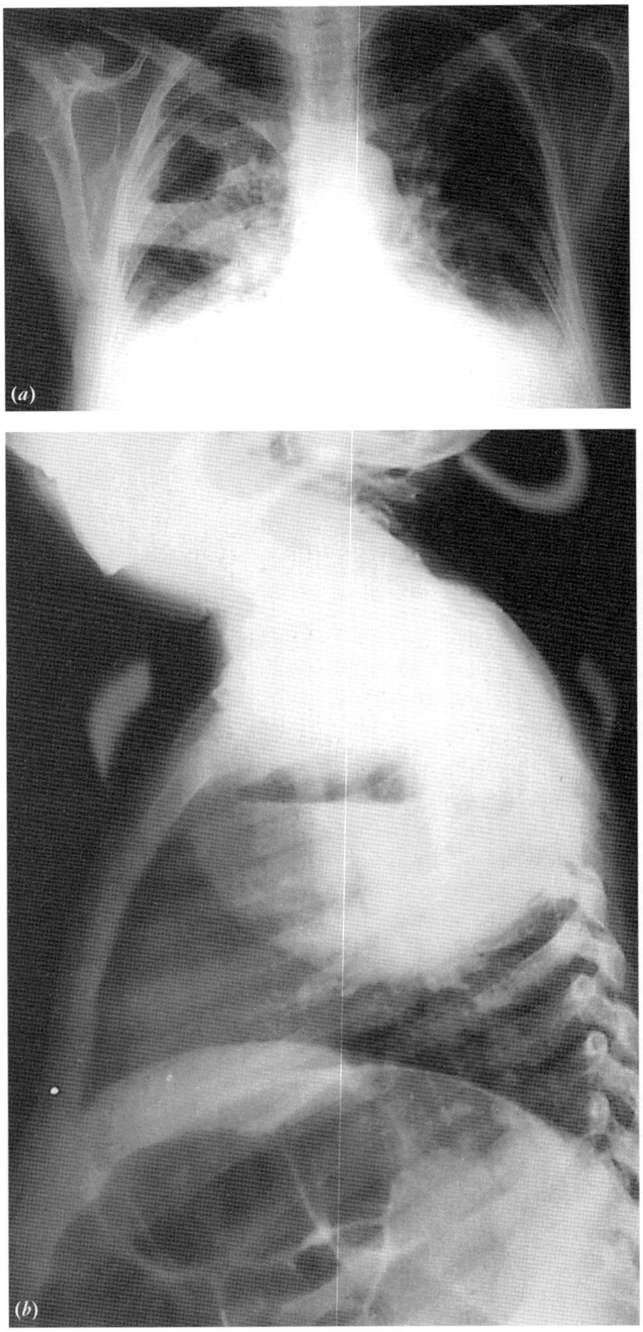

FIGURE 6.2 (*a*), (*b*) Bilateral pleural effusions, infiltrates, lobar consolidation and abscess cavity with fluid level.

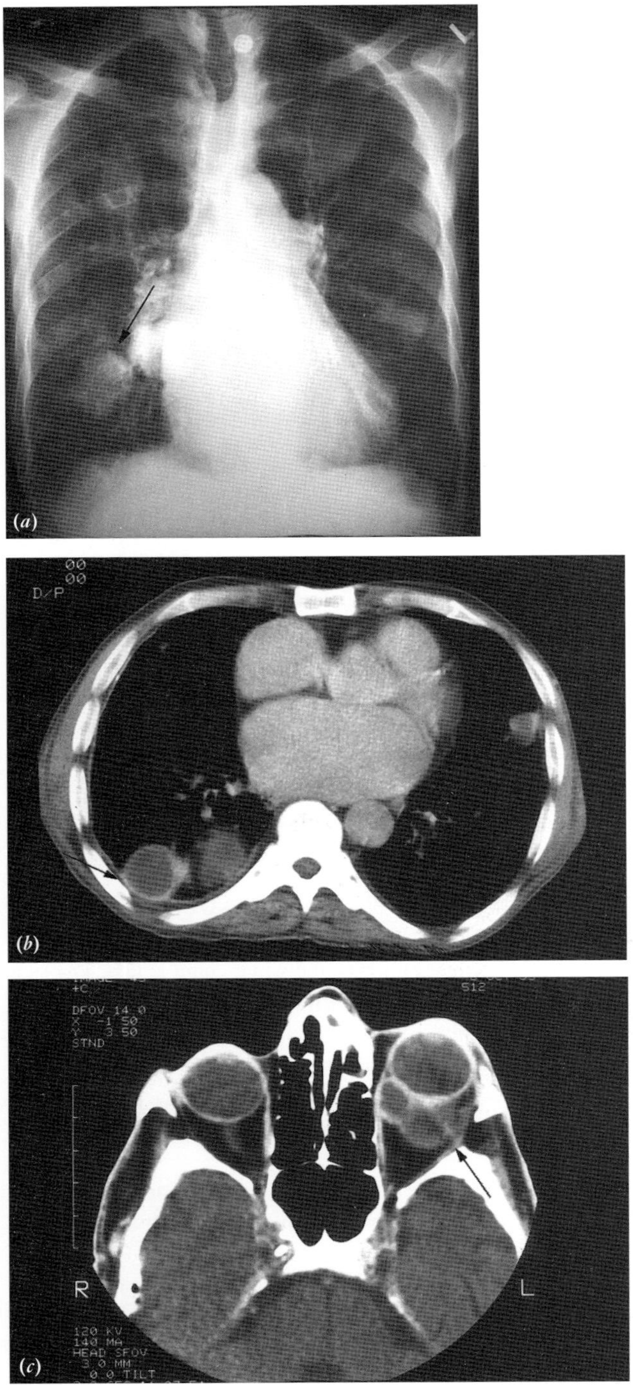

FIGURE 6.3 (*a*) Nodular lesions both lungs. (*b*) CT chest: hypodense nodules; ground glass appearances both lungs due to oedema. (*c*) CT orbit: multiloculated cystic lesions. L orbit with compression and displacement; L globe with proptosis. [Patient with primary *S. aureus* focus node, spreading to orbit and haematogeneous dissemination to lungs.]

Table 6.5. *Management*

Cloxacillin or clindamycin for MSSA
Vancomycin (or cotrimoxazole) for MRSA
Rifampicin/aminoglycoside for treatment failures
Drain empyema
Drain pneumothorax
Surgery for fistula
Ventilation

be useful if patients fail to respond to other therapy or microbial tolerance is suspected.

Addition of other antimicrobials with other actions, such as an aminoglycoside (ribosomal binding + unknown mechanisms) and rifampicin (inhibition of RNA polymerase) may be a further useful therapeutic manoeuvre in desperately ill or deteriorating patients. However, aminoglycosides may not be effective in the presence of large amounts of pus. These antimicrobials should not be used as the sole agents since they are relatively ineffective when used alone, for example, resistance with rifampicin rapidly develops. In particularly ill and septic patients, those with liver and renal insufficiency, aminoglycosides are more likely to be highly nephrotoxic and serum level monitoring is advised.

If infection with MRSA is suspected or proven, then vancomycin is the treatment of choice. However, treatment failures have been documented and the addition of a second drug such as rifampicin/ciprofloxacin is recommended in patients failing to respond to vancomycin alone. There is no hard data to support this approach in general, apart from anecdotal reports[49]. Antagonism of vancomycin/rifampicin has been seen in MRSA endocarditis[50]. Cotrimoxazole is an alternative antibiotic. Sensitivity reports should be used for guidance of treatment in difficult cases.

Alternative antimicrobials include first generation cephalosporins such as cefazolin, imipenem and fusidic acid.

In the situation of cystic fibrosis, the management is more aggressive and is discussed in further detail in Chapter 24.

The presence of infective foci, for example, long-term indwelling lines, suppurative thrombophlebitis, infected heart valves, should be ruled out and managed appropriately.

Pneumatoceles and pneumothoraces may develop and must be clearly differentiated from each other since the management is different for each. Pneumatoceles (usually in children), can be managed

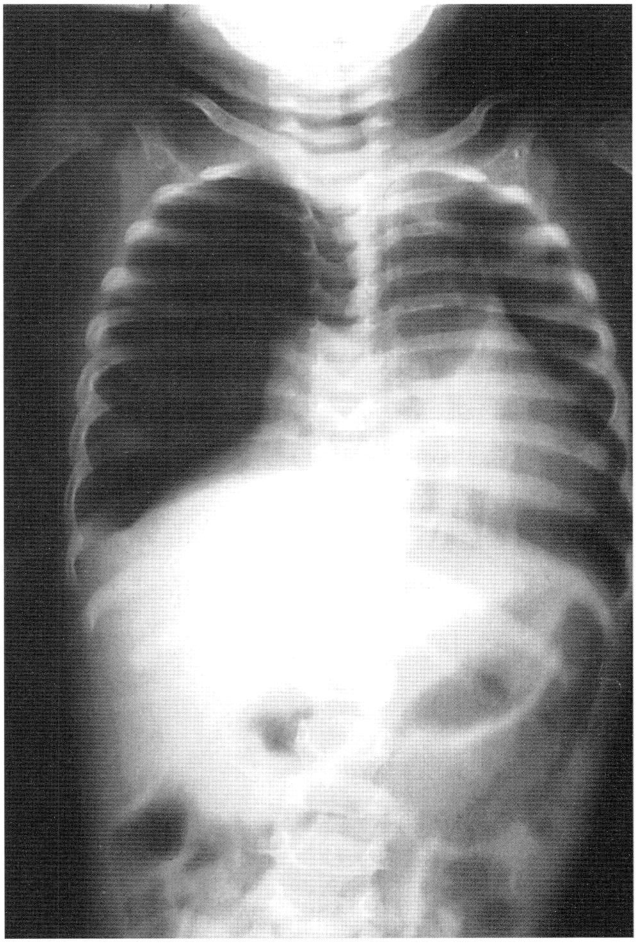

FIGURE 6.4 Large tension pneumothorax complicating *S. aureus* pneumonia.

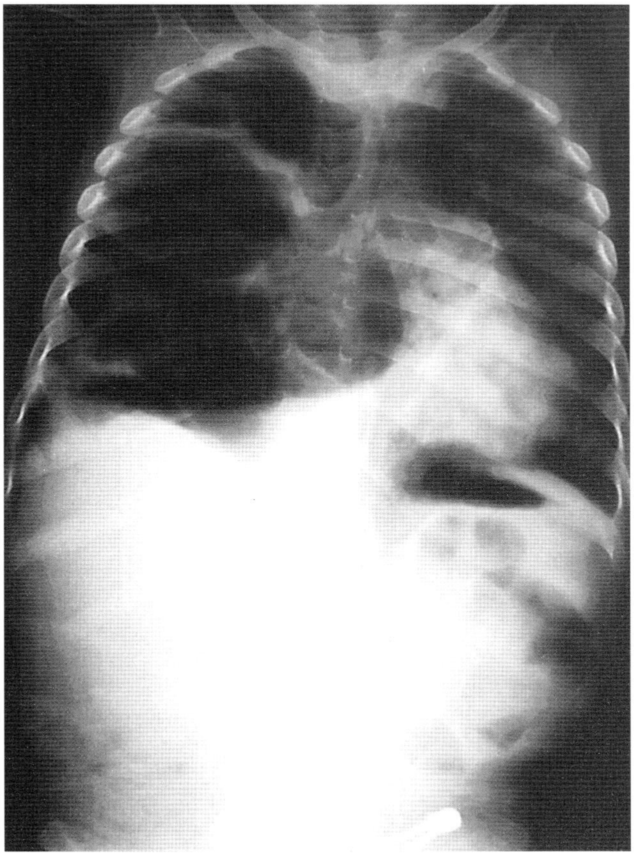

FIGURE 6.5 Multiple large pneumatocoeles with right peripheral pneumothorax producing mediastinal shift.

conservatively in most cases, since most do not cause tension or cardiopulmonary embarrassment, and most disappear within 6 weeks with few residual sequelae. Occasionally they may enlarge rapidly or rupture into the pleural space with pyopneumothorax formation. Although some cases of pneumothorax can also be managed conservatively if relatively asymptomatic, most will require either aspiration or formal intercostal intubation and underwater seal drainage. Empyema requires surgical drainage. The presence of a pyopneumothorax, particularly if complicated by bronchopleural fistula, will usually require drainage and possibly surgical excision of cysts, decortication, partial pleurectomy or even lobectomy in severe cases. Postoperative morbidity (bronchopleural fistula/empyema/pyopneumothorax) and mortality (cardiogenic shock/aspiration) can be high[51]. In some complicated cases, such as those with bilateral pneumothoraces with bronchopleural fistula, novel ventilatory support may be required, for example, synchronous independent lung ventilation may be necessary to reverse mediastinal shift and allow closure of fistulae[52].

Preventive measures

One of the concerns in the management of patients with *S. aureus* pneumonia is that the organism is an MRSA and that outbreaks within the hospital will occur as a result of the spread of the organism via the hands of health care workers[53,54]. Hence, preventative measures are of utmost importance. Segregation of patients with MRSA and elimination of carriage sites from particularly the nose with topical mupirocin is necessary[54]. Further measures include early discharge of such patients from hospital, screening of new hospital admissions for patients coming from a known MRSA source, culture surveillance of staff and patients and elimination of nasal carriage.

The use of antiseptic-impregnated intravascular devices has proved successful in reducing staphylococcal line infections[55].

No staphylococcal vaccine is currently available, but influenza vaccine is an indirect way of reducing staphylococcal pneumonia and will be indicated for patients at risk.

Summary

S. aureus pneumonia is an uncommon cause of community acquired pneumonia but has an increasingly important role in nosocomial acquired pneumonia particularly in the setting of the global increase in immunocompromised individuals. It often has a high mortality rate. Future areas of research include heightened epidemiological surveillance, more detailed analysis of avoidable mortality factors and comparative clinical trials for effective antimicrobial regimes not only for a regular staphylococcal infections but those which are resistant, particularly the MRSA organisms. A recent worrying trend has been the emergence of strains of both MSSA and MRSA with reduced susceptibility and resistance even to teicoplanin[56]. A number of other antimicrobials with good activity against MRSA are available; however, clinical studies are lacking. These antimicrobials include the fourth generation cephalosporins such as cefpirone and cefepine, the newer quinolones such as CP-99,219, fosfomycin and pristinamycin.

Adjunctive immodulatory therapy of staphylococcal infections is in its infancy, although preliminary animal studies, for example, with intranasal intravenous immunoglobulins, have demonstrated anti-staphylococcal activity[57].

References

1. HAWIGER J, TIMMONS S, STRONG DD, CONTRELL BA, RILEY M, DOOLITTLE RF. Identification of a region of human fibrinogen interacting with staphylococcal clumping factor. *Biochemistry* 1982; 21:1407–13.
2. MOREILLON P, ENTENZA J, FRANCIOLI P *et al.* Role of staphylococcal coagulase (Coa) and clumping factor (CIFA) in the pathogenesis of experimental endocarditis (EE) [abstract B63]. In *Proceedings and Abstracts of the Thirty-Fourth Interscience Conference on Antimicrobial Agents and Chemotherapy, October 1994* Orlando: American Society for Microbiology; 1994:149.
3. COSTERTON JW, CHENG KJ, GEESEY GG *et al.* Bacterial biofilms in nature and disease. *Ann Rev Microbiol* 1987; 41: 435–64.
4. DAROUICHE RO, DHIR A, MILLER AJ, LANDON GC, RAAD II, MUSHER D M Vancomycin penetration into biofilm covering infected prosthesis and effect on bacteria. *J Infect Dis* 1994; 170: 720–3.
5. CHUARD C, LUCET JC, ROHNER P *et al.* Resistance of *Staphylococcus aureus* recovered from infected foreign body *in vivo* to killing by antimicrobials. *J Infect Dis*ease 1991; 163: 1369–73.
6. SHAIO MF, YANG KD, BOHNSACK JF, HILL HR. Effect of immune globulin intravenous on opsonization of bacteria by classic and alternative complement pathways in premature serum. *Pediatr Res* 1989; 25: 643–40.
7. ZUMLA A. Superantigens. T cells, and microbes. *Clin Infect Dis* 1992; 15: 313–20.
8. HARTMANN BJ, TOMASZ A. Low-affinity penicillin-binding protein associated with β-lactam resistance in *Staphylococcus aureus*. *J Bacteriol* 1984; 158: 513–16.
9. HACKBARTH CJ, CHAMBERS HF. Methicillin-resistant staphylococci: genetics and mechanisms of resistance. *Antimicrob Agents Chemother* 1989; 33: 991–4.
10. MCDOUGAL LK, THORNSBERRY C. The role of β-lactamase in staphylococcal resistance to penicillinase-resistant penicillins and cephalosporins. *J Clin Microbiol* 1986; 23: 832–9.
11. TOMASZ A, DRUGEON HB, DELENCASTRE HM *et al.* New mechanism for methicillin resistance in *Staphylococcus aureus* Clinical isolates that lack the PBP2a gene and contain normal penicillin-binding proteins with modified penicillin-binding capacity. *Antimicrob Agents Chemother* 1989; 33: 1869–74.
12. YOUNG SEJ. Bacteraemia 1975–1980: a survey of cases reported to the PHLS Communicable Disease Surveillance Centre. *J Infect* 1982; 5: 19–26.
13. GRANSDEN WR, EYKYN SJ, PHILLIPS I. *Staphylococcus aureus* bacteraemia: 400 episodes in St Thomas's Hospital. *Br M J* 1984; 288: 300–3.
14. WOODHEAD MA, RADVAN J, MACFARLANE JT. Adult community-acquired Staphylococcal pneumonia in the antibiotic era: a review of 61 cases. *Quart J of Med*, New Series 64 1987; 245: 783–90.
15. FISHER AM, TREVER RW, CURTIN JA, SCHULTZE G, MILLER DF. Staphylococcal pneumonia: a review of 21 cases in adults. *New Engl J Med* 1958; 258: 919–28.
16. MUSHER DM, LAMM N, DAROUICHE RO,

YOUNG EJ, HAMILL RJ, LANDON GC. The current spectrum of *Staphylococcus aureus* infection in a tertiary care hospital. *Medicine* 1994; 73: 186–208.

17. TSAO TC, TSAI YH, LAN RS, SHIEH WB, LEE CH Pulmonary manifestations of *Staphylococcus aureus* septicemia. *Chest* 1992; 101: 574–6.
18. FANG G D, FINE M, ORLOFF J *et al.* New and emerging etiologies for community-acquired pneumonia with implications for therapy: a prospective multicenter study of 359 cases. *Medicine* 1990; 69: 307–16.
19. MARRIE TJ, DURANT H, YATES L. Community-acquired pneumonia requiring hospitalization: 5-year prospective study. *Rev Infect Dis* 1989; 11: 586–599.
20. HUI KP, CHIN NK, CHOW K *et al.* Prospective study of the aetiology of adult community acquired bacterial pneumonia needing hospitalisation in Singapore. *Singapore Med J* 1993; 34(4): 329–34.
21. CDC SURVEILLANCE SUMMARIES Nosocomial infection surveillance, 1993. *MMWR* 1984; 33(2SS): 9SS–21SS.
22. RAMIREZ JA. The choice of empirical antibiotic therapy for nosocomial pneumonia. *J Chemother* 1994; 6 Suppl 2: 47–50.
23. RELLO J, QUINTANA E, AUSINA V, PUZO C, NET A, PRATS G. Risk factors for *Staphylococcus aureus* nosocomial pneumonia in critically ill patients. *Am Rev Resp Dis* 1990; 142: 1320–4.
24. RELLO J, TORRES A, RICART M. *et al.* Ventilator-associated pneumonia by *Staphylococcus aureus*: comparison of methicillin-resistant and methicillin-sensitive episodes. *Am J Resp Crit Care Med* 1994; 150: 1545–9.
25. DICPINIGAITIS PV, LEVY D E, GNASS RD, BERNSTEIN RG. Pneumonia due to *Staphylococcus aureus* in a patient with AIDS: review of incidence and report of an atypical roentgenographic presentation. *South Med J* 1995; 88: 586–90.
26. THOMAS JC, BRIDGE J, WATERMAN S *et al.* Transmission and control of methicillin-resistant *Staphylococcus aureus* in a skilled nursing facility. *Infect Control Hosp Epidemiol* 1989; 10: 106–10.
27. EMORI TG, GAYNES RP An Overview of nosocomial infections, including the role of the microbiology laboratory. *Clin Microbiol Rev* 1993; 6: 428–42.
28. VOSS A, MILATOVIC D, WALLRAUCH-SCHWARZ C, ROSDAHL VT, BRAVENY I. Methicillin-resistant *Staphylococcus aureus* in Europe. *Eur J Clin Microbiol Infect Dis* 1994; 13: 50–5.
29. WATANAKUNAKORN C. Bacteremic *Staphylococcus aureus* pneumonia. *Scand J Infect Dis* 1987; 19(6): 623–7.
30. EMSON HE. *Staphylococci* in bronchi of hospital patients: an autopsy study. *Can Med Assoc J* 1964; 90: 1005–7.
31. SCRIMGEOUR EM, KAVEN J. Severe Staphylococcal pneumonia complicating pyomyositis. *Am J Trop Med Hyg* 1982; 31(4): 822–6.
32. INGLIS TJJ, SPROAT LJ, HAWKEY PM, GIBSON JS Staphylococcal pneumonia in ventilated patients: a twelve-month review of cases in an intensive care unit. *J Hosp Inf* 1993; 25: 207–10.
33. KAYE MG, FOX MJ, BARTLETT JG, BRAMAN SS, GLASSROTH J. The clinical spectrum of *Staphylococcus aureus* pulmonary infection. *Chest* 1990; 97: 788–92.
34. CHICKERING HT, PARK JH. *Staphylococcus aureus* pneumonia. *JAMA* 1919; 72: 617–26.
35. SCHWARZMANN SW, ADLER JL, SULLIVAN RJ, MARINE WM. Bacterial pneumonia during the Hong Kong influenza epidemic of 1968–1969. *Arch Intern Med* 1971; 127: 1037–41.
36. CONNOR E, POWELL K. Fulminant pneumonia caused by concomitant infection with influenza B virus and *Staphylococcus aureus*. *J Pediat* 1985; 106: 447–50.
37. JAKAB GJ. Sequential virus infections, bacterial superinfections, and fibrinogenesis. *Am Rev Resp Dis* 1990; 142: 374–9.
38. HENDERSON A, REID D, FREEMAN R. *Mycoplasma* pneumoniae infection predisposing to Staphylococcal pneumonia. *Br J Clin Pract* 1983; 37: 75–76.
39. LEVINE SJ, WHITE DA, FELS AOS The incidence and significance of *Staphylococcus aureus* in respiratory cultures from patients infected with the human immunodeficiency virus. *Am Rev Resp Dis* 1990; 141: 89–93.
40. FISH DN, DANZIER LH. Neglected pathogens: bacterial infections in persons with human immunodeficiency virus infection, a review of literature (second of two parts). *Pharmacotherapy* 1993; 13: 543–63.
41. MURPHY PM, LANE HC, FAUCI AS, GALLIN JI. Impairment of neutrophil bactericidal capacity in patients with AIDS. *J Infect Dis* 1988; 158: 627–30.
42. WHIMBEY E, GOLD JWM, POLKSY B *et al.* Bacteremia and fungemia in patients with AIDS. *Ann Intern Med* 1986; 104: 511–14.
43. DAVIDSON AC, CREACH M, CAMERON IR Staphylococcal pneumonia, pneumatoceles, and the toxic shock syndrome. *Thorax* 1990; 45: 639–40.
44. IWAHARA T, ICHIYAMA S, NADA T, SHIMOKATA K, NAKASHIMA N. Clinical and epidemiologic investigations of nosocomial pulmonary infections caused by methicillin-resistant *Staphylococcus aureus*. *Chest* 1994; 105: 826–31.
45. BATES I. Characteristic rash sssociated with staphylococcal pneumonia. *Lancet* 1987; 1026–7.
46. SILVERMAN MS, MACLEOD JP. Pancoast's syndrome due to staphylococcal pneumonia. *Can Med Assoc J* 1990; 142: 343–5.
47. GOLD W, VELLEND H, BRUNTON J. The air crescent sign caused by *Staphylococcus aureus* lung infection in a neutropenic patient with leukemia. *Ann Intern Med* 1992; 116: 910–11.
48. HERSHOW RC, KHAYR WF, SMITH NL. A comparison of clinical virulence of nosocomially acquired methicillin-resistant and methicillin-sensitive *Staphylococcus aureus* infections in a university hospital. *Infect Control Hosp Epidemiol* 1992; 13: 587–93.
49. FAVILLE JR RJ, ZASKE DE, KAPLAN EL *et al.* *Staphylococcus aureus* endocarditis: combined therapy with vancomycin and rifampicin. *JAMA* 1978; 240: 1963–5.
50. LEVINE DP, FROMM BS, REDDY BR Slow response to vancomycin or vancomycin plus rifampicin in methicillin-resistant *Staphylococcus aureus* endocarditis. *Ann Intern Med* 1991; 115: 674–80.
51. SINZOBAHAMVYA N. Emergency pulmonary resection for pneumonia. High morbidity and mortality. *Scand J Thor & Cardiovasc Surg* 1991; 25(1): 69–71.
52. LOHSE AW, KLEIN O, HERMANN E *et al.* Pneumatoceles and pneumothoraces complicating staphylococcal pneumonia: treatment by synchronous independent lung ventilation. *Thorax* 1993; 48(5): 578–80.
53. WENZEL RP, NETTLEMAN MD, JONES RN *et al.* Methicillin-resistant *Staphylococcus aureus*: Implications for the 1990s and effective control measures. *Am J Med* 1991; 91: 221S–7S.
54. EMMERSON AM, GARAU J Postoperative complications due to methicillin-resistant *Staphylococcus aureus* (MRSA) in an elderly patient: management and control of MRSA. *J Hosp Infect* 1992; 22: 43–50.
55. MAKI DG, STOLZ SM, WHEELER S, MERMEL LA. Clinical trial of a novel antiseptic coated central venous catheter. *Abstract No. 461. ICAAC.* October 1991, Chicago.
56. SHLAES DM, SHLAES JH, VINCENT S, ETTER L, FEY PD, GOERING RV. Teicoplanin-resistant *Staphylococcus aureus* expresses a novel membrane protein and increases expression of penicillin-binding protein 2 complex. *Antimicrob Agents Chemother* 1993; 37: 2432–7.
57. RAMISSE F, SZATANIK M, BINDER P, ALONSO JM. Passive local immunotherapy of experimental Staphylococcal pneumonia with human intravenous immunoglobulin. *J Infect Dis* 1993; 168: 1030–3.

7 *Haemophilus influenzae* and *Moraxella* infections

MATS KALIN
Karolinska Hospital, Sweden

HAEMOPHILUS INFLUENZAE

Microbiology

Haemophilus is a genus of aerobic non-motile, non-sporeforming, small Gram-negative rods with rather special growth requirements, including haem (X factor, protoporphyrin IX containing iron), for which there seems to be a special receptor[1]. *Haemophilus influenzae* is the *Haemophilus* species with the most significant impact on human health, but *Haemophilus parainfluenzae* and *Haemophilus aphrophilus* are responsible for rare cases of both invasive diseases such as endocarditis and for occasional cases of respiratory tract infection[2,3].

The cell wall of *H. influenzae* has the same structure as in other Gram-negative bacteria including an inner, cytoplasmic, phospholipid bilayer, a thin peptidoglycan layer, a periplasmic space and an outer membrane[4–7] (Fig. 7.1). The outer membrane is an asymmetric bilayer with proteins inserted. The outer membrane of *Haemophilus* is different from most other Gram-negative bacteria in so far as it is devoid of the long polysaccharide side chains of the lipopolysaccharide. These O-chains have distinct antigenic properties in other Gram-negative bacteria and confer some protection against the effect of antibiotics and the killing action of serum complement, actions to which *H. influenzae* is therefore more susceptible. The lipopolysaccharide of *Haemophilus*, most often designated lipooligosaccharide (LOS), is nonetheless, as other endotoxins, a structure with potent biological effects.

The major outer membrane protein (OMP) is the P2 protein, which is a porin and a target for human bactericidal antibodies[4–8]. This protein, which constitutes some 50% of the outer membrane's protein content, is strain-specific and a basis for subtyping, since the diversity is extensive. This variation is especially marked for non-encapsulated strains, while encapsulated type b strains form a more homogenous group. The P6 protein, on the other hand, accounts for less than 5% of the OMPs and is highly conserved in all *H. influenzae* strains. Three other OMPs are known, but are less well characterised.

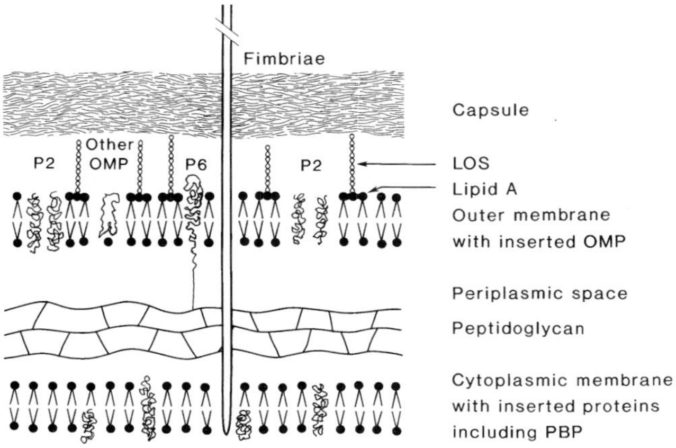

FIGURE 7.1 Schematic of cell wall structure in *Haemophilus influenzae*.

Most of the *H. influenzae* strains causing respiratory tract infections are unencapsulated, while those causing invasive disease, particularly meningitis are usually encapsulated[4,5,9–14]. There are six different capsular serotypes, but type b with a capsule consisting of polyribosyl-ribitol phosphate is by far the most common one in human disease. The capsule can be lost *in vivo* or *in vitro*, and it was previously believed that unencapsulated strains were encapsulated variants devoid of their capsules; today it is clear that the majority of non-encapsulated strains are genetically different from encapsulated ones.

In vivo a majority of *H. influenzae* strains, both encapsulated and unencapsulated, seem to be fimbriated, but the fimbriae are often lost after several *in vitro* passages[4,7,15,16]. The degree of fimbriation has been found to vary widely. The fimbriae often appear to have a polar distribution.

H. influenzae can be divided into seven biotypes on the basis of certain enzymatic and biochemical properties, specifically the ability to produce indole, urease and ornithine decarboxylase[5,11,17–23]. Eight biotypes are currently recognised. There is some correlation between biotype and pathogenicity; most invasive infections are caused by biotype I, and to a lesser degree type II and these strains are most often of capsular type (serotype) b (see below). However, today it is evident that the capsule is the important virulence factor. The other six biotypes are most often found in non-encapsulated strains. In some studies different biotypes have predominated in different clinical types of infections, i.e. type II in respiratory tract infections and type IV in genitourinary infections, but the findings have not been entirely consistent when different materials from different geographical sites have been compared.

Epidemiology and pathogenesis

H. influenzae and some other *Haemophilus* species, such as *H. parainfluenzae*, *Haemophilus haemolyticus*, and *Haemophilus parahaemolyticus*, are common inhabitants of the indigenous human pharyngeal flora[4]. Invasive *H. influenzae* type b disease is most commonly seen in small children, but may occasionally occur in adults. *Non-encapsulated* strains are considerably less virulent, but nevertheless are significant pathogens in respiratory tract diseases in both children and adults.

Carriership of *Haemophilus influenzae*

Carriage of *Haemophilus* species is very common both in children and adults; virtually all individuals are carriers of one or more *Haemophilus* strains, and up to 80% of healthy humans more than six months of age may be carriers of *H. influenzae*[4,6,22,24–26]. Nasopharyngeal colonisation in childhood is strongly correlated to development of acute otitis media[27,28]. Especially high carrier rates are seen in patients with chronic obstructive pulmonary disease (COPD), the organism being recovered from virtually all such patients when serial cultures are performed. Only 5% of strains found in healthy carriers are encapsulated, half of which are type b[29]. In association with cases of invasive *H. influenzae* type b disease the carriage rate of type b strains is considerably higher in close contacts in households and day-care centres. The risk of invasive disease in such close contacts is increased about 500 times compared to the endemic rate[4,30]. In developing countries carriage of *H. influenzae* seems to be still more frequent, contracted even earlier, and the rate of type b being higher than in Western countries[4,31,32]. It has now been shown that the type b capsular polysaccharide protein conjugate vaccines protect also against colonisation with *H. influenzae* type b[14,33]

The same strain of *H. influenzae* may be carried for several weeks or months, after which it is often replaced by a new strain with different antigenic properties[4,6,22]. Non-encapsulated strains adher more efficiently to pharyngeal cells and cause less serious disease with lower risk of host death and may therefore be said to be more adopted to the human host than the encapsulated variants. *H. influenzae* does not survive for long outside the human host, so pharyngeal colonisation is crucial for the survival of the species. Non-encapsulated *H. influenzae* strains have also been found to reside inside phagocytic cells in adenoid tissues of children[34]. This may be a mechanism of evading the human host defence, but the exact importance of this finding is not yet known.

Fimbriae or pili (Fig. 7.2), filamentous structures on the bacterial surface, with capacity to bind to specific receptors on the epithelial cells, seem to play an important role in the adherence of *H. influenzae* to pharyngeal cells. Cell receptors for *H. influenzae* become accessible only after damage to the cells, and viral infection is one factor that increases the binding of *H. influenzae*[4,7,16]. However, structural and functional damage can also occur if the respiratory epithelium is exposed to non-typable *H. influenzae* adhering to mucus[4,6,35,36]. Both encapsulated and non-encapsulated strains as well as pneumococci produce factors that causes slowed and disorganised ciliary beating and increased respiratory secretion of mucin.

The adhesion fimbriae are easily lost and are often not found in strains after isolation on culture media[15]. Fimbriae on *H. influenzae* type b enhance binding to pharyngeal cells, but organisms isolated from blood or CSF lack fimbriae, suggesting that fimbriae are important for the initiation of colonisation, but may be lost during invasion, when they confer no functional advantage[4,7]. In contrast, there is evidence that fimbriae may increase the susceptibility to phagocytosis, and the loss of fimbriae may then facilitate evasion of host defence mechanisms.

Invasive disease

H. influenzae is the most common cause of bacteraemic disease in children. The great majority of cases are caused by encapsulated strains of serotype b[4,5,9–14,37]. Meningitis is the most common clinical presentation of invasive *H. influenzae* type b disease in children, but epiglottitis, pneumonia, septic arthritis and cellulitis together account for almost half of the cases (Table 7.1, 7.2). Periorbital cellulitis is especially characteristic of *H. influenzae* aetiology, the pathogenesis probably being an extension from the respiratory tract; most cases seem to be caused by type b and bacteraemia may occur in one-third of the clinical cases[38,39]. Conjunctivitis is also a characteristic clinical presentation of *H. influenzae* disease[40]. Outbreaks with extension of the infection from the eye to cause life-threatening septicaemia with a rash resembling that caused by meningococci has recently been described as Brazilian purpuric fever[41].

The capsule is an important virulence factor, conferring protection against immediate phagocytosis in the absence of anticapsular antibodies and possibly protection against antibodies directed against underlying structures[4,5,9–12,14]. The type b capsule evidently confers the most efficacious protection against the host defence, since type b strains are responsible for more than 95% of the meningitis cases;

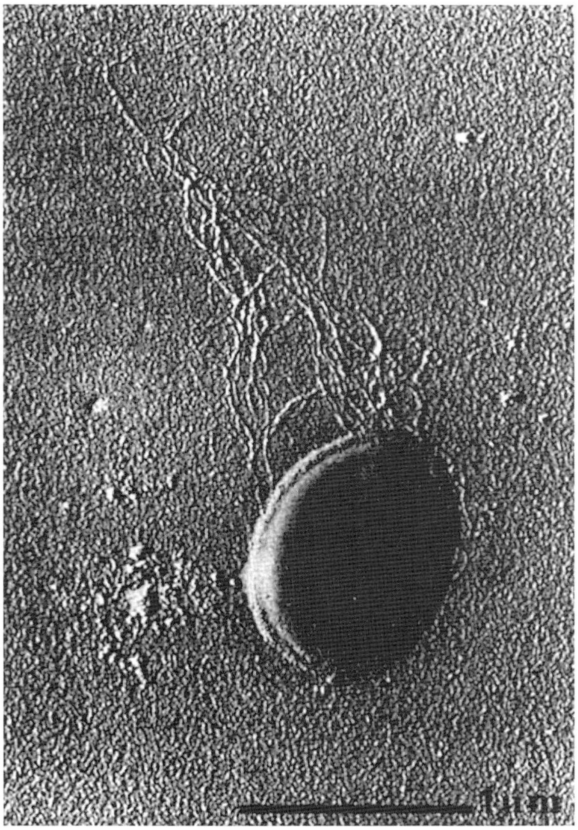

FIGURE 7.2 Electron micrograph of platinum–palladium shadowing of a non-typable strain of *H. influenzae*. (Reproduced from Apicella *et al.*, *J Infec Dis* 1984; 150: 40–3[15] by permission of The University of Chicago Press.)

Table 7.1. *Diseases caused by* Haemophilus influenzae: *some estimated incidences and frequencies of cases caused by all types of H. influenzae and by type b specifically in Western countries*

	Incidence of cases caused by *H. influenzae* per 100 000 individuals	Percentage of clinical cases with *H. influenzae* aetiology	Percentage of *H. influenzae* cases caused by type b[a]
Meningitis			
children <5 years	50[a]	30[a]	95
children ≥5 years and adults	0.2	5	50
Bacteraemia			
neonates	10		17
children	15		95
adults	1.5		30
Pneumonia			
adults	50	10	10
Epiglottitis			
children <5 y	10	97	95
adults		30	60
Sinusitis		25	5
Otitis media all ages	700	20	5
Conjunctivitis		40	5
Periorbital cellulitis in children		75	95
Brazilian purpuric fever			
Septic arthritis			
children < 5 y		30	95
adults		< 1	95
Osteomyelitis			
Peritonitis			
Pericarditis			
Endocarditis			
Soft tissue abscess			
Genitourinary infections			
Neonatal septicaemia			

[a] Now rapidly decreasing in areas with *H. influenzae* type b immunisation programmes.

Data from Carenfelt; Dajani, Asmar & Thirumoorthi; Falla *et al.*; Farley *et al.*; Gellady, Shulman & Ayoub; Gigliotti *et al*; Wald; Powell, K.R. *et al.*; Takala 1989; Takala, Eskola & van Alphen 1990[9–11, 13, 14, 38–40, 63].

Table 7.2. *Invasive* H. influenzae *disease in children and adults*

Presenting disease	Percentage of cases with respective clinical presentation			
	Type b		Non-typable	
	Children	Adults	Children	Adults
Meningitis	51	10	27	2
Epiglottitis	17	19		4
Pneumonia	15	23	27	72
Arthritis	8	7		
Cellulitis	6			
Osteomyelitis	2			
Otitis media			18	
Genitourinary infection				13
Septicaemia	2	42	27	9
Total	100	100	100	100
Total incidence per 100 000 person–years	10–20	0.2	0.5	0.2–0.8
Case fatality rate	6	26	10	28

Data from Dajani, Asmar & Thirumoorthi; Falla *et al.*; Farley *et al.*; Takala, Eskola & van Alphen, 1990[9–11, 14].

other capsular types and non-encapsulated strains cause invasive disease only occasionally. Also most other bacteraemic infections in children are caused by type b, an exception being the uncommon but well-documented neonatal *H. influenzae* infections of which some 80% are caused by non-typable strains[23].

It has long been known that protective antibody against the type b capsular polysaccharide develops in virtually all children before the age of 4–6 years[4,5,7,42]. Consequently the incidence of invasive *H. influenzae* type b disease declines rapidly from the age of 2, being less by a factor of almost 100 in individuals >10 years compared with those < 2 years of age[9]. *H. influenzae* type b disease is therefore an uncommon disease in older children and adults; most cases occur in elderly and those with underlying illnesses[14,43,44]. Septicaemia without evident focal infection, pneumonia, epiglottitis and meningitis are the most frequently encountered clinical presentations.

During the last 15 years it has become evident that also non-encapsulated *H. influenzae* may cause invasive disease. It appears to be especially common in neonates with an incidence of 3–14/100 000 person–years[10,23,45]. In older children and adults the incidence is considerably lower, approximately 0.5/100 000 person–years[10,11]. The majority of patients falling ill with invasive non-encapsualted *H. influenzae* disease have underlying predisposing conditions, but also previously healthy individuals may be affected. Pneumonia accounts for two-thirds of the adult cases and for almost all the cases in elderly[11], while in children only one-quarter of the cases are associated with pneumonia[10]. In total, bacteraemia may occur in up to 20% of the patients with *H. influenzae* pneumonia, whether caused by encapsulated or non-encapsulated strains[7,6,12]. Genitourinary infections, especially in pregnant women seem to be responsible for some 15% of adult *H. influenzae* bacteremias[11,23]. Other clinical entities encountered in patients with non-encapsulated *H. influenzae* bacteraemia include meningitis and also epiglottitis in adults. Septic arthritis in adults has been reported, but accounts for less than 1% of arthritis cases in adults; most cases have been caused by type b, but bacteraemic arthritis by non-encapsulated *H. influenzae* has also been reported[46]. *H. influenzae* may also cause pericarditis, endocarditis, primary peritonitis, mesenteric lymphadenitis, soft tissue abscesses and infected aortic grafts[11,23,43,46–51].

Respiratory tract infections

Severe *H. influenzae* disease is a significant threat to young children in developing countries (Table 7.3). It is estimated that about five million children below the age of five in developing countries each year die from pneumonia[31,52]. According to results obtained by percutaneous lung aspiration, one-quarter of the bacterial pneumonias in children in developing countries may be caused by *H. influenzae*, the same figure as for *Streptococcus pneumoniae*. At least half of the cases are caused by non-encapsulated strains and, among capsulated strains, the other five capsular types (a, c–f) together account for about as many cases as type b[31,32].

Table 7.3. *Approximate relative importance of different bacteria in severe pneumonia in children in developing countries*

Bacterial agent	%
Streptococcus pneumoniae, 83 serotypes	27
Haemophilus influenzae type b	5
other capsular types	7
non-encapsulated	15
Staphylococcus aureus	0–33
Branhamella catarrhalis	0–18
Other bacteria	20
Mixed infections	4–42

Data from Shann 1986[31] and Shann *et al.* 1984[32].

In developed countries pneumonia is a not uncommon presentation of serious *H. influenzae* type b infection in small children. However, the great majority of respiratory tract infections are caused by non-encapsulated strains. In small children acute otitis media (AOM) is the predominating clinical presentation and *H. influenzae* is the second most common aetiological agent, most often accounting for more than 20% of all cases of acute otitis media[53–56]. By outer membrane protein and lipooligosaccharide analysis as well as by DNA, fingerprinting of isolates from the nasopharynx and the middle ear, it has been clarified that AOM occurs when bacteria colonising the nasopharynx gain entrance to the middle ear[57,58]. Antecedent viral infection may be of importance in this process by damaging the respiratory epithelium in the Eustachian tube[59,60].

Acute epiglottitis (Fig. 7.3) is a rather unusual infection, but may account for 1 of every 1000 paediatric admissions[61]. Pathologically, it is a rapidly progressive cellulitis of the epiglottis. Typically, children below 5 years of age are affected and in this age-group *H. influenzae* is always found in blood cultures obtained before the start of antibiotic treatment[62]. In recent years, also, epiglottitis in older children and adults has been increasingly recognised[63–66]. In adults, the infection is most often not bacteraemic and in a significant proportion of cases caused by other bacteria than *H. influenzae*, notably *S. pneumoniae* and group A *streptococci*. Bacteria may be isolated from the epiglottic area in non-bacteraemic cases; the good correlation of such findings with those of blood cultures when they are positive, speak in favour of their significance in a majority of cases, though colonisation as a cause of false positive findings cannot be ruled out[63]. Also, viral infections have been suggested as aetiological agents in adult epiglottitis. The clinical picture in adults may be different from that in children with less dramatic symptoms and lower risk of airway obstruction.

In older children and young adults, *H. influenzae* is a rather unusual pathogen, although occasional cases of otitis media, sinusitis and severe *H. influenzae* type b disease do occur. In elderly adults the greatest impact of *H. influenzae* is as the predominating pathogen in COPD. However, pneumonia due to non-encapsulated *H. influenzae* has also been increasingly recognised during the last two decades. *H. influenzae* is probably second only to *S. pneumoniae* as a cause of bacterial pneumonia, accounting for about 10% of the cases[4,5,44,67–76]. It is especially prevalent in the elderly and in those with underlying illnesses, in particular those with chronic lung disease[14,44,77,78]. Bacteraemia is present in up to 20% of the cases of pneumonia[6,7,79].

In recent years it has become evident that *H. influenzae*, both type b and non-typable strains, may be an important cause of hospital-

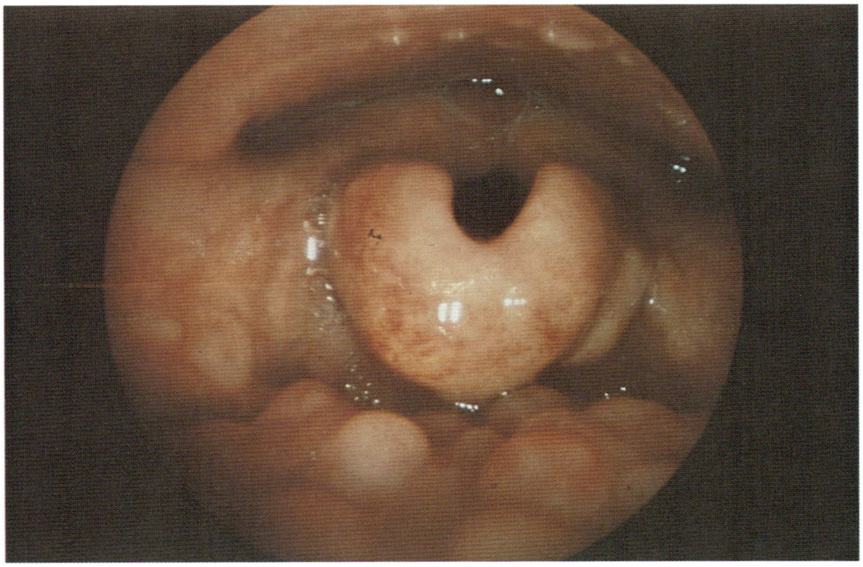

FIGURE 7.3 Acute epiglottitis. (Reproduced by permission of Dr Ove Söderberg, Department of Oto-rhino-laryngology, Umeå University Hospital.)

acquired pneumonia, accounting for up to more than 20% of the cases[51,80–84]. Spread within hospitals of specific strains has been indicated to occur from contaminated devices or by person-to-person transmission.

Host defence mechanisms

In healthy humans the filtering effect of the nose and the lower airways, as well as the barrier effect of the epiglottis, prevent bacteria of the abundant pharyngeal flora from invading and colonising the lower airways[85,86]. However, significant numbers of bacteria are nevertheless aspirated or inhaled into the bronchi even in healthy subjects; these bacteria are normally eliminated by the mucociliary transport system, by cough and by alveolar macrophages. As a response to larger numbers of aspirated bacteria an effective inflammatory response is initiated in the lung with complement and cytokine activation as well as recruitment of polymorphonuclear leukocytes, which may increase 100-fold in numbers during a few hours[86]. By these mechanisms alpha-streptococci may rapidly be eliminated, while *S. pneumoniae*, *H. influenzae* and *Moraxella catarrhalis* may survive somewhat longer, though normally eventually cleared from the lungs. These mechanisms are significantly less effective in patients with COPD and bacteria, including potentially pathogenic species such as *Pneumococci*, *H. influenzae* and *M. catarrhalis,* seem to colonise the lower airways more or less constantly in these patients[6,24,87,88]. Therefore, it has been difficult to clarify the role of bacterial infection in exacerbations of COPD. However, while non-infectious events may be responsible for a substantial part and viral and mycoplasmal infections for up to one-third of the episodes, several facts speak in favour of bacteria being the most significant factor in most episodes of acute exacerbation of chronic bronchitis[6,89,90]. Rise in antibody titres when adequate bacterial antigens have been used and significant response to antimicrobial chemotherapy directed at the isolated pathogen, support an aetiological role of bacteria[5,6,79]. By the use of transtracheal aspiration (TTA), it has been found that *Haemophilus* and *S. pneumoniae* dominate in the trachea during exacerbations in bronchitis patients, and although bacteria might also be present between exacerbations, their quantity increases during exacerbations[24,87,88,91–93]. Recently also *Moraxella (Branhamella) catarrhalis* has been found to be an important pathogen, and mixed infections involving two or even all three of these species are common.

Antibody and complement

As mentioned, protective antibody against the type b capsular polysaccharide develops in virtually all children before the age of 4–6 years leading to a dramatic reduction of the prevalence of *H. influenzae* type b infection beyond that age[4,5,42]. During infection and colonisation with non-encapsulated *H. influenzae,* an antibody response is elicited both in serum and on mucus membranes against the OMPs of the colonising strain. Individuals with defects in B-cell function are more prone to acquire *H. influenzae* infections[4,5]. However, the great heterogeneity in OMP 2 pattern exhibited by non-encapsulated *H. influenzae* strains precludes protection against newly acquired strains by previously developed antibodies. Moreover there seem to be a continuous minor alteration of the OMP 2 pattern during colonisation in COPD patients, possibly enabling the organisms to evade host defences[17,94]. Antibodies to the highly conserved P6 protein are protective[6], but thus seem not to develop in a way to confer sufficient protection against re-infection. The efficacy of the local IgA response on the mucous membranes has not been fully elucidated[7]. Oral vaccination of COPD-patients with formalin-killed non-typable *H. influenzae* induces a significant reduction of exacerbations, but only for one winter season[6].

Complement is important in the hosts defence against *H. influenzae* infection[85,95]. Both the classical and the alternative pathways can be activated by capsular substance of the type b capsule as well as by cell wall structures exposed on unencapsulated strains. Anticapsular antibody of the IgG1 subclass seems to be more efficient than IgG2 at promoting complement-dependent opsonisation or bactericidal activity. C3 deficiency is associated with an increased susceptibility to bacterial infections with *H. influenzae* being the most important pathogen beside *S. pneumoniae* and *Neisseria meningitidis*. Furthermore, C4 may play a certain role in the defence against infections with *H. influenzae*, since C4 deficiency, which is rather common, is more frequently seen in patients with invasive *H. influenzae* disease[95].

Functional asplenia and HIV

Asplenic individuals (splenectomised persons or those with a non-functioning spleen, for example patients with sickle cell anaemia) are at an increased risk of acquiring fulminant infections with encapsulated bacteria[96]. (For pathogenesis of infection in asplenic individuals, see Chapter 4.) *S. pneumoniae* predominates as the aetiological agent, while encapsulated *H. influenzae* is the second most frequent organism encountered, being responsible for roughly 10% of the cases. A reduction of the incidence of *S. pneumoniae* infections has been noted in individuals older than 2 years of age after the introduction of the 14-valent pneumococcal polysaccharide vaccine in 1978. With the recent introduction of polyribosyl–ribitol phosphate-protein conjugate vaccines (*H. influenzae* type b polysaccharide–protein conjugate), the incidence of invasive *H. influenzae* disease in asplenic individuals can be anticipated to become significantly reduced[33,97–101]. The conjugate vaccines are also immunogenic in children less than 2 years of age and in asplenic children, and these vaccines have decreased both the incidence of invasive disease and the carriage of *H. influenzae* type b.

Several studies have indicated that the risk of invasive *H. influenzae* disease is markedly increased in patients with human immunodeficiency virus (HIV) infection[77,78,102,103], in AIDS patients perhaps up to 100-fold compared with the rate in the general population, in HIV-patients without AIDS up to 20-fold. Pneumonia and septicaemia are the most common clinical presentations. As in other adults, at least half of the infecting strains seem to be non-encapsulated. Antibody titres against PRP are lower than in non-HIV-infected individuals; the antibody level may be below the putative protective level in as much as 40% of AIDS-patients[104]. Both symptomatic and asymptomatic HIV-infection are associated with an impaired antibody response to *H. influenzae* type b polysaccharide vaccine[104]. However, contrary to asymptomatic HIV-positive recipients of vaccine, AIDS-patients for unclear reasons, seem to respond better to pure polysaccharide than to protein-conjugated polysaccharide.

Clinical presentation

In pneumonia in children in developed countries an aetiological diagnosis is usually not obtained and it is therefore not possible to specifically characterise *H. influenzae* pneumonia. However, as in developing countries[31,52] *H. influenzae* is probably the second most common bacterial agent. Both encapsulated and non-encapsulated strains may be responsible. In the former case the presentation typically will be one of severe lower respiratory tract disease with rapid onset, and in the latter more insidious bronchitis-like. In the latter case, the illness often starts with coryza-like illness with gradually increasing symptoms of anorexia, malaise and tachypnoea. Pleuritic chest pain may occur.

Severe pneumonia with acute onset with high fever and pleuritic chest pain due to *H. influenzae* type b may occur also in adults (Fig. 7.4), but the vast majority of respiratory tract infections in adults are caused by non-encapsulated strains affecting primarily the elderly and those with underlying lung disease[11,14,43,44,105,106]. In many cases the patients have actually been treated for an underlying lung disease in hospital when *H. influenzae* pneumonia has developed. The onset of *H. influenzae* pneumonia is often more insidious than that seen in typical pneumococcal pneumonia. Pleuritic chest pain is common in *H. influenzae* pneumonia and haemoptysis has been noted in a significant proportion of cases in some series. However, in practice it is often impossible to differentiate beween different bacterial aetiologies on the basis of clinical presentation. The existence of underlying pulmonary illness should alert the physician to think of *H. influenzae* as the aetiological agent. The severity of the infectious event will, to a large extent, be dependent on the severity of the underlying lung disease. *H. influenzae* pneumonia, therefore, may be as severe a disease as *S. pneumoniae* pneumonia with a high percentage of cases requiring ICU admission[73].

In patients with COPD, acute exacerbation is often manifested by increased frequency of cough and increased amount and purulence of sputum[6,87]. The patient's own registration of the changes in sputum are important. Haemoptysis may occur and dyspnoea, wheezing and general malaise may be present. However, there is no accepted definition for an acute exacerbation of chronic bronchitis, and the diagnosis rests on the interpretation of the patient's history. Rigors, high fever and pleuritic chest pain suggest pneumonia.

On examination, dyspnea, cyanosis, tachypnoea, tachycardia, wheezing, rhonchi, decreased breath sounds and rales are found to varying degrees depending on the patient's previous condition and the severity of the current infection.

The chest radiographical findings in *H. influenzae* respiratory disease may be highly variable[5,44,105–109]. In severe bacteraemic *H. influenzae* type b pneumonia, the chest X-ray often shows segmental, lobar or even multilobar or bilateral infiltrates. In most cases of adult *H. influenzae* pneumonia, however, the appearance is typically one of bronchopneumonia with small patchy infiltrates. Even diffuse, interstitial or mixed alveolar – interstitial patterns of infiltrates may occur. Pleural involvement is common, being noted in at least half of the patients (Fig. 7.5), but frank empyema is uncommon. Lung abscesses may develop in up to 5% of the cases of *H. influenzae* pneumonia. In acute exacerbations of chronic bronchitis the chest X-ray often contributes little to the diagnosis: small, uncharacteristic infiltrates may be present, but are often absent despite existence of a bacterial aetiology.

Other laboratory parameters are usually non-characteristic. In bacteraemic infections, marked leukocytosis and high C-reactive protein levels are frequent, while in the majority of non-bacteraemic infections these parameters are only slightly abnormal. Hypoxia is

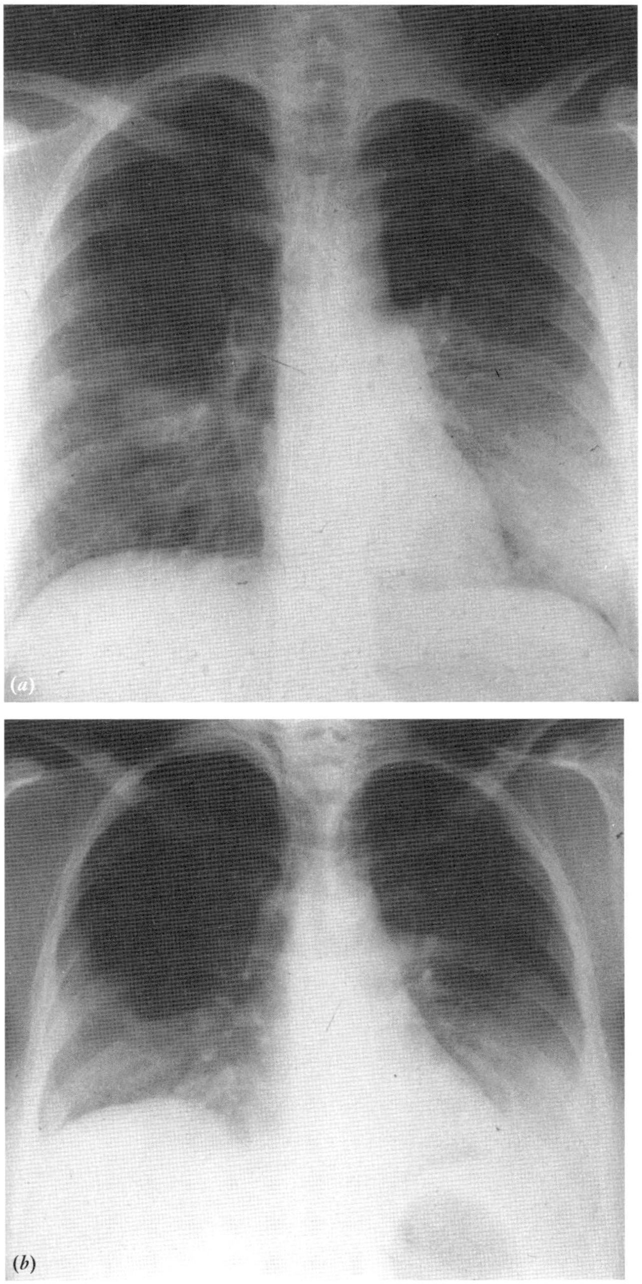

FIGURE 7.4 (*a*), (*b*) Pneumonia in a 22-year-old woman caused by a betalactamase-producing strain of *H. influenzae* serotype b. The patient was admitted because of deterioration on oral penicillin. She was given ampicillin when Gram's stain indicated small Gram-negative rods, but continued to deteriorate (790505 4a –790509 4b). She recovered when therapy was changed to chloramphenicol.

common in patients with moderate to severe chronic bronchitis and may occur also in patients with lobar pneumonia, most often due to *H. influenzae* type b.

Aetiological diagnosis

In epiglottitis, meningitis and other invasive infections in childhood, blood cultures are usually positive. In most other cases of respiratory tract infections due to *H. influenzae* type b or to unencapsulated types, blood cultures are positive in 10–20%[6,7,79]. Presence of *H. influenzae* bacteraemia was probably greatly underdiagnosed in many laboratories until the 1980s, since many broth culture systems used without routine subculturing produced little or no evidence of presence of bacteria in the broth[106].

There are conflicting reports on the usefulness of culture and direct Gram's stain of sputum specimes[44,67]. Growth of *Haemophilus* is often missed and bacteraemic patients have often been found negative by sputum culture. Moreover, contamination of the sputum specimen by oropharyngeal secretions is inevitable and since carriership is very common, the rate of false positive results will be very high with routine sputum procedures[110]. A concomitant positive Gram's stain with many (most often numerous) small Gram-negative rods in purulent parts of a sputum smear increases the likelihood of a positive culture being significant[68,71,77,79,111] (Fig. 7.6). However, sensitivity and specificity can be improved beyond that. Both Gram's stains and cultures are much easier interpreted if performed after washing the sputum specimen with tap water; the washing procedure eliminates more than 99% of the oropharyngeal flora; thus both sensitivity and specificity are increased[112–115]. Cultures performed quantitatively with a cut-off limit of 10^6 bacteria per ml of homogenised sputum further increases the specificity. With any procedure, only purulent specimens should be accepted for Gram's stain and culture, non-purulent specimens being too heavily contaminated by saliva. Sputum sampling by means of transtracheal aspiration avoids most, but not all, of the oropharyngeal contamination[93,110], but this procedure is today not well accepted by the patient. If an invasive method should be used, flexible bronchoscopy should probably be preferred, due to the acceptability to the patient, the very low risk of complications, the high sensitivity and specificity of cultures via a protected specimen brush, and finally due to the advantage of the possibility of direct inspection of the respiratory tree[116].

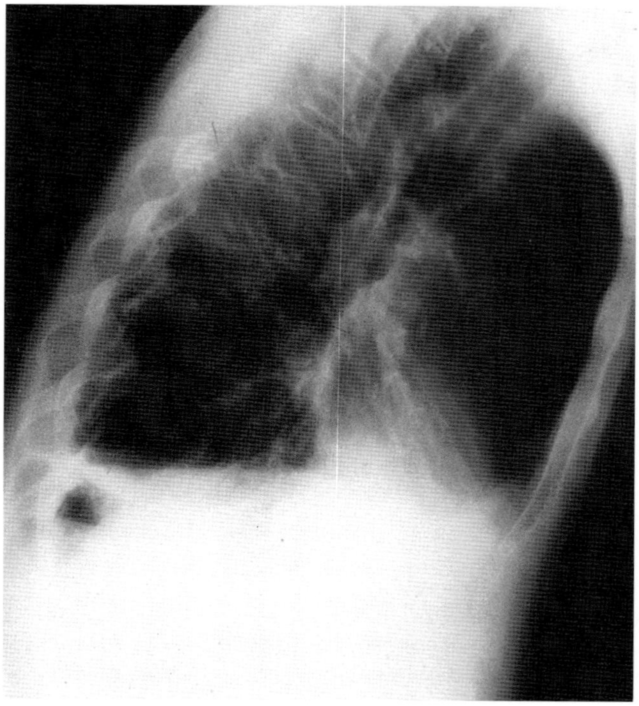

FIGURE 7.5 *H. influenzae* pneumonia with typical pleural effusion.

While quantitative bacterial cultures have been found less valuable in establishing the diagnosis of a bacterial infection in patients with COPD, Gram's stains by revealing increased number of polymorphonuclear leukocytes and bacteria have been found to be more reliable in suggesting a bacterial involvement[71,87,91]. The number of bacteria per oil immersion field is usually more than ten.

Type b capsular polysaccharide antigen may be detected in serum, urine or sputum by an immunological method such as counterimmunoelectrophoresis, latex agglutination or coagglutination[117–119]. However, due to the low prevalence of *H. influenzae* type b as the cause of pneumonia in most clinical settings, it is not a cost-effective test. In contrast, in bacterial meningitis *H. influenzae* type b antigen detection is well established for obtaining a rapid diagnosis and especially useful when the patient has received antibiotics prior to sampling, in which case cultures most often are negative. All the methods are almost 100% specific, but the latex agglutination method appears to be the most sensitive, detecting 90–100 % of cases of *H. influenzae* type b meningitis.

Complications

Children with bacteraemic non-meningitic disease usually have an uneventful recovery if they receive adequate and prompt antibiotic treatment[120,121]. This is true also in most of the cases with associated focal infections including otitis media, arthritis, cellulitis or pericarditis. With associated meningitis the prognosis is more serious, but the case fatality rate is only a few per cent in most settings today.

In previously healthy adults with bacteraemic *H. influenzae* type b pneumonia, the course resembles that of bacteraemic *S. pneumoniae* pneumonia; that is the prognosis is good in non-alcoholic young patients, but with a mortality rate of 20% or more in elderly patients and those with serious underlying conditions[105,106]. In contrast, many patients with severe underlying diseases and *H. influenzae* pneumonia will have a more serious course, and will depend on the underlying diseases rather than the *H. influenzae* infection *per se*. These patients may rapidly develop tachycardia, dyspnea, disorientation and septic shock. Respiratory and multi-organ failure may develop. The mortality in this patient group may be very high.

In patients with acute exacerbation of chronic bronchitis, the infectious episode may be minor and bacteraemia is uncommon. However, due to the pre-existing lung disease, the course may be serious. The lung capacity during the infection-free intervals is the most important determining factor for the development of respiratory failure. The prognosis is thus dependent on the nature of the advanced chronic pulmonary disease. The acute infectious event can often be brought under control, but if acceptable oxygenation cannot be maintained without artificial ventilation, other complications are likely to develop and the patients' chances of being weaned from the ventilator are guarded. The decision whether to put such a patient on a ventilator is therefore often difficult.

As mentioned, a pleural reaction indicated by symptomatic pleurisy and/or radiological evidence of pleural effusion has been noted in at least half of the patients with *H. influenzae* pneumonia[5,44,106–109]. Empyema with growth of *H. influenzae* from the pleural space and with requirement for drainage is, however, uncommon. Pulmonary abscess formation due to *H. influenzae* has been noted in rare cases, but appears to be uncommon and is seen only in the severest cases today[106]. It may have been more frequent in the beginning of the twentieth century[109].

Management

In patients with pneumonia prompt initation of effective antimicrobial chemotherapy may be life-saving, especially in the elderly and in those with debilitating underlying diseases. Ampicillin or amoxicillin were the drugs of choice before β-lactamase-producing strains became prevalent in cases when *H. influenzae* was identified as the incriminated pathogen for patients not allergic to penicillin. In geographical areas where the frequency of β-lactamase-producing strains is low, this may still be adequate in infections that are not life threatening. In areas with higher prevalence of β-lactamase-producing strains, amoxicillin may be used in combination with a β-lactamase-inhibitor such as clavulanate potassium. In patients allergic to penicillin cotrimoxazole, tetracyclines, or fluoroquinolones are alternatives to be used judiciously in view of the local resistance situation[89,122]. In patients with a history of non-anaphylactic reaction to penicillin, cephalosporins may also be used, and second or third generation cephalosporins are the main alternatives in most cases of serious *H. influenzae* disease.

In the acute stage of exacerbation of chronic bronchitis, appropriate antibiotic chemotherapy, oxygen and improvement of ventilatory

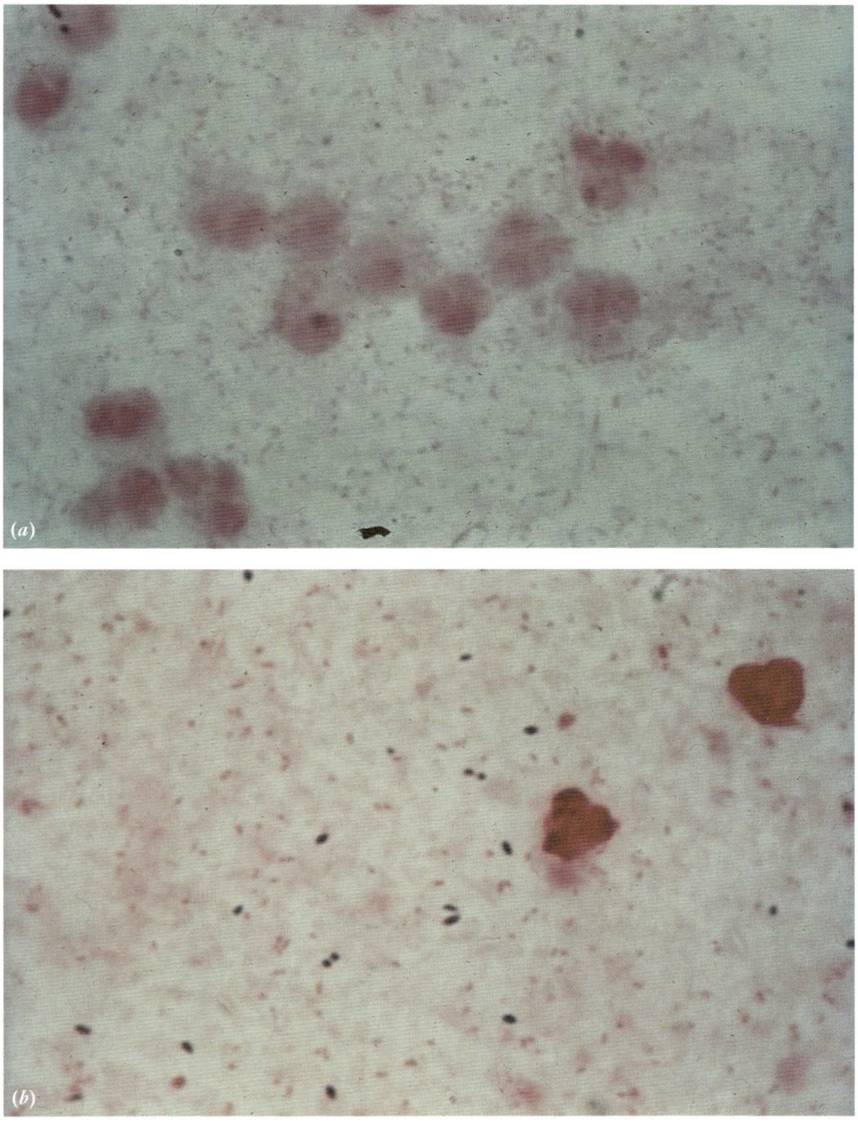

FIGURE 7.6 (*a*) Sputum Gram's stain with numerous small Gram-negative rods in purulent specimen. (*b*) Sputum Gram's stain with numerous small Gram-negative rods mixed with Gram-positive diplococci in purulent specimen.

function are the most important measures. Patients with hypoxia should, in general, be treated with oxygen to achieve oxygenation close to the degree the patient is accustomed to in the absence of acute infection (which is nevertheless often below the normal range), in order to reduce dyspnoea and to improve cardiac function and tissue oxygenation, and thus facilitate breathing. Pulmonary function tests to assess expiratory airflow and to determine whether the patient has a reversible component of bronchoconstriction may be valuable diagnostic procedures. If there is reversible bronchospasm, bronchodilator therapy may be effective for improvement of the ventilation. Steroids may sometimes be effective for relieving acute symptoms of dyspnoea, but their long-term use is controversial. Physiotherapy, supported if necessary by mucolytic agents, may be important in those cases where large amounts of secretions contribute to decreased ventilation[123,124]. In patients without copious sputum production, physiotherapy is often unhelpful and may even be harmful by inducing bronchospasm. Relief of acute infectious signs and symptoms or radiographic resolution may be delayed by physiotherapy. However, regaining lung volume by physiotherapy may sometimes be achieved when there is a lobar pneumonia without an air bronchogram, i.e. a mucus plug. Forced expiration without coughing may improve sputum production and ventilation in patients who produce copious sputum.

There are still many unresolved issues concerning the use of antibiotics in patients with COPD[6,87,89,122]. The role of acute infectious exacerbations in accelerating the decline of pulmonary function in patients with COPD is not yet defined[6]. While there are indications that frequent exacerbations may lead to a more rapid deterioration of lung function, which then might be prevented by antibiotic treatment of acute exacerbations[125], most investigators have been unable to confirm this. The role of prophylactic antibiotic treatment is also unsettled, but mucosal damage may be averted by sub-MIC concentration of antibiotics[36]. Patients with severe disease and many exacerbations may benefit from such a regimen, but for the great majority of patients there is probably no advantage of such a regimen. The risk of selecting bacteria with increased resistance to antibiotics must also be kept in mind.

The role of antibiotics during acute exacerbations has also been extensively debated. However, given several facts which suggest a causal role for bacteria in many of these episodes, and the benefit seen in large studies which have included patients with severe disease, the decision to treat moderately severe and severe episodes with adequate antimicrobial agents seems well founded[5,6,87]. In a recent meta-analysis, a small, but statistically significant, improvement was found to be due to antibiotic therapy during acute exacerbations[126]. Due to the frequent colonisation of these patients between exacerbations, sputum culture is not suitable for establishing an infectious diagnosis, but information of the susceptibility of bacteria identified in sputum specimens may be used for choosing the most appropriate antibiotic treatment. Since three species, *H. influenzae*, *S. pneumoniae*, and *M. catarrhalis,* predominate in these infections, standardised empiric treatment is often used.

The time-honoured regimen in these patients has been prompt initiation of antimicrobial chemotherapy with good activity against *H. influenzae* and *S. pneumoniae* (and recently against *M.catarrhalis*) in high dose for 10–14 days[6,67,87,122,125]. The ampicillin-group, the fluorinated quinolones, doxycycline and cotrimoxazole, have proved effective in the acute stage, while erythromycin, cephalexin, cephaclor and penicillin V have been associated with higher failure rates. Moreover, infection-free periods have been significantly longer with ampicillin, the quinolones, and doxycycline. The choice of antibiotic therapy must, of course, be influenced by the current information concerning antibiotic resistance among prevalent pathogens. In areas with a high frequency of β-lactamase-producing *H. influenzae*, ampicillin should probably not be used as a first-line drug. On the other hand, activity against *S. pneumoniae* has been unsatisfactory for ciprofloxacin[127], and, the extensive use of tetracyclines, as used in Spain, has led to a very high degree of resistance[128,129]. The concomitant use of several alternatives within a community is probably preferable from a resistance development point of view.

Antibiotic resistance in *H. influenzae*

The first ampicillin-resistant strains were described from Europe in 1972. Since then there has been a world-wide increase in the prevalence of resistance to ampicillin, today affecting 1–36% of strains isolated in different geographical areas[130–133]. The most common mechanism of ampicillin resistance is plasmid-mediated production of the TEM-1 β-lactamase, which is found in almost 20% of strains isolated in the USA and Canada and in some 10% in most European countries. Significantly higher prevalences may be seen in strains isolated from young children, especially with type b strains. Rare strains (in less than 1% of instances), are ampicillin-resistant but β-lactamase-negative. In such strains the affinity of two of the penicillin-binding proteins (PBP, i.e. the peptidoglycan-synthesising enzymes) is reduced for ampicillin[134]. The binding of penicillin is affected to the same degree as that of ampicillin. Also cephalosporin binding is reduced. In Canada altered PBPs have been found also in strains with only slightly increased MIC values for ampicillin, increasing the prevalence of such strains ten-fold to 2.6%[131,134].

Second- and particularly the third-generation parenteral cephalosporins show a very high activity against virtually all strains of *H. influenzae*. These drugs are very stable against the TEM-1 β-lactamases and their binding is only slightly affected by altered PBPs. Most oral cephalosporins, on the other hand, are less active, though significantly better alternatives are continously becoming available.

In the USA, resistance to non-betalactam drugs is uncommon, though approximately 6% may be resistant to tetracycline[130,131]. Resistance to tetracycline, chloramphenicol and trimethoprim-sulphamethoxazole and also multiple resistance, seem to be significantly more prevalent in Europe than in the USA. The proportion of isolates of *H. influenzae* resistant to antimicrobials also varies considerably among countries in Europe, the highest incidence being recorded in Spain[129,133]. Multiply-resistant strains of *H. influenzae* for the most part are susceptible to amoxycillin-clavulanate, second and third generation cephalosporins and fluoroquinolones. Strains resistant to erythromycin are also resistant to the newer macrolides.

Prophylaxis and control

The first licensed *H. influenzae* type b vaccine consisting of purified PRP was effective in certain settings, but to a very limited degree in the most important target group, namely children below the age of 18 months[98]. The second generation of vaccines consist of PRP conjugated to diphtheria or tetanus toxoid or *N. meningitides OMP*, or of *H. influenzae* oligosaccharide conjugated to diphtheria toxoid. All of these four conjugates are immunogenic in small children. These vaccines have proved very effective for protection against systemic *H. influenzae* type b disease in small children. In the US and in Finland, where they have been used for several years, the number of such infections has been reduced by 80–90% subsequent to the vaccine introduction[97–99,135,136]. *H. influenzae* type b conjugate vaccines are therefore now recommended for general use as early as possible in childhood. In addition, carriage rates of *H. influenzae* type b have been significantly reduced after vaccination, and this will contribute to the pace with which invasive *H. influenzae* type b disease will decrease when vaccination has been widely implemented[33,100,136]. For protection against non-encapsulated strains, no definitive vaccine candidate in the surface structure of *H. influenzae* is recognised at this time[4]. Outer membrane protein–lipo-oligosaccharide complex has been shown to produce antibodies and increase pulmonary clearance of *H. influenzae*[86]. The available vaccines composed of protein conjugated type b capsule polysaccharide, while very effective for the protection against systemic *H. influenzae* type b disease, do not confer any protection against disease with non-encapsulated strains.

Areas for research

It is important to follow the epidemiology of invasive *H. influenzae* disease after the introduction of the type b polysaccharide protein conjugate vaccines. It is at present uncertain as to the longevity of the protection and whether booster doses are necessary, particularly since the prevalence of *H. influenzae* type b seems to become very low after implementation of the vaccine, so that natural boostering will not take place.

It is vital to find ways of immunising persons with COPD against non-encapsulated *H. influenzae* strains and to elucidate the mechanisms by which the bacteria evade host defences. Mucosal immunisation may be one possible means of progress. The role of bacteria residing for long periods inside phagocytes should be further explored.

Management of patients with COPD may be improved by clarifying the relative roles of bacteria, other infectious agents and non-infectious factors in the progress of the chronic disease as well as in acute exacerbations. The use of antibiotics in these patients may subsequently be improved. This may be especially important considering the emergence of resistance in several geographical areas.

The epidemiology of antibiotic resistance has to be followed continously. The emergence of β-lactam-antibiotic resistance through changes in penicillin binding proteins is worrying and deserves special attention. The impact of PBP resistance is at this time unclear.

Methods for diagnosing bacterial lower respiratory tract infection will hopefully be improved. Polymerase chain reaction techniques may be applicable, but the very prevalent colonisation with *H. influenzae* in the upper airways will most probably cause problems with the specificity of that test. New approaches to circumvent this are needed.

Summary

H. influenzae is one of the most common inhabitants of the human oropharyngeal flora, where the bacteria adhere to epithelial cell receptors that become accessible after cell damage by virus or bacteria or other agents. Colonisation is especially common in small children and in people with COPD. Most strains, both those colonising and those causing disease are unencapsulated.

Encapsulated *H. influenzae* serotype b is the most important cause of invasive disease including meningitis, epiglottitis, arthritis, osteomyelitis, and cellulitis in small children. Protective antibodies against the polysaccharide capsule develop in the majority of humans within the first 5 years of life and therefore invasive *H. influenzae* disease is uncommon in older children and adults. However, such antibodies do not develop in small children owing to their immature immune system. Vaccines have recently been developed by conjugation of the type b polysaccharide with a protein carrier molecule, and confer a very high degree of protection in all age groups. *H. influenzae* type b disease and also carriage is therefore being almost eliminated in areas with a high degree of vaccination.

Unencapsulated strains cause primarily respiratory tract infections such as otitis media, sinusitis, bronchitis and pneumonia. In all these conditions *H. influenzae* is second in frequency only to *S. pneumoniae* in infections with a bacterial aetiology. *H. influenzae* is a particularly important pathogen in patients with COPD. The role of bacteria in this disease has been under debate for 40 years, but several facts speak in favour of an important role for *H. influenzae*, *S. pneumoniae* and *M. catarrhalis*, at least in the more severe episodes of acute exacerbations. *H. influenzae* may colonise patients with COPD continuously and seems to evade host defence mechanisms by a constant change of outer membrane proteins to which antibodies are directed.

Unencapsulated strains may also cause invasive disease, especially in neonates and in persons with predisposing underlying conditions. Pneumonia is the most common focal infection, especially in the elderly. Meningitis, septicaemia, and genitourinary infections account for most of the other cases, while other conditions constitute unusual clinical presentations.

Treatment success in *H. influenzae* infection is often dependent on the severity of the underlying condition, the most important being the severity of chronic lung disease. Ampicillin, second or third generation cephalosporins, tetracyclines, cotrimoxazole and fluoroquinolones are usually effective alternatives for antimicrobial therapy. However, in some areas up to 30% or more of the strains may produce β-lactamase, rendering them resistant to ampicillin. Emergence of resistance against all of the alternative drugs is today seen with increasing frequency, in most areas.

MORAXELLA (BRANHAMELLA) CATARRHALIS

Microbiology

The first report of bronchitis caused by *Moraxella (Branhamella) catarrhalis*, by then named *Micrococcus catarrhalis*, appeared in 1896[137].

It was subsequently classified in the genus Neisseria, and, despite a few reports on invasive infections, for most of this century was regarded as an apathogenic inhabitant of the oropharyngeal cavity[138]. In 1970 the species was reclassified, and transferred to another genus, *Branhamella* on the basis of DNA analysis[138,139]. However, from further studies, the close relationship to *Moraxella* became evident, and it is today classified as a subgenus within the genus *Moraxella*, rendering it the official name *Moraxella* (*Branhamella*) *catarrhalis* in the 1984 edition of *Bergey's Manual of Systematic Bacteriology*[138–140]. Today, the tendency is either to delete the subgenus name, i.e. *Moraxella catarrhalis*, or to keep the well-established name *Branhamella catarrhalis*. Despite the fact that the name *Branhamella catarrhalis* recently has gained widespread acceptance as the name of a clinically significant pathogen, the formally more correct *Moraxella catarrhalis* is being increasingly used and will be used here.

M. catarrhalis appears on Gram's stain as large kidney-shaped Gram-negative cocci. It grows on blood or chocolate agar media aerobically or under 10% CO_2. Colonies characteristically remain intact as they are dislodged and nudged across the agar surface. This phenomenon in conjunction with oxidase and catalase positivity and typical Gram's stain is in most settings appropriate for presumptive identification[139]. For definitive identification *M. catarrhalis* is differentiated from *Neisseriae* by its failure to ferment any of the common carbohydrates; it reduces both nitrates and nitrites and produces butyric acid esterase[138,139].

The cell wall of *M. catarrhalis* is composed of the two phospholipid bilayers characteristic of all Gram-negative bacteria with a periplasmic space and a thin peptidoglycan layer in-between[138]. The innermost layer, the cytoplasmic membrane carries the penicillin binding proteins. As with *H. influenzae*, the lipopolysaccharide structure of the outer membrane is devoid of the long O antigen polysaccharide chains characteristic of Gram-negative enteric bacteria and hence the term lipooligosaccharide (LOS) is used. The absence of long lipopolysaccharide chains renders the bacterial envelope more permeable, and is the reason for erythromycin and rifampicin susceptibility. In sharp contrast to *H. influenzae*, however, the eight identified outer membrane proteins of *M. catarrhalis* from diverse geographical and clinical settings have been found to be strikingly constant[141–143]. Also the lipooligosaccharide, consisting of lipid A and a seven-residue oligosaccharide, seems to be non-varying and appears to be unique to this organism.

Several phenotypic characteristics are consistent with the presence of pili or fimbriae, at least on some strains of *M. catarrhalis*[144]. Fimbriae seem to be involved in the adherence of *M. catarrhalis* strains to nasopharyngeal cells during colonisation; an epithelial receptor is indicated by the mode of adherence[138,145,146]. A substance consistent with a capsule outside the cell wall has been visualised by electron microscopy[138].

Epidemiology and pathogenesis

Moraxella species other than *catarrhalis*, for example, *Moraxella lacunata*, *Moraxella liquefaciens*, *Moraxella nonliquefaciens* and *Moraxella osloensis* have been reported as the cause of infections such as septicaemia and ophthalmitis as well as respiratory and urinary tract infections[147–152]. However, in the context of respiratory tract infections their importance is minor, while *M. catarrhalis* now appears as one of the predominating pathogens.

M. catarrhalis produces a spectrum of infectious diseases (Table 7.4). The first cases of septicaemia were described in the beginning of the twentieth century, and at present more than 30 cases have been reported[153–161]. Many, but not all, of the recent cases have occurred in patients with immunosuppressive diseases or treatments, and some have had focal infections identified. Rare cases of endocarditis, pericarditis, septic arthritis and meningitis have been reported[138,162]. *M. catarrhalis* is an established cause of ophthalmia neonatorum, and rare cases of conjunctivitis as well as keratitis have been described also in older children[138,147,150,162]. Also *M. lacunata* has been isolated from conjunctival infections[152], and epidemic conjunctivitis with this species, as well as with *M. catarrhalis*, have been described[151,163]. A few cases of genitourinary infections have been reported[138,162,164,165]. However, the importance of *M. catarrhalis* as a human pathogen is primarily due to its role in respiratory tract infections.

The pathogenetic role of *M. catarrhalis* in respiratory tract infections has been appreciated only during the last two decades, though as mentioned the first cases were described almost 100 years ago (Table 7.5)[161,162,166,167]. *M. catarrhalis* has in many centres in recent years emerged as the major respiratory tract pathogen alongside *S. pneumoniae* and *H. influenzae*, both in sinusitis and in otitis media[53,54,162,168,169]. It has also been implicated as a cause of bacterial tracheitis and laryngitis[162,170] *M. catarrhalis* has been implicated in a condition in children characterised by long-standing cough; in non-pertussis cases *M. catarrhalis* has been isolated significantly more often in cases than in controls, while the frequency of isolation of S. pneumoniae and *H. influenzae* has been the same in the two groups[171,172]. A pathogenetic role of *M. catarrhalis* is supported by the effectiveness of treatment directed against it[172,173].

In lower respiratory tract infections the use of invasive diagnostic methods such as TTA and percutaneous lung aspiration have helped to clarify the pathogenicity. *M. catarrhalis* has been isolated in pure culture in high counts or has been isolated together with an established chest pathogen, usually *S. pneumoniae* or *H. influenzae*, both in children and adults[32,91,112,162]. The demonstration of an antibody response in the majority of patients supports a pathogenetic role of *M.catarrhalis*.

Bactericidal antibodies against *M. catarrhalis* have been found in most of the patients recovering from an infection with this bacterial species[174]. With other immunological methods an antibody response has, in most studies, been demonstrated in approximately half of the patients[175–180]. *M. catarrhalis* therefore, may sometimes be isolated from respiratory secretions as a commensal or as a co-pathogen with minor importance. However, in children with *M. catarrhalis* isolated from the middle ear, an antibody response has often been lacking[178,180]. Alternative explanations may thus be that an antibody response fails to occur also in significant infections or that the most relevant antigens have not been used or been exposed in the test settings employed.

Other respiratory tract pathogens have been isolated concomitantly in at least a third of the *M. catarrhalis* chest infections[138,161,167,181,182].

Table 7.4. *Infections reported as due to* Moraxella catarrhalis

Septicaemia
Endocarditis
Pericarditis
Septic arthritis
Meningitis
Ophthalmia neonatorum
Conjunctivitis in older children
Keratitis
Urinary tract infection
Otitis media
Sinusitis
Bacterial tracheitis
Long-standing cough
Acute exacerbation of chronic bronchitis
Pneumonia
Empyema

Table 7.5. *Evidence of pathogenicity of* M. catarrhalis *in respiratory tract infections*

- More than 30 cases of bacteraemia have been described.
- *M. catarrhalis* has been isolated in pure culture from TTA material.
- *M. catarrhalis* has been isolated in combination with *H. influenzae* or *S. pneumoniae* from lung aspirates from children with pneumonia.
- *M. catarrhalis* has been isolated in pure culture from middle ear or maxillary sinus aspirates.
- *M. catarrhalis* has been isolated, recovered as the only pathogen from sputum in conjunction with direct Gram-stained smear showing numerous Gram-negative diplococci and no other bacteria within purulent parts of the smear. Also bacteria within leukocytes may be identified.
- An antibody response against *M. catarrhalis* specific antigens develops in a high percentage of cases when *M. catarrhalis* has been isolated.
- Clinical failure is common when inappropriate antibiotics have been used – but response when therapy has been changed to one directed against *M.catarrhalis*.
- Fatal cases of pneumonia in which *M. catarrhalis* was the only isolated pathogen have been described.

Previously healthy people seem to be uncommonly affected. Some 90% have had an underlying cardiopulmonary disease, usually chronic obstructive pulmonary disease (COPD)[70,114,138,161,167,182–184] (Table 7.6, 7.7). *M. catarrhalis* appears to be the third most prevalent aetiological agent in acute exacerbation of chronic bronchitis after *H. influenzae* and *S. pneumoniae*. It is probably responsible for 1–5% of the cases of community-acquired pneumonia. Interestingly, there are some indications that *M. catarrhalis* may act as an indirect pathogen in mixed infections through β-lactamase production which protects a co-pathogen, e.g. *S. pneumoniae*, from the killing effect of penicillin[114,138,166]. Recently, evidence for the importance of this mechanism has been acquired from infections in experimental animals[185].

Whether there has been a real increase during the last two decades is debatable[138,162,166–168]. Increased awareness of this pathogen no doubt is one factor for the increased number of cases diagnosed. It is also clear that an unknown number of *M. catarrhalis* strains isolated before 1980 were mis-identified as other *Neisseria* species. Antibiotic prescription routines may have been of importance for an increased incidence of *M. catarrhalis* infections, but can hardly be the only explanation, since there has been no dramatic change in the spectrum of drugs used during the time period when the increase has been noted. A change in virulence cannot be excluded, but there are no data supporting such a view. The increased number of immunosuppressed patients may be of some importance, since *M. catarrhalis* often affects people with underlying malignancies and only occasionally people without underlying chronic lung disease. A final point of possible

Table 7.6. *429 bronchopulmonary infections with* Moraxella catarrhalis

	%
Patients with COPD:	55
with a smoking history	77
without underlying cardiopulmonary disease	11
with immunocompromising disease	74
Pure cultures were obtained in	61
Mixed culture in	39
In the cases with mixed infections	
H. influenzae was isolated in	44
S. pneumoniae	29
Gram-negative enteric rods	18
Other bacteria	9

Adapted after Hager *et al.* 1987[167].

Table 7.7. *42 cases of pneumonia with* M. catarrhalis *as the sole pathogen*

	%
Age over 65 years	55
55 years	81
Malnourished	71
Patients in good health before *M. catarrhalis* infection	0
Chronic obstructive pulmonary disease	76
Current smokers or ex-smokers	83
Occurrence September – April	93
Chills	24
Pleuritic chest pain	33
Fever >100 °F (37.8 °C)	57
Leukocytosis	76
Chest X-ray	
consolidation	43
interstitial or diffuse infiltrates	38
mixed infiltrates	19
pleural effusion	5
cavitary lesions	5
Death	
of pneumonia	7
totally during hospitalisation	21
totally within three months of discharge	45

Adapted after Wright, Wallace & Shephard 1990[184].

importance is that the rapid increase in the frequency of β-lactamase-producing *M. catarrhalis* strains has changed a previously innocent pathogen, eradicated by almost any antibiotic regimen to a more important microorganism, which may be isolated even after treatment with commonly prescribed drugs.

The natural habitat of *M. catarrhalis* is the human pharyngeal cavity and it is frequently isolated from upper respiratory tract secretions of healthy children. Up to 50% of children, and sometimes still more in the youngest age-groups, may be carriers, while in healthy adults *M. catarrhalis* seems to be an uncommon commensal, though it tends be more commonly found in the elderly[138,162,170,171,186–189]. The mechanisms enabling *M. catarrhalis* to colonise the human nasopharyngeal mucus membranes are not fully elucidated, but adherence through pili is one means[138,144,146]. As with *H. influenzae*, cells that are damaged by chronic inflammation or other mechanisms permits adherence[138].

The isolation of *M. catarrhalis* from respiratory secretions has been consistently and very significantly higher during the winter and spring months in both children and adults, in both the northern and the southern hemispheres[138,161,181,190–192]. The same association has been seen for *S. pneumoniae*, but not for *H. influenzae*[181]. It is known that the spread of *S. pneumoniae* is increased during outbreaks of respiratory viral disease[25] and the same mechanism may be valid for *M. catarrhalis*, at least partially, explaining the winter–spring increase[190].

Person-to-person spread through inhalation is not considered to be a mode of transmission, while hand-to-hand nosocomial spread may be common in certain settings[191,192]. Up to half of the infections with *M. catarrhalis* have been diagnosed in hospitalised patients[166,192]. At least two outbreaks of respiratory tract nosocomial infection due to *M. catarrhalis* have been reported[166,193]. In one study, identity between several isolated strains was proved by restriction endonuclease typing of chromosomal DNA. This proved to be a useful tool for epidemiologic studies, in contrast to lipopolysaccharide or outer membrane protein typing, biotyping, or antibiograms[138,139]. Electrophoretic mobility profiles of a soluble protein has also been found useful for tracing the spread of strains between patients with nosocomial bronchopulmonary infections[194].

Clinical presentation

About 90% of patients contracting lower respiratory tract infection with *M. catarrhalis* have an underlying chronic lung disease[138,167,182,184] (Table 7.6, 7.7). Most patients are elderly and many have malignancies or other immunosuppressive diseases. Of patients with pneumonia due to *M. catarrhalis* only, almost half may have such severe underlying diseases that they will die during or soon after the *Moraxella* infection[184].

Only about one-third of the patients with *M. catarrhalis* chest infection have pulmonary infiltrates on CXR (Fig. 7.7), the rest of the patients have bronchitis. Infiltrates, when present, most often are unilateral or bilateral patchy, interstitial or mixed alveolar–interstitial[161,167,183,184]. However, in one report, six of 22 patients had lobar pneumonia[183]. Small pleural effusions may occur in about one-fourth of the patients[184]. Cavitary lesions have been described, but are uncommon.

Since most of the patients contracting *M. catarrhalis* chest infection have significant underlying chronic pulmonary disease, the presentation in most cases is one of acute exacerbation of chronic bronchitis, whether pulmonary infiltrates are present or not[138,161,167,183,184]. The onset of disease is seldom as acute as with pneumococcal infection , and many cases present without fever or other symptoms suggesting pneumonia, but with only increased amount and purulence of sputum or increased dyspnoea. Fever may be found in only half of the patients. Severe chest infections presenting with chills or pleuritic chest pain may occur, however, especially in patients with underlying immunosuppressive diseases. Moreover, at least 30 cases of bacteraemia have been described, most of them in conjunction with pneumonia[153,156,158–161].

The aetiology of acute exacerbation of chronic bronchitis seem to comprise more than one bacterial species particularly when *M. catarrhalis* is involved[167,181]. Usually *M. catarrhalis* is isolated together with *H. influenzae* or *S. pneumoniae*; sometimes all three species may be isolated at the same time.

By comparing the yield of sputum culture with that of transtracheal aspiration, it is clear that Gram's stain-directed quantitative culture, preferably from washed specimens is a reliable method for diagnosis with a specificity of more than 90% (Fig. 7.8)[112,114,138,161,167]. The presence of 10^7 cfu of *M.catarrhalis*/ml sputum in conjunction with a predominance of Gram-negative diplococci in purulent parts of a Gram-stained smear of the sputum specimen is diagnostic for *M. catarrhalis* infection. Moreover, since the carrier rate of *M. catarrhalis* in adults seems to be low, the risk of contamination of sputum with *M. catarrhalis* from the pharyngeal flora is considerably lower than previously believed[187].

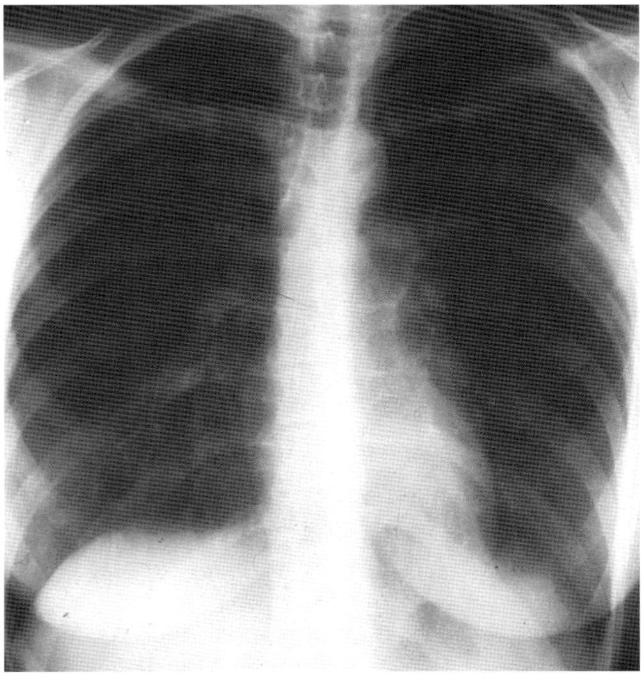

FIGURE 7.7 Pulmonary infiltrates are most often absent in *M. catarrhalis* chest infection. When present they are most often small and patchy and may even be interstitial.

Apart from chest X-ray and sputum examination, laboratory tests are most often of limited value[161]. A moderate leukocytosis is seen in many of the cases.

Complications

Pleural effusions occur occasionally[138,161,184,195]. A few cases of empyema have been described, one in conjunction with a bronchoalveolar fistula. Pericarditis is another uncommon complication[138,196]. Bacteraemia is uncommon, but at least 30 cases have been described[153–161]. Many of the bacteraemic patients have had underlying malignant or other debilitating diseases, but about half of the bacteraemias have been diagnosed in patients without immunosuppressive disorders. Petechial rash, ecchymoses or purpura fulminans have been noted in several bacteraemic cases. Disseminated intravascular coagulation and septic shock have occurred. Focal infections diagnosed in connection with bacteraemia include pneumonia, sinusitis, and endocarditis. A total of five cases of endocarditis have been described, four of which were fatal[160]. In one-third of the bacteraemic cases, no focus could be identified; most of these occurred in children with malignant diseases. Another three bacteraemic cases were noted among the total of 24 with *Moraxella* meningitis that have been described[160].

Management

Though many infections are mild, with patients improving without specific therapy, it is clear that this is not always the case[161,167,183,192]. Many series have reported fatal courses and patients failing to improve until antibiotics active against the isolated *M. catarrhalis* strain were given.

As mentioned, the pathogenicity of *M. catarrhalis* became evident in the 1970s, and by that time all the strains were sensitive to penicillin and ampicillin and most other antibiotics used for treatment of respiratory tract infections[138,197]. In 1976–7, β-lactamase-producing strains appeared in several European countries and in the US, and within four years three-fourths of strains isolated in many parts of the world were found to be β-lactamase-producing[130,138,186,197]. The explanation for this uniquely rapid spread of an important resistance mechanism soon after the appreciation of the significance of *M. catarrhalis* as a pathogen is not understood. It is clear that it is not due to dissemination of one highly communicable progenitor strain[138]. The policy of antibiotic usage has been discussed as a factor of possible importance; it has been shown that also a short oral course of β-lactam treatment leads to a significant increase in the percentage of β-lactamase-producing strains of different species in the upper respiratory tract and this effect prevails for several weeks after discontinuation of the treatment[198]. However, the same drugs had been in use for many years prior to 1976, so this explanation is only part of the explanation for the rapid spread of the β-lactamases.

Two phenotypically closely related β-lactamases, BRO-1 (produced by 90% of the β-lactamase-positive strains) and BRO-2 (produced by 10% of those strains) account for the resistance to penicillin and ampicillin[138,197]. The BRO designation reflects the fact that these enzymes may be produced by both subgenus *Branhamella* and subgenus *Moraxella*, but are unique to this genus. In fact, it has been found only in two commensal *Moraxella* species, but in no other bacteria. Despite the rapid spread of these enzymes, no plasmids have been detected. Instead, the BRO genes appear to be chromosomal, but are readily transferred within the *Moraxella* genus by conjugation. The source of these unique enzymes remains a mystery.

BRO-1 positive strains typically make significantly larger amounts of β-lactamase, and have higher ampicillin MICs than do strains that produce the BRO-2 enzyme[197]. Since it has been found that disease-causing strains have higher ampicillin MICs than commensals, it has been speculated that the BRO-1 is a virulence factor[139]. The BRO enzymes are broad spectrum β-lactamases, but relatively weak, presumably because of their strong cell association. They hydrolyse several of the oral cephalosporins including cephaclor, while parenteral second and third generation cephalosporins seem to be essentially stable and are considered to be very active drugs for infections due to *M. catarrhalis*[138,161,197]. However, despite the different susceptibility

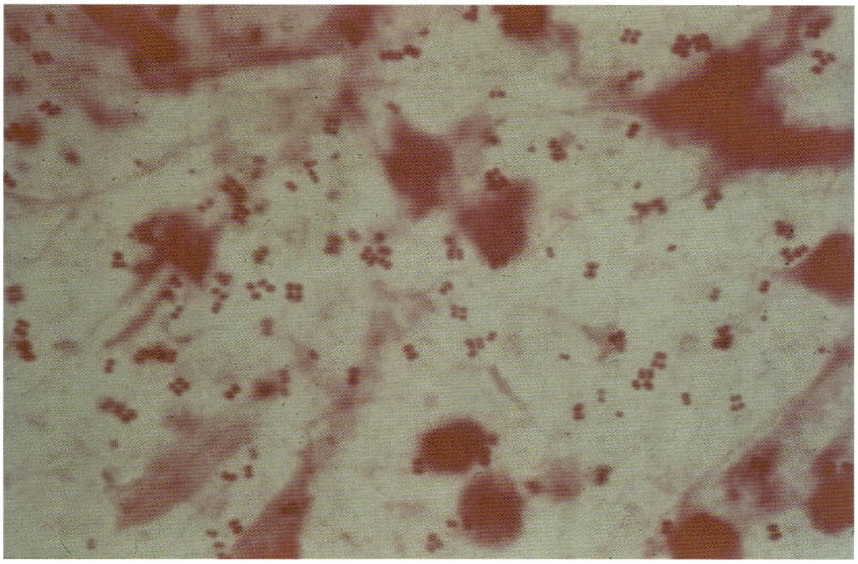

FIGURE 7.8 Gram's stain in *Moraxella catarrhalis* chest infections most often show numerous Gram-negative cocci in purulent parts of the smear.

to hydrolysis by the BRO β-lactamases, the MIC values for most cephalosporins seem to be only moderately affected by β-lactamase production. β-lactamase inhibitors like clavulanic acid, tazobactam and sulbactam inhibit the BRO enzymes effectively.

It has been questioned whether β-lactamase-production is always of significance; many enzyme-producing strains will have ampicillin MIC values that are only moderately raised[197]. However, several case reports on ampicillin failure and a clinical review reporting ampicillin failure in 40% of the cases infected with β-lactamase producing strains support the view, that all β-lactamase-producing strains should be regarded as resistant to penicillin and ampicillin[192,197]. Moreover, it has even been reported that the effect of β-lactamase produced by *M. catarrhalis* may prevent the eradication of respiratory tract co-pathogens like *S. pneumoniae* and *H. influenzae*[114,138,166,185,199,200]. To complicate things further, the MICs of ampicillin of non-β-lactamase producing strains can differ 42-fold, disease-causing strains being more sensitive than carrier strains[138]. The significance of these findings is at present not understood.

All *M. catarrhalis* strains are intrinsically resistant to vancomycin, clindamycin, and trimethoprim[138,166,197]. In spite of the trimethoprim resistance, most strains are highly susceptible to the combination of trimethoprim and sulfamethoxazole; only occasional reports of resistance to this combination have occurred. The same is true for erythromycin to which most strains are highly sensitive. *M. catarrhalis* strains are generally highly susceptible to fluorinated quinolones such as ciprofloxacin. Most strains are also susceptible to rifampicin and aminoglycosides. Tetracyclines have been clinically useful drugs for *M. catarrhalis* infections, especially since many of the infections occur in COPD patients and in conjunction with *H. influenzae*. However, spread of the Tet B resistance determinant has given rise to high frequency of resistance in several areas of the world and may reduce the appropriateness of these drugs when *M. catarrhalis* is involved[197]. The Tet B gene is also responsible for tetracycline resistance in many enteric Gram-negative rods and in *Haemophilus* species; the mode of transmission of this gene within the *M. catarrhalis* species is not known.

Prophylaxis and control

There is, at present, no vaccine available and there is no clear candidate for a vaccine from the bacterial structure, though both the outer membrane proteins and the lipo-oligosaccharides are remarkably stable. There are two possible target populations for a vaccine, namely small children with a high risk of acquiring otitis media, and the elderly with chronic lung disease at risk of severe chest infection with *M.catarrhalis*.

Areas for research

Further epidemiological studies are important. *M. catarrhalis* is today an established and important respiratory pathogen and this fact does not need any further confirmation. However, the prevalence appears to be different in different areas and also to differ from time to time. Factors influencing this variation should be further studied. The increased frequency during winter is of interest. Improved methods for strain typing would facilitate epidemiological studies. Furthermore, the prevalence in other clinical infections such as febrile infections in immunosuppressed patients does not appear to be fully clarified.

Adherence mechanisms including pili, their structure, frequency of occurrence and mode of action are important research objectives. The role of carriership and the importance of adherence in the pathogenesis of mucosal membrane as well as invasive disease needs further study.

Knowledge of other virulence mechanisms is also essential. The possible existence of a capsule should be elucidated and its composition and importance for virulence. The role of antibodies, mucosal as well as serum antibodies, for the host defence against *M. catarrhalis* needs further study. Reliable antibody assays would also be helpful for the continued study both of immunity and for epidemiological studies.

The factors behind the rapid spread of the two β-lactamases are puzzling; increased knowledge in this field could possibly influence strategies for reducing spread of resistance factors among other bacterial species.

The possible role of *M. catarrhalis* as an indirect pathogen, i.e. by protection of other pathogens, including pneumococci, from the lethal effect of β-lactam antibiotics by production of β-lactamase is another research area with conceivable impact on the study of other pathogens.

Summary

M. catarrhalis has been known as a human pathogen for almost 100 years, but its significance as a respiratory pathogen has been fully appreciated only during the last 10–20 years. The reason for this may be a real increase but whether such an increase has really occurred is not known. It appears to be the third most important pathogen after *S. pneumoniae* and *H. influenzae* in otitis media and sinuitis as well as in acute exacerbation of COPD. It also seems to be an important cause of long-standing cough in small children. *M. catarrhalis* may be responsible for 1–5% of the cases of community-acquired pneumonia and it has been described as a cause of hospital-acquired pneumonia.

M. catarrhalis is a very common inhabitant of the normal oropharyngeal flora of small children, but it seems to be an uncommon colonising agent in adults. It appears to adhere to pharyngeal epithelial cells by the use of fimbriae.

The most common clinical presentation of *M. catarrhalis* in chest infection is that of acute exacerbation of chronic bronchitis. Previously healthy people are uncommonly affected. Mixed infections, most often together with *S. pneumoniae* or *H. influenzae* are common. Pulmonary infiltrates are usually absent on chest X-ray and when they occur, are small, patchy or even interstitial. Gram's stain of sputum is the mainstay for aetiologicalal diagnosis and most often show numerous Gram-negative cocci.

Most strains of *M. catarrhalis* produce one of two β-lactamases rendering them resistant to penicillin, ampicillin and many oral cephalosporins. Second and third generation cephalosporins are, however, generally effective. The frequency of strains producing β-lactamase increased during a few years in the 1970s from 0 to more than 70% shortly after the appreciation of the significance of *M. catarrhalis* as an important respiratory pathogen. The reason is unclear. Likewise, the origin of the so-called BRO β-lactamases is enigmatic. A number of other drugs such as macrolides, cotrimoxazole and quinolones are generally effective for the treatment of *M. catarrhalis* infections.

References

1. LEE BC. Isolation of an outer membrane hemin-binding protein of *Haemophilus influenzae* type b. *Infect Immun* 1992; 60:810–16.
2. QILL PA, CHOW AW, GUZE LB. Adult bacteraemic *Haemophilus parainfluenzae* infections. Seven reports of cases and a review of the literature. *Arch Intern Med* 1979; 139:985–8.
3. TROLLFORS B, BRORSON J.-E, CLAESSON B, SANDBERG T. Invasive infections caused by *Haemophilus* species other than *Haemophilus influenzae. Infection* 1985; 13.12–14.
4. MOXON ER, WILSON R. The role of *Haemophilus influenzae* in the pathogenesis of pneumonia. *Rev Infect Dis* 1991; 13 (Suppl 6):S518–27.
5. MURPHY TF APICELLA MA. Nontypable *Haemophilus influenzae*: a review of clinical aspects, surface antigens, and the human immune response to infection. *Rev Infect Dis* 1987; 9:1–15.
6. MURPHY TF, SETHI S. Bacterial infection in chronic obstructive pulmonary disease. *Am Rev Resp Dis* 1992; 146:1067–83.
7. MÄKELÄ PH. Unencapsulated *Haemophilus influenzae* – what kind of a pathogen? *Eur J Clin Microbiol Infect Dis* 1988; 7:606–9.
8. BELL J, GRASS S, JEANTEUR D, MUNSON JR RS. Diversity of the P2 protein among nontypable *Haemophilus influenzae* isolates. *Infect Immun* 1994; 62:2639–43.
9. DAJANI AS, ASMAR BI, THIRUMOORTHI MC. Systemic *Haemophilus influenzae* disease: an overview. *J Pediatr* 1979; 94:355–64.
10. FALLA TJ, DOBSON SRM, CROOK DWM *et al.* Population-based study of non-typable *Haemophilus influenzae* invasive disease in children and neonates. *Lancet* 1993; 341:851–4.
11. FARLEY MM, STEPHENS DS, BRACHMAN PS, HARVEY RC, SMITH JD, WENGER JD, AND CDC MENINGITIS SURVEILLANCE GROUP. Invasive *Haemophilus influenzae* disease in adults. A prospective, population-based surveillance. *Ann Intern Med* 1992; 116:806–12.
12. MUSSER JM, BARENKAMP SJ, GRANOFF DM, SELANDER RK. Genetic relationship of serologically nontypable and serotype b strains of *Haemophilus influenzae. Infect Immun* 1986; 52:183–91.
13. TAKALA AK. Epidemiologic characteristics and risk factors for invasive *Haemophilus influenzae* type b disease in a population with high vaccine efficacy. *Pediatr Infect Dis J* 1989; 8:343–6.
14. TAKALA AK, ESKOLA J, VAN ALPHEN L. Spectrum of invasive *Haemophilus influenzae* type b disease in adults. *Arch Intern Med* 1990; 150:2573–6.
15. APICELLA MA, SHERO M, DUDAS KC. *et al.* Fimbriation of *Haemophilus* species isolated from the respiratory tract of adults. *J Infect Dis* 1984; 150:40–3.
16. PATEL J, FADEN H, SHARMA S, OGRA PL. Effect of respiratory syncytial virus on adherence, colonisation and immunity of nontypable *Haemophilus influenzae*: implications for otitis media. Int *J Pediat Otorhinolaryngol* 1992; 23:15–23.
17. GROENEVELD K, VALPHEN L, EIJK PP, JANSEN HM, ZANEN HC. Changes in outer membrane proteins of nontypable *Haemophilus influenzae* in patients with chronic obstructive pulmonary disease. *J Infect Dis* 1988; 158:360–5.
18. HARPER JJ, TILSE MT. Biotypes of *Haemophilus influenzae* that are associated with noninvasive disease. *J Clin Microbiol* 1991; 29:2539–42.
19. KILIAN M. A taxonomic study of the genus *Haemophilus*, with the proposal of a new species. *J Gen Microbiol* 1976; 93:9–62.
20. KILIAN M, SORENSEN I, FREDERIKSEN W. Biochemical characteristics of 130 recent isolates from *Haemophilus influenzae* meningitis. *J Clin Microbiol* 1979; 9:409–12
21. OBERHOFER TR; BACK AE. Biotypes of *Haemophilus* encountered in clinical laboratories. *J Clin Microbiol* 1979; 10:168–74.
22. TROTTIER S, STENBERG K, SVANBORG-EDEN C. Turnover of nontypable *Haemophilus influenzae* in the nasopharynges of healthy children. *J Clin Microbiol* 1989; 27:2175–9.
23. WALLACE RJJR, BAKER CJ, QUINONES FJ, HOLLIES DG, WEAVER RE, WISS K. Nontypable *Haemophilus influenzae* (Bitype 4) as a neonatal, maternal, and genital pathogen. *Rev Infect Dis* 1983; 5:123–36.
24. LEES AW, MCNAUGHT W. Bacteriology of lower respiratory tract secretions, sputum, and upper respiratory tract secretions in 'normals' and chronic bronchitis. *Lancet* 1959; 2:1112–15.
25. GWALTNEY JM, SANDE MA, AUSTRIAN R, HENDLEY JO. Spread of *Streptococcus pneumoniae* in families. II. Relation of transfer of *S. pneumoniae* to incidence of colds and serum antibody. *J Infect Dis* 1975; 132:62–8.
26. MILLER DL, JONES R. The bacterial flora of the upper respiratory tract and sputum of working men. *J Path Bacteriol* 1964; 87:182–6.
27. HARABUCHI Y, FADEN H, YAMANAKA N *et al.* Nasopharyngeal colonisation with nontypeable *Haemophilus influenzae* and recurrent otitis media. *J Infect Dis* 1994; 170:862–6.
28. SAMUELSON A, FREIJD A, RYNNEL-DAGÖÖ B. Treatment failure in otitis-prone children with prophylactic tympanostomy tubes is correlated with nasopharyngeal *Haemophilus influenzae* colonisation. *Acta Otolaryngol* (Stockh) 1991; 111:1090–6.
29. MOXON ER. The carrier state: *Haemophilus influenzae J Antimicrob Chemother* 1986; 18 (Suppl A):17–24.
30. GRANOFF DM, DAUM RS. Spread of *Haemophilus influenzae* type b: recent epidemiologic and therapeutic considerations. *J Pediat* 1980; 97:854–60.
31. SHANN F. Etiology of severe pneumonia in children in developing countries. *Pediatr Infect Dis J* 1986; 5:247–52.
32. SHANN F, GRATTEN M, GERMER S, LINNEMAN V, HAZLETT D, PAYNE R. Aetiology of pneumonia in children in Goroka Hospital, Papua New Guinea. *Lancet* 1984; 1:537–41.
33. MURPHY TV, PASTOR P, MEDLEY F, OSTERHOLM MT, GRANOFF DM. Decreased *Haemophilus* colonisation in children vaccinated with *Haemophilus influenzae* type b conjugate vaccine. *J Pediat* 1993; 122:517–23.
34. FORSGREN J, SAMUELSON A, AHLIN A, JONASSON J, RYNNEL-DAGÖÖ B, LINDBERG A. *Haemophilus influenzae* resides and multiplies intracellularly in human adenoid tissue as demonstrated by *in situ* hybridization and bacterial viability assay. *Infect Immun* 1994; 62:673–9.
35. READ RC, RUTMAN AA, JEFFERY PK. Interaction of capsulate *Haemophilus influenzae* with human airway mucosa *in vitro. Infect Immun* 1992; 60:3244–52.

36. TSANG K W, RUTMAN A, KANTHAKUMAR K *et al.* *Haemophilus influenzae* infection of human respiratory mucosa in low concentrations of antibiotics. *Am Rev Resp Dis* 1993; 148:201–7.
37. DYAS A, GEORGE RH. Ten years experience of *Haemophilus influenzae* infection at Birmingham children´s hospital. *J Infect* 1986; 13: 179–85.
38. GELLADY AM, SHULMAN ST, AYOUB EM. Periorbital and orbital cellulitis in children. *Pediatrics* 1978; 61:272–7.
39. POWELL KR, KAPLAN SB, HALL CB, NASELLO MA, ROGHMANN KJ. Periorbital cellulitis. Clinical and laboratory findings in 146 episodes, including tear countercurrent immunoelectrophoresis in 89 episodes. *Am J Dis Child* 1988; 142:853–7.
40. GIGLIOTTI F, WILLIAMS WT, HAYDEN FG *et al.* Etiology of acute conjunctivitis in children. *J Pediat* 1981; 98:531–6.
41. BRAZILIAN PURPURIC FEVER STUDY GROUP. Report of a symposium. *Pediat Infect Dis J* 1989; 8:237–49.
42. FOTHERGILL LD, WRIGHT J. Influenzal meningitis: the relation of age to the incidence of the bactericidal power against the causal organism. *J Immunol* 1933; 24:273–84.
43. KOSTMAN JR, SHERRY BL, FLIGNER CL *et al.* Invasive *Haemophilus influenzae* infections in older children and adults. *Clin Infect Dis* 1993; 17:389–96.
44. QUINONES CA, MEMON MA, SAROSI GA. Bacteremic *Haemophilus influenzae* pneumonia in the adult. *Sem Resp Infect* 1989;4:12–18.
45. KINNEY JS, JOHNSON K, PAPASIAN C, HALL RT, KURTH CG, JACKSON MA. Early onset *Haemophilus influenzae* sepsis in the newborn infant. *Pediat Infect Dis J* 1993; 12:739–43.
46. LESTER A, PEDERSEN PB. Serious systemic infection caused by non-encapsulated *Haemophilus influenzae* biotype III in an adult. *Scand J Infect Dis* 1991; 23:111–3.
47. ALBRITTON WL, HAMMOND GW, RONALD AR. Bacteremic *Haemophilus influenzae* genitourinary tract infections in adults. *Arch Intern Med* 1978; 138: 1819–21.
48. CSUKAS SR, ELBI F, MARSHALL GS. Type b and non-type b *Haemophilus influenzae* endocarditis. *Pediatr Infect Dis J* 1992; 11:1053–6.
49. KRAGSBJERG P, NILSSON K, PERSSON L, TÖRNQVIST E, VIKERFORS T. Deep obstetrical and gynecological infection caused by non-typable *Haemophilus influenzae. Scand J Infect Dis* 1993; 25:341–6.
50. NORDEN CW. *Haemophilus influenzae* infections in adults. *Med Clin North Am* 1978; 62:1037.
51. SIMON HB, SOUTHWICK FS, MOELLERING RC, SHERMAN E. *Haemophilus influenzae* in hospitalized adults: current perspectives. *Am J Med* 1980; 69:219–26.
52. MONTO AS. Acute respiratory infection in children of developing countries: challenge of the 1990s. *Rev Infect Dis* 1989; 11:498–505.
53. BLUESTONE D. Otitis media and sinusitis in children; role of *Branhamella catarrhalis. Drugs* 1988; 31(Suppl 3):132–141.
54. KAMME C, LUNDGREN K MÅRDH P-A. The aetiology of acute otitis media in children. *Scand J Infect Dis* 1971; 3:217–33.
55. VAN HARE GF, SHURIN PA. The increasing importance of *Branhamella catarrhalis* in respiratory infections. *Paediatr Infect Dis J* 1987; 6:92–4.
56. WALD ER. *Haemophilus influenzae* as a cause of acute otitis media. *Pediatr Infect Dis J* 1989; 8:28–30.
57. LOOS BG, BERNSTEIN JM, DRYJA DM, MURPHY TF, DICKINSON DP. Determination of epidemiology and transmission of nontypable *Haemophilus influenzae* in children with otitis media by comparison of total genomic DNA restriction analysis. *Infect Immun* 1989; 57:2751–7.
58. MURPHY TF, BERNSTEIN JM, DRYJA DM, CAMPAGNARI AA, APICELLA MA. Outer membrane protein and lipooligosacharide analysis of paired nasopharyngeal and middle ear isolates in otitis media due to nontypable *Haemophilus influenzae*: pathogenetic and epidemiologic observations. *J Infect Dis* 1987; 156:723–31.
59. RUUSKANEN O, HEIKKINEN T. Otitis media: etiology and diagnosis. *Pediatr Infect Dis J* 1994; 13:S23–S26.
60. SUZUKI K, BAKALETZ LO. Synergistic effect of adenovirus type 1 and nontypeable *Haemophilus influenzae* in a chinchilla model of experimental otitis media. *Infect Immun* 1994; 62:1710–18.
61. KESSLER A, WETMORE RF, MARSH RR. Childhood epiglottis in recent years. *Int J Pediatr Otolaryngol* 1993; 25:155–62.
62. SENDI K, CRYSDALE WS. Acute epiglottitis: decade of change – a ten-year experience with 242 children. *J Otolaryngol* 1987; 161:196–202.
63. CARENFELT C. Etiology of acute infectious epiglottitis in adults: septic vs. local infection. *Scand J Infect Dis* 1989; 21:53–7.
64. MAYOSMITH MF, HIRSCH PJ, WODZINSKI SF, SCHIFFMAN FJ. Acute epiglottitis in adults. An eight-year experience in the state of Rhode Island. *New Engl J Med* 1986; 314:1133–9.
65. MUSTOE T, STROME M. Adult epiglottitis. *Am J Otolaryngol* 1983; 4:393–9.
66. RYAN M, HUNT M SNOWBERGER T. A changing pattern of epiglottitis. *Clin Pediatr* 1992:532–5.
67. AMERICAN THORACIC SOCIETY. Guidelines for the initial management of adults with community-acquired pneumonia: diagnosis, assessment of severity, and initial antimicrobial therapy. *Am Rev Resp Dis* 1993; 148:1418–26.
68. BELLIVEAU P, HICKINGBOTHAM N, MADERAZO EG, MAZENS-SULLIVAN M, ROBINSON A. Institution-specific patterns of infection and Gram´s stain as guide for empiric treatment of patients hospitalized with typical community-acquired pneumonia. *Pharmacotherapy* 1993;13:396–401.
69. BURMAN LÅ, TROLLFORS B, ANDERSSON B. Diagnosis of pneumonia by cultures, bacterial and viral antigen detection tests, and serology with special reference to antibodies against pneumococcal antigens. *J Infect Dis* 1991; 163, 1087–93
70. FANG G-D, FINE M, ORLOFF J *et al.* New and emerging etiologies for community-acquired pneumonia with implications for therapy: a prospective multicenter study of 359 cases. *Medicine (Baltimore)* 1990; 69:307–16.
71. KALIN M, LINDBERG AA, TUNEVALL G. Etiological Diagnosis of bacterial pneumonia by Gram stain and quantitive culture of expectorates. *Scand J Infect Dis* 1983; 15:153–60.
72. LEHTOMÄKI K, LEINONEN M, TAKALA A, HOVI T, HERVA E, KOSKELA M. Etiological diagnosis of pneumonia in military conscripts by combined of bacterial culture and serological methods. *Eur J Clin Microbiol Infect Dis* 1988; 7:348–54.
73. POTGIETER PD, HAMMOND JMJ. Etiology and diagnosis of pneumonia requiring ICU admission. *Chest* 1992; 101:199–203.
74. MACFARLANE J. An overview of community acquired pneumonia with lessons learned from the British Thoracic Society study. *Sem Resp Infect* 1994; 9:153–65.
75. MOINE P, VERCKEN J-B, CHEVRET S, CHASTANG C, GAJDOS P. Severe community-acquired pneumonia. Etiology, epidemiology, and prognosis factors. *Chest* 1994; 105:1487–95.
76. WOODHEAD MA MACFARLANE JT. *Haemophilus influenzae* pneumonia in previously fit adults. *Eur J Resp Dis* 1987; 70:218.20.
77. SCHLAMM HT, YANCOVITZ SR. *Haemophilus influenzae* pneumonia in young adults with AIDS, ARC, or risk of AIDS. *Am J Med* 1991; 86:11–14.
78. STEINHART R, REINGOLD AL, TAYLOR F, ANDERSON G, WENGER JD. Invasive

Haemophilus influenzae infections in men with HIV infection. *JAMA* 1992; 268:3350–2.

79. MUSHER DM, KUBITSCHEK KR, CRENNAN J, BAUGHN RE. Pneumonia and acute febrile tracheobronchitis due to *Haemophilus influenzae. Ann Intern Med* 1983; 99:444–50.

80. GOUGH J, KRAAK, WAG, ANDERSON EC, NICHOLS WW, SLACK MPE, MCGHIE D. Cross-infection by non-encapsulated *Haemophilus influenzae*. *The Lancet* 1990; 336:159–60.

81. HEKKER TAM, VAN DER SCHEE AC, KEMPERS J, MNAMAVAR F, VAN ALPHEN L. A nosocomial outbrake of amoxycillin-resistant non-typable *Haemophilus influenzae* in a respiratory ward. *J Hosp Infect* 1991; 19:25–31.

82. HOWARD AJ. Editorial. Nosocomial spread of *Haemophilus influenzae. J Hosp Infect* 1991; 19: 1–3.

83. RELLO J, RICART M, AUSINA V, NET A, PRATS G. Pneumonia due to *Haemophilus influenzae* among mechanically ventilated patients. Incidence, outcome, and risk factors. *Chest* 1992; 102:1562–5.

84. STURM AW, MOSTERT R, ROUING PJE, VAN KLINGEREN B, VAN ALPHEN L. Outbrake of multiresistant non-encapsulated *Haemophilus influenzae* infections in a pulmonary rehabilitation centre. *Lancet* 1990; 335:214–16.

85. BUSSE WW. Pathogenesis and sequelae of respiratory infections. *Rev Infect Dis* 1991; 13 (Suppl 6), S477–85.

86. TOEWS GB, HANSEN EJ, STRIETER RM. Pulmonary host defenses and oropharyngeal pathogens. *Am J Med*, 1990; 88(Suppl5A):520–4

87. CHODOSH, S. Treatment of acute exacerbations of chronic bronchitis: state of the art. *Am J Med* 1991; 91(Suppl 6A), 87S–93S.

88. LAURENZI GA, POTTER RT, KASS EH. Bacteriologic flora of the lower respiratory tract. *New Engl J Med* 1961;265:1273–7

89. ANONYMOUS. Antibiotics for exacerbations of chronic bronchitis? [Editorial] *Lancet* 1987; 2:23–4.

90. GUMP DW, PHILLIPS CA, FORSYTH BR, MCINTOSH K, LAMBORN KR, STOUCH WH. Role of infection in chronic bronchitis. *Am Rev Resp Dis* 1976; 113:465–74.

91. BAIGLEMAN W, CHODOSH S, PIZZUTO D, SADOW T. Quantitative sputum Gram stains in chronic bronchial disease. *Lung* 1979; 156: 265–70.

92. BERK SL, HOLTSCLAW SA, WIENER SL, SMITH JK. Nontypable *Haemophilus influenzae* in the elderly. *Arch Intern Med* 1982; 142:537–9.

93. SCHREINER A, BJERKESTRAND G, DIGRANES A, HALVORSEN FJ, KOMMENDAL TM. Bacteriological findings in the transtracheal aspirate from patients with acute exacerbation of chronic bronchitis. *Infection* 1978; 6:54–6.

94. WEISER JN, LOVE JM, MOXON ER. The molecular mechanism of phase-variation of *H. influenzae* lipopolysaccharide. *Cell* 1989; 59:657–65.

95. WINKELSTEIN JA MOXON ER. The role of complement in the host´s defence against *Haemophilus influenzae. J Infect Dis* 1992; 165 (Suppl 1):S62–5.

96. WONG W-Y, OVERTURF GD, POWARS DR. Infection cad by *Streptococcus pneumoniae* in children with sickle cell disease: epidemiology, immunologic mechanisms, prophylaxis, and vaccination. *Clin Infect Dis* 1992; 14:1124–36.

97. PELTOLA H, KILPI T, ANTTILA M. Rapid disappearance of *Haemophilus influenzae* type b meningitis after routine childhood immunisation with conjugate vaccines. *Lancet* 1992; 340;592–4.

98. SANTOSHAM M. Prevention of *Haemophilus influenzae* type b disease. *Vaccine* 1993; 11(Suppl 1):S52–7.

99. SHAPIRO ED. Infections caused by *Haemophilus influenzae* type b. The beginning of the end? *JAMA* 1993; 269:264–6.

100. TAKALA AK, SANTOSHAM M, ALMEIDO-HILL J *et al.* Vaccination with *Haemophilus influenzae* type b meningococcal protein conjugate vaccine reduces oropharyngeal carriage of *Haemophilus influenzae* type b among American Indian children. *Pediatr Infect Dis J* 1993; 12:593–9.

101. WEBBER SA, SANDOR GGS, PATTERSON MWH *et al.* Immunogenicity of *Haemophilus influenzae* type b conjugate vaccine in children with congenital asplenia. *J Infect Dis* 1993; 167:1210–2.

102. CASADEVALL, A., DOBROSZYCKI, J., SMALL, C. & PIROFSKI, L.-A. *Haemophilus influenzae* type b bacteraemia in adults with AIDS and at risk for AIDS. *Am J Med* 1992; 92, 587–90.

103. POLSKY B, GOLD JWM, WHIMBERLEY E. Bacterial pneumonia in patients with the acquired immune deficiency syndrome. *Arch Intern Med* 1986; 104:38–41.

104. STEINHOFF MC, AUERBACH BS, NELSON KE *et al.* Antibody response to *Haemophilus influenzae* type b vaccines in men with human immunodeficiency virus infection. *New Engl J Med* 1991; 325:1837–42.

105. LEVIN DC, SCHWARTZ MI, MATTHAY RA, LAFORCE M. Bacteremic *Haemophilus influenzae* pneumonia in adults. A report of 24 cases and a review of the literature. *Am J Med* 1977; 62:219–24.

106. WALLACE RJJR, MUSHER D.M, MARTIN RR. *Haemophilus influenzae* pneumonia in adults. *Am J Med* 1978; 64:87–93.

107. PAZ HL, WOOD CA. Pneumonia and chronic obstructive pulmonary disease. *Postgrad Med J* 1991; 90:77–86.

108. SMITH AL. *Haemophilus influenzae* pneumonia. In Weinstein L, Fields BN eds. *Seminars in Infectious Diseases* New York: Thieme-Stratton Inc 1983: 56–70. .

109. VINIK M, ALTMAN DH, PARKS RE. Experience with *Haemophilus influenzae* pneumonia. *Radiology* 1986; 186:701–6

110. DAVIDSON M, TEMPEST B, PALMER DL. Bacteriologic diagnosis of acute pneumonia. Comparison of sputum, transtracheal aspirates, and lunaspirates. *JAMA* 1976; 235:158–63.

111. HEINEMAN HS, CHAWLA JK, LOFTON WM. Misinformation from sputum cultures without microscopic examination. *J Clin Microbiol* 1977; 6:518–27.

112. AITKEN JM, THORNLEY PE. Isolation of *Branhamella catarrhalis* from sputum and tracheal aspirates. *J Clin Microbiol* 1983; 18:1262–3.

113. BARTLETT JG, FINEGOLD SM. Bacteriology of expectorated sputum with quantitative culture and wash technique compared to transtracheal aspirates. *Am Rev Resp Dis* 1978; 117:1019–27.

114. DAVIES BI, MAESEN FPV. Epidemiological and bacteriological findings on *Branhamella catarrhalis* respiratory infections in the Netherlands. *Drugs* 1986; 31 (Suppl 3):28–33.

115. KALIN M. Bacteremic pneumococcal pneumonia: value of nasopharynx culture and examination of washed sputum specimens. *Eur J Clin Microbiol* 1:394–6.

116. BROUGHTON WA, MIDDLETON RM, KIRKPATRICK MB, BASS JB. Bronchoscopic protected specimen brush and bronchoalveolar lavage in the diagnosis of bacterial pneumonia. *Infect Dis Clin North Am* 1991; 5:437–452.

117. MARCON MJ, HAMOUDI AC, CANNON HJ. Comparative laboratory evaluation of three antigen detection methods for diagnosis of *Haemophilus influenzae* type b disease. *J Clin Microbiol* 1984; 19:333–7.

118. WELCH DF, HENSEL D. Evaluation of bactogen and phadebact for detection of *Haemophilus influenzae* type b antigen in cerebrospinal fluid. *J Clin Microbiol* 1982; 16:905–8.

119. WITT CS, MONTGOMERY JM, POMAT W, LEHMANN D, ALPERS MP. Detection of *Streptococcus pneumoniae* and *Haemophilus influenzae* type b antigens in the serum and urine of patients with pneumonia in Papua New Guinea: comparison of latex agglutination and

counterimmunoelectrophoresis. *Rev Infect Dis* 1990; 12 (Suppl 8):S1001–5.

120. GINSBURG CM, HOWARD JB, NELSON JD. Report of 65 cases of *Haemophilus influenzae* b pneumonia. *Pediatrics* 1979; 64:283–6.

121. JACOBS NM, HARRIS VJ. Acute *Haemophilus* pneumonia in childhood. *Am J Dis Child* 1979; 133:603–5.

122. AMERICAN THORACIC SOCIETY. Standards for the diagnosis and care of patients with chronic obstructive pulmonary disease (COPD) and asthma. *Am Rev Resp Dis* 1987; 136:225–44.

123. MURRAY JF. The ketchup-bottle method. *New Engl J Med* 1979; 300:1155–6.

124. SELSBY DS. Chest physiotherapy. May be harmful in some patients. *Br Med J* 1989; 298:541–2.

125. ANTHONISEN NR, MANFREDA J, WARREN CPW, HERSHFIELD ES, HARDING GKM, NELSON NA. Antibiotic therapy in exacerbations of chronic obstructive pulmonary disease. *Ann Intern Med* 1987; 106:196–204.

126. SAINT S, BENT S, VITTINGHOFF E, GRADY D. Antibiotics in chronic obstructive pulmonary disease exacerbations. A meta-analysis. *JAMA* 1995; 273:957–60.

122. THYS JP, JACOBS F, BYL B. Role of quinolones in the treatment of bronchopulmonary infections, particularly pneumococcal and community-acquired pneumonia. *Eur J Clin Microbiol Infect Dis* 1991; 10:304–15.

128. FENOLL A, BOURGON MC, MUNOZ R, VICIOSO D, CASAL J. Serotype distribution and antimicrobial resistance of *Streptococcus pneumoniae* isolates causing systemic infections in Spain, 1979–1989. *Rev Infect Dis* 1991; 13:56–60.

129. KAYSER FH, MORENZONI G, SANTANAM P. The second European collaborative study on the frequency of antimicrobial resistance in *Haemophilus influenzae. Eur J Clin Microbiol Infect Dis* 1990; 9:810–17.

130. JORGENSEN JH, DOERN GV, MAHER LA, HOWELL AW, REDDING JS. Antimicrobial resistance among respiratory isolates of *Haemophilus influenzae*, *Moraxella catarrhalis*, and *Streptococcus pneumoniae* in the United States. *Antimicrob Agents Chemother* 1990; 34:2075–80.

131. JORGENSEN JH. Update on mechanisms and prevalence of antimicrobial resistance in *Haemophilus influenzae. Clin Infect Dis* 1992; 14:1119–23.

132. MACHKA K, BRAVENY I, DABERNAT H *et al.* Distribution and resistance patterns of *Haemophilus influenzae*: a European cooperative study. *Eur J Clin Microbiol Infect Dis* 1988; 7:14–24.

133. POWELL M, FAH YS, SEYMOUR A, YUAN M, WILLIAMS JD. Antimicrobial susceptibility in *Haemophilus influenzae* from England and Scotland. *J Antimicrob Chemother* 1992; 29:547–54.

134. CLAIROUX N, PICARD M, BROCHU, A, *et al.* Molecular basis of the non-beta-lactamase-mediated resistance to beta-lactam antibiotics in strains of *Haemophilus influenzae* isolated in Canada. *Antimicrob Agents Chemother* 1992; 36:1504–13.

135. ANDERSON G, SMITHEE L, RADOS M, BOUGHAM W. Progress toward elimination of *Haemophilus influenzae* type b disease among infants and children – United States, 1987–1993. *Morb Mort Wkl Rep* 1994; 43, 144–8.

136. HALL CB, COMMITTEE ON INFECTIOUS DISEASE. *Haemophilus influenzae* type b conjugate vaccines: recommendations for immunization with recently and previously licensed vaccines. *Pediatrics* 1993; 92:480–8.

137. FROSCH P, KOLLE W. Die Mikrokokken. In: Flugge, ed: *Die Mikrokokken* 1896; 3, 154–5.

138. CATLIN BW. *Branhamella catarrhalis*: an organism gaining respect as a Pathogen. *Clin Microbiol Rev* 1990; 3:293–320.

139. DOERN GV. *Branhamella catarrhalis*: phenotypic characteristics. *Am J Med* 1990; 88 (Suppl 5A): 33S–35S.

140. BØVRE, K. GENUS II. *Moraxella* Lwoffi 1939. emend. Henriksen and Bøvre 1968. In Krieg NR, Holt JG, eds. *Bergey's Manual of Systematic Bacteriology*, vol 1. The Williams and Wilkins Company, Baltimore, 1984:296–303.

141. BARTOS LC, MURPHY TF. Comparison of the outer membrane proteins of 50 strains of *Branhamella catarrhalis. J Infect Dis* 1988; 158:761–5.

142. JÖNSSON I, HOLME T, KROOK A, RAHMAN M, THORÉN M. Variability of surface-exposed antigens of different strains of *Moraxella catarrhalis. Eur J Clin Microbiol Infect Dis* 1992; 11:919–22.

143. MURPHY TF. Studies of the outer membrane proteins of *Branhamella catarrhalis Am J Med* 1990; 88 (Suppl 5A):41S–45S.

144. MARRS CF, WEIR S. Pili (fimpriae) of *Branhamella catarrhalis. Am J Med* 1990; 88 (Suppl 5A):36S–40S.

145. AHMED K, RIKITOMI N, NAGATAKE T, MATSUMOTO K. Ultrastructural study on the adherence of *Branhamella catarrhalis* to oropharyngeal epithelial cells. *Microbiol Immunol* 1992; 36:563–73.

146. RIKITOMI N, ANDERSSON B, MATSUMOTO K, LINDSTEDT R, SVANBORG C. Mechanism of adherence of *Moraxella (Branhamella) catarrhalis. Scand J Infect Dis* 1991; 23:559–67.

147. ABBOTT M. Neisseriacae and *Moraxella* sp.: the role of related microorganisms associated with conjunctivitis in the newborn. *Internat J STD AIDS* 1992; 3:212–13.

148. COKER DM, GRIFFITHS LR. *Moraxella* urethritis mimicking gonorrhea. *Genitourin Med* 1991; 67:173–4.

149. GRÖSCHEL, D.H.M. *Moraxella catarrhalis* and other Gram-negative cocci. In: Mandell RG, Bennett JE, Dolin R eds. *Principles and Practice of Infectious Diseases* 3rd edn Principles and practice of infectious diseases. New York: Churchill Livingstone Press, 1994:1926–33.

150. KOWALSKI RP, HARWICK JC. Incidence of *Moraxella* conjunctival infection. *Am J Ophthalmol* 1986;101:437–40.

151. RINGVOLD A, VIK E, BEVANGER LS. *Moraxella* lacunata isolated from epidemic conjunctivitis among teenaged females. *Acta Ophthalmol* (Copenhagen) 1985; 63:427.

152. VAN BIJSTERVELD OP. The incidence of *Moraxella* on mucus membranes of the skin. *Am J Ophthalmol* 1972; 63:1702–5.

153. ALAEUS A, STIERNSTEDT G. *Branhamella catarrhalis* septicaemia in an immunocompetent adult. *Scand J Infect Dis* 1991; 23:115–16.

154. BONADIO WA. *Branhamella catarrhalis* bacteraemia in children. *Pediatr Infect Dis J* 1988; 10:738–9.

155. CIMOLAI N, ADDERLEY RJ. *Branhamella catarrhalis* bacteraemia in children. *Acta Pediatr Scand* 1989; 78:465–8.

156. COLLAZOS J, DE MIGUEL J, AYARZA R. *Moraxella catarrhalis* bacteraemic pneumonia in adults: two cases and review of the literature. *Eur J Clin Microbiol Infect Dis* 1992; 11:237–40.

157. DOERN GV, SCHMID RE. *Branhamella catarrhalis* pneumonia with bacteraemia. *Clin Microbiol Newslett* 1986; 8:34–6.

158. GUTRIE R, BAKENHASTER K, NELSON R, WOSKOBNICK R. *Branhamella catarrhalis* sepsis: a case report and review of the literature. *J Infect Dis* 1988; 158:907–8.

159. MALKAMÄKI M, HONKANEN E, LEINONEN M, MÄKELÄ PH. *Branhamella catarrhalis* as a cause of bacteraemic pneumonia. *Scand J Infect Dis* 1983; 15:125–6.

160. WALLACE MR OLDFIELD EC. *Moraxella (Branhamella) catarrhalis* bacteraemia. A case report and literature review. *Arch Intern Med* 1990; 150:1332–4.

161. WRIGHT PW, WALLACE JR RJ. Pneumonia due to *Moraxella (Branhamella) catarrhalis. Sem Resp Infect* 1989; 4:40–6.

162. MARCHANT CD. Spectrum of disease due to *Branhamella catarrhalis* in children with

particular reference to acute otitis media. *Am J Med* 1990; 88 (Suppl 5A):15S–19S.

163. SCHWARZ B, HARRISON LH, MOTTER JS. Investigation of an outbreak of *Moraxella* conjunctivitis at a Navajo boarding school. *Am J Ophthalmol* 1989; 107:341–7.

164. AHMAD F, CALDER MA, CROUGHAN MJ, MARSHALL TG. Urinary tract infections caused by *Branhamella catarrhalis*. *J Infect* 1985;10:176–7.

165. JACOBSSON SH, BJÖRKLIND A. Symptomatic bacteriuria caused by *Branhamella catarrhalis*. *J Infect* 1989; 18:192–3.

166. CALDER, M.A., CROUGHAN, M.J., MCLEOD, D.T. AHMAD, F. The incidence and antibiotic susceptibility of *Branhamella catarrhalis* in respiratory infections. *Drugs* 1986; 31(Suppl 3), 11–16.

167. HAGER H, VERGHESE A, ALVAREZ S, BERK SL. *Branhamella catarrhalis* respiratory infections. *Rev Infect Dis* 1987; 9:1140–9.

168. VAN HARE GF, SHURIN PA, MARCHANT CD *et al.* Acute otitis media caused by *Branhamella catarrhalis. Rev Infect Dis* 1987; 9:16–27.

169. WALD ED, MILMOE GJ, BOWEN AD, LEDESMA-MEDINA J, SALAMON N, BLUESTONE CD. Acute maxillary sinusitis in children. *New Engl J Med* 1981; 304:749–54.

170. SCHALÉN L, CHRISTENSEN P, KAMME C, MIÖRNER H, PETERSSON KI, SCHALÉN C. High isolation rates of *Branhamella catarrhalis* from nasopharynx in adults with acute laryngitis. *Scand J Infect Dis* 1980; 12:277–80.

171. BRORSON JE, MALMVALL BE. *Branhamella* catarrhlis and other bacteria in the nasopharynx of children with longstanding cough. *Scand J Infect Dis* 1981; 13:111–3.

172. DARELID J, LÖFGREN S, MALMVALL B-E Erythromycin treatment is beneficial for longstanding cough in children, *Scand J Infect Dis* 1993; 25:323–9.

173. GOTTFARB P, BRAUNER A. Children with persistent cough – outcome with treatment and role of *Moraxella catarrhalis. Scand J Infect Dis* 1994; 26:545–51.

174. CHAPMAN AJ, MUSHER DM, JOHNSON S, CLARIDGE JE, WALLACE RJ. Development of bactericidal antibody during *Branhamella catarrhalis* infection. *J Infect Dis* 1985; 152:878–82.

175. BLACK AJ, WILSON TS. Immunoglobulin G (IgG) serological response to *Branhamella catarrhalis* in patients with bronchopulmonary infections. *J Clin Pathol* 1988; 41:329–33.

176. CHI DS, VERGHESE A, MOORE C, HAMATI F, BERK SL. Antibody response to P-protein in patients with *Branhamella catarrhalis* infections. *Am J Med* 1990; 88 (Suppl5A):25S–27S.

177. ELIASSON I. Serological identification of *Branhamella catarrhalis* Serological evidence for infection. *Drugs* 1986; 31:7–10.

178. FADEN H, HONG J, MURPHY T. Immune response to outer membrane antigens of *Moraxella catarrhalis* in children with otitis media. *Infect Immun* 1992; 60:3824–9.

179. GOLDBLATT D, SEYMOUR ND, LIVINSKY RJ, TURNER MW. An enzyme linked immunosorbent assay for the determination of human IgG subclass antibodies directed against *Branhamella catarrhalis*. *J Immunol Meth* 1990; 128:219–25.

180. LEINONEN M, LUOTOTNEN J, HERVA E, MÄKELÄ H. Preliminary serologic evidence for a pathogenic role of *Branhamella catarrhalis*. *J Infect Dis* 1981; 144:570–4.

181. SARUBBI FA, MYERS JW, WILLIAMS JJ, SHELL CG. Respiratory infections caused by *Branhamella catarrhalis*: selected epidemiologic features. *Am J Med* 1990; 88 (5A):9S–14S.

182. SLEVIN NJ, AITKEN J, THORNLEY P. Clinical and microbiological features of *Branhamella catarrhalis* bronchopulmonary infection. *Lancet* 1984; 1:782–3.

183. NICOTRA B, RIVERA M, LUMAN JI, WALLACE JR RJ. *Branhamella catarrhalis* as a lower respiratory tract pathogen in patients with chronic lung disease. *Arch Intern Med* 1986; 146:890–3.

184. WRIGHT PW, WALLACE JR RJ, SHEPHARD JR. A descriptive study of 42 cases of *Branhamella catarrhalis* pneumonia. *Am J Med* 1990; 88 (5A):2S–8S.

185. HOL C, VAN DIJKE EEM, VERDUIN CM, VERHOEF J, VAN DIJK H. Experimental evidence for *Moraxella*-induced penicillin neutralization in pneumococcal pneumonia. *J Infect Dis* 1994; 170:1613–6.

186. EJLERTSEN T, SCHØNHEYDER HC, THISTED E. β-lactamase production in *Branhamella catarrhalis* isolated from lower respiratory tract secretions in Danish children: An increasing problem. *Infection* 1991; 19:328–30.

187. VANEECHOUTTE M, VERSCHRAEGEN G, CLAEYS G, WEISE B, VAN DEN ABEELE AM. Respiratory tract carrier rates of *Moraxella* (*Branhamella*) *catarrhalis* in adults and children and interpretation of the isolation of *M. catarrhalis* from sputum. *J Clin Microbiol* 1990; 28:2674–80.

188. FADEN H, HARABUCHI Y, HONG JJ. Epidemiology of *Moraxella catarrhalis* in children during the first 2 years of life: relationship to otitis media. *J Infect Dis* 1994;169:1312–7.

189. EJLERTSEN T, THISTED E, EBBESEN F, OLESEN B, RENNEBERG J. *Branhamella catarrhalis* in children and adults. A study of prevalence, time of colonisation, and association with upper and lower respiratory tract infections. *J Infect* 1994; 29:23–31.

190. DIGIOVANNI C, RILEY TV, HOYNE GF, YEO R, COOKSEY P. Respiratory infections due to *Branhamella catarrhalis*: epidemiological data from Western Australia. *Epidemiol Infect* 1987; 99:445–53.

191. MCLEOD DT, AHMAD F, CAPEWELL S, CROUGHAM MJ, CALDER MA, SEATON A. Increase in bronchopulmonary infection due to *Branhamella catarrhalis Br Med J* 1986; 292:1103–5.

192. MCLEOD DT, AHMAD F, CROUGHAM MJ, CALDER MA. Bronchopulmonary infection due to *Branhamella catarrhalis* clinical features and therapeutic response. *Drugs* 1986; 31 (Suppl 3):110–12.

193. PATTERSON TF, PATTERSON JE, MASECAR BL, BARDEN GE, HIERHOLZER WJJR, ZERVOS MJ. A nosocomial outbreak of *Branhamella catarrhalis* confirmed by restriction endonuclease analysis. *J Infect Dis* 1988; 157:996–1001.

194. PICARD B, GOULLET P, DENAMUR E, SUERMONDT G. Esterase electrophoresis: a molecular tool for studying the epidemiology of *Branhamella catarrhalis* nosocomial infection. *Epidemiol Infect* 1989; 103:547–54.

195. EJLERTSEN T, SCHØNHEYDER HC. *Branhamella catarrhalis* as a cause of multiple subpleural abscesses. *Scand J Infect Dis* 1991; 23:117–8.

196. KOSTIALA AAI, HONKANEN T. *Branhamella catarrhalis* as a cause of acute purulent pericarditis. *J Infect*, 1989; 19:291–2.

197. WALLACE RJJR, NASH DR, STEINGRUBE VA. Antibiotic susceptibilities and drug resistance in *Moraxella* (*Branhamella*) *catarrhalis*. *Am J Med* 1990; 88 (Suppl 5A): 46S–50S.

198. ELIASSON I, HOLST E, MÖLSTAD S, KAMME C. Emergence and persistence of beta-lactamase-producing bacteria in the upper respiratory tract in children treated with beta-lactam antibiotics. *Am J Med* 1990; 88 (5A):51S–55S.

199. BROOK I. Direct and indirect pathogenicity of *Branhamella catarrhalis Drugs* 1986; 31(Suppl 3): 97–102.

200. WARDLE JK. *Branhamella catarrhalis* as an indirect pathogen. *Drugs* 1986; (Suppl 3): 93–6.

8 Gram-negative bacillary pneumonia

MICHAEL E. ELLIS

King Faisal Specialist Hospital and Research Centre, Riyadh, Saudi Arabia

Introduction

Although aerobic Gram-negative rod pneumonia was first recognised over a century ago, aetiological agents other than *Klebsiella pneumoniae* did not feature until the last three decades. Their entrance into the pulmonary arena was heralded by the evolution of health care, particularly the vast explosion in high technology medical practice such as intensive care, the paraphernalia of invasive procedural devices such as endotracheal intubation and intravascular devices, iatrogenic immunosuppressive therapy for malignancy, use of antimicrobials and the ever-increasing population of the elderly with their relatively immunocompromised status. This scenario has permitted expression of the opportunistic potential of many commensal organisms. It is impossible to present precise incidence figures, as these vary from centre to centre and are influenced by diagnostic sensitivity, patient populations, etc. However, the figures quoted are generally taken from larger or more representative sources. In contrast to the fall in the aetiological contribution of the pneumococcus to community acquired pneumonia which now stands at approximately 30–40%, compared to over 80% 30 years ago, the incidence of Gram-negative bacillary pneumonia has increased from between 0.65 to 8.5% before the mid-1960s up to at least 20% since that time[1–3]. In hospital-acquired pneumonia, the contribution is even more striking, with enteric Gram-negative bacilli causing between 50 and 60% of all nosocomial pneumonias[4,5] and contributing substantially to the 15.5% of hospital deaths caused by nosocomial pneumonia[4]. This chapter will review in detail the more frequently found Gram-negative bacillary organisms namely the *Pseudomonads*, the important *Enterobacteriaceae* (tribes *Klebsiella*, *Escherichia* and *Enterobacter*) and will comment briefly on the other uncommon or rarely found organisms. Anaerobic bacteria, *Legionella* spp., *Haemophilus* spp., *Branhamella/Moraxella* spp. and other Gram-negative organisms are covered elsewhere.

Pseudomonas infection

The pseudomonads are Gram-negative, aerobic, straight/curved bacilli; moving by a single polar flagellum. They are oxidase and catalase positive and have a wide temperature growth spectrum of between 4 °C and 43 °C, and simple growth requirements. On the basis of RNA analysis, there are five groups containing 15 species. Most often these free living bacteria are found in damp environments and have the propensity for causing a wide spectrum of human disease ranging from bacteraemia, soft tissue infection such as malignant otitis externa, corneal infection, osteomyelitis, endocarditis, meningitis, urinary infection and pneumonia. Whilst *Pseudomonas aeruginosa* respiratory infection can occur in immunocompetent hosts, it is the predilection for the immunocompromised that usually produces serious infections. *P. aeruginosa* is by far the most important of species. Aspects of pneumonia due to *P. aeruginosa* will be described here – the reader is encouraged also to read the chapter on cystic fibrosis.

Pseudomonas aeruginosa

The organism is approximately 0.7 × 2.0 μ in size and certain biochemical features differentiate it from other species. These include oxidation of specific sugars such as glucose but not maltose, ability to grow at 37/42 °C rather than 4 °C and the presence of pyocyanic pigment. This pigment is responsible for the green colour imparted to *Pseudomonas* pus. Some strains possess a pathogenic polysaccharide capsule which produces alginate. The strains from patients with cystic fibrosis have particularly large capsules.

In nature, it is ubiquitous wherever there is a suitable moist environment such as the soil, water, plants, and this property permits growth in the hospital environment such as sinks, water reservoirs, ventilatory equipment, whirlpools, endoscopes, pacing wires, mattresses and aqueous medicines. In man, it can colonise the gut in up to 24% of healthy people, less frequently the skin and upper respiratory tract. It may colonise and infect wounds, ulcers, burns and the instrumented/catheterised urinary tract[6,7]. It is therefore a major cause of nosocomial infection, particularly hospital-acquired pneumonia with attendant serious morbidity, mortality and cost implications[6].

Host–parasite interactions

In the context of a healthy individual, *P. aeruginosa* is saprophytic. Deterioration of the host's defence mechanisms permits expression of the organism's pathogenic virulence factors. *P. aeruginosa* produces much of the devastating critical-organ pathology through the elaboration of toxins, but prior to this, colonisation of crucial epithelial receptors must occur.

P. aeruginosa possesses pili (adhesins), the terminal peptide of which allows adherence of the bacteria to respiratory epithelial cells – this is an important mechanism in non-mucoid strains. The central importance of these has been shown by elegant experiments where adhesiveness could be reduced by pili antibodies[7]. In the case of mucoid strains, alginate may be a more important adhesin. The receptors for the *P. aeruginosa* pili include mucins which may be more important for mucoid strains, and epithelial cilia.

It is not sufficient that these adhesins exist – the host must be primed to be receptive. For example, damage to the airways from viral tracheitis or endotracheal intubation enhances binding of *P. aeruginosa*, for example by removing the surface defensive layer of the respiratory tract[8]. In addition, the normally protective fibronectin which is removed as a result of various illnesses, and by some strains of *P. aeruginosa per se*, exposes epithelial cell receptors. Mannose also protects these receptors by acting as an adhesin analogue.

In the case of the mucin-producing strains, the mannuronic/glucuronic structure of the alginate appears to coat *Pseudomonas* and offers defence against phagocytosis, removal by the muco-ciliary elevator, aminoglycoside action and antibody/complement attachment.

Additional properties of *P. aeruginosa* which assist the organism in making successful colonisation of the respiratory tract include production of at least seven ciliastatic agents such as pyocyanic and hydroxyphenazine pigments. These permit increased duration of contact with respiratory epithelium. Other properties include the stimulation of, and modification of, the structure of respiratory mucins, which presumably leads to increased adherence, production of elastase which removes protective IgA and possibly digestion of fibronectin, allowing for ease of the epithelial cell attachment[9].

A number of factors exist on the host side of the host–parasite equation to facilitate colonisation and invasion of the respiratory tract. Underlying disease in the host will place the oropharynx and tracheo-bronchial airways in a vulnerable state, with replacement of the normal resident bacterial flora by various gut Gram-negative bacteria (GGNB) usually present in the enteric tract, or acquired from the hospital environment. GGNB constitute no more than a few per cent of the normal oral flora but with illness or hospitalisation, this figure rises to approximately 20% for patients with malignancy and far exceeds 50% with increasing duration of hospitalisation[10,11] – and many, if not the majority, of these are *Pseudomonas* spp. The predisposing factors are similar to those described for *Klebsiella* spp. and other GGNBs (see relevant sections, this chapter). These include neutropenia and immune suppression associated with organ transplantation and chemotherapy, and HIV infection. Others include the use of H_2 blockers (stomach pH rises and no longer inhibits GGNB growth), pre-existing lung disease, smoking and endotracheal intubation (mechanical bypassing of the upper airways defences leading to direct tracheal access). Tracheostomy or endotracheal intubation are particularly important especially if the tubes are not changed frequently. Colonisation by bacteria occurs in a biofilm which can become dislodged during suctioning[12]. *Pseudomonas* spp. may preferentially colonise the lower rather than the upper respiratory tract in some of these patients. Important humoral and cell-mediated immunity (CMI) factors in the host are crucial in defence against *Pseudomonas* spp. For example, an ability to mount an antibody response, particularly to exotoxin-A[13]; an effective T-cell-mediated response[14], and an adequate white blood cell response which governs both susceptibility to *P. aeruginosa* disease[6] and predicts survival[15]. The elderly are prone to *P. aeruginosa*, as a result of age-related changes in immune function. Uraemia predisposes to increased adherence to buccal epithelial cells[16]. Malnutrition is a particularly important factor, which can result in diminished intestinal cell integrity, alteration in CMI, reduced defence by the reticulo-endothelial system with consequent translocation of GGNB to regional lymph nodes and thereby to the circulation[17,18]. It also increases adherence of *P. aeruginosa* to buccal and tracheal cells[19]. Total parenteral nutrition *per se* can also lead to an increased risk of Gram-negative septic complications. Although enteric feeding via nasogastric intubation preserves intestinal structure and function, it has itself a definite risk for infectious complications[20,21], through increasing the risk for gastric aspiration and by contamination of feeds.

Other factors include malignancy, acidosis, hypotension, post-surgery antibiotic use, steroids, coma, chronic ambulatory peritoneal dialysis, lung injury, cystic fibrosis and bronchiectasis. Viral infection is said to be a factor in predisposing to *P. aeruginosa* infection. For example, cytomegalovirus has been shown to diminish CMI and to predispose animal models to subsequent *P. aeruginosa* disease[22]. Certain patients with excess iron and saturated transferrin levels may show increased susceptibility to pseudomonal disease – an indication of the importance of free iron for this organism.

There has been much debate on whether colonisation of the oropharynx/upper respiratory tract with *P. aeruginosa* itself directly leads to pneumonia or whether this is merely a surrogate marker reflecting the increased risk of the patient to Gram-negative sepsis. Although GGNB can appear in the oropharyngeal cavity prior to lower respiratory tract colonisation and pneumonia, there is evidence that in the case of *P. aeruginosa* the trachea can be infected without oropharyngeal colonisation or by strains different from those present in the more proximal airways[23,24]. This may be related to more avid binding of *P. aeruginosa* to ciliated tracheal epithelium than to non-ciliated oropharyngeal epithelium, particularly in the case of mucoid strains. It is also known that *P. aeruginosa* can reach the lungs via a haematogenous route from patients with a primary source, for example, in patients with thermal burns or other integument breakdown situations, or in patients with indwelling IV catheters. Some recent studies, using plasmid, biochemical, antibiotic resistance patterns, DNA fingerprinting and repetitive extragenic palindromic sequence analysis demonstrated that bacteria from the stomach of ICU ventilated patients were identical to those from the lower respiratory tract in 11/19 patients – duodenogastric reflux and subsequent aspiration of stomach contents was the postulated mechanism. No oropharyngeal isolate was identical to that in the lower respiratory tract[24].

Aspiration of the patient's own flora directly into the lungs has been postulated as the mechanism in cases of community-acquired *P. aeruginosa* pneumonia. Various hospital reservoirs of *P. aeruginosa*, and other *Pseudomonas* spp. have been identified, from which patients have been infected, including respiratory nebulisers, 'sterile' water, hydrotherapy equipment and flowers. It has been assumed to be transmitted on the hands of hospital personnel[25,26]. Some nebulisation equipment not only harbours reservoirs of *P. aeruginosa* but can disperse aerosols containing *P. aeruginosa* several feet distant. Ventilators, particularly the tubing and condensates can become colonised with GGNB even within a few hours of change of this equipment.

P. aeruginosa has a number of important additional properties to facilitate tissue invasion, lung damage and multiorgan failure. The enzyme elastase inactivates C3b and C5a complement components, thus inhibiting opsonisation and chemotaxis. Elastase has been postulated as responsible for tissue necrosis, and by destroying the elastic lamina of blood vessels produces necrotising pneumonia associated with alveolar and arterial wall necrosis and ecthyma gangrenosum characteristic of *P. aeruginosa* septicaemia. Elastase antibodies can be detected in patients with pneumonia. Cleavage of type III and IV collagen and activation of lysosyme are further mechanisms. There are other proteases which directly attack host tissue as well as inactivating complement. Other products include cytotoxin – its action on cell membranes leads directly to diminished polymorph function and peripheral vascular injury, and haemolysins which destroy lipids, such as lung surfactant.

There are, in addition, two other major toxins – lipopolysaccharide endotoxin, and exotoxin A. The lipopolysaccharide can cause complement activation, trigger cytokine responses, e.g. tumour necrosis factor, activate the clotting cascade, and stimulate prostaglandin release. No doubt these biological activities have an important role in the production of fever, DIC, leukopenia, hypotension and other features constituting the Gram-negative sepsis syndrome. Exotoxin A has been identified, the responsible gene isolated, its structure elucidated, and has been cloned. Its major function is to inhibit protein synthesis. It has necrotising properties in the lung and in extrapulmonary sites, is cytotoxic for polymorphs and can enhance bacterial invasiveness. Toxin-producing strains have enhanced invasiveness; an effective exotoxin A antibody response appears to correlate with survival in cases of *P. aeruginosa* septicaemia[13]. Another toxin called exoenzyme S has also been identified which plays a role in producing local lung damage and in dissemination of the bacterium.

Epidemiological highlights

Pneumonia caused by *P. aeruginosa* is almost exclusively restricted to individuals who have endogenous or iatrogenic disturbance of local/systemic immune defences. It is therefore not surprising that reports of community-acquired pneumonia do not commonly include *Pseudomonas* spp. In a 5-year prospective study of patients with community-acquired pneumonia requiring hospitalisation, *P. aeruginosa* was not listed among 588 patients with community-acquired pneumonia or 131 with nursing home acquired pneumonia and among 48 patients with bacteraemia and community-acquired pneumonia who had blood cultures performed, *P. aeruginosa* was present in only one[28]. Another study, however, quoted an approximately 5% incidence from nursing homes[29]. Some reviews do not specify *Pseudomonas* spp. but these organisms may be hidden in the grouping 'aerobic Gram-negative bacteria'[30,31]. Elderly patients, particularly those from nursing homes, might be expected to be at greater risk from GGNB pneumonia, since these persons usually have chronic illness, or are diabetic or have received antibiotics[30]. Nevertheless, there have been isolated reports of community-acquired pneumonia due to *P. aeruginosa* in the absence of any recognised immunodeficiency although many of these patients have a history of smoking[31,32]. *P. aeruginosa* pneumonia is therefore largely a disease arising in hospitalised patients[33]. In a hospital setting, approximately 15% of all nosocomial pneumonias are due to *P. aeruginosa*[34]. In a recent study *Pseudomonas* spp. or *Acinetobacter* spp. accounted for over 40% of Gram-negative nosocomial pneumonias in patients ventilated on an ICU[35]. An entity of recurrent *P. aeruginosa* pneumonia occurring among ICU patients, particularly those who have chronic lung disease and despite adequate antibiotic treatment has been recently described. This carries a particularly unfavourable prognosis[36]. The majority of these pneumonias arise in patients on an ICU, or who have cancer or neutropaenia[35,37–39]. Among bacteraemic patients with malignancy in general, *P. aeruginosa*, together with *Klebsiella* spp. contribute the majority of Gram-negative isolates[40,41]. Of all bacteraemic episodes in such patients, 14% are associated with a respiratory tract source[41]. The mortality in patients with *P. aeruginosa* is high (50–80%) and appears to be higher than other Gram-negative pneumonias[38] and in excess of that resulting from the patients' underlying disease[35].

Clinical presentation, radiological and histological features and management

The presentation and course of patients with *Pseudomonas* pneumonia takes three forms depending on the clinical setting and underlying risk factors. One manifestation, that of chronic *Pseudomonas* infection, occurs in patients with cystic fibrosis or with chronic pulmonary disease (Fig. 8.1 (*a*), (*b*), (*c*)). This has been addressed in Chapters 24 and 29.

The term 'primary' or 'non-bacteraemic pneumonia' is used to describe the pneumonia which occurs in patients usually without neutropenia, in which aspiration from prior colonisation of the pharynx or upper respiratory tract has occurred (Fig. 8.2). However, the causal relationship between upper respiratory tract colonisation and lower respiratory infection has not been clearly established. This term covers both patients admitted from the community (rarely) and also hospital patients. If the patient is from the community, the patient will probably be a smoker or alcoholic and from a nursing home. More commonly, however, the patient will be critically ill in hospital, possibly ventilated on an ICU with some of the risk factors for *Pseudomonas* colonisation alluded to previously. Chills, fever, dyspnoea and cough productive of yellow or green sputum will be present. Substantial toxicity, marked cyanosis, confusion or fear will be present. Relative bradycardia and the reversal of the usual diurnal temperature pattern has been described[42].

The chest radiograph shows diffuse bilateral bronchopneumonia with small nodular infiltrates; some of the nodules may have small lucencies which may coalesce. Pleural effusions may occur. Histologically, alveolar wall necrosis, macro- and micro- abscesses are found, and focal pulmonary haemorrhage is present without evidence of Gram-negative bacillary vasculitis[42].

The third form is called bacteraemic *Pseudomonas* pneumonia. This usually occurs in patients rendered neutropenic by leukaemia or by the use of cytotoxic chemotherapy. Although there is presumed to be an element of upper respiratory tract colonisation and distal aspiration as suggested for primary *P. aeruginosa* pneumonia, haematogenous invasion occurs producing diffuse pneumonia and extrapulmonary metastatic infective foci. These patients usually present abruptly with high fever, confusion and tachypnoea. There may be pleuritic chest pain. Chest findings include widespread crepitations, usually basal, and occasionally a pleural rub. Skin manifestations of *P. aeruginosa* pneumonia may also be present[43]. The most frequently described is ecthyma gangrenosum, a round erythematous macule which rapidly enlarges to form a blue–black necrotic centre (Fig. 8.3). Over a quarter of all patients with *Pseudomonas*

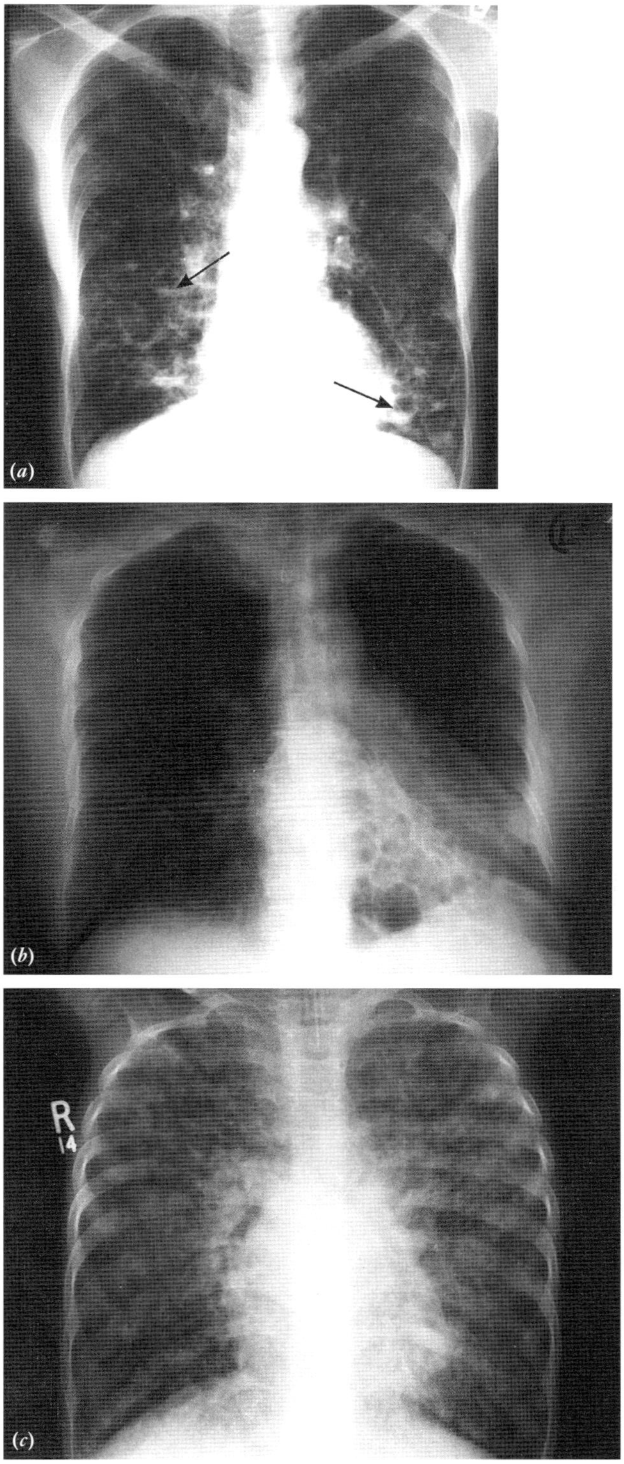

FIGURE 8.1 (*a*) 47 male with COAD and bilateral bronchiectasis. Infective exacerbation with *P. aeruginosa*. Extensive cystic changes throughout lower and mid lung zones. Note fluid levels in cysts. (*b*) 75-year-old patient with COAD. *Pseudomonas* spp. exacerbation of respiratory failure. Marked cystic bronchiectasis with peribronchiectactic infiltrates left lower lobe. (*c*) 5-year-old child with cystic fibrosis chronically infected with *Pseudomonas* spp. Bilateral gross alveolar/interstitial infiltrates with little apparent normal functioning lung parenchyma.

bacteraemia have this lesion, which usually occurs singly in the perineum, on extremities or occasionally on mucous membranes. It has histological features similar to those seen in the lung. It is highly suggestive but not pathognomonic of *Pseudomonas*: fungi particularly *Aspergillus*, *Serratia* spp. are other causative agents. Other lesions found in bacteraemic *P. aeruginosa* pneumonia include cellulitis, petechiae, subcutaneous nodules and rose spots, similar to those found in typhoid fever. The bacteraemic process may lead to *Pseudomonas* pneumonia, or alternatively, it could occur as a secondary haematogenous spread from a primary lung focus. There may be other features of haematogenously directed extrapulmonary metastatic manifestations including panophthalmitis, cutaneous pustules, endocarditis, meningitis, brain abscess, osteomyelitis and other major organ involvement[31].

An early chest radiograph of bacteraemic *Pseudomonas* pneumonia will usually be non-specific with features of pulmonary venous congestion and pulmonary oedema, although a normal pulmonary artery wedge pressure excludes left heart failure as the cause. Serial radiographs will often show a diffuse mixed alveolar interstitial infiltrate pattern (Fig. 8.4) of bronchopneumonia which progresses to cavitation. Histologically, necrotising vasculitis is present in which *Pseudomonas* is seen to invade both the arterial and venous vessel walls. This feature is often found in areas of microabscesses with plentiful leukocytes and in haemorrhagic necrotic areas[44]. Some lesions similar to those found in primary pneumonia as described above may also be present.

Local pulmonary complications include pleural effusion, cavitation and abscess formation and Pancoasts' syndrome[45,46].

Systemic features directly related to sepsis include DIC, respiratory distress syndrome and multiorgan failure, and indirectly, additional problems arise from intensive care manipulations which all interact to produce a complex presentation of illness[47].

Pseudomonas infections in patients with HIV

Previously, *Pseudomonas* was not considered an important or common pathogen in patients with HIV. Recent reports, however, indicate the

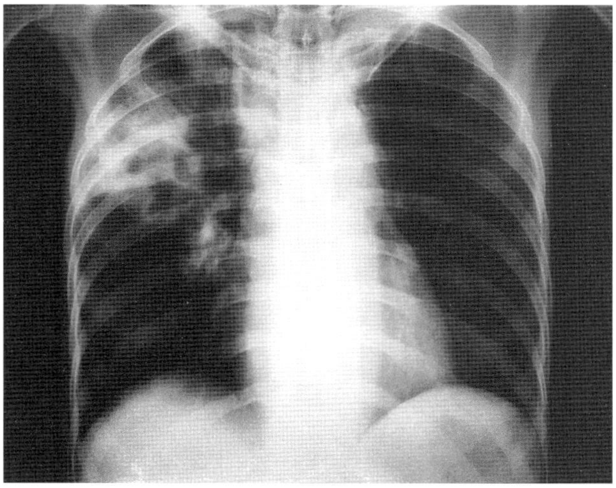

FIGURE 8.2 Patient with hypopharyngeal carcinoma; aspiration pneumonia right upper lobe showing consolidation and cavities due to *Pseudomonas* spp.

contrary. For example, it was found to be responsible for significant clinical infection in 15% of adults[48] which may not be diagnosed until post-mortem. In some series, *P. aeruginosa* was the most common Gram-negative organism among bacteraemias in HIV patients[49]. Among children with HIV, the rate of *Pseudomonas* bacteraemia appears to be even higher than that seen among paediatric patients with cancer[50]. Four of six patients reported by Flores had pulmonary infection: one had severe pulmonary necrosis and all had skin lesions. Neutropenia was only present in two of four patients; however, there may have been subtle defects in neutrophil function and specific antibody production[50,51]. Similar reports appear from the adult HIV population which includes both community-acquired *Pseudomonas* pneumonia and hospital acquired *Pseudomonas* pneumonia[52]. A recent study from Milan has indicated that *Pseudomonas* spp. were responsible for over 40% of all nosocomial pneumonias in ARC/AIDS patients[53]. The clinical presentation of *P. aeruginosa* pneumonia in HIV-infected patients may display some features distinct from that in other immunocompromised hosts. For example, patients may have lobar consolidation, in others the radiological appearance may be indistinguishable from *Pneumocystis carinii* pneumonia. The clinical course tends to be less fulminant. Coexisting opportunistic lung disease due to *Mycobacterium* spp., CMV, KS, cryptococcosis, non-Hodgkin's lymphoma, and *P. carinii* pneumonia was found to be common in nosocomial cases[53].

Treatment

Management of *P. aeruginosa* pneumonia involves directed antimicrobial therapy, adjunctive immunomodulatory therapy, supportive and intensive care aspects. The management of cystic fibrosis patients is covered in Chapter 24.

Antibiotic treatment

The approach to antibiotic treatment is complicated by the immunocompromised host status, some conflicting literature results from antibiotic trials and emergence of resistant organisms. Most physicians would treat *P. aeruginosa* pneumonia with an antipseudomonal penicillin such as piperacillin, mezlocillin, azlocillin or ticarcillin ± a β-lactamase inhibitor such as clavulanic acid, or an antipseudomonal third-generation cephalosporin such as ceftazidime, plus an aminoglycoside. The rationale behind the concomitant use of an aminoglycoside is (i) more rapid bacterial killing by the aminoglycoside; (ii) synergistic effect of the combination; (iii) the significant aminoglycoside post antibiotic effect; (iv) lack of an inoculum effect; (v) reduction of the emergence of resistant organisms or superinfections.

There are some *in vivo* studies which support the clinical use of combination therapy with aminoglycoside and antipseudomonal β-lactam treatment. One of these major studies, which did not address *Pseudomonas* pneumonia specifically, showed that a long rather than a short course of antimicrobial combination therapy with amikacin and ceftazidime was more beneficial[54]. Other studies confirm that mortality and clinical success from *P. aeruginosa* pneumonia with proven bacteraemia could be halved by using combination rather than single agent treatment[55,56]. Combination therapy in severe immunocompromised hosts with Gram-negative sepsis which include *Pseudomonas* spp. have a greater survival in general if combination rather than monotherapy is used[57].

Dosing of the aminoglycoside has to be adequate whilst minimising toxicity. Attaining a serum peak level as rapidly as possible is achieved with an appropriate loading dose and this is followed by twice daily or once daily dosing rather than the traditional three times daily dosing. This results in high serum peak levels which are associated with a better outcome. Ideally, the peak serum concentration should be at least ten times greater than the MIC of the organism, but there should be a sufficient time interval between dosing to allow the bacteria to recover. Another advantage of less frequent dosing is a lower incidence of aminoglycoside related nephrotoxicity. A concern is that there may not be therapeutically acceptable levels of aminoglycosides in pulmonary secretions when it is given by the intravenous route. One approach therefore has been to instill the aminoglycoside locally via the endotracheal tube. Two studies have indicated either an improved outcome in patients receiving local aminoglycoside (Sisomicin)[58] or a superior bacterial eradication rate

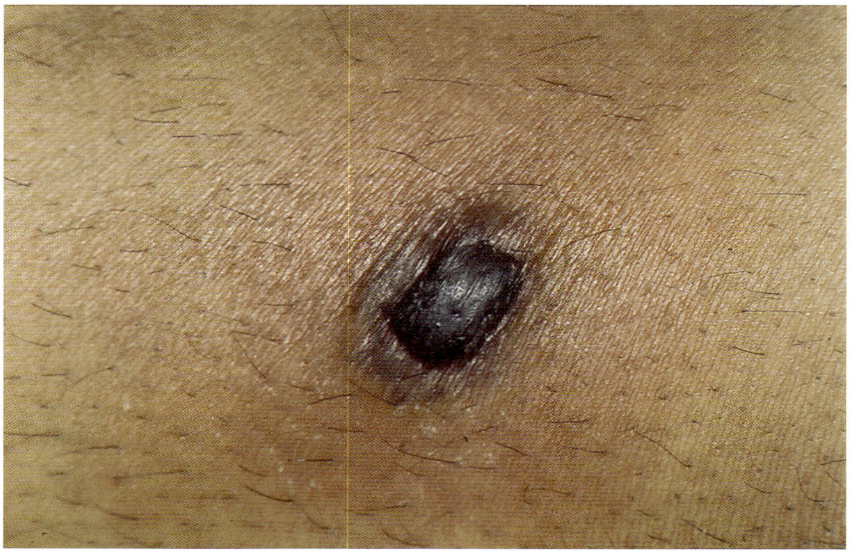

FIGURE 8.3 Ecthyma gangrenosum.

without effect on clinical outcome (Tobramycin)[59]. However, this mode of administration is rarely practised. Often the patients in whom *P. aeruginosa* pneumonia occurs are critically ill with pre-existing renal disease and who have other factors which appear to enhance aminoglycoside nephrotoxicity, for example, older age, liver disease, hypotension. Optimal dosing should be directed in collaboration with a clinical pharmacokineticist and the microbiology laboratory. The duration of antimicrobial therapy is also an important issue and will to an extent depend on the underlying neutrophil status. In a patient with a normal neutrophil count, 7 to 10 days of therapy should be adequate. However, in patients with persistent neutropenia, treatment should be continued until the neutrophil count exceeds 500 and the clinical response is adequate. The possibility of other infections, for example, Gram-positive cocci or fungi should be borne in mind if the patient remains febrile despite antibiotics. Resistant *Pseudomonas* spp. may also be an explanation for this and knowledge of the antibiotic sensitivity is crucial.

Other alternative therapies to the β-lactam aminoglycoside regimen include monotherapy or combination therapy with other agents such as imipenem, aztreonam, or ciprofloxacin. However, as previously mooted, monotherapy may not be advisable and clinical failures have indeed been documented, whilst some trials have documented good clinical outcomes[60,61]. Clearly, the issue of efficacy of monotherapy with newer antibiotic agents remains at this time to be clarified.

The problem of antibiotic resistance

All the major antimicrobials that have been used for treating *P. aeruginosa* pneumonia have resulted in the emergence of resistant organisms. Aminoglycoside treatment has led to plasmid-mediated aminoglycoside modifying enzymes and differential resistance (gentamicin > tobramycin > amikacin). Plasmid-mediated *Pseudomonas*-specific enzymes are largely responsible for the high incidence of β-lactamase resistant *P. aeruginosa*, whereas chromosomal enzymes mediate the cephalosporin resistant strains. Traditionally, sensitivity to the carbapenem imipenem has been found in the face of resistance to other β-lactams, since a specific outer membrane porin (protein D2) exists through which imipenem penetration occurs; furthermore, imipenem is usually highly resistant to β-lactamases. Recently, however, imipenem resistance, largely due to lack of D2 protein has been documented in about 25% of cases Interestingly, imipenem resistant strains still remain sensitive to piperacillin and ceftazidime. They are also sensitive to meropenem, a newer carbapenem. Addition of rifampicin to an antipseudomonal β-lactam and aminoglycoside regime has been associated with a more substantial bacteriological cure and with less incidence of relapse in bacteraemia[62]. This therapeutic manipulation, however, has not so far influenced survival. Quinolones are alternative therapeutic agents but resistance is now well documented and increasing in frequency. Both DNA gyrase and fluoroquinolone-specific porin defective mutants are recognised. The complexity and increased seriousness of the situation has been documented by the emergence of quinolone imipenem cross-resistance[63].

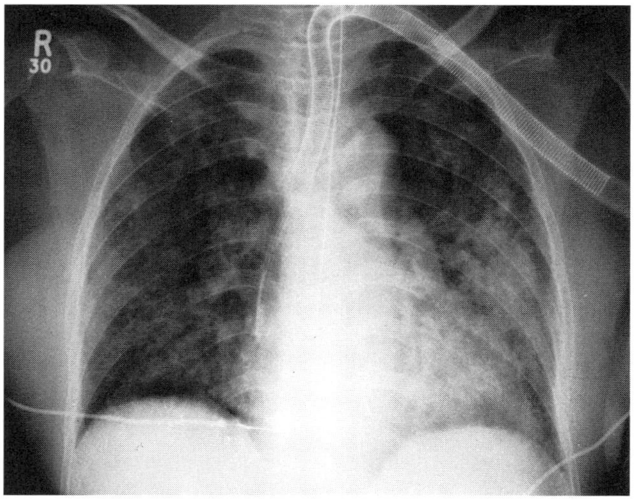

FIGURE 8.4 Patient with scleroderma, renal failure and severe brain damage. Extensive alveolar and interstitial infiltrates.

Immunomodulatory therapy

Immunomodulatory therapy has attracted considerable attention in recent years because of the unacceptably high mortality rate of *P. aeruginosa* pneumonia despite antimicrobial therapy. Experimental treatment modalities have included administration of antibodies to Gram-negative organisms and immunomodifying agents. A number of animal studies have demonstrated that passive administration of serum immunoglobulins conveys protection against *Pseudomonas* infections including pneumonia[64]. These have included antibodies directed towards the bacterial cell wall O side chain lipopolysaccharides[65]. IgG antibodies to *P. aeruginosa* have been shown to modify the acute lung and pleural injury in a sheep model of *P. aeruginosa* pneumonia[66]. A pseudomonas vaccine in which the toxic lipid A component had been removed has been shown to produce IgG antibodies to *P. aeruginosa* in healthy human volunteers, and to a level found in survivors from *P. aeruginosa* sepsis[67,68]. Recently, however, efforts have been directed towards the development of human monoclonal antibodies to the more important *P. aeruginosa* antigens, and a protective effect against lethal infections of *P. aeruginosa* in animal models has been demonstrated[69,70]. It has also been shown that human monoclonal antibodies directed towards *P. aeruginosa* flagella are effective in a mouse model of pneumonia[71]. The synergistic effect with sparfloxacin reported in that paper suggests that future therapeutic interventional investigations will have to explore antimicrobial – immunomodifier interactions. Of some interest is the finding that antibodies raised to other Gram-negative organisms will cross-protect to *P. aeruginosa*, for example, *E. coli* J5 antibodies. However, there is a need for controlled studies to investigate the clinical efficacy of these various preparations in humans.

Other experimental strategies include modulating the host response to the infection, by directing therapies towards various mediators including the cytokines. Many of these are of course not specific for *Pseudomonas*. They include the use of pentoxifylline (augments intracellular cAMP) to reduce lung injury, nitric oxide synthetase inhibitors (reduces production of nitric oxide in septic shock), antioxidants (reduces reactive oxygen metabolite-mediated cellular injury), protein C (as an anticoagulant in the DIC cascade mechanism), monoclonal antibodies against CD18 (an important leukocyte surface integrin) in neutrophil–endothelial– interaction mediated vascular injury, and antibodies towards cytokines, particularly tumour necrosis factor (a key mediator in sepsis). Few clinical human trials, however, have yet been performed and the complexity of pseudomonal-directed sepsis syndromes pose major problems for constructing appropriately designed human clinical trials.

The use of white cell colony stimulating factors has generated much interest in attempts to prevent and control sepsis in the types of patients in whom severe pseudomonas sepsis occurs. There have been some encouraging preliminary reports, for example, in terms of the efficacy of GCSF in shortening neutropenia and duration of fever, and possibly reducing the number of infections[72,73] but far more studies need to be done to assess efficacy in the treatment of established pseudomonal infection.

Non-aeruginosa *Pseudomonas* organisms

The non-aeruginosa organisms other than *Pseudomonas* spp. cause pneumonia much less frequently. However, there has been a noticeable trend in increased frequency of reporting in recent years[74]. The majority of these are *Pseudomonas pseudomallei*, *Pseudomonas fluorescens*, *Pseudomonas (Burkholderia) cepacia*, *Pseudomonas alcaligenes*, and *Xanthomonas maltophilia*.

Xanthomonas (Pseudomonas) maltophilia

Since the first clear description of this organism in 1960, evidence of its nosocomial role and pathogenicity has accrued[75,76]. It is now the most common Pseudomonad after *P. aeruginosa* identified in patients, accounting for approximately 50% of the non-aeruginosa spp.[39,77]. The organism is usually hospital acquired – in patients who have severe underlying illness, endotracheal intubation or tracheostomy, have received prior antibiotics or who have prolonged hospital stay[39]. *X. maltophilia* is found in wet environments such as sinks, respirators but the mode of transmission has not yet been clarified. The respiratory tract is the major site from which *X. maltophilia* is isolated[78] and this can be the source of bacteraemia[76]. Most isolates occur in the setting of colonisation rather than infection. However, pneumonia accounted for 5/17 patients (30%) who had *X. maltophilia* isolated from the respiratory tract in one series[76]. It is not uncommon for other organisms to be present, particularly *Staphylococcus aureus*. In patients with haematological malignancy, particularly those with neutropenia, the presence of *X. maltophilia* is more likely to be associated with infection rather than colonisation[79].

A worrying phenomenon is its multiple antibiotic resistance to aminoglycosides and to third generation cephalosporins, aztreonam and even imipenem. To date, most isolates are sensitive to cotrimoxazole, moxolactams, ciprofloxacin, chloramphenicol andticarcillin/clavulanic acid.

Pseudomonas (Burkholderia) cepacia

This is a highly unusual cause of pneumonia although there is no doubt that it can produce pulmonary disease in cystic fibrosis and in non-cystic fibrosis patients, including patients with chronic granulomatous disease[80,81]. Community-acquired bacteraemic pneumonia in an immunocompetent host is described[82]. Outbreaks have been linked to contaminated fluids and other hospital equipment[83,84]. Multiple antibiotic resistance including imipenem, ticarcillin and ceftazidime is described, as is failure of clinical treatment even if the organism is sensitive *in vitro*[83,85]. *P. (B.) cepacia* and cystic fibrosis is covered in Chapter 24.

Pseudomonas mallei

This usually produces the disease 'glanders' in equine animals and others, but on rare occasions has spread to humans[86], who have been in close contact with the animal source. It is reported sporadically from patients who have been to Asia/Africa/Central and South America. Infection can manifest as skin nodules or abscesses, lymphangitis and lymphadenopathy, splenomegaly, ulcerating lesions of the mucous membranes, generalised pustular eruption and multisystem involvement, and a severe pneumonic illness. Chest radiological findings are variable but multiple rounded opacifications are common. Diagnosis is based on the exposure history, methylene blue staining and culture of abscess/exudate material or agglutination titres. The outcome is good for local manifestations of the disease but for septicaemic illness the mortality rate approaches 100%. Treatment is with sulphadiazine.

Other pseudomonads

There are several other pseudomonads which have been isolated from sputum but whose exact role in the pathogenesis of lower respiratory tract infection is not always clear. Nevertheless, community-acquired pneumonia has been described in the case of *Pseudomonas stutzeri*[87]. Another organism which is isolated from sputum is *Pseudomonas putida*[78]. *Pseudomonas paucimobilis* has been implicated in empyema in a cardiac transplant recipient[88].

Pseudomonas pseudomallei, the causative agent of melioidosis is discussed in Chapter 26.

A newly recognised pseudomonad with phenotypic similarities to *P. (B.) cepacia* and biochemical resemblance to *Pseudomonas pickettii* was implicated in pneumonia in a child with chronic granulomatous disease[89].

Enterobacteraeciae

Klebsiella spp.

Klebsiella pulmonary infection was first described by Friedlander in 1882. Initially, the presentation of Friedlander's pneumonia was described in terms of what were considered to be rather specific clinico-radiological features appropriate to a susceptible host profile recognised in the early/mid -1900s. The advent of high technology medicine, resulting in the immunocompromised host has had an impact on the presentation, morbidity and mortality in patients with this pathogen.

The *Klebsiella* genus has three species, namely, *Klebsiella pneumoniae*, *Klebsiella oxytoza* and *Klebsiella rhinoscleromatis*, of which *K. pneumoniae* is the one most often associated with pulmonary disease, in hosts usually having some degree of immunocompromisation. The organism is a Gram-negative, non-motile, encapsulated, mucoid-producing bacterium which normally colonises the human gastrointestinal tract, but is also present in vegetation and the soil. Characteristically, it is thick, its dimension varies from approximately 0.3–1.5 μ by 0.6 – 6 μ. The presence of the polysaccharide capsule can be specified by the Quellung reaction. Capsular types 1, 3, 4 and 5 are particularly associated with respiratory infection. The somatic O antigen can also be utilised for classification. Biochemical properties include lactose fermentation, hydrogen sulphide and indole non-production, and ability to grow in KCN.

K. oxytoza and *K. rhinoscleromatis* are rare aetiological agents of lower respiratory tract infection. Their role in chronic upper airway sinusitis and chronic pseudo-tumour-like granulomatous disease is covered in Chapter 25.

The precise contribution of *Klebsiella* spp. to community-acquired pneumonia is difficult to ascertain, because of diagnostic limitations. Over-reliance on sputum culture alone might overestimate the incidence, since colonisation of the upper respiratory tract is well known to occur in alcoholics, debilitated individuals and others. An appropriate sample of sputum, i.e. one free of oropharyngeal epithelial cells with no other pathogens is preferred. Ideally, a quantitative culture from a protected bronchial brush specimen, which is not usually practically feasible or a positive blood culture would leave no doubt as to the correct diagnosis. Recent studies have implicated Gram-negative organisms in-between approximately 3 and 35% of all community-acquired bacterial pneumonias[90–92] but *Klebsiella* spp. feature rather uncommonly among these compared to *Haemophilus influenzae* and accounts for a few per cent only. This rather low incidence is confirmed in a review of US hospitals between 1900 and 1987[93], the average number of cases of *Klebsiella* pneumonia seen from 22 institutions was approximately four per year, or only two bacteraemic proven cases/year. Among over 1000 cases of community-acquired pneumonias reported from six centres, 51 (4%) were thought to be due to *Klebsiella* spp. of which only nine were bacteraemic confirmed. A 5-year prospective study of community-acquired pneumonia also confirmed this low incidence: 4/588 cases of community-acquired pneumonia, though the organism accounted for 2/48 bacteraemic patients with community-acquired pneumonia[28]. It has been suggested, however, that *Klebsiella* spp. occur relatively more frequently among the elderly, particularly those in institutions such as nursing homes[29,91] where it contributes 5–13% of all cases of pneumonia[91]. Certainly among patients with hospital-acquired pneumonia, *Klebsiella* spp. are commoner compared to community-acquired pneumonia: approximately 10% of all nosocomial pneumonia is due to *Klebsiella* spp. Among cancer patients and other seriously immunocompromised hosts, Gram-negative pneumonia and septicaemia due to *Klebsiella* spp./*Escherischia coli*/*Pseudomonas* spp. is a major cause of morbidity and mortality[5,37,39]. *K. pneumoniae* and *E. coli* were the predominant organisms in one study among cancer patients, and 25% of all episodes of *Klebsiella* spp. bacteraemia were associated with pulmonary infection[95].

Important inanimate sources of *Klebsiella* spp. in hospital environments include urinary catheters, endotracheal tubes and IV lines. Recently, ventilator condensates were identified as a probable source of cross-infection in an ICU[96]. Since *Klebsiella* spp. can colonise hands of staff after minimal patient contact and survive thereon for some hours, correct handwashing procedure of all patient care attenders is central in reducing spread of this organism in a hospital environment.

An important virulence factor appears to be the polysaccharide capsule which can reduce phagocyte migration and activity. The mechanism is unclear, it may be mechanical, or the capsule may inhibit attachment of C3b. *Klebsiella* spp. possess adhesive properties in the form of type 1 fimbriae which permits attachments to phagocytes, epithelial and other cell surfaces, thus, aiding colonisation. The number of fimbriae expressed at any given time varies with the bacterial generation. However, lack of fimbriae correlates with increased pathogenicity. D-mannose and derivatives can inhibit this attachment by binding to the epithelial cell or to the bacteria which then facilitates uptake of the organism by polymorphonucleocytes. The fimbriae bind to epithelial cell receptors probably glycoproteins which may be expressed in certain underlying disease. Fibronectin is normally present which serves to prevent these surface sugar receptors from complexing with the bacteria and its removal by polymorphonuclear produced elastase makes the host cells more vulnerable to adherence by *K. pneumoniae*.

It is unusual for *Klebsiella* spp. to produce pneumonia in persons who are otherwise well – a background of alcoholism is the classical association often mentioned in earlier descriptions of the disease. In addition to the deleterious effects of alcohol/chronic liver disease on immune function, alcohol may enhance the upper airway epithelial binding of *Klebsiella* spp. Normally, the upper respiratory tract does not harbour *Klebsiella* spp. Diabetes mellitus, chronic renal disease, chronic pulmonary disease and neoplasia may also enhance the susceptibility to *K. pneumoniae*. In a hospital setting, the colonisation of the upper airway is also increased by such factors as endotracheal intubation, malnutrition, use of H2 blocking agents, antimicrobial use, steroid administration and surgery. Enhanced adhesion to epithelial cells occurs in some of these situations, permitting increased colonisation of the respiratory tract. It is not clear whether colonisation of the upper respiratory tract *per se* leads to pneumonia via aspiration or is merely a surrogate marker of significantly impaired pulmonary and systemic defence mechanisms. A number of mechanisms exist whereby *Klebsiella* spp. may reach the respiratory tract. Transfer of infected body secretions and excretions such as faecal, urine, tracheo-bronchial, on the hands of hospital personnel and from contaminated ventilatory assist devices are extremely important. There is no evidence that person-to-person transmission occurs by the airborne-route. Other modes of transfer include transfer from the GI tract via naso-intestinal intubation devices, particularly in patients with gastric acid neutralising medications, and bypassing of the upper respiratory tract defences by endotracheal intubation.

The highly virulent nature of the organism results in substantial lung destruction due to inflammatory alveolar wall necrosis and arterial vessel thrombosis resulting in infarction of lung tissue. Local pulmonary complications include abscess formation, cavitation, empyema, pleural adhesions and lung haemorrhage, pericarditis, pyopneumothorax and pneumopericardium. An antigenic relationship between *Klebsiella* spp. and HLA-B27 antigen has been postulated, and incriminated *Klebsiella* spp. as a trigger of disease activity in patients with ankylosing spondylitis but this has been challenged on epidemiological grounds[97].

Clinical/radiological features and management

The presentation is of abrupt onset with profound toxicity. Often the patient is a male alcoholic, of late middle age, who may have had a recent seemingly insignificant upper respiratory tract infection. Recent reviews, however, have indicated a change in the patient population. Although a history of alcohol abuse is present in just under a half of all patients, immunosuppression such as corticosteroid therapy, neutropenia, chemotherapy, transplantation or haematological malignancy is now almost as common, being present in a third of all patients at presentation[98]. Prominent features include fever, rigors, productive cough, haemoptysis, and prolific chest pain. The sputum is substantial and mucoid (said to resemble red-currant jelly).

The patient is ill, highly febrile, and may have cyanosis. Accompanying herpes labialis is uncommon. Auscultatory and percussion findings reveal features usually of lobar consolidation, most often in the right upper lobe[98]. Radiographically, in the acute stage, lobar consolidation of at least two lobes in approximately 50% of patients at presentation, with bulging interlobar fissures are the most commonly observed findings[93] (Fig. 8.5). However, diffuse infiltrates may be found in as many 50% of patients[98] particularly in those with granulocytopenia[99]. Abscess formation, cavitation and increase in lung volume may be present. Later, residual pulmonary fibrosis, pleural thickening and chronic cavitation may occur. Rarely, pneumopyopericardium occurs[100].

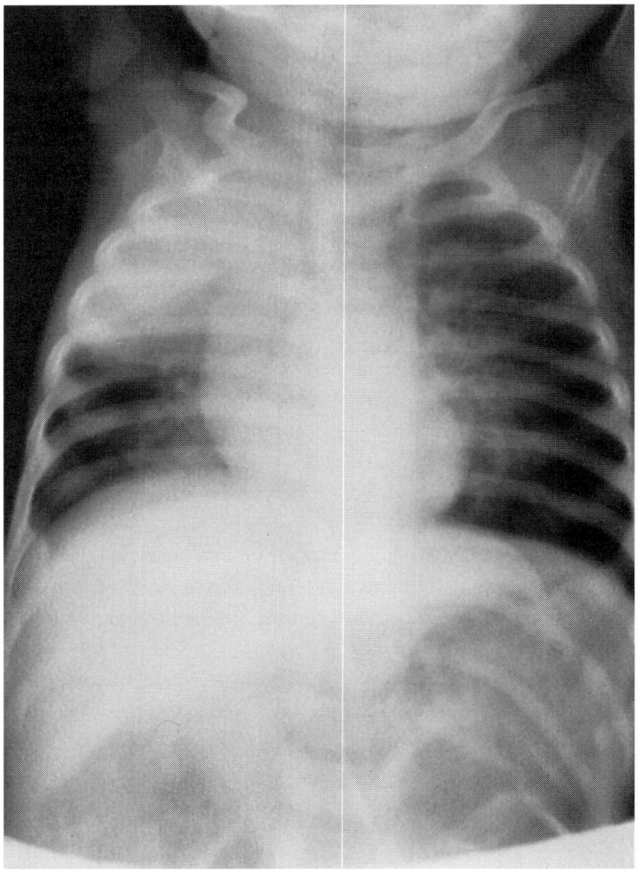

FIGURE 8.5 *Klebsiella pneumoniae* pneumonia.

Complications include abscess formation and chronic pulmonary disease. Early abscess formation is particularly suggestive of *K. pneumoniae*[93]. It occurs in up to 50% of cases and as early as the first week of the illness. An unusual variant of abscess formation is termed massive pulmonary gangrene, consequent on extensive vascular involvement. Several cavities develop in the pneumonic lung which coalesce and contain necrotic lung at the base of the large cavity[93]. A chronic form of *K. pneumoniae* in which cough, anaemia, fatigue and upper lobe cavitation are found has been described[93,101,102].

Certain of these features, particularly upper lobe distribution, cavitation and the chronic syndrome may suggest alternative diagnoses including tuberculosis, necrotising pulmonary aspergillosis and anaerobic infection. Furthermore, the exact role of *Klebsiella* spp. in the aetiology of some of these presentations may not always be easy to define with certainty[93]. It is important to remember that the clinico-radiographic features of *Klebsiella* spp. pneumonia seen nowadays may be quite different from those described more than 50 years ago, and that several of the so-called 'classical' clinico-radiological features can also be found in pneumonia due to other aetiological agents. Therefore, they should be really considered as suggestive, rather than pathognomonic of *Klebsiella* spp. pneumonia. Extrapulmonary complications may be found which include osteomyelitis, sinusitis, meningitis, and prostatitis. Ventilatory failure requiring assisted ventilation may be necessary and the mortality is substantial with an approximate survival rate of 50% at 14 days[62].

The diagnosis is confirmed by the finding of the organism in a satisfactory respiratory specimen or from blood culture. A positive blood culture is said to be found in 70% or more of cases[62,93] though some series report a much lower incidence. A satisfactory sputum culture, that is with no contamination of oropharyngeal epithelial cells and large numbers of bacteria alone, is crucial to avoid including cases of colonised patients. There is a high degree of oropharyngeal colonisation which occurs in certain individuals without pneumonia such as the debilitated, alcoholic or following viral upper respiratory tract infection.

Management of *Klebsiella* spp. pneumonia is a multi-faceted approach involving (i) reduction of any immunosuppression and avoiding factors responsible for continuing Gram-negative colonisation of the airway; (ii) ventilatory support; (iii) antimicrobial therapy; (iv) management of complications; and (v) non-antimicrobial drug therapeutic support.

In practice, inappropriate use of broad spectrum antibiotics should be avoided. Judicious control of diabetes, use of a mucosal coating agent such as sucralfate in preference to H2 blockers in ICU patients, maintenance of an adequate nutritional status, reduction of excessive steroid dosage and correction of neutropenia are some general manipulations that should be adopted wherever possible.

A common antimicrobial choice is either a third-generation cephalosporin such as ceftazidime or a ureidopenicillin such as piperacillin together with an aminoglycoside. However, resistance is an increasing and complex problem and it is mandatory to direct therapy according to the hospital's known antimicrobial susceptibility patterns and of course the particular isolate in question. Imipenem and aztreonam are alternative therapies that could be used if susceptibility patterns are appropriate. Furthermore, it is permissible to alter antimicrobial therapy from one third generation cephalosporin to another should clinical failure occur, e.g. from ceftazidime to cefotaxime.

In the past, most isolates of *Klebsiella* spp. have been sensitive to first generation cephalosporins such as cefazolin. An aminoglycoside was often added, despite its poor penetration and activity in purulent secretions, though rapid bacterial killing of the circulating organism in bacteraemic patients may have occurred. *Klebsiella* spp. are intrinsically resistant to ampicillin and carbenicillin, and in addition there is an increasing incidence of acquired resistance to many antimicrobials which has been reported in the last decade or so. Recently, increased use of second- and third-generation cephalosporins such as cefuroxime and cefotaxime have been used in managing these infections. However, their widespread use inevitably has led to an increasing frequency of reporting of strains resistant even to these antimicrobials[103]. Ceftazidime resistance is now well documented. Almost one-fifth of all *K. pneumoniae* isolates in a recent nosocomial outbreak in a North American hospital were resistant to the bactericidal activity of *all* cephalosporins and cephamycins – a situation possibly precipitated by the increasing use of ceftazidime for the treatment of multi-resistant acinetobacter infections[104]. The widespread use of this same antibiotic in managing cancer patients has also resulted in a similar outbreak of ceftazidime resistant *K. pneumoniae* infection[105]. Extended spectrum β-lactamases, for example, SHV-2, 4, 5, TEM 3, 6, 10 and 12 which have evolved from earlier plasma derived β-lactamases such as TEM 1/2 and SHV 1[106] have been reported from several countries and have been shown to be responsible for this phenomenon. Aminoglycoside resistance is often co-present. Of considerable concern is the development of virtual total multiresistant *Klebsiella* spp. isolates mediated by an extreme extended spectrum β-lactamase (MRI-1)[107]. Novel extended spectrum β-lactamases produced by *K. pneumoniae* are continually being reported, for example, with resistance to aztreonam[108]. Early detection of bacterial isolates genuinely responsible for pneumonia, early reporting of susceptibilities, meticulous control/selection of appropriate antimicrobial therapy and barrier precautions are important measures which will reduce the spread of resistant organisms.

The limitations of antibiotics in managing some patients with *Klebsiella* spp. infection has lead to the search for alternative treatment modalities. Salicylates are known to suppress capsular polysaccharide synthesis and this results in increased phagocytosis of *Klebsiella* spp. This has been translated to the *in vivo* situation where, in a mouse lethality pneumonia model, it has been shown that salicylate potentiated the antimicrobial activity of amikacin possibly by enhancing phagocytosis rather than antibiotic action[109]. Increased understanding of the pathogenic mechanisms involved in severe *Klebsiella* spp. sepsis may provide the basis for other therapeutic interventions in the future. For example, it has been shown that reduction in plasma antithrombin III levels correlates with bacterial septicaemia. Antithrombin III is necessary to control thrombin and other coagulation factors which are responsible for DIC. In a rat model of *Klebsiella* spp. pneumonia, Gram-negative sepsis, administration of antithrombin III both prophylactically and therapeutically reduces mortality to approximately 50% of the control group[110].

Escherichia coli

E. coli was first isolated from the intestinal tract by Escherisch in 1885 and, in fact, is normally present there. Nevertheless, specific enteropathogenic, enterotoxigenic and enteroinvasive strains are major causes of enteritis among infants and children and in travellers. The organism usually ferments lactose, and may be motile/non-motile. Like all enterobacteriaciae, it possesses O (somatic) antigens (polysaccharide side chains of lipopolysaccharide envelopes responsible for smooth colonies, which are associated with virulence and adhesion), H (flagellar) antigens (motility properties, variably expressed as type I fimbriae) and K (capsular) antigens. K1 is particularly associated with virulence and with bacteraemia, neonatal meningitis and urinary tract infections. Adhesins permit the organisms to successfully colonise the gastrointestinal tract and these and other aspects of virulence/pathogenicity for non-pulmonary *E. coli* infections have been exhaustively studied.

In contrast, in strains producing respiratory disease, although they may originate from the gut, the role of the virulence factors associated with the pathogenesis of pneumonia remain to be elucidated, and may not be the same virulence factors as those described in the production of non-pulmonary disease. For example, K1+ strains are usually associated with pyelonephritis. Both K1+ and K1– strains are present in cases of pneumonia – the clinical outcome appears to be the same irrespective of the strain type. It is known, however, that *E. coli*, like *P. aeruginosa* and other gut Gram-negative bacteria can also attach to upper respiratory epithelial receptors and this can be blocked with mannose which complexes with *E. coli*[111].

E. coli strains responsible for invasive infection outside the gastrointestinal tract possess an iron chelating mechanism (enterobactin) and, in keeping with other enterobacteriaciae, this appears to increase virulence.

E. coli is more commonly associated with hospital-acquired pneumonia due to the much higher frequency of immunocompromisation (both mechanical and systemic) which is found in hospital patients. However, community-acquired pneumonia cases with a background of debilitation and risk factors such as diabetes mellitus, alcohol abuse, chronic obstructive airways disease and other chronic lung disease do occur[112]. Occasional cases occurring in otherwise perfectly normal individuals have been reported[114]. Of the 20% of patients with Gram-negative community-acquired pneumonia admitted to a City county hospital in Atlanta, *E. coli* was the responsible pathogen in approximately one-fifth of these (3.6% of the total)[1]. A similar proportion (23%) of *E. coli* contributed to Gram-negative community-acquired pneumonia in a series by Tillotson[112]. Other studies rate *E. coli* lower than these figures, for example, 1–2% of all community-acquired admissions[92,115]. In patients with nosocomial pneumonia, the frequency of isolation of *E. coli* is slightly higher – of the order of 6%[3,34]. Approximately 28% of nosocomial pneumonias were caused by *E. coli* in Tillotson's series[42,112]. An interesting trend reported from some centres is that there is a decline in the overall incidence of *E. coli* hospital infections over recent years[39].

The lungs of patients who have died from *E. coli* pneumonia usually show a mononuclear and sometimes a haemorrhagic infiltrate in the alveoli, which are usually lined with fibrin and show cuboidal metaplasia and alveolar necrosis. Septal oedema and abscess formation (unusual) may be present. The reason for a predominantly mononuclear cell infiltrate which is quite unlike the mixed mononuclear/polymorphonuclear infiltrate in other Gram-negative pneumonias is unclear. There is usually no involvement of the pulmonary vasculature, unlike *P. aeruginosa* pneumonia. The pathogenesis is presumed to be bacteraemic from foci in the gastrointestinal tract or urinary tract, or occasionally from direct aspiration of colonised pharyngeal contents.

The typical patient with *E. coli* pneumonia is a male of 50 years with a background of chronic illness or haematological malignancy or cancer; urinary infection or diarrhoea may also be present. Respiratory symptoms and signs are not specific for *E. coli* pneumonia. However, undue tachycardia and hypotensive shock may be notable features. Most patients have right lower lobe bronchopneumonia; empyema may be present[112]. Cold agglutinaemia, a finding usually associated with mycoplasma pneumonia has been described for *E. coli* pneumonia and has produced fulminant gangrene[116].

Diagnosis is made on the basis of a positive culture of the organism from urine/blood/pleural fluid/respiratory secretions in an appropriate clinical setting. The mortality rate is of the order of 60%. Antimicrobial treatment of choice is a third-generation cephalosporin, together with an aminoglycoside. A significant number of isolates are resistant to ampicillin and multiresistant strains are described[117]. Many of these are sensitive to third-generation cephalosporins and to ciprofloxacin. Appropriate management of complications such as draining of an empyema, and treatment of the primary source of the sepsis is mandatory to effect cure.

Enterobacter spp.

The pathogenic *enterobacter* spp. comprise *Enterobacter aerogenes*, *Enterobacter cloacae*, *Enterobacter agglomerans*, *Enterobacter gergoviae*, and *Enterobacter sakazakii*, of which *E. cloacae* and *E. aerogenes* are the organisms most frequently implicated in pneumonia[118]. The species are motile, lightly encapsulated thin rods. Differential decarboxylation of some diamino acids serves to distinguish them. In the past, little effort was made to differentiate them from *Klebsiella* spp. and reports on their specific clinical pathological features have been scanty.

Enterobacter spp. can colonise hospitalised patients including those with burns. Hospital personnel can transmit the organism from patient to patient through improper hand care. Community acquired pneumonia and nosocomial pneumonia associated with *Enterobacter* spp. is uncommon/rare – overall, the incidence is less than with *Klebsiella* spp.[3,92,115], and accounts for between 5 and 11% of all Gram-negative pneumonias[118], though some series report unusually high figures, for example, 10% of all community-acquired pneumonias[1]. In cancer patients from the Memorial Sloan Kettering Cancer Center, *Enterobacter* spp. ranked sixth after *E. coli* in frequency[39]. They accounted for 9.4% of all nosocomial pneumonias according to the nosocomial infections surveillance published in 1984[34]. The vast majority of the cases have underlying disease including alcohol abuse, diabetes mellitus, carcinoma, chronic obstructive airways disease and burns. In some cardiac surgery intensive care units, *E. cloacae* was the most common *Enterobacter* pathogen and associated with pneumonia in about 50%[119]. Males in their early 50s predominate. The route of infection is presumed to be from endogenous aspiration though haematogenous spread is well documented.

The clinical features of cough, yellow sputum, fever and dyspnoea are not specific for *Enterobacter* spp. pneumonia. However, patients with *Enterobacter* pneumonia are often said to be less ill than those with other pneumonias – that is with less sputum, absence of haemoptysis and fewer patients have shock. The overall mortality rate at about 15% is generally lower than with other Gram-negative pneumonias. However, the mortality rate can be as high as 45%[118]. Chest radiology shows bronchopneumonic changes sometimes bilateral; dense consolidation is uncommon as is abscess formation and cavitary lesions. Pleural effusions are unlikely to be seen. Nevertheless, *E. cloacae* necrotising pneumonia does occur[120].

Enterobacter spp. are usually resistant to first- and second-generation cephalosporins, but retain sensitivity to third-generation cephalosporins, imipenem, cotrimoxazole, and ciprofloxacin. The antimicrobial regime commonly used is a third-generation cephalosporin together with an aminoglycoside.

Serratia spp.

These are other important pathogens recognised since 1960 and almost entirely confined to hospitalised immunocompromised patients. The most frequent species found are *Serratia marcescens*, *Serratia liquefaciens* and *Serratia rubidaea*. A new species, *Serratia proteamaculans*, has been found to cause fatal community-acquired pneumonia in an alcoholic[121]. Originally, these were believed to be avirulent, and testimony to this was the fact that they were used as tracer organisms to study a population's susceptibility to airborne bacteria. Their unique biochemical feature is an extracellular DNAse. The production of red pigment by a few strains coloured sputum red and this has been mistaken for haemoptysis. Like other Gram-negative bacteria, their affinity for moist environments has led to nosocomial outbreaks associated with bronchoscopes, respiratory treatment equipment including nebulisers, intravascular devices, ECG bulbs, total artificial hearts and sterile water sources[122–125]. *Serratia* spp. can also be found in the soil, water and food. Colonisation of hospital personnel is an important mode of transmission. Colonisation of the gut is uncommon unlike the other enterobacteriaciae but when this does occur this can be a reservoir for important nosocomial outbreaks[126]. Colonisation of the respiratory tract is more likely and can lead to pneumonia. Recently an outbreak of chest infections associated with a common source of a diluent of saline used for nebulisers was described[127]. *Serratia* spp. are thought to be responsible for approximately 7% of all nosocomial pneumonias[34]. In recent years, *Serratia* spp. bacteraemia was found to be associated with pneumonia in 13%–38% of patients[123,128] and the respiratory tract was a common portal of entry[123]. Patients are predominantly middle aged or elderly with cardiopulmonary disease or malignancy, particularly solid tumours or acute leukaemias[123,129]. A history of prior antimicrobial use is common. Chest radiology shows interstitial infiltrates, sometimes with fine nodularity. Cavitation and abscess is distinctly unusual but pleural effusion or empyema may occur. The radiological pattern may mimic that of *Pneumocystis carinii* pneumonia[99]. The mortality rate is in excess of 50%; prognostic factors include persistent bacteraemia, use of inappropriate antibiotics, e.g. an aminoglycoside alone and shock[123]. The organism is usually antibiotic multiply resistant, particularly to aminoglycosides (least of all to amikacin), cephalosporins such as cefoxitin and cefotaxime. It is usually susceptible to imipenem, later generation cephalosporins, aztreonam, and cotrimoxazole. Combination of an extended penicillin such as ticarcillin with amikacin may prove synergistic. Other combinations in difficult to treat situations include polymyxin + rifampicin or cotrimoxazole + polymyxin.

Proteae

This tribe comprises three genera, namely, *Proteus*, *Morganella* and *Providencia*, biochemically characterised by a positive methyl red reaction, negative VP reaction, and indole positivity, apart from *Proteus mirabilis*. *Proteus* spp. swarm on agar media since they possess unduly high numbers of flagellae. *Proteus* spp. contribute between 2% and 4% of all hospital-acquired pneumonias, mainly, *P. mirabilis* – they are the least commonly found among pneumonias due to Gram-negative bacteria[1,3] and exceedingly rare in community-acquired pneumonia[92,115]. Patients usually have a background of chronic pulmonary disease and may be alcoholic; a background of haematological malignancy may also be present. Cough, thick purulent sputum and dyspnoea are the major findings. The mortality rate is of the order of 20%.

As with *K. pneumonia*, right upper lobe infiltrates are common and abscess formation cavities or larger pneumatoceles are common features[99,130,131]. Ipsilateral tracheal shift and loss of lung volume are not unusual features.

P. mirabilis is generally susceptible to most antimicrobials. Other species – the indole positive species – have a high degree of aminoglycoside resistance. A third-generation cephalosporin with amikacin is a commonly used antimicrobial regime.

Exceptionally uncommon are pneumonias caused by *Providentia* spp.[132]. During a 5-year prospective study of bacteraemia in a long-care hospital facility, in which many patients had chronic underlying conditions such as cerebral vascular disease, chronic obstructive airways disease, malignancy and immunosuppression, although there was a 13% incidence of *Providentia stuartii* bacteraemia, only one patient had pneumonia due to this organism from among 207 blood isolates from 144 patients[133]. The organism is usually resistant to second-generation cephalosporins, ampicillin, and cotrimoxazole but usually sensitive to cefoxitin, extended penicillins, and amikacins but less so to gentamicin.

Salmonella spp.

It is perhaps not surprising that multiorgan disease typical of invasive *Salmonella* spp., can include pleuro-pulmonary disease. In an evaluation of 7779 cases at the New York Salmonella Center, due to virulent but not typhoidal *Salmonella* spp., such as *Salmonella paratyphi* and *Salmonella cholerasuis*, 85 (1%) had lobar/bronchopneumonia[134]. In a review of 585 South African children with typhoid fever, 21% had abnormal chest auscultatory findings and 57% had abnormal chest radiography[135]. Other series report an 11% incidence of pneumonia[136]. The true incidence is possibly underestimated since gastrointestinal symptoms may be absent and *Salmonella* spp. are not looked for routinely in respiratory secretions or tissues. Many patients with microbiologically proven salmonella pleuro-pulmonary infection have a major underlying disease such as malignancy, chronic renal failure, diabetes mellitus, chronic lung disease, and the patients are characteristically male, aged over 60 years[134,137,138].

Clinical presentation and the chest radiology is not specific for *Salmonella* spp. Sputum is not always positive, and blood, lung tissue or pleural fluid are the usual sources of the bacteria. The peripheral white cell count is characteristically normal or low. Mortality tends to be high, of the order of 60%[137]. Complications include lung abscess and empyema[134,137,139–141]. The route of spread is not understood, but gastric aspiration, extension from a nearby focus, and haematogenous spread from a dormant focus in the reticulo-endothelial system have been suggested. Patients with underlying T-cell defects are particularly vulnerable to disseminated salmonellosis, which includes pneumonia. The increasing incidence of resistant *Salmonella* spp. is now widespread. Although ampicillin, cotrimoxazole and chloramphenicol were the antibiotics of choice in the past, oral or intravenous ciprofloxacin is now considered the first line drug particularly in patients coming from known areas of resistance.

Citrobacter spp.

Citrobacter spp., previously classified with the *Salmonellae*[142] occasionally produce pneumonia usually in patients with cancer. In a 16-year review of *Citrobacter* spp. bacteraemia in cancer patients, 38% of patients had pneumonia and this carried a poor prognosis[143].

Other miscellaneous Gram-negative organisms

Acinetobacter spp.

These are actually Gram-negative encapsulated cocco-bacilli normally found in the soil and water and are usually commensal in the throat, skin and gastrointestinal tract in up to 25% persons. They may be confused with *Gonococcus* spp., *Meningococcus* spp. and *H. influenzae*. They have been well established as a cause of nosocomial pneumonia in the prolonged ventilated patient, often on an ICU, who characteristically has received prior broad spectrum antibiotic therapy and has a previous history of chronic obstructive pulmonary disease[144,145]. Underlying malignancy and immunosuppressive treatment may be additional factors. In a hospital setting, as for *Pseudomonas* spp., ventilator circuits, patient's secretions and the hands of personnel are sources leading to nosocomial infection[146]. Using protective specimen brush catheters, transtracheal aspiration, and fluid aspiration, *Acinetobacter* spp. were found to be as common as *P. aeruginosa* in one series of such patients, giving an incidence of 6/14 patients with nosocomial pneumonia[145]. Radiologically, multilobar bronchopneumonic infiltrates are found in over a half of patients; abscess formation/pleural effusion occurs in approximately a quarter. The organism may well be resistant to a number of antibiotics including ceftazidime, gentamicin and cefotaxime[147]. Mortality is of the order of 36%, a figure that has not changed over at least a decade[144,145].

Community-acquired *Acinetobacter* pneumonia has also been described but this appears to be much less common than nosocomial pneumonia. In this setting, alcoholism, smoking, and chronic debilitation seem to be common accompanying features. This may have a rapidly fatal course possibly due to the too frequent use of inappropriate antibiotic therapy since the organism may be resistant to several antibiotics. However, the antibiotic of choice is an aminoglycoside – tobramycin or amikacin should be used initially until gentamicin resistance is ruled out, together with a β-lactam. Imipenem and piperacillin are also usually active.

Brucella spp.

This bacterium, as with *Salmonella* spp., can produce multisystem disease, often mimicking other pathological processes. Lobar or bronchopneumonic pulmonary changes, hilar/mediastinal lymphadenopathy and pleural effusions have all been described[148]. The diagnosis should be thought of in patients living in an endemic area such as the Middle East or who have close contact with an animal or laboratory source. Laboratory diagnosis is based upon a standard agglutination test in which a titre of well in excess of 1/320 is diagnostic (see Chapter 26).

Aeromonas spp.

Aeromonas spp. are usually found in the soil, fresh and salt water. They cause disease in sea creatures. In the hospital setting, they can contaminate water and medicinal supplies[149]. Medicinal leeches and contaminated soil or aquatic trauma have been the source of severe soft tissue infections. They can also cause gastroenteritis and bacteraemia. Pneumonia caused by *Aeromonas hydrophila* is rare, usually occurring in the immunocompromised host, or in patients with chronic disease such as those with alcohol abuse, chronic liver disease, chronic obstructive airways disease, congestive cardiac failure and in patients with a tendency to aspiration pneumonia, e.g. those with cerebral vascular disease or patients who have been immersed in water[150]. Occasionally, *A. hydrophila* pneumonia occurs in previously healthy individuals, e.g. after swimming in sea water[151]. Thus exposure to contaminated water, such as may occur in patients experiencing near drowning is often documented. Onset is sudden, and the course often fulminant. Radiographical changes of bilateral pulmonary infiltrates, lobar consolidation and cavitation occur. ARDS may be present in patients with near drowning. Survival is of the order of 50%. Resistance to penicillin, ampicillin, first- and second-generation cephalosporins is common. Most isolates are sensitive to aminoglycosides, to third-generation cephalosporins, imipenem and aztreonam.

Eikenella spp.

Eikenella corrodens is a fastidious, facultative anaerobic Gram-negative bacillus, normally present throughout the gastrointestinal and upper respiratory tracts. In patients with underlying immunodeficiency, most commonly pulmonary malignancy or patients with chronic lung disease, alcoholism and an aspiration tendency, the organism assumes pathogenicity. The fact that the organism may fail to grow on routine culture suggests that some cases in the past may have been missed. Cutaneous infections from human bites, head and neck and respiratory tract infections are the commonest manifestations. Situations which predispose to aspiration such as epilepsy, alcoholism or oesophageal cancer are often associated with pleuro-pulmonary infections. Empyema is a particularly common complication; cavitation and abscess formation also occur[152]. There is an association with other microorganisms, particularly *Streptococcal* spp. which includes *Streptococcus viridans* and *Streptococcus anginosis*[152–154]. Provided appropriate antibiotic treatment is given, recovery is usual. The organism is normally resistant to clindamycin, metronidazole and to penicillin but sensitive to ampicillin and susceptible to first-, second- and third-generation cephalosporins, antipseudomonal penicillins, quinolones and aminoglycosides. Hence, it should be considered as the aetiological agent in a high risk patient with a clinically suspected staphylococcal or Gram-negative pneumonia, particularly if it is complicated by abscess, cavity or pleural effusion and who fails to respond to initial antibiotic treatment.

Flavobacterium spp.

These Gram-negative rods are found in salt and fresh water and the soil but they do not usually contribute to the normal human microflora. Some of them have been reclassified into the *Weeksella* genus. The can contaminate water and disinfectants and thrive in humidifiers and ventilatory circuits. In the past, *Flavobacterium* spp. like many other less common Gram-negative rods have been dismissed as non-pathogenic. They are nevertheless highly pathogenic in vulnerable hosts and they have been most often implicated in neonatal and infant meningitis, soft tissue infections, endocarditis and less commonly in nosocomial pneumonia in the immunocompromised host particularly those with underlying reticulo-endothelial or haematological or solid tumour malignancies[155–157]. Rare cases have been described from the community[158]. The organisms are usually multiply resistant to most antimicrobials that would be prescribed for the initial treatment of Gram-negative pneumonia. These include aminoglycosides, third-generation cephalosporins and imipenem. They are usually sensitive to ciprofloxacin, rifampicin, and clindamycin. Hence, sensitivity testing is mandatory.

Campylobacter spp.

Campylobacter spp. (now called *Helicobacter* spp.) are comma-shaped Gram-negative rods, occasionally producing extragastrointestinal disease in the case of *C. jejuni* (*Helicobacter pylori*). Bacteraemia is highly unusual for these species but it does occur occasionally in the immunocompromised host. *Campylobacter fetus*, on the other hand produces a systemic bacteraemic illness usually in the immunocompromised host and lung abscess has been described[159]. *Campylobacter sputorum* is also a causative agent of lung abscess. The management of pneumonia and pleuro-pulmonary problems caused by these organisms include parenteral antibiotics (usually erythromycin, ampicillin or imipenem) and appropriate surgical management such as drainage of the abscess.

Miscellaneous organisms – The remainder
Of the remaining organisms, only a few have been found in respiratory secretions. In the majority of these, clinical significance remains difficult to establish. All the literature relating to pulmonary infection consists of isolated case reports. Among these organisms include *Citrobacter* spp. from the *enterobacteriaciae* previously classified with *Salmonella* spp.[142]; *Citrobacter erwiniae*[160]; *Citrobacter hafnia*[161]; *Citrobacter ewingella*[162], *Actinobacillus* spp. and *Actinomycetemcomitans* spp. The latter is a cocco-bacillus slowly growing – 25 days – and usually associated with oro-dental bacteraemia or endocarditis, and having the propensity to penetrate tissue barriers such as the chest wall. It has a narrow spectrum of antimicrobial susceptibility including rifampicin, chloramphenicol and cephalosporins. Prolonged treatment is often necessary[163]. *Chromobacterium violaceum*, CDC group DF2, probably including some *Flavobacterium* spp., and *Achromobacter* spp. are further organisms whose role in respiratory colonisation and infection requires to be clarified. A previously unrecognised bacterium has recently been identified – *Balneatrix alpica* – and caused an outbreak of pneumonia and meningitis in a spa centre[164].

References

1. SULLIVAN RJ JR, DOWDLE WR, MARINE WM, HIERBOLZER JC Adult pneumonia in a general hospital: aetiology and host risk factors. *Arch Int Med* 1972;129:935–42.
2. PIERCE AK, SANFORD JP. Aerobic gram-negative bacillary pneumonia. *Am Rev Resp Dis* 1974;110:647–58.
3. KAYSER FSH. Changes in the spectrum of organism causing respiratory tract infections: a review. *Postgrad Med J* 1992;68(Suppl 3): S17–23.
4. LAFORCE FM. Hospital-acquired gram-negative rod pneumonias: an overview. *Am J Med* 1981;70:669–4.
5. SCHELD WM, MANDELL GL. Nosocomial pneumonia: pathogenesis and recent advances in diagnosis and therapy. *Rev Infect Dis* 1991;13(Suppl 9):S743–51.
6. MORRISON AJ JR, WENZEL RP. Epidemiology of infections due to *Pseudomonas aeruginosa*. *Rev Infect Dis* 1984;6(Suppl):S627–S42.
7. ROSENTHAL S, TAGER IB. Prevalence of Gram-negative rods in the normal pharyngeal flora. *Ann Intern Med* 1975;83:355–7.
7. WOODS DE, STRAUSS DC, JOHANSON WG, BERRY VK, BASS JA. Role of pili in adherence of *Pseudomonas aeruginosa* to mammalian buccal epithelial cells. *Infect Immun* 1980;29:1146–51.
8. RAMPHAL R, PYLE M. Adherence of mucoid and non-mucoid *Pseudomonas aeruginosa* to acid-injured tracheal epithelium. *Infect Immun* 1983;41:345–51.
9. MORIHARA K. Production of elastase and proteinase by *Pseudomonas aeruginosa*. *J Bacteriol* 1964;88:745–50.
10. SCHIMPFF SC, YOUNG VM, GREENE WH, VERMEULEN GD, MOODY MR, WIERNIK PH. Origin of infection in acute non-lymphocytic leukemia: significance of hospital acquisition of potential pathogens. *Ann Intern Med* 1972;77:707–14.
11. SCHWARTZ SN, DOWLING JN, BENKOVIC C, DEQUITTNER-BUCHANAN M, PROSTKO T, YEE RB. Sources of Gram-negative bacilli colonising the trachea of intubated patients. *J Infect Dis* 1978;138:227–31.
12. SOTTILE FD, MARRIE TJ, PROUGH DS *et al.* Nosocomial pulmonary infection: possible etiologic significance of bacterial adhesion to endotracheal tubes. *Crit Care Med* 1986;14:265–70.
13. POLLACK M, YOUNG LS. Protective activity of antibodies to exotoxin A and lipopolysaccharide at the onset of *Pseudomonas aeruginosa* septicaemia in man. *J Clin Invest* 1979;63:276–86.
14. MARKHAM RB, PIER GB, SCHREIBER JR. The role of cytophilic IgG3 antibody in T cell-mediated resistance to infection with the extracellular bacterium, *Pseudomonas aeruginosa*. *J Immunol* 1991;146:316–20.
15. BISBE J, GATELL JM, PUIG J, MARTINEZ JA, DE ANTA JIMENEZ M, SORIANO E. *Pseudomonas aeruginosa* bacteraemia: univariate and multivariate analyses of factors influencing the prognosis in 133 episodes. *Rev Infect Dis* 1988;10:629:35.
16. HIGUCHI JH, JOHANSON WG. The relationship between adherence of *Pseudomonas aeruginosa* to upper respiratory cells *in vitro* and susceptibility to colonization *in vivo*. *J Lab Clin Med* 1980;95:698–705.
17. BERG RD. Bacterial translocation from the gastrointestinal tract. *Trends Microbiol* 1995; 3:149–54.
18. DIETCH EA, WINTERTON J, BERG R. The gut as a portal of entry for bacteraemia – role of protein malnutrition. *Ann Surg* 1987;205: 681–92.
19. SKERRETT SJ, NIEDERMAN FS, FEIN AM. Respiratory infections and acute lung injury in systemic illness. *Clin Chest Med* 1989;10:469–502.
20. LO CW, WALKER NA. Changes in the gastrointestinal tract during enteral or parenteral feeding. *Nutrit Rev* 1989;47: 193–8.
21. PINGLETON SK, HINTHOR ND, LUI C. Enteral nutrition in patients receiving mechanical ventilation. *Am J Med* 1986;80:827–32.
22. HAMILTON JR, OVERALL JC JR. Synergistic infection with murine cytomegalovirus and *Pseudomonas aeruginosa* in mice. *J Infect Dis* 1978;137:775–82.
23. NIEDERMAN MS, MANTOVANI R, SCHOCH P, PAPAS J, FEIN AM. Patterns and routes of tracheobronchial colonization in mechanically ventilated patients. The role of nutritional status in colonization of the lower airway by *Pseudomonas* species. *Chest* 1989; 95:155–61.
24. INGLIS TJJ, SHERRATT MJS, SPROAT LJ, GIBSON JS, HAWKEY PM. Gastroduodenal dysfunction and bacterial colonization of the ventilated lung. *Lancet* 1993;341:911–3.
25. LACEY S, WANT SV. *Pseudomonas pickettii* infections in a paediatric oncology unit. *J Hosp Infect* 1991;17:45–51.
26. TREDGET EE, SHANKOWSKY HA, JOFFE AM *et al.* Epidemiology of infections with *Pseudomonas aeruginosa* in burn patients: the role of hydrotherapy. *Clin Infect Dis* 1992;15:941–9.
27. WIDMER AF, WENZEL RP, TRILLA A, BALE MJ, JONES RN, DOEBBELING BN. Outbreak of *Pseudomonas aeruginosa* infections in a surgical intensive care unit: probable transmission via hands of a health care worker. *Clin Infect Dis* 1993;16:372–6.
28. MARRIE TJ, DURANT H, YATES L. Community-acquired pneumonia requiring hospitalization: 5-year prospective study. *Rev Infect Dis* 1989;11:586–99.
29. GARB JL, BROWN RB, GARB JR, TUTHILL RW. Differences in aetiology of pneumonias in nursing home and community patients. *J Am Med Assoc* 1978;240:2169–72.
30. BROWN RB. Community-acquired pneumonia: diagnosis and therapy of older adults. *Geriatrics* 1993;48:43–50.
31. FILE TM JR, TAN JS. Community-acquired

pneumonia – the changing picture. *Postgrad Med* 1992;92:197–214.

31. QUIRK JA, BEAMAN MH, BLAKE M. Community-acquired *Pseudomonas* pneumonia in a normal host complicated by metastatic panophthalmitis and cutaneous pustules. *Aust NZ J Med* 1990;20:254–6.

32. HOOGWERF BJ, KHAN MY. Community-acquired bacteraemic *Pseudomonas* pneumonia in a healthy adult. *Am Rev Resp Dis* 1981;123:132–4.

33. PENNINGTON JE, REYNOLDS HY, CARBONE PP. *Pseudomonas* pneumonia; a retrospective study of 36 cases. *Am J Med* 1973;55:155–60.

34. HORANT C, WHIE JW, JARVIS WR, EMORI TG. Nosocomial infection surveillance 1984. *MMWR CDC Surveillance Summaries* 1986;35:17SS–29SS.

35. FAGON J-Y, CHASTRE J, HANCE AJ, MONTRAVERS P, NOVARA A, GIBERT C. Nosocomial pneumonia in ventilated patients: a cohort study evaluating attributable mortality and hospital stay. *Am J Med* 1993;94:281–8.

36. SILVER DR, COHEN IL, WEINBERG PF. Recurrent *Pseudomonas aeruginosa* pneumonia in an intensive care unit. *Chest* 1992;101:194–8.

37. VALDIVIESO M, GIL-EXTREMERA B, ZORNOZA J, RODRIGUEZ V, BODEY GP. Gram negative bacillary pneumonia in the compromised host. *Medicine* 1977;56:241–54.

39. KOLL BS, BROWN AE. The changing epidemiology of infections at cancer hospitals. *Clin Infect Dis* 1993;17(Suppl 2):S322–8.

40. WHIMBEY E, KIEHN TE, BRANNON P, BLEVINS A, ARMSTRONG D. Bacteremia and fungemia in patients with neoplastic disease. *Am J Med* 1987;82:723–30.

41. EHNI WF, RELLER LB, ELLISON III RT. Bacteremia in granulocytopenic patients in a tertiary-care general hospital. *Rev Infect Dis* 1991;13:613–19.

42. TILLOTSON JR, LERNER AM. Characteristics of non-bacteraemic *Pseudomonas* pneumonia. *Ann Intern Med* 1986;68:287–294.

43. FORKNER CE, FREI E, EDGCOMB JH. *Pseudomonas* septicemia. *Am J Med* 1958;25:877–89.

44. FETZER AE, WERNER AS, HAGSTROM JWC. Pathologic features of pseudomonal pneumonia. *Am Rev Resp Dis* 1967;12:757–9.

45. LUBITZ RM. Resolution of lung abscess due to *Pseudomonas aeruginosa* with oral ciprofloxacin: case report. *Rev Infect Dis* 1990;12:757–9.

46. VANDENPLAS O, MERCENIER C, TRIGAUX J-P, DALAUNOIS L. Pancoast's syndrome due to *Pseudomonas aeruginosa* infection of the lung apex. *Thorax* 1991;46:683–4.

47. STRIETER RM, LYNCH III JP, BASHA MA, STANDIFORD TJ, KASAHARA K, KUNKEL SL. Host responses in mediating sepsis and adult respiratory distress syndrome. *Sem Resp Infect* 1990;5(3):233–47.

48. NICHOLS L, BALOGH K, SILVERMAN M. Bacterial infections in the acquired immune deficiency syndrome. Clinicopathologic correlations in series of autopsy cases. *Am J Clin Pathol* 1989;92:787–90.

49. RONSTON KV, URIBE-BOTERO G, MANSELL WA. Bacterial infections in adult patients with the acquired immunodeficiency syndrome (AIDS) and AIDS-related complex. *Am J Med* 1987;83:604–5.

50. FLORES G, STAVOLA JJ, NOEL GJ. Bacteremia due to *Pseudomonas aeruginosa* in children with AIDS. *Clin Infect Dis* 1993;16:706–8.

51. ELLIS M, GUPTA S, GALANT S *et al.* Impaired neutrophil functions in patients with AIDS or AIDS-related complex: a comprehensive review. *J Infect Dis* 1988;158:1268–76.

52. KRUMHOLZ HM, SANDE MA, LO B. Community acquired bacteraemia in patients with acquired immunodeficiency syndrome: clinical presentation, bacteriology and outcome. *Am J Med* 1989;86:776–9.

53. FRANZETTI F, CERNUSCHI M, ESPOSITO R, MORONI M. Pseudomonas infections in patients with AIDS and AIDS-related complex. *J Intern Med* 1992;231:1692–8.

54. EORTC INTERNATIONAL ANTIMICROBIAL THERAPY COOPERATIVE GROUP. Ceftazidime combined with a short or long course of amikacin for empirical therapy of Gram-negative bacteraemia in cancer patients with granulocytopenia. *New Engl J Med* 1987;317:1692–98.

55. HILF M, YU VL, SHARP J, ZURAVIEFF JJ, KORVICK JA, MUDER RR. Antibiotic therapy for *Pseudomonas aeruginosa* bacteraemia: outcome correlations in a prospective study of 200 patients. *Am J Med* 1989;87:540–6.

56. YOUNG LS. Treatment of respiratory infections in the patient at risk. *Am J Med* 1984;77 (Suppl):S61–S68.

57. LOVE LJ, SCHIMPFF SC, SCHRIFFER CA, WIERNIR PH. Improved prognosis for granulocytopenic patients with Gram-negative bacteraemia. *Am J Med* 1980;68:643–8.

58. KLASTERSKY J, CARPENTIER-MEUNIER F, KAHAN-COPPENS L, THYS JP. Endotracheally administered antibiotics for Gram-negative bronchopneumonia. *Chest* 1979;75:586–91.

59. BROWN RB, KRUSE JA, COUNTS GW, RUSSEL JA, CHRISTAU NV, SANDS ML. Double-blind study of endotracheal tobramycin in the treatment of Gram-negative bacterial pneumonia. *Antimicrob Agents Chemother* 1990;34:269–72.

60. BODEY GP. Empirical antibiotic therapy for fever in neutropenic patients. *Clin Infect Dis* 1993;17(Suppl 2):S378–S384.

61. PIZZO PA, HATHORN JW, HIEMENZ J *et al.* A randomized trial comparing ceftazidime alone with combination antibiotic therapy in cancer patients with fever and neutropaenia. *N Engl J Med* 1986;315:552–8.

62. KORVICK JA, PEACOCK JE JR, MUDER RR, WHEELER RR, YU VL. Addition of rifampicin to combination antibiotic therapy for *Pseudomonas aeruginosa* bacteraemia: prospective trial using the zelen protocol. *Antimicrob Agents Chemother* 1992;36:620–5.

63. AUBERT G, POZZETTO B, DORCHE G. Emergence of quinolone-imipenem cross-resistance in *Pseudomonas aeruginosa* after fluoroquinolone therapy. *J Antimicrob Chemother* 1992;29:307:12.

64. MILLICAN RC, RUST J, ROTHENTAL SM. Gammaglobulin factors protective against infections from *Pseudomonas* and other organisms. *Science* 1957;126:509:11.

65. PENNINGTON JE. Efficacy of lipopolysaccharide *Pseudomonas* vaccine for pulmonary infection. *J Infect Dis* 1979;140:73–80.

66. PITTET JF, MATTHAY MA, PIER G, GRADY M, WIENER-KRONISH JP. *Pseudomonas aeruginosa*-induced lung and pleural injury in sheep. Differential protective effect of circulating versus alveolar immunoglobulin G antibody. *J Clin Invest* 1993;92:1221–8.

67. POLLACK M, HUANG AI, PRESCOTT RK, YOUNG LS, HUNTER KW, CRUESS DF, TSAI CM. Enhanced survival in *Pseudomonas aeruginosa* septicemia associated with high levels of circulating antibody to *Escherichia coli* endotoxin core. *J Clin Invest* 1983;72:1874–81.

68. PIER GB. Structural analysis and immunogenicity of *Pseudomonas aeruginosa* immunotype 2 high-molecular weight polysaccharide. *J Clin Invest* 1986;77:491–5.

69. HECTOR RF, COLLINS MS, PENNINGTON JE. Treatment of experimental *Pseudomonas aeruginosa* pneumonia with a human IgM monoclonal antibody. *J Infect Dis* 1989;160:483–9.

70. O'OKA H, CHONAN E, MIZUTANI K *et al.* Establishment of stable cell lines producing anti-*Pseudomonas aeruginosa* monoclonal antibodies and their protective effects for the infection in mice. *Microbiol Immunol* 1992;36:1305–16.

71. OISHI K, SONODA F, IWAGAKI A *et al.* Therapeutic effects of a human antiflagella

monoclonal antibody in a neutropenic murine model of *Pseudomonas aeruginosa* pneumonia. *Antimicrob Agents Chemother* 1993;37:164–70.

72. CRAWFORD J, OZER H, STOLLER R *et al.* Reduction by granulocyte colony-stimulating factor of fever and neutropaenia induced by chemotherapy in patients with small-cell lung cancer. *New Engl J Med* 1991;325:164–70.

73. OHNO R, TOMONAGA M, KOBAYASHI T *et al.* Effect of granulocyte colony-stimulating factor after intensive induction therapy in relapsed or refractory acute leukemia. *New Engl J Med* 1990;3223:871–7.

74. ELTING LS, BODY GP. Septicemia due to *Xanthomonas* species and non-*aeruginosa Pseudomonas* species: increasing incidence of catheter-related infections. *Medicine* 1990;69:296–3076.

75. KHARDORI N, ELTING L, WONG E, SCHABLE B, BODEY GP Nosocomial infections due to *Xanthomonas maltophilia* (*Pseudomonas maltophilia*) in patients with cancer. *Rev Infect Dis* 1990;12:997–1002.

76. AOUN M, VAN DER AUWERA P, DEVLEESHOUWER C *et al.* Bacteraemia caused by non-*aeruginosa Pseudomonas* species in a cancer centre. *J Hosp Infect* 1992;22:307–16.

77. HOLMES B, LAPAGE SP, EASTERLING BG. Distribution in clinical material gram-negative bacilli of nosocomial interest. *Am J Med* 1979;48:735–49.

79. KERR KG, CORPS CM, HAWKEY PM. Infections due to *Xanthomonas maltophilia* in patients with hematologic malignancy. *Rev Infect Dis* 1991;13:762.

80. POE RH, MARCUS HR, EMERSON GL. Lung abscess due to *Pseudomonas cepacia*. *Am Rev Resp Dis* 1977;115:861–5.

81. O'NEIL KM, HERMAN JH, MODLIN JF *Pseudomonas cepacia*: an emerging pathogen in chronic granulomatous disease. *J Pediat* 1986;108:940–2.

82. KAUFFMAN CA, BAGNASCO FA. Community-acquired bacteraemic *Pseudomonas cepacia* pneumonia in an immunocompetent host. *Clin Infect Dis* 1992;15:887–8.

83. PEGUES DA, CARSON LA, ANDERSON RL *et al.* Outbreak of *Pseudomonas cepacia* bacteraemia in oncology patients. *Clin Infect Dis* 1993;16:407–11.

84. HOLMES B. The identification of *Pseudomonas cepacia* and its occurrence in clinical material. *J Appl Bacteriol* 1986;61:299–314.

85. TAYLOR RFH, GAYA H, HODSON ME. *Pseudomonas cepacia*: pulmonary infection in patients with cystic fibrosis. *Resp Med* 1993;87:187–92.

86. HOWE C, MILLER WR. Human glanders: report of six cases. *Ann Intern Med* 1947;26:93–8.

87. CARRATALA J, SALAZAR A, MASCARO J, SANTIN M. Community-acquired pneumonia due to *Pseudomonas stutzeri*. *Clin Infect Dis* 1992;14:792.

88. COVER TL, APPELBAUM PC, ABER RC. *Pseudomonas paucimobilis* empyema after cardial transplantation. *South Med J* 1988;81:796–8.

89. TROTTER JA, KUHLS TL, PICKETTE DA, DE LA ROCHA SR, WELCH DF. Pneumonia caused by a newly recognized pseudomonad in a child with chronic granulomatous disease. *J Clin Microbiol* 1990;28:1120–4.

90. MACFARLANE JT, FINCH RG, WARD MJ, MACRAE AD. Hospital study of adult community-acquired pneumonia. *Lancet* 1982;2:255–8.

91. VERGHESE A, BERK SL. Bacterial pneumonia in the elderly. *Medicine* 1983;62:271–85.

92. KARALUS NC, CURSONS RT, LENG RA *et al.* Community acquired pneumonia: aaetiology and prognostic index evaluation. *Thorax* 1991;46:413–18.

93. CARPENTER JL. *Klebsiella* pulmonary infections: occurrence at one Medical Center and review. *Rev Infect Dis* 1990;12:672–82.

95. BODEY GP, ELTING LS, RODRIGUEZ S, HERNANDEZ M. *Klebsiella* bacteraemia. A 10-year review in a cancer institution. *Cancer* 1989;64:2368–76.

96. GORMAN LJ, SANAI L, NOTMAN AW, GRANT IS, MASTERON RG. Cross infection in an intensive care unit by *Klebsiella pneumoniae* from ventilator condensate. *J Hosp Infect* 1990;23:27:34.

97. VAN KREGTEN E, HUBER-BRUNING O, VANDENBROUCKE JP, WILLERS JMN. No conclusive evidence of an epidemiological relation between *Klebsiella* and ankylosing spondylitis. *J Rheumatol* 1991;18:384–8.

98. KORVICK JA, HACKETTE AK, YU VL, MUDER RR. *Klebsiella* pneumonia in the modern era: clinicoradiographic correlations. *South Med J* 1991;84:200–4.

99. ZORNOSA J, GOLDMAN AM, WALLACE S, VALDIVIESO M, BODEY PG. Radiologic features of gram-negative pneumonias in the neutropenic patient. *Am J Roentgenol* 1976;127:989–96.

100. SASTRY CF, SCRIMGEOUS EM. Pneumopyopericardium in a Zimbabwean man with *Klebsiella* pneumonia. *Resp Med* 1991;85:427–9.

101. LIMSON BM, ROMANSKY MJ, SHEA JG. An evaluation of twenty-two patients with acute and chronic pulmonary infection with Friedlander's bacillus. *Ann Intern Med* 1956;44:1070–81.

102. DOMENICO P, JOHANSON WG JR, STRAUSS DC. Lobar pneumonia in rats produced by clinical isolates of *Klebsiella pneumoniae*. *Infect Immun* 1982;37:327–35.

103. KNOTHE H, SHAH P, KREMERY V, ANATAL M, MITSUHASHI S. Transferable resistance to cefotaxime, cefoxitin, cefamandole and cefuroxime in clinical isolates of *Klebsiella* pneumoniae and *Serratia marcescens*. *Infection* 1983;11:315–17.

104. MEYER KS, URBAN C, EAGAN JA, BERGER BJ, RAHAL JJ. Nosocomial outbreak of *Klebsiella* infection resistant to late-generation cephalosporins. *Ann Intern Med* 1993;119:353–8.

105. NAUMOVSKI L, QUINN JP, MIYASHIRO D *et al.* Outbreak of ceftazidime resistance due to a novel extended spectrum beta-lactamase in isolates from cancer patients. *Antimicrob Agents Chemother* 1992;36:1991–6.

106. LIU PY, GUR D, HALL LM, LIVERMMORE DM. Survey of the prevalence of beta-lactamases amongst 1000 gram-negative bacilli isolated consecutively at the Royal London Hospital. *J Antimicrob Chemother* 1992;30:429–47.

107. PAPANICOLAOU GA, MEDEIROS AA, JACOBY GA. Novel plasmid-mediated beta-lactamase (MIR-1) conferring resistance to oxyimino- and alpha-methoxy beta-lactams in clinical isolates of *Klebsiella* pneumoniae. *Antimicrob Agents Chemother* 1990;34:2200–9.

108. ARLET G, ROUVEAU M, FOURNIER G, LAGRANGE PH, PHILIPPON A. Novel, Plasmid-encoded, TEM-derived extended-spectrum β-lactamase in *Klebsiella* pneumoniae conferring higher resistance to aztreonam than to extended-spectrum cephalosporins. *Antimicrob Agents Chemother* 1993;37:2020–3.

109. DOMENICO P, STRAUS DC, WOODS DE, CUNHA BA. Salicylate pontentiates amikacin therapy in rodent models of *Klebsiella pneumoniae* infection. *J Infect Dis* 1993;168:766–9.

110. DICKNEITE G, PÂQUES E-P. Reduction of mortality with antithrombin III in septicemic rats: a study of *Klebsiella pneumoniae* induced sepsis. *Thrombo Haemo* 1993;69:98–102.

111. OFEK I, MIRELMAN D, SHARON N. Adherence of *Escherichia* coli to human mucosal cells mediated by mannose receptors. *Nature* 1977;263:623–5.

112. TILLOTSON JR, LERNER AM. Characteristics of pneumonia caused by *Escherichia coli*. *N Engl J Med* 1967;277:115–22.

114. BLIGH J, EMMANUEL FX, JONES ME *Escherichia coli* lobar pneumonia [letter]. *J Infect* 1990;21:321–2.

115. THE BRITISH THORACIC SOCIETY RESEARCH COMMITTEE AND THE PUBLIC HEALTH LABORATORY SERVICE. The aetiology, management and outcome of severe

community-acquired pneumonia on the intensive care unit. *Resp Med* 1992;86:7–13.

116. POLDRE P, PRUZANSKI W, CHIU HM, DOTTEN DA. Fulminant gangrene in transient cold agglutinemia associated with *Escherichia coli* infection. *Can Med Assoc J* 1985;132:261–3.

117. PHILLIPS I, EYKYN S, KING A *et al.* Epidemic multiresistant *Escherichia coli* infection in West Lambeth health district. *The Lancet* 1988;1:1038–41.

118. KARNAD A, ALVAREZ S, BERK SL. *Enterobacter* Pneumonia. *South Med J* 1987;80:601–4.

119. FLYNN DM, WEINSTEIN RA, KABINS SA. Infections with gram-negative bacilli in a cardiac surgery intensive care unit: the relative role of *Enterobacter. J Hosp Infect* 1988;11(suppl. A): 367–73.

120. BROUGHTON WA, KIRKPATRICK ME. Acute necrotizing pneumonia caused by *Enterobacter cloacae. South Med J* 1988;81:1061–2.

121. BOLLET C, GRIMONT P, GAINNIER M, GEISSLER A, SAINTY J-M., DE MICCO P. Fatal pneumonia due to *Serratia proteamaculans* subsp. quinovora. *J Clin Microbiol* 1993;31:444–5.

122. RINGROSE RE, MCKOWN B, FELTON FG, BARCLAY BO. A hospital outbreak of *Serratia marcescens* associated with ultrasonic nebulizers. *Ann Intern Med* 1968;69:719–29.

123. SAITO H, ELTING L, BODEY GP, BERKEY P. *Serratia* bacteraemia: review of 118 cases. *Rev Infect Dis* 1989;2:912–20.

124. GRIFFITH BP, KORMOS RL, HARDESTY RL, ARMITAGE JM, DUMMER JS. The artificial heart: infection-related morbidity and its effect on transplantation. *Ann Thorac Surg* 1988;45:409–13.

125. SOKALSKI SJ, JEWELL MA, ASMUS-SHILLINGTON AC, MULCAHY J, SEGRETI J. An outbreak of *Serratia marcescens* in 14 adult cardiac surgical patients associated with 12-lead electrocardiogram bulbs. *Arch Int Med* 1992;152:841–4.

126. NEWPORT MT, JOHN JF, MICHEL YM, LEVKOFF AH. Endemic *Serratia marcescens* infection in a neonatal intensive care nursery associated with gastrointestinal colonization. *Pediat Infect Dis* 1985;4:160–7.

127. CHAUDHURI AK, BOOTH CF. Outbreak of chest infections with *Serratia marcescens* [letter]. *J Hosp Infect* 1992;22:169–70.

128. WONG WW, WANG LS, CHENG DL *et al.* *Serratia marcescens* bacteraemia. *J Formosan Med Assoc* 1991;90:88–93.

129. BODEY GP, RODRIGUEZ V, SMITH JP. *Serratia* sp infections in cancer patients. *Cancer* 1970;25:199–205.

130. SALOMON PF, TAMLYN TT, GRIECO MH. *Escherichia coli* pneumonia -case report. *Am Rev Resp Dis* 1970;102:248–57.

130. TILLOTSON JR, LERNER AM. Characteristics of pneumonias caused by *Bacillus proteus. Ann Intern Med* 1986;68:295–307.

131. THAPA BR, KUMAR L, MITRA SK *Proteus mirabilis* pneumonis with giant pneumatocele. *Ind J Pediat* 1987;54:593–7.

132. SOLBERG C, MATSIN JM. Infections with *Providencia bacilli*: a clinical bacteriologic study. *Am J Med* 1971;50:241–6.

133. MUDER RR, BRENNEN C, WAGENER MM, GOETZ AM. Bacteremia in a long-term-care facility: a five-year prospective study of 163 consecutive episodes. *Clin Infect Dis* 1992;14:647–54.

134. SAPHRA I, WINTER JW. Clinical manifestations of salmonellosis in man. An evaluation of 7779 human infections identified at the New York Salmonella Center. *N Engl J Med* 1957;256:1128–34.

135. ELLIS ME, MOOSA A, HILLIER V. A review of typhoid fever in South African black children. *Postgrad Med J* 1990;66:1032–6.

136. STUART BM, PULLEN RL. Typhoid : clinical analysis of three hundred and sixty cases. *Arch Intern Med* 1946;78:629–61.

137. AGUADO JM, OBESO G, CABANILLAS JJ, FENDANDEZ-GUERRERO ALES J. Pleuropulmonary infections due to nontyphoid strains of salmonella. *Arch Intern Med* 1990;150:54–6.

138. BRYAN CS, REYNOLDS KL. Bacteremic nosocomial pneumonia: analysis of 172 episodes from a single metropolitan area. *Am Rev Resp Dis* 1984;129:668–71.

139. LEONG KH, BOEY ML, FENG PH. Coexisting *Pneumocystis carinii* pneumonia, cytomegalovirus pneumonitis and salmonellosis in systemic lupus erythematosus. *Ann Rheum Dis* 1991;50:811–12.

140. ANKOLABIAH WA, SALEHI F. Salmonella lung abscess in a patient with acquired immunodeficiency syndrome. *Chest* 1991;100:591.

141. CHAN JC, RAFFIN TA. Salmonella lung abscess complicating Wegener's granulomatosis. *Resp Med* 1991;85:339–41.

142. MURDOCH MB, PETERSON LR. Nontyphoidal salmonella pleuropulmonary infections. *Arch Intern Med*; 151:196.

143. LIPSKY BA, HOOK III ER, SMITH *et al.* Citrobacter infection in humans: experience at the Seattle Veterans Administration Medical Center and a review of the literature. *Rev Infect Dis* 1980;2:746–60.

144. SAMONIS G, ANAISSIE E, ELTING L, BODEY GP. Review of *Citrobacter* bacteraemia in cancer patients over a sixteen-year period. *Eur J Clin Microbiol Infect Dis* 1991;10(6):479–85.

145. GLEW RH, MOELLERING RC JR, KUNZ LJ. Infections with *Acinetobacter calcoaceticus* (*Herellea vaginicola*): clinical and laboratory studies. *Medicine* 1977;56:79–97.

146. JIMENEZ P, TORRES A, RODRIGUEZ-ROISIN R, DE LA BELLACASA JP, AZNAR R, GATELL JM, AGUSTI-VIDAL A. Incidence and aetiology of pneumonia acquired during mechanical ventilation. *Crit Care Med* 1989;17:882–5.

147. WISE KA, TOSOLINI FA. Epidemiological surveillance of *Acinetobacter* species. *J Hosp Infect* 1990;16:319–29.

148. ANSTEY NM, CURRIE BJ, WITHNALL KM. Community-acquired *Acinetobacter* pneumonia in the Northern territory of Australia. *Clin Infect Dis* 1992;14:83–91.

149. GELFAND MS, KAISER AB, DALE WA. Localized brucellosis: popliteal artery aneurysm, mediastinitis, dementia, and pneumonia. *Rev Infect Dis* 1989;11:783–8.

150. GAYNES RP, CULVER DH. The National Sosocomial Infections Surveillance System. Resistance to imipenem among selected gram-negative bacilli in the United States. *Infect Cont Hosp Epidemiol* 1992;13:10–14.

151. GOLD WL, SALIT IE. *Aeromonas hydrophila* infections of skin and soft tissue: report of 11 cases and review. *Clin Infect Dis* 1993;16:69–74.

152. BADDOUR LM, BASELSKI VS. Pneumonia due to *Aeromonas hydrophila*-complex: epidemiologic, clinical, and microbiologic features. *South Med J* 1988;88: 461–3.

153. GONCALVES JR, BRUM G, FERNANDES A, BISCAIA I, CORREIA MJS, BASTARDO J. *Aeromonas hydrophila* fulminant pneumonia in a fit young man. *Thorax* 1992;47:482–3.

154. JOSHI N, O'BRYAN T, APPELBAUM PC. Pleuropulmonary infections caused by *Eikenella corrodens. Rev Infect Dis* 1991;13: 1207–12.

155. STONE DR. *Eikenella corrodens* and group C *Streptococci. Clin Infect Dis* 1992;14:789.

156. JACOBS JA, ALGIE GD, SIE GH, STOBBERINGH EE. Association between *Eikenella corrodens* and *Streptococci. Clin Infect Dis* 1993;16:173.

157. TERES D. ICU-acquired pneumonia due to *Flavobacterium meningosepticum. J Am Med Assoc* 1974;228:732.

158. TAM AYC, YUNG RWH, FU K-H. Fatal pneumonia caused by *Flavobacterium meningosepticum. Pediat Infect Dis J* 1989;8:252–4.

159. FUJITA J, HATA Y, IRINO S. Respiratory infection caused by *Flavobacterium meningosepticum* [letter]. *Lancet* 1990;335:544.

160. ASHDOWN LR, PREVITERA S Community acquired *Flavobacterium meningosepticum* pneumonia and septicaemia. *Med J Aust* 1992;156:69–70.

161. LAWRENCE R, NIBBE AF, LEVIN S. Lung abscess secondary to vibrio fetus, malabsorption syndrome and acquired agammaglobulinemia. *Chest* 1971;60:191–4.

162. MEYERS BR, BOTTONE E, HIRSCHMAN SZ, SCHNEIERSON SS. Infections caused by micro-organisms of the genus *Erwinia*. *Ann Intern Med* 1972;76:9–14.

163. BERGER SA, EDBERG SC, KLEIN RS. *Enterobacter hafnia* infection: report of two cases and review of the literature. *Am J Med* Sci 1977;273: 101–4.

164. DEVREESE K, CLAEYS G, VERSCHRAEGEN G. Septicemia with *Ewingella americana*. *J Clin Microbiol* 1992;30:2746–7.

165. YUAN A, YANG P-C, LEE L-N, CHANG D-B, KUO, S-H, LUH K-T. *Actinobacillus actinomycetemcomitans* pneumonia with chest wall involvement and rib destruction. *Chest* 1992;101:1450–2.

166. DAUGA C, GILLIS M, VANDAMME P *et al.* (1993). *Balneatrix alpica* gen. nov., sp. now., a bacterium associated with pneumonia and meningitis in a spa therapy centre. *Res Microbiol* 1993;144:35–46.

9 Viral lower respiratory tract infections

MICHAEL E. ELLIS

King Faisal Specialist Hospital and Research Centre, Riyadh, Saudi Arabia

Introduction

Respiratory viruses in general produce relatively trivial disease, localised to the upper respiratory tract resulting in such syndromes as the common cold, pharyngitis/sore throat, tracheitis and otitis media. Viral pneumonia or other lower respiratory tract infections are relatively uncommon, but when they do occur are often severe, sometimes fulminant and not infrequently fatal. Unlike the situation with bacterial infections the antimicrobial drug armamentarium is limited in numbers and effectiveness. This chapter will focus on lower respiratory infections in adults. Paediatric lower respiratory tract infections are covered in Chapter 23 and further aspects in the immunocompromised host setting in Chapter 21. Cytomegalovirus because of its special relationship to the compromised host is covered in Chapter 10.

Only a few pathogenic viruses have a potential for invasion of the lower respiratory tract (Table 9.1). Among these the Orthomyxoviridae (notably influenza) are the most prominent in terms of numbers of young and elderly people infected, disabled or dying. A pandemic of influenza A is predicted for the near future. Among the Paramyxoviridae, respiratory syncytial virus is of importance for the severity of the illness it can produce, its possible underestimated role in the elderly and modern assessment of ribavirin therapy. The remaining viruses include parainfluenza (Paramyxoviridae), herpes simplex and Epstein–Barr virus (DNA Herpesviridae), and Adenoviridae. In addition, there are a few other viruses which invade the respiratory tract as part of a more generalised viraemic syndrome, such as measles and varicella.

Table 9.1. *Major respiratory viruses causing pneumonia in adults*

Influenza
Parainfluenza
Respiratory syncytial virus
Cytomegalovirus
Adenovirus
Measles
Varicella zoster
Herpes simplex
Epstein–Barr
Human herpes virus 6
Sin nombre

Virology and pathology: general comments

Viral infections of the respiratory tract depend upon the organism's ability to attack and penetrate the host cell and to utilise the host's replicative machinery in order to reproduce. Attachment to the host's ciliated epithelial cells of the airways is a prerequisite for disease. First the virus has to overcome the host mucus barrier. The molecular adherence of the virus to the protective mucus of airways secretion is caused by viral sialic acid receptors linking to the mucus glycoproteins. Viral neuraminidase activity co-present with haemagglutinin antigen results in severing this attachment and permits direct attachment of virus to the host cell. This mechanism also frees the virus from host infected cells at the stage of terminal replication. Mutations in viral surface antigens render the human population constantly susceptible to reinfection by influenza viruses and accounts for the pattern of epidemics and pandemics[1]. Other viruses have less well-defined attachment mechanisms. Recently, the finding that secretion of blood group antigens is associated with respiratory virus diseases suggests that these antigens might act as receptors for certain viruses[2]. Some viruses have specific identifiable subunits which bind to cell receptors. In the case of the influenza virus, combination of surface haemagglutinin antigen to specific host cell receptors is necessary. Receptor specificity of host ciliated cells is governed by their affinity for well-defined neuraminic acid on the influenza virus surface.

Cell entry is the next mandatory step and this usually occurs by pinocytosis. Uncoating of the genomic material follows by a mechanism which may include a fusion process between the viral membrane and the host lipid bilayer in the case of the Orthomyxoviridae, or by pH-dependent structural surface alterations in the case of the picornaviruses. The RNA respiratory viruses undergo replication, nucleocapsid and virion assembly in the cytoplasm (apart from the Orthomyxoviridae in which case genomic replication and nucleocapsid assembly occurs in the nucleus). In the case of the DNA viruses, all three processes occur in the nucleus. Replication of the viral genome proceeds via synthesis of viral mRNA from viral mDNA in the case of the adenoviruses, from viral mRNA primed by host cell mRNA in the case of Orthomyxoviridae and from viral mRNA *per se* for the other RNA viruses. Structural viral proteins are translated from the RNA on ribosomes, the process inhibiting or replacing host cell protein synthesis. Viral antigens may appear on the surface of the infected cells early in the replication processes, which can be detected by immunofluorescent techniques and permits immune recognition and response by the host. Viral assembly occurs in the nucleus/cytoplasm as appropriate. Virus release from the cell occurs by budding off from cellular nuclear membranes or by cell lysis. Infectivity of Orthomyxoviridae is conferred by host cell-mediated proteolysis of haemagglutinin and heightened by a disaggregative neuraminidase activity.

Pathology and the immune response: general comments

Infection results from entry of aerogenous infectious particles into the respiratory tract of a susceptible (nonimmune) individual, Cytomegalovirus can also spread haematogenously, and via organ transplants. The smaller the particles, the more distally they travel into the respiratory tract and the more likely they are to produce infection. Target cells are mainly the ciliated columnar epithelial cells of the respiratory tract. Following cell entry, viral replication occurs within approximately 8 hours, each cell releasing of the order of 100 virions which reinfect neighbouring cells. Infected cells become dysmorphic, swollen – the nucleus fragments and cell death occurs. The infective process provokes an intense host immune response[3]. Initially, a polymorphonuclear infiltrate of the peribronchiolar submucosal regions of the airways occurs, compounded or replaced later by a mild lymphocytic/mononuclear cell reaction. Parallel with increasing clinical severity the histological changes quicken and intensify. Increased vessel permeability is seen with submucosal oedema and epithelial necrosis. Mucus production is increased resulting in inspissation of bronchioles and bronchi and attendant atelectasis. However, distal hyperinflation secondary to airway trapping may also occur. Progressive lymphocytic infiltration of the adjacent alveoli and the interstitial tissues of the lung parenchyma occurs. Intranuclear inclusion bodies and multinucleate giant cells may be found, particularly in patients with parainfluenza and measles. In severe instances, pulmonary haemorrhage may be present. In most cases, repair of respiratory epithelium is rapid provided the infection has been abated by a protective host response. Occasionally, a chronic increase in mucus secreting goblet cells occurs with evolution to chronic bronchitis. Permanent destructive sequelae, particularly bronchiectasis, can also result, particularly among children who survive severe viral pneumonia.

The immunological response to viral infection involves the augmentation of cell-mediated activities and antibody production. The early appearance of cytotoxic T-cell activities, humoral antibodies and interferon production are three key events essential for overcoming the virus infection. However, the increased monocyte macrophage activity may actually cause tissue damage through the release of toxic oxygen radicals. In addition, there is an overwhelming commitment of host immune function to protection against viruses and this may result in downgrading protective efficiency against secondary bacterial sepsis. T-cell cytotoxic activity is crucial, particularly in terminating established advanced viral infection. Thus, animal studies have shown that persistent influenzal viral infection occurs in conditions of T-cell depletion[4], and in humans T-cell cytotoxic activity parallels viral activity[5]. Humoral antibody responses have been studied largely in connection with influenza virus infection[6]. For example, serum haemagglutinin and neuraminidase IgA, IgG and IgM appear within 2 weeks of infection. Thereafter, IgA and IgM levels decline within 2 weeks but raised IgG levels persist for a longer period. Nasal IgA response by contrast is short lived. Haemagglutinin specific antibody in the acute phase is neutralising, protects an infected cell against virus attachment, and participates in cellular cytotoxic functions. Antibody to neuraminidase is important in preventing virus release. In the long term, IgG persistence probably diminishes the chance of type specific viral recurrence, whereas IgA, being totally produced in the respiratory mucosa, is not as effective in the prevention of virus reinfection. Some viruses produce IgE which has been found to be associated with the ongoing pathogenesis of the disease[7], namely, the appearance of bronchospasm and hypoxia in patients with respiratory syncytial virus infection. Several respiratory viruses, notably rhinoviruses, coronaviruses, influenza B, respiratory syncytial virus and parainfluenza virus are all associated with exacerbation of asthma in adults[8].

The role of interferon has been studied extensively, and it is thought to play a key role in host events. Interferon levels are highest at the height of maximal viral replication, and recovery from serious virus infection parallels interferon production – overwhelming virus infection has been associated with low or undetectable levels of interferon. The host mononuclear cells contain genes coding for interferon production. Following the initial viral stimulus, the interferon genes are derepressed, interferon mRNA is produced and interferon protein is released from infected cells and binds to interferon receptors on non-infected cell surfaces. Transmembrane signalling triggers the synthesis of more than two dozen interferon-directed proteins, which mediate the antiviral and immunomodulatory actions of interferon. For example, MX protein inhibits transcription of viral nucleic acid, 2'5' oligo-synthetase degrades mRNA and protein kinase inhibits RNA translation to polypeptides. Interferon has additional deleterious effects on cell membranes, therefore, preventing virion assembly and release. Interferon also augments the production and display of HLA major histocompatibility proteins thereby facilitating lysis of infected cells by cytotoxic T-cells. It also increases the activity of non-virus specific natural killer cell activity and macrophage function. Many of the symptoms and signs attributed to viral infection such as myalgia, chills and fever occur as a result of interferon's regulation of cytokine production, for example, interleukin and tumour necrosis factor, as well as hypothalamic-induced prostaglandin E2 release.

Bacterial superinfection is a common accompaniment to viral respiratory tract infection as a direct result of diminished host responsiveness or defence to bacteria[9]. Likely mechanisms include an increased affinity of virus-infected cells for bacterial attachment as a result of induction of bacterial surface receptors and abnormalities in cell surfaces. In addition, there is diminished mucociliary clearance early in virus infection. Furthermore, diminished phagocytic function of alveolar macrophages and neutrophils, reduced chemotaxis and bactericidal activity have been documented.

Specific viral lower respiratory tract infections of adults

Influenza

Virology, immunology and pathology

The influenza viruses are single-stranded RNA viruses with the segmented genome complexed with nuclear protein (NP) contained within a host-derived cell membrane. Differences in the NP produce types A, B and C. Most cases of influenza are due to types A and B, type C being rarely pathogenic. Ten proteins are encoded by the genome. Of these, the haemagglutinin (HA) and neuraminidase (NA) are projecting surface glycoproteins. HA is responsible for cellular attachment via sialic acid structures and thereafter facilitating endocytosis. NA facilitates virus release from the cell with subsequent spread, via enzymic cleavage of the sialic acid–HA and sialic acid–cell surface bonds. The HA can be partially split by exogenous proteases into HA1 and HA2 chains. The actual cellular attachment site is located at HA2. This area is subject to amino acid mutations leading to antigenic changes which are associated with epidemics and pandemics. NA changes are also associated with this phenomenon. Actual entry of the viral genome into the host cell is possible through the formation of ionic channels under the control of M1 matrix protein. The M_2 membrane sparing protein controls resistance to the antivirals amantadine and rimantadine, via amino acid mutation.

Protection against influenza *infection* is essentially mediated via antibodies directed against HA. Cytotoxic T-cells do little to protect against infection but play a role in modulating *disease* and governing recovery from disease. The viral RNA after entry into the cell nucleus requires host mRNA primers to switch on the viral polymerase (PA, PB1 and PB2) to produce viral mRNA. This is then translated into viral protein in the host cell cytoplasm, which encloses the complementary viral RNA templates produced in the host cell nucleus. Viral budding incorporates a portion of the host cell membrane for the viral envelope.

Cleavage of HA is necessary to generate infectious virus and for its spread. This is accomplished either by host-derived endoproteases, or by exoproteases provided by bacteria. Thus, plasminogen activating streptococci and staphylococci produce streptokinase and staphylokinase respectively, and by amplifying the plasminogen/plasmin system facilitate viral replication and this leads to viral pneumonia[10]. *Aeromonas viridans* also produces a protease which activates HA. On the other hand, *Pseudomonas aeruginosa* although producing a protease cannot activate HA *in vitro* but a combination of virus and the protease in animal models does cause increased pulmonary viral titres and extensive pneumonia[10].

There are a number of pathological effects of the influenza virus on the targeted host respiratory epithelium. In the upper respiratory tract desquamation of nasal ciliated cells, together with creation of large interbasal pores leads to rhinorrhoea. Impaired mucociliary clearance occurs as a result of diminished ciliary beat frequency, and this continues even into the recovery phase of the illness. Tracheal toiletting is therefore severely impaired leading to retention of secretions. These alterations in ciliary functions, extravasation of culture-rich fluids, alteration in polymorph function and increased tendency for bacterial adherence lead to secondary bacterial sepsis.

More distally in the bronchopulmonary tree, the influenza virus appears to destroy alveolar epithelial cells, removes alveolar surfactant and produces capillary leak. Patients with mitral stenosis or others with pre-existing pulmonary hydrostatic pressure, are at risk for pulmonary oedema. Should viral receptors be present on only one type of alveolar cell, then regeneration of the other type may be advantageous to the host if the patient can be maintained by extracorporeal membrane oxygenation during pneumonia. The likelihood and severity of influenza pneumonia can be governed by the size of the infectious dose, site of initial infection (upper or lower airways as determined by large or small droplet transmissions) and existing host immunity profile. Thus, the presence of heterotypic immunity – that is previous exposure to the same type but different strain of influenza virus – will not prevent infection but will contain the influenzal infection to the original site of the infecting virus. Systemic antibodies to HA, mediated by T-cells plays an important role as indicated in a ferret study[11]. Upper respiratory tract locally secreted IgA prevents upper respiratory tract infection due to influenza. Systemic cell-mediated immunity, on the other hand is more important in modulating the disease course, having little effect in preventing infection[12]. Specific cytotoxic CD8 lymphocytes appear to be important for the clearance of virus and recovery of lung histology[13].

Histological changes of influenzal lower respiratory tract infection present a wide spectrum ranging from necrosis, ulceration of bronchial mucosa, shrunken ciliated columnar cells without cilia, through mild lung injury such as mild alveolar damage, focal inflammatory cell infiltrates, BOOP pattern, fibrinous exudates, alveolar septal oedema and type 2 cell metaplasia, to severe changes characterised by necrotising tracheobronchitis, diffuse alveolar damage, peribronchiolar squamous metaplasia, fibrosis and secondary bacterial pneumonic changes[14].

At a systemic level the influenza virus triggers the release of cytokines such as TNF-α which are responsible for the prominent systemic symptoms.

Epidemiology

Influenza infection and disease is characterised by yearly, usually winter, outbreaks and less frequent irregular cycles of pandemics. There is a constantly occurring mutation-driven antigenic variation in the amino acid composition of HA and NA. Epidemics occur if the strains are grossly different from those previously seen in a particular population.

Mild outbreaks are characterised by up to 10% of the general population being infected; 20–30% are infected in severe epidemics and at least 50% in pandemics. Colder winter months are the usual times for outbreaks, due to closer person proximity and lower humidity favouring increased survival of the influenza virus.

Early in an influenza season which usually occurs in mid- or late December, sporadic cases are noted and are usually due to one predominant subtype, followed by a rapid increase in the numbers of children and workers attending family physicians. Paralleling these reports are increased incidences of school and work absenteeism, and once an outbreak or epidemic is established, admissions to hospital of more severe influenza cases occur. Peaking of the cases occurs at about 6 weeks into the outbreak; a rapid fall off in numbers occurs thereafter. There may be a second or herald wave of a new subtype of influenza strain late in the season – this may indicate the predominant strain for the next season[15]. Finally, the season terminates during early March.

Attack rates for influenza are highest in young children, and decrease with age. This is due to the older population having been previously exposed and also probably they have less exposure to school children and less crowding. Hospital admissions on the other hand for severe influenza or complicated influenza are more frequent in the very young or the very old, whilst the incidence of influenza related deaths increases substantially with age[16], being even greater in elderly patients with certain chronic conditions[17]. These include chronic obstructive airways disease, cardiovascular disease and to a lesser extent endocrine disturbances such as diabetes mellitus, anaemia and immunosuppression.

The devastating Spanish influenza pandemic of 1918–1919 claimed more than 20 million deaths worldwide. The influenza A subtype H1N1 strain responsible for this disappeared for over half a century but reappeared in 1977 causing a further (and the latest) pandemic. In the meantime, pandemics caused by other strains appeared in 1957 and 1968. The next pandemic is predicted within the next two decades. The mechanisms of why, how and where the strains move to or disappear and re-emerge has only begun to be clarified. It has been established that several animal species harbour influenza viruses. Ducks, shorebirds and gulls have been found to be infected with strains, some of which closely relate to those found in humans. Analysis of both avium and human influenza virus has indicated cross-reactivity of avium H_2 strains with human H_2 strains from the 1957 pandemic[18] and suggest that the pandemic may have originated as a result of avium–human interactions. The recent documentation of a fatal case of influenza in a 27-year animal caretaker due to influenza A/Maryland/12/91 (A/MD) with a high level of identity (based on HA, NP and matrix gene homologies) to contemporary swine virus, further highlights the importance of the animal–human interface[19]. It also indicates that the avium reservoir is not the only source. In fact, the pig population may function as an interchange to permit genetic reassortment between avium and human like viruses[20]. These observations may provide important strategies for future control of epidemics and pandemics, for example, by eradication of pig influenza through vaccination, or modification of farming practices in those parts of the world where pandemics appear to originate, for example, in China.

Influenza still continues to claim substantial deaths particularly in infants and the elderly. In the US, during the 11 influenzal seasons from 1977 to 1988, more than 10 000 excess deaths ascribed to pneumonia and influenza were reported during each of seven seasons, rising to 45 000 in each of two seasons[21]. Twenty-six thousand people died in England and Wales in 1989 to 1990 from influenza[22]. From 1934 to 1972, influenza pneumonia deaths in the USA averaged around 50/100 000[23]. The presence of underlying medical conditions and increasing age (possibly due to a decline in T-cell function) dramatically increase influenza related mortality. Thus, in the very elderly (> 75 years) mortality is 31/100 000 compared to only 0.44 for persons aged 45–54[16]. The presence of at least one underlying medical condition increases the mortality by a factor of at least 40[17].

Host risk factors for influenza

Risk factors for the acquisition of influenza have been identified. In the first instance, diminished host defences may predispose to infection. Thus, in the non-immune, immunocompromised or even in individuals with past exposure to influenza having detectable antibodies, lack of *specific* antibodies to haemagglutinin or neuraminidase is a major factor in establishment of infection[24]. As a corollary of the role of defective immunity, extremes of age, malnutrition and possibly vitamin A deficiency[25] are particular risk factors for severe disease. Protein-calorie malnutrition causes thymic atrophy and consequently quantitative and qualitative dysfunction of T-cell lymphocytes as well as impaired neutrophil phagocytosis. Although vitamin A deficiency can lead to mechanical disintegrity of the respiratory tract lining in addition to having a direct depression on humoral and cell-mediated immune functions, the relation to severity of the influenza remains speculative. Influenza is a contender for the cause of the sudden infant death syndrome (SIDS) – possibly through the heightened mucosal reactivity and virus load which characterises the disease in the young and could produce upper respiratory tract obstruction[26]. It has been known for some time that rheumatic valvular heart disease and chronic pulmonary disease in pregnancy predispose to severe influenzal illness; possibly because of limited cardiopulmonary reserve due to pulmonary hypertension, obstructive airways disease and chronic bacterial sepsis, the latter of which leads to bacterial superinfection. Exposure to environmental air pollutants probably influence the host's susceptibility to influenza A. This has been shown for nitrogen dioxide[27] and it is reasonable to postulate that others such as cigarette smoke may do the same possibly through damage to the mucociliary escalator, increased bronchial reactivity and effects on selective macrophage function, e.g. diminished bacterial adherence.

Clinical

Influenza actually produces significant lower respiratory tract infection in the minority of cases. There are five categories of illness (Table 9.2): (i) most people experience mild symptoms such as the common cold and pharyngitis characterised by sneezing, headache, nasal discharge, myalgia and photophobia; (ii) lower respiratory tract but non-pneumonic manifestations occur such as laryngo-tracheobronchitis or bronchitis (more common in children); (iii) influenza followed by bacterial pneumonia; (iv) primary influenzal pneumonia; and (v) concomitant bacterial and viral pneumonia. Categories (ii) and early category (iv) may sometimes be difficult to differentiate clinically and radiographically as both may include patients who present with rhonchi/crepitations, and the presence of so-called alveolar infiltrates which favour (iv) may in reality be peribronchial inflammation. Influenza accounts for up to 5–10% of all cases of community-acquired pneumonia[28].

Transmission of the virus occurs as a result of close contact with cough-generated small particulate aerosols. Symptoms occur following an incubation period of between 1 and 4 days.

Uncomplicated influenza is manifested by an abrupt onset of fever, chills, malaise, myalgia, which involves the ocular muscles particularly, substernal discomfort (which may be prominent), sneezing, nasal discharge and non-productive cough. In the majority of cases,

Table 9.2. *Disease spectrum of influenza*

Common cold symptoms
Laryngo-tracheo-bronchitis
Bronchitis
Primary influenzal pneumonia
Secondary bacterial pneumonia
Concomitant influenzal and bacterial pneumonia
Meningococcal sepsis
Exacerbation of asthma, bronchitis, CF
Deterioration of COAD
Transverse myelitis
Encephalopathy
Guillain–Barré syndrome
Myositis
Toxic shock syndrome (secondary bacteria sepsis with *S. aureus*)
Schizophrenia
SIDS

these are self-limiting, and most symptoms clear by approximately 5 days, although cough and malaise can persist for several days or more.

In a few people, there is progression to lower respiratory tract involvement. There are few specific clinical and radiographical features which serve to make an unequivocal diagnosis of influenzal pneumonia. The diagnosis, therefore, is often presumptive. For example, if a patient with lower respiratory tract signs presents during an influenza outbreak or epidemic, then influenza pneumonia has to be a differential diagnosis. Although the absence of an outbreak does not preclude the diagnosis of influenza (or indeed any other viral) pneumonia, the patient will have had prior symptoms suggesting 'flu'. Features of established influenza pneumonia include cough, chest pain which may be pleuritic, haemoptysis, breathlessness, unremittent fever and wheeze due to bronchospasm produced by release of inflammatory cell mediators and by certain neuro-reflexes. Occasionally, a differential diagnosis of pulmonary embolism is entertained. Cyanosis often occurs. Pre-existing pulmonary and valvular heart disease are major risk factors for such cases. A chest radiograph will show the typical appearance of bilateral perihilar interstitial and alveolar infiltrates. This chest radiographic appearance is highly suggestive of viral infection, particularly if auscultatory signs are relatively scant. Acute overwhelming diffuse pneumonia due to either influenza *per se* or to a mixed influenzal and bacterial infection is a frightening phenomenon. High risk patients (see Table 9.5) are particularly prone to this presentation. The chest radiograph features may mimic pulmonary oedema. Leukopenia may occur.

Secondary bacterial pneumonia is a severe complication[29] particularly in patients over the age of 65 or those with cardiopulmonary, metabolic or other disease. The patient may exhibit a biphasic pattern in the illness. There may be an initial partial recovery from the influenza then sudden deterioration with relapse of fever, the emergence of severe cough, productive of purulent and perhaps blood-stained sputum. The clinical, radiographical and diagnostic features of staphylococcal pneumonia which is the major bacterial cause in this situation have already been described in this setting (see Chapter 6). Staphylococcal toxic shock syndrome has been described. Infection with *Streptococcus pneumoniae* and *Haemophilus* spp may also occur. However, this biphasic pattern of presentation does not always present, and the features of bacterial sepsis may complicate the influenzal illness at a much earlier stage. *S. aureus* pneumonia is believed to be a major contributor to influenza mortality with up to one-third of patients who develop this complication dying[29]. Occasionally other bacterial opportunists such as *Pseudomonas* spp. can cause superinfection.

Secondary bacterial infection is not only confined to pulmonary involvement. It appears that influenza (and other common upper respiratory infections) may act as a cofactor for meningococcal meningitis[30,31]. The mechanism for this is unclear, but may include increased aerosol transmission of meningococci through coughing, viral-mediated meningococcal invasion of the upper respiratory tract mucosa, and inhibition of bacterial phagocytosis.

In the absence of chronic pulmonary disease influenza, even if uncomplicated, produces abnormal small airways function, diminished DLCO, abnormal perfusion and increased alveolar arterial oxygen gradients – many of these changes taking weeks to resolve after clinical recovery. Other pulmonary complications include exacerbation of asthma and chronic bronchitis due to influenza-related bronchial reactivity[8,32–34]. Permanent deterioration of the underlying chronic respiratory problem may occur. Pulmonary function testing has revealed chronic deterioration of alveolar/arterial gas exchange and other abnormalities[35].

Otitis media is a common complication of influenza particularly in children and association also noted for RSV, adenovirus, rhinovirus, and parainfluenza virus. Of some interest is that influenzal vaccination has produced a parallel decline in the incidence of otitis media and influenza[36]. In patients with cystic fibrosis, some studies have shown that respiratory viral infections are capable of producing pulmonary deterioration[37]. Others have not confirmed such a strong association[38]. Invasive aspergillosis following influenzal pneumonia has been documented, possibly a consequence of viral induced T-cell depression[39].

Involvement outside the respiratory tract is rare. When it does occur, the central nervous system is the most frequently involved[40,41], and includes transverse myelitis, encephalopathy (sometimes as part of Reye's syndrome and occurring usually but not exclusively in children) and the Guillain-Barré syndrome. An association between exposure to influenza in the second trimester of pregnancy and schizophrenia in the baby has been mooted but is a subject to controversy[42]. Myositis has also been described. The toxic shock syndrome occurs mainly with influenza A/B due to secondary staphylococcal infections[43]. The plague of Athens was thought to be caused by this complication of influenza[44]. In immunocompromised patients such as renal transplants, bone marrow transplants, patients with graft vs. host disease or haematological malignancy, the course of influenza A is in general mild and self-limiting, similar to that described in the majority of immunocompromised patients. Occasional severe complications are seen, particularly in patients with severe combined immune defects[45]. Non-survivors of proven influenza tend to exhibit on admission confusion, uraemia, lack of focal chest signs and symptoms and not to have been treated with antistaphylococcal therapy[46].

The peripheral white cell count may not distinguish influenzal from bacterial pneumonia. A neutrophil leukocytosis is often seen initially, and may reach up to $20 \times 10^9/l$. Later leukoneutropenia will become the predominant haematological response. Laboratory confirmation of diagnosis can be made by culture of appropriately obtained, and correctly transported, respiratory specimens from throat, nasopharynx, sputum, bronchial washings and sometimes by transbronchial biopsy. Inoculated onto kidney tissue culture cell lines, or chicken embryo amniotic cavities, a cytotoxic effect due to the influenza virus will be seen well within 1 week. Guinea pig erythrocyte absorption or agglutination effects are also used diagnostically.

Direct detection of viral antigen expressed in naso-pharyngeal cells is possible with monoclonal antibody ELISA techniques. Rapid, highly specific and sensitive diagnosis using an immunocaptive ELISA test against NP antigen is possible[47]. The polymerase chain reaction has also been used for a rapid diagnostic service. A four-fold rise in the convalescent serum antibody titre from that taken on admission is also diagnostic. A single 'high' IgM titre in the correct clinical setting may also be taken as presumptive or supportive data. Often the serum antibody results are returned well after the clinical event. Complement fixation or haemagglutination inhibition tests are available but are less sensitive than the ELISA test. Routine laboratory diagnosis during an epidemic is not usually indicated in every patient suspected of having influenza. However, it is justified at the beginning of a suspected epidemic for differentiation from other viral infections particularly RSV and for unusual presentations.

Management

Table 9.3 summarises the treatment of influenza. The management of uncomplicated influenza involves symptomatic relief which includes rest, ensuring adequate oral fluids, regular soluble aspirin to relieve systemic viral effects such as fever, paracetamol for pain, oxymetazoline locally for nasal discharge, and cough suppressants (See Chapter 9). Aspirin should not be used in children because of the risk of Reye's syndrome. Antihistamines may increase the risk of amantadine's central nervous system side effects. The prognosis for uncomplicated influenza without pulmonary involvement is excellent.

In patients desperately ill with influenzal pneumonia who require artificial ventilation, the use of extracorporeal membrane oxygenation (ECMO) may be considered in an attempt to permit the regeneration of alveolar cells.

Antiviral drugs used in the management of influenza

Antiviral drugs are available, and are probably underused, in the management of acute influenza. However, their use in a treatment mode is probably less effective than when used for prophylaxis.

Amantadine long known as 'Symmetrel' for the treatment of extrapyramidal neurological diseases such as Parkinson's disease has been recognised since 1964 as having virustatic properties against a broad range of RNA viruses, particularly influenza A. Rimantadine is a similar drug. Most subtypes are inhibited by amantadine. Influenza B strains are resistant and certain influenza A, HA and NA subtypes are less susceptible. Amantadine is a three-ringed amine, first manufactured in 1941. The usual adult oral dose for patients with normal renal function when given as a treatment modality is 100 mg Q12 hourly. It is continued for approximately 5 days or until symptoms begin to abate. A more prolonged course may lead to the emergence of resistant mutants. Although these can emerge as early as 3 days into treatment (rimantadine)[48] in a prophylactic setting, a 2–3 week course is usually given to adequately protect over the ongoing exposure period. Peak serum levels are attained by 4 hours following oral dosing with a half-life of approximately 16 hours. Dose modification is needed in patients with renal failure in which the dose is reduced progressively when the creatinine clearance is < 80 ml min^{-1}. It is not removed by haemodialysis. Dose reductions are also needed in the elderly or in children. Amantadine is widely distributed in tissues, including the lungs, by the second day of administration. Alternatively, it may be administered by the aerosol route producing higher levels in nasal wash samples than corresponding oral doses, with little systemic absorption and toxicity.

Table 9.3. *Treatment of influenza*

Symptomatic
Amantadine/rimantadine for high risk patients[a], or for influenza pneumonia
Early institution antibacterial including antistaphylococcal therapy for
prolonged or severe illness
biphasic illness
pneumonia
bacterial bronchitis
ECMO
? Ribavirin
Investigational drugs, e.g. neuraminidase inhibitors

[a] Definition : see Table 9.5.

The mode of action is not clear, but a postulated mechanism is an amantadine-directed pH buffering effect which inhibits fusion of the virus envelope with the endosome membrane thereby preventing viral uncoating. Additional mechanisms include blocking the assembly of viral particles.

Dose-related side-effects of oral amantadine and to a lesser extent rimantadine occur in approximately 10% of patients, and are mainly neurological (Table 9.4). These are catecholamine-release-mediated in the case of amantadine, but not in the case of rimantadine, and include motor incoordination, conscious level alterations, insomnia, headache, concentration problems, convulsions (and is therefore relatively contraindicated in patients with convulsive tendencies). A dose reduction of 50% may be tried. The CNS effects may be potentiated in patients receiving antihistamines/anticholigenic and psychotropic drugs. Mild anticholinergic side-effects such as dry mouth and urinary difficulties may also occur. Less commonly, self-limiting gastrointestinal intolerance (the drug is contraindicated in patients with gastric ulceration) has been documented and rarely leukopenia, hypotension, livido reticularis and other skin rashes. Since amantadine is excreted in breast milk, it is contraindicated in nursing mothers. It is not approved for use in pregnancy, since it is teratogenic in rats although it should be used in life threatening situations.

Concern over the possibility of these relatively uncommon side-

Table 9.4. *Amantadine/rimantadine side-effects*

Neurological[a]	
	motor incoordination
	depressed level of consciousness
	insomnia
	headache
	inability to concentrate
	convulsions
	dry mouth micturition
	slow/difficult inclination
Leukopenia	
Hypotension	
Livido reticularis/other rashes	

[a] Increase in side-effects in elderly, patients on antihistamines/anticholinergics/psychotropic drugs/impaired renal function.

effects has unfortunately precluded the appropriate use of these antimicrobials. Widespread unavailability of laboratory diagnostic techniques to make a rapid and specific diagnosis of influenza A is another. The side-effects are particularly common among certain groups of patients who are *per se* more vulnerable to severe influenza namely, the elderly who have diminished renal function or who may be more prone to neuropsychiatric disturbances.

As previously mentioned there is some evidence to suggest that resistant strains to rimantadine (and which are also usually cross resistant to amantadine) can emerge during the course of treatment with this drug[48,49] and are due to mutation of the M2 gene. Despite the recovery of drug-resistant virus from 33% of patients with influenza A when given rimantadine for 10 days, the overall improvement in symptom duration compared to placebo was unaffected, although illness resolution tended to be slower in those with resistant mutants when compared to those with sensitive mutants[48]. However, despite the transmissibility and pathogenicity of the resistant mutants[50] no evidence has so far emerged to suggest a major clinical impact from such strains in a community or even within groups where the antiviral drugs are being used. This has been supported by the finding that widespread use of the drugs in the former Soviet Union[51] has not been associated with any reduction in their efficacy. Nevertheless, resistance is a serious concern and requires close monitoring. Spread of resistant organisms following amantadine treatment has been observed in a nursing facility[52]. Patients receiving amantadine or rimantadine should therefore be nursed in an appropriate respiratory isolation facility to reduce this risk of spread of resistant organisms to others. In addition, clearer guidelines for the use of amantadine and rimantadine for patients with influenza are needed.

Ribavirin has also been used to treat influenza. This nucleoside analogue has a fairly broad antiviral spectrum which includes influenza A and B, parainfluenza 1,2,3, RSV, adenovirus and others including measles and arena viruses such as Lassa fever. It can be administered orally, intravenously and by aerosol. Provided it is given within 24 hours of onset of symptoms, case reports suggest a therapeutic effect on influenza A and B[53] but it is only effective if given by the aerosol route.

Interferon does not appear to be useful. Other investigational drugs include neuraminidase and sialidase inhibitors. Crystallographic visualisation of the influenza virus is proving instrumental in a search for novel compounds[54].

Indications for amantadine/rimantadine

When given to patients with established but uncomplicated influenza, oral amantadine has demonstrable activity in terms of significantly reducing the duration of both local and systemic clinical viral symptomatology and the degree of fever, and probably has an effect on viral shedding. There is a high therapeutic index[55,56]. There are also benefits in terms of a significant reduction in time lost from work and school as a result of illness. However, loss of therapeutic efficacy becomes apparent when it is given later than 48 hours after established viral infection or if the virus load is high. In comparative clinical trials comparing amantadine to rimantadine, efficacy is similar but side-effects appear to be less common with rimantadine.

In patients with established influenza pneumonia, there have been no unequivocal reports of efficacy, though it is logical to administer in this situation as the mortality is up to 90%, particularly in patients with diffuse pneumonia. Aerosol-administered amantadine at a dose of 4 mg/kg/day appears to have similar efficacy, apart from resolution of fever. A collision generator[57] provides aerosol particles between 1 and 6 Mu which when equilibrated at high humidity provide a 40% deposition rate in the nose and 40% in the distal bronchial/alveolar ducts.

Therefore, rimantadine or amantadine should be seriously considered in patients with symptoms of influenza at risk for complications, or who hold important social and other positions (Table 9.5). In patients with established influenza pneumonia, it should also be given.

There is a strong recommendation to use antistaphylococcal agents during influenza epidemics[58] due to the high mortality associated with this complication. However, the precise indications and benefits have yet to be clarified. One study of proven influenza showed that non-survivors were less frequently given antistaphylococcal treatment[46]. Certainly antistaphylococcal drugs should be used in influenza pneumonia where it may not be possible to exclude staphylococcal etiology. Antimicrobial therapy should be modified according to the results of cultures. Other bacterial etiologies which should be considered include *S. pneumoniae* which may be penicillin resistant, *Hemophilus* spp and *Pseudomonas* spp. Appropriate antibiotic therapy is indicated for these pathogens.

Prophylaxis of influenza

Influenza is, at the very least, a miserable illness and, at worst, carries a risk of substantial mortality. For these reasons, effective prophylaxis is a worthy goal. This may be achieved with antiviral agents or with vaccines.

Antiviral medications

Amantadine and rimantadine have been widely studied as prophylactics in the settings both of artificial challenge and natural exposure. Protection against influenza A is immediate, unlike the situation with vaccination in which 2–3 weeks are required to build up protective

Table 9.5. *Indications for amantadine/rimantidine*

Treatment	
	High risk patients[a] with early (≤ 48 h) uncomplicated influenza (apart from pregnancy unless severe disease)
	Established influenza pneumonia
Prophylaxis during influenzal epidemic	
	High risk unvaccinated patients
	Unvaccinated health professionals
	Unvaccinated non-health professionals in important social positions
	High risk vaccinated patients if known influenza strain different from vaccine strain
	Residents and staff (vaccinated and unvaccinated)
	Local institutional outbreaks
	Persons who have a contraindication to vacccination

[a] High risk patients:
Chronic pulmonary disease (asthma, COAD, CF).
Cardiac disease (coronary artery disease, CCF, MV disease).
Endocrine disorder (including diabetes mellitus).
Haemoglobinopathy.
Iatrogenic immunosuppression.
HIV infection.
Malignancy.
Pregnancy.

antibody levels. It may therefore be given at the same time as an active vaccine is given, to provide protection in the initial 2-week window phase. The majority of studies have shown significant protection both against infection and clinical disease in 70–100% of cases[59,60]. Some reports suggest that patients with pre-existing immunity and those patients undergoing concomitant active influenza vaccination appear to fare better. The indications for prophylaxis include individuals at high risk for influenza complications or key social and other personnel (Table 9.5). The usual course is between 2 and 3 weeks given to an individual over the ongoing exposure period. It is, of course, necessary to vaccinate an unvaccinated person because a longer course of prophylaxis with amantadine/rimantadine would otherwise be required. In individuals who have a contraindication to vaccination, the course of prophylaxis will have to be longer.

Vaccination

Two major types of killed vaccine currently exist: the subunit vaccines, either composed of haemagglutinin and neuraminidase antigens or split virions (disrupted), and whole viral vaccines. These vaccines offer similar protection against influenza A and B. The earlier whole viral vaccines contained large quantities of egg antigen and were associated with a high incidence of adverse reactions. Modern vaccines are highly purified with carefully quantified constituent components. They are revised annually to contain the more likely strains to be encountered during the next imminent outbreak. This means that the manufacturing of vaccines has to start at the end of the previous influenza season and is based upon the strains known at that time from global surveillance. Occasionally, a new strain emerges in the interim period and rapid efforts have to be made to cover this. The vaccine is administered during the autumn months, ensuring that the few weeks needed for antibodies to peak just precede the start of the influenza season. The vaccine needs to be administered annually.

In terms of an antibody response, in younger healthy vaccinees efficacy is estimated to be in excess of 80% with 75% of vaccinees being protected against symptomatic disease and nearly all protected against influenzal death[61].

In immunocompromised patients, for example, those with HIV or patients with chronic illness, antibody production is diminished[62]. Despite widespread claims of a reduced antibody response in the elderly, a literature review has not provided conclusive evidence for this[63]. In terms of prevention against influenzal illness, approximately 75% of young healthy adults are protected. A positive protective effect is seen in the elderly against serious influenzal morbidity, hospitalisation and death but the magnitude of the results are variable. Protective efficacy has varied between 19% and 75%[64]. Many of the results are based upon observational studies with inclusion of different epidemic years and hence different strains. In addition there were various other methodological differences. Influenza vaccine nevertheless is strongly recommended for people of all ages but particularly those from high risk groups (Table 9.6). Cost-effective issues have also been addressed. For example, it was found that net *savings* accrued to a hospital management organization for non-institutional high risk elderly (> 65 years) patients. On the contrary net *costs* accrued for non-high risk elderly patients. However, for all elderly patients vaccinated there was still a net *savings* on direct medical care costs[65]. Similar findings were reported in another study[66]. Unfortunately, immunisation rates in the general population are extremely low possibly reflecting (unreal) concern over vaccine side-effects and uncertainties over efficacy.

Placebo-controlled studies with the modern vaccines have shown that local side-effects are mild and occur in 17.5% compared to 7.3% in placebo[67]. Systemic side-effects consisting of fever, myalgia and malaise occur in 6–11% of patients and no more frequently than placebo[67,68]. More severe side-effects are exceptionally rare, provided the vaccine is not administered to patients with known egg hypersensitivity (since the vaccine contains traces of chicken egg protein), a history of antibiotic anaphylaxis (since the vaccine has trace quantities of aminoglycosides and polymyxin). Other side-effects include a direct-type hypersensitivity reaction to thimerosal preservative, and an uncertain relation to the Guillain–Barré syndrome which was noted in an immunisation programme directed against swine influenza. However, even if there was a risk of Guillain–Barré syndrome, this risk is much less than the predicted risk of influenza complications[69]. There was one case report suggesting recurrent uveitis. The vaccine is not contraindicated in pregnancy. Concerns over increase in theophylline and warfarin levels mediated through depressed hepatic cytochrome p450 activity are largely theoretical. Temporary false positive ELISA tests for HIV and HCV can occur[70].

The responsibility for strategies to improve the uptake of influenza vaccine lies primarily with family physicians. Reminders on patient's scheduled lists, availability of vaccination sessions at the surgery, or home-mobile units for the elderly are possible approaches. Another possibility is for hospitals to vaccinate all elderly high risk outpatients and inpatients. The Minneapolis Flu

Table 9.6. *Indications for vaccination*

Persons, particularly elderly, with high risk conditions (see Table 9.5)	annually
Residents of long-stay institutions	annually
Above persons at start of influenzal epidemic receiving amantadine prophylaxis	

Shot Program achieved almost 80% vaccination uptake of discharged elderly patients[71].

Novel experimental vaccines are being developed in an attempt to improve efficacy particularly in the high risk patients. These include combined live reassortant intranasally administered and inactivated vaccines[72], further subunit vaccines such as HAI, vaccines with potential to preferentially induce high levels of saliva antibodies, for example, orally administered, microencapsulated antigen within biodegradable microspheres[73], genetically manipulated NM/HA to heighten immunogenicity and the use of liposomal delivery systems.

Parainfluenzal infection

Parainfluenza viruses (PIV) also belong to the family *Paramyxoviridae*, genus *paramyxovirus*. They are 150–300 nm, single-stranded RNA viruses consisting of a nucleocapsid which contains the genome, there are P, L and NP proteins. The envelope contains the haemagglutinin-neurominadase and F fusion protein (this is activated via proteases to F_1 and F_2), and its fatty acid composition is derived from the host cell. Interaction between nucleic capsid and the glycoproteins occurs via the hydrophobic M protein.

PIV_1, PIV_2, PIV_3, and PIV_4 are the four human pathogens producing common cold symptoms, flu-like symptoms, laryngo-tracheobronchitis, bronchiolitis and pneumonia. The vast majority of infections occur in children usually aged < 2 years and reinfection is common. PIV_1, PIV_2, and PIV_3 mainly cause croup and laryngitis, whereas pneumonia or bronchiolitis is associated mainly with PIV_3[74]. Otitis media can also occur with PIV. PIV can rarely cause extra-respiratory infections including viraemia, parotitis and meningitis. PIV contribute 8–16% of all viral isolates in the respiratory tract infectious spectrum[75]. There is inconsistency of the seasonal distribution of these viruses. For example, PIV_3 has been found to cause summer epidemics in England and Wales, spring epidemics in Finland, late winter/spring outbreaks in Houston or consistent monthly cases in Michigan[76].

It is rare for PIV to cause respiratory infection in adults despite decay of antibodies with time[77]. PIV antibodies are absent in one-quarter of young adults. When PIV infection does occur the disease is usually mild and cannot be distinguished from uncomplicated influenza. Severe lower respiratory tract infection in immunocompetent adults has rarely been documented[78], including pneumonia which can be associated with pleural effusion. Among immunocompromised adults it has been increasingly documented, for example, in cancer patients and BMT recipients[79]. Approximately 3–10% of such high risk patients develop PIV infection[80]. Lower respiratory tract infection occurs in approximately three-quarters of those infected. The overall mortality rate in such patients is between 30% and 50%, being higher if other concomitant pathogens are present, for example, fungi[79].

Diagnosis can be achieved by culture of respiratory tract samples onto the monkey kidney, LLC-MK2 and mucoepidermoid human lung cancer cell lines, when the cytopathic effect can be demonstrated. Alternatively, monoclonal antibody/immunoperoxidase staining of the earlier expressed antigen on the cell culture samples permits detection of PIV sooner. Other diagnostic tests include antigen detection using radioimmunoassay, or enzyme immunoassays including europium-labelled detector antibody incubation immunoassay methods. Serum antibodies may be demonstrated by haemagglutination inhibition and enzyme immunoassays.

Treatment is similar to that described for influenza. Amantadine and rimantadine have activity against PIV but there is limited experience. Ribavirin, interferon, protease inhibitors are candidate antiviral drugs.

Vaccination efforts include inactivated vaccines which are so far ineffective. Experimental or novel vaccines include the use of bovine PIV_3, cold adapted temperature sensitive mutants of PIV_3, F glycoprotein defective mutants, recombinant vector virus and PIV_3 subunit vaccines. The use of the cotton-rat model is a significant advance in pre-human testing of some of these vaccines. This will do much to allay the fears of inducing atypical or severe forms of post-vaccination disease that have been observed in, for example, RSV vaccine preparations.

Respiratory syncytial virus

Virology and epidemiology

Human Respiratory Syncytial Virus (RSV) is a single-stranded negative sense RNA virus (family *Paramyxoviridae*, genus *Pneumovirus*). Two subgroups A and B are identified. Of the ten virus proteins coded by the RSV genome, the cellular attachment glycoprotein (G) and the fusion protein (F) – important for subsequent cellular entry – are important in governing infection/replication. Both RSV-A and RSV-B have stable F-glycoproteins (50% related for the two) and are conserved among isolates seen over many years, but they are only less than 5% related in G-glycoprotein. This significant antigenic heterogeneity in the major RSV groups[81,82] could explain the occurrence of repeated RSV infections and lack of protection despite high levels of neutralising antibodies to surface glycoproteins and specific IgA nasal antibodies[83]. Similar respiratory syncytial viruses responsible for respiratory disease are found in other animal species including cattle particularly calves, sheep, goats and monkeys. Despite their similarity, there does not appear to be any instance of non-human RSV transmitted from animals to humans.

Outbreaks of RSV occur in autumn/winter/spring with major peaking in the winter months and minor peaks in the spring[84,85], in temperate zones and at the times of the rains[86] in tropical countries. Transmission is believed to be via large rather than small aerosol droplets, facilitated by damp conditions either by direct inoculation contact or inhalation.

Following infection, shedding of RSV lasts for a mean of approximately 1 week (range 2–10 days), being slightly less in adults compared to children. Some believe that RSV transmission occurs within rather than between communities or regions[85]. However, the existence of a persistently infected carrier has not been identified. Other explanations include a low background rate of infection in summer months or reintroduction of RSV into communities. The majority of RSV infections occur in children < 2 years of age. In fact, over 90% of children have serological evidence of previous RSV infection. It is thought that 1% of all infants in the general population will be hospitalized for RSV infection during their first year of life[87]. Therefore, only a few older children, adults and elderly, are vulnerable to primary RSV infection. Reinfection with RSV is common in the first 4 years of life[88]. Previous exposure appears to reduce the severity of any subsequent RSV disease.

RSV is the most frequently isolated virus in children with respiratory infections particularly those under 3 years of age. One-half of all paediatric pneumonias are due to RSV. Aspects of paediatric RSV have been reviewed in Chapter 23.

There is increasing evidence that RSV can produce both infection and disease in adults[89–91]. In families where RSV is introduced by older siblings, the attack rate among adults is of the order of 17%[90] and associated respiratory tract clinical illness occurs in many of those infected. Among hospital personnel caring for infected patients with RSV, respiratory illness can occur in approximately 50%[92] and underscores the increasing role RSV is playing in nosocomial acquired respiratory tract infections. RSV outbreaks have also been described among the elderly in chronic care institutions[92,93]. Infections can be life threatening among immunocompromised patients[94,95]. It seems that RSV is often overlooked and contributes far more to acute respiratory disease in the elderly than was formally recognised. It may be as important as influenza in this age-group. Thus, in a report by a network of sentinel general practitioners increases in adult respiratory diseases, deaths, RSV or influenza isolates in elderly people showed strong similarities in timing[96]. In the elderly age-group it may not be possible to clinically differentiate influenza from RSV infection[93]. Furthermore, virological investigations are infrequently performed in that group, contrary to the situation in children. More epidemiological–virological data are needed to clarify the picture. Although the illness is generally mild in the elderly, severe manifestations and death have been described[93].

Clinical manifestations

Although the majority of illness is confined to the upper respiratory tract as indicated by predominant symptoms such as rhinitis and earache, moderately severe lower respiratory tract involvement has been documented. Pneumonia and bronchiolitis are the most frequent presentations of lower respiratory tract infection in children (see Chapter 23). Clinical features in adults may simulate influenza particularly in the elderly[97]. Other characteristic features are nasal congestion, otitis media, sinusitis, fever, dry irritative cough, chest pain, tachypnea, sore throat and hoarseness. There is associated heightened airways reactivity and a significantly increased airways resistance which may be prolonged for several weeks. This may clinically manifest as wheeze; rhonchi or crepitations may also be auscultated. These changes may be related to sensitisation of airways receptors induced by epithelial viral damage and resultant production and persistence of respiratory epithelial bound IgE[98].

In immunocompromised adults including those with cardiac transplantation[99], HIV[100] and bone marrow transplantation[101], RSV can assume a more virulent role with an appreciable mortality[101]. RSV was an unexpected finding among several immunocompromised adults (bone marrow transplant, renal transplant, renal and pancreas transplant and T-cell lymphoma). Four of 11 patients died, despite aerosolized ribavirin[95].

The chest radiograph may be normal but bilateral interstitial infiltrates, lobar infiltrates or pleural effusions may occur.

The diagnosis is made by detection of early viral antigen expressed on naso-pharyngeal epithelial cells after culture of nasal washings (best yield), naso-pharyngeal aspiration, pulmonary secretions or bronchoalveolar lavage specimens. Rapid detection immunoassay tests are available with sensitivity and specificity in excess of 90%[102]. Serological diagnosis is a much less sensitive diagnostic tool due to lack of production of complement fixating antibodies.

Most experience in the specific treatment of RSV has been gained in the paediatric population. Ribavirin, a nucleoside analogue, is the treatment of choice. It has to be administered by aerosol. Earlier mechanical problems in patients on ventilators have been overcome. It is not clear just how beneficial this treatment is when administered to all paediatric patients with RSV, and some selective targeting appears justified, for example, those patients with underlying immune deficiency or cardiac disease[103]. Some investigations have been performed in young adult volunteers with aerosolized ribavirin at a dose of 0.8 mg/kg body weight which has been shown to diminish systemic symptoms and viral shedding[104].

Other treatment modalities under investigation include capsid binding agents such as the pyridazinamine R61837 and pirodavir which have been shown in experimental rhinoviral infections to be safe and efficacious in prophylaxis[104,105]. Other experimental treatment modalities include intravenous high titre anti-RSV globulin, aerosolized anti-RSV antibodies with/without corticosteroids and combinations of aerosolized ribavirin and immunoglobulin[106].

Nasal inflammation and cold symptoms, if troublesome, may be suppressed by combination intranasal and systemic glucocorticoids[107].

Initial studies with inactivated vaccine and to some extent with subunit vaccines not only fail to prevent RSV infection but increase the severity of the illness of the subsequently contracted natural RSV infection. This may have occurred either through failure to produce neutralising antibodies or by inadvertent stimulation of host cytotoxic CD4 cells[87,106]. Attention is therefore now focused on using live attenuated vaccines. Initial animal studies suggest safety and efficacy against subsequent RSV challenge. Novel approaches using vaccinia or adenoviral RSV recombinant vectored vaccines as well as peptide vaccines are being explored[108]. If vaccines prove successful and safe, then the target risk population has to be defined.

Adenovirus infections

Virology, immunology and pathology

Adenoviruses are 70 nm non-enveloped double-stranded DNA viruses with over 200 hexons (these produce type specific neutralising antibodies) composing the outer shell. Cellular attachment occurs by means of vertex situated penton (group-specifying antigens) fibres (which give rise to haemagglutinin inhibiting antibodies). Only a few of the 50 human types produce disease. Different types are associated with particular disease manifestations, ranging from paediatric diarrhoea, haemorrhagic cystitis, pharyngocon junctival fever to laryngotracheo-bronchitis and pneumonia. In immunocompromised patients, disseminated disease may occur.

In cases of lower respiratory tract infection, the virus appears to replicate in bronchiolar epithelial cells but there is gene expression in alveolar macrophages, monocytes and hilar lymph nodes[109]. The pathogenesis of adenoviral pneumonia has been investigated in a mouse model. Early phase infection involves induction of TNF-α, IL1 and IL6 which recruits lymphocytes and the late phase consists of a lymphocytic perivascular/peribronchial infiltration possibly mediated by cytotoxic T-cell responses following signalling by viral expressed proteins[110].

There is a tendency for the virus to persist in lymphoid tissues through viral driven inhibition of lysis of the infected cells and inhibition of interferon, natural killer cell and cytotoxic T-cell functions which would normally destroy the virus.

Epidemiology and clinical manifestations

Adenoviruses are responsible for approximately 3% of all pneumonias in children. In adults, pneumonia has been documented rarely in healthy individuals. Infections occur either sporadically (types 11, 14, 16, and 21)[111–113] or in outbreaks either in the community such as those occurring among military recruits or in hospitals (types 3, 4, 7, 19, 35)[114,115].

Spread from person to person occurs via inhalation, faecal–oral contamination or direct inoculation of the conjunctival sacs.

The illness is often severe with one-third of all cases requiring hospitalisation. Severe illness usually occurs more often in children than in adults. Adults usually have a self-limiting course. Mortality is substantially high in children with up to 20% dying. Nevertheless, fatalities have been described in otherwise healthy adults[114]. However, in the immunocompromised host a severe illness can occur particularly in recipients of bone marrow and renal transplantation[116].

Specific pathognomonic clinical features are not often present. However, preceding rhinitis, pharyngitis, hoarseness, cervical lymphadenopathy, maculopapular rash, insidious onset, rhabdomyolysis, myoglobulinuria, DIC, and multiorgan failure have all been described[112]. Characteristic of the disease appears to be a prolonged post-infective impaired pulmonary function profile, particularly restrictive disease.

Sputum, conjunctival secretions, throat or rectal swabs can be used for viral isolation. Tissue culture on human epithelial cell/embryonic kidney lines produces bunches of round cells. Electron-microscopical appearances are diagnostic. Since the virus can be excreted in an asymptomatic person a positive conjunctival isolate is more suggestive of acute infection than a positive isolate from the other sources. Detection of viral antigens from tissue culture or from exfoliated conjunctival or respiratory cells by immunofluorescence provides an alternative early diagnostic mode. Biopsy may show intranuclear inclusions and adenovirus can be confirmed by immunofluorescence staining. Serological diagnosis is accomplished by demonstrating a four-fold rise in haemagglutination inhibition or neutralising antibodies from the baseline levels.

There are no effective antiviral agents and treatment is largely supportive. Secondary bacterial infection is treated with antibiotics.

A safe and 95% effective vaccine is available and has been used extensively in American service men[117]. Adenovirus types 4 and 7 have been partially attenuated in human diploid fibroblast cell lines and administered as an enteric coated tablet[118]. Some intrafamilial spread, however, of the virus has been documented. There is no substantial ongoing vaccine programme in this field.

Measles

Virology, immunology and pathology

This section will focus on measles in adults.

The measles virus, a member of the *Paramyxoviridae* family and genus *Morbillivirus*, has produced widespread disease in childhood before the advent of vaccination. Vaccination programmes have resulted in a substantial decline in paediatric measles.

Measles pneumonitis is a severe complication characterised histopathologically by multinucleated giant cells with eosinophilic cytoplasmic and intranuclear inclusions. Other changes include diffuse alveolar damage, interstitial pneumonitis without giant cells and necrotising bronchiolitis. This indicates a spectrum of histology depending on the degree of immunocompetence, duration and tempo of the disease[119]. The primary reaction in measles virus-infected lungs is thought to be an increase in CD8+ and CD8+ CD11b – cells seen in BAL fluid[120].

There has been a resurgence in preschool measles in recent years in children who had never been vaccinated. The lack of full vaccination coverage has also been responsible for an increase in cases among adults. In New York city in 1991, for example, 15% of the confirmed measles cases occurred in persons > 20 years of age[121]. The CDC has reported that 40% of cases of measles between 1988 and 1990 occurred in individuals of reproductive age[122]. Measles pneumonitis occurred in 72% of South Indian children in a recent survey[123]. Other reports indicates pneumonia complications in between 3% and 65% of patients[124–126].

The mortality in adult measles pneumonitis in general appears to be lower than that in children. However, mortality rates reported vary considerably between 1%[123] up to 36%[124,127]. Although it is suggested that adult measles pneumonitis is mild and usually nonfatal[125,126] recent publications have suggested that life-threatening measles pneumonitis in adults may be more common than previously appreciated regardless of the patient's immune status[121]. Nevertheless in patients with malignancy or immunocompromisation, mortality is usually high[124]. One of the six patients who died in Forni's series had presumed HIV infection[121]. Pregnancy also carries a significant risk factor for measles mortality[128], although that has not always been reported or appreciated.

Clinical

Patients with measles pneumonitis usually develop the pulmonary complication against the clinical background of classical measles. However, atypical presentations of measles pneumonitis without rash or other manifestation of measles does occur usually in the setting of patients with cell-mediated immune defects[121]. This poses a dilemma for diagnosis.

Following an incubation period of approximately 14 days and a prodrome of fever, upper respiratory tract congestion, rhinitis, conjunctivitis (Fig. 9.1 (*a*)) and cough, the exanthem appears. This is a maculopapular blotchy papular rash appearing first on the face (Fig. 9.1 (*a*), (*b*)) and behind the ears and spreading within 3 days to involve the remainder of the body. Koplik spots on the buccal mucosa appear at this time (Fig. 9.2). Natural resolution of the rash and symptoms is the norm for most patients, but clinical encephalopathy, enteritis, subacute combined sclerosing panencephalitis and tuberculosis reactivation occur in some patients.

Measles pneumonia is characterised by continued fever, increased cough, and progressive respiratory failure. The onset usually coincides with the rash. Secondary superinfection with bacterial pneumonia is uncommon unlike the situation in children where *Staphylococcus* is a particularly frequent secondary invader in which case toxic shock syndrome is a definite possibility[129].

Chest radiographical findings may show bilateral interstitial infiltrates, focal or diffuse reticulo/nodular shadows/alveolar infiltrates or bilateral severe alveolar opacification suggesting adult respiratory distress syndrome[121]. CT scanning appears to be much more sensitive and can detect pulmonary radiographical abnormalities in twice as many patients as plain radiology, even in patients with suspected pneumonia whose plain radiographs are clear. Ground glass opacifications, nodular opacities and consolidation can be revealed by CT scanning[130].

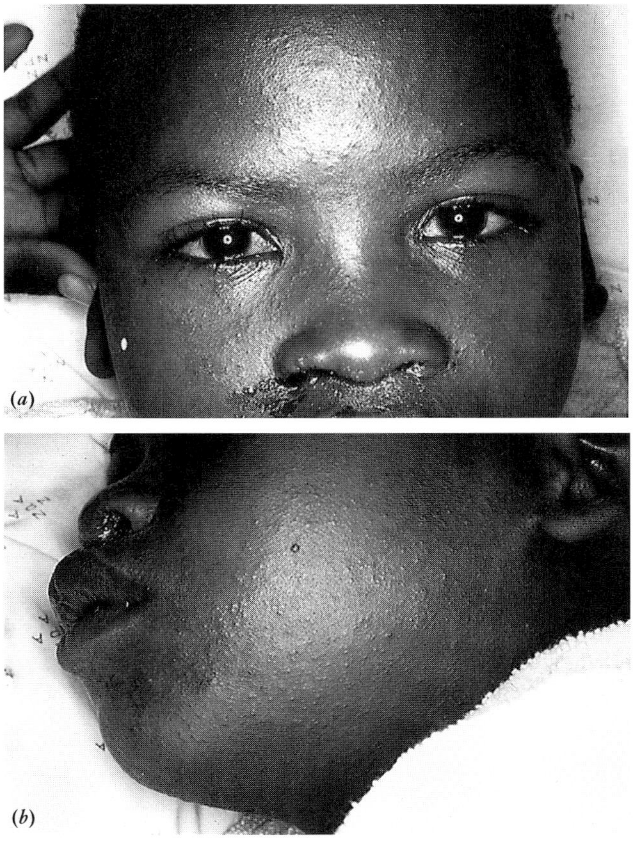

FIGURE 9.1 (*a*) Young adult with conjunctivitis, rhinitis of measles. (*b*) The papular nature of measles rash is best appreciated in side-lighting.

Profound hypoxemia and substantive alveolar-arterial oxygen gradients are found. Increases in ALT, thrombocytopenia, hypocalcaemia, ECG evidence of myocarditis and raised CPK levels may also be present[121].

Current experience suggest that many patients with adult measles pneumonitis will require mechanical ventilation. Should measles complicate pregnancy, then premature labour and spontaneous abortion are additional complications[128].

The diagnosis is made from the typical clinical presentation. Serological confirmation is with ELISA. Tissue biopsy may be necessary. Multinucleate giant cells may also be observed in the sputum.

Recently, the use of intravenously administered ribavirin to achieve high plasma levels has been suggested as efficacious. Thus, five of six patients with severe measles pneumonitis promptly improved with all abnormal parameters returning to baseline[121]. When given by the aerosol route, although it may at best attenuate symptoms, it does not appear to be very effective[121]. The use of high dose corticosteroids with vitamin A has been reported effective in one near fatal case of adult measles pneumonitis[131]. Based on the knowledge that vitamin A deficiency is common in severe measles[123], possibly due to an effect on epithelial cell maturation, and that vitamin A appears to diminish mortality and morbidity from measles[132], this potential mode of treatment in the setting of measles pneumonitis requires further evaluation.

In the meantime, live attenuated vaccine should continue to be administered as a routine to preschool children. Revaccination of older children and adults should be considered as a future strategy. In addition, the live attenuated vaccine can be administered as prophylaxis at-risk adults in specific situations. High dose measles immunoglobulin can also be administered to contacts of measles cases to prevent the natural illness.

Varicella zoster

This virus produces either chickenpox or herpes zoster. Chickenpox is usually recognised by its typical exanthematous presentation of

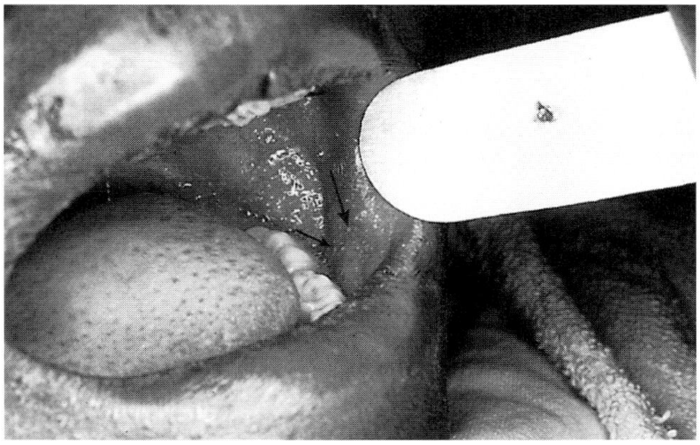

FIGURE 9.2 Koplik's spots.

sequentially occurring erythema, vesicles, pustules and crusts. Herpes zoster displays the same spectrum of rash but in a dermatomal distribution. Occasionally, the varicella zoster virus (VZV) can produce pneumonia. In healthy children pneumonia is rare. In children with cancer, leukaemia and with solid organ transplantations, the risk for pneumonia which is often fatal, is increased[133,134]. In adults, even if they are otherwise healthy, pneumonia can complicate chickenpox in as many as 50%[135–137], although recent series suggest a lower incidence of < 5%[138]. In addition, there is a substantial risk for ventilatory failure in adults with chickenpox pneumonia of the order of 10% and a mortality rate of around 20%[139]. This is even higher in pregnancy and other immunocompromised situations[140]. Although chickenpox *per se* occurs much less frequently in adults than children, 25% of all chickenpox deaths (mainly due to pneumonia) occur in adults[141]. In addition, mild or asymptomatic pulmonary involvement is common. Although zoster is a viraemic illness like chickenpox, pneumonia seems to complicate this expression of VZV less frequently than primary chickenpox. It is crucial for the physician not to dismiss chickenpox as a mild self-limiting disease even in previously normal individuals particularly healthy adults, but rather to recognize the potential for pneumonia, since effective antiviral treatment is available.

Several reports of primary pulmonary chickenpox have appeared since 1942 and a detailed review was published by Knyvit in 1966[142]. The pathogenesis is not clear. Inhalation from oropharyngeal mucosal lesions has been postulated, although it is more likely that pneumonia occurs as part of the generalised secondary viraemic phase following the intense replication in the reticuloendothelial system after the primary viraemia. Vesicles may be found throughout the trachea and bronchi and the pleural surface in the early stage; later scattered necrotic and haemorrhagic lesions are present in a peribronchiolar distribution. An interstitial pneumonitis characterised by mononuclear cell infiltration together with eosinophilic intranuclear inclusion bodies and syncytial giant cells is found. Thickening of the alveolar membrane is also common and intra-alveolar fibrin exudates may be found. Necrotising bronchitis/ bronchiolitis may occasionally be present. Pulmonary hypertension is a possible sequel of arteriolitis. Survivors of chickenpox pneumonia may develop multiple calcified pulmonary nodules.

Risk factors for the development of this complication of varicella-zoster infection include adult age-group and smoking[143,144]. Up to 50% of smokers who have varicella develop varicella pneumonia compared to < 5% of non-smokers[143,145]. Smoking is known to increase the susceptibility of alveolar macrophages to herpes viruses. Pregnancy is another well-recognised predisposition[146], possibly associated with the altered immune status of the mother, for example, thymic involution, pregnancy associated disturbance of immunoregulatory proteins, hormones and enzymes. Other factors which increase the risk for VZV pneumonia include patients with severe immunocompromised states such as cancer, bone marrow transplantation, solid organ transplantation, systemic topical or inhaled steroid usage and acquired congenital immunodeficiencies. Among these, bone marrow transplantation[147] and children with cancer[134] represent some of the highest categories.

Clinically patients present with the typical chickenpox rash, namely centripetally distributed vesicles which evolve to pustules and crusts, appearing in crops waves with each viraemic pulse. New lesions appear for up to 5 days in immunocompetent adults and for up to 14 days in immunocompromised hosts. There is usually a history of exposure to chickenpox within the previous 2–3 weeks. Cough, largely dry (though haemoptysis may be present) dyspnoea and pleuritic chest pain often severe and unremitting, signal the development of pneumonic complications which characteristically develops within 1 week of the rash – slightly longer in the immunocompromised host. Examination usually reveals tachypnea and signs of airways obstruction, namely, intercostal recession and prolonged high pitched expiratory rhonchi. Diffuse crepitations are found. Cyanosis may be present. In milder cases, respiratory examination maybe unremarkable despite radiological abnormalities. Secondary pulmonary bacterial sepsis may be suspected if the sputum is disproportionately purulent. Frank and severe pulmonary haemorrhage and haemothorax may complicate the course of the disease[148]. The rash is often widespread and severe (Fig. 9.3). The occurrence of chickenpox in early pregnancy is associated with a small risk of congenital herpes zoster (Fig. 9.4).

A chest radiograph will reveal diffuse usually bilateral and lower zone 2–5 mm nodular or reticular densities. These may later coalesce

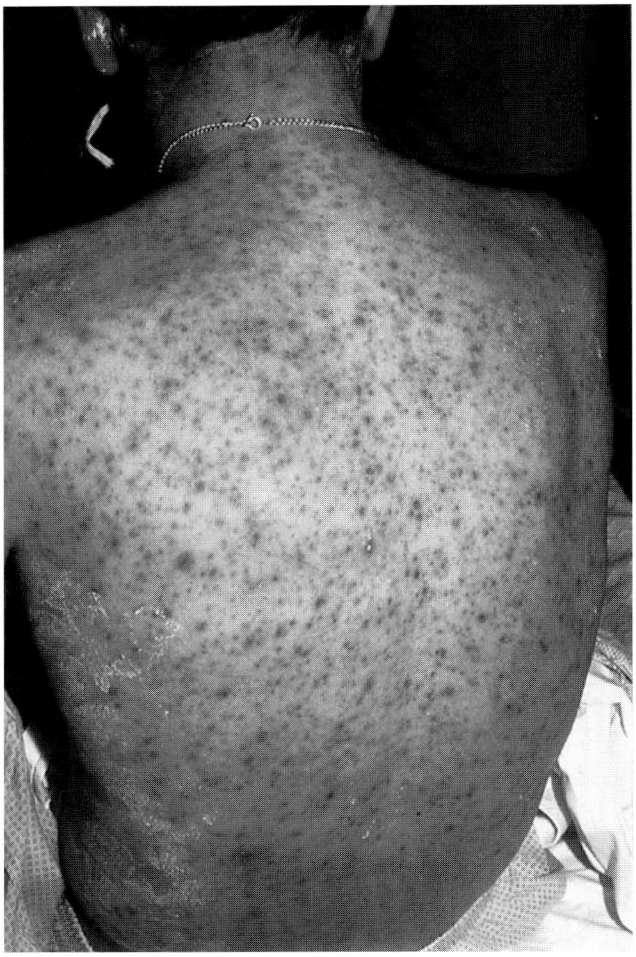

FIGURE 9.3 Chickenpox.

(Fig. 9.5). Occasionally, pleural effusion develops. Residual radiological changes may be present for several months and multiple lower zone small calcified nodules may appear later.

In children with cancer the degree of lymphopenia at the beginning of the chickenpox infection predicts for the development of pneumonitis[134].

Pulmonary function tests reveal profound hypoxaemia and hypocapnia[148,149], reduced peak expiratory flow and reduced FEF25-75, indicating airways obstruction; there is a significant reduction in the carbon monoxide (CO) transfer factor. It is of some interest that the CO transfer factor can be abnormally low in some adults with chickenpox but without clinical signs of pneumonia. It can also remain depressed for several weeks and occasionally for up to 2 years after clinical recovery[143,150].

Treatment

Any adult and any immunocompromised person of whatever age with chickenpox who develops a cough should have a chest radiograph to exclude pneumonia. In established pneumonia, it is common and correct practice to administer intravenous acyclovir despite the absence of prospective controlled studies to confirm an impact on the course of the disease[151,152]. However, a maternal mortality rate of 13% for acyclovir-treated cases of VZV during pregnancy was reported compared to 36% deduced from a review of a series of patients who did not receive antiviral therapy[153]. Retrospective controlled data do suggest that early intravenous acyclovir has a positive effect on clinical recovery and promotes oxygenation in adults with VZV[154]. Anecdotal evidence suggests that, since intravenous acyclovir has been in use since the early 1980s, there has been a fall in the number of patients with established chickenpox pneumonia and who have required ventilation. Others have suggested that the mortality rate of chickenpox pneumonia has not changed since the advent of acyclovir[155]. However, the effect of acyclovir in other severe VZV infections, for example, shingles in the immunocompromised host, has shown statistically significant benefits on viral shedding, dissemination, resolution of rash and acute pain. Recent studies have confirmed the efficacy in paediatric cutaneous chickenpox[156]. It should be instituted early in the course of the disease to optimise the chance of therapeutic success[157].

Acyclovir is a nucleoside analogue in which the deoxyribose moiety of deoxyguanosine has been substituted by an hydroxyethoxymethyl component, and thereby inhibits viral DNA replication. It is active against herpes simplex and VZV. The usual intravenous dosage is

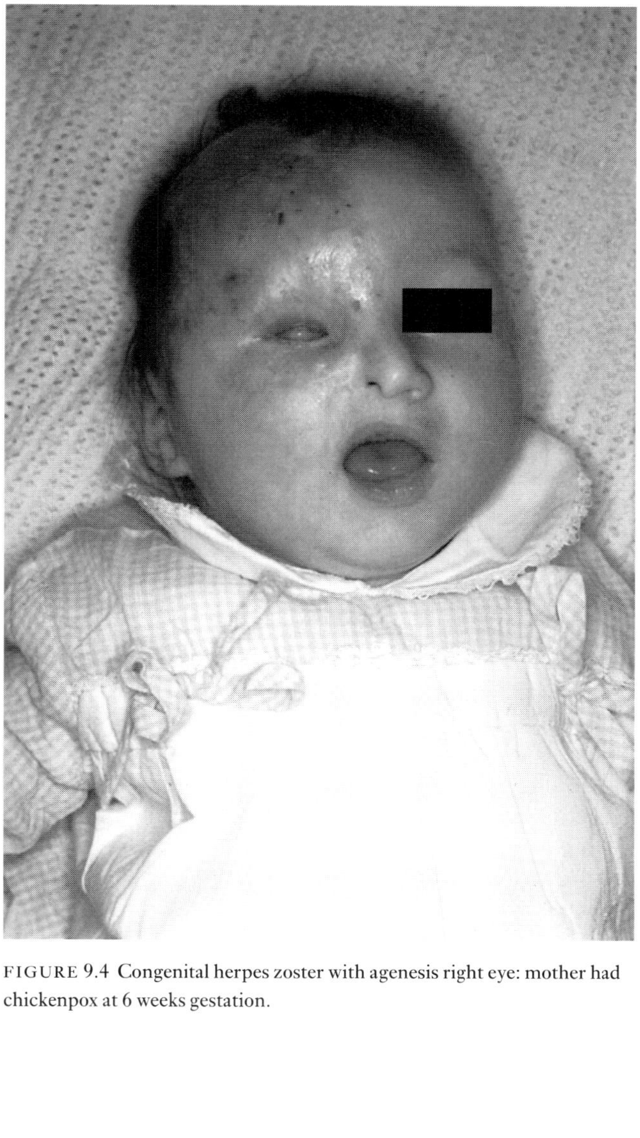

FIGURE 9.4 Congenital herpes zoster with agenesis right eye: mother had chickenpox at 6 weeks gestation.

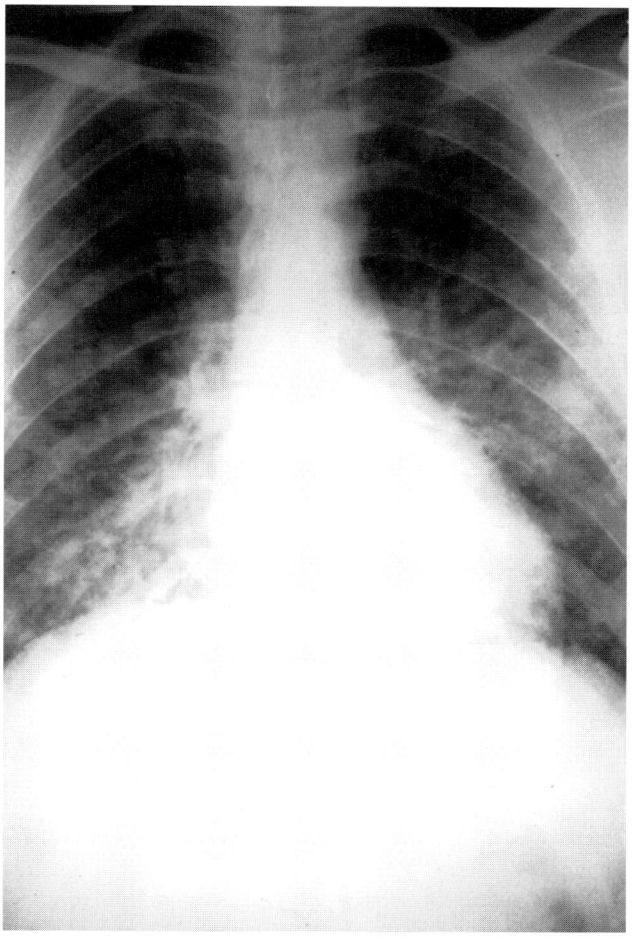

FIGURE 9.5 Chickenpox pneumonia.

10–15 mg/kg Q 8 hourly given for 7–10 days for established chickenpox pneumonia. Toxicity of acyclovir is limited and uncommon – including nausea, vomiting, abdominal pain, impaired renal function (which can be reduced by adequate hydration and slowing the infusion rates) and rarely temporary paresis/neurotoxic side-effects.

Its use in pregnant women is a cause for concern which poses a dilemma since this group of individuals are at a particular risk for chickenpox pneumonia, but acyclovir crosses the placenta and mutagenicity is possible. However, chickenpox acquired in early pregnancy *per se* can also result in foetal malformation (Fig. 9.4). Limited data on its use in mid-trimester has not so far indicated adverse foetal effects[140,153,158]. Although further information is needed, it should be offered to such patients who have symptomatic chickenpox pneumonia.

Although acyclovir resistant mutants (thymidine kinase defective, or altered DNA polymerase strains) of VZV can be raised *in vitro*, clinical instances of resistant strains have not yet been seen[159].

Vidarabine used in a dosage of 10 mg/kg daily intravenously is an alternative nucleoside analogue agent which is also effective but has a greater incidence of and more serious toxic side-effects, including bone marrow suppression and neurological problems such as seizures. In cases not responding to acyclovir, it may be justified to switch to vidarabine. Foscarnet has also been used in therapy but experience is limited. The role of corticosteroids, α-interferon and transfer factor remains controversial.

Some patients may require ventilatory support either with CPAP or with intubation and IPPV. Recently, extracorporeal membrane oxygenation has been used with some success[160].

Appropriate antibiotic administration is also indicated for patients who develop secondary bacterial superinfection, which may occur in approximately 25% of patients with chickenpox pneumonia.

Prophylaxis

The potential for the prevention of chickenpox in those individuals who are at high risk for subsequent chickenpox pneumonia may be addressed by consideration of passive immunisation with VZV immunoglobulin (VZIG) active immunisation or with prophylactic acyclovir.

VZIG has some benefit in protecting susceptible individuals following contact with chickenpox cases. Preparations containing antibody titres of approximately 1/2048 are available and if administered within 96 hours of exposure can reduce the frequency and severity of infection. It is indicated for nonimmune individuals who are exposed to chickenpox and who are at high risk for severe chickenpox, for example, children with immunosuppression and pregnant women. It is also indicated at birth (particularly the premature baby) for the infant born to her mother who develop chickenpox up to 5 days prior or 2 days after delivery since maternally acquired antibodies will not have been passed to the baby transplacentally – this gives passive immunity to the foetus at that time.

Certain susceptible high risk adults may be offered active vaccination against varicella. The vaccine strain has been available for over 20 years and this live attenuated vaccine has been subject to extensive testing in normal and immunocompromised children where it has been found to be safe and effective. In normal adults, an immediate antibody response of 70% occurs which can be boosted to over 90% with second doses, but later falls to 80% and is maintained at about 70% for up to 6 years[161,162]. However, *protection* may be higher than these antibody titres reflect. Clinical studies demonstrate a protective efficacy against attack of about 64% and breakthrough disease appears to be mild. In children the efficacy is higher[162]. Side-effects are mild. Vaccine virus person to person transmission is rare, and emergence of vaccine-associated herpes zoster is a concern. Potential vaccine recipients include nurses and physicians (to prevent nosocomial transmission), and nonimmune females of child-bearing age (to reduce foetal morbidity and maternal morbidity and mortality). Its role in protecting susceptible adult contacts soon after exposure remains to be explored – this has been successful in children. The FDA has recently approved Varivax – chickenpox vaccine.

One study has suggested that oral acyclovir may prevent varicella if started on day 7–9 of the incubation period and continued for 1 week[163]. Another study suggested that oral acyclovir given to immunocompromised children with varicella prevented the development of varicella pneumonitis compared to historical controls[164]. However, its exact role and efficacy in the different risk groups has yet to be precisely determined.

Herpes simplex

Herpes simplex (HSV) is a double-stranded DNA virus, with an icosahedral capsid and a lipid envelope and has an approximate diameter of 180 nm. In common with all other herpes viruses latency is a key feature. HSV1 and HSV2 are differentiated clinically, epidemiologically, biochemically and biologically.

Infection of the local epithelial cells with cell lysis, followed by lymphatic drainage to regional lymph nodes and thence viraemia with distant dissemination is the proposed mechanism of infection and disease. The likelihood of viraemia is dependent upon the host immune integrity. Cell-mediated immunity through macrophages, natural killer cells as well as cytokine production for example interferons, are felt to be the major factors in controlling disease dissemination. Antibodies are felt to play a lesser role.

Superior cervical, trigeminal, vagal and sacral ganglia are sites of latency. Reactivation of the latent virus results in viral replication in the neurones without neuronal lysis, travel along the sensory nerve pathway and viral assembly in the anatomically appropriate and predominantly squamous epithelial cells.

HS viruses are ubiquitous. Spread is by person-to-person through mucosal, corneal, or skin abrasion contact with infected secretions.

Clinical

Primary herpetic gingivostomatitis, genital infection, ocular infections and encephalitis are the most common manifestations of herpes simplex infections in both the immunocompetent and immunocompromised host. In the immunocompromised host including the neonate severe local mucocutaneous disease or generalised/disseminated infections can occur. The respiratory tract is a rather uncommon site of involvement.

In the neonate, severe bilateral HSV pneumonia can occur as a result of passage through the infected birth canal and aspiration by the baby. Respiratory distress presents at approximately 4–9 days postpartum.

The precise role of HSV in producing lower respiratory infection in general is often difficult to delineate. The relation between a positive identification in respiratory secretions, pulmonary function and clinical outcome is not always clear. Nevertheless, herpetic tracheobronchitis has been documented in otherwise normal persons or following surgery[165,166].

The first time HSV pneumonitis was documented was in the early 1980s[167]. Since then only approximately 70 such cases have been documented and most cases have been diagnosed based on post-mortem demonstration of HSV inclusion bodies. Most cases of HSV pneumonitis occur in severely immunocompromised patients or in patients with extensive burns or in patients with adult respiratory distress syndrome[167]. In an extensive review of over 500 patients with allogeneic bone marrow transplantation over a 10-year period, HSV pneumonitis was found to account for 5% of nonbacterial pneumonias[168]. The incidence and occurrence therefore of HSV pneumonitis is rather uncommon and occurs usually in critically ill or severely immunocompromised patients.

In a study of 308 patients with severe respiratory distress, HSV was the most commonly found pathogen in lower respiratory secretions and was present in 12% (mainly ventilated patients)[169].

The major problem therefore centres on the interpretation of a positive finding of HSV in respiratory secretions in a patient with respiratory distress, because asymptomatic upper respiratory tract HSV shedding occurs in up to 10% of normal individuals[170]. This rate is considerably increased, up to 80%[171], by such factors as trauma of the airways, for example, intubation, burns, radiotherapy, chemotherapy, surgery, and immunocompromisation – through reactivation of latent virus[172]. Reactivation is postulated to occur through mechanical stimulation of relevant ganglia – postulated to be the vagal ganglia in the case of HIV lower respiratory infections, or mediated through fall-off in cell mediated immunity. HSV can also be aspirated into the more distal parts of the respiratory tree. Alternatively, HSV can invade lung tissue from a hematogenous route outside of the pulmonary source.

In patients with a positive isolate from respiratory secretions, demonstrable cytopathic effects, herpes simplex antigens, nucleic acid sequencing and quantitation of HSV cultures in bronchial washes or in BAL analogous to bacterial infections have not been systematically evaluated in patients with lower respiratory tract infections. However, in patients with ARDS – particularly the severely immunocompromised such as leukaemics on chemotherapy, organ transplant recipients and patients with cancer – from whom no other pathogen apart from herpes simplex has been found, and in whom there is bronchoscopical evidence of herpetic tracheobronchitis, it is currently generally accepted that HSV is a likely cause of the pneumonia. Herpetic tracheobronchitis is characterised by the presence of oedema, erythema, mucosal friability, ulcerations, vesicles and grey membranes[172].

Histologically proven parenchymal involvement on tissue biopsy due to HSV demonstrated by direct immunofluorescence staining is therefore helpful in establishing a firm diagnosis of disease rather than infection. Thus, in one series of HSV in lower respiratory tract secretions in patients with adult respiratory distress syndrome HSV could not be demonstrated on lung biopsy[167]. However, sampling error could have led to non-pathogenic areas being biopsied.

Bronchial HSV infection has been associated with fever, wheeze, cough, and bronchospasm[165]. Dyspnoea and diffuse infiltrates suggest HSV parenchymal involvement. The finding of concomitant pathogens such as bacteria, CMV and fungi which occurs in approximately half of all patients with HSV[173], again poses a dilemma for the interpretation of the precise role of HSV. The presence of associated mucocutaneous lesions in many patients with a pneumonia may be helpful in making a diagnosis of HSV pneumonia[173].

Treatment of established HSV pneumonitis is with acyclovir, foscarnet, or vidarabine. The use of prophylactic acyclovir in severely immunocompromised patients appears to be effective in reducing the incidence of reactivation of herpes simplex infections, e.g. following bone marrow transplantation[174] or in patients with solid organ transplantations including heart–lung transplantations[175].

Epstein–Barr virus

This double-stranded DNA virus is 200 nm in diameter, composed of an enveloped hexagonal nucleocapsid. In contrast to its established role in infectious mononucleosis, an association with Burkett's lymphoma and other proliferative disorders, nasopharyngeal carcinoma and possibly associated with the chronic fatigue syndrome, its role in pulmonary disease appears to be somewhat unclear but probably rare.

Nevertheless, Epstein–Barr virus (EBV) has been detected using specific monoclonal antibodies extensively in the lungs of 7/61 patients dying with diffuse interstitial pneumonia secondary to malignancy, leukaemia, collagen vascular disease and immunosuppression compared to none in the controls[176]. The alveolar lining pneumocytes, intra-alveolar cells, bronchial and bronchiolar epithelial cells were mainly involved. Unlike HSV and CMV, however, cytological transformation or inclusion bodies were not observed and raises questions concerning the role of EBV in pneumonia.

The frequency of pulmonary involvement in patients with infectious mononucleosis varies between 0% and 5%[177,178]. Even in those patients with pulmonary infiltrates, other aetiological agents have not always been ruled out. A few cases in which the association was circumstantially strong have been described[178,179]. However, definitive diagnosis requires tissue evidence of pathological invasion by the virus. In Schooley's two cases, although extremely high titre of antibody to replicative antigen of EBV were described and transbronchial lung biopsy showed an interstitial infiltrate of intra-alveolar mature lymphocytes with involvement of the peribronchioles and veins, definitive proof of lung tissue involvement by EBV, for example, using DNA hybrid analysis was lacking. However, there was a clear response to acyclovir.

EBV has been implicated in the aetiology of lymphocytic interstitial pneumonitis (LIP)[180] – a disorder associated with hypergammaglobulinaemia, autoimmune disorders particularly Sjögren's syndrome and malignancy. Archival lung tissue samples of such patients with LIP has revealed a B lymphocyte interstitial infiltrate, and *in situ* hybridisation studies revealed EBV genome in 9/14 patients[181]. EBV may provoke the proliferation of B lymphocytes in a number of patients with LIP.

An association has also been shown between paediatric HIV-associated LIP and EBV. Lung biopsies of such patients have shown the presence of EBV DNA[182]. The presence of HIV RNA in lung biopsy specimens[183] and the understanding that EBV cells have increased susceptibility to HIV, raises the possibility of EBV/HIV interaction in the genesis of AIDS related LIP. Symptoms of LIP include dyspnoea, cough, sweats, hepatosplenomegaly, parotid gland enlargement and Sicca syndrome. Chest radiography shows diffuse (including lower lobar), reticular nodular shadowing/infiltrates. BAL may indicate lymphocytosis with CD_8 cells. Steroids may prove effective[184].

The diagnosis of EBV infection can be made by demonstrating heterophile antibodies by the monospot test. EBV specific antibodies should be measured in cases of suspected pneumonia: IgM viral capsid antibodies appear at clinical presentation and last for up to 2 months, followed by anti-D/anti-R at 2–4 weeks, then EBV nuclear antibody and soluble complement fixating antigens at 4 weeks. DNA hybridisation/monoclonal antibodies will detect virus in tissue.

Although acyclovir appears to diminish oropharyngeal shedding of EBV, no clinical effect has been documented on the clinical course of interstitial pneumonia. It appears to inhibit EBV specific DNA replication in cell lines but has no effect on the latent EBV genome[185]. Although it had no effect on two paediatric patients with life threatening EBV infection (both had underlying immune disorders)[185] it did appear useful in two other patients with suspected EBV pneumonia who were apparently immunocompetent[179]. Despite the absence of controlled studies designed to test efficacy, acyclovir should currently be administered to patients with suspected/proven EBV pneumonia.

Steroids appear to be useful in some cases of LIP[184].

Other experimental modalities of treatment include drugs known to inhibit EBV *in vitro* including desciclovir, sorivudine, interferons and phosphonoacetic acid.

Human herpes virus 6

Virology, immunology and pathology

In 1986 a new virus with morphological characteristics of the herpes viruses was discovered in patients with lymphoproliferative disorders[186] and termed human B lymphotropic virus, and later human herpes virus 6 (HHV6). It is an enveloped double-stranded virus of approximately 180 nm. There is marked tropism for CD_4 cells, monocytes, macrophages, glial cells, fibroblasts and epithelial cells (being found in salivary glands, bronchial glands and pneumocytes)[187–189]. It is now recognised that HHV-6A and HHV-6B variants exist[190].

The precise role of HHV6 in cases of pneumonia with which it is associated is not known. The pathogenic mechanisms remain unclear at this stage but epithelial cell lysis, pulmonary macrophage damage, induction of co-infection or damage by other pathogens such as CMV, and cytokine induction have been postulated.

There is an increasing frequency of seropositivity to HHV6 from 6 months of age to 3 years when almost 100% of children have antibodies. Thereafter this falls to about 65% in adults[191,192].

Decline in transplacentally acquired antibodies is thought to be responsible for the fall in levels of neonatal HHV6 antibodies down to 6 months of age and thereafter increasing. Respiratory transmission may be one route of infection although little is known of precise mechanisms of transmission.

Clinical

A number of clinical syndromes have been associated (but not necessarily causal) with HHV6. These include exanthema subitum – an infectious mononucleosis like syndrome – histiocytic necrotising lymphadenopathy (Kikuchi's lymphadenitis), chronic fatigue syndrome, lymphoproliferative disease, erythrophagocytic syndrome, hepatitis and pneumonia.

The association of HHV6 with pneumonia in otherwise healthy individuals appears rare. The consensus of opinion is that it is not often associated with lower respiratory tract infection in infants, although exanthema subitum when associated with upper respiratory tract involvement such as rhinitis is generally accepted as being due to HHV6[193]. It has been described in association with Legionnaire's disease in adults[194].

In HIV-infected persons HHV6 has been postulated both to suppress HIV replication[195] and to increase HIV expression in T-cells[196].

In patients with bone marrow transplantation, HHV-6 associated pneumonia has been described[197,198], sometimes in association with other pathogens which include CMV, adenovirus and aspergillus[188,199]. Its role in other immunocompromised hosts remains unclear at this time. These findings together with the detection of HHV6 in normal tissue[199] demand further clarification as to whether HHV-6 can be primarily pathological, indirectly or directly co-pathological with other organisms or be merely a passenger virus in cases of pneumonia.

Methods for the diagnosis of HHV6 infection include IgG/IgM antibody determination, culture (which is insensitive and lengthy) or nucleic acid/viral antigen detection. In lung tissue from patients with interstitial pneumonitis, HHV6 can be documented using monoclonal antibody stains, and without any cross-reactivity to other viruses such as cytomegalovirus and adenovirus, although these may also be present in the lung tissue[88]. However, HHV6 can be found in the lung tissue of normal individuals[199] suggesting the lung may be a site of latency for subsequent HHV6 reactivation.

HHV6 is sensitive *in vitro* to ganciclovir or foscarnet though proof of *in vivo* therapeutic efficacy is difficult to establish in view of the uncertainties of its precise role in pneumonia. Methylprednisolone had appeared to be highly successful in one case of coinfection of Legionella/HHV6[194].

Hantavirus pulmonary syndrome

Hantaviruses (HTV) are negative-sense RNA viruses belonging to the *Bunyaviridae* family. Transmission to humans from different primary rodents results in a haemorrhagic fever with renal syndrome. This syndrome has a number of clinical variants ranging from a mild HTV illness caused by Puumala virus called nephropathia epidemica (fever, acute renal failure, thrombocytopenia, with or without ophthalmological complications), a more severe form (SEO) virus most frequently found in Asia to the most severe and often fatal forms of haemorrhagic fever due to Hantaan virus found, for example, in Korea, Japan and China. However, pulmonary involvement is not a feature of the previously recognised causes of haemorrhagic fever with renal syndrome.

In 1993, several deaths characterised by adult respiratory distress syndrome occurring in previously healthy individuals were reported in the four corners region of Arizona, Colorado, New Mexico and

Utah[200,201]. Clinical characteristics included an influenza-like illness with fever and myalgia, followed several days later by dyspnoea, hypoxia, pulmonary oedema, hypotension and death in 50% of those infected. Laboratory findings included thrombocytopenia, haemoconcentration, neutrophil leukocytosis and atypical lymphocytosis.

Initial laboratory testing failed to reveal a known specific causal agent, although there appeared to be an active immune response to HTV[202]. However, the pattern of reactivity was irregular for the different known HTVs. PCR amplification of RNA extracted from lung/liver tissues demonstrated that patients were infected with the same virus that had been found in rodents of the area and this subsequently proved to be a new species of HTV[203].

The major reservoir for the virus is the deer mouse *Peromyscus maniculatus*. The virus has been named the Sin Nombre virus[204]. In fact, this virus has been known for many years and it is of some interest and concern that severe human disease associated with it has only recently emerged. Genetic mutation or increase in the rodent population are possible mechanisms for this phenomenon[202].

The virus appears to be particularly trophic for the lung, endothelial cell and pulmonary macrophages. In most cases an interstitial pneumonitis characterised by a variable mononuclear cell infiltrate, oedema, focal hyaline membrane formation, and to a lesser extent diffuse alveolar damage and airspace disorganisation. Hantaviral antigens are detected in the endothelial cells[204]. Increased vascular permeability results from cytokine recruitment (e.g. TNF-α, interleukin-1, monocyte chemoattractant protein-1 and lipid mediators)[202], and leads to lethal pulmonary oedema.

This newly emerged human disease is being closely monitored. No effective known therapy currently exists.

Table 9.7. *Efficacy of specific antiviral management*

	Antiviral treatment	Antiviral prophylaxis	Active vaccination	Passive vaccination
Influenza	$++^{1}$	$++^{1}$	$++$	0
Parainfluenza	$\pm^{1}$	$\pm^{1}$	$-$	0
RSV	$+^{2}$	0	0	$\pm$
Adenovirus	0	0	$+$	$-$
Measles	$+^{3}$	0	$++$	$++$
VZV	$++^{4/5}$	$\pm^{4}$	$++$	$++$
Herpes simplex	$\pm^{4/5}$	$+^{4}$	0	0
EBV	$\pm^{4}$	0	0	0
HHV6	$\pm^{6}$	0	0	0
Sin Nombre	0	0	0	0

Efficacy:
0 = no evidence/not available.
– = no benefit.
± = possible benefit.
\+ = some benefit.
++ = good beneficial effect.

Drugs:
1 = amantadine/rimantadine.
2 = ribavirin aerosol.
3 = ribavirin IV.
4 = acyclovir.
5 = vidarabine.
6 = ganciclovir.

References

1. LEIGH MW, CARSON JL, DENNY FW. Pathogenesis of respiratory infections due to influenza virus: implications for developing countries. *Rev Inf Dis* 1991;13 (Suppl 6):5501–8.
2. RAZA MW, BLACKMORE CC, MOLYNEAUS P *et al.* Association between secretor status and respiratory viral illness. *Br Med J* 1991;303:815–18.
3. AHERNE W, BIRD T, COURT SDM *et al.* Pathological changes in virus infections of the lower respiratory tract in children. *J Clin Path* 1970;23:7–12.
4. SULLIVAN JL, MAYNER RE, BARRY DW, ENNIS FA. Influenza virus infection in nude mice. *J Infect Dis* 1976;133:91–7.
5. ENNIS FA. Some newly recognised aspects of resistance against and recovering from influenza. *Arch Virol* 1982;73:207–12.
6. ADA GL, JONES PD. The immune response to influenza infection. *Curr Top, Microbiol Immunol* 1986;128:1–54.
7. IDA S, HOOK JJ, SIRAGANIAN RP, NOTKINS AL. Enhancement of IgE mediated histamine release from human basophils by viruses: role of interferon. *J Exp Med* 1977;145:892–906.
8. NICHOLSON KG, KENT J, IRELAND DC. Respiratory viruses and exacerbations of asthma in adults. *BMJ* 1993;307:982–6.
9. COUCH RB. Effects of influenza and host defence. *J Infect Dis* 1981;144:284–91.
10. SCHEIBLAUER H, REINACHER M, TASHIRO M, ROTT R. Interactions between bacteria and influenza A virus in the development of pneumonia. *J Infect Dis* 1992;166:783–91.
11. BARBER WH, SMALL PA JR. Local and systemic immunity to influenza infections in ferrets. *Infect Immun* 1978;21:221.
12. ASKONAS BA, TAYLOR PM, ESQUIVEL F. Cytotoxic T cells in influenza infection. *Ann NY Acad Sci* 1988;532:230.

13. MACKENZIE CD, TAYLOR PM, ASKONAS BA. Rapid recovery of lung histology correlates with clearance of influenza virus by specific CD8+ cytotoxic T cells. *Immunology* 1989;67:375–81.

14. YELDANDI AV, COLBY TV. Pathologic features of lung biopsy. Specimens from influenza pneumonia cases. *Hum Pathol* 1994;25:47–53.

15. CENTERS FOR DISEASE CONTROL AND PREVENTION. Influenza – United States, 1987–88 season. *MMWR* 1988;37:497–503.

16. NICHOLSON KG. Influenza vaccination and the elderly. *Br Med J* 1990;301:617.

17. BARKER WH, MULLOOLY JP. Pneumonia and influenza deaths during epidemic. Implications for prevention. *Arch Intern Med* 1982;142:85–9.

18. SCHÄFER JR, KAWOKA Y, BEAN WJ, SÜSS J, SENNE D, WEBSTER RG. Origin of the pandemic 1957/H2 influenza A virus and the persistence of its possible progenitors in the Avaian reservoir. *Virology* 1993;194:781–88.

19. WENTWORTH DE, THOMPSON BL, XU X *et al.* An influenza (H1N1) virus, closely related to swine influenza virus, responsible for a fatal case of human influenza. *J Virol* 1994;68:2051–8.

20. WEBSTER RG, WRIGHT SM, CASTRUCCI MR, BEAN WJ, KAWAOKA Y. Influenza – a model of an emerging virus disease. *Intervirology* 1993;35:16–25.

21. CDC. Update: influenza activity – United States, 1991–92 season. *MMWR* 1992;41–63–5.

22. CURWEN M, DUNNELL K, ASHLEY J. Hidden influenza death. *Br Med J* 1990;118:139–43.

23. CENTERS FOR DISEASE CONTROL. Influenza – Respiratory Disease Surveillance Report No. 88. Department of Health, Education and Welfare Public Health Service 1973.

24. KILBOURNE ED. Influenza in Man. In Kilbourne ED, ed. *Influenza*. New York: Plenum Medical Book Co.; 1987:157–218.

25. WEST KP, HOWARD GR, SOMMER A. Vitamin A and infection: Public Health implications. *Ann Rev Nutr* 1989;9:63–86.

26. SWEET C, JAKEMAN KJ, RUSHTON DI *et al.* Role of upper respiratory tract infection in the deaths occurring in neonatal females infected with influenza virus. *Microbiol Pathog* 1988;5:121–5.

27. GOINGS SAJ, KULLE TJ, BASCOM R *et al.* Effects of nitrogen dioxide exposure on susceptibility to influenza A virus infection in healthy adults. *Am Rev Resp Dis* 1989;139:1075–81.

28. MACFARLANE J. Community-acquired pneumonia. *Br J Dis Chest* 1987;81:116–27.

29. SCHWARZMANN SW, ADLER JL, SULLIVAN RJ *et al.* Bacterial pneumonia during the Hong Kong influenza epidemic of 1968–1969. *Arch Int Med* 1971;127:1037–42.

30. CARTMIGHT KAC, JONES DM, SMITH AJ *et al.* Influenza A and meningococcal disease. *Lancet* 1991;338:554–7.

31. MOORE PS, HIERHOLZER J, DE WITT W *et al.* Respiratory viruses and *Mycoplasma* as cofactors for epidemic group A meningococcal meningitis. *JAMA* 1990;264:1271–5.

32. LOURIA DB, BLUMENFIELD HL, ELLIS JT *et al.* Studies on influenza in the pandemic of 1957–58 II. Pulmonary complications of influenza. *J Clin Invest* 1959;38:213–25.

33. BUSCHO RO, SAXTON D, SCHULTZ PS *et al.* Infections with viruses and *Mycoplasma pneumoniae* during exacerbation of chronic bronchitis. *J Infect Dis* 1978;137:377–83.

34. BEASLEY R, COLEMAN ED, HERMON Y, HOLST PE, O'DONNELL TV, TOBIAS M. Viral respiratory tract infection and exacerbations of asthma in adult patients. *Thorax* 1988;43:679–83.

35. HALL WJ, DOUGLAS RG, HYDE RW *et al.* Pulmonary mechanics following uncomplicated influenza A infection. *Am Rev Resp Dis* 1976;113:141–50.

36. HEIKKINEN T, WARIS M, RUUSKANEN O. Efficacy of influenza vaccination in reducing otitis media in children. In Hannoun C, Kendal AP, Klenk HD, Ruben FL, eds. *Options for the Control of Influenza* II. Amsterdam: Elsevier;1993:431–4.

37. CONWAY SP, SIMMONDS EJ, LITTLEWOOD JM. Acute severe deterioration in cystic fibrosis associated with influenza A virus infection. *Thorax* 1992;47:112–14.

38. ONG EL, ELLIS ME, WEBB AK *et al.* Infective respiratory exacerbations in young adults with cystic fibrosis: role of viruses and atypical microorganisms. *Thorax* 1989;44:739–42.

39. KOBAYASHI O, SEKIYA M, SAITOH H. A case of invasive bronchopulmonary aspergillosis associated with influenza A (H3N2) infection. *Jap J Thorac Dis* 1992;30:1338–44.

40. WELLS CEC. Neurologic complications of so-called influenza: a winter study in Southeast Wales. *Br Med J* 1971;1:369–74.

41. LENEMAN F. The Guillain Barré syndrome. *Arch Intern Med* 1966;118:139–43.

42. WRIGHT P, GILL M, MURRAY RM. Schizophrenia: genetics and the maternal immune response to viral infection. *Am Med Genet* 1993;48:40–6.

43. TOLAN RW JR. Toxic shock syndrome complicating influenza A in a child: case report and review. *Clin Infect Dis* 1993;17:43–5.

44. LANGMUIR AD, WORTHEN TD, SOLOMON J, RAY CG, PETERSEN E. The Thucydides syndrome: a new hypothesis for the cause of the plague of Athens. *N Engl J Med* 1985;313:1027–30.

45. LJUNGMAN P, ANDERSON J, ASCHAN J *et al.* Influenza A in immunocompromised patients. *Clin Infect Dis* 1993;17:244–7.

46. JONES A, MACFARLANE J, PUGH S. Antibiotic therapy, clinical features and outcome of 36 adults presenting to hospital with proven influenza: do we follow guidelines? *Postgrad Med J* 1991;67:988–90.

47. CHOMEL JJ, THOUVENOT D, ONNO M, KAISER C, GOURREAU JM, AYMARD M. Rapid diagnosis of influenza infection of NP antigen using an immunocapture ELISA test. *J Virol Meths* 1989;25:81–91.

48. HAYDEN FG, SPERBER SJ, BELSHE RB, CLOVER RD, HAY AJ, PYKE S Recovery of drug-resistant influenza A virus during therapeutic use of rimantadine. *Antimicrob Agents Chemother* 1991;35:1741–7.

49. BELSHE RB, BURK B, NEUMAN F, CERRITI RM, SINI IS. Resistance of influenza A virus to Amantadine and Rimantadine: results of a decade of surveillance. *J Inf Dis* 1989;159:430–5.

50. HAYDEN FG, HAY AJ. Emergence and transmission of influenza A viruses resistant to amantadine and rimantadine. *Curr Top Microbiol Immunol* 1992:176:119–30.

51. NIKITANA LE, ZLYDNITOV DM. The importance of drug resistance in the treatment of influenza with rimantidine. *Antiviral Res* 1989;11:313–16.

52. DEGELAU J, SOMANNI SK, COOPER SL, GUAY DRP, CROSSLEY KB. Amantadine-resistant influenza A in a nursing facility. *Arch Intern Med* 1992;152:390–2.

53. KNIGHT V, GILBERT BE. Chemotherapy of respiratory viruses. *Adv Int Med* 1986;31:95–118.

54. VON ITZTEIN M, WU WY, KOK GB *et al.* Rational design of potent sialidase-based inhibitors on influenza virus replication. *Nature* 1993;363:418–23.

55. WINGFIELD WL, POLLACK D, GRUNERT RR. Therapeutic efficacy of amantadine HCl and rimantidine HCl as naturally occurring influenza A2 respiratory illness in man. *N Engl J Med* 1969;281:579–84.

56. VAN VORIS LP, BELTS RF, HAYDEN FG, CHRISTMAS WA, DOUGLAS RG. Successful treatment of naturally occurring influenza A/USSR/77/H1N1. *JAMA* 1981;245:1128–31.

57. KNIGHT LV, GILBERT BE, WIBA SZ. Ribavirin small particle aerosol treatment of influenza and respiratory syncytial virus infections. In Stapleton T, ed. *Studies with a*

Broad Spectrum Antiviral Agent. Royal Soc Med London 1986;37–56.

58. SCIENTIFIC COMMITTEE OF THE BRITISH THORACIC SOCIETY. Community acquired pneumonia in adults in British hospitals in 1982–83: a survey of aetiology, mortality, prognostic factors and outcome. *Quart J Med* 1987;62:195–220.

59. DELKER LE, MOSER RH, NEBAR JD *et al.* Amantadine – does it have a role in the prevention and treatment of influenza? A National Institutes of Health Consensus Development Conference. *Ann Int Med* 1980;92:256–61.

60. TOMINACH RL, HAYDEN FG. Rimantidine HCl and Amantadine HCl use in influenza A infections. *Inf Dis Clin N Am* 1987;1:459–78.

61. GARDNER P, SCHAFFNER W. Immunization of adults. *N Engl J Med* 1993;328:1252–8.

62. MIOTTI PG, NELSON KE, DALLABETTA GA, FARZADEGAN H, MARGOLICK J, CLEMENTS ML. The influence of HIV infection on antibody responses to a two-dose regimen of influenza vaccine. *JAMA* 1989;262:779–83.

63. BEYER WE, PALACHE AM, BALJET M, MASUREL N. Antibody induction by influenza vaccines in the elderly: a review of the literature. *Vaccine* 1989;7:385–94.

64. FIEBACH N, BECKETT W. Prevention of respiratory infections in adults. *Arch Intern Med* 1994;154:2545–57.

65. MULLOLLY JP, BENNETT MD, HORNBROOK MC *et al.* Influenza vaccination programmes for elderly persons: cost-effectiveness in a health maintenance organization. *Ann Intern Med* 1994;121:947–52.

66. NICHOL KH, MARGOLIS KL, WUORENMA J, VON STERNBERG T. *N Engl J Med* 1994;331:778–84.

67. GOVAERT TM, DINANT GJ, ARETZ K, MASUREL N, SPRENGER MJW, KNOTTNERUS JA. Adverse reactions to influenza vaccine in elderly people: randomised double blind placebo controlled trial. *Br Med J* 1993;307:988–90.

68. MARGOLIS KL, NICHOL KL, POLAND GA, PLUHAR RE. Frequency of adverse reactions to influenza vaccine in the elderly: a randomized, placebo-controlled trial. *JAMA* 1990;264:1139–41.

69. CENTERS FOR DISEASE CONTROL AND PREVENTION. Prevention and control of influenza, part I: vaccines: recommendations of the Advisory Committee on Immunization Practices. *MMWR* 1993;42:1–14.

70. MACKENZIE WR, DAVIS JP, PETERSON DE, HIBBARD AJ, BECKER G, ZARVAN BS. Multiple false-positive serologic tests for HIV, HTLV-1, and hepatitis C following influenza vaccination. *JAMA* 1992;268:1015–17.

71. NICHOL KL. Improving influenza vaccination rates for high-risk inpatients. *Am J Med* 1991;91:584–8.

72. TREANOR JJ, MATTISON HR, DUMYATI G *et al.* Protective efficacy of combined live intranasal and inactivated influenza A virus vaccines in the elderly. *Ann Intern Med* 1992;117:625–33.

73. MOLDOVEANU Z, NOVAK M, HUANG WO *et al.* Oral immunisation with influenza virus in biodegradable microspheres. *J Infect Dis* 1993;167:84–90.

74. MURPHY BR, PRINCE GA, COLLINS PL *et al.* Current approaches to the development of vaccines effective against parainfluenza and respiratory syncytial viruses. *Virus Res* 1988;11:1–15.

75. PUTTO A, RUUSKANEN O, MEURMAN O. Fever in respiratory virus infections. *Am J Dis Child* 1986;140:1159–63.

76. VAINIONPÄÄ, HYYPIÄ T. Biology of parainfluenza viruses. *Clin Microbiol Rev* 1994;7:265–75.

77. WENZEL RP, MCCORMICK DP, BEAM WE. Parainfluenza pneumonia in adults. *JAMA* 1972;221:294–5.

78. AKIZUKI S, NASU N, SETOGUCHI M, YOSHIDA S, HIGUCHI Y, YAMAMOTO S. Parainfluenza virus pneumonitis in an adult. *Arch Pathol Lab Med* 1991;115:824–6.

79. WHIMBEY E, VARTIVARIAN SE, CHAMPLIN RE, ELTING LS, LUNA M, BODEY GP. Parainfluenza virus infection in adult bone marrow transplant recipients. *Eur J Clin Microbiol Infect Dis* 1993;12:699–701.

80. LJUNGMAN P, GLEAVES CA, MEYERS JD. Respiratory virus infections in immunocompromised patients. *Bone Marrow Transpl* 1989;4:35–40.

81. STORCH GA, ANDERSON LJ, PARK CS, TSOU C, DOHNER DE. Antigenic and genomic diversity within Group a respiratory syncytial virus. *J Infect Dis* 1991;163:858–61.

82. ANDERSON LJ, HENDRY RM, PIERIK LT, TSOU C, MCINTOSH K. Multicenter study of strains of respiratory syncytial virus. *J Infect Dis* 1991;163:687–92.

83. HALL CB, WALSH EE, LONG CE, SCHNABEL KC. Immunity to and frequency of reinfection with respiratory syncytial virus. *J Infect Dis* 1991;163:693–8.

84. WARIS M. Pattern of respiratory syncytial virus epidemics in Finland: two-year cycles with alternating prevalence of groups A and B. *J Infect Dis* 1991;163:464–9.

85. GILCHRIST S, TÖRÖK TJ, GARY HE JR, ALEXANDER JP, ANDERSON LJ. National surveillance for respiratory syncytial virus, United States, 1985–1990. *J Infect Dis* 1994;170:986–90.

86. NWANKO MU, DYM AM, SCHUIT KE, OFFOR E, OMENE JA. Seasonal variation in respiratory syncytial virus infections in children in Benin-city, Nigeria. *Trop Geogr Med* 1988;40:309–13.

87. TRISTRAM DA, WELLIVER RC. Respiratory syncytial virus vaccines: can we improve on nature? *Pediatr Ann* 1993;22:715–18.

88. COLOCHO ZELAYA EA, PETTERSSON CA, FORSGREN M, ORVELL C, STRANNEGARD O. Respiratory syncytial virus infection in hospitalized patients and healthy children in El Salvador. *Am J Trop Med Hyg* 1994;51:577–84.

89. HALL WJ, HALL CB, SPEERS DM. Respiratory syncytial virus infection in adults. Clinical, virologic, and serial pulmonary function studies. *Ann Int Med* 1978;88:203–5.

90. HALL CB, GEIMAN JM, BIGGAR R, KOTOK DI, HOGAN PM, DOUGLAS RG JR. Respiratory syncytial virus infections within families. *New Engl J Med* 1976;294:414–9.

91. FEKETY FR JR, CALDWELL J, GUMP D *et al.* Bacteria, viruses, and mycoplasmas in acute pneumonia in adults. *Am Rev Resp Dis* 1971;104:499–507.

92. MATHUR U, BENTLEY DW, HALL CB. Concurrent respiratory syncytial virus and influenza A infections in the institutionalized elderly and chronically ill. *Ann Int Med* 1980;93:49–52.

93. GARVIE DG, GRAY J. Outbreak of respiratory syncytial virus infection in the elderly. *Br Med J* 1980;281:1253–4.

94. HARRINGTON RD, HOOTON TM, HACKMAN RC *et al.* An outbreak of respiratory syncytial virus in a bone marrow transplant center. *J Infect Dis* 1992;165:987–93.

95. ENGLUND JA, SULLIVAN CJ, JORDAN C *et al.* Respiratory syncytial virus infection in immunocompromised adults. *Ann Intern Med* 1988;109:203–8.

96. FLEMING DM, CROSS KW. Respiratory syncytial virus or influenza? *Lancet* 1993;342:1507–10.

97. AGIUS G, DINDINAUD RJ, BIGGAR RJ *et al.* An epidemic of respiratory syncytial virus in elderly people: Clinical and serological findings. *J Med Virol* 1990;30:117–27.

98. WELLIVER RC, KAUL TN, OGRA PL. The appearance of cell-bound IgE in respiratory tract epithelium after respiratory-syncytial-virus infection. *N Engl J Med* 1980;303:1190–1202.

99. SINNOTT JT IV, CULLISON JP, SWEENEY MS, HAMMON M, HOLT DA. Respiratory syncytial virus pneumonia in a cardiac transplant recipient. *J Infect Dis* 1988;158:650–1.

100. MURPHY D, ROSE RC III. Respiratory syncytial virus pneumonia in a human immunodeficiency virus–infected man. *JAMA* 1989;261:1147.
101. HARRINGTON RD, HOOTON TM, HACKMAN RC *et al.* An outbreak of respiratory syncytial virus in a bone marrow transplant center. *J Infect Dis* 1992;165:987–93.
102. KRILOV LR, LIPSON SM, BARONE SR, KAPLAN MH, CIAMICIAN Z, HARKNESS SH. Evaluation of a rapid diagnostic test for respiratory syncytial virus (RSV): potential for bedside diagnosis. *Pediatrics* 1994;93:903–6.
103. COMMITTEE ON INFECTIOUS DISEASES, AMERICAN ACADEMY OF PAEDIATRICS. Use of ribavirin in the treatment of respiratory syncytial virus infection. *Pediatrics* 1993;92:501–3.
104. HALL CB, WALSH ED, HOUSKA JF *et al.* Ribavirin treatment of experimental respiratory syncytial viral infection. A controlled double-blind study in young adults. *JAMA* 1983;249:2666–74.
105. HAYDEN FG, ANDRIES K, JANSSEN PJ. Safety and efficacy of intranasal pirodavir (R77975) in experimental rhinovirus infection. *Antimicrob Agents Chemother* 1992;36:727–32.
106. LEVIN MJ. Treatment and prevention options for respiratory syncytial virus infections. *J Pediatr* 1994;124:S22–S27.
107. FARR BM, GWALTNEY JM JR, HENDLEY JO *et al.* A randomized controlled trial of gluococorticoid prophylaxis against experimental rhinovirus infection. *J Infect Dis* 1990;162:1173–7.
108. MURPHY BR, HALL SL, KULKARNI AB *et al.* An update on approaches to the development of respiratory syncytial virus (RSV) and parainfluenza virus type 3 (PIV3) vaccines *Virus Res* 1994;32(1):13–36.
109. GINSBERG HS, PRINCE GA. The molecular basis of adenovirus pathogenesis (review). *Infect Agents Dis* 1994;3(1):1–8.
110. GINSBERG HS, MOLDAWER LL, SEHGAL PB *et al.* A mouse model for investigating the molecular pathogenesis of adenovirus pneumonia. *Proc Natl Acad Sci USA* 1991;88:1651–5.
111. PEASON RD, HALL WJ, MENEGUS MA, DOUGLAS RG. Diffuse pneumonitis due to adenovirus type 21 in a civilian. *Chest* 1980;78:107–9.
112. WRIGHT J, COUCHONNAL G, HODGES GR. Adenovirus type 21 infection. Occurrence with pneumonia, rhabdomyolysis and myogloginuria in adult. *JAMA* 1979;241:2420–1.
113. FERSTENFELD E, SCHULUETER P, RYTEL W, MOLLOY P. Recognition and treatment of adult respiratory distress syndrome secondary to viral interstitial pneumonia. *Am J Med* 1975;58:709–18.
114. DUDDING BA, WAGNER SC, ZELLER JA, GMELICH JT, FRENCH GR, TOP FH JR. Fatal pneumonia associated with adenovirus type 7 in three military trainees. *N Engl J Med* 1987;24:1289–92.
115. ELLENBOGEN C, GRAYBILL JR, SILVA J JR, HOMME PJ. Bacterial pneumonia complicating adenoviral pneumonia. A comparison of respiratory tract bacterial culture sources and effectiveness of chemoprophylaxis against bacterial pneumonia. *Am J Med* 1974;56:169–78.
116. RODRIGUEZ FH JR, LIUZZA GE, GOHD RH. Disseminated adenovirus serotype 3 infection in an immunecompromised host. *Am J Clin Pathol* 1984;82:615–18.
117. TOP FH, GROSSMAN RA, BARTELLORI PJ *et al.* Immunisation with live types 7 and 4 vaccines – I. Safety, infectivity and potency of adenovirus type 7 vaccine in humans. *J Infect Dis* 1971;12:148–54.
118. TOP FH JR. Control of adenovirus acute respiratory disease in US Army trainees. *Yale J Biol Med* 1975;48:185–95.
119. RADOYCICH GE, ZUPPAN CW, WEEKS DA, KROUS HF, LANGSTON C. Patterns of measles pneumonitis. *Ped Pathol* 1992;12:773–86.
120. MYOU S, FUJIMURA M, YASUI M, UENO T, MATSUDA T. Bronchoalveolar lavage cell analysis in measles viral pneumonia. *Eur Resp J* 1993;6:1437–42.
121. FORNI AL, SCHLUGER NW, ROBERTS RB. Severe measles pneumonitis in adults: evaluation of clinical characteristics and therapy with intravenous ribavirin. *Clin Infect Dis* 1994;19:454–62.
122. CENTERS FOR DISEASE CONTROL. Summary – cases of specified notifiable diseases, United States. *MMWR* 1991;39:936.
123. DEIVANAYAGAM N, MALA N, AHAMED SS, SHANKAR VJ. Measles associated diarrhea and pneumonia in South India. *Ind Pediat* 1994;31:35–40.
124. KERNAHAN J, MCQUILLIN J, CRAFT AW. Measles in children who have malignant disease. *Br Med J* 1987;295:15–18.
125. GREMILLION DH, CRAWFORD GE. Measles pneumonia in young adults: an analysis of 106 cases. *Am J Med* 1981;71:539–42.
126. MOUALLEM M, FRIEDMAN E, PAUZNER R, FARFEL Z. Measles epidemic in young adults: clinical manifestations and laboratory analysis in 40 patients. *Arch Intern Med* 1987;147:1111–13.
127. DOVER AS, ESCOBAR JA, DUENAS AL, LEAF EC. Pneumonia associated with measles. *JAMA* 1975;234:612–14.
128. ATMAR RL, ENGLUND JA, HAMMILL H. Complications of measles during pregnancy. *Clin Infect Dis* 1992;4:217–26.
129. SWIFT JD, BARRUGA, MC, PERKIN RM, VAN STRALEN D. Respiratory failure complicating rubeola. *Chest* 1993;104:1786–7.
130. TANAKA H, HONMA S, YAMAGISHI M *et al.* Clinical features of measles pneumonia in adults: usefulness of computed tomography. *Jap J Thorac Dis* 1993;31:1129–33.
131. RUPP ME, SCHWARTZ ML, BECHARD DE. Measles pneumonia. Treatment of a near-fatal case with corticosteroids and vitamin A. *Chest* 1993;103:1625–6.
132. HUSSEY GD, KLEIN M. A randomised controlled trial of vitamin A in children with severe measles. *N Engl J Med* 1990;323:160–4.
133. WACKER P, HARMANN O, BEHNAMOU E, SALLOUM E, LEMERLE J. Varicella-zoster virus infections after autologous bone marrow transplantation in children. *Bone Marrow Transpl* 1989;4:191–4.
134. FELDMAN S, LOTT L. Varicella in children with cancer: impact of antiviral therapy and prophylaxis. *Pediatrics* 1987;80:465–72.
135. WEBER DM, PELLECHIA JA. Varicella pneumonia. Study of prevalence in adult men. *J Am Med Assoc* 1965;192:572–3.
136. HOCKBERGER RS, ROTHSTEIN RJ. Varicella pneumonia in adults: a spectrum of disease. *Ann Emerg Med* 1986;15:931–4.
137. TRIEBWASSER JH, HARRIS RE, BRYANT RE, RHOADES ER. Varicella pneumonia in adults. *Medicine* 1967;46:409–23.
138. WALLACE MR, BOWLER WA, MURRAY NB, BRODINE SK, OLDFIELD EC III. Treatment of adult varicella with oral acyclovir: a randomized, placebo-controlled trial. *Ann Intern Med* 1992;117:358–63.
139. TRIEBWASSER JH, HARRIS RE, BRYANT RE, RHOADES ER. Varicella pneumonia in adults: report of seven cases and a review of literature. *Medicine* 1967;46:409–23.
140. SMEGO RA JR, ASPERILLA MO. Use of acyclovir for varicella pneumonia during pregnancy. *Obstet Gynecol* 1991;78:1112.
141. PREBLUD SR, D'ANGELO LJ. Chickenpox in the United States, 1972–1977. *J Infect Dis* 1979;140:257–60.
142. KNYVETT AF. The pulmonary lesions of chickenpox. *Quart J Med* 1966;139:313–23.
143. ELLIS ME, NEAL KR, WEBB AK. Is smoking a risk factor for pneumonia in adults with chickenpox? *Br J Med* 1987;294:1002.
144. KNYVETT AF. The relation between tobacco smoking and pulmonary chickenpox. *Med J Aust* 1967;2:1197.
145. GRAYSON ML, NEWTON-JOHN H.

Smoking and varicella pneumonia [letter]. *J Infect* 1988;16:312.

146. ESMONDE TF, HERDMAN G, ANDERSON G. Chickenpox pneumonia: an association with pregnancy. *Thorax* 1989;44:812–15.

147. LOCKSLEY RM, FLOURNOY N, SULLIVAN KM, MEYERS JD. Infection with varicella-zoster virus after marrow transplantation. *J Infect Dis* 1985;152:1172–81.

148. RODRIGUEZ E, MARTINEZ J, JAVALOYAS M, NONELL F, TORRES M. Haemothorax in the course of chickenpox. *Thorax* 1986;41:491–2.

149. BOCLES JS, EHRENKRANZ NJ, MARKS A. Abnormalities of respiratory function in varicella pneumonia. *Ann Intern Med* 1964;60:183–95.

150. BOCLES JS, EHRENKRANZ NJ, MARKS A. Abnormalities of respiratory function in varicella pneumonia. *Ann Intern Med* 1964;60:183–5.

151. DAVIDSON RN, LYNN W, SAVAGE P, WANSBOROUGH-JONES MH. Chickenpox pneumonia: experience with antiviral treatment. *Thorax* 1988;43:627–30.

152. BALFOUR HH. Intravenous acyclovir therapy for varicella in immunocompromised children. *J Pediat* 1984;104:134–6.

153. BROUSSARD RC, PAYNE DK, GEORGE RB. Treatment with acyclovir of varicella pneumonia in pregnancy. *Chest* 1991;99:1045–7.

154. HAAKE DA, ZAKOWSKI PC, HAAKE DL, BRYSON YJ. Early treatment with acyclovir for varicella pneumonia in otherwise healthy adults: retrospective controlled study and review. *Rev Infect Dis* 1990;12:788–98.

155. JOSEPH CA, NOAH ND. Epidemiology of chickenpox in England and Wales 1967–85. *Br Med J* 1988;296:673–6.

156. DUNKLE LM, ARVIN AM, WHITLEY RJ *et al.* A controlled trial of acyclovir for chicken pox in normal children. *N Engl J Med* 1991;325:1539–44.

157. DAVIDSON RN, LYNN W, SAVAGE P, WANSBROUGH-JONES MH. Chickenpox pneumonia: experience with antiviral treatment. *Thorax* 1988;43:627–30.

158. LEEN CL, MANDAL BK, ELLIS ME. Acyclovir and pregnancy. *Br Med J* 1987;294–308.

159. COLE NL, BALFOUR HH. Varicella zoster virus does not become more resistant to acyclovir during therapy. *J Infect Dis* 1986;153:605–8.

160. CLAYDON AH, NICHOLSON KG, WISELKA MJ, FIRMIN RK. Varicella pneumonitis: a role for extra-corporeal membrane oxygenation? *J Infect* 1994;28:65–7.

161. GERSHON AA, STEINBERG SP, LA RUSS P *et al.* Immunization of healthy adults with live attentuated varicella vaccine. *J Infect Dis* 1988;158:132–46.

162. GERSHON AA, LARUSSA P, HARDY I, STEINBERG S, SILVERSTEIN S. Varicella vaccine: the American experience. *J Infect Dis* 1992;166 (Suppl 1):S63–68.

163. ASANO Y, YOSHIKAWA T, SUGA S *et al.* Postexposure prophylaxis of varicella in family contact by oral acyclovir. *Pediatrics* 1993;92:219–22.

164. MESZNER Z, NYERGES G, BELL AR. Oral acyclovir to prevent dissemination of varicella in immunocompromised children. *J Infect* 1993;26(1):9–15.

165. SHERRY MK, KLAINER AS, WOLFF M, GERHARD H. Herpetic tracheobronchitis. *Ann Intern Med* 1988;109:229–33.

166. PORTEOUS C, BRADLEY JA, HAMILTON DN, LEDINGHAM IM, CLEMENTS GB, ROBINSON CG. Herpes simplex virus reactivation in surgical patients. *Crit Care Med* 1984;12:626–8.

167. TUXEN DV, CADE JF, MCDONALD MI, BUCHANAN MRC, CLARK RJ, PAIN MCF. Herpes simplex virus from the lower respiratory tract in adult respiratory distress syndrome. *Am Rev Resp Dis* 1982;126:416–19.

168. MEYERS JD, FLOURNOY N, THOMAS ED. Non-bacterial pneumonia after allogeneic marrow transplantation : a review of ten year's experience. *Rev Infect Dis* 1982;4:1119–32.

169. PRELLNER T, FLAMHOLC L, HAIDL S, LINDHOLM K, WIDELL A. Herpes simplex virus – the most frequently isolated pathogen in the lungs of patients with severe respiratory distress. *Scand J Infect Dis* 1929;24:283–92.

170. COREY L, SPEAR PG Infections with herpes simplex viruses. *N Engl J Med* 1986;314:749–57.

171. TUXEN DV. Prevention of lower respiratory herpes simplex virus infection with acyclovir in patients with adult respiratory distress synrome. *Chest* 1994;106(Suppl 1):28S–33S.

172. KLAINER AS, OUD L, RANDAZZO J, FREIHEITER J, BISACCIA E, GERHARD H. Herpes simplex virus involvement of the lower respiratory tract following surgery. *Chest* 1994;106(Suppl 1):8S–14S.

173. RAMSEY PG, FIFE KH, HACKMAN RC *et al.* Herpes simplex virus pneumonia: Clinical, virologic and pathologic features in 20 patients. *Ann Intern Med* 1982;97:813–20.

174. WADE JC, NEWTON B, FLOURNOY N, MEYERS JD. Oral acyclovir for prevention of herpes simplex virus reactivation after marrow transplantation. *Ann Intern Med* 1984;100:823–8.

175. SMYTH RL, HIGENBOTTAM TW, SCOTT JP *et al.* Herpes simplex virus infection in heart–lung transplant recipients. *Transplantation* 1990;49:735–9.

176. ODA Y, OKADA Y, KATSUDA S, NAKANISHI I. Immunochemical study on the infection of herpes simplex virus, human cytomegalovirus, and Epstein–Barr virus in secondary diffuse interstitial pneumonia. *Hum Pathol* 1994;25:1057–62.

177. DUNNET WN. Infectious mononucleosis. *Br Med J* 1963;1:1187–91.

178. MUNDY GR. Infectious mononucleosis with pulmonary parenchymal involvement. *Br Med J* 1972;1:219–20.

179. SCHOOLEY RT, CAREY RW, MILLER G *et al.* Chronic Epstein–Barr virus infection associated with fever and interstitial pneumonitis. *Ann Intern Med* 1986;104:636–43.

180. LIEBOW AA, CARRINGTON CB. Diffuse pulmonary lymphoreticular infiltrations associated with dysproteinemia. *Med Clin North Am* 1973;57:809–43.

181. BARBERA JA, HAYASHI S, HEGELE RG, HOGG JC. Detection of Epstein-Barr virus in lymphocytic interstitial pneumonia by *in situ* hybridization. *Am Rev Resp Dis* 1992;145:940–6.

182. ANDIMAN WA, EASTMAN R, MARTIN R *et al.* Opportunistic lymphoproliferation associated with Epstein–Barr viral DNA in infants and children with AIDS. *Lancet* 1985;2:1390–3.

183. CHAYT KJ, HARPER ME, MARSELLE LM *et al.* Detection of HTLV-III RNA in lungs of patients with AIDS and pulmonary involvement. *JAMA* 1986;256:2356–9.

184. TEIRSTEIN AS, ROSEN MJ. Lymphocytic interstitial pneumonia. *Clin Chest Med* 1988;9:467–71.

185. SULLIVAN JL, BYRON KS, BREWSTER FE, SAKAMOTO K, SHAW JE, PAGANO JS. Treatment of life-threatening Epstein-Barr virus infections with acyclovir. *Am J Med* 1982;73(1A):262.

186. SALAHUDDIN SZ, ABLASHI DV, MARKHAM PD *et al.* Isolation of a new virus (HBLV) in patients with lymphoproliferative disorders. *Science* 1986;234:596–601.

187. KRUEGER DG, WASSERMANN K, DE CLERCK *et al.* Latent herpesvirus-6 in salivary and bronchial glands. *Lancet* 1990:336:1255–6.

188. PITALIA AK, LIU-YIN JA, FREEMONT AJ, MORRIS DJ, FITZMAURICE RJ. Immunohistological detection of human herpes virus 6 in formalin-fixed, paraffin-embedded lung tissues. *J Med Virol* 1993;41:103–7.

189. LUSSO P, SALAHUDDIN SZ, ABLASHI DV *et al.* Diverse tropism of human B-lymphotropic virus (HHV-6). *Lancet* 1987;2:743–4.

190. ABLASHI D, AGUT H, BERNEMAN Z *et al.*

Human herpesvirus 6 (HHV-6) variant B accounts for the majority of symptomatic primary HHV-6 infections in a population of US infants. *J Clin Microbiol* 1993; 129:363–6.

191. BRIGGS M, FOX JD, TEDDER RS. Age prevalence of antibody to human herpesvirus 6. *Lancet* 1988;1:1058–9.

192. BROWN NA, SUMAYA CV, LIU CR *et al.* Fall in human herpesvirus 6 seropositivity with age. *Lancet* 1988;2:396.

193. ENDERS G, BIBER M, MEYERS G *et al.* Prevalence of antibodies to HHV-6 in different age-groups, in children with exanthema subitum, other acute exanthematous childhood diseases, Kawasaki syndrome and acute infection with other herpes viruses and HIV. *Infection* 1990;18:12–15.

194. RUSSLER SK, TAPPER MA, KNOX KK, LIEPINS A, CARRIGAN DR. Pneumonitis associated with coinfection by human herpesvirus 6 and Legionella in an immunocompetent adult. *Am J Pathol* 1991;138:1405–11.

195. CARRIGAN DR, KNOW KK, TAPPER MA. Suppression of human immunodeficiency virus type 1 replication by human herpes virus 6. *J Infect Dis* 1990;162:844–51.

196. ENSOLI B, LUSSO P, SCHACHTER F *et al.* Human herpes virus-6 increases HIV-1 expression in co-infected T-cells via nuclear factors binding to the HIV-1 enhancer. *EMBO J* 1989;8:3019–27.

197. CARRIGAN DR, DROBYSKI WR, RUSSLER S, TAPPER MA, KNOX KK, ASH RC. Interstitial pneumonitis associated with human herpesvirus-6 infection after marrow transplantation. *Lancet* 1991;338:147–9.

198. CONE RW, HACKMAN RC, HUANG MLW *et al.* Human herpesvirus 6 in lung tissue from bone marrow transplant patients with pneumonia. *N Engl J Med* 1993;329:156–61.

199. CONE RW, HUANG MW, HACKMAN RC. Human herpesvirus 6 and pneumonia. *Leukemia and Lymphoma* 1994;15:235–41.

200. CENTERS FOR DISEASE CONTROL, 1993. Outbreak of acute illness – Southwestern United States, 1993. *MMWR* 42:421–4.

201. DUCHIN JS, KOSTER F, PTERS CJ *et al.* Hantaviral pulmonary syndrome: a clinical description of 17 patients with a newly recognised disease. *N Engl J Med* 330;949–55.

202. KSIAZEK TG, PETERS CJ, PIERRE E *et al.* Identification of a new North American hantavirus that causes acute pulmonary insufficiency. *Am J Trop Med Hyg* 1995;52:117–23.

203. NICHOL ST, SPIROPOULOU C, MORZUNOV S *et al.* Genetic identification of a hantavirus associated with an outbreak of acute respiratory illness. *Science* 1993;262:914–17.

204. ZAKI SR, GREER PW COFFIELD LM *et al.* Hantavirus pulmonary syndrome. Pathogenesis of an emerging infectious disease. *Am J Pathol* 1995;146:552–79.

10 Cytomegalovirus pneumonia

MICHAEL E. ELLIS

King Faisal Specialist Hospital and Research Centre, Riyadh, Saudi Arabia

Introduction

This chapter will deal with cytomegalovirus (CMV) pulmonary disease in the immunocompromised host.

The expression of CMV disease is heavily dependent on the immune integrity of the host (Table 10.1). In the immune competent person it rarely poses clinical problems of significance[1]. The most frequently encountered manifestation in older children and adults is a glandular fever-like syndrome. Fever (sometimes as a fever of unknown origin), malaise, pharyngitis, headache, mild diffuse erythematous rash, lymphadenopathy and splenomegaly may also be present. Manifestations usually associated with immunocompromised patients, can be found, but these are rare. They include pneumonitis, meningoencephalitis, Guillain–Barré syndrome, severe thrombocytopenia, haemolysis and hepatitis. Atypical mononucleosis with negative serology for EBV and various immunological epiphenomena such as cryoglobulinaemia, cold agglutinins and positive rheumatoid factor are highly suggestive of CMV disease. In the majority of cases, recovery is usually complete, though deaths have been described.

Infection in pregnancy is a hazard to the foetus and transmission transplacentally or during the second stage of labour (in the case of maternal cervical infections) occurs in approximately 1% of deliveries. It can also be transmitted through breast milk. Transplacental infection causes a substantial risk of the order of 20% for infected neonates for the congenital CMV syndrome characterised by multisystem involvement including particularly microcephaly, mental retardation, chorioretinitis, sensorineural hearing loss, motor disability and hepatosplenomegaly[2]. Risk for disease is governed to an extent by timing of infection during pregnancy and maternal immune status. Young infants may have a variety of upper and lower respiratory manifestations which include pharyngitis, bronchitis, and pneumonia. The majority of infections in any age group of immune competent people, however, are asymptomatic. CMV has been incriminated in the genesis of atherosclerosis, and tumors. It appears to be immunosuppressive. It may also play a role in the wasting syndrome of HIV.

It is, however, the setting of the immunocompromised patient that presents the greatest potential for severe disease with high mortality. This arena has also posed enormous challenges for swift diagnosis, effective treatment and prophylaxis.

The concept that there can be CMV infection (positive culture of blood, urine, throat swab and of other secretions or tissues, or the documentation of a fourfold rise in serological titres) without disease (as defined by appropriate clinical symptoms and signs due to CMV) is important to grasp. For example, 50% of bone marrow transplant recipients will yield a positive CMV culture from routine bronchoalveolar lavage but the majority do not develop CMV pneumonitis[3]. At the Royal Free Hospital, London, CMV infection was documented between 1.5 and 6 times more frequently than CMV disease in patients with renal or bone marrow transplantation[4].

Table 10.1. *CMV infection – disease spectrum*

	Immune competent	Immune compromised
Asymptomatic infection	++	+
Pyrexia unknown origin	++	+
Mononucleosis syndrome	++	+
Invasive target organ disease	±	+ (+)
CMVIP	±	+ (± in HIV)
Rejection	NA	+
Atherosclerosis	? ±	? ±
Malignancy	±	±
Obliterative bronchiolitis	?	? ±
Immunosuppression	?	+

CMVIP, CMV interstitial pneumonitis.
++ common.
+ sometimes.
± rare/possible association.
? uncertain.
NA not applicable.

The routes of transmission include blood, sexual intercourse, intrauterine and peripartum, organ transplantation and close physical contact, for example, at day nurseries. Body secretions such as those from the oropharynx, vagina or cervix, urine, breast milk and seminal fluid contain virus. Asymptomatic excretion occurs in a few per cent of individuals. The risk of acquisition of infection from a blood transfusion for a susceptible individual is approximately 2%. In comparison, for all susceptible (i.e. non-immune, seronegative recipients) transplantation recipients in general it is of the order of 60% with clinical disease occurring in approximately two-thirds of those infected. For CMV seronegative bone marrow transplant recipients the risk of CMV infection from a seropositive donor varies between 14% and 57%, CMV disease between 0% and 20%, the incidence depending on seropositivity of the blood and blood products, use of IVIG, acyclovir and other factors[5].

The seroprevalence of CMV infection varies with geography, socioeconomic class, sexual habits, obstetric history and age (prevalence rising with age). In the USA, 40%–70% of the general population have CMV antibodies, in parts of Africa it is 100%, in Saudi

Arabia 80%, and in Europe 40%[6,7]. Almost all homosexual men with HIV infection also have recently acquired/activated CMV infection.

Virology and general aspects of immunopathology

CMV is a 180 nm double-stranded DNA herpes virus, discovered in the 1950s by Weller, Rowe *et al.* It is composed of a 64 nm core of nucleic acid within a multiple capsomere structured icosahedral capsid, all contained within a host-derived glycoprotein/protein/lipid envelope. The CMV genome, although large, encodes for only approximately 30 known proteins. Early immediate (α) genes control the expression of early (β) and late (γ) genes. Following initial cellular infection which include steps of adsorption and uncoating, the viral genome is rapidly incorporated into the host-cell nucleus. Replication of the virus involves the synthesis of nuclear capsids derived from the host-cell nucleus and directed by viral coded polymerase, and the envelope is formed from the host-cell membrane. It is the envelope which elicits important antibody responses, though the early immediate or α gene products are important in cytotoxic T-cell reactions. Effective host containment of CMV is mediated by both cellular and humoral mechanisms. These include cytotoxic NK and macrophage cells, cytokines (particularly alpha interferon) and immunoglobulins IgG and IgM. Direct cell-to-cell spread of the virus renders some protection of CMV from neutralising antibodies, elevating cell-mediated immune mechanisms in their importance. Probably intact cytotoxic T-lymphocyte HLA governed function is the supreme protective mechanism against CMV disease and CMV specific cytotoxic responses have been correlated with patient survival[8]. Intact natural killer cell activity has also been shown to parallel improvement in CMV disease and Graft vs. Host Disease (GVHD). Deficiencies in these two cellular immune functions are caused by transplant immunosuppressive drugs.

A major property of CMV is its subsequent lifelong latency in the infected host. Immortalised in the host-cell nucleus, subsequent appropriate immunosuppression triggers recrudescence of infection. The viral reservoirs are polymorphs, peripheral monocytes and lymphocytes both circulating and tissue bound. Hepatocytes, cardiac muscle and renal tubules, glomeruli and endothelial cells are further extravascular sources. Thus, multiple sites are involved in which the virus is present but dormant. No doubt some of these cells are responsible for the organ associated transmission of CMV.

There is some evidence that CMV can enhance the immunosuppressive status of patients[9]. It is known to depress monocyte and lymphocyte functions via formation of IgM lymphocytotoxic complexes and by induction of metabolic changes, and in addition can lower CD4 levels and increase CD8 levels[10]. Bronchoalveolar macrophages are also affected. The absence of HLA class II antigens on infected alveolar epithelial cells may account in part for the secondary immunosuppression associated with CMV pneumonia[11]. These immunomodulatory actions of CMV may explain the increased potential for the development of other opportunistic infections which are known to occur in patients with CMV, particularly *Pneumocystis carinii* pneumonia, gram negative sepsis, *Listeria* spp., *Aspergillus* spp., *Candida* spp. and cryptococcal infections[12,13]. In HIV patients with CMV not only does the HIV predispose to CMV infection through severe CD4 depletion but CMV may well drive HIV replication through cytokine release, transactivation of HIV genomes and facilitation of HIV cell entry[4]. CMV may also increase the possibility for graft rejection[14]. For example, it has been shown that renal transplant recipients with CMV have a much higher risk of rejection in the absence of direct viral invasion of the graft. This is associated with a unique histological glomerulopathy, possibly related to CMV induced interferon release, inversion of the CD4 CD8 status and increased expression of HLA Type II antigens[15]. Primary and secondary CMV infection has been found to be linked to chronic liver graft rejection (vanishing bile duct syndrome)[16]. It is also associated with obliterative bronchiolitis in lung transplant patients[17].

The oncogenic potential of CMV is realised in its association with Kaposi's sarcoma[18], though this association with malignancy is not as strong as that for EBV with nasopharyngeal carcinoma. Association with colonic adenocarcinoma has also been described[19].

The histological hallmark of CMV disease (Figs. 10.1 (*a*), (*b*)) is giant cell formation composed of intranuclear eosinophilic single membrane and intracytoplasmic basophilic double membrane inclusion bodies containing viral DNA. Cytomegalic or giant cell formation was first noted in 1881 but the virus was not identified in human tissue until 1956[20]. Depending on the clinical setting, these changes are variably found in most tissues. In CMV pneumonia, a variety of inflammatory infiltrates may be found which include polymorphs and monocytes and alveolar filling with haemorrhage and protein. Fibrin deposition, septal oedema or obliteration may also be present. Increase in pneumocytes and their desquamation and hyaline membrane formation may be found. Alveolar wall dysfunction is a constant finding in CMV interstitial pneumonitis (CMVIP). Occasionally, CMV inclusion bodies without an obvious inflammatory reaction may also occur and suggest infection rather than disease.

The immunocompromised host and transmission of CMV

The immunocompromised host population at risk from CMV infection includes patients with solid organ and bone marrow transplantation, patients with malignant disease and those with HIV infection. In these patients, CMV infection is the most common viral pathogen. However, it is the transplant patient who is the most vulnerable to CMV infection with an overall incidence in excess of 50%. The subsequent discussion will focus on this risk group. Although many of these infections are mild and in addition in recent years, the incidence is falling in transplant centres, severe disease such as pneumonia occurs in up to 30%[21–25]. In these patients, primary reactivation and superinfection can occur.

The risk of primary infection exists when a seronegative recipient is exposed to blood/blood products/tissue from a seropositive donor. Reactivation occurs in a known seropositive patient who is subjective to intense immunosuppression. Superinfection by a strain different from that dormant in a seropositive recipient has been documented in immunocompromised hosts by restriction endo-nuclease techniques and this is the third mode of infection. The source of virus is most often the organ transplanted for renal, heart, heart–lung and bone marrow transplantations, whereas blood or blood products present an additional hazard for liver and bone marrow transplants.

Disease severity and frequency appear to be partially modulated by the pre-existing CMV immune status of the patient, the nature of the transplant and the particular immunocompromised setting (Table 10.2). Seronegative recipients of seropositive sources pose a higher risk for infection compared to seropositive recipients[24]. Thus, a seronegative recipient of a seropositive transplanted kidney or other solid organs has a 90% chance of being infected if the donor is cadaveric non-related, compared to 70% for a living related donor[22,26]. It is curious that if one seropositive kidney does not transmit CMV to a particular seronegative recipient, the other kidney also usually does not so that unknown donor factors operate[27]. Among bone marrow transplant recipients factors governing risk of infection include CMV status of the donor and recipient and whether the transplant is allogeneic or autologous. Thus, for allogeneic bone marrow transplants approximately 70% of positive recipients develop CMV infection irrespective of donor serology and are due to reactivation or superinfection. The relative importance of each remains to be determined. Of seronegative recipients, 60% develop CMV infection if the donor is CMV positive and these are due to primary infections but only 30% develop CMV infection if both the donor and recipient are seronegative – this suggests primary infection from seropositive blood and seropositive blood product supports[28]. In the case of bone marrow autografts the risk for CMV infection appears to be lower than for allografts being approximately 60% for seropositive recipients and 35% for seronegative recipients[29]. Assiduous application of sensitive laboratory diagnostic techniques indicate that the majority of patients who are seropositive before transplantation will display at least some evidence of CMV infection after transplantation.

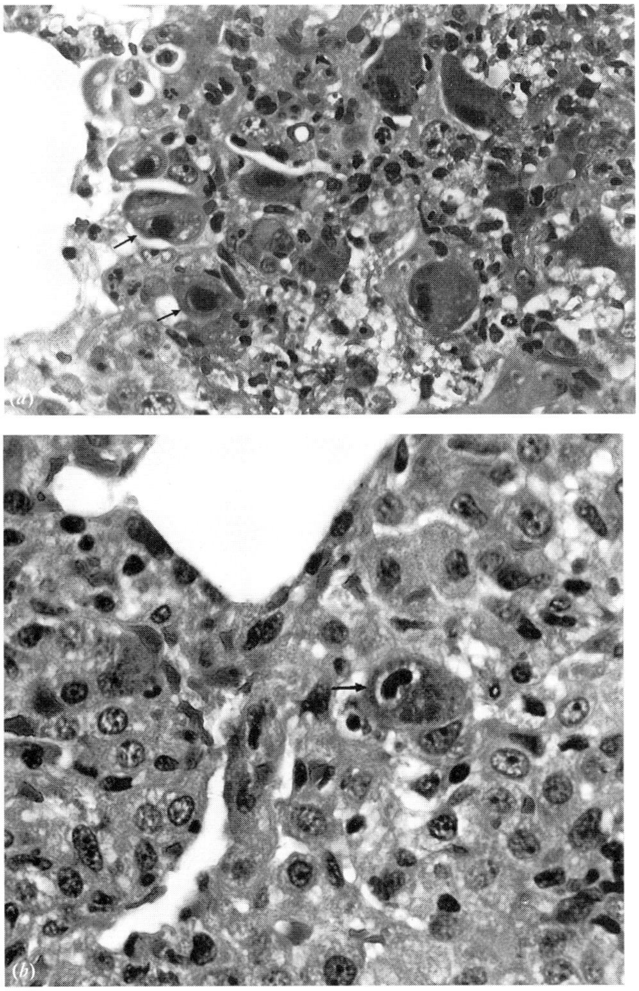
FIGURE 10.1 (*a*) CMV pneumonia : many cells containing cytomegalic inclusions at the edge of microabscess. (*b*) CMV pneumonia : characteristic enlarged cell with prominent nuclear and cytoplasmic inclusions ('Owl's eye' (arrowed)) (Courtesy of Dr Fouad Dayel.)

Table 10.2. *Risk factors for CMV infection and disease in transplant patients*

D– R–	+	
D+ R–	+++	
D+ R+	++	
D– R+	++	
BM allogeneic	++	
BM autograft	+	
Sero + blood/products	+ (+)	
Corticosteroids	+	
ALG, ATG, ALS, OKT_3	+++	
Cyclosporin	++ (for disease)	
GVHD	+ (+)	}
Age ↑	++	}
Cyclophosphamide	++	}
CMV viremia	++	} *
Total body irradiation	++	}
Abnormal pretransplant lung function	+	}

Relative risk:
\+ small.
++ moderate.
+++ large.
* for CMVIP in bone marrow transplants.
D donor.
R recipient.
– seronegative.
\+ seropositive.
BM, bone marrow transplant.
ALG, ATG, ALS, OKT_3, see text.

Frequency of disease as opposed to infection to some extent depends upon the source of the CMV, with 70% of primary infections, 40% of superinfections and 15% of reactivations displaying CMV disease features. However, severity of disease may be accentuated in patients whose CMV is of superinfection origin. In addition, bone marrow transplant recipients are at risk from more severe CMV disease than renal transplantation. CMV has been documented as the commonest infectious cause of death in allogeneic marrow transplants. Thus, CMVIP carries a mortality of up to 50%

in bone marrow allogeneic transplants[30,31] but is much lower in solid organ transplants[32]. Heart–lung transplants also have a high risk of invasive CMV disease[33].

Development of CMV infection and CMV pulmonary disease

The mechanisms which permit CMV to exert a pulmonary pathogenic role are not fully comprehended but certain key features are understood (Table 10.2). Immunosuppressive therapy including azathioprine, cyclophosphamide, corticosteroids and antilymphocytic globulins (ALG) have been variably associated with CMV infection reactivation, and increased CMV morbidity. This is mediated through their direct depressive effects on cell-mediated immune functions particularly the natural killer and cytotoxic T-cell functions. Of all the immunosuppressive agents used in transplant patients steroids are the least CMV-reactivating. Thus, in the pre-cytotoxic era, CMV infection or disease was uncommon and not until azathioprine and cyclophosphamide were introduced did CMV emerge as a significant cause of morbidity and mortality in transplant patients. However, high dose methylprednisolone is in fact known to impair cytotoxic T-cell responses in renal and bone marrow transplant recipients and prednisolone therapy does occasionally predispose to CMVIP which however usually responds to prednisolone withdrawal[34,35]. Polyclonal antilymphocytic globulins (ATG), antithymocyte globulins, antilymphocytic serum (ALS) and monoclonal antilymphocytic preparations (such as those directed against human CD3 – OKT_3) have the most potent effects on CMV reactivation. These are used for managing transplant rejection and carry a high risk for CMV disease[36,37]. Cyclosporin, although less able to cause CMV reactivation than antilymphocytic preparations, may have a profound dampening effect on the host response to replicating virus and may result in increased severity of CMV disease if it occurs. This has been demonstrated in a murine model[38]. Cyclosporin with ALG or with azathioprine/ALG, by combining maximal viral replication with suppression of host responsiveness are thus potential lethal combinations[7,10]. Another significant risk factor for CMVIP is GVHD. Thus, in patients with GVHD the risk of CMVIP is higher, compared to transplants with a low risk for GVHD, such as those occurring between identical twin donors or autografts[28,39–42]. The incidence in allogeneic bone marrow transplants is of the order of 20% compared with less than 5% in autografts or other low risk populations[40–42]. However, the precise relation of CMV and GVHD, however, remains unclear. An additional risk factor for CMVIP appears to be the use of total body irradiation[17] particularly if the dose rate exceeds 0.06 gy/minute. Other risk factors for CMVIP in marrow transplant recipients include increased age, treatment with cyclophosphamide, CMV viraemia and of course CMV seropositivity[28,43]. Of some interest is that certain pretransplant lung functions namely, FEV1, FVC, and TLC strongly predict for the subsequent development of CMVIP in bone marrow transplantation recipients[44]. This supports the suggestion that preexisting lung damage sets the scene for more frequent and more severe CMVIP. CMV releases interferon which enhances the expression of HLA antigens[45]. This could result in an amplification of mismatch and hence GVHD.

However, clinical epidemiological information relating CMV directly to rejection is weak.

The exact mechanism (cytopathic or immune-mediated) by which CMV induces interstitial pneumonitis is a subject of intense debate[46,47]. In certain types of transplant recipients, CMV pneumonia may be much more due to a direct viral cytopathic effect and hence response to antivirals alone might be effective. In others, particularly bone marrow transplant recipients there is evidence to suggest that the CMV triggered altered immune reactions may play an important role in ongoing pulmonary injury. Hence, antiviral agents alone are less effective therapeutically. One hypothesis, therefore, of CMVIP is that of an immunopathological process rather than a direct effect of viral replication within the lung tissue[10,46,48]. Mouse models have shown that although CMV *per se* can lead to interstitial pneumonia there appears to be a cellular pulmonary response involving THY1–2 lymphocytes and a Graft vs. Host reaction[49,50]. The resultant pneumonitis can proceed despite ganciclovir control of viral replication[51,52]. A possibility is that viral antigens or CMV enhanced HLA antigens are continually expressed to provide the basis for the ongoing pneumonitis. CMV has also been shown to encode a glycoprotein homologous to MHC class I antigens and cross reactivity of CMV with HLA DR β chains may occur[53,54]. The immunopathological basis for CMV is supported by clinical observations that autologous BMT patients have lower rates of CMVIP than allogeneic BMT patients[55]. Furthermore, severe CMV pneumonia is rare in patients with DiGeorge's syndrome who have T-cell deficiency. CMVIP, although rare in HIV patients, is more often severe in those patients whose CD4 counts are relatively preserved, the disease being mild in those whose CD4 count is lower[56]. Nevertheless, CMV viral inclusions do occur in pneumocytes and CMV antigens have been detected in BAL cells[57]. Any functional damage at alveolar level due directly to CMV could be worsened in the face of recent interstitial pneumonitis induced by chemotherapy.

Antibodies play an unclear role in CMVIP – endogenous levels are high during disease and there are conflicting reports over their efficacy in treatment. However, some studies have suggested that they may play a role in conjunction with ganciclovir in reducing the mortality rate from CMVIP possibly by blocking expressed CMV antigens in pulmonary tissues and hence reducing lymphocyte mediated cell damage.

In several patients with CMV disease, other pathogens may also be present. For example, fungi, protozoa particularly *Pneumocystis carinii* and bacteria[12]. Whether these are found as as a result of the immunosuppressive properties of CMV is a moot point. The contribution/collaboration of all these pathogens to overall morbidity and mortality is often difficult to delineate. Certainly in HIV patients the presence of CMV is more often interpreted as a 'passenger' and the lung disease ascribed to other pathogens or to nonspecific interstitial pneumonitis.

A rather facile synthesis of this conglomeration of observations with respect to the pathogenesis of CMVIP might be as follows. A viremic driven subclinical pulmonary infection occurs which in the face of depression of natural killer, cytotoxic and other immune responses fails to contain the infection. This results in widespread pneumocyte infection. BAL performed at this time will recover CMV in asymptomatic persons. Possibly aided by pre-existing lung damage, CMV then causes overt pneumonia, either due to a direct cytopathy or due to an immunopathological mechanism or to both.

Clinical presentation of CMV pulmonary disease

Fever, dry cough, and tachypnoea associated with hypoxaemia are commonly found, accompanied by fatigue, myalgia, and anorexia. Typically, the symptoms occur between 1 and 3 months after transplantation, although they can occur much later. Against these organ-specific features, a number of other manifestations of CMV may be present. These include hepatitis (raised ALT without hyperbilirubinaemia), gastrointestinal involvement (solitary or diffuse mucosal ulcerations, diarrhoea, cholecystitis and pancreatitis), retinitis (with characteristic perivascular exudates and flame-shaped haemorrhages), myocarditis with cardiac dysfunction, meningo-encephalitis, endocrine disturbance (particularly hypoadrenalism but also thyroiditis and parathyroid disturbance) and skin manifestations (petechiae, rubella-like or maculopapular rashes). In addition, thrombocytopaenia, leukopaenia, and atypical lymphocytosis may be found. The presence of hepatitis with this blood picture and fever completes a triad called the CMV syndrome. It is of some interest that extrapulmonary manifestations of CMV, such as retinitis, are not as commonly observed in bone marrow transplant patients as in other immunocompromised hosts (particularly HIV patients or those with renal transplantation). This may occur as a result of non-viral contributory aetiologies in this setting. CMV disease is often rapidly progressive but occasionally it can be stable and even self-resolving. CMV disease is usually more severe in primary infections and in bone marrow transplant recipients.

It is also important to remember that CMV is an immunosuppressive agent, and that this can lead to the emergence of superinfection with other opportunistic pathogens such as *Pneumocystis carinii*, *Aspergillus*, *Candida* and other fungi, *Listeria*, etc. Other features that should be looked for include the expression of the CMV graft interaction including features of CMV glomerulopathy in kidney transplantation[15], myocarditis and graft atherosclerosis in cardiac transplantation[58] and a unique CMV associated pseudorejection hepatitis picture in liver transplantation[26].

Radiographic abnormalities include diffuse lower lobe interstitial infiltrates (which is the most frequently observed pattern) (Fig. 10.2 (*a*), (*b*)) although a focal consolidation pattern multiple nodules (Fig. 10.3 (*a*)) or even solitary nodules or mass lesions have been described[59,60] (Fig. 10.4). Rapid progression to total lung opacification should indicate the need to rule out superinfection with other organisms such as *Pneumocystis carinii* (Figs. 10.5 (*a*), (*b*), (*c*)). Unusually, the chest radiograph may be normal.

Obviously, the differential diagnosis of interstitial pneumonia in these patients is wide and includes lung infiltration by recurrence of underlying disease, treatment toxicity (for example, radiochemotherapy), leukoagglutination reaction, pulmonary oedema, and other opportunistic infections including *Pneumocystis carinii* and mycobacterium tuberculosis.

Survival in patients with CMVIP is guarded but varies with the risk population and treatment modality. Solid organ transplant recipients generally fare better (Fig. 10.6 (*a*), (*b*)). Mortality is related to the severe respiratory distress of CMVIP, complications of GVHD and disseminated bacterial/fungal infections. Even in those who survive initially the outcome is not good. Significant long-term sequelae in BMT patients include restrictive lung disease and relapse of malignancy[61]. The use of CMV polymerase chain reaction techniques may predict the efficacy of antiviral therapy better than culture or clinical assessment[62].

Diagnosis

The laboratory diagnosis of CMV infection can be accomplished in a number of ways (Table 10.3). Histological demonstration of a cytopathic effect with CMV basophilic intranuclear/intracytoplasmic inclusion bodies called owl's eyes, stained by haematoxylin/eosin/Papanicolau/Wright–Giemsa in tissue culture or tissue biopsy is too time consuming. Concern arises from the fact that, by the time end organ pathology is microscopically evident, therapeutic opportunities may have passed by. Tissue sampling areas also severely hamper this diagnostic approach. Electronmicroscopy, similarly, appears to be of limited usefulness.

Serological methods include antibody detection based upon IgG (lifetime persistence) and IgM (persisting for up to 9 months but in some patients for more than 1 year) response to infection. Antibodies can usually be detected after a few weeks following initial viral infection and these are usually IgM. The presence of antibodies may provide information relating to the patient's immune status,

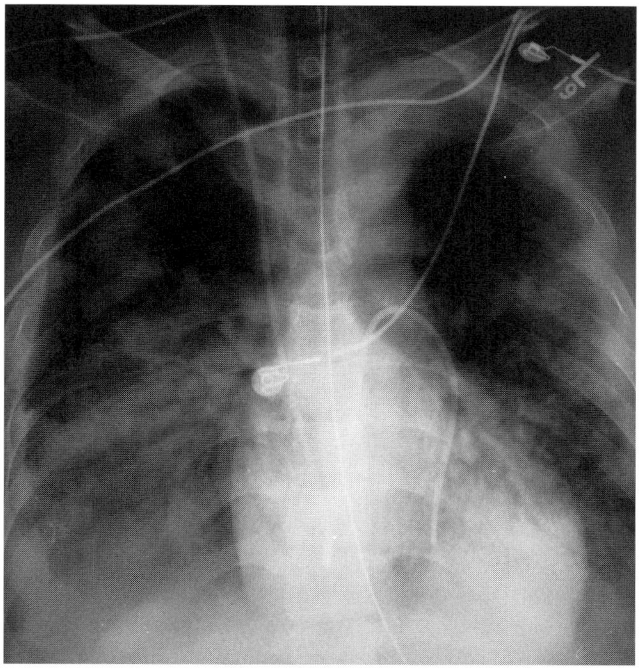

FIGURE 10.2 Patient received cadaveric renal transplant 3 years previously; developed chronic rejection and recent increasing dyspnoea. Chest radiograph shows widespread alveolar lower zone densities. Open lung biopsy indicated CMV by immunofluorescence.

indicating previous exposure to CMV or alternatively susceptibility to infection. If this is the situation pretransplant, it indicates that the patient is at risk from infection. The presence of IgM may suggest recent infection. However, development of antibodies may take some weeks and the uncertainty over their precise interpretation limits their utility in a patient whose symptoms may or may not be due to CMV infection. Seroconversion i.e. the development of antibodies in a patient previously documented as seronegative is usually indicative of primary infection. However, fluctuation in antibody levels as measured by complement fixation poses a problem. For example, an immune person on one occasion may have complement fixating titres of < 1 in 4, and > 1 in 1024 on a different occasion, but with no evidence of symptoms[63]. Thus, this considerable variability can provide dilemmas for interpretation. Hence, immune haemagglutination, immune fluorescent antibody determination (using an anticomplement method to diminish non-specific IgG binding) and latex agglutination tests are preferred. ELISA latex agglutination tests are useful in emergency situations since the result can be determined within an hour but suffer from 5% false negative and some false positive returns due to cross-reaction with other herpes viruses and with hepatitis B. More specific ELISA tests are being developed which no longer react against up to a hundred different viral antigens but are targeted toward detecting specific CMV antigens including pp150 and pp65[64]. The detection of neutralising antibodies gives an indication not of protection against CMV infection but of protection against more severe disease. Methodology involves a plaque reduction assay, however, is extremely time consuming and hampered by the necessity to obtain *in vitro* CMV strains with good plaque-forming properties. Hence, their determination is not of great clinical relevance[65].

In individuals who were previously seronegative the appearance of CMV-specific IgM is a specific and sensitive indicator of primary

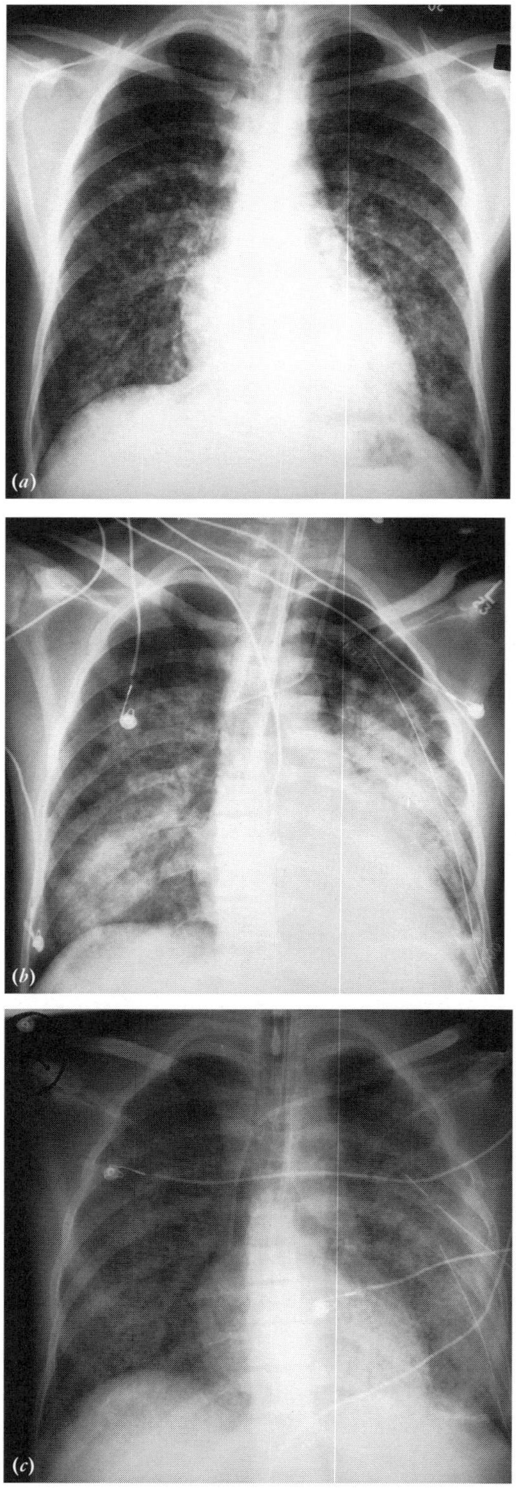

FIGURE 10.3 (*a*) Six weeks after cadaveric renal transplant; fever dyspnoea. (*b*) Same patient 2 days later. (*c*) Same patient 3 weeks later with ARDS.

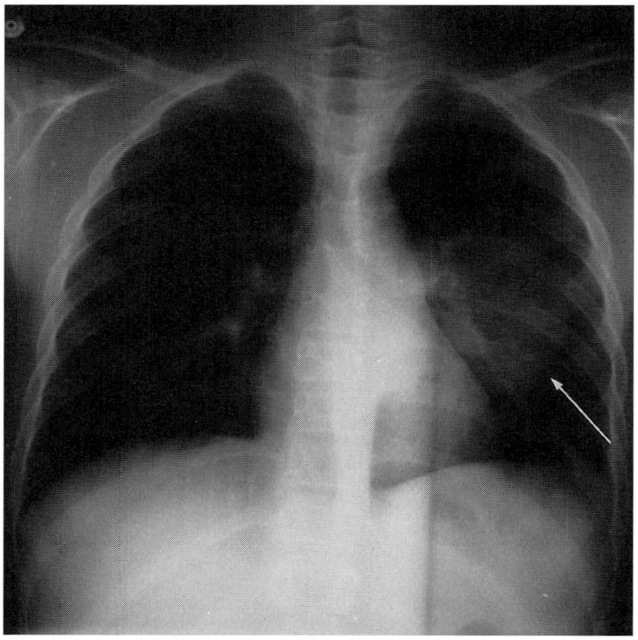

FIGURE 10.4 14-year bone marrow transplant allograft for AML, 6 weeks of hypoxia, cough, and Graft vs. Host disease. CMV cultured from throat and urine. CMV index increased from 2.57 to 5.30 (≅ ≥ four-fold titre increase). Chest radiograph showed large rounded mass, left mid-zone (arrow) which diminished on ganciclovir.

infection. It can be detected by RIA, immunofluorescence or ELISA methods. However, these tests have the same limitations as indicated for IgG. The presence of CMV IgM as detected by ELISA kits, however, may also indicate reactivation or superinfection. By targeting more specific antibodies associated with response to primary infection, for example, cytolytic IgM, IgM to infected fibroblasts, rp52, mp60, etc., a primary infection may be diagnosable[64]. Some immunocompromised hosts may not be able to mount an IgM response. Furthermore, rheumatoid factor interaction with IgG have to be eliminated by technical manoeuvres if these tests are to be reliable. Another problem is that the absence of CMV IgM in tissue/organ donors is no guarantee of non-infectiousness for CMV negative recipients. In summary, the presence of IgM or a fourfold rise in IgG or seroconversion is suggestive but not conclusive of active ongoing infection with CMV.

The use of traditional fibroblast culture techniques and observation of specific cytopathic effects is not a clinically useful method for the detection of CMV since it takes far too long (1–6 weeks) to provide information.

However, it is possible to detect CMV antigen much earlier than the cytopathic effects develop in tissue culture, a result being obtainable within days. This was originally performed using fluorescent antibody staining. Later the technique evolved into a super rapid or overnight cell culture method the shell-vial assay[66]. Increased intercellular contact using centrifugation, heat shock treatment of the cell monolayer, use of MRC-5 cells and monoclonal antibodies with power to detect immediate early or early antigen are important technical factors governing sensitivity of the assay. Detection of CMV antigen with the shell-vial assay system can be accomplished in bronchoalveolar lavage, tissue biopsies, blood leukocytes and other specimens and can provide a positive answer within 48 hours[67,68]. It may be necessary to use several antibodies towards both early and late antigens to detect the majority of strains[65]. Recently, it has been shown that a rapid centrifugation method using murine monoantibodies applied to BAL specimens in BMT patients with pneumonia was 96% sensitive and 100% specific for detecting CMV within 16 hours[67]. Furthermore, this method is much more sensitive than immunofluorescence antibody staining (sensitivity 59%) or observation of cytopathic changes (sensitivity 29%)[69]. Nevertheless, a few strains of CMV may go undetected by these methods. Viraemia as detected by shell-vial assay although having a high (60–70%) positive

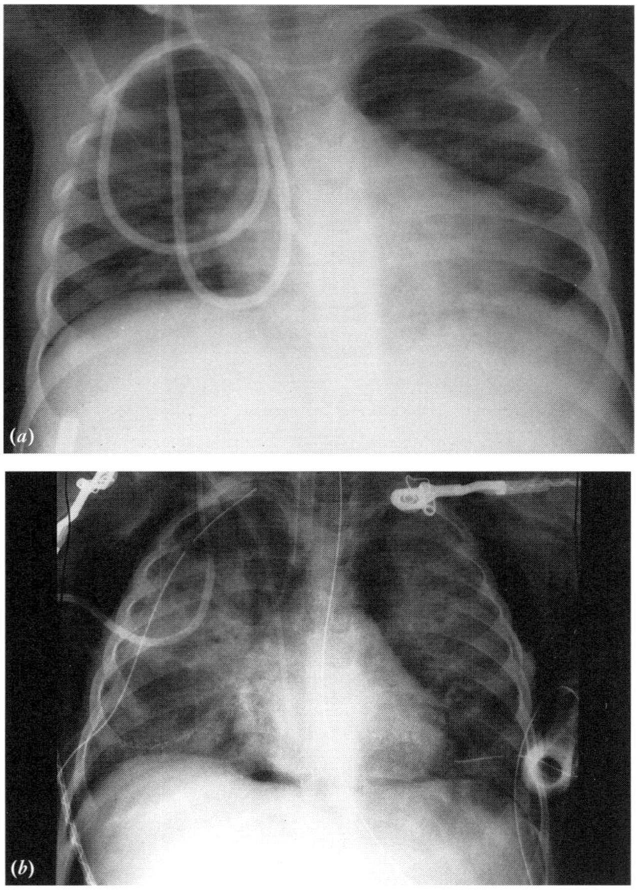

FIGURE 10.5 (*a*) Day 35 allograft bone marrow transplant. Mild dyspnoea and cough, subtle bilateral mainly lower zone infiltrates. (*b*) One week later, extensive bilateral dense infiltrates, left pneumothorax, mediastinal and subcutaneous emphysema. Open lung biopsy revealed both *Pneumocystis carinii* and CMV.

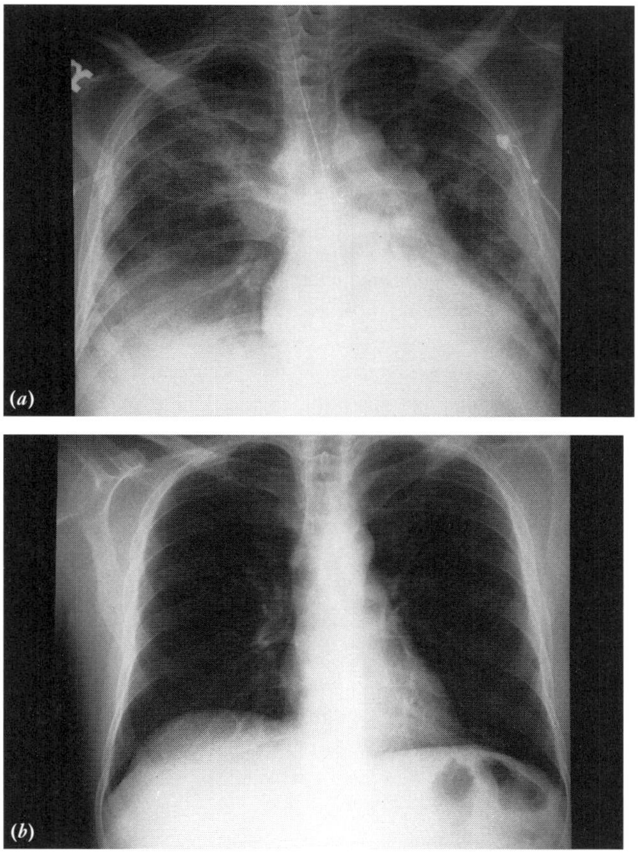

FIGURE 10.6 (*a*) 6 months liver transplant for cirrhosis maintained on azathioprine, prednisolone and FK506. 2 weeks of non-resolving pneumonia. Bilateral infiltrates with bilateral lower lobe atelactasis. Most open lung biopsy revealed *Pneumocystis carinii* and CMV. (*b*) Following treatment with ganciclovir and septrin for 6 weeks, patient recovered with a normal chest radiograph.

Table 10.3. *CMV detection methods*

Visualisation	
	histology inclusions
	electronmicroscopy
CMV antibodies	
	IgM
	IgG
	seroconversion
	fourfold rise in titre
Isolation of virus	
	traditional culture
	shell-vial assay
Direct detection of viral antigens	
	blood
	secretions
	tissue
Detection viral nucleic acid	
	Hybridisation
	PCR
	mRNA

predictive value for disease[43], nevertheless may be absent in as many as 50% of patients who have CMV disease[43]. Its value as an early predictor, therefore, is because of the rapidity with which a positive *in vitro* result is obtained. Such cultures become negative following treatment irrespective of clinical outcome and their use for monitoring therapy is therefore very limited[43].

Direct detection of circulating CMV antigen (CMV antigenaemia) has become very popular in recent years and is a landmark in CMV diagnostics[70]. An immunoperoxidase or immunofluorescence technique is used to stain for the lower matrix glycoprotein pp65 Ag in peripheral blood leucocytes. There is a positive correlation between the degree of antigenaemia and occurrence or severity of CMV disease. Thus, high level antigenaemia defined as > 50 antigen positive cells per 2×10^5 neutrophils is more likely to be seen with severe clinical disease[71,72]. Of great clinical importance is the finding that CMV antigenaemia occurs at a significant interval before clinical signs become evident. Thus, in a recent series of lung and heart transplant recipients, CMV antigenaemia occurred at a median of 35 days posttransplant whereas overt CMVIP occurred at 65 days. Although CMV antigenaemia is highly sensitive and specific for the detection of CMV infection, its positive predictive and negative predictive values for disease are of the order of 50% and 100% respectively. It therefore, provides an opportunity to identify patients likely to develop CMV disease and provide an early therapeutic opportunity[72]. CMV antigenaemia persists for some weeks after clinical recovery[73] Whether this could provide the basis for monitoring treatment and outcome remains to be clarified. The usefulness of this diagnostic approach in predicting CMV disease has also been seen for renal transplant patients[74] and for bone marrow transplant patients[75]. Currently, its detection represents one of the earliest means of diagnosing CMV infection. In BMT patients, it was suggested that even low grade antigenaemia may be predictive of disease and some such patients when retested showed rising antigen levels[75].

Direct determination of CMV antigen can also be performed in specimens other than blood leukocytes such as bowel, saliva, urine and lung biopsy[68,76,77]. Its usefulness, for example, in detecting asymptomatic CMV infection within lung tissue even before cytopathic changes occur has been demonstrated[77]. Logistic problems in performing the assay include the need for rapid processing (within 5 hours), the use of high grade microbiological safety cabinets, the need for improvement in standardisation techniques and selection of patients in whom it would be of greatest cost benefit.

Direct detection of part or whole of the viral genome sequences by polymerase chain reaction amplification techniques (PCR) or directly by hybridisation techniques has emerged and attracted considerable attention. *In situ* hybridisation detects DNA within organs. It is very sensitive and positive findings without obvious CMV disease are reported. Dot–blot hybridisation probe technique sensitivity is probably on a par with culture techniques. However, there are reports of discrepancies compared with tissue culture results, problems with false positivity possibly due to contamination (nested PCR reduces this) and how exactly to interpret the results. In bone marrow transplant and other transplant recipients, when compared to antigenaemic and shell-vial antigen techniques, CMV-DNA detected in peripheral blood lymphocytes or in serum is currently the earliest indicator of CMV infection[78,79]. It is more sensitive, but of lower specificity compared to culture and has a low positive but a high negative predictive value for disease[80]. For lung and heart–lung transplantation patients in whom BAL and peripheral blood samples were investigated, PCR was more sensitive and became positive earlier than tissue culture, cytology and histology in those who subsequently developed CMVIP[81]. In a comparison of PCR, CMV culture and hybridisation techniques for detecting CMV in the BAL of patients with CMVIP, PCR was at least as sensitive as CMV culture, and provided results faster and was superior to hybridisation techniques[82]. The relatively low positive predictive values for CMVIP using PCR can be improved by combining PCR testing with staining for CMV antigen in alveolar cells. Sensitivity, specificity, positive and negative predictive values for CMV disease using such strategies can then approach 100%[83,84]. Alternative approaches for maximising positive predictivity include the utilisation of two positive PCR signals, PCR quantitation, m-RNA measurement and use of plasma rather than peripheral blood leukocytes[80]. Detection of CMV mRNA (replicating CMV) may prove to be more indicative of active infection than CMV DNA. The concomitant presence of GVHD in BMT patients may also strengthen the significance of a positive PCR representing CMV disease[80].

CMV diagnostic possibilities – disease/infection

A plethora of diagnostic techniques are therefore now available for determining exposure/infection with CMV. The newer molecular biological techniques identify with the greatest rapidity evidence of CMV infection well before histological evidence of CMV disease has become established. Yet the gold standard for CMV disease to which all tests are compared is the isolation of the virus and of course demonstration of clinical, histological, and radiological evidence of disease. Hence, the PCR and peripheral antigen tests alone have a low positive predictive value for CMV disease. In an analysis of current practices for the diagnosis of CMV disease conducted by members of the European Bone Marrow Transplant Group, 57/70 centres used standard or rapid isolation techniques and 37/70 employed one of the newly developed techniques such as detection of antigen in peripheral blood leukocytes or PCR. Standard or rapid isolation as a sole technique was used by only 9 of 70 centres[85]. Clearly, there is a need to clarify the role of these various diagnostic tests in different immunocompromised populations, in the context of cost effectiveness, ease of performance, result interpretation and influence on prophylactive/ preemptive measures. Currently meanwhile, CMV antigenaemia assays rather than viraemic assays appear to be the preferred option for many patients for the prediction of CMVIP and CMV disease should more invasive techniques be considered inappropriate for particular patients. Certain features might prove useful in the dilemma of distinguishing infection from disease. These include (i) a compatible clinical presentation with detectable CMV as the sole pathogen (ideally from tissue or a positive blood culture or by the presence of CMV antigen); (ii) GVHD in transplant patients; and (iii) subsequent resolution of clinical features on specific treatment. The presence of all three features is highly indicative of CMV disease. Failure to fulfil *all* these requirements equates with a presumptive diagnosis only.

Specific management of CMV pneumonia

A number of antiviral drugs are available with variable activity against CMV. These include the nucleoside analogues idoxuridine, floxuridine, cytarabine, vidarabine, acyclovir and ganciclovir, the pyrophosphate analogue foscarnet, CMV immunoglobulin, interferon and growth factors.

The first four nucleoside compounds mentioned have not been adequately tested in controlled trial situations because of either lack of obvious clinical benefit in smaller pilot studies or unacceptable toxicities.

Acyclovir (a 2-deoxyguanosine analogue) requires three crucial metabolic steps to become an active antiherpes viral agent. The drug has to be converted to acyclovir monophosphate (by a cellular induced virus thymidine kinase), then acyclovir diphosphate (by cellular guanylate kinase) and finally to acyclovir triphosphate. In cells infected by herpes simplex and herpes zoster, large amounts of acyclovir triphosphate are formed. Since CMV does not induce thymidine kinase, only small amounts of acyclovir triphosphate are produced by the host cell which nevertheless may be sufficient to partly inhibit CMV viral DNA polymerase. However, clinical studies have not demonstrated a definite clinical advantage of acyclovir over placebo in patients with proven CMV pneumonia, for example, in bone marrow recipients[86]. However, there have been some encouraging results with prophylaxis studies (see later).

Ganciclovir, a deoxyguanosine analogue has up to 100 times more activity against CMV than acyclovir. This is related to the fact that the triphosphorylated form is readily produced in virus-infected cells, and this acts as an alternative substrate for CMV DNA polymerase, leading to termination of viral CMV DNA production. Although it can be administered orally, absorption is poor although some anti-CMV activity is detectable in serum. It is, therefore, usually administered intravenously, reaching peak levels at 2.5 hours, with $t_{\frac{1}{2}}$ of 2.5 hours and distribution to most body tissues and organs (which include the CNS, retina, liver, kidney, and lungs). It undergoes more than 90% renal elimination with virtually non-extrarenal metabolism. The dosage for established infection is 2.5 – 5 mg/kg Q8–Q12 hourly intravenously given for 3 weeks. Dosage is reduced in patients with diminished renal function: for patients with a creatinine clearance of 50–79 ml/min dosage is 2.5 mg/kg 12 hourly, 25–49 is 2.5 mg/kg 24 hourly and less than 25 is 1.25 mg/kg 24 hourly. Haemodialysis removes 50% of the drug and appropriate adjustments and supplementations have to be made.

As ganciclovir is also incorporated into host cell DNA, it is not surprising that toxicity occurs. However, as this drug is usually always used in patients with other concurrent severe illnesses, on multiple drugs, identification of specific ganciclovir toxicity is not easy. Nevertheless, leukopenia/thromboctypenia occurs in between 20% and 45% set of patients, usually after the first week of treatment. Neutropenia may be particularly problematic with concomitant administration of azidothymidine in HIV patients. Less commonly reported are associated symptoms of a neuro-psychiatric nature (confusion, headache, tremor, somnolence), gastrointestinal disturbances (nausea and diarrhoea), anaemia, rash, and phlebitis. Reproductive toxicity, teratogenicity and carcinogenicity have been observed in animals. Apart from reversible decreased spermatogenesis and increases in levels of FSH, LH and testosterone (which may or may not be related), no other side-effects have been documented in humans.

Despite effective *in vitro* activity of ganciclovir against CMV and very good virological responses *in vivo*, well-documented clinical responses are variable and depend on such factors as the primary risk/setting of the patient group being treated, and illness severity and duration. Unfortunately, there is a dearth of well-controlled clinical studies. Nevertheless, certain pertinent general conclusions can be drawn. In patients with solid organ transplants, clinical cure or improvement of CMV pneumonia has been documented in between 17% and 100% (overall approximately 79%)[87]. In some patients, early initiation of ganciclovir treatment after CMV pneumonia has been associated with a better outcome. This contrasts with previous mortality rates in patients not treated with ganciclovir of between 25% and 95%, for example, in renal and liver transplant recipients; in heart and heart–lung transplant recipients, the historical mortality rate from CMV pneumonia is 75%. The mortality rate from untreated bone marrow transplant recipients is between 80% and 100%[24,28,88].

In bone marrow transplant recipients, there appears to be a lesser therapeutic impact of ganciclovir with survival rates of between 10% and 45% being documented from uncontrolled studies[89,90]. Although these figures are not impressive, the overall picture is of improvement compared to historical controls or to patients treated with other nucleoside analogues or interferon. Initial animal studies demonstrated that although neither ganciclovir nor immunoglobulin alone was effective in the management of CMVIP, the combination was[91].

Some human studies using combined therapy with ganciclovir and intravenous immunoglobulin (IVIG) (usually with high titre for

CMV) have indicated that a better survival is achieved compared to historical series using ganciclovir or other therapies alone. CMV often persists in the lungs of BMT patients despite GCV treatment of the CMVIP. Although resistance to GCV has been described this does not always appear to explain its persistence in the lung[92]. Therefore, survival has been documented of the order of 70%[30,93] by some, others have reported a more modest response (approximately 30–50%[31,94]. The two most recent studies reported survivals of 52% and 70% using ganciclovir at 2.5 mg/kg Q8 hourly with IVIG at a dose of either 400 or 500 mg/day given in different regimes. Historical controls from these 2 centres were composed of patients who had been previously treated with ganciclovir or IVIG alone, or with other antivirals, and had survival rates which were significantly lower at 0–15%[30,93]. The reason for the variation in survival rates reported between different centres is not all clear but may include different diagnostic criteria and different patient population selection, which includes varying conditioning regimes (for example, total body irradiation has been shown to have a deleterious impact on survival)[94]. Other factors may include the timing with respect to the transplant at which the pneumonia occurs. The closer to the time of transplantation, the less likely is recovery, which is possibly related to the integrity of the host immune function. Early initiation of ganciclovir treatment may well be expected to be another factor although it remains unproven[95]. It has also been noted in some centres that the incidence of fatal CMV interstitial pneumonia in BMT patients has fallen significantly following the introduction of IVIG[96]. Improved survival in other patients (non-bone marrow transplant recipients) with CMV pneumonia treated with both ganciclovir and IVIG has not yet been documented. The mechanism for the apparent improved survival among BMT patients remains conjectural. One theory is that IVIG blocks the T-cell response to viral-induced antigen or HLA expressed antigens on lung cells, thereby reducing the cytotoxic reaction. Ganciclovir would meantime reduce viral replication and ultimately the expression of viral antigen might be diminished.

Foscarnet (trisodium phosphonophormate) is a pyrophosphate analogue that inhibits herpes DNA polymerase. Like ganciclovir it has to be administered intravenously and has a toxic spectrum. This includes nephrotoxicity, nausea and vomiting, anaemia, neuropsychiatric changes (tremors, seizures, headaches), phlebitis, hepatitis and electrolyte disturbances which include hypocalcaemia. Its major use has been in CMV disease (particularly retinitis) in AIDS patients, though it has been used in BMT and renal transplant recipients. It is difficult to draw conclusions over its effectiveness in CMV pneumonia in non-HIV immunocompromised hosts. However, in patients who have serious adverse reactions to ganciclovir, or in patients who have persistence of clinical symptoms and perhaps persistent viral excretion, then foscarnet treatment can be considered.

Studies using single or combination treatment with alpha interferon, acyclovir, vidarabine or corticosteroids have not shown any clinical benefit.

CMV PCR appears to predict the efficacy of antiviral treatment[62].

The management of CMV disease in the immunocompromised host should not only involve an aggressive attitude towards achieving early diagnosis but early instigation of specific anti-CMV treatment. It is not clear whether such an approach would really improve survival although there is some circumstantial evidence[95]. Thus, treatment should not be delayed because evidence of CMV disease has not been firmly established. It should be instigated on suspicion and continued, pending response and diagnostic results. For example, in patients with fever, unexplained thrombocytopaenia and cough in which other pathogens have been reliably excluded, CMV disease should be seriously entertained.

The question arises as to the need for secondary prophylaxis against CMV once the initial infective episode has been controlled, since relapse can occur particularly in BMT patients with Graft vs. Host disease or immunosuppressive therapy. Some continue with maintenance ganciclovir given daily for 5 days a week, together with IVIG given weekly after the initial treatment phase, either until the GVHD or immunosuppressive therapy is reduced/discontinued or for an empirical period of between 2 and 4 weeks.

The current status of management of CMVIP is summarised in Table 10.4.

CMV prophylaxis

Given the devastating course of established CMVIP in many transplant patients, currently most effort and emphasis is given to its prevention. Certain measures apart from the use of antivirals may prove useful to achieve this goal. Reduction in the intensity and type of immunosuppressive therapy may reduce the impact from CMV, for example, reduction of the dose and use of antilymphocytic globulin and OKT_3, but not cyclosporin, which is known to be associated with an increased incidence of CMV disease[70,97–99]. The use of seronegative blood/blood products for seronegative recipients has been shown to be highly effective in reducing the incidence of primary CMV infection in bone marrow transplant kidney and heart transplant recipients[100–104]. A sufficiently sensitive CMV antibody assay is crucial to identify those who are seropositive[105]. Serious supply problems can occur as seronegative donors are scarce and HLA matching for BMT is crucial. Leukocyte depletion of blood from seropositive donors for example by the use of blood filters is an alternative approach which is successful[106]. This strategy is of no use in preventing CMV infection in seropositive recipients[103].

Interferon has been used in renal transplant recipients. It may have some effect on CMV reactivation and CMV excretion in urine/saliva, but significant diminution in CMV disease is difficult to prove[107]. Concern over graft rejection (not seen in all studies) is a major disadvantage.

Active immunisation of seronegative recipients is another possibility. Studies using the life-attenuated Towne vaccine have shown that the immune response in immunocompromised patients is reduced although the vaccine is safe. It appears to offer some protection against the development of severe CMV disease but not of infection and it also improves graft survival, for example in renal transplant patients[108]. Concerns have been generated over the potential oncogenicity of the live vaccine and inadequate coverage of all CMV strains.

Use of immunoglobulins and antivirals in a prophylactic role has generated much attention in recent years. Passive immunisation

Table 10.4. *Management of CMVIP: synopsis*

IV GCV 5 mg/kg Q12 hrly × 3 weeks		
and		
CMVIVIG 500 mg/kg alternate days × 3 weeks		
If neutropenia	→	hold GCV growth factors foscarnet
If no response by 7 days		
	→	repeat BAL open lung biopsy cover other opportunistic infection change treatment, e.g. add foscarnet
Consider assisted ventilation (but poor outcome)		
Follow-up maintenance with GCV 5 mg/kg alternate days and CMVIVIG 500 mg/kg weekly until immunosuppressive therapy (for GVHD/rejection) curtailed		

using preparations of intravenous immunoglobulin of variable anti-CMV activity have tended to show a reduction in the severity of CMV disease and frequency of symptomatic disease in renal, marrow, liver and heart transplants[109–115]. In some patients concomitant reduction in fungal infection has also been documented[116]. However, results are conflicting and randomised controlled studies have only been consistently performed in bone marrow transplant recipients. Initial studies in seronegative BMT recipients suggested that CMV specific intravenous immunoglobulin (CMVIVIG) added little benefit in the prevention of CMV infection or disease over and above that of using screen blood products[117–119]. However, one controlled study did confirm a reduction in primary CMV infection but not of CMV disease[119]. Other studies have investigated the effect of pooled intravenous immunoglobulin (IVIG) when given to seronegative BMT recipients. The results indicate a significant reduction in CMVIP which is not clearly related to reduction in CMV infection[120–123]. This apparent paradoxical dissociation of the effect of CMV infection from CMV disease is not clearly understood. It could be due to a primary effect on the reduction of GVHD with a reduction in CMV disease as secondary phenomenon[123]. Possible contaminants such as CD4, CD8 and HLA molecules within IVIG might be responsible for the effect on CMV disease[124]. A meta analysis of 12 published studies involving 1282 patients indicated that both CMVIVIG and IVIG significantly reduce fatal CMV infection, CMVIP and total mortality in BMT recipients. Effects were seen for both CMV negative and CMV positive recipients[125]. In addition to these somewhat unclear results immunoglobulin preparations are expensive. The precise role of passive immunisation therefore still requires more elucidation although the current evidence suggests that it is of use in bone marrow transplant recipients, in renal transplant recipients at risk from primary CMV infection[109] and in liver transplant recipients at risk from secondary CMV infection[126].

Despite the poor activity of acyclovir against established CMV disease, it appears to have protective efficacy. Earlier reports investigating the prophylactic efficacy of oral acyclovir for herpes simplex virus infections in bone marrow transplant recipients also indicated that protection against CMV occurred[127]. In renal transplant recipients, controlled studies indicate that oral acyclovir 800 mg Q6 hourly (reduced in patients with diminished renal function) significantly reduces the rate of CMV infection and disease including CMVIP particularly in patients at risk of primary CMV disease[128]. In other solid organ transplants, namely, lung, heart–lung and in some other kidney transplant studies, high dose oral acyclovir with/without other CMV prophylaxis was not beneficial[129,130]. However, in BMT recipients IV acyclovir at a dose of 500 mg/sq m Q8 hourly resulted in significant reduction in rates of CMV infection, disease including pneumonia, mortality, and CMV excretion as well as delaying the time to onset of infection[131]. Other studies did not find acyclovir beneficial but this may be due to different dosages used[132]. The most recent study investigated 310 bone marrow transplant recipients at risk from CMV infection[133]. The three treatment arms were intravenous acyclovir 500 mg/sq m Q8 hourly for one month followed by either oral acyclovir 800 mg 4 times per day for 6 months (Group A) or placebo (Group B) and low dose oral acyclovir (200 to 400 mg 4 times per day) followed by placebo (Group C). Survival was significantly increased in Group A. The frequency of CMV infection was diminished and the time to occurrence of viraemia increased in patients in Group A. However, criticisms were raised concerning the concomitant use of ganciclovir, different treatments for CMV disease and rates of non-herpetic severe infectious complications. In liver transplant patients, low dose acyclovir with immunoglobulin was very successful in preventing primary infection[134]. This could not be confirmed in a recent study, where oral acyclovir was found to be inferior compared to preemptive short course ganciclovir[135]. Acyclovir therefore, though not totally efficacious has made a significant impact on CMV disease in some patients. Future studies with oral acyclovir pro-drugs which should increase the serum levels of acyclovir to well above the MICs for CMV, may produce some interesting results.

Ganciclovir has been used in two major disease preventative modes, namely, (i) prophylactically in all patients at risk from active CMV infection but without disease, and (ii) preemptively in patients who have documented laboratory evidence of active infection but without disease.

Use of ganciclovir in all patients at risk from active CMV infection

To date, five studies have addressed the issue of universal ganciclovir prophylaxis in allogeneic seropositive BMT recipients[136–140]. There was variation in study design -historical controls, double-blindedness, time of initiation and duration of prophylaxis, concomitant acyclovir treatment, dosages, study population, and the incidence of GVHD and CD8 profile in the control group were not uniform. Nevertheless, all the studies agree that there was a significant reduction in CMV infection and CMV disease but not all reported improvement in survival. Ganciclovir associated haematological toxicity was notable in some studies and associated with a high risk for bacterial infection. When used in heart transplant recipients sometimes with acyclovir and sometimes with immunoglobulin, GCV reduced CMV morbidity in seropositive recipients[141,142] but had no significant effect in seronegative recipients[33,142,143]. Since viraemia appeared to have been delayed in the patients who were on ganciclovir, it may be that ganciclovir needs to be given for a longer period of time to be more effective in heart/heart–lung transplant patients. The benefit of GCV in solid organ transplant patients may also have been ascribed to the group who would have been expected to have milder CMV disease anyway namely, the seropositive recipients. The general opinion is that ganciclovir used in solid organ transplant recipients should be targeted for those at higher risk for CMV disease, namely, those who are receiving OKT_3 or those who are seronegative.

Foscarnet has not been studied so intensively. Preliminary results from an open study among BMT patients suggest some efficacy in reducing CMV infection but at the risk of nephrotoxicity[144] and it cannot be recommended at this stage.

Pre-emptive therapy with ganciclovir

One of the concerns of the universal prophylactic approach as outlined above is overuse of ganciclovir with haematological toxicity, emergence of superinfections and resistant strains of CMV. In an attempt to reduce this, patients who develop early infection with CMV have been selected for intravenous ganciclovir treatment in an attempt to prevent CMV disease. This is known as preemptive therapy. There have been two major studies at the time of writing using this approach[145,146]. In Schmidt's study[145], allogeneic bone marrow transplant patients underwent bronchoalveolar lavage on day 35. Those who had a positive CMV culture on BAL received ganciclovir or placebo. A significant reduction (of 93%) in CMVIP occurred in those given ganciclovir at 5 mg/kg IV twice daily for 14 days then daily to day 120. Survival was not improved. In the Goodrich study[146], all patients underwent regular weekly surveillance screening of throat, urine and blood. Those who had a positive CMV culture at any site received ganciclovir 5 mg/kg intravenous twice daily for 7 days then daily to day 100. High dose acyclovir was also permitted in this study. A significant reduction (77%) of CMVIP and mortality was documented. In both studies, ganciclovir-associated neutropenia developed in 35% leading to ganciclovir dose modification. Approximately 12% of patients in either study who had negative surveillance cultures developed CMV disease indicating that more rapid and sensitive methods for CMV detection (such as CMV antigenaemia or PCR) are required to heighten the efficacy of ganciclovir pre-emptive therapy. Viraemia was found to be a predictor for CMV disease in both studies.

It therefore appears that, by monitoring bone marrow transplant patients for the occurrence of early CMV infection and then instituting early treatment with ganciclovir, a significant impact on CMV disease can be made. This is to be preferred to the concept of universal prophylaxis. Issues requiring clarification include an improvement in early and rapid diagnostic methods, clarification of dose and duration of preemptive therapy which may be monitored by serial quantitation of CMV antigen for example, reduction in frequency of ganciclovir toxicity, for example, by the use of growth factors, monitoring for emergence of ganciclovir resistance and the role of additional prophylaxis such as low dose acyclovir in combination with ganciclovir.

The role of such preemptive therapy in solid organ transplant recipients remains to be clarified. However, in one study of liver transplant recipients, it has been shown that a 7-day course of ganciclovir pre-emptive therapy for patients shedding virus in urine or blood significantly reduced the likelihood of progression to CMV disease[135].

Recently it has been shown that the administration of low-dose pre-emptive gancicovir to seropositive renal transplant recipients during periods of heightened intense immunosuppression during ALG therapy, irrespective of detection of CMV antigen or virus, decreased the incidence of CMV disease[147].

The current practices of preventing CMV infection/disease are summarised in Table 10.5.

Table 10.5. *CMV infection/disease preventative strategies*

	Bone marrow	Kidney	Heart/lung	Liver
Seroneg blood/ products/matching/ filters	+++[a]	+++[a]	+++[a]	+++[a]
CMVIVIG	++[b]	++[c]	NA	++[a]
IVIG	++[d]	NA	NA	NA
Acyclovir	++	++[c]	0	(+) +[c]
Ganciclovir[e]	++(+)	NA	+++[a]	NA

Efficacy NA = Little/no data from controlled studies available.
0 = None.
\+ = Controversial/conflicting.
++ = Effective.
+++ = Highly effective.

[a] = Only for seronegative recipients at risk from primary CMV disease, no effect in seropositive recipients.
[b] = CMV infection prevented but not CMV disease.
[c] = Has also been used as a moderate dose acyclovir/CMVIVIG combination.
[d] = CMV disease prevented but not CMV infection.
[e] = Effective also in pre-emptive mode.

Other prophylactic measures

Newer antivirals include valaciclovir, an acyclovir pro-drug providing higher serum levels, is undergoing trials. HPMPC, a cytosine nucleotide analogue, which does not require a viral directed phosphorylation step is also undergoing early studies. By infusing cloned CMV specific cytotoxic lymphocytes prepared *in vitro* to seronegative BMT patients it may be possible to restore CMV immune competency and to protect the patient from CMV infection and disease. Phase 1 studies have already indicated the feasibility of this approach[148]. Development of a safer active vaccine than the present Towne preparation, for example, by the use of immunogenic CMV subunit preparations or suicide programmed live recombinant vaccines are further possibilities.

Final comments

CMV lung disease still presents a major challenge in the immunocompromised host. Better diagnostic techniques are needed which will increase the sensitivity for detecting CMV infection and to reliably differentiate between infection and disease. Unfortunately, no controlled studies have been done using ganciclovir for treatment and as many physicians now believe that since the introduction of this drug survival from CMV pneumonia has improved that it may be unethical to conduct such studies. However, improvement in other aspects of care of the immunocompromised host has occurred over the same period that ganciclovir was introduced, and confuses this issue. Comparative studies of different modalities of treatment, for example, combination foscarnet with ganciclovir need to be undertaken. These studies also need to address response predictors. Newer anti-CMV drugs require development. These should have greater activity, less toxicity, and should be available for oral administration. Already there is some progress on the horizon with the development of oral preparations, e.g. oral ganciclovir.

As immunocompromised pathogenic mechanisms for CMV pneumonia become further clarified, unique modalities of treatment may become available to supplement antiviral therapy. These could include, for example, immunomodulatory approaches using cytotoxic T-cells, adjuvant cytokine therapy and newer vaccine treatments, for example, subunit vaccines.

References

1. COHEN JI, COREY GR. Cytomegalovirus infection in the normal host. *Medicine* 1985; 64:100–14.
2. PASS RF, STAGNO S, MYERS GJ *et al.* Outcome of symptomatic congenital CMV infection: results of long-term longitudinal follow up. *Pediatrics* 1980;66:758–62.
3. RUUTU P, RUUTU T, VIOLON L *et al.* Cytomegalovirus is frequently isolated in bronchoalveolar lavage fluid of bone marrow transplant recipients without pneumonia. *Ann Intern Med* 1990;112:913–16.
4. GRIFFITHS PD. Current management of cytomegalovirus disease. *J Med Virol* Suppl 1993;1:106–11.
5. GOODRICH JM, BOECKH M, BOWDEN R. Strategies for the prevention of cytomegalovirus disease after marrow transplantation. *Clin Infect Dis* 1994;19:287–98.
6. KRECH U. Complement-fixing antibodies against cytomegalovirus in different parts of the world. *Bull WHO* 1973;49:103–6.
7. HO M. Epidemiology of cytomegalovirus infections. *Rev Infect Dis* 1990:12(57)S701–10.
8. REUSSER P, RIDDELL SR, MEYERS JD, GREENBERG PD. Cytotoxic T-lymphocyte response to cytomegalovirus after human allogeneic bone marrow transplantation: pattern of recovery and correlation with cytomegalovirus infection and disease. *Blood* 1991;78:1373–80.
9. GRIFFITHS PD, GRUNDY JE. Molecular biology and immunology of cytomegalovirus. *Biochem J* 1987;241:313–24.
10. RUBIN RH. Impact of cytomegalovirus infection on organ transplant recipients. *Rev Infect Dis* 1990;12:S754–66.
11. NG-BAUTISTA, CL, SEDMAK DD. Cytomegalovirus infection is associated with absence of alveolar epithelial cell HLA class II antigen expression. *J Infect Dis* 1995;171(1):39–44.
12. RAND KH, POLLARD RB, MERIGAN TC. Increased pulmonary superinfections in cardiac transplant recipients undergoing primary cytomegalovirus infection. *N Engl J Med* 1978;298:951–3.
13. RUBIN RH, WOLFSON JS, COSIMI AB *et al.* Infection in the renal transplant recipient. *Am J Med* 1981;70:405–11.
14. FRYD DS, PETERSON PK, FERGUSON RM *et al.* Cytomegalovirus as a risk factor in renal transplantation. *Transplantation* 1980;30:436–9.
15. RICHARDSON WP, COLVIN RB, CHEESEMAN SH *et al.* Glomerulopathy associated with cytomegalovirus viraemia in renal allografts. *N Engl J Med* 1981;305:57–63.
16. O'GRADY JG, ALEXANDER GJM, SUTHERLAND S *et al.* Cytomegalovirus infection and donor recipient HLA antigens: interdependent co-factors in pathogenesis of vanishing bile duct syndrome after liver transplantation. *Lancet* 1988;1:302–5.
17. DUNCAN SR, PARADIS IL, YOUSEM SA *et al.* Sequelae of cytomegalovirus pulmonary infection in lung allograft recipients. *Am Rev Resp Dis* 1992;146:1419–25.
18. GIRALDO G, BETH E, COEUR P *et al.* Kaposi's sarcoma – new model in the search for viruses associated with human malignancies. *JNCI* 1972;49:1495–507.
19. HUANG ES, ROCHE JK. Cytomegalovirus adenocarcinoma of the colon: evidence for latent virus infection. *Lancet* 1978;1:957–60.
20. SMITH MG. Propagation in tissue cultures of a cytopathogenic virus from human salivary gland virus (SGV) disease. *Proc Soc Exp Biol Med* 1956;92:424–30.
21. WINGARD JR, PIANTADOSI S, BURNS WH *et al.* Cytomegalovirus infections in bone marrow transplant recipients given intensive cytoreductive therapy. *Rev Infect Dis* 1990;12:S793–804.
22. PETERSON RD, BALFOUR HH JR, MARKER SC *et al.* Cytomegalovirus disease in renal allograft recipients: a prospective study of the clinical features, risk factors and impact on renal transplantation. *Medicine* 1980;59:283–300.
23. RUBIN RH. Impact of cytomegalovirus infection on organ transplant recipients. *Rev Infect Dis* 1990;12:S754–66.
24. DUMMER JS, WHITE LT, HO M *et al.* Morbidity of cytomegalovirus infection in recipients of heart or heart–lung transplants who received cyclosporine. *J Infect Dis* 1985;152:1182–91.
25. JACOBSON MA, MILLS J. Serious cytomegalovirus disease in the acquired immunodeficiency syndrome (AIDS). Clinical findings diagnosis and treatment. *Ann Intern Med* 1988;108:585–94.
26. PAYA CV, HERMANS PE, WIESNER RH *et al.* Cytomegalovirus hepatitis in liver transplantation: prospective analysis of 93 consecutive orthotopic liver transplantations. *J Infect Dis* 1989;160:752–8.
27. CHAN SW, NORMAN DJ. The influence of donor factors other than serologic status on transmission of cytomegalovirus to transplant recipients. *Transplantation* 1988;46:89–93.
28. MEYERS JD, FLOURNEY N, THOMAS ED. Risk factors for cytomegalovirus infection after human marrow transplantation. *J Infect Dis* 1986;153:478–88.
29. REUSSER P, FISHER LD, BUCKNER CD, THOMAS ED, MEYERS JD. Cytomegalovirus infection after autologous bone marrow transplantation: occurrence of cytomeglovirus disease and effect on engraftment. *Blood* 1990;75:1888–94.
30. EMANUEL D, CUNNINGHAM I, JULES-EYSEE K *et al.* Cytomegalovirus pneumonia after bone marrow transplantation successfully treated with the combination of ganciclovir and high-dose intravenous immune globutus. *Ann Intern Med* 1988;109:777–82.
31. REED EC, BOWDEN RA, DANDLIKER PS *et al.* Treatment of cytomegalovirus pneumonia with ganciclovir and intravenous cytomegalovirus immunoglobulin in patients with bone marrow transplants. *Ann Intern Med* 1988;109:783–8.
32. JORDAN ML, HREBINKO RL JR, DUMMER JS *et al.* Therapeutic use of ganciclovir for

invasive cytomegalovirus infection in cadaveric renal allograft recipients. *J Urol* 1992;148:1388–92.

33. ETTINGER NA, BAILEY TC, TRULOCK EP *et al.* Cytomegalovirus infection and pneumonitis. Impact after isolated lung transplantation. *Am Rev Resp Dis* 1993;147(4):1017–23.
34. MORRIS DJ, LONGSON M, POSLETHWAITE R, MALLICK NP, JOHNSON RWG. Donor seropositivity and maintenance prednisolone therapy as determinants of the incidence of cytomegalovirus infection in cyclosporin-treated renal allograft recipients. *Quart J Med* 1990;77:1165–73.
35. JEFFREY JR, GUTTMAN RD, BECKLAKE MR, BEAUDOIN JG, MOREHOUSE DD. Recovery from severe cytomegalovirus pneumonia in a renal transplant patient. *Am Rev Resp Dis* 1974;109:129–33.
36. BAILEY TC, POWDERLEY WG, STORCH GA *et al.* Symptomatic cytomegalovirus infection in renal transplant recipients given either Minnesota antilymphoblast globulin (MALG) or OKT_3 for rejection prophylaxis. *Am J Kidney Dis* 1993;21:196–201.
37. CALHOON JH, LARHEA N, DAVIS R *et al.* Single lung transplantation. Factors in postoperative cytomegalovirus infection. *J Thoracic Cardiovasc Surg* 1992;103:21–6.
38. RUBIN RH, PASTERACK MS, MEDEARIS DN, LYNCH P, SMITH S, AUCHINCLOSS H. The effects of different immunosuppressive regimens on the course of murine cytomegalovirus infection. *Transplantation* 1990 (in press).
39. MEYERS JD, FLUORNOY N, THOMAS ED. Non-bacterial pneumonia after allogeneic marrow transplantation. A review of ten years' experience. *Rev Infect Dis* 1982;4:1119–1132.
40. WINGARD JR, CHEN DY, BURNS WH *et al.* Cytomegalovirus infection after autologous bone marrow transplantation with comparison to infection after allogeneic bone marrow transplantation. *Blood* 1988;71:1432–7.
41. APPELBAUM FR, MEYERS JD, FEFER A *et al.* Non-bacterial non-fungal pneumonia following marrow transplantation in 100 identical twins. *Transplantation* 1982;33:265–8.
42. WINGARD JR, SOSTRIN MB, VRIESENDORP HM *et al.* Interstitial pneumonitis following autologous bone marrow transplantation. *Transplantation* 1988;46:61–5.
43. MEYERS JD, LJUNGMAN P, FISCHER LD. Cytomegalovirus excretion as a predictor of cytomegalovirus disease after marrow transplantation: importance of cytomegalovirus viremia. *J Infect Dis* 1990;162:373–80.
44. HORAK DA, SCHMIDT GM, ZAIA JA, NILAND JC, AHN C, FORMAN SJ. Pretransplant pulmonary function predicts cytomegalovirus-associated interstitial pneumonia following bone marrow transplantation. *Chest* 1992;102(5):1484–90.
45. GRUNDY JE, AYLES HM, MCKEATING JA *et al.* Enhancement of class I HLA antigen expression by cytomegalovirus: role in amplification of virus infection. *J Med Virol* 1988;25:483–95.
46. GRUNDY JE, SHANLEY JD, AND GRIFFITHS PD. Is cytomegalovirus interstitial pneumonitis in transplant recipients an immunopathological condition? *Lancet* 1987;2:996–9.
47. MORRIS DJ. Cytomegalovirus pneumonia – a consequence of immunosuppression and pre-existing lung damage rather than immunopathology? *Resp Med* 1993;87:345–9.
48. WINSTON DJ, HO WG, AND CHAMPLIN RE. Cytomegalovirus infection after allogeneic bone marrow transplantation. *Rev Infect Dis* 1990;12:S776–92.
49. SHANLEY JD, VIA CS, SHARROW SO *et al.* Interstitial pneumonitis during murine cytomegalovirus infection and graft versus host reaction. Characterisation of bronchoalveolar lavage cells. *Transplantation* 1987;44:658–62.
50. GRUNDY JE, SHANLEY JD, SHEARER GM. Augmentation of graft versus host reaction by cytomegalovirus infection resulting in interstitial pneumonitis. *Transplantation* 1985;39:548–53.
51. SHANLEY JD AND JODRON MC. Viral pneumonia in the immunocompromised patient. *Semin Resp Infect* 1986;1(3):193–201.
52. SHEPP DH, DANDLIKER PS, DE MIRANDAP *et al.* Activity of 9-[2-hydroxy-1 (hydroxymethyl) ethoxymethyl] guanine in the treatment of cytomegalovirus pneumonia. *Ann Intern Med* 1985;103:368–73.
53. FUJINAMI RS, NELSON JA, WALKER L, OLDSTONE MBA. Sequence homology and immunologic cross-reactivity of human cytomegalovirus with HLA-dr β chains: a means for graft rejection and immunosuppression. *J Virol* 1988;62:100–5.
54. BECK S, BARRELL BG. Human cytomegalovirus encodes a glycoprotein homologous to MHC class I antigens. *Nature* 1988;331:269–72.
55. GRUNDY JE. Virologic and pathogenic aspects of cytomegalovirus infection. *Rev Infect Dis* 1990;12:S711–S19.
56. SQUIRE SB, LIPMAN MC, BAGDADES EK *et al.* Severe cytomegalovirus pneumonitis in HIV infected patients with higher than average CD4 counts. *Thorax* 1992;47(4):301–4.
57. DEGRÉ M, BUKHOLM G, HOLTER E, MÜLLER F, ROLLAG H. Rapid detection of cytomegalovirus infection in immunocompromised patients. *Eur J Clin Microbiol Infect Dis* 1994;13:668–70.
58. GRATTAN MT, MORENO-CABRAL CE, STARNES VA *et al.* Cytomegalovirus infection is associated with cardiac allograft rejection and atherosclerosis. *JAMA* 1989;261:3561–6.
59. RUBIN RH, COSIMI AB, TOLKOFF-RUBIN NE *et al.* Infectious disease syndromes attributable to cytomegalovirus and their significance among renal transplant patients. *Transplantation* 1977;24:458–64.
60. RAVIN CE, SMITH GW, AHERN MJ *et al.* Cytomegalovirus Infection presenting as a solitary pulmonary nodule. *Chest* 1977;71:220–2.
61. CHIEN SM, CHAN CK, KASUPSKI G, CHAMBERLAIN D, FYLES G, MESSNER H. Long-term sequelae after recovery from cytomegalovirus pneumonia in allogeneic bone marrow transplant recipients. *Chest* 1992;101(4):1000–4.
62. EINSELE H, EHNINGER G, STEIDLE M *et al.* Polymerase chain reaction to evaluate antiviral therapy for cytomegalovirus disease. *Lancet* 1991;338(8776):1170–2.
63. WANER JL, WELLER TH, KEVY SV. Patterns of cytomegalovirus complement-fixing antibody activity: a longitudinal study of blood donors. *J Infect Dis* 1973;127:538–43.
64. LANDINI MP. New approaches and perspectives in cytomegalovirus diagnosis. Melnick JL, ed. *Progress in Medical Virology*, Basel: Karger 1993;40:157–77.
65. PLUMMER G AND BENYESH-MELNICK M. A plaque reduction neutralisation test for human cytomegalovirus. *Proc Soc Exp Biol Med* 1964;117:145–50.
66. GLEAVES CA, SMITH TF, SHUSTER EA, PEARSON GR. Rapid detection of cytomegalovirus in MRC-5 cells inoculated with urine specimens by using low-speed centrifugation and monoclonal antibody to an early antigen. *J Clin Microbiol* 1984;19:917–19.
67. PAYA CW, WOLD AD, SMITH TF. Detection of cytomegalovirus infections in specimens other than urine by the shell vial assay and conventional tube cultures. *J Clin Microbiol* 1987;25(5):755–7.
68. EMANUEL D, PEPPARD J, STOVER D *et al.* Rapid immunodiagnosis of cytomegalovirus pneumonia by bronchoalveolar lavage, using human and murine monoclonal antibodies. *Ann Intern Med* 1986;104:476–81.
69. CRAWFORD SW, BOWDEN RA, HACKMAN RC *et al.* Rapid detection of cytomegalovirus pulmonary infection by bronchoalveolar lavage and centrifugation culture. *Ann Intern Med* 1988;108:180–5.
70. BIJ W VAN DER, SCHIRM J, TORENSMA R

et al. Comparison between viremia and antigenaemia for detection of cytomegalovirus in blood. *J Clin Microbiol* 1988;26:2531–5.

71. GERNA G, ZIPETO D, PAREA M *et al.* Monitoring of human cytomegalovirus infections and ganciclovir treatment in heart transplant recipients by determination of viremia, antigenaemia and DNAemia. *J Infect Dis* 1991;164;488–98.

72. EGAN JJ, BARBER L, LOMAX J *et al.* Detection of human cytomegalovirus antigenaemia: a rapid diagnostic technique for predicting cytomegalovirus infection/pneumonitis in lung and heart transplant recipients. *Thorax* 1995;50:9–13.

73. THE TH, BIJ VANDER W, BERG VANDEN AP *et al.* Cytomegalovirus antigenaemia. *Rev Inf Dis* 1990;12:S737–44.

74. KLAUSER R, KOTZMANN H, WAMSER P *et al.* Is determination of pp65 useful for early diagnosis of cytomegalovirus infection in renal transplant recipients. *Transpl Proc* 1992;24:2628–30.

75. BOECKH M, BOWDEN RA, GOODRICH J, PETTINGER M, MEYERS JD. Cytomegalovirus antigen detection in peripheral blood luekocytes after allogeneic bone marrow transplantation. *Blood* 1992;80:1358–64.

76. CORDONNIER C, ESCUDIER E, NICOLAS JC *et al.* Evaluation of three assays on alveolar lavage fluid in the diagnosis of cytomegalovirus pneumonias after bone marrow transplantation. *J Infect Dis* 1987;155:495–500.

77. SOLANS EP, GARRITY ER, MCCABE M, MARTINEZ R, HUSAIN AN. Early diagnosis of cytomegalovirus pneumonitis in lung transplant patients. *Arch Pathol Lab Med* 1995;119:33–5.

78. WOLF DG, SPECTOR SA. Early diagnosis of human cytomegalovirus disease in transplant recipients by DNA amplification in plasma. *Transplantation* 1993;27:1802.

79. ISHIGAKI S, TAKEDA M, KURA T *et al.* Cytomegalovirus DNA in the sera of patients with cytomegalovirus pneumonia. *Br J Haematol* 1991;79(2):198–204.

80. BOECKH M, MYERSON D, BOWDEN RA. Early detection and treatment of cytomegalovirus infections in marrow transplant patients: methodological aspects and implications for therapeutic interventions. *Bone Marrow Transpl* 1994;14(Suppl):S66–70.

81. BUFFONE GJ, FROST A, SAMO T *et al.* The diagnosis of CMV pneumonitis in lung and heart/lung transplant patients by PCR compared with traditional laboratory criteria. *Transplantation* 1993;56:342–7.

82. LIESNARD C, DE WIT L, MOTTE S, BRANCART F, CONTENT J. Rapid diagnosis of cytomegalovirus lung infection by DNA amplification in bronchoalveolar lavages. *Mol Cell Probes* 1994;8(4):273–83.

83. CATHOMAS G, MORRIS P, PEKLE K, CUNNINGHAM I, EMANUEL D. Rapid diagnosis of cytomegalovirus pneumonia in marrow transplant recipients by bronchoalveolar lavage using the polymerase chain reaction, cirus culture, and the direct immunostaining of alveolar cells. *Blood* 1993;81(7):1909–14.

84. ERIKSSON BM, BRYTTING M, ZWEYGBERG-WIRGART B *et al.* Diagnosis of cytomegalovirus in bronchoalveolar lavage by polymerase chain reaction, in comparison with virus isolation and detection of viral antigen. *Scand J Infect Dis* 1993;25(4):421–7.

85. LJUNGMAN P, DE BOCK R, CORDONNIER C *et al.* Practices for cytomegalovirus diagnosis, prophylaxis and treatment in allogeneic bone marrow transplant recipients: a report from the Working Party for Infectious disease of the EBMT. *Bone Marrow Transpl* 1993;12:399–403.

86. WADE JC, HINTZ M, MCGUFFIN RW *et al.* Treatment of cytomegalovirus pneumonia with high dose acyclovir. *Am J Med* 1982;73 (Suppl 1A):249–56.

87. SNYDMAN DR. Ganciclovir treatment of solid organ transplant recipients with cytomegalovirus disease. In Spector SA, ed. *Ganciclovir Therapy for Cytomegalovirus Infection* . New York, Basel, Hong Kong; Marcel Dekker Inc. 1991: 145–54.

88. JENSEN WA, ROSE RM, HAMMER SM *et al.* Pulmonary complications of orthotopic liver transplantation. *Transplantation* 1986;42(5):484–90.

89. SHEPP DH, DANDLIKER PS, DE MIRANDA P *et al.* Activity of 9-[2-hydroxy-1(hydroxymethyl) ethoxymethyl] guanine in the treatment of cytomegalovirus pneumonia. *Ann Intern Med* 1985;103:368–73.

90. WINSTON DJ, HO WG, BARTONI K *et al.* Ganciclovir therapy for cytomegalovirus infections in recipients of bone marrow transplants and other immunosuppressed patients. *Rev Infect Dis* 1988;10:S547–53.

91. WILSON EJ, MEDEARIS DN JR, HANSEN LA, RUBIN RH. 9-(1-3-dihydroxy-2-propoxymethyl) guanine prevents death but not immunity in murine cytomegalovirus-infected normal and immunosuppressed BALB/c mice. *Antimicrob Agents Chemother* 1987;31:1017.

92. SLAVIN MA, BINDRA RR, GLEAVES CA, PETTINGER MB, BOWDEN RA. Ganciclovir sensitivity of cytomegalovirus at diagnosis and during treatment of cytomegalovirus pneumonia in marrow transplant recipients. *Antimicrob Agents Chemother* 1993;37(6):1360–3.

93. BRATANOW NC, ASH RC, TURNER PA *et al.* Successful treatment of serious cytomegalovirus (CMV) disease with 9 (1,3-dihydroxy-2-propoxymethyl) guanine (ganciclovir, DHPG) and intravenous immunoglobulin (IVIG) in bone marrow transplant (BMT) patients [abstract n. 254]. *Exp Hematol* 1987;15:541.

94. LJUNGMAN P, ENGELHARD D, LINK H *et al.* Treatment of interstitial pneumonitis due to cytomegalovirus with ganciclovir and intravenous immune-globulin: experience of European Bone Marrow Transplant Group. *Clin Infect Dis* 1992;14:831–5.

95. HECHT DW, SNYDMAN DR, CRUMPACKER CS *et al.* Ganciclovir for treatment of renal transplant-associated primary cytomegalovirus pneumonia. *J Infect Dis* 1988;157:187–90.

96. ZAIA J, SCHIMDT GM. Ganciclovir treatment of bone marrow transplant recipient with cytomegalovirus disease. In *Ganciclovir Therapy for Cytomegalovirus Infection* New York, Basel, Hong Kong: Marcel Dekker; 1991: 155–83.

97. SINGH N, DRUMMER JS, KUSNE S *et al.* Infections with cytomegalovirus and other herpes viruses in 121 liver transplant recipients: transmission by donated organ and the effect of OKT_3 antibodies. *J Infect Dis* 1988;158:124–31.

98. OH CS, STRATTA RJ, FOX BC *et al.* Increased infections associated with the use of OKT_3 for treatment of steroid resistant rejection in renal transplantation. *Transplantation* 1988; 45(1):68–73.

99. WEIR MR, IRWIN BC, WATERS AW *et al.* Incidence of cytomegalovirus disease in cyclosporin treated renal transplant recipients based on donor/recipient pretransplant immunity. *Transplantation* 1987;43(2):187–93.

100. BOWDEN RA, SAYERJ M, FLUORNOY N *et al.* Cytomegalovirus immune globulin and seronegative blood products to prevent primary cytomegalovirus infection after marrow transplantation. *NEJM* 1986;314:1006–10.

101. NOVICK RJ, MENKIS AH, MCKENZIE FN *et al.* Should heart–lung transplant donors and recipients be matched according to cytomegalovirus serologic status? *J Heart Transpl* 1990;9:699–706.

102. ELFENBEIN GJ, SIDDIQUI T, RAND KH *et al.* Successful strategy for prevention of cytomegalovirus interstitial pneumonia after human leucocyte antigen-identical bone marrow transplantation. *Rev Infect Dis* 1990;12:S805–10.

103. MILLER WJ, MCCULLOUGH J, BALFOUR HH JR *et al.* Prevention of cytomegalovirus infection following bone marrow transplantation: a randomized trial of blood

product screening. *Bone Marrow Transpl* 1991;7:227–34.

104. SAYERS MH, ANDERSON KC, GOODNOUGH LT *et al.* Reducing the risk for transfusion-transmitted cytomegalovirus infection. *Ann Intern Med* 1992;116:55–62.

105. PREIKSAITIS JK, ROSNO S, GRUMET C, MERIGAN TC. Infections due to herpes viruses in cardiac transplant recipients: role of the donor heart and immunosuppressive therapy. *J Infect Dis* 1983;147:974–81.

106. BOWDEN RA, SAYERS MH, CAYS M, SLICKNER SJ. The role of blood product filtration in the prevention of transfusion associated cytomegalovirus (CMV) infection after marrow transplant. *Transfusion* 1989;29:5205–8.

107. LUI SF, ALI AA, GRUNDY JE, FERNANDO ON, GRIFFITHS PD, SWENY P. Double-blind, placebo-controlled trial of human lymphoblastoid interferon prophylaxis of cytomegalovirus infection in renal transplant recipients. *Nephrol, Dialysis, Transpl* 1992;7(12):1230–7.

108. PLOTKIN SA, STARR SE, FRIEDMAN HM *et al.* Vaccines for the prevention of human cytomegalovirus infection. *Rev Infect Dis* 12;S827–38.

109. SNYDMAN DR, WERNER BG, HEINZE-LACEY B *et al.* Use of cytomegalovirus immunoglobulin to prevent cytomegalovirus disease in renal transplant recipients. *N Engl J Med* 1987;317:1049–54.

110. ELFENBEIN G, KRISCHER J, RAND K *et al.* Preliminary results of multicenter trial to prevent death from cytomegalovirus pneumonia with intravenous immunoglobulin after allogeneic bone marrow transplantation. *Transpl Proc* 1987;19 (Suppl 7):138–43.

111. KUBANEK B, ERNST P, OSTENDORF P *et al.* Preliminary data of a controlled trial of intravenous hyperimmune globulin in the prevention of cytomegalovirus infection in bone marrow transplant recipients. *Transpl Proc* 1985;17:468–69.

112. FASSBINDER W, ERNST W, HANKE P *et al.* Cytomegalovirus infections after renal transplantation: effect of a prophylactic hyperimmunoglobulin. *Transpl Proc* 1986;18:1393–6.

113. SALIBA F, GUGENHEIM J, SAMUEL D *et al.* Incidence of cytomegalovirus infection and effects of cytomegalovirus immune globulin prophylaxis after orthotopic liver transplantation. *Transpl Proc* 1987; 19:4081–2.

114. CONDIE RM AND O'REILLY RJ. Prevention of cytomegalovirus infection by prophylaxis with an intravenous hyperimmune native unmodified cytomegalovirus globulin. Randomised trial in bone marrow transplant recipients. *Am J Med* 1984;76 (Suppl 3A):134–41.

115. METSELAAR HJ, BALK AHMM, MOCHTAR B *et al.* Cytomegalovirus seronegative heart transplant recipients. Prophylactic use of anti-CMV immunoglobulin. *Chest* 1990;97:396–9.

116. SNYDMAN DR. Prevention of cytomegalovirus-associated diseases with immunoglobulin. *Transpl Proc* 1991;23(Suppl 3):131–5.

117. MEYERS JD, LESZCZYNSKI J, ZAIA J *et al.* Prevention of cytomegalovirus infection by cytomegalovirus immune globulin after marrow transplantation. *Ann Intern Med* 1983;928:442–6.

118. BOWDEN RA, SAYERS M, FLOURNOY N *et al.* Cytomegalovirus immunoglobulin and seronegative blood products to prevent primary cytomegalovirus infection after marrow transplantation. *N Engl J Med* 1986;314:1006–10.

119. BOWDEN RA, FISHER LD, ROGERS K, CAYS M, MEYERS JD. Cytomegalovirus (CMV)-specific intravenous immunoglobulin for the prevention of primary CMV infection and disease after marrow transplant. *J Infect Dis* 1991;164:483–7.

120. O'REILLY RJ, REICH L, GOLD J *et al.* A randomized trial of intravenous hyperimmune globulin for the prevention of cytomegalovirus (CMV) Infections following marrow transplantation: preliminary results. *Transpl Proc* 1983;15:1405–11.

121. KUBANEK B, ERNST P, OSTENDORF P, SCHÄFER U, WOLF H. Preliminary data of a controlled trial of intravenous hyperimmune globulin in the prevention of cytomegalovirus infection in bone marrow transplant recipients. *Transpl Proc* 1985;17:468–9.

122. WINSTON DJ, HO WG, LIN C-H *et al.* Intravenous immune globulin for prevention of cytomegalovirus infection and interstitial pneumonia after bone marrow transplantation. *Ann Intern Med* 1987;106:12–18.

123. SULLIVAN KM, KOPECKY KJ, JOCOM J *et al.* Immunomodulatory and antimicrobial efficacy of intravenous immunoglobulin in bone marrow transplantation. *N Engl J Med* 1990;323:705–12.

124. BLASCZYK R, WESTHOFF U, GROSSE-WILDE H. Soluble CD4, CD8, and HLA molecules in commercial immunoglobulin preparations. *Lancet* 1993;2:789.

125. BASS EB, POWE NR, GOODMAN SN *et al.* Efficacy of immune globulin in preventing complications of bone marrow transplantation: a meta-analysis. *Bone Marrow Transpl* 1993;12:273–82.

126. SNYDMAN DR, WERNER BG, DOUGHERTY NN *et al.* Cytomegalovirus immune globulin prophylaxis in liver transplantation. A randomized, double-blind, placebo-controlled trial. The Boston Center for Liver *Transplantation* CMVIG Study Group. *Ann Intern Med* 1993;119:984–91.

127. GLUCKMAN E, DEVERGIE A, MELO R *et al.* Prophylaxis of herpes infections after bone marrow transplantation by oral acyclovir. *Lancet* 1983;2:706–8.

128. BALFOUR HH, CHACE BA, STAPLETON JT *et al.* A randomised placebo-controlled trial of oral acyclovir for the prevention of cytomegalovirus disease in recipients of renal allografts. *N Engl J Med* 1989;321:1381–7.

129. BAILEY TC, TRULOCK EO, ETTINGER NA *et al.* Failure of prophylactic ganciclovir to prevent cytomegalovirus disease in recipients of lung transplants. *J Infect Dis* 1992;165:548–52.

130. BAILEY TC, ETTINGER NA, STORCH GA *et al.* Failure of high dose oral acyclovir with or without immune globulin to prevent primary CMV disease in solid organ transplant recipients. *Am J Med* 1993;95:273–8.

131. MEYERS JD, REED EC, SHEPP DH *et al.* Acyclovir for prevention of cytomegalovirus infection and disease after allogeneic marrow transplantation. *N Engl J Med* 1988;318:70–5.

132. LUNDGREN G, WILCZEK H, LÖNNQVIST B, LINDHOLM A, WAHREN B, RINGDÉN O. Acyclovir prophylaxis in bone marrow transplant recipients. *Scand J Infect Dis* 1985 (Suppl 47):137–44.

133. GRANT PRENTICE H, GLUCKMAN E, POWLES RL *et al.* Impact of long-term acyclovir on cytomegalovirus infection and survival after allogeneic bone marrow transplantation. *Lancet* 1994;343:749–53.

134. SCHMIDT GM, HORAK DA, NILAND JC *et al.* A randomized, controlled trial of prophylactic ganciclovir for cytomegalovirus pulmonary infection in recipients of allogeneic bone marrow transplants. *N Engl J Med* 1991;324;1005–11.

135. SINGH N, YU VL, MIELES L, WAGENER MM *et al.* High-dose acyclovir compared with short-course preemptive ganciclovir therapy to prevent cytomegalovirus disease in liver transplant recipients. *Ann Intern Med* 1994;120:375–81.

136. ATKINSON K, DOWNS K, GOLENIA M *et al.* Prophylactic use of ganciclovir in allogeneic bone marrow transplantation: absence of clinical cytomegalovirus infection. *Br J Haematol* 1991;79:57–62.

137. YAU JC, DIMOPOULOS MA, HUAN SD *et al.* Prophylaxis of cytomegalovirus infection with ganciclovir in allogeneic marrow transplantation. *Eur J Haematol* 1991;47:371–6.

138. VON BUELTZINGSLOEWEN A, BORDIGONI P, WITZ F *et al.* Prophylactic use of ganciclovir for allogeneic bone marrow transplant recipients. *Bone Marrow Transpl* 1993;12:197–202.

139. GOODRICH JM, BOWDEN RA, FISHER L, KELLER C, SCHOCH G, MEYERS JD. Ganciclovir prophylaxis to prevent cytomegalovirus disease after allogeneic marrow transplant. *Ann Intern Med* 1993;118:173–8.

140. WINSTON DH, HO WG, BARTONI K *et al.* Ganciclovir prophylaxis of cytomegalovirus infection and disease in allogeneic bone marrow transplant recipients: results of a placebo-controlled, double-blind trial. *Ann Intern Med* 1993;118:179–84.

141. ZAMORA MR, FULLERTON DA, CAMPBELL DN *et al.* Use of cytomegalovirus (CMV) hyperimmune globulin for prevention of CMV disease in CMV-seropositive lung transplant recipients. *Transpl Proc* 1994; 26(5 Suppl 1):49–51.

142. MERIGAN TC, RENLUND DG, KEAY S *et al.* A controlled trial of ganciclovir to prevent cytomegalovirus disease after heart transplantation. *N Engl J Med* 1992;326:1182–6.

143. BAILEY TC, TRULOCK EP, ETTINGER NA *et al.* Failure of prophylactic ganciclovir to prevent cytomegalovirus disease in recipients of lung transplants. *J Infect Dis* 1992;165:548–52.

144. REUSSER P, GAMBERTOGLIO JG, LILLEBY K, MEYERS JD. Phase1-II trial of foscarnet for prevention of cytomegalovirus infection in autologous and allogeneic marrow transplant recipients. *J Infect Dis* 1992;166:473–9.

145. SCHMIDT GM, HORAK DA, NILAND JC *et al.* A randomized, controlled trial of prophylactic ganciclovir for cytomegalovirus pulmonary infection in recipients of allogeneic bone marrow transplants. *N Engl J Med* 1991;324:1005–11.

146. GOODRICH JM, MORI M, GLEAVES CA *et al.* Early treatment with ganciclovir to prevent cytomegalovirus disease after allogeneic bone marrow transplantation. *N Engl J Med* 1991;325:1601–7.

147. HIBBERD PL, TOLKOFF-RUBIN NE, CONTI D *et al.* Preemptive ganciclovir therapy to prevent cytomegalovirus disease in cytomegalovirus antibody-positive renal transplant recipients. *Ann Intern Med* 1995; 123:18–26.

148. RIDDELL SR, WATANABE KS, GOODRICH JM, LI CR, AGHA ME, GREENBERG PD. Restoration of viral immunity in immunodeficient humans by the adoptive transfer of T cell clones. *Science* 1992;257:238–41.

11 Non-tuberculous mycobacteria

MICHAEL E. ELLIS* and R. FROTHINGHAM†

**King Faisal Specialist Hospital and Research Centre, Riyadh, Saudi Arabia; †Duke University Medical Center, Durham, USA*

Introduction

Non-tuberculous mycobacteria (NTM) are unique from the amount of controversy generated over nomenclature, classification, exact role in disease and appropriate treatments. The archetype of mycobacterial disease – tuberculosis – has been recognised since neolithic times; Villemin in 1865 demonstrated its infectious aetiology 27 years prior to the discovery of the tubercle bacillus by Koch. There has never been any doubt that the isolation of *Mycobacterium tuberculosis* from any body secretion/tissue is synonymous with disease. Following the description of *Mycobacterium avium* by Nocard and Roux in 1887, the occasional finding of other mycobacterial species from clinical specimens had been largely dismissed as contamination for many years despite reports of apparent clinical disease[1,2]. Obsession with the requirement that the organism should produce disease in guinea pigs in order to be considered significant undoubtedly contributed to under-diagnosis of disease due to NTM, until Timpe and Runyon in 1954 drew attention to disease caused by NTM[3]. Since then there has been increasing recognition that NTM can produce significant human disease, both before and during the AIDS pandemic. This is reflected in, for example, the increase in notifications of NTM to the Communicable Disease Surveillance Centre and the reporting of cases of apparent pulmonary tuberculosis due to NTM[4,5]. There are a number of controversial areas in the field of non-tuberculous mycobacteriology including nomenclature, differentiation between diagnosis of disease and colonisation and drug regimens including the relationship of *in vitro/in vivo* drug activities. In addition, the literature is changing continually and dramatically. A number of key reviews in the field have appeared, the reader is referred particularly to those of Wolinsky[4,5].

A nomenclature which embraces all of the differences between the classical pathogenic species of mycobacteria, namely *M. tuberculosis/Mycobacterium bovis/Mycobacterium leprae* and the other mycobacterial spp has not been agreed. The term 'atypical', originally applied by Pinner in 1935 and later utilised by Timpe and Runyon, is unacceptable (because each atypical species can be characterised) and is no longer utilised. The following terminologies are also strongly and widely disfavoured: anonymous or unclassified (since many are now speciated), or opportunistic (since most have caused infection in immunocompetent hosts in addition to the immunocompromised). Mycobacteria other than tuberculosis (MOTT) is inaccurate since a mycobacterium is a micro-organism whereas tuberculosis is a disease. Absence of contagiousness from host to host, ability to live and survive in non-human environmental habitats and restricted susceptibility to antimycobacterial agents have led some to coin the term 'potentially pathogenic environmental mycobacteria' or PPEM. However, the current most commonly used term is 'non-tuberculous mycobacteria' (NTM) and has been adopted by the American Society of Microbiology and the Centers for Disease Control and we will use this throughout this chapter. Yet these organisms can indeed mimic histological *M. tuberculosis* tubercles in tissue and so even this term fails to underscore the essential differences between *M. tuberculosis/M. bovis/M. leprae* and the remainder. For the purpose of the clinical approach, the NTM will be considered in the following groups: (i) potentially pathogenic species in humans; (ii) saprophytic species rarely causing human disease (a) slow growers and (b) intermediate/rapid growers.

There are some 19 NTM organisms which can cause human disease, and numerous new mycobacterial species have been described in the past decade[5]. *M. avium* complex, *Mycobacterium kansasii* and *Mycobacterium xenopi* are the most frequently incriminated potential pulmonary pathogens. There is a spectrum of pathogenicity (Table 11.1).

Microbiology

The NTM are acid and alcohol fast, sometimes weakly Gram-positive, aerobic, non-motile bacilli, which on Ziehl–Neelsen (ZN) or Kinyoun staining are usually indistinguishable from *M. tuberculosis*; rarely peculiar morphological characteristics and direct smear may suggest certain species[6], e.g. the long, tapered cells of *M. xenopi* and *M. kansasii* have thick, cross-barred cells[4]. NTM are usually distinguished by a profile of optimal growth temperature, rate of growth, gross colony characteristics and biochemical characteristics (niacin accumulation tests, nitrate reduction, catalase production and heat lability, urease activity, arylsulphatase activity, growth in sodium chloride, susceptibility to Tween hydrolysis and ability to take up iron). A good in-depth summary of the microbiology characteristics is available in the *Manual of Clinical Microbiology*[7].

Until recently, the most frequently used classification for NTM was based on that of Runyon[8]: Groups I – IV depending on the colour and morphological characteristics alluded to previously: Group I, the photochromogens (i.e. they form yellow/orange/red pigmented, usually smooth colonies on light exposure; Group II, the scotochromogens (i.e. yellow/orange pigmented, smooth colonies in the dark, red pigment in the light); Group III, the non-chromogens (i.e. no such intense colour production and smooth circular colonies); Group IV, rapidly growing (3–7 days compared to 7–60 days for Groups I–III), usually non-pigmented either producing rough and

Table 11.1. *Pathogenicity for humans of mycobacteria encountered in pulmonary specimens*

Group	Species
Pathogenic	*M. tuberculosis* complex (*M. tuberculosis, M. bovis*)
Potentially pathogenic	*M. avium* complex (*M. avium, M. intracellulare*, others), *M. kansasii, M. xenopi, M. scrofulaceum, M. marinum, M. szulgai, M. simiae, M. fortuitum complex (M. chelonae, M. fortuitum), M. malmoense, M. asiaticum, M. shimoidei, M. celatum*
Rarely pathogenic	*M. gordonae, M. gastri, M. terrae* complex (*M. terrae, M. nonchromogenicum, M. triviale*), rapidly growing mycobacteria other than the *M. fortuitum* complex

From Refs. 4, 5 and 14.

cord-like or smooth colonies which can sometimes resemble those of *M. tuberculosis*). However, some NTM cannot be readily classified into Runyon groupings, for example, *M. xenopi* shows characteristics of Groups II/III and *M. kansasii* usually placed in Group I may on occasions be scotochromogenic. Mycobacteria should be identified to the species level since this predicts their pathogenicity (Table 11.1) and is a guide to therapy. Hence, the Runyon system is no longer used by clinical laboratories. Other methods of classification and description include the potential for human pathogenicity[4], seroagglutination characteristics, antibiogram and chromatography of surface lipids.

The past decade has brought significant advances in clinical mycobacteriology. The changes have largely been driven by the important clinical and infection control implications of rapid identification of *M. tuberculosis*. Thus, the use of fluorescing dyes to detect acid-fast bacilli on smears such as auramine O rather than basic fuschin (ZN/Kinyoun) is more rapid. Cytocentrifugation (CYTOTEK, Ames Division, Miles Laboratories, Inc., Elkhart, Ind) techniques also increase the detection of mycobacteria. The use of the BACTEC liquid radiometric media (BACTEC, Becton Dickinson, Towson, Md) results in more rapid culture positivity and a higher rate of positive cultures as compared with conventional solid media[7]. Thus, the average detection time for *M. tuberculosis* and for NTM is reduced 2.5 and 3.5-fold, respectively, compared to conventional methods. Complete identification and drug susceptibility testing can be reduced to a little over 2 weeks. The SEPTICHEK AFB system has also been shown to be at least as sensitive as BACTEC[8].

Once mycobacteria are isolated, they can be rapidly identified using nucleic acid probes (e.g. AccuProbe, Gen-Probe, San Diego, California). Probes are currently available for the *M. tuberculosis* complex, the *M. avium* complex, *M. gordonae*, and *M. kansasii*, the species most commonly isolated in clinical microbiology laboratories[9]. However, the genetic heterogeneity of some NTM species leading to failure of hybridisation with probes may result in a low sensitivity for detection[10]. Recently, detection and identification of mycobacteria directly from BACTEC bottles has been possible using a DNA – RNA probe, hence producing considerable time saving since colony production is not necessary[11]. Alternatively, the NAP test can be used in conjunction with the BACTEC system for rapid differentiation of the *M. tuberculosis* complex from NTM[7]. Some reference laboratories are using high performance liquid chromatography (HPLC) to rapidly identify most mycobacterial species[7]. When liquid media (e.g. BACTEC) are used for culture, and one or more rapid methods (probes, NAP test, or HPLC) is used for species identification, the species *M. tuberculosis* can be identified in an average of 22 days from specimen collection[12]. In the case of *M. avium* complex the interval to detection can be decreased to 5–12 days with BACTEC TB and to 12–19 days with Septi-check AFB, compared to 4 to 8 weeks with conventional methods[13] yet less than one-third of all US state PHLS use a more rapid radiomimetric culture method[12,13]. It was common previously for NTM infections to be presumptively treated as *M. tuberculosis* for weeks or months while clinicians waited for species identification. Of all US state public health laboratories, 72% use modern microbiological techniques[12] thus, rendering presumptive treatment unnecessary or needed for only brief durations.

Standardised methods have been developed to test the susceptibility of *M. tuberculosis* isolates to antibiotics (usually streptomycin, isoniazid, rifampicin, and ethambutol). Many isolates of NTM are found to be highly resistant to these antituberculous medications when tested by the same methodologies. These *in vitro* susceptibility results for NTM have not been shown to correlate with *in vivo* clinical response to therapy. One reason for this may be that certain antimycobacterial agents are highly concentrated into cells, whereas *in vitro* testing uses cell-free systems. Use of the J774 macrophage live/immunocompromised beige mouse may be more indicative of the human *in vivo* situation[13]. The American Thoracic Society has therefore recommended that routine susceptibility testing should not be done for *M. avium* complex isolates[14]. The one exception is clarithromycin, for which a clear correlation has been demonstrated between the minimum inhibitory concentration and the response to therapy for disseminated *M. avium* complex infection[15]. Isolates of rapidly growing mycobacteria (especially the *M. fortuitum* complex) should be tested for susceptibility to clarithromycin, doxycycline and amikacin, but not to traditional antituberculous agents[14].

Epidemiology and role in human disease: general

The majority of NTM are ubiquitous and free living in nature: soil, dust, water, milk, food, fish and animals are worldwide sources. Growth requirements of certain species have led to geographical clustering of species and cases, for example, the requirement of fresh water for *M. avium* complex is thought to be responsible for clustering of patients around river estuaries[16], whereas the natural habitat of *Mycobacterium marinum*, namely marine life and water, gives rise to suppurative soft tissue lesions following appropriate trauma[17].

Nevertheless, it is the widespread distribution of these organisms that has contributed to the major problem of distinguishing contamination, colonisation (infection in the absence of disease) and disease. It is common to isolate NTM in the absence of clinical disease. Thus, of 168 cases of sputum positive cultures for NTM in Hong Kong, 80% were thought to be transient colonisers and clinically insignificant[18]. NTM have been also known to be easily introduced into, and contaminate, laboratory agents, diagnostic equipment and specimens and this has led to incorrect diagnosis of infection and disease[19]. Laboratory contamination of mycobacterial cultures appears to be reasonably common and has been confirmed by strain differentiation techniques including phage typing, restriction fragment length polymorphism and DNA sequencing[20–23]. *M. xenopi* in the tap water contaminated bronchoscopes and resulted in an excessive isolation of *M. xenopi* (35% of all mycobacterial isolates)[24]. Even glutaraldehyde and disinfection of bronchoscopes failed to eradicate *M. chelonae* in one 'outbreak'[25]. Gargling with tap water prior to sputum collection, rinsing bed pans with tap water and using tap water to irrigate per-colonoscopy resulted in misdiagnosis of *M. xenopi* infection rather than diagnosing colonisation[26]. Contamination of BACTEC TB systems by an antimicrobial solution BACTEC PANTA PLUS due to ineffective sterilisation of water used in the manufacturing process led to inappropriate diagnosis of *Mycobacterium gordonae* infection and unnecessary treatment[27]. Furthermore, NTMs are found in human faeces, a finding which could complicate interpretation of their role in gastrointestinal tract disease, and can colonise skin and the respiratory tract[28] presumably from dust[29], again making the separation of colonisation/disease difficult.

There are important gaps in our understanding of the distribution and transmission of NTM infection due in part to uncertainty over their role as pathogens, absence of statutory reporting requirements and apparent paradoxes, for example, non-concordance of serotypes in the environment and from patients[30].

The mode of transmission of NTM is not clear, presumably those which cause pulmonary disease gain primary entry into the respiratory tract. Direct inoculation is the route with certain other NTM species[17], and ingestion may be the primary route of entry for some forms of *M. avium* complex. There is lack of epidemiological evidence for human/human or animal/human transmission.

Although NTM are found worldwide, concentration of cases associated with specific NTM are described, for example, *Mycobacterium malmoense* is more common in the UK and Scandinavia compared to the USA[31,32].

Many cases of pulmonary disease due to NTM occur in older smoking males, often with a background of chronic pulmonary or other disease such as chronic obstructive airways disease, silicosis, neoplasia, and cystic fibrosis. The association with HIV infection will be described later in this chapter. Other immunocompromised patients are also at risk for NTM disease. For example, infections due to NTM in solid organ transplants are unusual but cause significant morbidity. Immunosuppressive treatment appears to be the key risk factor[33]. Generally, in these patients, NTM occurs late in the post-transplant period at around 48 months. Pulmonary manifestations occur in approximately a quarter of patients (of whom half will have concomitant NTM extrapulmonary disease). The most common pulmonary organism is *M. kansasii*. Particular problems of management are posed by this group of patients. For example, reduction in immunosuppressive therapy may be unrealistic in heart and liver transplants, significant adverse drug interactions may occur, for example, rifampicin increasing the catabolism of cyclosporin A leading to allograft rejection risk[33].

Guidelines for diagnosis and pitfalls

Guidelines have been published[14,34–6] (Tables 11.2, 11.3) to assist in deciding whether an NTM is playing a pathogenic role (i.e. disease producing) in a patient with pulmonary symptoms or whether the NTM is colonising or has been introduced as a contaminant. There is a broad consensus that a number of clinical, radiological and microbiological factors are important in diagnosing disease. The same single NTM spp should be isolated on repeated occasions and in heavy growth and despite bronchial toiletting; acid-fast smear positivity; no other known pathogen should be identified; isolation from a closed or normally sterile source such as lung tissue/lung abscess is highly suggestive; and dentification of a species that is more often associated with disease. The presence of certain underlying conditions that have been associated with NTM pulmonary disease, including immunosuppression, cancer, transplant patients, previous *M. tuberculosis* infection, chronic obstructive airways disease (COAD) and silicosis are helpful features[37–39]. A recent survey indicated that pre-existing chronic lung disease was present in 84% of patients with NTM pulmonary disease[40]. The diagnostic implications of an NTM isolate may also depend on the species isolated. Whereas a single colony of *M. tuberculosis* is diagnostic, the isolation of one of the rarely pathogenic NTM should be treated with caution unless tissue involvement (histological evidence of a mycobacterial process such as caseating necrosis, the presence of Langhan's giant cells associated with granulomas) is demonstrated by biopsy. However, in highly immunocompromised patients, the classical histological response may not occur. In solid organ transplant patients, for example, a predominant polymorponuclear infiltrate mimicking bacterial sepsis may be found[41]. The cellular response and granuloma formation in HIV positive patients may be extremely scant. Again, the guideline that the NTM should be the sole pathogen is difficult to adhere to in immunocompromised patients where multiple pathogens are a distinct possibility. Another group of patients, in whom the role of NTM is difficult to decide, is that with chronic suppurative lung disease. In patients with cystic fibrosis it is of interest that approximately 10% have positive smears or cultures of NTM[42,43]. In some cases, it was proposed that deterioration in pulmonary function may occur secondary to these infections[42]. Similarly, in patients with pre-existing bronchiectasis, the isolation of NTM may, in the setting of clinical or radiological deterioration, merit treatment[44]. Conservative observation may be a useful strategy in some patients as NTM pulmonary disease often progresses slowly over months or years. A negative tuberculin skin test is very soft evidence against *M. tuberculosis* infection. A therapeutic trial of antimycobacterial therapy may be another soft indicator of NTM disease particularly when there are objective signs such as fever, weight loss, cough and radiological infiltrates to follow. The choice, however, of antimicrobial drugs to use in NTM infections is difficult. Often there is little correlation between frequently observed *in vitro* resistance and clinical outcome with more patients actually responding to standard antituberculous drugs than would be predicted from the *in vitro* results[40].

Although these are useful guidelines, they are indeed guidelines and each patient has to be assessed individually and a clinical decision

Table 11.2. *American Thoracic Society diagnostic criteria for pulmonary disease caused by non-tuberculous mycobacteria*

I. For patients with cavitary lung disease
   1. Presence of two or more sputum specimens (or sputum and a bronchial washing) that are acid-fast bacilli smear-positive and/or result in moderate to heavy growth of NTM on culture
   2. Other reasonable causes for the disease process have been excluded (e.g., tuberculosis, fungal disease, etc.)

II. For patients with noncavitary lung disease
   1. Presence of two or more sputum specimens (or sputum and a bronchial washing) that are acid-fast bacilli smear-positive and/or produce moderate to heavy growth on culture
   2. If the isolate is *M. kansasii* or *M. avium* complex, failure of the sputum cultures to clear with bronchial toilet or within 2 weeks of institution of specific mycobacterial drug therapy (although only studied for these two species, this criteria is probably valid for other species of NTM)
   3. Other reasonable causes for the disease process have been excluded

III. For patients with cavitary or noncavitary lung disease whose sputum evaluation is nondiagnostic or another disease cannot be excluded
   1. A transbronchial or open lung biopsy yields the organism and shows mycobacterial histopathologic features (i.e. granulomatous inflammation, with or without acid-fast bacilli). No other criteria needed
   2. A transbronchial or open lung biopsy that fails to yield the organism but shows mycobacterial histopathologic features in the absence of a prior history of other granulomatous or mycobacterial disease plus: (i) presence of two or more positive cultures of sputum or bronchial washings; (ii) other reasonable causes for granulomatous disease have been excluded.

From Ref. 14.

Table 11.3. *Practical guidelines for diagnosing NTM pulmonary disease*

Clinical features compatible with mycobacterial disease[a]
Radiological features compatible with mycobacterial disease[a,e]
Single NTM species isolated on ≥ two occasions[b]
Heavy growth NTM species[b]
Absence of other pathogens[b]
Acid-fast smear positivity[b]
Isolation from a normally sterile source[c,d]
An NTM species most often associated with pulmonary disease[b]
Histological evidence of mycobacterial disease (granuloma inflammation)[c,d]
Underlying host predisposing conditions (COAD, neoplasia, immuncompromisation, etc), negative tuberculin reaction[b]
Therapeutic trial[b]
Modification of the histologic/radiologic findings may occur in highly immunocompromised patients.

[a]Mandatory.
[b]Supportive.
[c]Virtually diagnostic.
[d]Diagnostic.
[e]Certain radiological features may suggest NTM > *M. tuberculosis*, e.g. thin-walled cavities, prominent pleural disease (see text).

Table 11.4. *Treatment guidelines for pulmonary disease due to potentially pathological NTM*

Organism	Drug treatment regimens/antimycobacterials
M. avium complex	[a]R E I S [a]Clar E R/Rb/Clof/Am Clof ± Az ± R ± Cip ± liposomal Gm/Cap/Dap R E I Clof R E Am Cip R E Cip Clof
M. kansasii	[a]R E I ± Cy/Ethion R E Clar Cip E/Cotrim/Rif/Am
M. xenopi	[a]R I E ± S
M. scrofulaceum	[a]R I E S Cy, Ethion, Am, Cip, Clof, Clar
M. marinum	[a]R E Dox Tc Cotrim Dox [a]Cotrim Cip
M.szulgai	[a]R E I ± Cap
M. simiae	R E I/Clar
M. fortuitum complex	[a]Am Cef → Dox/Sulph/Em/Rif/Eth Cef/Im/Cip/Olflox/Clar
M. malmoense	[a]R I E
M. asiaticum	R I E + Cap/PAS/Cip
M. shimoidei	R I E/Cip/Oflox
M. celatum	- unclear

AM	= Amikacin.	S	= Streptomycin.
AZ	= Azithromycin.	Tz	= Tetracycline.
Cap	= Capreomycin.	[a]	= Recommended or established regimens. See text for details and references. Note that the ideal regimen for most NTM infections is not known. Clarithromycin has recently been shown to have *in vitro* activity against most NTM[101]. There is limited clinical efficacy observed in the few reports to date. It could be included in a multidrug regimen for most NTM. However, the *M. tuberculosis* complex and *M.simiae* are resistant *in vitro* to clarithromycin.
Cep	= Cefixime.		
Cip	= Ciprofloxacin.		
Clar	= Clarithromycin.		
Clof	= Clofazimine.		
Cotrim	= Cotrimoxazole.		
Cy	= Cycloserine.		
Dap	= Dapsone.		
Dox	= Doxycycline.		
E	= Ethambutol.		
Ethion	= Ethionamide.		
Gm	= Gentamicin.		
I	= Isoniazid.		
Im	= Imipenen.		
Oflox	= Ofloxacin.		
PAS	= Para-aminosalicylic acid.		
Rb	= Ribabutin.		

made. For example, *M. gordonae* is often and probably correctly dismissed as a contaminant, yet obvious cases of pulmonary disease have been reported[45,46]. In some cases of disease, NTM have been found scantily or infrequently even from specimens collected from closed or normally sterile sources[47] (see also the comments under *M. xenopi*). However, it is generally accepted that even a scanty growth from such a source is diagnostic of disease. A recent report suggested that even a single isolation of *M. avium* complex from sputum, in the context of appropriate clinical and radiological findings, was sufficient to make a diagnosis of infection in one patient[47]. The case illustrated by Fig. 11.1 underscores this point. Although the patient had only one of several sputa positive for *M. avium* complex, tissue biopsy grew *M. avium* complex. It also illustrates the usefulness of tissue biopsy in clarifying ambiguous cases. Furthermore, radiological changes may also be subtle, stable or change slowly and clustered fibroproductive nodules are commonly found[48]. In one study of patients from whom NTM had been isolated, the physician had initially suspected tuberculosis on clinical grounds and many patients had apparently responded to treatment with antibiotics given prior to their identification of the NTM. Many of the prescribed antibiotics had some antimycobacterial activity and a low grade pathogenic role in many patients could not be excluded[49]. The presence of acid-fast bacilli on direct smear has been shown to be a useful indicator as to whether the subsequently isolated NTM represent true infection or colonisation namely, contamination is associated with a 2% smear positivity rate if compared with over 80% for infection/colonisation[18].

Radiographical appearances of NTM are highly variable and can range from a classical tuberculosis-like appearance, namely, upper lobe apical opacities with cavitation to non-specific lower zone infiltrates or isolated nodules. To a limited extent, some aspects of these features may point towards NTM disease, for example, cavitary disease is particularly common in *M. malmoense* in which the cavities are unusually large (> 6 cm)[50]. In contrast, *M. kansasii* infection, the cavities are usually much smaller (< 2 cm)[51]. Others have commented that cavitary disease is less common in NTM infections compared to *M. tuberculosis*[52,53]. In the presence of cavitary disease, other findings which would tend to suggest NTM are thin-walled cavities, less association with parenchymal infiltrates, less bronchogenic spread but more continguous spread of disease and the more intense pleural reaction[14]. Other common radiological manifestations of NTM, which may be better visualised on CT scanning, include multifocal bronchiectasis, air space disease, nodules, scarring and/or volume loss[53]. It is of some interest that bronchiectasis may result from NTM infection rather than pre-existing prior to the NTM disease[53]. Recently, Miller classified NTM disease into five types[54]. These included 'classical' tuberculosis-like, occurring in male patients with COAD, nodular infiltrative/bronchiectasis in otherwise well elderly females, asymptomatic nodules, aspiration pneumonitis associated with achalasia and disseminated disease with variable chest manifestations. Nevertheless, no radiological feature is diagnostic or pathognomonic of NTM disease.

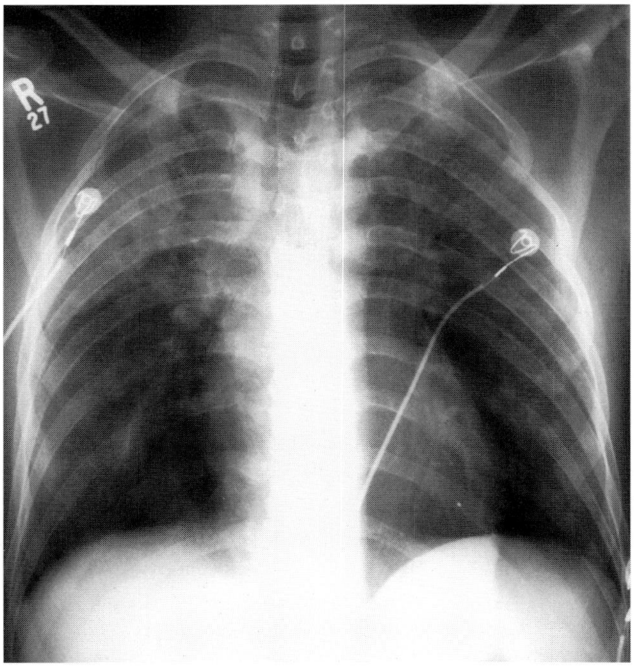

FIGURE 11.1 Right upper lobe infiltrate of a 27-year-old male with acute myeloid leukaemia, cough and green sputum. Only one colony of *M. avium* complex was isolated.

Skin testing is of very limited use for the diagnosis of NTM infection because of limited and unstandardised species specific antigen availability, cross-species reactivity due to antigen similarities, false-negative results, unpredictable reactions and the inability to distinguish past infection from current active disease. Current serological testing for precipitating antibodies or antigen determination is also rather limited but specific antigens may become available in the future. ELISA testing for IgA against *M. avium* complex antigens has had some success in differentiating *M. avium* complex from *M. tuberculosis* disease[55]. It remains to be seen whether the application of molecular methodology, for example, polymerase chain reaction or DNA probing will clarify the situation.

An approach to the patient with acid-fast bacilli seen and/or NTM isolated from sputum

The physician is often confronted with the patient from whom acid-fast bacilli have been identified in the sputum. What is the significance and how to manage the patient? There are four major scenarios that will present to the physician.

A patient with clinical and radiological features strongly suggestive of mycobacterial disease

A full history and physical examination will reveal whether the patient does indeed have an infectious respiratory disease strongly indicative of mycobacteriosis such as cough, fever, weight loss and haemoptysis together with appropriate physical signs. Radiology in these patients will show upper lobe cavitary disease. Further sputum specimens should be obtained from these patients and their initial management should be as a case of pulmonary tuberculosis, entailing quadruple therapy with rifampicin, isoniazid, ethambutol and pyrazinamide. In addition, appropriate infection control and Public Health measures should be adopted. In the meantime, the organism should be identified to species level. If *M. tuberculosis* is confirmed, antituberculous therapy is continued. If the organism is identified as a non-tuberculous mycobacterium, efforts should be made to establish its pathogenicity using the guidelines summarised in Tables 11.1–11.3. If the patient is already on standard antituberculous therapy and improving by the time of NTM species identification, this alone is a strong pointer towards its pathogenic role. If the NTM cannot be speciated, but the patient is responding, the treatment should be continued. However, pyrazinamide should be discontinued as it rarely appears to be beneficial in NTM disease. If the NTM is speciated, a therapeutic regime appropriate for that species should be instigated (see details for each species). Changes in therapy will be dictated by the NTM species, patient response, and toxicity occurrence or potential. For patients who are failing to respond, or if the organisms are resistant, usually an empirical change in medications is indicated (see relevant species). *In vitro* susceptibility testing is a complex and controversial issue, and has not been shown to correlate with clinical outcome, and therefore is not routinely indicated. It is important to exclude *M. tuberculosis* in all of the sputum specimens collected as its presence has important Public Health implications, whereas NTM is not generally thought to be transmissible from person to person.

A patient with clinical and radiological disease compatible with an acute respiratory tract infection but not classical of mycobacterial disease

Often a patient will have scattered infiltrates or nodules or bronchiectasis but not classical upper lobe infiltrates with cavities, i.e. the patient has respiratory tract infection and NTM has been isolated. In this situation, if there is isolation from multiple specimens, a heavy growth of a single NTM species, a positive direct smear for acid-fast bacilli in a setting of an appropriate risk factor category for NTM, NTM disease can be presumed and treated appropriately.

If the microbiological criteria cannot be fulfilled, for example, only one specimen has grown NTM, an attempt to demonstrate tissue involvement histologically and microbiologically by transbronchial biopsy or open lung biopsy should be done, if the patient continues to be symptomatic. If the histological and microbiological findings from the sterile tissue source is compatible with mycobacterial disease, appropriate treatment should be given.

A patient with chronic lung disease such as chronic obstructive airways disease, bronchiectasis, cystic fibrosis, etc. whose clinical and radiological features are 'chronic'

In this setting, NTM may merely be colonisers. This would be suggested first by the stability of the patient's clinical condition. However, many patients have a very slow disease progression over several years and others may have exacerbations in an otherwise chronic course. If there is a clear, pyogenic bacterial cause for exacerbations such as sudden onset of high fever, increase of purulent secretions from which pathogenic bacteria are isolated which responds to antibiotic treatment, the NTM may not be playing a role. In this situation, a prolonged period of observation without specific NTM treatment followed by reassessment is indicated. Despite this, if the clinical and radiological condition does not improve during the exacerbation or appears to be relentlessly progressive over the period of observation, in the face of repeated isolation of NTM from sputum which fails to clear with bronchial hygiene techniques, the trial of treatment directed towards the NTM is reasonable. The patient's overall condition, age and frailty have to be taken into consideration and benefits of antimycobacterial treatment vs. toxicity/compliance, weighed up.

Patients who are highly immunosuppressed

Each patient has to be assessed in the light of the likelihood that the immunosuppression grossly downgrades the classical microbiological, radiological and immunopathological hallmarks of NTM disease. In this situation, the finding of any NTM species should be regarded with extreme suspicion before being dismissed as a coloniser.

Pulmonary disease due to specific NTM: potentially pathogenic

M. avium complex

M. avium was first incriminated in disease of chickens at the end of the nineteenth century. Closely related to *M. avium* is *M. intracellulare* also called the Battey bacillus after a hospital in which it was incriminated in pulmonary disease during the 1950s. *M. avium* and *M. intracellulare* complex were formerly distinguished by their differing degrees of virulence in rabbits, chickens, and guinea pigs. *M. avium* is more virulent for birds than *M. intracellulare* and is the predominant cause of disseminated NTM in humans. However, the two species cannot be distinguished on the basis of biochemical reactions, pigmentation, colony morphology or optimal growth requirements. This has led to the term *M. avium* complex which includes the four species *M. avium, M. intracellulare, Mycobacterium paratuberculosis* (possibly related to Crohn's disease) and *Mycobacterium lepraemurium* (pathogenic only for rodents), as well as strains which do not fit into any recognised species. The most widely used nucleic acid probe (Accu Probe, Gen Probe, San Diego, California) identifies all the members of the complex. *M. avium* and *M. intracellulare* are genetically distinct and can be identified using species specific nucleic acid probes, serology, DNA–DNA homology, DNA sequence analysis, high pressure liquid chromatography of mycolic acid *p*-bromophenacyl esters, and *M. avium* complex A-catalase. However, clinical laboratories usually identify only to the level of the *M. avium* complex. Some 28 serovars of the *M. avium* complex are recognised. Serovars 1 to 6 and 8 to 11 are usually associated with *M. avium*. Serovars 7, 12 to 20, and 25 are usually associated with *M. intracellulare*. Strains belonging to other serovars often cannot be assigned to either species. It is likely that one or more new species remain to be defined within the *M. avium* complex.

Species from the *M. avium* complex are widely distributed in food, soil, water, birds, cattle, rabbits and man. Extensive epidemiological work has indicated that the waters, soils and aerosols of the acid brown water swamps of the Southeast in the United States coastal plain yield high *M. avium* complex numbers[56] and are likely to represent major environmental sources connected to the higher incidence of human infection in that region. Following the discovery of a number of clinical cases of *M. avium* complex, a US-wide survey of over a quarter of a million lifetime one-county resident naval recruits, using skin test reactivity to *M. avium* complex antigen (PPD-Battey) culminated in a US atlas of positive skin test prevalence[57]. This indicated that the highest percentage of positive skin reactions were found in the Southeast/Gulf coast states and that approximately three-quarters of those tested had positive reactions. This distribution approximated to the swamp area distribution[56]. Indeed, in some areas of the USA, *M. avium* complex is found more frequently than *M. tuberculosis* in patients with pulmonary infiltrates.

Work on plasmid profiles suggest that aerosols may be the source of infection[58]. Subsequent colonisation of respiratory and gastrointestinal tracts provide a later entry portal for disease[59].

It is not entirely clear what factors operate to permit these ubiquitous organisms to cause disease. However, *M. avium* complex virulence is linked to smooth–transparent colony morphological forms since these replicate more avidly, are more resistant to antibiotics, and induce less host protective tumor necrosis factor[60]. Underlying host disease which may alter local or systemic immunity is often present. For example, in a series from a tertiary care hospital, underlying malignancy (solid tumours, lymphoma, leukaemia) was found in 47%, organ transplantation in 12%, chronic lung disease in 22% and diabetes mellitus in 11% of patients with *M. avium* complex infection[49]. Others have noted the high incidence of chronic lung disease such as bronchiectasis, pulmonary fibrosis and pneumoconiosis in these patients. Perhaps these patients who have defects in mucociliary function producing for example excessive or tenacious sputum of chronic bronchitis or in cystic fibrosis or who have failure of clearance of sputum, for example, in bronchiectasis create a suitable milieu to allow replication and pathogenicity of *M. avium* complex. Ankylosing spondylitis, rheumatoid arthritis and chronic oesophageal regurgitation are other common associated factors, but are not found in all individuals. Pectus excavatum and scoliosis have been identified by some workers as phenotypic markers, associated with some connective tissue disorders, for increased risk of *M. avium* complex[61]. These, and other anomalies (including mitral valve prolapse), are interesting but, as yet, unexplained associations. *M. avium* complex (and also *M. kansasii*, *M. gordonae* and *M. tuberculosis*) have been associated with cystic fibrosis and should be considered as a possible cause for otherwise unexplained pulmonary deterioration in these patients[42]. *M. avium* complex has also been added to the list of infectious pathogens that can infect allogeneic bone marrow transplantation recipients[62]. The key immunological and host defence defects underscoring the above mentioned susceptible hosts are beginning to emerge. Structural pulmonary abnormalities, for example, in cystic lung disease is one possibility. Cytokine disregulatory functions may permit macrophage growth of *M. avium* complex, for example, diminished TNF, diminished GMCSF and increased interleukin-6 levels. Patients with HIV infection are at particular risk from disseminated *M. avium* complex because of their low CD4 counts (possibly mediated by cytokine abnormalities) and defects in sera which decrease macrophage resistance to *M. avium* complex[63]. Pulmonary disease caused by *M. avium* complex can also affect patients with no predisposing conditions, particularly elderly females, in whom the diagnosis it is often delayed[38]. Some series report an absence of obvious risk factors in as many as 50% of adult patients with pulmonary *M. avium* complex[64].

The symptoms of *M. avium* complex pulmonary disease are variable. On the one hand, the presentation may be so remarkably similar to that of pulmonary tuberculosis that the latter diagnosis often heads the differential list. In this situation, patients are often male in their 50s–60s. Cough, sputum, sweats, weight loss, fatigue and haemoptysis are found. However, other presentations are characterised by simple cough and sputum, whilst other patients may have disseminated disease. In recent years, there has been an increase in cases associated with females. In the series described by Prince[38] the females with no underlying predisposing condition presented with persistent cough and troublesome purulent sputum in the absence of fever or weight loss in which the radiological abnormality was one of progressive nodular opacifications. Another presentation in females has been characterised by saccular bronchiectasis (possibly the cause of which was the *M. avium* complex itself) in which cough and purulent sputum were the main features[65]. A further female dominated syndrome has been recently described termed the Lady Windermere Syndrome. This occurs in elderly women with no past pulmonary disease who developed distinctive clinical and radiological features of *M. avium* complex disease. They voluntarily suppressed cough and had dependent lingula/middle lobar disease[66].

Radiological findings include unilateral/bilateral apical infiltrates (Fig. 11.2 (*a*), (*b*)), cavitation, diffuse nodular infiltrates (particularly in women), patchy interstitial infiltrates or sometimes a miliary pattern indistinguishable from *M. tuberculosis* (Fig. 11.3). Pulmonary nodules (tuberculomas) indistinguishable from neoplasia is not an uncommon presentation[67]. Pleural effusions and mediastinal lymphadenopathy, however, are infrequently seen. If cavities are thin-walled with sparse surrounding inflammation, this may favour NTM rather than *M. tuberculosis*.

Associated extrapulmonary disease with extrapulmonary lymphadenopathy and other soft tissue and bone manifestations are extremely unusual. Disseminated disease is common in HIV-infected patients but otherwise rare and should suggest significant underlying immunosuppression particularly HIV but hairy cell leukaemia, lymphoma or reticulo endothelial malignancies, corticosteroid administration should also be considered.

Most patients have stable or slowly progressive disease compared to infection with *M. tuberculosis*. Some patients do have, however, a rapidly progressive and sometimes fatal outcome particularly in those with significant underlying disease.

By utilising the criteria for diagnosis referred to previously, and considering various clinical factors, a reasonably confident diagnosis can be made in most cases. One approach to management is simply to observe the patient if his condition is stable, and symptoms are mild. However, the patient with significant clinical disease or significant immunosuppression requires prompt treatment. There is no uniform agreement over treatment regimes and no controlled studies have been undertaken.

Most strains of *M. avium* complex are resistant *in vitro* to first-line antimycobacterial drugs when tested singly. Therapy for *M. avium* complex (as for other slowly growing mycobacteria) should always include multiple drugs since resistance develops on monotherapy and needs to be given for long periods of time. Most clinicians agree that ethambutol and a rifamycin (rifampicin or rifabutin) should be included in regimens. The role of isoniazid in *M. avium* complex is particularly controversial, despite one set of recommendations for its use in *M. avium* complex[14]. There are many physicians who argue against the use of isoniazid; their evidence has been based upon *in vitro* studies which indicate high MICs. However, there is often poor correlation between *in vitro* findings and *in vivo* responses. When the drug is used as part of combination chemotherapy, synergism can sometimes be demonstrated both *in vitro* and *in vivo*[68]. In contrast, the Public Health Service Task Force, writing in 1993, made the statement that 'isoniazid and pyrazinamide have no role in the therapy of *M. avium* complex disease', though the focus of that report was on disseminated disease[15]. Nevertheless, isoniazid has been a component of many multidrug regimes which were clinically successful, but the degree of contribution of isoniazid is not really known for several mycobacteria. Evidence for combination synergistic activity *in vitro*[69, 70] for different antimycobacterial drugs, possibly due to the different sites of drug action has accrued and this is translated into effective *in vivo* activity[71].

On the basis of these findings, a common practice, at least until relatively recently, is to treat pulmonary *M. avium* complex with a regime consisting of isoniazid, rifampicin and ethambutol for between 18 and 24 months with the optional addition of streptomycin for the initial 3 months[72]. Patients generally respond better if more than two different drugs are used. Should there be no improvement over the first 3 months, then an alternative selection of drugs or additional drugs based on *in vitro* sensitivities may be added. If the patient has severe and progressive symptoms from presentation, then further drugs which include cycloserine, ethionamide, kanamycin (if streptomycin has not been used) and capreomycin may be added on an entirely empirical basis[72]. Duration of therapy is usually until the patient has improved and sputum is negative, and has had treatment for 12 months after sputum conversion, following which continuation with at least 4 drugs for another 12 months is suggested. Overall, most patients respond reasonably satisfactorily with sputum conversion in

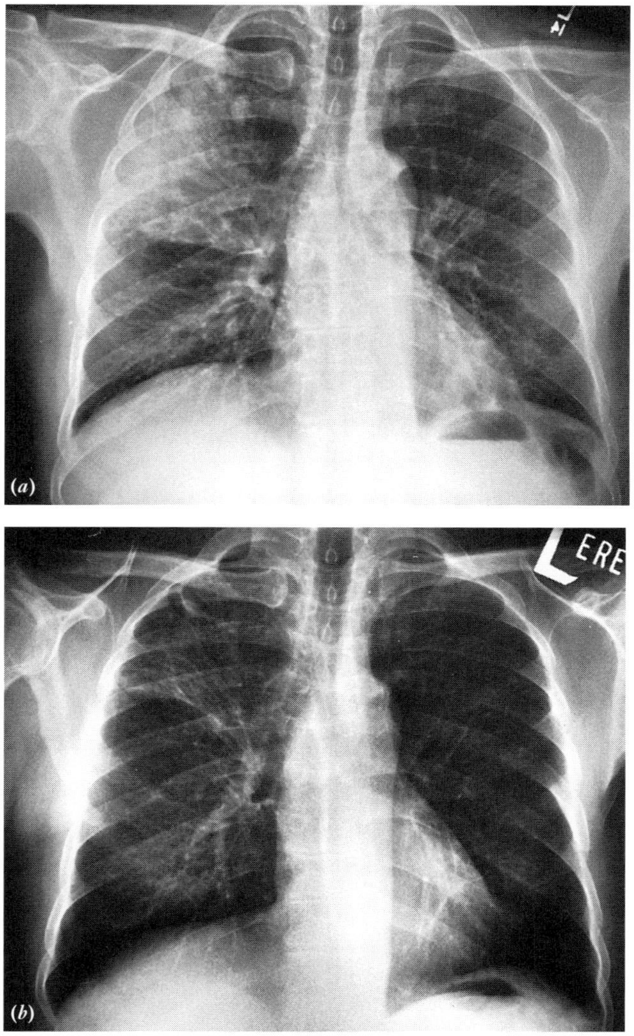

FIGURE 11.2 (*a*) 53-year-old male with non-Hodgkin's lymphoma, insulin-dependent diabetes, on steroids, received recent chemotherapy. Presents with cough, sputum and sweats. Right upper lobe infiltrate – sputum grew *M. avium* complex. (*b*) Note improvement of chest radiograph concomitant with improvement of symptoms on ciprofloxacin as monotherapy.

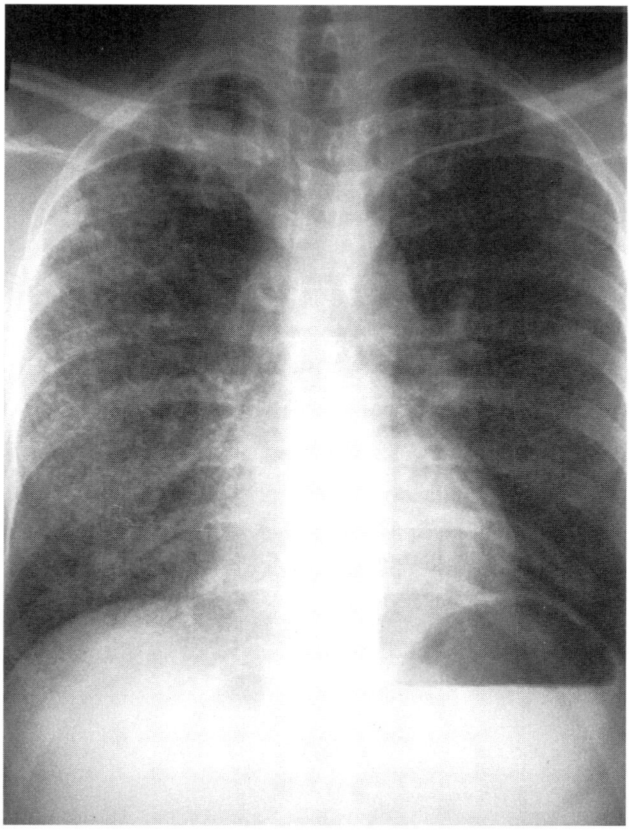

FIGURE 11.3 33-year-old male renal transplant recipient, diabetic, on cyclophosphamide and steroids presents with headache, fever and sweats. Note widespread miliary nodularity of both lungs. CSF and sputum grew *M. avium* complex. Cure achieved with rifampicin, isoniazid, pyrazinamide, and ethambutol.

up to 80%, clinical cure in up to 60%, although bacteriological and clinical relapse may occur in approximately 20%[72–74].

There is now considerable interest in the use of the new macrolides, clarithromycin and azithromycin for the treatment of NTM disease including *M. avium* complex. Heavily concentrated into phagocytes, their *in vitro* activity has been remarkable. The MICs of clarithromycin were found to be less than 4 µg/ml for 90% of isolates of *M. avium* complex in one study[75]. A recent open controlled non-comparative study using low dose (500 mg twice daily) of clarithromycin given for four months as monotherapy for *M. avium* complex lung disease in 30 HIV negative patients resulted in conversion to sputum negative/significant reduction in sputum positive in 79% and almost all evaluable patients showed improvement in sputum culture and/or chest radiographs[76]. Clarythromycin resistance developed in 3 out of 19 patients (16%) during the four months of therapy. The resistant post-treatment isolate from each patient had an identical DNA large restriction fragment pattern to the initial susceptible isolate, indicating acquired resistance, not reinfection. Another patient who had previously received clarithromycin entered this trial with an isolate resistant to clarithromycin. Clarithromycin resistance was strongly associated with a poor clinical outcome. Though demonstrating the short-term efficacy of clarithromycin alone, the authors recommended multidrug therapy, including clarithromycin as one of the agents. They suggested ethambutol and rifampicin or rifabutin as additional agents, but the optimal combination has not been defined in a controlled study. A higher dosage of clarithromycin in elderly patients is associated with unacceptable drug toxicity[77]. Clearly, clarithromycin presents a significant potential in treatment. The role of clarithromycin and other agents in HIV-associated disseminated *M. avium* complex is discussed later.

A number of other drugs that could be used in *M. avium* complex infection are under investigation. Many of these have been tested in HIV-associated disseminated *M. avium* complex or in animal models and their role in human or non-HIV and pulmonary *M. avium* complex disease remains to be clearly elucidated. Clofazimine is one such drug but its pulmonary distribution is poor. Other drugs include azithromycin, rifabutin, quinolones including ciprofloxacin, liposomal preparations of gentamicin and capreomycin and dapsone, given either alone or in various combinations.

Surgical resection of localised disease up to a maximum of two adjacent lobes may be considered in selected patients with adequate cardiopulmonary reserve who fail to respond, relapse after a reasonable period of chemotherapy, develop multiple drug resistance or severe drug toxicity or intolerance[72]. Lobectomy is associated with a better outcome than sublobar resection[78]. Timing of surgery may be crucial to reduce complications such as bronchopleural fistula and secondary infections, with resection being advocated by some as early as 3 months after a trial of drug therapy has failed[79]. Following surgery, it may be prudent, though not proven necessary, to continue chemotherapy in patients who can tolerate it for 6 months.

M. kansasii

M. kansasii was first identified by Haundoroy in 1955; the organism is usually recoverable from human sources rather than alternative reservoirs such as water, pig and cattle. The presence of *M. kansasii* in specimens unlike most other NTM should carry a high degree of suspicion for disease owing to the relative infrequency with which it is found in the environment. It has unique staining characteristics (cross-bars) as well as β-carotene crystal formation in light, which may distinguish it from other NTM. The disease incidence is higher in the UK and Europe, particularly in coal mining areas, than the USA, for example, in South Carolina, *M. kansasii* accounted for only 4% of infections due to NTM[80] compared to approximately 33% in the UK[81]. Over a 10-year period *M. kansasii* accounted for 65% of all cases of pulmonary disease due to NTM in Merseyside UK[82] and 1.2% of all pulmonary mycobacterial infections in Wales[83]. In Western Australia the average incidence rate for *M. kansasii* infections (of which 90% were pulmonary) was 0.14/100 000[84]. Geographical clustering of human cases is recognised. Nowadays the sex distribution is almost equal[85], probably as a result of the increasing population of females with chronic pulmonary disease. The usual age is 30–60 years.

A pulmonary presentation for *M. kansasii* is the most frequent observed. Pre-existing lung disease is present in about two-thirds of patients, mainly chronic bronchitis or emphysema or coal workers pneumoconiosis (Fig. 11.4). There may be a past history of pulmonary tuberculosis. Extrapulmonary disease may also be present, particularly of the head and neck (Fig. 11.5). In a 10-year review of 55 patients with *M. kansasii* infections, the majority had underlying pulmonary disease, and 70% had systemic predisposing factors particularly immunocompromisation[85]. Although COPD is particularly

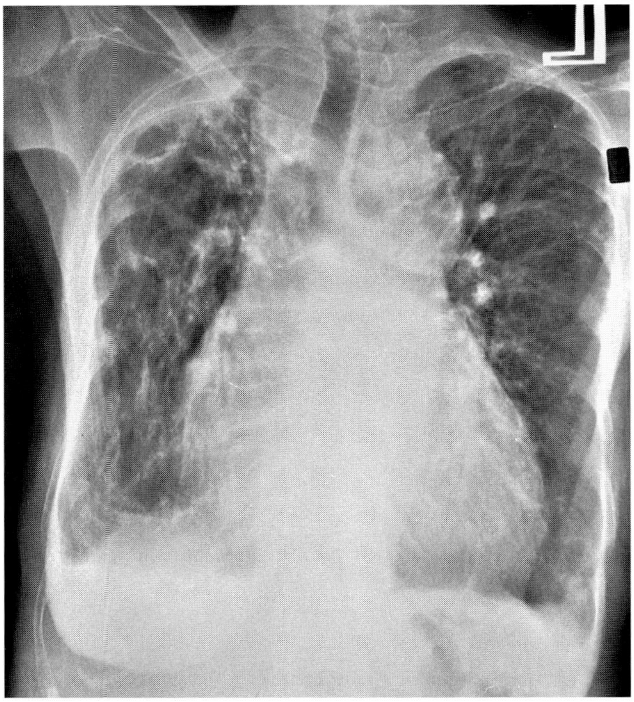

FIGURE 11.4 Chronic pulmonary changes in 84-year-old female with chronic asthma and chronic respiratory failure showing bronchiectatic cavities and compensatory emphysema. Sputum grew *M. kansasii* during this exacerbation with cough and yellow sputum. Unresponsive to cotrimoxazole but settled on rifampicin, ethambutol, isoniazid.

common other rarer chronic pulmonary predisposing conditions are described including the Swyer–James syndrome (reduced ciliary function with abnormal ventilation and perfusion in the lung)[86] and Bechterew's disease (ankylosing spondylitis associated with upper lobe fibrocystic disease)[87]. Recently, an association has been described between primary pulmonary malignancy, radiotherapy and *M. kansasii* disease[88].

Extrapulmonary disease is well described for *M. kansasii*, such as inoculation associated cutaneous abscesses, cellulitis, osteomyelitis, fascitis, tendinitis, lymphadenopathy, GI tract involvement and renal granulomatous disease. Disseminated disease also occurs and is associated with leukaemoid or cytopenic reactions. Bacteraemia has been described in immunosuppressed patients[89].

Presenting symptoms are usually impossible to differentiate from those of the underlying associated disease, though many patients have some exacerbation of chronic cough, etc. Haemoptysis occurs. Obstructing endobronchial mass lesions can occur[90]. Studies on the natural history of the infection suggest a slowly progressive course in about 40% of patients, resulting in progressive lung destruction[91]. Other patients, however, may have minimal disease. An association with previous spontaneous pneumothorax has been recognised[92]. The symptoms are generally non-specific for *M. kansasii*. However, in a direct comparison to patients with other NTM, *M. kansasii* infections were significantly less likely to have a history of diabetes, heavy alcohol intake, and more likely to experience haemoptysis[93]. In general, the prognosis of patients with *M. kansasii* pulmonary disease is determined by the concomitant underlying diseases.

Radiographically, the features are similar to those described in pulmonary tuberculosis but with thin wall cavitation being particularly

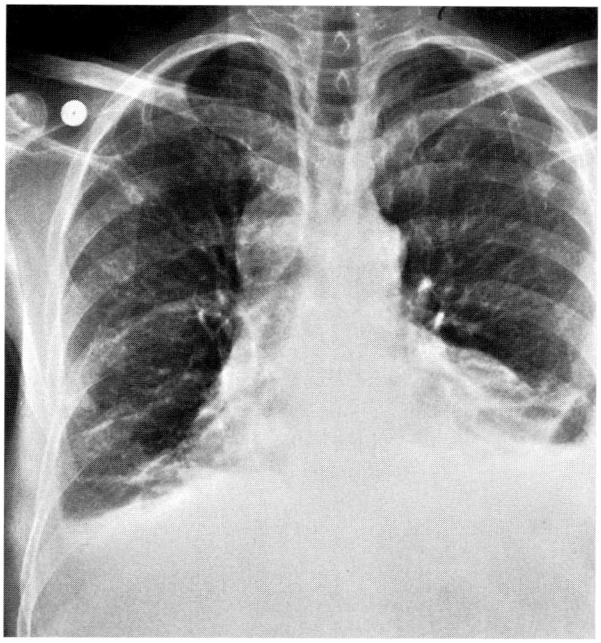

FIGURE 11.5 60-year-old male farmer with 3 months of fever, sweats, weight loss and pericardial tamponade. Pericardial fluid, mediastinal lymph node and sputum grew *M. kansasii*. Chest radiograph shows large right paratracheal lymph node.

common, in up to 70–90% of cases. Patients with *M. kansasii* compared with TB were significantly less likely to have middle/lower lobe involvement, air space shadowing in more than one bronchopulmonary segment, cavities larger than 2 cm, intracavitary air fluid levels and pleural effusions and more likely to have disease confined to the upper lobes[51]. However, individual patients cannot be distinguished on the basis of the radiological findings.

The organism is usually sensitive to rifampicin and ethambutol and has intermediate sensitivity or resistance to isoniazid, pyrazinamide and streptomycin. However, these isolates may be susceptible to higher drug concentrations. Treatment regimes employing rifampicin and ethambutol are usually successful[84,85], producing up to 100% sputum conversion with no long term relapses[83]. A combination of rifampicin, ethambutol and isoniazid (with the option of three months' streptomycin given initially) for 18–24 months has been used commonly, though there have been some successes with 12-month regimes[94]. High dose isoniazid (potentially toxic at 600–900 mg daily) has been recommended by some[94]. The use of at least three drugs is suggested to diminish the emergence of rifampicin resistance which occurs if only two drugs are used[95]. Addition of cycloserine or ethionamide might be pertinent since almost one-fifth of strains in some areas may be resistant to ethambutol[84]. A retrospective study indicated that there was no significant difference in the outcome of patients with *M. kansasii* or *M. tuberculosis* when given standard antituberculous drugs (rifampicin, isoniazid, ethambutol, pyrazinamide)[96]. A recent publication on the chemotherapy of *M. kansasii* came from the Research Committee of the British Thoracic Society. In a prospective study of 9 months of rifampicin + ethambutol in patients with *M. kansasii* a good response rate was obtained[97]. However, relapse or reinfection was approximately 10% and therefore perhaps 12 months treatment with or without newer drugs is more appropriate. Relapsing disease may be due to acquired resistance particularly to rifampicin/ethambutol/isoniazid and can be successfully treated with at least three drugs not used in the previous courses, for example, ethionamide, cycloserine or capreomycin[98]. Rifampicin-resistant *M. kansasii* is being increasingly recognised[99]. For these patients, drug regimens which include clarithromycin, ciprofloxacin, ethambutol, sulfamethoxazole-trimethoprim, rifampicin or aminoglycoside can offer useful therapeutic alternative. *In vitro* studies indicate ethambutol/ciprofloxacin erythromycin synergisms[100]. Isolates of *M. kansasii* are highly susceptible to clarithromycin[101], though there is limited clinical experience with this drug for such infections. Recourse to surgical resection for localised disease or for complications or for antimicrobial non-response occurs less commonly than with other NTM.

M. xenopi

This NTM was first described by Schwabacher in 1959. ZN staining may reveal unique morphological characteristics: long, slender and tapered and palisaded. It was originally isolated from the skin of the toad *Xenopus laevis*, though it has an avian reservoir and can also be found in hot and cold water sources. Water, for example, showers, may be the source of infection[102]. Contamination of diagnostic instruments and specimens may initially suggest an outbreak of infection[26]; care is needed to recognise and differentiate contamination from infection. In the USA, *M. xenopi* accounts for less than 1% of all mycobacterial isolates which is in strong contrast to reports from the UK and Europe. For example, Smith and Citron found that *M. xenopi* comprised 56% of all NTM isolated at the Brompton Hospital over a 6-year period and accounted for pulmonary disease in 15/23 patients reviewed[103]. A similar finding was reported from Canada, where approximately 40% of pulmonary NTM disease was due to *M. xenopi*[104]. Clustering of cases has been described and in association with biochemical, cultural and antimicrobials sensitivity homologies suggest endemic foci[105].

M. xenopi usually causes pulmonary infections and many individuals have similar underlying diseases to those described for *M. avium* complex. Malnutrition, for example, secondary to anorexia nervosa possibly via diminution in cell mediated immunity is another risk factor[106]. *M. xenopi* can produce severe disease in renal allograft recipients[107]. Symptomatology is also similar to that described in other NTM; some individuals have an indolent, others a subacute course. Haemoptysis may be a feature. Radiological findings include multiple thin-walled cavities, apical infiltrates, nodules, fibrosis and consolidation. The disease is often bilateral, posterior upper lobar in distribution[104]. Cavitation, often multiple and thin-walled, is common as it is with *M. kansasii*.

Extrapulmonary disease does occur though rarely. Epididymitis, synovitis, cuneiform bone abscess, tonsillar infection, endocarditis, bone graft infection and disseminated disease (in HIV and in immune competent patients) have all been described. Obvious clinical disease was found in two patients described by Smith and Citron, yet these patients had single positive cultures only[103], an example of the limited usefulness of the diagnostic criteria in common use.

Antibiotic sensitivity testing gives variable results even to first line drugs[103,108,109] but the clinical response has little relation to this[103]. Previously, it was thought that pulmonary disease due to *M. xenopi* was mild and relatively easy to manage. This has not been substantiated by recent studies[104,108], with relapse (sometimes occurring several years later) and progressive disease being increasingly documented. Only 23% in one series were cured (as defined by a satisfactory clinical and radiological improvement and sputum conversion) by chemotherapy[108]. Serious underlying disease and short course chemotherapy of less than 9 months may contribute to the poor outcome. Nevertheless, many patients do experience an increase in well-being, sputum conversion and radiological improvement including cavitary closure, e.g. 8 out of 11 responding[103]. A combination of rifampicin, isoniazid and ethambutol with/without streptomycin is the most frequently advocated regime. These drugs are given for at least 9 months[108] and in many case for 18–24 months[103,109]. The threshold for surgical intervention in patients with *M. xenopi* pulmonary disease appears to be lower compared to *M. avium* complex because of the unpredictable outcome and progressive nature of the illness in many patients[108]. As mentioned previously, there is a dearth of comparative treatment studies and reports are mainly retrospective descriptions of relatively small numbers of patients. Newer antimycobacterial agents such as clarithromycin require evaluation.

Mycobacterium scrofulaceum

This NTM is found in milk, cheese, soil, water and oysters. It has biochemical and antibiotic sensitivity patterns closely resembling *M. avium* complex but morphological distinctions include coarse staining and buttery consistency of the colonies. Also, it does not react to the nucleic acid probe for *M. avium* complex (Accu Probe, Gen Probe). In children, high cervical lymphadenopathy and paramandibular abscesses secondary to an oropharyngeal focus are common. Disseminated disease includes osteomyelitis, granulomatous hepatitis and meningitis. Pulmonary manifestations are rare, occurring in individuals with preexisting chronic pulmonary disease[110], including silicosis, arc-welding fume disease and other dust associated diseases. Recently, a pulmonary nodular presentation of *M. scrofulaceum* complicating heart transplantation was described[111]. Resistance to several antituberculous drugs is not uncommon, though limited experience suggests a clinical response if a combination of isoniazid, rifampicin, ethambutol and streptomycin is used. Cycloserine, ethionamide, amikacin, ciprofloxacin, clofazimine and clarithromycin are alternative agents. If anything less than total excision of associated lymph nodes is performed, persistent sinus formation complicates recovery.

M. marinum

M. marinum usually produces superficial skin infections secondary to aquatic trauma such as Fish fancier's finger or Surfer's nodules. However, deeper soft tissue infections including osteomyelitis and tenosynovitis have been described particularly in patients with antigen specific T-cell anergy[112]. Non-caseating granulomas characterise the histology. Rarely, disseminated disease occurs. Involvement of the respiratory tract is confined to a few patients who have laryngeal lesions[113]. Although infections usually respond to rifampicin and ethambutol, the tetracyclines and cotrimoxazole have also been used. Often single agent therapy with doxycycline or cotrimoxazole or ciprofloxacin has been successful. *M. marinum* isolates are susceptible to clarithromycin[101]. Clarithromycin has been used successfully for *M. marinum* skin disease, alone or in combination with ethambutol, though experience is limited[114]. Localised disease can be treated with cryotherapy, steroids or surgery although chemotherapy alone is often successful even with deep infections[115].

Mycobacterium szulgai

Marks *et al.* were the first to implicate this organism in human disease in 1972[116]. It is scotochromogenic at 37 °C, but photochromogenic at 25 °C. Snails and tropical fish harbour the organism. Most clinical reports originate from the USA, Japan, Australia, Portugal and UK. It is a relatively uncommon NTM, accounting for less than 1% of all NTM isolations, but most cases of disease are pulmonary. Cervical lymphadenopathy, carpal tunnel syndrome, cutaneous infections, osteomyelitis and disseminated disease are less common manifestations. Its presence in secretions has a high prediction for disease rather than colonisation (this is akin to the situation with *M. kansasii* and *M. xenopi*). In keeping with other NTMs there is usually a background of chronic pulmonary disease. Presentation is indistinguishable from pulmonary tuberculosis but radiologically thin wall cavities is the predominant finding[117]. The pulmonary and radiological course can be rapid. Although the organism shows a variable antibiotic sensitivity pattern, most strains are only fractionally more resistant than *M. tuberculosis*. A combination of rifampicin, isoniazid and ethambutol given for 18–24 months is usually effective. However, treatment failures have been described. One case of a dual infection of *M. tuberculosis*/*M. szulgai* failed to respond to rifampicin and isoniazid. In vitro testing showed the organism to be resistant to these drugs but sensitive to capreomycin and ethambutol to which the patient responded[118].

Mycobacterium simiae

M. simiae is an unusual cause of chronic pulmonary disease occurring in male, middle-aged, or elderly patients who often have a history of pulmonary tuberculosis. As its name suggests, the organism is also found in monkeys but is widespread environmentally particularly in water and in human faeces. Close contact with monkeys has been documented as producing infection with *M. simiae*[119]. Many cases of infection originate from Israel. A characteristic mycolic acid profile demonstrated by thin layer chromatography methylated lipids, is a point of differentiation from *M. avium complex*. It is usually resistant *in vitro* to most antituberculous drugs. This includes clarithromycin which is somewhat unusual for the NTM. Clinical response to these drugs has been demonstrated, however.

M. fortuitum complex

The *M. fortuitum* complex includes *M. fortuitum*, *M. chelonae* (formerly *M. chelonae* subsp. *chelonae*) and *M. abscessus* (formerly *M. chelonae* subsp. *abscessus*). They are found in soil, water, marine life (*M. chelonae* was in fact first discovered in turtles) and domestic animals, and can survive extremes of temperature and dryness. Visible growth on culture is detected by 7 days and a positive aryl-sulphatase test occurs by day 3, they are rapid growers. Regular ZN/Kinyoun staining techniques may not be sensitive enough to detect *M. fortuitum* complex. As these organisms may be Gram's stain positive and are beaded rods, they can be mistaken for diphtheroids. Colonial morphology may be mistaken for *Nocardia*. In addition, overlapping characteristics have resulted in the *M. fortuitum* and *M. chelonae* organisms being grouped together. However, nitrate reduction and iron uptake can be used to differentiate the two species. This is of some clinical importance as *M. fortuitum* associated disease may be managed more successfully with drugs alone than *M. chelonae* associated disease which is most likely to relapse after medical treatment and requires surgery at an early stage. Three biovariants of *M. fortuitum* and three subspecies of *M. chelonae* are recognised. They produce different disease manifestations, for example, respiratory infections due to *M. fortuitum* complex are usually associated with *M. abscessus* (approximately 85% of the respiratory isolates).

Respiratory disease is somewhat unusual in the disease spectrum due to *M. fortuitum* complex. In a series of 125 cases of *M. fortuitum complex* infections, only 19% had pulmonary manifestations, the majority being associated with iatrogenic soft tissue infections secondary to inoculation and surgery[120]. These include injection abscesses and wound infections after, for example, silicone implant mammoplasty and cosmetic surgery. Sometimes there are associated chronic draining sinuses. Rare manifestations of *M. fortuitum* complex infections are peritoneal dialysis induced peritonitis, prosthetic valve endocarditis, cervical lymphadenopathy, hepatitis, meningitis, urinary tract infection and disseminated disease)[14] (Fig. 11.6). *M. fortuitum* complex has also been found in patients with cystic fibrosis[121]. The true incidence and role in cystic fibrosis patients may be underestimated because of the propensity of sputum from cystic fibrosis patients to liquidise Löwenstein–Jensen medium[121]. Megaoesophagus or achalasia has also been identified as a predisposing factor, presumably due to aspiration pneumonia. Rheumatoid arthritis, a past history of pulmonary disease including tuberculosis and carcinoma, and lipoid aspiration pneumonia[122] are other associated factors (Fig. 11.7). It had previously been thought that patients with immunosuppression are no more prone to develop or to have worse disease. Recently, however, *M.chelonae* infection has been described in neutropenic patients in whom response to antimicrobials did not occur until the neutrophil count had recovered[123]. Right

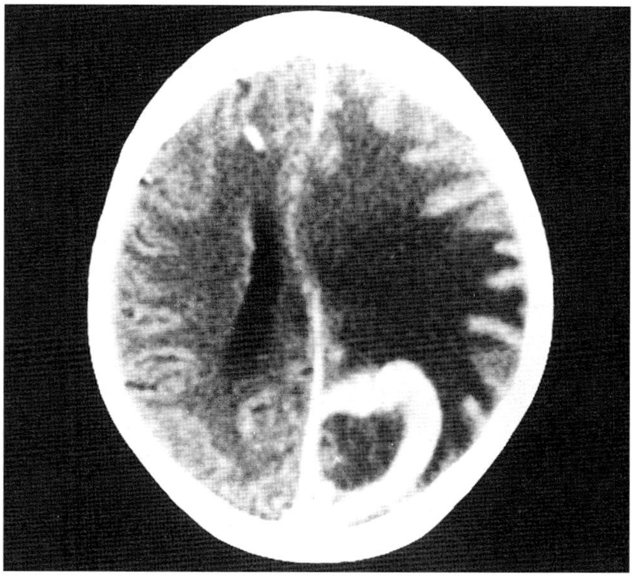

FIGURE 11.6 44-year-old female, non-Hodgkin's lymphoma and headache. CT head shows enhancing lesion in parieto-occipital area with oedema, compressing left lateral ventricle and shifting midline to the right. CSF grew *M. fortuitum* complex.

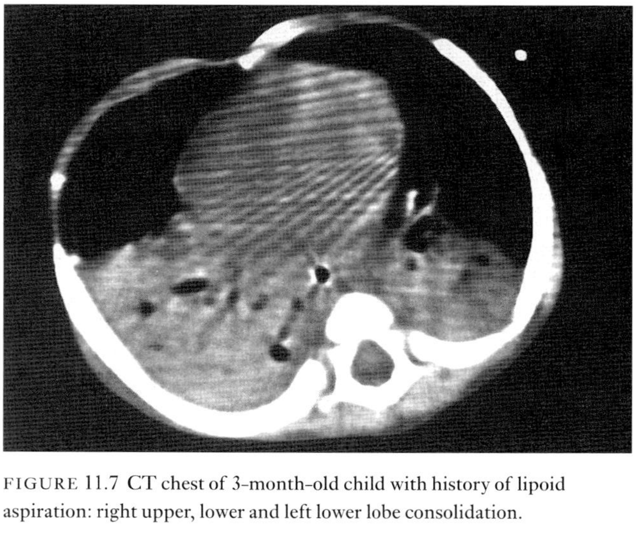

FIGURE 11.7 CT chest of 3-month-old child with history of lipoid aspiration: right upper, lower and left lower lobe consolidation.

middle lobe syndrome in HIV-positive patients has been reported[124]. Cases have been described of immunocompetent patients with pulmonary disease and mycobacteraemia due to *M. fortuitum* complex which proved fatal[125–127]. It is currently thought that up to 60% of patients with *M. fortuitum* complex lung disease have no recognised underlying abnormalities[128]. This highlights the need to be cautious in dismissing the organisms as medically unimportant. In fact, the presence of *M. fortuitum* complex usually indicates disease. Colonisation is not common. However, contamination of diagnostic specimens from water has been described leading to erroneous diagnosis of outbreaks[129].

Most cases occur in late middle age (approximately 60 years) female non-smokers, something of a distinction from the majority of the other NTMs.

The characteristics of the disease due to *M. fortuitum* complex have been difficult to describe accurately but most patients have mild but chronic and relapsing symptomatology including intermittent productive cough, fever, and fatigue. Haemoptysis can occur. Rarely severe and progressive disease or fatality has been described[121,123–125,126,130], particularly in association with lipid pneumonia, or achalasia. In immunocompromised patients, the disease may be aggressive and relapse unless long-term suppressive therapy is given[123].

M. fortuitum complex is the only NTM in which radiographical appearances may be sufficiently unique to suggest differentiation from other mycobacteria. Diffuse or patchy interstitial/alveolar infiltrates, and bilateral upper or lower lobe, reticulo-nodular infiltrates with lack of cavitation is usual. It may produce solitary pulmonary nodules or mimic carcinoma[131] (Fig. 11.8).

Although fatalities have been described, the generally good clinical outcome in most patients with *M. fortuitum* complex has not necessarily been ascribed to antimicrobial treatment, since some cases appear to resolve spontaneously and others deteriorate slowly over many years. Indications for treatment therefore, have to be individualised and degree of symptomatology and disease progression have to be considered. Conversion of sputum positive cases may not occur with antimicrobial treatment.

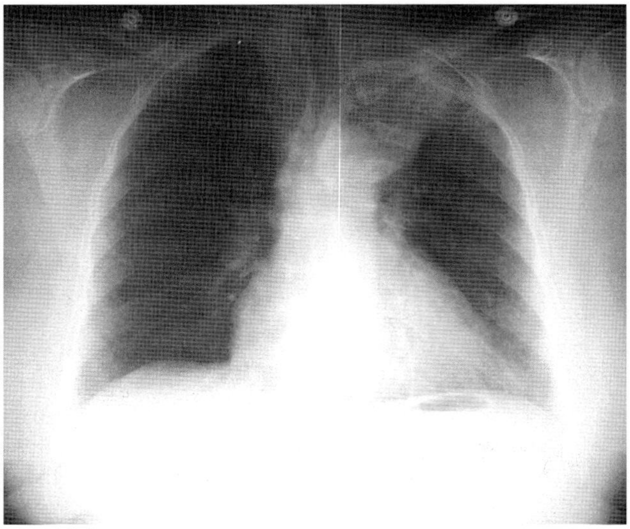

FIGURE 11.8 64-year-old female with chronic obstructive pulmonary disease and cough. Bronchoscopy indicated inflammatory stenosis left upper lobe. Chest radiograph indicates soft tissue mass in the left upper lobe ? carcinoma. Sputum grew *M. chelonae*. X-ray became normal after 4 months of rifampicin, isoniazid and ethambutol.

The management includes surgical drainage of abscesses, removal of any foreign bodies and antibiotics. *In vitro* testing usually indicates that *M. chelonae* is resistant to most conventional oral antituberculous drugs. Cefoxitin and amikacin usually have good *in vitro* activity and imipenem shows fair activity. Susceptibility of these strains to erythromycin occurs in about a third of cases. For these reasons, standard antituberculous regimes are not usually used despite apparent clinical and radiological success when such combinations are given[132]. Instead, a commonly used regimen has been extrapolated from the experience with extrapulmonary infections. This is amikacin at a dose of 15 mg/kg/day together with cefoxitin 3 gm Q6 hourly for 6 weeks. If there is good response, oral therapy (doxycycline or sulphonamides or erythromycin or rifampicin or ethambutol) is substituted for at least a further 6 weeks. Recently, the use of cefoxitin, imipenem, ciprofloxacin and ofloxacin proved successful in treating pulmonary disease including cases of pulmonary abscess due to *M. fortuitum* complex[133–135]. Relapse appears to be common following discontinuation of therapy. The place of surgical resection is not established, but some authors suggest that this is a therapeutic option that should be employed early on, even in patients with organisms susceptible to the antimicrobials used, because of the high rate of relapse. *M. chelonae* is susceptible to clarithromycin. A very good short-term clinical response was seen in a small trial using clarithromycin monotherapy for cutaneous disease in patients on immunosuppressive therapy[136]. Further experience with clarithromycin is needed in patients with pulmonary disease.

M. malmoense

M. malmoense is an emerged pathogen in both normal and immunocompromised hosts, mainly found in the UK and Northern Europe. First recognised as a human pathogen as such in 1977 in Malmö[137], it may have escaped prior recognition because of its slow growth on Löwenstein–Jensen medium (cultures may not be positive for 3 months) and confusion with other NTM, e.g. *M. terrae*/*M. avium* complex. Tween hydrolysis, catalase, β-galactosidase, arylsulphatase, acid phosphatase and urease testing are key features which may help to differentiate *M. malmoense* from *M. terrae*/*M. avium* complex[138]. The presence of a distinctive surface lipid pattern in addition to the aforementioned biochemical phenomena as well as the determination of the base sequence of a selected region of PCR amplified r-RNA gene has been used in its definitive identification[139]. Retrospective analysis of stored previously unspeciated strains of NTM held at the Mycobacteriological Reference Laboratory, Cardiff indicated that 61 isolates over a 21-year period were, in fact, *M. malmoense*[140]. The year of the first isolate that could be identified was 1954.

In the UK, after *M. avium* complex and *M. kansasii*, *M. malmoense* is the third most common NTM reported, whilst in Sweden it ranks second to *M. avium* complex. In Nottingham, *M. malmoense* accounts for 7% of all mycobacterial and 23% of all NTM pulmonary infections between 1980 and 1991[50]. It has also been described in the USA but the incidence among NTM is much less than 1%[141]. Furthermore, the frequency of cases is increasing which may be due to improved isolation techniques, better awareness and possibly a true increase in the incidence[5,142]. *M. malmoense* has only recently been identified from inanimate sources[142]. It is known to colonise the gastrointestinal tract but the epidemiology (particularly the enormous disparity of incidence between Europe and the USA) and treatment aspects are not clear.

An extensive review of *M. malmoense* in Sweden was recently published[142]. 171/221 cases were pulmonary (all except one were adults) whilst 36/221 cases affected the cervical lymph nodes (all except one were children). This pulmonary bias is also reflected in other series and reports[5,143]. There is also a relatively high affinity for the respiratory tract when compared to other NTM[81]. For respiratory infections, the sex difference in Henriques' series was 99/72 male to female and the mean age 62 years. Underlying pulmonary disease appears in 80 of the 131 evaluable patients and included a past history of tuberculosis, lung cancer, chronic bronchitis, and silicosis. Other non-pulmonary identifiable possible risk factors included malignancy, leukaemia, alcoholism, immunological treatment and smoking. There was no underlying disease in approximately a third of the patients. It is only rarely found in patients with HIV unlike *M. avium* complex which may reflect the fact that the intracellular growth of *M. malmoense* is not enhanced by HIV. Other reports indicate a similar profile of underlying pulmonary and extrapulmonary associated diseases.

The retrospective nature of Henriquez's study makes it difficult to be precise about the pathogenic role of *M. malmoense* in all patients. However, 'many' patients with respiratory tract symptoms were thought likely to have disease due to *M. malmoense*. Cough, sputum, haemoptysis and weight loss are commonly present in patients with pulmonary *M. malmoense* and this makes differentiation from pulmonary tuberculosis or diseases due to other NTM difficult.

There is a dearth of information gathered prospectively on the significance of isolates as well as treatment impacts on the natural history and outcome. Nevertheless, the current information strongly supports the contention that progressive pulmonary disease due to *M. malmoense* does occur. Approximately 70% of the patients in Henriques's series received antimycobacterial treatment for progressive radiological changes, pneumonectomy was indicated in between 5% and 10% of patients and mortality ascribed to *M. malmoense* was 2% at least[142]. Recently, three patients with chronic obstructive airways disease on steroids with coexisting *Aspergillus* infection had progressive *M. malmoense* lung disease from which they died but without proof of invasive aspergillosis at post-mortem[144].

Radiographically, cavitary lesions are found in at least 70% of patients, together with air space shadowing, bronchopulmonary spread, and volume loss being the most common features[143,50]. Circumscribed opacities are relatively uncommon but a pseudo tumour presentation has been described[145]. Pulmonary radiographic differences from patients with *M. tuberculosis* have been described. Therefore, cavities > 6 cm, intracavity air fluid levels, lung volume loss, coexistent pneumoconiosis and air space shadow involving no more than one bronchopulmonary segment were found significantly more frequently in *M. malmoense* patients[50]. However, these features are not sufficient to permit a confident differentiation from *M. tuberculosis*.

Uncommonly, extrapulmonary infection sites include the skin, lymph nodes, and bursae; disseminated disease also occurs but only in patients with severe immunodeficiency[146].

The optimum therapeutic regime remains unclear. *In vitro*, the organism is sensitive to rifampicin and resistant to isoniazid, there is variable resistance to other antimycobacterials. Isoniazid has actually been shown to increase *in vitro* growth[147]. However, discordance between *in vitro* testing and *in vivo* clinical response is noted[143], since good results were obtained with the regimen of rifampicin, isoniazid and ethambutol for 18–24 months of treatment. Omission of ethambutol or discontinuation of the triple regimen before 18 months were completed leads to poor outcome[143,148]. Surgery may be required for failure of medical therapy – it may be life saving in the face of progressive disease[149]. However, its precise role in the overall management remains unclear.

Clearly, there are a number of important and interesting unexplained phenomena relating to this relatively recently identified pathogenic NTM which require urgent clarification.

M. asiaticum

M. asiaticum is found in healthy monkeys. It was first described as a human pulmonary coloniser or pulmonary pathogen in three or two Australian patients, respectively, in 1983[150]. Another case of human pulmonary disease due to *M. asiaticum* was described in the USA in 1990[151]. Antimycobacterial drugs to which the organism appears to respond include combinations of isoniazid, ethambutol, rifampicin, streptomycin, with capreomycin, PAS and ciprofloxacin.

M. shimoidei

This highly unusual NTM was first described in 1975. Subsequently, there was little interest in it until 1988 when it was formally recognised as a distinct NTM species[5]. It may have been formerly confused with *M. terrae* complex. It appears to be globally distributed and possibly more prevalent as a pathogen than previously realised. It is found usually in association with pulmonary disease. It may be resistant to isoniazid and rifampicin; the quinolones, ciprofloxacin/ofloxacin have good *in vitro* activity.

M. celatum

This is one of the newest NTM associated with human disease to be described. Isolates are difficult to differentiate from *M. avium* complex or *M. xenopi*. In a series described by Butler, all but 1 of 24 patients (some with HIV infection) had their organisms isolated from respiratory tract. The exact significance remains unclear. The organism is resistant *in vitro* to most of antituberculous medications[152]. One case of bilateral cavitary pulmonary disease has been described in an HIV-negative patient[23].

Pulmonary disease due to specific NTM: rarely pathogenic

A few other NTMs have on rare occasions been incriminated in the pathogenesis of human pulmonary disease.

M. thermoresistibile

M. thermoresistibile[153] can grow in temperatures exceeding 50 °C. It can produce cavitary lung disease, pulmonary abscesses or solitary nodules.

M. gordonae

Distinct laboratory characteristics of this NTM include absence of tuberculostearic acid. It is curious that it grows optimally over a narrow pH range, a feature found more often with pathogenic than saprophytic NTM. It is found naturally and extremely commonly in the soil, milk and water. It can be isolated commonly from clinical specimens. For example, it was reported almost as commonly (15% of total isolates) as the *M. avium* complex (17% of total isolates)[154]. However, the number of confirmed disease cases appears to be very small compared to the apparent high rate of contamination or colonisation. Even the reported cases are suspect in their authenticity due to lack of supportive evidence of disease-producing features[155]. In addition, it is possible that organisms said to be *M. gordonae* may be other closely related NTM. Specific nucleic acid probing could clarify these situations.

There are several reports of water-borne contamination of diagnostic tissue instruments -particularly bronchoscopes – laboratory agents, etc. which have lead to initial erroneous diagnoses of *M. gordonae* outbreaks[27,156,157]. In addition to contamination, chronic colonisation appears to be common and hence the guidelines for diagnosing true infection should be utilised during clinical decision-making. Colonisation rather than infection is suggested by cases whose clinical course appears to be unaffected by successful eradication of the *M. gordonae* with antimycobacterial treatment[158]. Nevertheless, solid clinical cases have been well documented. It was Douglas in 1986 who described two cases of pulmonary disease and suggested that *M. gordonae* could play a pathogenic role[159]. A recent case of pulmonary and disseminated *M. gordonae* in a non-immunocompromised host documented with liver biopsy histology and response to antimycobacterial therapy strengthens the view that *M. gordonae* can indeed be pathogenic on occasions and even in patients with normal host defences[160]. A recent review describes several more cases, thus consolidating the suspicion of the pathogenic potential for *M. gordonae*[158]. Therefore, not every patient who has a positive isolate of *M. gordonae* is merely colonised.

A variety of extrapulmonary presentations have also been documented and include shunt associated meningitis, prosthetic valve endocarditis, olecranon bursitis, localised skin granulomas and other soft tissue infections (sometimes related to previous trauma), corneal infection, peritonitis and disseminated disease (in immunocompromised hosts but not exclusively).

Pulmonary disease accounts for approximately one-third of all cases and usually occurs in males in their 60s with pre-existing pulmonary disease including chronic bronchitis, past history of tuberculosis, pulmonary Hodgkins and carcinoma (Figs. 11.9,11.10). Pulmonary disease can occur as the sole presentation or as part of a disseminated picture. The presentation is characterised by cough, weight loss, increasing dyspnoea, haemoptysis and fever[158]. Patients with pulmonary infections have the poorest outcome.

The organism shows case-to-case variation with regards to *in vitro* sensitivity to first and second line antituberculous drugs, but clinical response is seen with regimens containing rifampicin (usually in combination with isoniazid and ethambutol) given for 18 months[159]. There is, however, sometimes a discrepancy observed between sputum conversion and clinical response in some cases[158]. Surgical resection is sometimes performed, usually for extrapulmonary localised soft tissue disease[158]. If the infection is associated with intravascular or intraventricular foreign bodies, removal of these is usually necessary for cure[158].

M. ulcerans, *M. gastri*, *M. terrae*, *M. triviale*, *M. paratuberculosis* and the most recently documented *M. haemophilum*

These NTM have been rarely identified with pulmonary disease, and also extrapulmonary disease. An interesting example of upper respiratory tract (sinusitis) disease associated with *M. terrae* is shown in Fig. 11.11. Nevertheless, occasional cases are increasingly being reported, e.g. *M. terrae* miliary pulmonary disease associated with bone marrow transplantation[161] and in apparently normal competent or mildly immunocompromised hosts[162,163]. *M. haemophilum* pneumonia has recently been described in a BMT recipient[164] – the significance of its recovery in BAL specimens was previously uncertain[165]. Specific growth requirements of haemin or ferric ammonium citrate are necessary for diagnosis – cases could well have been overlooked[164]. More often *M. haemophilum* produces disseminated skin lesions.

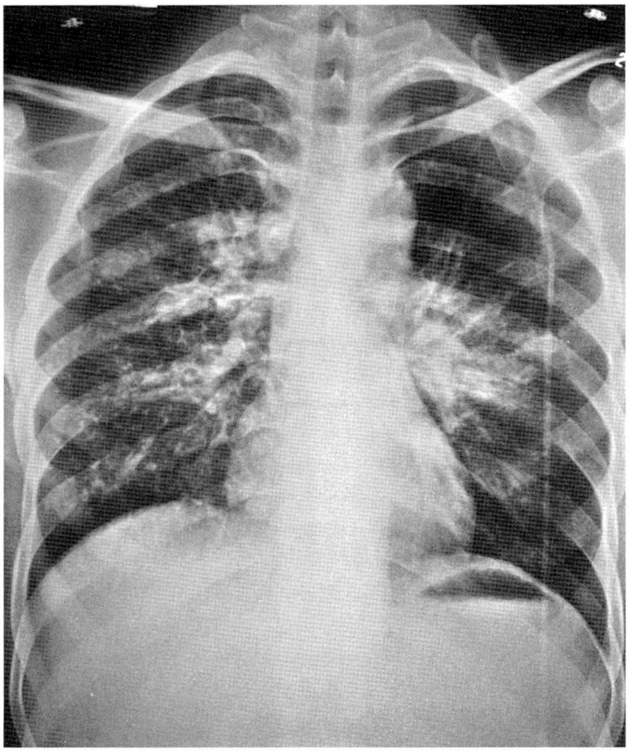

FIGURE 11.9 40-year-old policeman with acute myeloid leukaemia, fever and cough. Left perihilar infiltrate, right lung scattered infiltrates. Sputum grew *M. gordonae*.

Response to therapy is slow, the organism being susceptible only to rifampicin/PAS among the 'classical' antimycobacterial drugs.

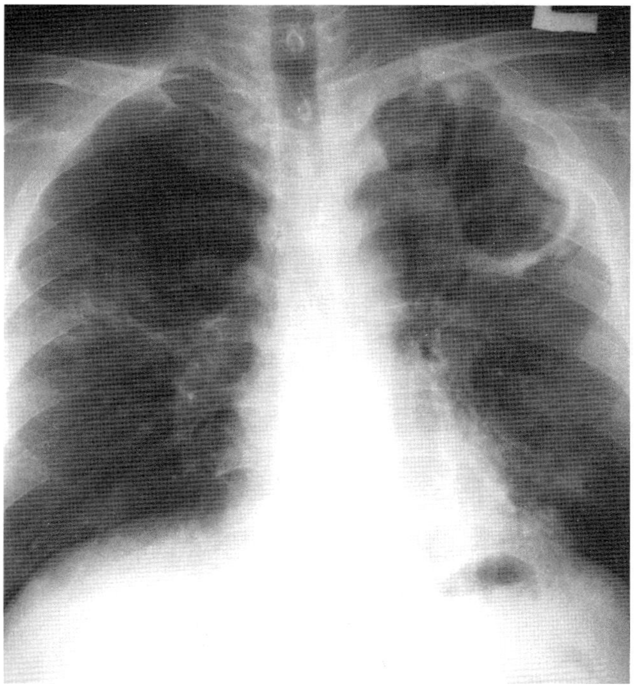

FIGURE 11.10 46-year-old male, smoker, insulin-dependent diabetic with chronic cough and cavity left upper lobe with diffuse pulmonary infiltrates. Sputum grew *M. gordonae*.

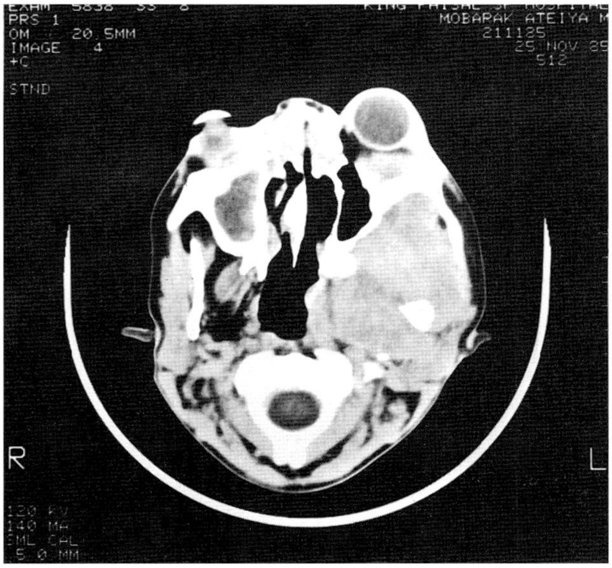

FIGURE 11.11 16-year-old female with penetrating injury to face 11 years previously. Now has left-sided facial swelling. Computerised tomography indicates large mass invading soft tissues of left face and skull, orbit and cavernous sinus. Biopsy showed epithelioid histocyte infiltrates with focal non-caseating granulomas. The ZN stain was positive, culture grew *M. terrae*. Cure achieved in 3 months with ethambutol, isoniazid and rifampicin.

M. flavescens

M. flavescens is usually considered a rapid grower and is extremely rarely pathogenic. Cavitary lung disease has been rarely described in association with *M. flavescens* and clinical response is documented with rifampicin, isoniazid and ethambutol[166]. It is also susceptible to amikacin, cefoxitin, imipenem, sulphonamides, ciprofloxacin, doxycycline and minocycline.

M. smegmatis

This NTM is a rare cause of pulmonary infection; nevertheless it has been described in association with lipoid pneumonia[167]. More often it is associated with soft tissue infections secondary to surgery/trauma.

Pulmonary disease in patients infected with the human immunodeficiency virus (HIV) (See also Chapter 22)

This subsection will address some of the aspects of pulmonary manifestations of NTM in the setting of HIV disease. Disseminated non-tuberculous mycobacteriosis is well described but specific aspects of pulmonary disease are less well reported.

The immunological dysfunction in patients with HIV permits infection with a range of NTM and unique clinical features. The case definition for AIDS has undergone revision to include NTM infections as marker diseases, paralleling our increasing knowledge of the role of these organisms. Some mycobacterial diseases were not eligible as an indicator diagnosis for AIDS in the earliest definitions[168]. However, the 1993 AIDS surveillance case definition includes not only *M. tuberculosis* but *M. avium* complex, *M. kansasii*, and other species[169,170]. HIV has been one factor resulting in a reversal of the progressive decline of *M. tuberculosis* in the USA[89] as well as the increasing widespread prevalence of NTM infections in these patients. The exact prevalence of infection with NTM is unknown – rates for *M. avium* complex have been reported at between 5% and 56% with many cases only being diagnosed postmortem[171–174]. Nevertheless, disseminated disease caused by NTM mainly *M. avium* complex or disseminated *M. avium* complex is now acknowledged to be the most common bacterial infection in North American and European patients who have AIDS[175]. The most frequently isolated NTM is *M. avium* complex, but *M. kansasii*, *M. gordonae*, *M. fortuitum* complex, *M. malmoense*, *M. celatum*, and *M. xenopi* have all been described in patients with HIV.

Pulmonary disease in the setting of disseminated *M. avium* complex infection

Following environmental exposure the respiratory and gastrointestinal tracts become colonised with *M. avium* complex. As qualitative and quantitative impairment of CD4 lymphocytes occurs, *M. avium* complex bacteraemia ensues, presumably from the respiratory and gastrointestinal tract entry portals. Thus, in those patients colonised, *M. avium* complex bacteraemia or disseminated *M. avium* complex usually only occurs when the mean CD4 count is low (of the mean order of 10/mm^3) whereas in patients whose mean CD4 count is considerably higher (some eightfold) disseminated *M. avium* complex does not occur[176]. However, by no means do all patients with disseminated *M. avium* complex have prior documented colonisation. Thus, the use of such colonisation as a predictive indicator for disseminated *M. avium* complex is highly controversial at this time[175,176]. Nevertheless, disseminated *M. avium* complex is unlikely in patients with CD4 counts above 0.2×10^9/cells/L[177], the incidence rising as the CD4 count falls, for example, 39% if the CD4 count is < 10/mm^3 and 3% at 100–199/mm^3 [178]. The risk of disseminated *M. avium* complex increases therefore with time in any particular cohort. For example, in one prospective study of 1000 patients with AIDS the incidence of disseminated *M. avium* complex was approximately 5% at entry, quadrupled by 12 months and doubled to over 40% at 2 years follow-up[178]. Patients are usually therefore already far advanced in their HIV disease at the time of risk for disseminated *M. avium* complex with many already having had episodes of other severe opportunistic infections. The sparse host cellular reaction to *M. avium* complex seen in many organs and tissues is a direct consequence of the low CD4 count and other aspects of the depressed immune status (Fig. 11.12). The immunopathological response is not clearly understood, though there are differences from that due to infection with *M. tuberculosis*. Macrophage activity, cytokine responses and humoral mechanisms appear to differ in the two infections – defective macrophage killing is one such identified factor. The importance of disseminated *M. avium* complex lies in the fact that it is a significant source both of morbidity – fever, sweats, diarrhoea and weight loss being particularly prominent. Disseminated *M. avium* complex also has a significant effect on survival, although the precise mechanism of the terminal stages in these patients is unknown – with most AIDS patients surviving for only half as long if they had disseminated *M. avium* complex[176].

M. avium complex in patients with AIDS is usually manifest as disseminated disease with multiorgan involvement, accompanied by continuous mycobacteremia. The features of disseminated disease include fever, malaise, profound weight loss, abdominal pain, diarrhoea, lymphadenopathy, hepatosplenomegaly, anemia and a raised alkaline phosphatase[179]. The non-specific nature of the presentation may lead to delay in diagnosis unless the organism can be demonstrated in the blood or other normally sterile body tissues. *M. avium* complex can be detected by culture of buffy coat preparations or the slightly less sensitive lysated cell pellet method from peripheral blood with adjunctive microscopical examination of blood smears. This is a fairly sensitive diagnostic tool for detecting disseminated disease[180]. Fluorochrome staining is the most sensitive method for microscopical identification. Although conventional culture will detect *M. avium* complex in 4 weeks, detection by radiometric BACTEC TB system is possible in 5–12 days and by the SEPTICHEK AFB system in 12–19 days. Specific identification by conventional biochemistry takes weeks and DNA probes or chromatography take a matter of hours[13]. Tissue such as bone marrow, liver, lymph nodes may be positive for *M. avium* complex before it can be isolated or detected in peripheral blood[181]. However in most patients with disseminated *M. avium* complex disease, mycobacteraemia is eventually diagnosed, and blood culturing is of course much less invasive than other methods[182].

Pulmonary disease in patients with disseminated *M. avium* complex is a minor contribution to the overall presentation profile. Thus, only 9% of 114 patients with disseminated *M. avium* complex had pulmonary symptoms and signs suggestive of clinical *M. avium* complex disease[183]. *M. avium* complex disease localised to the lungs either as the sole presentation or as part of the disseminated picture is highly unusual in patients with HIV infection. Ruf found that only 4% of AIDS patients with *M. avium* complex disease had pulmonary manifestations[184]. Among 650 HIV positive patients, 46 had positive sputum culture for *M. avium* complex of whom only two could be diagnosed confidently as having pulmonary disease[185]. *M. avium* complex pulmonary disease has been reported in approximately 16% of patients with AIDS and pulmonary disease[186]. However, post-mortem examination reveals that as many as one-third of patients with disseminated *M. avium* complex have *M. avium* complex in the lungs[187]. Another problem in patients with *M. avium* complex disease is the not infrequent finding of the concurrent presence of other pathogenic

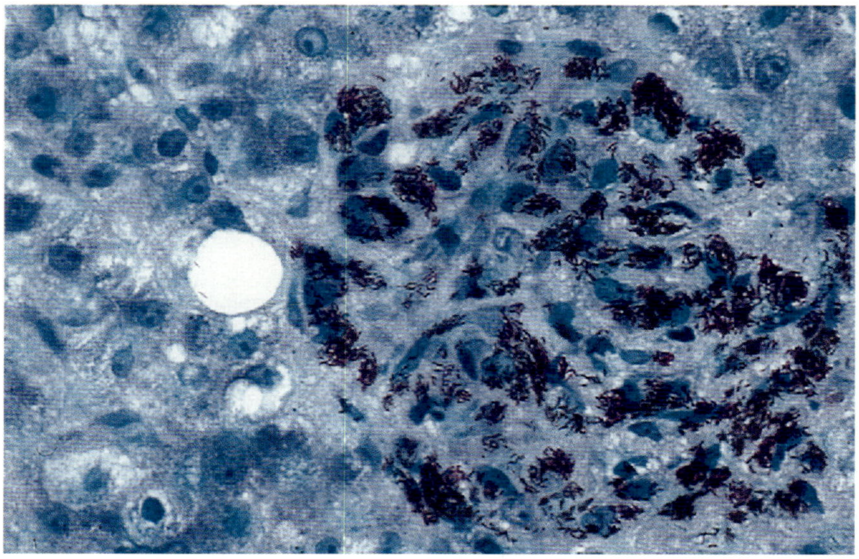

FIGURE 11.12 Liver biopsy from an HIV patient with disseminated *M. avium* complex infection. Note numerous mycobacteria with no apparent cellular reaction.

organisms particularly *Pneumocystis carinii*, making it difficult to ascribe with certainty that the pulmonary disease is due to *M. avium* complex[188].

Given the inherent difficulties, therefore, in making a confident diagnosis of pulmonary *M. avium* complex, the clinical features may be hard to define. With this proviso, it is generally accepted that the clinical features of *M. avium* complex pulmonary disease include intermittent fever, dry cough, night sweats, malaise, anorexia and weight loss. In addition, extrapulmonary findings including diarrhoea, emaciation, lymphadenopathy, hepatosplenomegaly and anaemia may be present. Plain chest radiographic appearances are non-specific and vary from complete normality to patchy interstitial infiltrates, diffuse interstitial disease, solitary nodules, and upper lobe apical infiltrates mimicking TB[189]. Many of these features cannot be differentiated from pulmonary tuberculosis and resemble those seen in reactivation TB with mainly bilateral, symmetrical course nodular densities, having no predisposition for upper lobe distribution[190]. Cavitary lesions are distinctly unusual, in contrast to *M. kansasii* pulmonary disease. They have, however, been described, inferring that *M. avium* complex should be included in the differential diagnosis of cavitary lung disease in AIDS patients[191].

Gallium scans have been shown to have positive and negative predictive values for any lung pathology in over 90% in patients with HIV. A more heterogenous diffuse uptake pattern suggests *P. carinii*[192], whilst focal uptake particularly in intrathoracic and supra-diaphragmatic lymph nodes is found with *M. avium* complex[193]. However, concomitant opportunistic and neoplastic pulmonary processes may cloud the interpretation of these results. Quantitative gallium-67 scintigraphy studies have shown positive results (a diffuse or focal pulmonary uptake) in the presence of a normal plain chest radiograph in approximately half of all patients with opportunistic pneumonias[194].

There should be a low threshold for diagnosis in these patients. The finding of acid-fast bacilli on direct smear of sputum, bronchial washings and broncho-alveolar lavage in a patient with compatible symptoms and signs should suggest a diagnosis of pulmonary tuberculosis or NTM infection. However, initial therapy should be directed towards tuberculosis rather than NTM infection, pending definitive culture results. This approach is supported by the finding that the presence of acid-fast bacilli on staining of any pulmonary secretion is highly suggestive of tuberculosis rather than *M. avium* complex infection[195]. Should *M. avium* complex be cultured from bronchial secretions, the recurrent problem of distinguishing colonisation from infection occurs, and this is even more of a dilemma in the face of unusual cellular responses and non-specific clinical features. In normal hosts, the presence of NTM cannot usually be guaranteed to cause disease unless a significant tissue reaction is demonstrable. However, in immunocompromised hosts and particularly in HIV, the tissue reaction may be scant despite the presence of numerous NTM. The presence of minimal tissue changes or poorly formed granulomas has been noted by several others[196]. Ideally, however, one would like to demonstrate a cellular/tissue reaction in such patients, and lung biopsy should be attempted if feasible and safe. However, in view of the diminished cellular response in patients with advanced HIV, modification of the classical diagnostic criteria for NTM infection may be necessary. There is no clear consensus on this but three positive sputum cultures or NTM in lung tissue or evidence of dissemination were used as criteria to define pulmonary *M. avium* complex in one centre[189]. Certainly, the presence of *M. avium* complex on culture of transbronchial biopsy, even in the absence of significant tissue reaction in the correct clinical setting, should make one very suspicious of NTM disease. Bronchoscopical appearances are not helpful though endobronchial lesions (seen much more commonly in M. tuberculosis in non-AIDS patients) have been described[197].

Because there is a paucity of patients with HIV-associated pulmonary *M. avium* complex compared to disseminated *M. avium* complex, comments on survival treatment modalities and their impact are difficult to assess. Hence, the following comments apply mainly to patients with disseminated *M. avium* complex infections. Some of these patients will also have pulmonary manifestations. Although the prognosis of patients with AIDS and low CD4 counts is poor, concurrent disseminated *M. avium* complex shortens the survival even further by a factor of 2–3[176,198,199] so that the median survival is of the order of 3 months. The presence of pulmonary manifestations does not appear to alter survival prospects[183]. High level mycobacteraemia and anaemia are independent poor prognostic factors[183]. Until recently, there was no concrete evidence that treatment influenced this abysmal survival rate. Two recent studies, however, have shown a significant survival advantage of the order of 2–4-fold using antimycobacterial treatment[183,200]. In addition, antiretroviral therapy provided a survival advantage.

Antimycobacterial agents used to treat pulmonary *M. avium* complex in patients without HIV have been discussed previously. In the setting of HIV, treatment of disseminated *M. avium* complex poses a different therapeutic challenge and standard drug regimens have not always been successful. *In vitro* resistance to isoniazid and rifampicin is common; ethambutol shows some bactericidal activity; rifabutin, clofazimine and cycloserine show good *in vitro* activity. *In vitro* synergy may occur, even when susceptibility cannot be shown for agents tested individually. Recently, the quinolones, macrolides such as erythromycin, and other antibiotics such as ampicillin and imipenem have shown *in vitro* activity. The beige mouse model has been used to demonstrate reductions in mortality using amikacin/ciprofloxacin/imipenem regimens[201]. In fact, macrophage and animal models are good systems for testing drug susceptibilities, since *M. avium* complex is an intracellular pathogen. Often these patients with advanced HIV disease have other opportunistic infections and are receiving other antimicrobials, and antiretroviral therapy, all of which complicate assessment of treatment efficacy. Combinations that have been explored include, for example, a three to four drug regime selected from rifabutin, isoniazid, ethambutol, ethionamide or clofazimine. In general, the response to treatment in humans is disappointing. One representative review concluded that mycobacteraemia persisted in the vast majority of patients treated and clinical improvement did not occur in any patient[180]. Recent studies, however, have suggested symptomatic improvement and reduction in mycobacteraemia using four-drug regimes, for example, isoniazid, ethambutol, rifampicin and clofazimine[202] or with the addition of quinolones, for example, amikacin, ethambutol, rifampicin and ciprofloxacin[203] or ethambutol, rifampicin, ciprofloxacin and clofazimine[204]. However, antimycobacterial drug toxicity can be formidable in AIDS patients[205]. The use of ethambutol is of some interest. Although *in vitro* tests usually indicate rather poor activity against *M. avium* complex, recent beige mouse model studies show that used alone, it does have significant activity. In the human situation, the use of ethambutol has led to some 37% reduction in mycobacteraemia whilst clofazimine or rifampicin showed no reduction; the addition of rifampicin or clofazimine to ethambutol did not produce any further reduction but clofazimine, rifampicin, ethambutol and ciprofloxacin together led to an 80% reduction[204].

The use of clarithromycin as a single agent therapy has been shown markedly to reduce bacteraemia[179,206,207] and to eradicate it in almost all patients receiving high doses (1500–2000 mg/day)[207]. Other workers have demonstrated similar microbiological effects accompanied by improvement in quality of life scores and survival benefits[208,209]. GI tracts side-effects are extremely common particularly with the high doses which may lead to patient non-compliance. A further problem is the high frequency (nearly 50%) of bacteriological resistance arising during therapy. This has also been noted when other NTM such as *M. chelonae*[210] have been treated with clarithromycin alone. Azithromycin has also been used but there are few reports to date.

Combination therapy regimens in which clarithromycin is used with other drugs are popular. For example, 54% of the patients in Chin's study and 90% in Horsburgh's study received combination therapy in this way[200,183]. Other modalities of treatment being investigated include the use of sparfloxacin and liposomal gentamicin. Patients with refractory disseminated NTM (including *M. avium* complex) who have idiopathic CD4 penia but without HIV are known to have a subnormal production of gamma interferon and these patients appear to respond to exogenous gamma interferon[211]. It remains to be seen whether such adjunctive therapy has a place in HIV infected disseminated *M. avium* complex patients.

Where can recommendations be made from the bewildering choice of antimycobacterial agents? At the moment, clarithromycin + ethambutol (used in combination to reduce the risk of emergence of resistance) with an optional third or fourth drug chosen from rifampicin/ rifabutin/clofazimine/ciprofloxacin/ amikacin is advocated[15].

It appears that patients with pulmonary *M. avium* complex also respond to appropriate therapy but there is sparse detailed information in this area.

A detailed discussion of the issue of *M. avium* complex prophylaxis is outside the scope of this chapter, but see Chapter 22. Based on studies which documented efficacy in reducing the incidence of *M. avium* complex bacteraemia and subsequent symptoms of breakthrough of mycobacteraemia, it is recommended that rifabutin at 300 mg/day should be given to HIV patients whose CD4 count is $< 100/mm^3$, for life[15,212]. Clarithromycin prophylaxis 500 mg twice daily has also been shown to significantly reduce disseminated *M. avium* complex by 68% and significantly improve survival in AIDS patients with a CD4 count of $< 100/mm^3$ [213].

Other pulmonary NTM infections in HIV patients

M. kansasii, *M. xenopi*, *M. gordonae*, *M. fortuitum* complex, *M. malmoense*, *M. haemophilum* and *M. celatum* have also been reported to cause pulmonary and extrapulmonary disease in patients with HIV, although much less frequently, accounting for between 1.4% and 8% of all HIV associated NTM infections[214].

M. kansaii has been the subject of some reviews with conflicting conclusions. In one series, *M. kansasii* accounted for 9/219 patients with mycobacterial infections (9 *M. kansasii*, 160 disseminated *M. avium* complex, 50 *M. tuberculosis*) – seven of the nine had pulmonary disease[215]. Carpenter and Parks found that approximately 50% of patients with pulmonary *M. kansasii* had concomitant extrapulmonary disease. The pulmonary disease was diffuse, non-specific, non-cavitary and refractory to treatment, although some patients did respond quite favourably[215]. Levine and Chaisson also reported a pulmonary bias in *M. kansasii* disease, with 14/19 patients having a sole pulmonary presentation and three others having prominent pulmonary features in an otherwise disseminated presentation. Several patients had concomitant *P. carinii* pneumonia[216]. Upper lobe infiltrates with thin-walled cavitary lesions in the majority were found. There was also a good response to drug therapy. The overall disease profile resembled that of *M. tuberculosis*[216]. Subacute cough, fever, shortness of breath, sweats, pleural pain and haemoptysis predominated. Isoniazid, rifampicin and ethambutol are frequently used to treat *M. kansasii* infection with good effect[216] despite *in vitro* resistance to isoniazid. Cotrimoxazole, ciprofloxacin and clarithromycin are alternative agents which could be used in patients with failure or toxicity from standard antituberculous therapy.

In patients with *M. xenopi*, 50% had either concurrent *P. carinii* or *M. tuberculosis* infections posing a dilemma for the role of *M. xenopi* in those patients[217].

M. genavense is a recently recognised fastidious pathogen[218–220]. It appears to produce a spectrum of illness similar to *M. avium* complex, in patients whose median CD4 counts are $15/mm^3$. Patients in whom this organism is found appear to survive longer than patients with *M. avium* complex, and treatment with multiple drug regimens including amikacin, rifampicin, clofazimine, ethambutol, a quinolone, an amide, may increase survival.

Final comments

Since the classical paper by Timpe and Runyon in 1954 when the idea of human disease due to NTM was first established, there has been an increasing awareness of their role in several situations. Nevertheless, challenges remain for the immediate future. First, a rapid means of laboratory identification is required, both to avoid unnecessary contact tracing manoeuvres and to select particular treatment regimes. This is especially important in HIV patients and other immunocompromised hosts, where the patient presents with fever of unknown origin and other non-specific symptoms and signs, and where early specific treatment is the goal. The current status of differential skin testing is rather crude although improvements are to be expected in this area. Results of culture in the past have often been delayed, although there have been important improvements, for example, the use of lysis centrifugation, now largely replaced by radiomimetric methodology. Serological testing largely has still to be explored, but there have been some advances in this field, for example, the detection of IgA antibody against *M. avium* complex antigen by ELISA, which has been shown to have a sensitivity of 69% and specificity of 90%[105]. Molecular biological tools may prove useful; for example, the application of DNA probes and amplification techniques such as the polymerase chain reaction. Secondly, the guidelines for clinical diagnosis of disease rather than colonisation are useful but by no means infallible. The criteria for diagnosis should not be applied rigidly, since there are considerable clinical variations of cases with NTM disease. This is supported by the finding that NTM are being increasingly implicated in disease, even with previously described 'non-pathogenic' varieties and even among immunocompetent hosts. Each patient has to be carefully and individually assessed; care must be taken to ensure that cases are not dismissed as NTM colonisation simply because there is a sparse growth of NTM from non-sterile sites. Clarification over the clinical significance of colonisation is necessary. Wherever possible, tissue sampling should be pursued to provide a solid diagnosis. Thirdly, large prospective randomised studies are urgently needed to address the problem of drug regimens and to provide answers to the apparent disparity between *in vitro* and *in vivo* activities. Fourthly, drug resistance, clinical failure, drug toxicity and the need to simplify therapy are factors which stimulate the need for research and development into new antimycobacterial drugs and newer formulations of existing drugs. The development of long-lasting rifamycins such as rifapentin could result in once weekly dosage administrations which would considerably improve compliance. Novel delivery systems such as polylactic and polyglycolic co-polymer release systems may also prove useful in this area though the mass of the drug required appears to be high. Liposomal formulations of existing agents might provide for more effective targeting and delivery of antimycobacterial drugs. Some new antibiotic classes have shown promise in terms of *in vitro* and *in vivo* antimycobacterial activity; for example, combination of β-lactamase inhibitors with β-lactams such as amoxycillin/ticarcillin with clavulanic acid, imipenem, and the DNA gyrase inhibitors – the new quinolones such as ofloxacin. Preliminary testing of the new drugs require a suitable animal model and the beige mouse model, being defective in T and natural killer cells, is an appropriate model for NTM infections in HIV patients. The issues surrounding the evaluation of new drugs in the management of NTM disease have been discussed[221]. However, and fifthly, it is important to elucidate the structure of the NTM-cell wall, subcellular components and biochemical pathways in order to develop new antimycobacterial antimicrobials. Knowledge of the immune mechanisms is crucial if we are to apply adjunctive therapeutic manoevres such as growth factors, interferons, and other cytokines.

References

1. OHLMACHER AP An atypical acid and alcohol pro-fungus from the sputum of a case clinically resembling pulmonary tuberculosis. *Trans Chicago Path Soc* 1901;5:33.
2. DUVALL CW. Studies in atypical forms of tubercle bacilli isolated directly from the human tissues in cases of primary surgical adenitis. *J Exp Med* 1908;9:403–29.
3. TIMPE A, RUNYON EH. Relationship of 'atypical' acid-fast bacilli to human disease: preliminary report. *J Lab Clin Med* 1954;44:202–9.
4. WOLINSKY E. Nontuberculous mycobacteria and associated diseases. *Am Rev Resp Dis* 19:1979;107–59.
5. WAYNE LG, SRAMEK HA. Agents of newly recognised or infrequently encountered mycobacterial diseases. *Clin Microbiol Rev* 1992;5:1–25.
6. RUNYON EH. Identification of mycobacterial pathogens utilising colony characteristics. *Am J Clin Pathol* 1970;54:578–86.
7. NOLTE FS, METCHOCK B. *Mycobacterium* In Murray PR, *Manual of Clinical Microbiology* Washington DC: ASM Press, 6th ed, 1995: 400–37.
8. WHITTIER PS, WESTFALL K, SETTERQUIST S, HOPFER RL. Evaluation of the Septi-Chek AFB system in the recovery of *Mycobacteria*. *Eur J Clin Microbiol Infec Dis* 1992;11:915–18.
8. RUNYON EH. Anonymous *Mycobacteria* in pulmonary disease. *Med Clin N Am* 1959;43:273–90.
9. LEBRUN L, ESPINASSE F, POVEDA JD, VINCENT-LEVY-FREBAULT V. Evaluation of nonradioactive DNA probes for identification of *Mycobacteria*. *J Clin Microbiol* 1992;30(9):2476–8.
10. TORTOLI E, SIMONETTI MT, LACCHINI C, PENATI V *et al.* Evaluation of a commercial DNA probe assay for the identification of *Mycobacterium kansasii Eur J Clin Microbiol Infect Dis* 1994;13:264–7.
11. CHAPIN-ROBERTSON K, DAHBERG S, WAYCOTT S, CORRALES J, KONTNICK C, EDBERG SC. Detection and identification of *Mycobacterium* directly from BACTEC bottles by using a DNA-rRNA probe. *Diag Microbiol Infec Dis* 1993;17(3):203–7.
12. HUEBNER RE, GOOD RC, TOKARS JI. Current practices in mycobacteriology: results of a survey of state public health laboratories. *J Clin Microbiol* 1993;31(4):771–5.
13. WOODS GL. Disease due to the *Mycobacterium avium* complex in patients infected with human immunodeficiency virus: diagnosis and susceptibility testing. CID 1994;18(Suppl 3):S227–32.
14. WALLACE JM *et al.* Diagnosis and treatment of disease caused by nontuberculous *Mycobacteria Am Rev Resp Dis* 1990;142:940–53.
15. MASUR H. Recommendations on prophylaxis and therapy for disseminated *Mycobacterium avium* complex disease in patients infected with the human immunodeficiency virus. *N Engl J Med* 1993;329(12):898–904.
16. GRUFT H, FALKINHAM JO III, PARKER BC. Recent experience in the epidemiology of disease caused by atypical *Mycobacteria*. *Rev Infect Dis* 1981;3:990–6.
17. BROWN JW, SANDERS CV. *Mycobacterium marinum* infection – a problem of recognition, not therapy. *Arch Intern Med* 1987;147:817–18.
18. HOSKER HSR, LAM CQ, NG TK, MA HK, CHAN SL. The prevalence and clinical significance of pulmonary infection due to non-tuberculous *Mycobacteria* in Hong Kong. *Resp Med* 1995;89:3–8.
19. GUBLER JG, SALFINGER M, VON GRAEVENITZ A pseudoepidemic of non-tuberculous *Mycobacteria* due to a contaminated bronchoscope cleaning machine. Report of an outbreak and review of the literature. *Chest* 1992;101:1245–9.
20. JONES WD JR. Bacteriophage typing of *Mycobacterium tuberculosis* cultures from incidents of suspected laboratory cross-contamination. *Tubercle* 1988;69:43–6.
21. DAS S, CHAN SL, ALLEN BW, MITCHISON DA, LOWRIE DB. Application of DNA fingerprinting with IS986 to sequential mycobacterial isolates obtained from pulmonary tuberculosis patients in Hong Kong before, during, and after short-course chemotherapy. *Tubercle Lung Dis* 1993;74:47–51.

22. SMALL PM, SHAFER RW, HOPEWELL PC *et al.* Exogenous reinfection with multidrug resistant *Mycobacterium tuberculosis* in patients with advanced HIV infection. *N Engl J Med* 1993;328:1137–44.

23. FROTHINGHAM R, WILSON KH Molecular phylogeny of the *Mycobacterium avium* complex demonstrates clinically meaningful divisions. *J Infect Dis* 1994;169:305–12.

24. BENNETT SN, PETERSON DE, JOHNSON DR, HALL WN, ROBINSON-DUNN B, DIETRICH S. Bronchoscopy-associated *Mycobacterium xenopi* pseudoinfections. *Am J Resp Crit Care Med* 1994;150(1):245–50.

25. FRASER VJ, JONES M, MURRAY PR, MEDOFF G, ZHANG Y, WALLACE RJ. Contamination of flexible fiberoptic bronchoscopies with *Mycobacterium chelonae* linked to an automated bronchoscope disinfection machine. *Am Rev Resp Dis* 1992;145(4 Pt 1):853–5.

26. SNIADACK DH, OSTROFF SM, KARLIX MA, SMITHWICK RW, SCHWARTZ B, SPRAUER MA. SILCOX VA. A nosocomial pseudo-outbreak of *Mycobacterium xenopi* due to a contaminated potable water supply: lessons in prevention. *Infect Control Hosp Epidemiol* 1993;14(11):636–41.

27. TOKARS JI, MCNEIL MM, TABLAN OC, CHAPIN-ROBERTSON K, PATTERSON JE, EDBERG SC, JARVIS WR. *Mycobacterium gordonae* pseudoinfection associated with a contaminated antimicrobial solution. *J Clin Microbiol* 1990;28(12):2765–9.

28. KIEWIET AA AND THOMPSON JE. Isolation of 'atypical' mycobacteria from health individuals in tropical Australia. *Tubercle* 1970;5:296–9.

29. REZNIKOV M, LEGGO JH, DAWSON DJ. Investigation by seroagglutination of strains of the *mycobacterium intracellulare – M. scrofulaceum* group from house dusts and sputum in S.E. Queensland. *Am Rev Resp Dis* 1974;104:951–3.

30. WENDT SL, GEORGE KL, PARKER BC, GRUGT H, FALKINHAM JO III. Epidemiology of infection by non-tuberculous mycobacteria III. Isolation of potentially pathogenic *Mycobacteria* from aerosols. *Am Rev Resp Dis* 1980;122:259–63.

31. JENKINS PA. *Mycobacterium malmoense. Tubercle* 1985;66:193–5.

32. WARREN NG, BODY BA, SILCOX VA *et al.* Pulmonary disease due to *Mycobacterium Malmoense. J Clin Microbiol* 1984;20:245–7.

33. PATEL R, ROBERTS GD, KEATING MR, PAYA CV. Infections due to nontuberculous mycobacteria in kidney, heart, and liver transplant recipients. *Clin Infect Dis* 1994;19:263–73.

34. YAMAMOTO M, OQURE YI, SUDO K *et al.* Diagnostic criteria for disease caused by atypical *Mycobacteria. Am Rev Resp Dis* 1967;96:773–8.

35. AHN CH, CHAI H, MCLARTY JW *et al.* Diagnostic criteria for pulmonary disease caused by *mycobacterium kansasii* and *Mycobacterium intracellulare Am Rev Resp Dis* 1982;125:388–91.

36. ANONYMOUS. Diagnostic standards and classification of tuberculosis and other mycobacterial diseases. *Am Rev Resp Dis* 1981;123:343–58.

37. ISEMANN MD, CORPE RF, O'BRIEN RJ, ROSENZWIEG DY, WOLINSKY E. Disease due to *Mycobacterium avium-intercellulare. Chest* 1985;87(2):139S–49S.

38. PRINCE DS, PETERSON DD, STEINER RM, GOTTLIEB JE *et al.* Infection with *Mycobacterium avium* complex in patients without predisposing conditions. *N Engl J Med* 1989;321(13):863–8.

39. WOLINSKY E. Mycobacterial diseases other than tuberculous. *Clin Infect Dis* 1992;15:1–12.

40. AL JARAD N, DEMERTZIS P, BARNES NC, WEDZICHA JA *et al.* Characteristics of patients with atypical mycobacterial disease. (Abstr British Thoracic Society Meeting.) *Thorax (Proc)* 1994;49:10.

41. FRASER DW, BAXTON AE, NAJI A, BARKER CF, RUDNICK M, WEINSTEIN AJ Disseminated *Mycobacterium kansasii* infection presenting as cellulitis in a recipient of a renal homograft. *Am Rev Resp Dis* 1975;112:299–300.

42. HJELTE L, PETRINI B, KALLENIUS G, STRANDVIK B. Prospective study of mycobacterial infections in patients with cystic fibrosis. *Thorax* 1990;45:397–400.

43. AITKEN ML, BURKE W, MCDONALD G, WALLIS C, RAMSEY B, NOLAN C. Nontuberculous mycobacterial disease in adult cystic fibrosis patients. *Chest* 1993;103(4):1096–9.

44. CHAN CHS, HO AKC, CHAN RCY, CHEUNG H, CHENG AFB. *Mycobacteria* as a cause of infective exacerbaction in bronchiectasis. *Postgrad Med J* 1992;68:896–9.

45. DOUGLAS JG, CALDER MA, CHOO-KANG YFJ *et al. Mycobacterium gordonae*: a new pathogen? *Thorax* 1986;41:152–3.

46. WEINBERGER M, BERG SL, FEUERSTEIN IM, PIZZO PA, WITEBSKY FG Disseminated infection with *Mycobacterium gordonae*: report of a case and critical review of the literature. *Clin Infect Dis* 1992;14:1229–39.

47. TSUKAMARA M. Diagnosis of disease caused by *Mycobacterium avium* complex. *Chest* 1991;99:667–9.

48. WOODRING JH, VANDIVIERE HM. Pulmonary disease caused by non-tuberculous *Mycobacteria. J Thorac Imaging* 1990;5:64–76.

49. ELLIS ME, QADRI SMH. Mycobacteria other than tuberculosis producing in a tertiary referral hospital in Saudi Arabia. *Ann Saudi Med* 1993;13:508–15.

50. EVANS AJ, CRIPS AJ, COLVILLE A, EVANS SA, JOHNSTON IDA. Pulmonary infections causes by *Mycobacterium malmoense* and *Mycobacterium tuberculosis*: comparison of radiographic features. *AJR* 1993;161:733–7.

51. CRISP AJ, EVANS AJ, COLVILLE A, EVANS SA, JOHNSTON IDA. Comparison of the radiographic features of pulmonary infections with *Mycobacterium kansasii* and *Mycobacterium tuberculosis. Thorax (Proc)* 1992;347(10):876.

52. ALBEDA SM, KERN JA, MARINELLI DL, MILLER WT. Expanding spectrum of pulmonary disease caused by nontuberculous *Mycobacteria. Radiology* 1985;157:289–96.

53. MOORE EH. Atypical mycobacterial infection in the lung: CT appearance. *Radiology* 1993;187:777–82.

55. AMANO H, MIZOGUCHI K, TSUKAMARA M *et al.* Enzyme-linked immunosorbent assay for the differential diagnosis of pulmonary tuberculosis and pulmonary diseases due to *Mycobacterium avium intracellulare* complex. *Jpn J Med* 1989;28:196–201.

56. KIRSCHNER RA, PARKER BC, FALKINAAM J Epidemiology of infection by non-tuberculous *Mycobacteria. Am Rev Resp Dis* 1992;145:271–5.

57. EDWARDS LB, ACQUAVIVA FA, LIVESAY VT, CROSS FW, PALMER CE. An atlas of sensitivity to tuberculin, PPD-B and histoplasmin in the United States. *Am Rev Resp Dis* 1969;99:1–132.

58. MEISSNER PS, FALKINHAM JO III. Plasmid DNA profiles as epidemiological marker from clinical and environmental isolates of *Mycobacterium avium, Mycobacterium intracellulare* and *Mycobacterium scrofulaceum. J Infect Dis* 1986;153:325–31.

59. HORSBURGH CR JR, METCHOCK B GORDON SM, HAVLIK JA JR, MCGOWAN JE JR, THOMPSON SE III. Predictors of survival in patients with AIDS and disseminated *Mycobacterium avium* complex disease. *J Infec Dis* 1994;170:573–7.

60. FURNEY SK, SKINNER PS, ROBERTS AD, APPLEBERG R, ORME IM. Capacity of *Mycobacterium avium* isolates to grow well or poorly in immune macrophages resides in their ability to induce secretion of tumor necrosis factor. *Infect Immun* 1992; 60:4410–13.

61. ISEMAN MD, BUSCHMAN DL, ACKERSON LM. Pectus excavatum and scoliosis. Thoracic anomalies associated with pulmonary disease

caused by *Mycobacterium avium* complex. *Am Rev Resp Dis* 1991;144:914–16.

62. OZKAYNAK MF, LENARSKY C, KOHN D *et al. Mycobacterium avium–intracellulare* infections after allogeneic bone marrow transplantation in children. *Am J Pediatr Hematol-Oncol* 1990;12:220–4.

63. CROWLE AJ, COHN DL, POCHE P. Defects in sera from acquired immunodeficiency syndrome (AIDS) patients and from non-AIDS patients with *Mycobacterium avium* infection which decrease macrophage resistance to *Mycobacterium avium. Infect Immun* 1989;57:1445–51.

64. ROSENWEIG DY. Pulmonary mycobacterial infections due to *Mycobacterium avium-intercellulare avium* complex. *Chest* 1979;75:115–19.

65. ISEMAN MD. Nontuberculous mycobacterial infections. In eds. Gorbach Sl, Bartlett JG, Blacklow NR. *Infectious Diseases* W.B. Saunders Co. 1992: 1246–56.

66. REICH JM, JOHNSON RE. *Mycobacterium avium* complex pulmonary disease presenting as an isolated lingular or middle lobe pattern. The Lady Windermere Syndrome. *Chest* 1992;101:1605–9.

67. TEIRSTEIN AS, DAMSKER B, KIRSCHNER PA *et al.* Pulmonary infection with *Mycobacterium avium–intracellulare*: diagnosis, clinical patterns, treatment (clinical conference). *Mt Sinai J Med* 1990;57:209–15.

68. REDDY MV, SRINIVASAN S, GANGADHARAM PRJ *In vitro* and *in vivo* synergistic effect of isoniazid with streptomycin and clofazimine against *Mycobacterium avium* complex (MAC). *Tubercle Lung Dis* 1994;75:208–12.

69. ZIMMER BL, DEYOUND DR, ROBERTS GD. *In vitro* synergistic activity of ethambutol, isoniazid, kanamycin, rifampicin and streptomycin against *mycobacterium avium–intracellulare* complex. *Antimicrob Agents Chemother* 1982;22:148–50.

70. BANKS J, JENKINS PA Combined versus single antituberculous drugs on the *in vitro* sensitivity patterns of non-tuberculous *Mycobacteria*. *Thorax* 1987;42:838–42.

71. BANKS J. Treatment of pulmonary disease caused by opportunistic mycobacteria. *Thorax* 1989;44:449–54.

72. ISEMAN MD, CORPE RF, O'BRIEN RJ *et al.* Disease due to *Mycobacterium avium-intracellulare*. *Chest* 1985;87(Suppl):139–49.

73. DUTT AK, STEAD WW. Long term results of medical treatment in *Mycobacterium intracellulare* infection. *Am J Med* 1979;67:445–52.

74. AHN CH, AHN SS, ANDERSON RA *et al.* A four drug regime for initial treatment of cavitary disease caused by *Mycobacterium avium* complex. *Am Rev Resp Dis* 1986;134:438–41.

75. BROWN BA, WALLACE RJ JR, ONYI GO Activities of clarithromycin against eight slowly growing species of nontuberculous *Mycobacteria*, determined by using a broth microdilution MIC system. *Antimicrob Agents Chemother* 1992;36(9):1987–90.

76. WALLACE RJ JR, BROWN BA, GRIFFITH DE, GIRARD WM *et al.* Initial clarithromycin monotherapy for *Mycobacterium avium–intracellulare* complex lung disease. *Am J Resp Crit Care Med* 1994;149:1335–41.

77. WALLACE RJ JR, BROWN BA, GRIFFITH DE. Drug intolerance to high-dose clarithromycin among elderly patients. *Diag Microbiol Infec Dis* 1993;16:215–21.

78. MORAN JF, ALEXANDER LG, STAUB EW *et al.* Long term results of pulmonary resection for atypical mycobacterial disease. *Am Thorax Surg* 1983;35:597–604.

79. POMERANTZ M, MADSEN L, GOBLE M *et al.* Surgical management of resistant *Mycobacterial tuberculosis* and other mycobacterial pulmonary infections. *Ann Thorac Surg* 1991;52:1108–11.

80. KRAJNACK MA, DOWDA H Non-tuberculous *Mycobacteria* in South Carolina. 1971–1980. *J Sc Med Assoc* 1981;77:551–5.

81. ELLIS ME. Mycobacteria other than *Mycobacterium tuberculosis. Curr Opin Infect Dis* 1988;1:252–71.

82. CLAGUE HW, EL-ANSARY EH, HOPKINS CA *et al.* Pulmonary infection with opportunistic *Mycobacteria* on Merseyside. 1974–1983. *Postgrad Med J* 1986;62:363–8.

83. BANKS J, HUNTER AM, CAMPBELL IAA *et al.* Pulmonary infection with *Mycobacterium kansasii* in Wales 1970–9: a review of treatment and response. *Thorax* 1983;38:271–4.

84. PANG SC *Mycobacterium kansasii* infections in Western Australia (1962–1987). *Resp Med* 1991;85:213–18.

85. LILLO M, ORENGO S, CERNOCH P *et al.* Pulmonary and disseminated infection due to *Mycobacterium kansasii*: a decade of experience. *Rev Infect Dis* 1990:12:760–7.

86. MATTHIESSEN W, SCHONFELD N, MAUCH H, WAHN U, GRASSOT A Nontuberculous mycobacteriosis as a complication of the Swyer–James syndrome. *Deutsch Med Wochenschr* 1993;118(5):139–44.

87. SCHONFELD N, MATTHIESSEN W, GRASSOT A. Complications of pulmonary involvement in Bechterew's disease. *Aktuelle Radio.* 1991;1(5):249–52.

88. ZVETINA JR, MALIWAN N, FREDERICK WE *et al. Mycobacterium kansasii* infection following primary pulmonary malignancy. *Chest* 1992;102(5):1460–3.

89. VEALE D, FISHWICK D, WHITE JE, GASCOIGNE AD *et al.* Culture of *Mycobacterium kansasii* in the blood of an HIV negative patieant. *Thorax* 1993;48(6):672–3.

90. CONNOLLY MG JR, BOUGHMAN RP, DOHN MN *Mycobacterium kansasii* presenting as an endobronchial lesion. *Am Rev Resp Dis* 1993;148(5):1405–7.

91. JOHANSON WG JR, NICHOLSON DP. A follow-up of ninety-nine patients with pulmonary disease caused by *Mycobacterium kansasii. Am Rev Resp Dis* 1968;98:141–6

92. GALE GL. Atypical mycobacteria in a tuberculosis hospital. *Can Med Assoc* 1976;114:612–14.

93. EVANS SA, COLVILLE A, EVANS AJ, CRISP AJ, JOHNSTON IDA. Comparison of the clinical features of pulmonary infections with *Mycobacterium kansasii* and *Mycobacterium tuberculosis. Thorax (Proc)* 1992;47(10):876.

94. AHN CH, LOWELL JR, AHN SS. Short course chemotherapy for pulmonary disease caused by *Mycobacterium kansasii. Am Rev Resp Dis* 1983;128:1048–50.

95. AHN CH, WALLACE RJ JR, AHN SS *et al.* Sulfonamide containing regimes for disease caused by rifampicin resistant *Mycobacterium kansasii Am Rev Resp Dis* 1987;135:10–16.

96. COLVILLE A, EVANS SA, EVANS AJ, CRISP AJ. Comparison of treatment and outcome in pulmonary infections with *Mycobacterium kansasii* and *Mycobacterium tuberculosis* in Nottingham. *Thorax (Proc)* 1993;48:423.

97. RESEARCH COMMITTEE OF THE BRITISH THORACIC SOCIETY. *Mycobacterium kansasii* pulmonary infections: a prospective study of the results of nine months of treatment with rifampicin and ethambutol. *Thorax* 1994;49:442–5.

98. DAVIDSON PT. Treatment and long-term follow-up of patients with atypical mycobacterial infections. *Bull Int Union Tuberc Lung Dis* 1976;51:257–61.

99. WALLACE RJ JR, DUNBAR D, BROWN BA, ONYI G, *et al.* Rifampin-resistant *Mycobacterium kansasii. Clin Infect Dis* 1994;18(5):736–43.

100. HJELM U, KAUSTOVA J, KUBIN M, HOFFNER SE. Susceptibility of *Mycobacterium kansasii* to ethambutol and its combination with rifamycins, ciprofloxacin and isoniazid. *Eur J Clin Micro Infect Dis* 1992;11:51–4.

101. BROWN BA, WALLACE RJ JR, ONYI GO. Activities of clarithromycin against eight slowly growing species of nontuberculous *Mycobacteria*, determined by using a broth microdilution MIC system. *Antimicrob Agents Chemother* 1992;36(9):1987–90.

102. COSTRINI AM, MAHLER DA, GROSS WM

et al. Clinical and roentgenographic features of nosocomial pulmonary disease due to *Mycobacterium xenopi Am Rev Resp Dis* 1981;123:104–19.

103. SMITH MJ, CITRON KM. Clinical review of pulmonary disease caused by *Mycobacterium xenopi*. *Thorax* 1983;38:373–7.

104. CONTRERAS MA, CHEUNG OT, SANDERS DE, GOLDSTEIN RS. Pulmonary infection with the non-tuberculous *Mycobacteria*. *Am Rev Resp Dis* 1988;137:149–52.

105. TORTOLI E, SIMONETTI MT, LABARDI C, LOPES PEGNA A *et al. Mycobacterium xenopi* isolation from clinical specimens in the Florence area: review of 46 cases. *Eur J Epidemiol* 1991;7(6):677–81.

106. TENHOLDER MF, PIKE JD Effect of anorexia nervosa on pulmonary immunocompetence. *South Med J* 1991;84(10):1188–91.

107. WEBER J, METTANG T, STAERZ E *et al.* Pulmonary disease due to *Mycobacterium xenopi* in a renal allograft recipient: report of a case and review. *Rev Infect Dis* 1989;11:964–9.

108. BANKS J, HUNTER AM, CAMPBELL IA *et al.* Pulmonary infection with *Mycobacterium xenopi*: review of treatment and response. *Thorax* 1984;39:376–82.

109. COSTRINI AM, MAHLER DA, GROSS WM *et al.* Clinical and roentgenographic features of nosocomial pulmonary disease due to *Mycobacterium xenopi Am Rev Resp* 1981;123:104–9.

110. AIKEN KR, JOHNSON RF. Tuberculous-like disease produced by *M. scrofulaceum*. *Pennsylvania Med* 1978;81:38–41.

111. LEMENSE GP, VANBAKEL AB, CRUMBLEY AJ III, JUDSON MA. *Mycobacterium scrofulaceum* infection presenting as lung nodules in a heart transplant recipient. *Chest* 1994;106(6):1918–20.

112. DATTWYLER RJ, THOMAS J, HURST LC. Antigen-specific T-cell anergy in progressive *Mycobacterium marinum* infection in humans. *Ann Intern Med* 1987;107:675–7.

113. GOULD WM, MCMEEKIN DR, BRIGHT RD. *Mycobacterium marinum (balaei)* infection. Report of a case with cutaneous and laryngeal lesions. *Arch Dermatol* 1968;97:159–62.

114. BONNET E, DEBAT-ZOGUEREH D, PETIT N, RAVAUX I, GALLAIS H Clarithromycin: a potent agent against infections due to *Mycobacterium marinum*. *Clin Infect Dis* 1994;18:664–6.

115. IREDELL J, WHITBY M, BLACKLOCK Z. *Mycobacterium marinum* infection: epidemiology and presentation in Queensland 1971–1990. *Med J Aust* 1992;157(9);569–568.

116. MARKS J, JENKINS PA, TSUKAMURA M. *Mycobacterium szulgai*: a new pathogen. *Tubercle* 1972;53:210–4.

117. DYLEWSKI JS, ZACKON HM, LATOUR AH, BERRY GR. *Mycobacterium szulgai*: an unusual pathogen. *Rev Infect Dis* 1987;9:578–80.

118. OLMOS JM, PERALTA FG, MELLADO A, GONZALEZ-MACIAS J. Infection by *Mycobacterium szulgai* in a patient with pulmonary tuberculosis. *Eur J Clin Microbiol Infect Dis* 1994;13:689–90.

119. DONOVAN WN, KRASNOW I, DONOWHO EM, JOHANSON WG JR *Mycobacterium simiae* (abstract). *Am Rev Resp Dis* 1976;113:55.

120. WALLACE RJ JR, SWENSON JM, SILCOX VA, GOOD KC, TSCHEN JA, STONE MS. Spectrum of disease due to rapidly growing mycobacteria. *Rev Infect Dis* 1983;5:657–79.

121. SMITH MJ, EFTHIMIOU J, HODSON ME *et al.* Mycobacterial isolations in young adults with cystic fibrosis. *Thorax* 1984;39:369–75.

122. ANNOBIL SH, JAMJOOM GA, BOBO R, IYENGAR J. Fatal lipoid pneumonia in an infant complicated by *Mycobacterium fortuitum* infection. *Trop Geogr Med* 1992;44(1–2):160–4.

123. MCWHINNEY PH, YATES M, PRENTICE HG *et al.* Infection caused by *Mycobacterium chelonae*: a diagnostic and therapeutic problem in the neutropaenic patient. *Clin Infect Dis* 1992;14(6):1208–12.

124. LAMBERT GW, BADDOUR LM. Right middle lobe syndrome caused by *Mycobacterium fortuitum* in a patient with human immunodeficiency virus infection. *South Med J* 1992;85(7):767–9.

125. PAUL J, BAIGRIE C, PARUMS DV. Fatal case of disseminated infection with the turtle bacillus *Mycobacterium chelonae J Clin Pathol* 1992;45(6):528–30.

126. BURNS DN, ROHATGI PK, ROSENTHAL R *et al.* Disseminated *Mycobacterium fortuitum* successfully treated with combination therapy including ciprofloxacin. *Am Rev Resp Dis* 1990;142:468–70 and 1235.

127. LESSING MP, WALKER MM Fatal pulmonary infection due to *Mycobacterium fortuitum*. *J Clin Pathol* 1993;46(3):271–2.

128. GRIFFITH DE, GIRARD WM, WALLACE RJ JR. Clinical features of pulmonary disease caused by rapidly growing mycobacteria. *Am Rev Resp Dis* 1993;147:1271–8.

129. HOY J, ROLSTON K AND HOPFER RL. Pseudoepidemic of *Mycobacterium fortuitum* in bone marrow cultures. *Am J Infect Contr* 1987;15:268–71.

130. PAONE RF, MERCER LC, GLASS BA. Pneumonectomy secondary to *Mycobacterium fortuitum* in infancy. *Ann Thorac Surg* 1991;51:1010–11.

131. PESCE RR, FEJK ES, COLODNY SM. *Mycobacterium fortuitum* presenting as an symptomatic enlarging pulmonary nodule. *Am J Med* 1991;91(3):310–12.

132. TANAKA H, KURIHARA M, TAKAHASHI K, HONDA Y, ASAKAWA M, OSHIMA S. *Mycobacterium fortuitum* pulmonary infection in a healthy 17-year-old man. *Kekkaku* 1992;67(9)613–19.

133. SINGH N, YU VL. Successful treatment of pulmonary infection due to *Mycobacterium chelonae*: case report and review. *Clin Infect Dis* 1992;14(1):156–61.

134. VADAKEKAZAM J, WARD MJ. *Mycobacterium fortuitum* lung abscess treated with ciprofloxacin. *Thorax* 1991;46(10):737–8.

135. YEW WW, KWAN SY, WONG PC *et al.* Ofloxacin and imipenem in the treatment of *Mycobacterium fortuitum* and *Mycobacterium chelonae* lung infections. *Tubercle* 1990;71:131–3.

136. WALLACE RJ JR, TANNER D, BRENNAN RJ, BROWN BA. Clinical trial of clarithromycin for cutaneous (disseminated) infection due to *Mycobacterium chelonae Ann Intern Med* 1993;119:482–6.

137. SCRODER KH, JUHLIN I. *Mycobacterium malmoense* sp nov. *Int J Syst Bacteriol* 1977;27:241–6.

138. WAYNE LG, SRAMEK HA. Agents of newly recognised or infrequently encountered mycobacterial diseases. *Clin Microbiol Rev* 1992;5:1–25.

139. ROGALL T, FLOHR T, BOTTGER EC. Differentiation of mycobacterium species by direct sequencing of amplified DNA. *J Gen Microbiol* 1990;136:1915–20.

140. JENKINS PA, TSUKAMURA M Infections with *Mycobacterium malmoense* in England and Wales. *Tubercle* 1979;60:71–6.

141. O'BRIEN RJ, GEITER LJ, SNIDER DE JR. The epidemiology of non-tuberculous mycobacterial diseases in the United States. *Am Rev Resp Dis* 1987;135:1007–14.

142. HENRIQUES B, HOFFNER SE, PETRINI B, JUHLIN I *et al.* Infection with *Mycobacterium malmoense* in Sweden: report of 221 cases. *Clin Infect Dis* 1994;18:596–600.

143. BANKS J, JENKINS PA, SMITH AP. Pulmonary infection with *Mycobacterium malmoense* – a review of treatment and response. *Tubercle* 1985;66:197–203.

144. BOLLERT FGE, SIME PJ, MACNEE W, CROMPTON GK. Pulmonary *Mycobacterium malmoense* and aspergillus infection: a fatal combination? *Thorax* 1994;49:521–2.

145. YOGANATHAN K, ELLIOTT MW, MOXHAM J, YATES M, POZNIAK AL. Pseudotumor of the lung caused by *Mycobacterium malmoense* infection in an HIV positive patient. *Thorax* 1994;49(2):179–80.

146. ZAUGG M, SALFINGER M, OPRAVIL M, LUTHY R. Extrapulmonary and disseminated infections due to *Mycobacterium malmoense*: case report and review. *Clin Infect Dis* 1993;16:540–9.

147. HOFFNER SE, HJELM U. Increased growth of *Mycobacterium malmoense in vitro* in the presence of isoniazid. *Eur J Clin Microbiol Infect Dis* 1991;10:787–8.

148. FRANCE AJ, MCLEOD DT, CALDER MA, SEATON A. *Mycobacterium malmoense* infections in Scotland: an increasing problem. *Thorax* 1987;42:593–5.

149. BARCLAY J, STANBRIDGE TN, DOYLE L. Pneumonectomy for drug resistant *Mycobacterium malmoense. Thorax* 1983;38:796–7.

150. BLACKLOCK ZM, DAWSON DJ, KANE DW, MCEVOY D. *Mycobacterium asiaticum* as a potential pulmonary pathogen for humans. A clinical and bacteriologic review of 5 cases. *Am Rev Resp Dis* 1983;127:241–4.

151. TAYLOR LQ, WILLIAMS AJ, SANTIAGO S. Pulmonary disease caused by *Mycobacterium asiaticium Tubercle* 1990;71:303–5.

152. BUTLER WR, O'CONNOR SP, YAKRUS MA *et al. Mycobacterium celatum* sp. nov. *Int J Syst Bacteriol* 1993;43:539–48.

153. WEITZMAN I, OSADCZYI D, CORRADO MC, KARP D. *Mycobacterium thermoresistibile*: a new pathogen for humans. *J Clin Microbiol* 1981;14:593–5.

154. GOOD RC AND SNIDER DE JR. Isolation of non-tuberculous *Mycobacteria* in the United States 1980. *J Infect Dis* 1982;146:829–33.

155. TSUKAMURA M. Infections due to *Mycobacterium gordonae IRYO* 1983;37:456–62.

156. STEER AC, CORRALES J, VON-GRAEVENITZ A. A cluster of *Mycobacterium gordonae* isolates from bronchoscopy specimens. *Am Rev Resp Dis* 1979;120:214–16.

157. GUBLER JG, SALFINGER M, VON GRAEVENITZ A. Pseudoepidemic of nontuberculous *Mycobacteria* due to a contaminated bronchoscope cleaning machine. Report of an outbreak and review of the literature (review). *Chest* 1992;101(5):1245–9.

158. WEINBERGER M, BERG SL, FEUERSTEIN IW *et al.* Disseminated infection with *Mycobacterium gordonae*: report of a case and critical review of the literature. *Clin Infec Dis* 1992;14:1229–39.

159. DOUGLAS JG, CALDER MA, CHOO-KANG YFJ *et al. Mycobacterium gordonae*: a new pathogen? *Thorax* 1986;41:152–3.

160. JARIKRE LN. Case report: disseminated *Mycobacterium gordonae* infection in a nonimmunocompromised host. *Am J Med Sci* 1991;302(6):383–4.

161. PETERS EJ, MORICE R. Miliary pulmonary infection caused by *Mycobacterium terrae* in an autologous bone marrow transplant patient. *Chest* 1991;100:1449–50.

162. PALMERO DJ, TERRES RI, EIGUCHI K Pulmonary disease due to *Mycobacterium terrae. Tubercle* 1989;70:301–3.

163. TONNER JA, HAMMOND MD. Pulmonary disease caused by *Mycobacterium terrae* complex. *South Med J* 1989;82:1279–82.

164. KIEHN TE, WHITE M, PURSELL KJ, BOONE N *et al.* A cluster of four cases of *Mycobacterium haemophilum* infection. *Eur J Clin Microbiol Infect Dis* 1993;12:114–18.

165. ROGERS PL, WALKER RE, LANE HC *et al.* Disseminated *Mycobacterium haemophilum* infection in two patients with the acquired immunodeficiency syndrome. *Am J Med* 1988;84:640–2.

166. CASIMIR MT, FAINSTEIN V, PAPADOPOLOUS N. Cavitary lung disease caused by *Mycobacterium flavescens. South Med J* 1982;75:253–4.

167. COX EG, HEIL SA, KLEIMAN MB. Lipoid pneumonia and *Mycobacterium smegmatis. Ped Infect Dis J* 1994;13(5):414–15.

168. CENTERS FOR DISEASE CONTROL: Update on acquired immune deficiency syndrome (AIDS) – United States. *MMWR* 1982;31:507–14.

169. CENTERS FOR DISEASE CONTROL: 1993 Revised clarification system for HIV infection and expanded surveillance case definition for AIDS among adolescents and adults. *MMWR* 1992;41:1–19.

170. CHAISSON RE, SLUTKIN G. Tuberculosis and human immunodeficiency virus infection. *J Infect Dis* 1989;159:96–100.

171. MILLAR AB. Respiratory manifestations of AIDS. *Br J Hosp Med* 1988;39:204–13.

172. HELBERT M, ROBINSON D, BUCHANAN D *et al.* Mycobacterial infection in patients infected with the human immunodeficiency virus. *Thorax* 1990;45:45–8.

173. GUTHERZ LS, DAMSKER B, BOTTONE EJ *et al. Mycobacterium avium* and *Mycobacterium intracellulare* infections in patients with and without AIDS. *J Infect Dis* 1989;160:1037–41.

174. FAUCI, AS, MACHER AM, LONGO DL *et al.* Acquired immunodeficiency syndrome: epidemiologic, clinical, immunologic, and therapeutic considerations. *Ann Intern Med* 1984:100:92–106.

175. HAVLIK JA JR, METCHCOCK B, THOMPSON SE III, BARRETT K, RIMLAND D, HORSBURGH CR JR. A prospective evaluation of *Mycobacterium avium* complex colonisation of the respiratory and gastrointestinal tracts of persons with human immunodeficiency virus infection. *J Infect Dis* 1993;168:1045–8.

176. JACOBSON MA, HOPEWELL PC, YAJKO DM *et al.* Natural history of disseminated *Mycobacterium avium* complex infection in AIDS. *J Infect Dis* 1991;164:994–8.

177. MASUR H, OGNIBENE FP, YARCHOAN R *et al.* CD4 counts as predictors of opportunistic pneumonias in human immunodeficiency virus (HIV) infection. *Ann Intern Med* 1989;111:223–31.

178. NIGHTINGALE SD, BYRD LT, SOUTHERN PM *et al.* Incidence of *Mycobacterium avium–intracellulare* complex bacteremia in human immunodeficiency virus – positive patients. *J Infect Dis* 1992;165:1082–5.

179. BENSON CA. Disease due to the *Mycobacterium avium* complex in patients with AIDS: epidemiology and clinical syndrome. CID 1994;18(Supp 3):S218–22.

180. HAWKINS CC, GOLD JW, WHIMBEY E *Mycobacterium avium* complex infections in patients with the acquired immunodeficiency syndrome. *Ann Intern Med* 1986;105:184–8.

182. YAGUPSKY P, MENEGUS MA. Cumulative positivity rates of multiple blood cultures for *Mycobacterium avium–intercellulare* and *Cryptococcus neoformans* in patients with acquired immunodeficiency syndrome. *Arch Pathol Lab Med* 1990;114(9):923–5.

183. HORSBURGH CR JR, METCHOCK B, GORDON SM, HAVLIK JA JR, MCGOWAN JE, THOMPSON SE III. Predictors of survival in patients with AIDS and disseminated *Mycobacterium avium* complex disease. *JID* 1994;170:573–7.

184. RUF B, SCHUERMANN D, BREHMER W, POHLE HD. Pulmonary manifestations due to *Mycobacterium avium–intercellulare* in AIDS patients (abst) *Am Rev Resp Dis* 1990;141(Supp):A611.

185. RIGSBY MO, CURTIS AM. Pulmonary disease from nontuberculous mycobacteria in patients with human immunodeficiency virus. *Chest* 1994;106(3):913–19.

186. NATIONAL HEART, LUNG AND BLOOD INSTITUTE WORKSHOP. Pulmonary complications of the acquired immunodeficiency syndrome. *N Engl J Med* 1984;310:1682–8.

187. WALLACE JM, HANNAH JB. *Mycobacterium avium* complex infection in patients with the acquired immunodeficiency syndrome. *Chest* 1988;93:926–32.

188. WELCH K, FINKBEINER W, ALPERS CI, BLUMFELD W, DAVIS RL *et al.* Autopsy pathology in the acquired immunodeficiency syndrome. *JAMA* 1984;252:1152–9.

189. TERSTEIN AS, PAMSKSER B, KIRSCHNER PA, KRELLENSTEIN DJ, ROBINSON B, CHUANG MT. Pulmonary infection with *Mycobacterium*

avium–intercellulare: diagnosis, clinical patterns, treatment (clinical conference). *Mt Sinai J Med* 1990;57:209–15.

190. GOODMAN PC. Mycobacterial disease in AIDS. *J Thorac Imaging* 1991;6:22–7.

191. MILLER RF, BIRLEY HDL, FOGARTY P *et al.* Cavitary lung disease caused by *Mycobacterium avium–intracellulare* in AIDS patients. *Resp Med* 1990;84:409–11.

192. KRAMER EL, SANGER JH, GARAY SM. Diagnostic implications of Ga-67 chest-scan patterns in human immunodeficiency virus sero-positive patients. *Radiology* 1989;170:671–6.

193. KRAMER EL, SANGER JJ, GARAY SM *et al.* Gallium 67 scans of the chest in patients with acquired immunodeficiency syndrome. *J Nucl Med* 1987;28:1107–14.

194. MOSER E, TATSCH K, KIRSH CM *et al.* Value of 67 gallium scintigraphy in primary diagnosis and follow-up of opportunistic pneumonia in patients with AIDS. *Lung* 1990;168 Suppl:692–703.

195. SALZMAN SH, SCHINDEL ML, ARANDAL CP *et al.* The role of bronchoscopy in the diagnosis of pulmonary tuberculosis in patients at risk for HIV infection. *Chest* 1992;102:143–6.

196. MURRAY JF, GARAY SM, HOPEWELL PC, MILLS J, SNIDER GL, STOVER DE. Pulmonary complication of the acquired immunodeficiency syndrome: an update: report of the Second National Heart Lung and Blood Institute Workshop. *Am Rev Resp Dis* 1987;135:504–9.

197. MEHLE ME, ADAMO JP, MEHTA AC *et al.* Endobronchial *Mycobacterium avium-intracellulare* infection in a patient with AIDS. *Chest* 1989;96:119–200.

198. HORSBURGH CR JR, HAVLIK JA, ELLIS DA *et al.* Survival of patients with acquired immune deficiency syndrome and disseminated *Mycobacterium avium* complex infection with and without antimicrobial chemotherapy. *Am Rev Resp Dis* 1991;144:557–9.

199. SATHES S, GASCON P, LO W, PINTO R, REICHMAN LB. Severe anemia is an important negative predictor for survival with disseminated *Mycobacterium avium–intercellulare* in acquired immune deficiency syndrome. *Am Rev Resp Dis* 1990;142:1306–12.

200. CHIN DP, REINGOLD AL, STONE EN, VITTINGHOFF E *et al.* The impact of *Mycobacterium avium* complex bacteremia and its treatment survival of AIDS patients – a prospective study. *JID* 1994;170:578–84.

201. YOUNG LS, INDERLIED CB, BERLIN OG *et al.* Mycobacterial infections in AIDS patients with an emphasis on the *Mycobacterium avium* complex. *Rev Infect Dis* 1986;8:1024–33.

202. HOY J, MIJCHA S, ANDLAND M *et al.* Quadruple-drug therapy for *Mycobacterium avium–intracellulare* bacteremia in AIDS patients. *J Infect Dis* 1990;161:801–5.

203. CHIU J, NUSSBAUM J, BOZZETTE S *et al.* Treatment of disseminated *Mycobacterium avium* complex infection in AIDS with amikacin, ethambutol, rifampicin and ciprofloxacin. *Ann Intern Med* 1990;113:358–61.

204. KEMPER CA, HAVLIR D, HAGHIGHAT D, DUBE M *et al.* The individual microbiologic effect of three antimycobacterial agents, clofazimine, ethambutol, and rifampin, on *Mycobacterium avium* complex bacteremia in patients with AIDS. *JID* 1994;170:157–4.

205. LEE BL, SAFRIN S. Interactions and toxicities of drugs used in patients with AIDS. *Clin Infect Dis* 1992;14:773–9.

206. DAUTZENBERG B, TRUFFOT C, LEGRIS S, MEYOHAS MC *et al.* Activity of clarithromycin against *Mycobacterium avium* infection in patients with acquired immune deficiency syndrome. *Am Rev Resp Dis* 1991;144:564–9.

207. DAUTZENBERG B, SAINT MARC T, MEYOHAS MC, ELIASZEWITCH M *et al.* Clarithromycin and other antimicrobial agents in the treatment of disseminated *Mycobacterium avium* infections in patients with acquired immunodeficiency syndrome. *Arch Intern Med* 1993;152:368–72.

208. GUPTA S, BLAHUNKA K, DELLERSON M, CRAFT JC, SMITH T. Interim results of safety and efficacy of clarithromycin in the treatment of disseminated *M. avium* complex infection in patients with AIDS. Abstract 892. In *Interscience Conference on Antimicrobial Agents and Chemotherapy*, Washington DC; 1992.

209. CHAISSON RE, BENSON C, DUBE M *et al.* Clarithromycin therapy for bacteremic *Mycobacterium avium* complex disease. A randomised double-blind, dose ranging study in patients with AIDS. ACTG protocol 157 study. *Ann Intern Med* 1994;121:905–11.

210. TEBAS P, SULTAN F, WALLACE RJ JR, FRASER V. Rapid development of resistance to clarithromycin following monotherapy for disseminated *Mycobacterium chelonae* infection in a heart transplant patient. *CID* 1995;20:443–4.

211. HOLLAND SM, EISENSTEIN EM, KUHNS B, TURNER ML *et al.* Treatment of refractory disseminated nontuberculous mycobacterial infection with interferon gamma. *NEJM* 1994;330(19):1348–55.

212. GORDIN F, MASUR H. Prophylaxis of *Mycobacterium avium* complex B bacteremia in patients with AIDS. CID 1994;18(Suppl 3):S223–6.

213. PIERCE M, LAMARCA A, JABLONOWSKI H *et al.* A Placebo controlled trial of clarithromycin prophylaxis against MAC infection in AIDS patients. A/2 ICAAC, 1994.

214. HORSBURGH CR JR, SELIK RM. Microbiology of disseminated non-tuberculous mycobacterial infection in the acquired immunodeficiency syndrome (AIDS). *Am Rev Resp Dis* 1989;139:4–7.

215. CARPENTER JL, PARKS JM. *Mycobacterium kansasii* infections in patients positive for human immunodeficiency virus. *Rev Infect Dis* 1991;13:789–96.

216. LEVINE B, CHAISSON RE. *Mycobacterium kansasii*: a cause of treatable pulmonary disease associated with advanced human immunodeficiency virus (HIV) infection. *Ann Intern Med* 1991;114:861–8.

217. SHAFER RW, SIERRA MF. *Mycobacterium xenopi*, *Mycobacterium fortuitum*, *Mycobacterium kansasii*, and other nontuberculous mycobacteria in an area of endemicity for AIDS. *CID* 1992;15:161–2.

218. BÖTTGER EC, TESKE A, KIRSCHNER P *et al.* Disseminated '*Mycobacterium genavense*' Lancet 1992;340:76–80.

219. PECHERE M, EMLERS, WALD A *et al.* Infection with *Mycobaterium genavense*: clinical features in 44 cases. *Abstr WS B10–2* IXth International Conference on AIDS, Berlin, 1993.

220. NADAL D, CADUFF R, KRAFT R, SALFINGER M *et al.* Invasive infection with *Mycobacterium genavense* in three children with acquired immunodeficiency syndrome. *Eur J Clin Microbiol Infect Dis* 1993;12:37–43.

221. HOPEWELL P, CYNAMON M, STARKE J, ISEMAN M, O'BRIEN R. Evaluation of new anti-infective drugs for the treatment of disease caused by *Mycobacterium kansasii* and other mycobacteria. *CID* 1992;15(Suppl 1); S307–12.

12 Actinomycosis and nocardiosis

MICHAEL E. ELLIS
King Faisal Specialist Hospital and Research Centre, Riyadh, Saudi Arabia

The order of actinomycetales comprises a number of different human pathogens, including the families actinomycetaceae, nocardiaceae and mycobacteriaceae. Mycobacterial diseases have been presented in Chapters 11 and 15. Diseases due to Nocardia spp. are described in the second part of this chapter. The aerobic actinomycetes such as Actinomadura madurale and Streptomyces somalienses produce progressive destructive infections usually in peripheral soft tissues called madura foot.

This chapter will describe respiratory infections due to *Actinomyces* spp. producing actimycosis and pulmonary infections due to *Nocardia* spp.

Actinomyces spp. and actinomycosis

Bacteriology, immunopathogenesis and epidemiology

The actinomycetaceae family has a variable tendency to form filaments as a result of failure to separate with growth. The higher actinomycetes are characterised by extensive branching filaments which may project above the colony (aerial forms). These appearances are termed hyphae/mycelia and the ray-like appearances of the sulphur granules of *Actinomyces israelii* led to previously erroneous classification as fungi. Actinomyces means ray fungus. However, lack of sporulation, budding, absence of chitin and glucan in the cell wall, lack of a nuclear membrane, non-response of infections to antifungal agents, replication by bacterial fission and response to penicillin/tetracycline reclassified them as higher bacteria.

The organism responsible for actinomycosis was recognised when the disease 'lumpy jaw' in cattle was described, and was named *Actinomyces bovis* by Bollinger. The organism does not produce human disease. *A. israelii* was then found in 1885 to be the causative agent of human disease and is the species most often implicated among the six of the 13 recognised species causing human disease. *A. israelii* is an anaerobic micro-aerophilic Gram-positive bacterium measuring approximately 13 $\mu \times 0.5$ μ, fastidious, slowly growing and showing filamentous branching morphology. *Actinomyces* spp. are best visualised using a tissue Gram's stain or modified Gomori's methenamine-silver stain rather than the regular haematoxylin and eosin stain. The organism may appear beaded due to the irregularity of the staining (Fig. 12.1). The main *Actinomyces* spp. can be differentiated using a fluorescein labelled antibody stain. Some degree of pleomorphism is common.

Initially, spider-like colonies form in culture at 3–7 days and these later become heaped up and rough to form 'molar tooth' colonies[1]. An alternative form is coccoid/diphtheroid like. Culture should continue for 3 weeks to ensure maximum yield. In early lesions the organism is free but, as the infection becomes more established, conglomerations of the bacteria form, bound by a phosphatase-mediated immunoglobulin and calcium matrix, into round/oval, basophilic/amphophilic masses with an eosinophilic fringe (clubs), measuring approximately 290 μ in diameter (Fig. 12.2). PAS staining reveals these 'sulphur' granules, which are only formed *in vivo*. They occur in about a quarter of patients with actinomycosis. The term 'sulphur' refers to the colour and not to the sulphur content which is very low. The organisms often extend through the fringe. A curious observation is that the

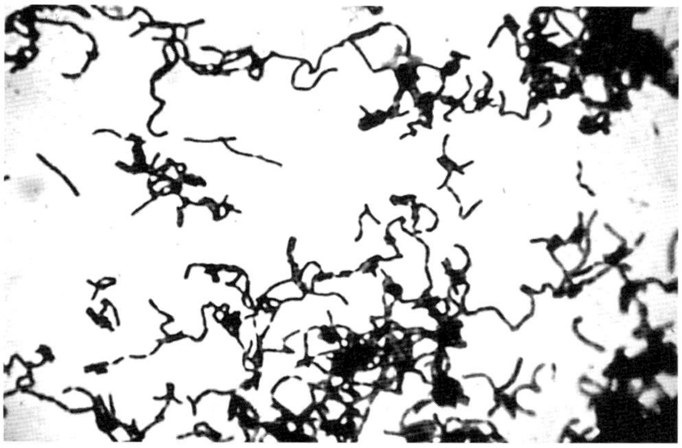

FIGURE 12.1 Gram-positive branching filaments of *A. israelii*. Note beading irregularity. (Courtesy of Dr S. M. Hussein Qadri.)

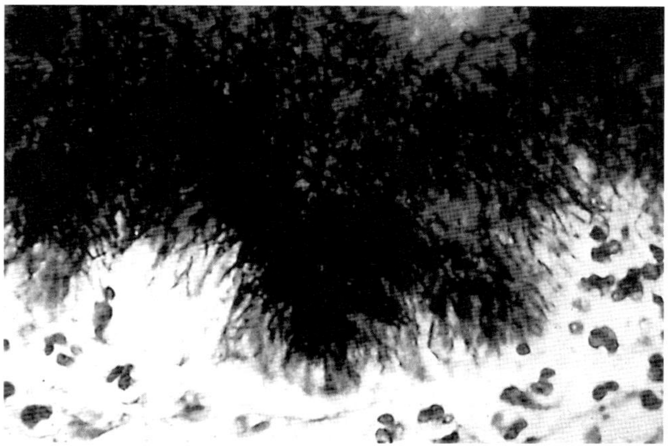

FIGURE 12.2 Sulphur granule: basophilic centre and peripheral eosinophilic clubs. (Courtesy of Dr S. M. Hussein Qadri.)

organisms are rarely found in pus – rather they tend to be associated with the granule – their presence being revealed by crushing the granule before staining. Granules may themselves be difficult to find. Sulphur granules represent a host reaction to foreign material which is called the Splendore–Hoeppli phenomenon and this can also be found in fungal diseases, nocardiosis, streptomyces, botromycosis and staphylococcal infections. Their presence, therefore, is suggestive rather than pathognomonic of actinomycosis. However, the distinctive clubbed boundary is said to be present only in actinomycosis. It has been hypothesised that granules offer some protection from antimicrobials, effect of oxygen and host defence mechanisms[1]. Polymicrobial infection with other bacteria is found in most lesions of actinomycosis[1] – it is possible that some advantageous synergistic interaction occurs.

The gross appearance of infected tissues is of an inflammatory process extending through and across anatomical boundaries, for example, across lung fissures into the ribs, or invading the chest wall. Microscopically there are areas of dense fibrous tissue within which are islands of pus containing active inflammatory cells such as foamy macrophages, neutrophils and, uncommonly, eosinophils. Ill-defined granulomas but without giant cells may be present. A non-specific inflammatory reaction in the interstitium or alveoli contiguous to the major infective focus may be found. There is relatively little blood supply. Multiple sinus tracks form and interconnect from these areas and penetrate anatomical tissue planes and barriers to exit onto the skin or into various organs.

The organism is normally present in the mouth, particularly around the gums, in the gingival sulci, tonsillar crypts and dental caries – they are more commonly found in patients whose dental hygiene is poor. The organism can also be found in the lower respiratory tract of patients with COAD, gastrointestinal tract and vagina. The majority of cases of actinomycosis arise in a setting where the host's mechanical defence barrier has been breached as a result of trauma, surgery or invasive infection, thereby allowing direct implantation of the organism. Aspiration from an oral reservoir can lead to lower respiratory tract infection. Spread can occur from contiguous sites, for example, arising from the face and extending to the thorax. Molecular mechanisms of host predisposition to actinomycosis are largely unknown. The precise mechanisms for tissue invasion are not understood but proteolytic enzymes may be involved. However, actinomycosis has been reported sometimes in patients with humoral or cell-mediated immune defects, for example, patients undergoing radiotherapy treatment, with cancer, patients on steroids or those with HIV disease[1–3]. Unusually actinomycosis can be found in patients with no recognisable pre-disposing factors, so-called primary lesions.

A. israelii has the propensity to involve any site but the most commonly involved are the cervico-facial (32–48% of cases), abdominal (22–63%), thoracic (15–30%) and miscellaneous, such as the heart, brain and skin (10%)[1,2]. There is some evidence that thoracic disease may have become less prevalent in some areas; for example, only 19 cases were identified from the hospital records of five UK health regions from 1974 to 1990, possibly due to the increased standard of dental care and the widespread use of penicillin[4]. The lungs can act as an initial focus for disseminated actinomycosis with metastatic foci particularly in the brain, liver, skin, heart and muscle.

It is difficult to be precise over mortality. In the pre-antibiotic era, thoracic disease carried a mortality rate of up to 80%. More recent experience with antibiotics and appropriate surgery have considerably improved on this. In a study of 181 patients published in 1973 (which did not only involve thoracic sites) death directly due to actinomycosis was 16%[1]. In the series of Weese and Smith in 1975, the mortality was 11%, which included some cases, including extrapulmonary disease, undiagnosed antemortem[2].

Clinical features of thoracic actinomycosis

Men are three times more frequently affected than women. Late teens/early adult and 30–50 years are the two peak age-groups involved. There may be a background history of bronchiectasis or chronic airways disease[1]. The disease can involve any part of the thoracic cage, bronchi, mediastinum, lungs or pleura. Often, it is insidious in onset and slowly progressive. There may be an antecedent event such as dental surgery, aspiration or penetrating trauma, often not recognised at the time of the initial presentation.

Initial features are mild or non-specific such as cough or fever. When fully established, however, features of actinomycosis often mimic other conditions such as carcinoma of the bronchus and alveolar cell carcinoma, and this results in delayed diagnosis. For example, 8 of 17 patients seen at a large referral hospital in Taipeh were initially referred as having a primary lung malignancy[5]. Other conditions with which it is confused include tuberculosis, aspergilloma, bronchiectasis, lung abscess, cryptococcosis, histoplasmosis and non-infectious conditions such as Wegener's granulomatosis. Occasionally, actinomycosis can coexist with pulmonary tuberculosis and bronchial carcinoma.

Chronic cough is invariably present and associated with haemoptysis, which can be massive in up to 50%[5–7]. Weight loss and malaise are common features. Pleuritic chest pain occurs in early pleural involvement. Later the development of cavitary lesions, empyema and invasion of the chest wall is found[4,5,7], and may cause more constant chest wall pain. Other presenting symptoms include night sweats and localised chest wall swelling. Vertebral involvement leads to nerve root or back pain. Systemic features of chills and fever may not always be found, perhaps in only between 20 and 50% of cases[2,4]. Subcutaneous abscesses and discharging chest wall sinuses which may be tender are frequently reported in the earlier literature[7] but are not so commonly represented in more recent reviews[4,5]. Mediastinal or pleural involvement as a result of oesophageal perforation, penetrating chest trauma, tracheal/bronchial perforation or spread from a primary pulmonary source, is said to be rather uncommon. In such cases the presentation may be of pericardial involvement or superior veno-caval obstruction or can be non-specific[1,2,8,9]. CT scanning may reveal hilar or mediastinal lymphadenopathy in approximately one-third of those cases of thoracic actinomycosis[10] which do not have obvious clinical features of such involvement. Endobronchial mass lesions associated with recurrent pneumonia or wheeze may simulate bronchial carcinoma[11–13]. Apical lesions with brachial plexus signs may mimic a Pancoast's tumor. Recurrent aspiration pneumonia or choking dysphagia may suggest tracheo-oesophageal fistula. Occasionally, primary or secondary pulmonary involvement may be diagnosed as part of the diagnostic work-up in a patient whose presenting features are those of extra-pulmonary lesions. Associated extra-pulmonary lesions may be present (Fig. 12.3) or disseminated disease occurs in thoracic actinomycosis[14] with central nervous system (e.g. subdural abscess and meningitis), musculo-skeletal and cardiac involvement.

Early radiographical findings often show non-specific pulmonary infiltrates in the lower lobes, limited by segment or lobe boundaries. Cavitation (mimicking TB), which is often multiple or lung abscess may be present. Mass lesions simulate neoplasia. Occasionally, coin lesions are found. Pleural involvement is found in over 50% of cases of thoracic actinomycosis, often with loculated effusions.

However, there are certain features which should increase the level of suspicion, such as bone changes, e.g. periostitis, bone destruction and transfissural or transthoracic masses. The plain chest radiograph may be normal. Assessment by CT scanning in general is superior to plain radiology. This may reveal the nodular nature of the consolidation, transfissural involvement, air space consolidation in association with adjacent pleural thickening, and hilar or mediastinal lymphadenopathy[10,15].

Usually, the peripheral white count is normal or slightly elevated, but in approximately one-third it will be $> 15 \times 10^9$/l (polymorph predominance in most cases). One-half of the patients show a mild anaemia of < 12 gm/dl, and an ESR elevated to >30 mm/h (occasionally to 100) in about a half[2,4].

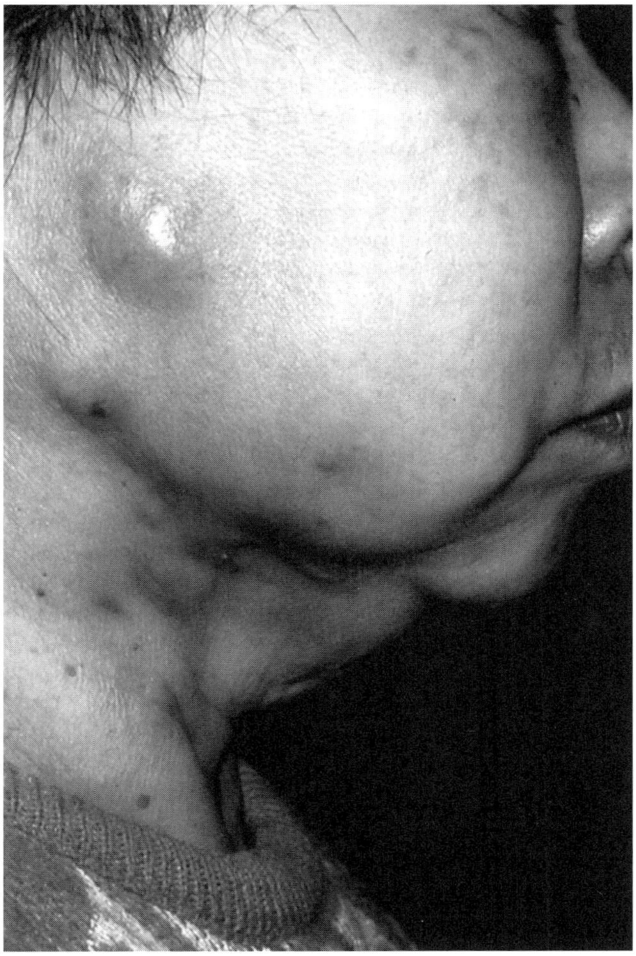

FIGURE 12.3 Subcutaneous masses of cervicofacial actinomycosis.

The diagnosis is made on the basis of the clinical findings and demonstration of the organism. Since *Actinomyces* spp. contribute towards the normal oral flora, a single positive sputum sample is not enough for the diagnosis. The organism has to be demonstrated repeatedly or in histological sections or grown from tissue (although *Actinomyces* spp. can also colonise necrotic tissue), or demonstrated in material from closed spaces. Pleural effusions may be lymphocytic if sympathetic or less commonly purulent if infected. The presence of sulphur granules is highly suggestive but not pathognomonic. Biopsy on occasions may be negative due to sampling error. Tuberculosis, histoplasmosis, nocardiosis, sporotroichosis, tumour, etc have to be ruled out by appropriate means. Serological diagnosis is neither sensitive nor specific enough currently.

Association with other organisms

Concomitant infection with other organisms is common, occurring in some 60% of patients[2]. These include *Actinobacillus actinomycetemcomitans*, *Streptococcus* spp., *Staphylococcus* spp., *Enterobacteriaceae* spp., *Bacteroides* spp., *Pseudomonas* spp., *Streptomyces* spp., *Hemophilus* spp., *Fusobacterium* spp. and *Eikenella* spp. The particular association is dependent on the anatomical location of the actinomytosis. *A. actinomycetencomitans* is found in approximately one-quarter of all cases of actinomycosis in which *A. israelii* is found[16]. It is believed *A. actinomycetencomitans* and other organisms are synergistic with *A. israelii*, enhancing invasiveness. They may be responsible for relapse or non-response to treatment for *A. israelii* since the organism is resistant to clindamycin, penicillins, erythromycin and vancomycin[16–18]. *A. actinomycetencomitans* can also act as a solitary pathogen *per se*[18,19] producing pneumonia, osteomyelitis, endocarditis, soft tissue infections, urinary tract infection, pericarditis and mediastinal abscess.

Management of actinomycosis

The mainstay of treatment is antimicrobials and surgery. Penicillin G in large doses of up to 20 mega units/day, to ensure adequate antimicrobial penetration into the relatively avascular tissue, given for approximately six weeks followed by oral penicillin V for another 6–12 months at 4 g/day has been and remains the initial drug regimen of choice[7]. A prolonged course may be needed for a particularly deep seated site, for example, the heart or central nervous system. The majority of patients, including those with extensive disease, respond dramatically to penicillin alone. Failure of response to penicillin has been reported however. This may be due to (i) persistent abscess, (ii) large, extremely avascular inflammatory areas, (iii) non-responding associated organisms, (iv) non-compliance, for example, due to penicillin allergy or (v) primary resistant or secondarily resistant *A. israelii* organisms. The last option is highly unlikely as sensitivity testing over the years has shown little variation in susceptibility. However, on occasions, MICs to penicillin have been known to increase during a course of therapy but *in vivo* resistance is not recognised. Alternative antimicrobials include first-generation parenteral cephalosporins, imipenem, clindamycin, chloramphenicol, erythromycin, tetracycline, co-trimoxazole, azithromycin, rifampacin, streptomycin or ciprofloxacin[18]. *A. actinomycetemcomitans* is much less sensitive to penicillin and clindamycin. Other appropriate antimicrobials are indicated depending on the particular associated organism present and the response to penicillin. An alternative therapeutic approach is to give ampicillin with metronidazole or clindamycin to cover both *A. israelii* and the possibility of the other associated organisms. Since there is also some response to rifampicin/isoniazid, the use of these antibiotics in the setting of a therapeutic trial for a possible TB diagnosis poses a dilemma.

Surgical intervention, if technically feasible, should be undertaken in patients who fail medical treatment, those with lung abscess or empyema, devitalised lung tissue, chronic sinus discharge, haemoptysis or for diagnostic purposes[20]. Pericardicentesis is necessary for cardiac tamponade secondary to a contiguous thoracic lesion[21]. Non-loculated, sterile pleural effusions may respond to antimicrobials alone – infected effusions require drainage. An alternative to surgery in, for example, patients at high risk, e.g. those with lung cancer or poor cardiorespiratory reserve and for haemoptysis,[15] is selective arterial embolisation[6].

Since a high oxygen tension is lethal for *Actinomyces* spp., hyperbaric oxygen, providing a high pO_2 at the point of tissue infection, has been shown to be an effective adjunctive therapy[22].

Other *Actinomyces* spp. involved in actinomycosis

Although *A. israelii* is the most frequently implicated species, others, namely, *A. naeslundii*, *Actinomyces viscosus*, *Actinomyces odontolyticus*, *Actinomyces meyeri* and *Actinomyces eriksonii* (now *Bifidobacterium adolescentis*) all give rise to actinomycosis. They display several biochemical and cultural differences from *A. israeli*, including variable oxygen tolerance (*A. israelii* is anaerobic, *Actinomyces odontolyticus* is facultatively anaerobic), carbon dioxide requirements and frequency of granule formation (not produced by *A. odontolyticus*). *Arachnia proprionica*, an organism belonging to another genus, can also produce actinomycosis. It is actually more common than the non-*israelii* *Actinomyces* spp. Morphologically and physiologically very similar to *A. israelii*, it produces propionic acid, has a different cell wall chemotype, and forms somewhat smoother colonies. Species identification can be accomplished by fluoroscein-labelled specific antibody staining techniques[23]. Actinomycosis due to the non-*israelii* strains normally show the same response to penicillin.

Actinomyces pyogenes

This organism was, until recently, called *Corynebacterium pyogenes*. It is a Gram-positive pleomorphic rod/coccus. It can haemolyse 5% horse blood, produces β glucuronidase, hydrolyses starch and gelatine, and produces acid from various sugars. Veterinary infections are more common than human. Nevertheless, it has on occasions been implicated in human pneumonia, lung abscess and empyema[24]. The possibility remains that the organism might on occasions have been confused with *Arcanobacterium haemolyticum*[25].

Nocardiosis

Nocardial infections are said most often to affect the immunocompromised host, although perhaps 30% or more of infections occur in the immunocompetent. The majority of patients present with pulmonary symptoms.

The organism

Nocardia was first discovered by Nocard in 1888 as the causative agent of disease in cattle. *Nocardia* unlike *Actinomyces* spp. is exclusively aerobic and partially acid fast, though not in older cultured strains. This Gram-positive variably weakly acid-fast facultative intracellular rod shares the morphological characteristics of branching filamentous bacteria. *Nocardia* spp. produce characteristic beading. Sputum has to be stained with Gram's and ZN/Kinyoun stains as haematoxylin/eosin is not satisfactory. Acid fastness occurs in most *N. asteroides* isolates, less so with other species. This property can serve to differentiate *Nocardia* spp. from *Actinomyces. Nocardia* forms spore-like cells which are capable of aerolisation. Colony formation is characteristically large (several mm) and coloured white/yellow/red. Its property of digesting paraffin provides the laboratory basis for separation from similar organisms (paraffin baiting). Culture may take up to 4 weeks before a specific microbiological diagnosis can be made. Multiple specimen collection whilst patients do not receive antibiotics is generally necessary to optimise the diagnostic sensitivity. Of the nine species, the most frequently isolated human pathogen is *Nocardia asteroides* (85% of cases) followed by *Nocardia brasiliensis*. *Nocardia otitidiscavarium* (*Nocardia caviae*), *Nocardia farcinica*, *Nocardia nova* and *Nocardia transvalensis* have been less frequently cited as causative agents. *N. asteroides* is usually responsible for pulmonary disease, whereas *N. brasiliensis* is mainly associated with soft tissue infections.

Epidemiology

The organisms are ubiquitous in soil. They are generally not considered to be commensal in humans. They can cause infection, mainly local skin disease, but some patients have pulmonary disease. Patients may be immunocompetent[26,27] or immunocompromised (usually pulmonary and systemic disease)[26,27]; particularly those with disturbed cell-mediated immunity. Nocardial infection is acquired mainly through inhalation, although direct inoculation for example, at surgery, trauma via tick bites, and intravenous injections are less common means. Haematogenous dissemination can occur from the primary pulmonary site in up to 45% of cases. Evidence for patient to patient transmission has not been fully substantiated but nosocomial outbreaks or clustering of cases have been documented[28,29]. Other such documented instances include an outbreak of nocardial infection on a liver unit from brick/plaster dust during hospital renovation[30] and spread in a renal unit from a patient with urinary excretion[31]. These phenomena suggest that person to person transmission may occur and that patients with *Nocardia* should be isolated to prevent spread to immunocompromised patients. In 1976, up to 1000 cases of nocardiosis per year occurred in the USA[32]. This number has now been superseded because of the growing population of immunocompromised patients and the global pandemic of HIV. In Queensland alone, over a 5-year period ending 1988, 102 isolates from 93 patients were reported[27] with an increasing number of referred strains occurring since 1983. Considerable under-reporting almost certainly occurs because of confusion with other diseases such as TB, the need for prolonged growth requirements and in addition, failure or inability to look for the organism in laboratory specimens. Pulmonary nocardiosis may occur and be overlooked in a substantial number of patients with chronic respiratory tract disease in developing countries, for example, parts of Africa[33].

As mentioned previously, many nocardial infections occur in patients with at least some degree of immunosuppression or predisposing factors. Of 29 cases of pulmonary/systemic infection, 20 had underlying chronic pulmonary disease, mainly chronic obstructive airways disease, bronchiectasis and pulmonary fibrosis, sometimes in association with immunosuppressive treatment – mainly steroids or cytotoxic drugs[27]. Nocardiosis is particularly well documented in solid organ transplants. For example, approximately 6–13% of cardiac transplant recipients and 0.7–3% of renal transplant recipients develop *Nocardia* infection[34–37]. It is recognised in other transplant populations, for example, bone marrow transplant recipients[38]. The occurrence of nocardiosis in these patients is highest at the peak of immunesuppressive therapy, usually within the first year and at times of anti-rejection therapy. However, as cyclosporin A has become more commonly used for immunosuppressive therapy, there appears to have been a decrease in the number of *Nocardia* cases, which may explain the unusually high incidence in some centres prior to cyclosporin use, for example, a 37% incidence[39]. An incidence of 0.7% among renal transplant recipients was documented in patients given cyclosporin A–prednisone compared to 2.6% given anzathioprine–prednisone. Approximately one-fifth of the patients with *Nocardia* have cancer[32] and many of these have reticulo-endothelial malignancies or haematological cancers[40]. Other risk factors for *Nocardia* include patients receiving cytotoxic therapy, steroid use, alcoholism, alveolar proteinosis, diseases with an autoimmune basis such as rheumatoid arthritis, pemphigus, glomerulo-nephritis and chronic liver disease. HIV infection has recently been added to the list of antecedent conditions[41]. Chronic granulomatous disease and patients with immunoglobulin disorders are also at risk. Rarely, nocardiosis can produce chronic pulmonary disease in the absence of risk factors – this may sometimes assume a life-threatening illness[42].

Nocardiosis can present with pulmonary, cutaneous, central nervous system and other system involvement. The relative frequency of reporting of a specific system or organ involvement depends upon the clinical practice observed. For example, in relatively unselected data from the Queensland State Health Laboratory, the frequency of pulmonary/systemic infection was roughly similar to that of skin and soft tissue infections[27] whereas in cancer patients approximately three-quarters of cases are pulmonary[43] and in solid organ transplant patients it accounts for up to 90% of cases[34]. In a comprehensive review of the English literature from 1961–1972, 73% of 243 cases had lung involvement[44].

Simultaneous infection with *Nocardia* and *Mycobacterium tuberculosis* or non-tuberculosis mycobacteriosis has been described in both HIV positive and HIV negative patients[41].

Virulence – host factors and pathogenesis

Although cell-mediated immune mechanisms are the most important in regulating infection, neutrophil and immunoglobulin defects are also thought to be contributory predisposing factors. In general, phagocytosis by neutrophils and the alveolar macrophage is the first line of defence against this organism in the lung. For example, infection in laboratory animals is worse if phagocytosis is inhibited by mucin coating of the organism. Lack of production of toxic oxygen radicals, for example, in patients with chronic granulomatous disease is a predisposition to nocardiosis. Nevertheless, even in patients with normal neutrophil function, the organism produces catalase and superoxide dismutase enzymes to resist intracellular killing following phagocytosis by the alveolar macrophage. The neutrophil response appears only to inhibit *Nocardia*, whilst intact cell-mediated immunity is necessary to complete cure via lymphocyte-directed killing effects. The secondary role of the neutrophil in patients with *Nocardia* infections is exemplified by the finding that only 25% of cancer patients with *Nocardia* are neutropenic[43]. Virulence of *Nocardia* is related to cell mycolic acid composition – organisms in an active peak growth phase have an advantageous mycolic acid profile, which produces cord factor, and gives rise to calcium-dependent inhibition of macrophage lysosome and phagosome fusion. This virulence factor leads to increased bacterial growth in the host, and increased tropism for tissues, including the brain. The interdependence of the various arms of the immune system is demonstrated by the finding that splenectomized patients are vulnerable to nocardiosis, more so if there is an associated underlying haematological malignancy[45].

Pulmonary lesions are typified by multiple pyogenic abscesses with central necrosis and polymorph infiltration. Granulomas similar to those in TB may occasionally occur. It is unusual for these inflammatory tissues to have a firm boundary or to be associated with a distinct fibrotic reaction – extension of the inflammatory edges of the lesion to breach adjacent anatomical boundaries usually occurs, for example, to the pleura, ribs and vertebrae or chest wall with sinus formation. Sulphur granules may be found in draining sinuses. Extra pulmonary dissemination to the central nervous systems, skin, kidneys, etc, may occur. Later, lung volume loss, cavity formation and pulmonary fibrosis may be found. There is an association with bronchiolitis obliterans[46]. In highly immune suppressed individuals *Nocardia* may be particularly aggressive, leading to pulmonary necrosis.

Clinical features

Patients are usually male, aged between 20 and 50 years, with an antecedent risk factor. However, an age range of 4 weeks to over 80 years has been reported. Presentation is typically with a productive cough of some weeks' duration associated with fatigue, weight loss, fever, dyspnoea and thoracic chest pain[26]. Haemoptysis may occur, particularly in patients with cavitation. Sometimes the presentation is virtually asymptomatic and abnormal chest radiograph findings may be discovered as part of a routine work-up. Unusually, the disease can present in an acute fashion which may be fatal[45]. The most common presentation, however is chronic, of some weeks' duration and often mimicking other chronic lung diseases such as pneumonia, fungal disease or pulmonary neoplasm. It may resolve spontaneously. Extrapulmonary manifestations may be present as secondary phenomena following dissemination, which occurs in 50% of patients with pulmonary *Nocardia*, or as a primary inoculation event. These include most commonly skin lesions with firm, subcutaneous nodules or abscesses, cellulitis, pyoderma and lympho-cutaneous manifestations. Local skin primary infection include cellulitis, lymphangitis and mycetoma. Headaches, confusion, convulsions, focal neurological signs and neck stiffness all suggest meningitis or an intracerebral abscess. Up to 25% of patients with pulmonary *Nocardia* have CNS involvement. Virtually any organ can be involved, including the eyes, heart valves, kidneys, mediastinum, bones, testicles and ilio-psoas muscles. A miliary picture can also present. Disseminated disease is particularly common in transplant recipients[34]. Fistula formation and necrotising pneumonia can also occur, mimicking actinomycosis, tuberculosis and fungal disease.

A form of chronic lung disease due to *Nocardia* occurring in patients without substantial immunosuppression, but who abuse alcohol, has been described in Africa and may be undiagnosed in other developing countries[33]. Haemoptysis appears to be a prominent feature in these patients. Most of these have been suspected to have had TB but the absence of *M. tuberculosis*, and the positive response to sulphonamides has supported the causal role for *Nocardia* in these patients.

Nocardiosis can be recurrent or relapsing, even on treatment, particularly so if secondary antibacterial prophylaxis is not given[45,47]. Association with *M. tuberculosis* and with *Aspergillus*[48] has been described. Not all presentations are florid and it is quite possible that nocardiosis may also present with mild upper respiratory tract infections such as pharyngitis or bronchitis[49].

Radiological abnormalities (Fig. 12.4) are highly variable and include unilateral or bilateral segmental infiltrates, lobar infiltrates, necrotising pneumonia, solitary and multiple nodules, honeycombing, miliary pattern, abscesses, pleural effusion, hilar/mediastinal lymphadenopathy and cavitation (in up to 60% in some series)[26,49,50]. Fungal balls may be observed.

The mortality in patients with pulmonary and disseminated disease is of the order of 25%, rising to over 40% in patients with central nervous system disease. Poor prognostic factors include acute onset disease, patients receiving cytotoxic therapy, patients with high levels of endogenous/exogenous steroids and those with dissemination, particularly to the brain[51]. Prompt recognition and treatment of *Nocardia* will achieve mortality rates well under 10%[36].

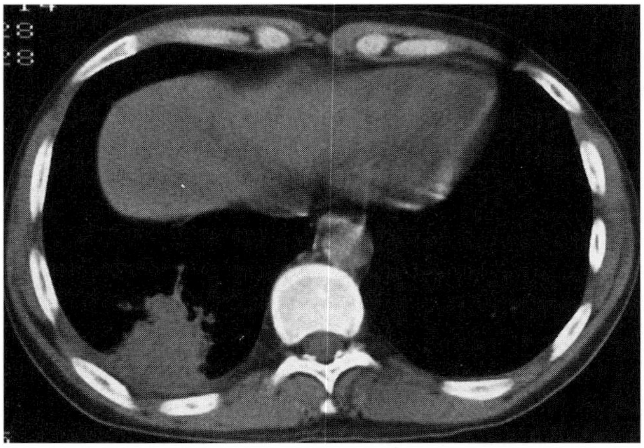

FIGURE 12.4 Renal transplantation, Hodgkin's disease. 'Triangular'-shaped density right lower lobe: *Nocardia*.

HIV and *Nocardia*

Nocardiosis has recently been recognised in patients with advanced HIV[3,41]. The incidence may be underestimated for reasons of lack of reporting, widespread use of cotrimoxazole prophylaxis and low diagnostic threshold. Presumably the profound loss of CD4 lymphocytes is the key predisposing immunological event, since most infections occur in patients with a CD4 count of $< 0.2 \times 10^9$/l. In 42% of such patients *Nocardia* was the initial major infection, despite not being listed as an indicator disease for AIDS. Although pulmonary symptoms are the most common presenting feature, evidence of dissemination is present in more than 80% of cases. The clinical features of *Nocardia* infection *per se* are similar to those in non-HIV patients, although primary extrapulmonary disease as well as dissemination tend to be more severe[41] and the patients may have an increased incidence of radiological evident cavitation[50]. Adverse reactions to co-trimoxazole are common in HIV patients and alternative antimicrobial therapy is necessary. Relapse is common and indicates the need for lifelong secondary prophylaxis.

Diagnosis and management

Diagnosis in patients without underlying disease is often delayed and unsuspected though nocardiosis should be among the differential diagnoses in patients with the chronic pneumonia syndrome. It should be part of the differential diagnosis of chronic and acute pulmonary disease in immunosuppressed patients. A combination of pneumonia, subcutaneous nodules and CNS disease requires that nocardiosis be excluded[51,52].

There may be associated mild leukocytosis; mild anaemia of chronic illness is common. There has been debate over the significance of a positive sputum examination since this finding could reflect colonisation from environmental inhalation. Nine of 25 patients in one series with positive sputum samples had no active clinical/radiological disease and did not progress[53]. However, observations of large numbers of sputum specimens submitted for mycological examination have not supported this supposition, so that the finding of *Nocardia* on sputum culture is virtually pathognomonic of disease[54]. Other workers have suggested that a positive stain rather than culture, and prior steroid use favours infection rather than colonisation[55]. In addition, care over the use of decontamination agents in sputum is necessary to avoid destroying *Nocardia*. If sputum proves negative, invasive diagnostic techniques are indicated, particularly BAL, transbronchial biopsy or open lung biopsy. Blood cultures are rarely positive. Serological confirmation tests are of limited use but an enzyme immunoassay test detecting antibody to a specific nocardial antigen is available[56]. Other means for diagnosis include detection of metabolites by frequency-pulsed electron capture gas–liquid chromatography of serum and other fluids[57].

Sulphonamides remain the mainstay of treatment for *N. asteroides* infections. Although sulphamethoxazole and trimethoprim are synergistic *in vitro*, measurement of serum levels has indicated that subtherapeutic amounts of the trimethoprim component are often present. Evidence for a heightened clinical therapeutic response of co-trimoxazole compared to sulphamethoxizole is lacking. Despite this, co-trimoxazole is widely used for the treatment of *Nocardia*. More than 90% of clinical isolates of *N. asteroides* currently remain susceptible to co-trimoxazole or sulphamethoxizole[57]. The dosage of sulfadiazine is between 4 and 9 g/day and that of co-trimoxazole is 640–1920 mg trimethoprim plus 3200–9600 mg sulphamethoxizole. Co-trimoxazole penetrates well into most body tissues, including the brain, and this property may be useful for the treatment of subclinical and extra-pulmonary metastatic foci. Ideally, sulphonamide blood levels should be maintained between 10 and 20 mgs/l. Treatment should continue for at least 6 weeks and longer courses of at least 3–6 months are probably necessary to prevent relapse[47]. Patients who are immunosuppressed or who have CNS disease should receive treatment for 12 months. Highly immunosuppressed patients may need indefinite therapy. Toxicity with co-trimoxazole, particularly in HIV patients, can be troublesome and leads to discontinuation of the drug in some 50% of patients[3]. In bone marrow transplant recipients, marrow suppression occurs in up to 20%. Furthermore, there have been some treatment failures with co-trimoxazole. Multiple drug-resistant *N. asteroides* infections are described[58]. Therefore, alternative effective antimicrobial regimes are necessary. Minocycline, amikacin, ceftriaxone, imipenem and cefotaxime have proven *in vitro* activity[59]. Combinations of antimicrobials such as minocycline with co-trimoxazole, amikacin with imipenem, cefotaxine or amikacin plus cefuroxime, ampicillin with erythromycin, show excellent activity *in vitro* and in animal models[60]. Ampicillin-clavulanic acid may prove useful in the face of betalactamase-producing strains. Other agents which may be used include cycloserine and ciprofloxacin. Some new quinolones have shown improved activity against *N. asteroides* compared with the relatively poor activity of norfloxacin and ciprofloxacin. Two new aminoglycosides have been shown to exhibit potent *in vitro* inhibitory effects[61]. Rifampicin resistance is usual.

In addition to antimicrobial therapy, surgical resection or drainage of thoracic abscesses or empyema is necessary. Non-response to treatment may indicate resistant strains, subtherapeutic levels of antibiotics, abscess formation or a coexisting pathogen, e.g., *Aspergillus*, *Pneumocystis carinii*, *Cryptococcus* spp. or *M. tuberculosis*.

Other nocardial species implicated in pulmonary disease

N. asteroides

This is the predominant human pathogen in *Nocardia* infections in general and pulmonary disease in particular. *N braziliensis* accounts for approximately 20% of all Nocardial infections which are mainly non-pulmonary and *N cavii* for less than 5%[59,62]. Pulmonary disease expression and response to antibiotics are indistinguishable between the species. In addition, there have been two recently described *Nocardia* spp., namely, *N. transvalensis* and *N. farcinica*.

N. transvalensis

This species had been formerly thought only to be associated with mycetoma. However, it appears to have acquired a niche in the immunocompromised population where it can produce pulmonary and disseminated disease similar to that caused by *N. asteroides*. It has been described particularly in the south-west USA and north-east Australia. A recent review has described ten patients with confirmed infection and the biochemical characteristics of the isolates have been documented[63]. The clinical outcome was generally good but one patient with disseminated disease and one patient with a brain abscess died. Most isolates of *N. transvalensis* appear to be more resistant than *N. asteroides* to antibiotics, particularly to augmentin, doxycycline and third generation cephalosporins. Nevertheless, co-trimoxazole remains the first line antimicrobial agent.

N. farcinica

Infection with this organism may well have been underdiagnosed formerly since up to one-fifth of isolates previously classified as *N. asteroides* were in fact *N. farcinica*[59]. However, *N. farcinica* appears to produce a similar profile of disease to that caused by *N. asteroides*, the species appears to be more virulent, and resistance to cefotaxime, ceftriaxone, ampicillin and aminoglycosides is virtually 100%, but they usually remain sensitive to co-trimoxazole[64].

References

1. BROWN JR. Human actinomycosis: a study of 181 subjects. *Hum Pathol* 1973;4:319–30.
2. WEESE WC, SMITH LC, STUNTER G, SMITH JM. Antimicrobial susceptibility patterns of *Nocardia asteroides. Antimicrob Agents Chemother* 1988;32:1776–9.
3. JAVALY K, HOROWITZ HW, WORMSER GP Nocardiosis in patients with human immunodeficiency virus infection: report of 2 cases and review of the literature. *Medicine* 1992;71:128–38.
4. KINNEAR WJM, MACFARLANE JT. A survey of thoracic actinomycosis. *Resp Med* 1990;84:57–9.
5. HSIEH MJ, LIU HP, CHANG JP, CHANG CH. Thoracic actinomycosis. *Chest* 1992;104:366–70.
6. HAMER DH, SCHWAB LE, GRAY R. Massive haemoptysis from thoracic actinomycosis successfully treated by embolization. *Chest* 1992;101:1442–3.
7. PRATHER JR, EASTRIDGE CE, HUGHES JR FA, MCCAUGHAN JR JJ. Actinomycosis of the thorax. *Ann Thorac Surg* 1970;9:307–12.
8. O'SULLIVAN RA, ARMSTRONG JG, RIVER JT, MITCHELL CA. Pulmonary actinomycosis complicated by effusive constrictive pericarditis. *Aust NZ J Med* 1991;21:879–80.
9. MORGAN DE, NATH H, SANDERS C, HASSON JH. Mediastinal actinomycosis. *Am J Radiol* 1990;155:735–7.
10. KWONG JS, MULLER NL, GODWIN JD, ABERLE D, GRYMALOSKI MR. Thoracic actinomycosis: CT findings in eight patients. *Radiology* 1992;183:189–92.
11. LAU K-Y. Endobronchial actinomycosis mimicking pulmonary neoplasm. *Thorax* 1992;47:664–5.
12. DICPINIGAITIS PV, BLEIWEISS IJ, KRELLENSTEIN DJ, HALTON KP, TEIRSTEIN AS. Primary endobronchial actinomycosis in association with foreign body aspiration. *Chest* 1992;101:283–5.
13. LENOIR P, GILBERT L, GOOSSENS A, TEMPELS D, ALEXANDER M, DAB I. Bronchoscopic diagnosis of an unusual presentation of pulmonary actinomycosis. *Pediat Pulmonol* 1993;16:138–40.
14. WEBB AK, HOWELL R, HICKMAN JA. Thoracic actinomycosis presenting with peripheral skin lesions. *Thorax* 1978;33:818–19.
15. MAJID AA, RATHAKRISHNAN V, ALHADY SF. Computed tomography as an aid to diagnosis of early pulmonary actinomycosis. *J Roy Soc Med* 1991;84:686–7.
16. TYRRELL J, NOONE P, PRICHARD JS. Thoracic actinomycosis complicated by

Actinobacillus actinomycetem comitans: case report and review of literature. *Resp Med* 1992;86:341–3.

17. ZIJLSTRA EE, SWART GR, GODFROY FJM, DEGENER JE. Pericarditis, pneumonia and brain abscess due to a combined *Actinomyces – Actinobacillus actinomycetemcomitans* infection. *J Infect* 1992;25:83–7.

18. MORRIS JF, SEWELL DL. Necrotizing pneumonia caused by mixed infection with *Actinobacillus actinomycetemcomitans* and *Actinomyces israelii:* case report and review. *Clin Infect Dis* 1994;18:450–2.

19. PAGE MI, KING EO. Infection due to *Actinobacillus actinomycetemcomitans* and *Haemophilus aphrophilus. N Engl J Med* 1966;275:181–8.

20. JARA FM, TOLEDO-PEREYRA LH, MAGILLIGEN DJ Surgical implications of pulmonary actinomycosis. *J Thorac Cardiovas Surg* 1979;78:600–4.

21. SLUTZKER AD, CLAYPOOL WD. Pericardial actinomycosis with cardiac tamponade from a contiguous thoracic lesion. *Thorax* 1989;44:442–3.

22. MADER JT, WILSON KJ. Actinomycosis. A review of utilization of hyperbaric oxygenation. *Hyper Oxy Rev* 1981;2:177–88.

23. HAPPONEN RP, VIANDER M. Comparison of fluorescent antibody technique and conventional staining methods on diagnosis of cervico-facial actinomycosis. *J Oral Pathol* 1982;11:417–25.

24. DRANCOURT M, OULÈS O, BOUCHE V, PELOUX Y. Two cases of *Actinomyces pyogenes* infection in humans. *Eur J Clin Microbiol Infect Dis* 1993;12:55–7.

25. GAHRN-HANSEN B, FREDERIKSEN W. Human infections with *Actinomyces pyogens (Corynebacteriumpyogenes). Diag Microbiol Infect Dis* 1992;15:349–54.

26. CURRY WA. Human nocardiosis: a clinical review with selected case reports. *Arch Intern Med* 1980;140:818–26.

27. GEORGHIOU PR, BLACKLOCK ZM. Infection with *Nocardia* species in Queensland. *Med J Aust* 1989;156:692–7.

28. BADDOUR LM, BASELSKI VS, HERR MJ *et al.* Nocardiosis in recipients of renal transplants: evidence for nosocomial acquisition. *Am J Infect Control* 1986;14:214–9.

29. HELLYAR AG. Experience with *Nocardia asteroides* in renal transplant recipients. *J Hosp Infect* 1988;12:13–8.

30. SAHATHEVAN M, HARVEY FAH, FORBES G *et al.* Epidemiology, bacteriology and control of an outbreak of *Nocardia asteroides* infection on a liver unit. *J Hosp Infect* 1991;18:473–80.

31. HOUANG ET, LOVETT IS, THOMPSON FD, HARRISON AR, JOEKES AM, GOODFELLOW M. *Nocardia asteroides* infection – a transmissible disease. *J Hosp Infect* 1980;1:31–40.

32. BEAMAN BL, BURNSIDE J, EDWARDS B, CAUSEY W. Nocardial infections in the United States, 1972–1974. *J Infect Dis* 1976;134:286–9.

33. BAILY GG, NEILL P, ROBERTSON VJ. Nocardiosis: a neglected chronic lung disease in Africa? *Thorax* 1988;43:905–10.

34. WILSON JP, TURNER HR, KIRCHNER KA, CHAPMAN SW. Nocardial infections in renal transplant recipients. *Medicine* 1989;68:38–57.

35. KIRKLIN JK, NAFTEL DC, MCGOFFEN DC *et al.* Analysis of morbid events and risk factors for death after cardiac transplantation. *J Am Coll Cardiol* 1988;11:917–24.

36. SIMPSON GL, STINSON EB, EGGER MJ *et al.* Nocardial infections in the immunocompromised host: a detailed study in a defined population. *Rev Infect Dis* 1981;3:492–507.

37. ARDUINO RC, JOHNSON PC, MIRANDA AG. Nocardiosis in renal transplant recipients undergoing immunosuppression with cyclosporin. *Clin Infect Dis* 1993;16:505–12.

38. HODOHARA K, FUJIYAMA Y, HIRAMITU Y *et al.* Disseminated subcutaneous *Nocardia asteroides* abscesses in a patient after one marrow transplantation. *Bone Marrow Transpl* 1992;11:341–3.

39. MAMMANA RB, PETERSEN EA, FULLER FK, SIROKY K, COPELAND JG. Pulmonary infections in cardiac transplant patients: modes of diagnosis, complications and effectiveness of therapy. *Ann Thorac Surg* 1983;36:700–5.

40. BERKEY P, BODEY GP. Nocardial infection in patients with neoplastic disease. *Rev Infect Dis* 1989;11:407–12.

41. KIM J, MINAMOTO GY, GRIECO MH. Nocardial infection as a complication of AIDS: report of six cases and review. *Rev Infect Dis* 1991;13:624–9.

42. BRECHOT JM, CAPRON F, PRUDENT J, ROCHEMAURE J. Unexpected pulmonary nocardiosis in a non-immunocompromised patient. *Thorax* 1987;42:479–80.

43. BODEY OP. Infections in cancer patients. *Cancer Treatment Rev* 1975;2:89–95.

44. PALMER DL, HARVEY RL, WHEELER JK. Diagnostic and therapeutic considerations in *Nocardia asteroides* infection. *Medicine* 1974;53:391–401.

45. ABDI EA, DING JC, COOPER IA Nocardia infection in splenectomized patients: case reports and a review of the literature. *Postgrad Med J* 1987;63:455–8.

46. CAMP M, MEHTA JB, WHITSON M. Bronchiolitis obliterans and *Nocardia asteroides* infection of the lung. *Chest* 1987;92:1107–8.

47. KING CT, CHAPMAN SW, BUTKUS DE. Recurrent nocardiosis in a renal transplant recipient. *South Med J* 1993;86:225–8.

48. MONTEFORTE JS, WOOD CA. Pneumonia caused by *Nocardia nova* and *Aspergillus fumigatus* after cardiac transplantation. *Eur J Clin Microbiol Infect Dis* 1993; 12:112–14.

49. YOUNG LS, ARMSTRONG D, BLEVINS A, LIEBERMAN P. *Nocardia asteroides* infection complicating neoplastic disease. *Am J Med* 1970;50:356–67.

50. KRAMER MR, UTTAMCHANDANI RB The radiographic appearance of pulmonary nocardiosis associated with AIDS. *Chest* 1990;98:382–5.

51. PREASANT CA, WIERNIK PH, SERPICK AA. Factors affecting survival in nocardiosis. *Am Rev Resp Dis* 1973;108:1444–8.

52. FRAZIER AR, ROSENOW III EC, ROBERTS GD. Nocardiosis. A review of 25 cases occurring during 24 months. *Mayo Clin Proc* 1975;50:657–63.

53. RAICH RA, CASEY F, HALL WH. Pulmonary and cutaneous nocardiosis. *Am Rev Resp Dis* 1961;83:505–11.

54. ROSETT W, HODGES GR. Recent experience with nocardial infections. *Am J Med* 1978;276:279–85.

55. ANGELES AM, SUGAR AM. Rapid diagnosis of nocardiosis with an enzyme immunoassay. *J Infect Dis* 1987;155:292–6.

56. BROOKS JB, KASIN JV, FAST DM, DANESHUAR MI. Detection of metabolites by frequency-pulsed electron capture gas-liquid chromatography in serum and cerebrospinal fluid of a pateint with *Nocardia* infection. *J Clin Microbiol* 1987;25:445–8.

57. MCNEIL MM, BROWN JM, JARVIS WR, AJELLO L. Comparison of species distribution and antimicrobial susceptibility of aerobic actinomycetes from clinical specimens. *Rev Infect Dis* 1990;12:778–83.

58. JOSHI N, HAMORY BH Drug-resistant *Nocardia asteroides* infection in a patient with acquired immunodeficiency syndrome. *South Med J* 1991;84:1155–6.

59. WALLACE RJ, STEELE LC, SUMTER G, SMITH JM. Antimicrobial susceptibility patterns of *Nocardia asteroides. Antimicrob Agents Chemother* 1988;32:1776–9.

60. GOMBERT ME, BERKOWITZ LB, AULICINO TM, DU BOUCHET L. Therapy of pulmonary nocardiosis in immunocompromised mice. *Antimicrob Agent Chemother* 1990;34:1766–8.

61. KHARDORI N, SHAWAR R, GUPTA R, ROSENBAUM B. *In vitro* antimicrobial susceptibilities of *Nocardia* species. *Antimicrob Agent Chemother* 1993;37:882–4.
62. SATH B, FREGAN C, HUSSAIN A, JAULIM A, WHALE K, WEBB A. Pulmonary infection with *Nocardia caviae* in a patient with diabetes mellitus and liver cirrhosis. *Thorax* 1988;43:933–4.
63. MCNEIL MM, BROWN JM, GEORGHIOU PR *et al.* Infections due to *Nocardia transvalensis:* clinical spectrum and antimicrobial therapy. *Clin Infect Dis* 1992;15:453–63.
64. SCHIFF TA, MCNEIL MM, BROWN JM. Cutaneous *Nocardia farcinica* infeciton in a nonimmunocompromised patient: case report and review. *Clin Infect Dis* 1993;16:756–60.

13 Pneumonia due to small bacterial organisms

J. GRAHAM DOUGLAS
Aberdeen Royal Infirmary, Scotland, UK

Introduction

Mycoplasma pneumoniae, Chlamydia psittaci and *Chlamydia pneumoniae* and *Coxiella burnetti* are now widely recognised as causes of lower respiratory tract infection and pneumonia. They are all relatively small bacterial organisms which do not have effective cell walls and are resistant to the action of β-lactam antibiotics. They are, therefore, grouped together in this chapter under the heading of 'small bacterial organisms'.

Mycoplasma pneumoniae

Mycoplasmas are ubiquitous pathogens in the plant and animal kingdoms. They represent the smallest known free-living forms being prokaryotes that lack a cell wall. They are bounded by a cell membrane containing sterols, substances not found in either other bacteria or viruses. Because of their small size (150–250 nm) when first discovered they were thought to be viruses.[1] However, their ability to grow in cell-free media and the fact that they contain both RNA and DNA clearly sets them apart from viruses. In addition, DNA homology studies have failed to demonstrate any significant relationship between mycoplasmas and known bacteria. As a result, mycoplasmas have now been assigned taxonomically to their own class, Mollicutes, within which the family, Mycoplasmataceae, contains the genus subgroup, *M. pneumoniae,* which can cause respiratory tract infection and pneumonia. This organism is primarily an extracelluar parasite which attaches to the surface of ciliated and non-ciliated epithelial cells and causes cell damage by elaboration of substances such as hydrogen peroxide and by initiation of an inflammatory response through chemotaxis of mononuclear cells.[2]

History

In 1944 Eaton and his colleagues described an agent that passed through virus filters and caused focal areas of pneumonia when inoculated into several species of rodent.[3] The relationship of this agent to the human primary atypical pneumonia syndrome was suggested by the fact that serum from some patients recovering from this pneumonia neutralised the agent.[4] In 1946, the disease could be transmitted to human volunteers by ultrafiltrates from patients[5] and in 1961 convalescent serum from volunteers inoculated with ultrafiltrate from patients with atypical pneumonia was shown to neutralise Eaton's chick embryo 'virus'.[6] The ultimate proof of the role of this Eaton agent in atypical pneumonia was the demonstration that the organism isolated in cell-free culture produced the syndrome in volunteers.[7]

Microbiology

M. pneumoniae is capable of growth on cell-free defined media, setting it apart from all but one (*Legionella*) of the common causes of pneumonia. Unlike most other mycoplasmas, it grows well aerobically and ferments glucose as its primary energy source producing acid. As previously mentioned, it is an extremely small organism, a short rod about 10 × 200 nm and has, at one end, an organelle that is responsible for attachment of the organism to cell membranes. The major protein of this organelle has been purified and it has been suggested that this peptide would serve well as an antigen for a vaccine.

Immunology

Mycoplasmas are active in stimulating cell components of the immune system. They can act as polyclonal T-cell and B-cell activators[8] and can cause capping of lymphocytes.[9] They are capable of inducing several cytokines including granulocyte-macrophage stimulating factor[10] and interferon[11] but not cytokine IL-2.[12]

In the course of infection, several classes of antibody are produced. Some of these neutralise the organism while others appear to be autoantibodies. The best known of these autoantibodies are the cold isohaemagglutinins first described by Finland and colleagues in 1943.[13] These cold agglutinins are found in 50–70% of patients with mycoplasma pneumonia. They are capable of clumping erythrocytes at 4 °C and agglutination can be reversed by warming the serum-erythrocyte mixture to 37 °C. These antibodies have been shown to be oligoclonal IgM antibodies directed against an altered I antigen on the surface of erythrocytes of infected patients.[14] The I antigen is one of the blood group antigens, but unlike A and B isoantigens seems to be common to almost all mature erythrocytes. Like other IgM antibodies, these mycoplasma induced cold agglutinins develop early in the disease at 7–10 days. They tend to peak at 2–3 weeks and persist for 2–3 months. The role of these antibodies in the pathogenesis of mycoplasma infection remains unclear. High titres of cold agglutinins in mycoplasma infection have been associated with Coomb's positive haemolytic anaemia,[15] chronic renal failure[16] and Raynaud's phenomenon.

M. pneumoniae infection also leads to production of complement fixing antibodies. These arise at 2–3 weeks after infection and persist for 2–3 months. Assay for *M. pneumoniae*-specific complement fixing antibodies has been the standard method for detection of infection.

It was hoped that the detection of IgM against *M. pneumoniae* would lead to more rapid and early diagnosis of infection. However, specific IgM is usually only detectable in children during a primary infection with *M. pneumoniae* and in contrast, many adults with this infection do not produce an IgM response. In addition, some methods of detection of specific IgM antibodies, particularly the particle agglutination assay tend to produce false-positive results. Therefore, unfortunately, serological tests for IgM against *M. pneumoniae* cannot be relied on particularly in adults. Development of assays for detection of IgA against *M. pneumoniae* are currently being assessed.

Epidemiology

M. pneumoniae infection is acquired by inhalation of respiratory droplets from an infected coughing individual. In closed populations such as military recruit camps or boarding schools, mycoplasma can cause mini-epidemics.[17] Serologically based epidemiological studies throughout the world have documented the high incidence of mycoplasma respiratory infection.[18,19] In the United States it is estimated that at least one case of mycoplasmal pneumonia occurs for each 1000 population per year and the incidence of non-pneumonic respiratory infection may be 10–20 times higher.[20] Although infection can occur at any age, the highest incidence is in those aged 5–20 years and mycoplasmal pneumonia is unusual over those aged 45 years. Younger children tend to develop upper respiratory tract symptoms while teenagers and young adults may develop pneumonia. Although 25% of *M. pneumoniae* infections are thought to be symptomless, about 75% of reported cases are of lower respiratory tract infections.[21]

Since the mid-1970s epidemics of infection due to mycoplasma pneumoniae have been observed in approximately 4-yearly cycles. Statistics from the Communicable Diseases Surveillance Centre of the Public Health Laboratory Service, UK, have shown peaks of infection in England and Wales in 1979, 83, 87, 91 and in Spring 1995 (Fig. 13.1). The reasons behind this cyclical pattern remain obscure.[22]

Table 13.1. *Clinical features of small bacterial pneumonias*

Characteristics	*Mycoplasma pneumoniae*	*Chlamydia psittaci*	*Chlamydia pneumoniae*	*Coxiella burnetti*
Symptoms				
Cough	+	+	+	+
Confusion	±	±	–	–
Headache	+	+	–	+
Myalgira	+	+	±	+
Ear pain	±	–	–	–
Meningism	–	+	–	–
Pleuritic pain	±	–	–	+
Abdominal pain	–	–	–	–
Diarrhoea	+	–	–	+
Signs				
Fever	+	+	+	+
Rash	E. multiforme	Horder's spots	–	–
Pharyngitis	+	+	+	–
Haemoptysis	–	±	–	–
Lobar consolidation	±	±	–	±
Splenomegaly	–	+	–	–
Rel. bradycardia	–	+	–	–

Key: – = not present.
± = occasionally reported.
+ = commonly reported.

Clinical features

The major clinical features of small bacterial pneumonias are summarised in Table 13.1. Symptoms develop 1–3 weeks after infection. There is usually an insidious onset of fever, malaise, headache and cough. The frequency and severity of cough increase over the next few days. This gradual onset of symptoms is in contrast to the more abrupt presentation of symptoms due to influenza and adenovirus infections.

In up to 25% of patients the illness progresses to tracheobronchitis or pneumonia. The cough becomes more severe, is usually non productive but may yield white sputum in about 30% of cases. Gram's staining of sputum reveals inflammatory cells but no organisms. With prolonged coughing, parasternal chest soreness can occur but pleuritic chest pain is rare. A mild fever continues but rigors are unusual.

In those who develop pneumonia, examination of the chest reveals localised crackles and wheeze but usually no signs of consolidation. There is often a disparity between the physical findings on chest examination and the chest X-ray evidence of pneumonia. While most cases of pneumonia due to mycoplasma are benign and self-limiting, severe disease can occur with multi-lobed consolidation, lung abscesses, pneumatocoeles, development of adult respiratory distress syndrome, chronic interstitial pulmonary fibrosis and Macleod's syndrome.[23,24] Although pleuritic chest pain is unusual, small pleural effusions occur in 5–20% of patients with mycoplasmal pneumonia.[25] Fever, headache and malaise usually resolve in 3–10 days but respiratory symptoms and signs take longer.

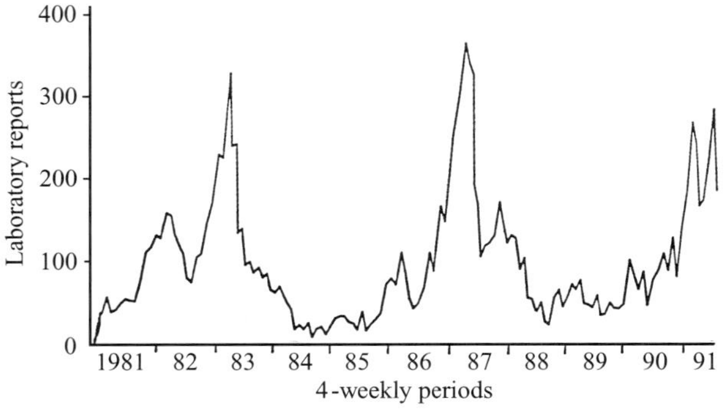

FIGURE 13.1 Variation in mycoplasma infection in England and Wales between 1981 and 1991.

Extrapulmonary manifestations

Abnormalities in almost every organ system have been described in *M. pneumoniae* infection (Table 13.2). The pathogenesis of these extrapulmonary sequelae is unclear, but severe complications have been reported in 2–10% of all confirmed mycoplasmal infections.[26] Extrapulmonary manifestations develop within 21 days of onset of the respiratory illness, although in some patients there is no history

Table 13.2. *Extra-pulmonary complications of Mycoplasma pneumoniae infection*

Blood	
	Cold agglutinins (50–70%)
	Haemolytic anaemia
	Disseminated intravascular coagulation
Central nervous system (1–7%)	
	Meningoencephalitis
	Aseptic meningitis
	Cerebellar ataxia
	Transverse myelitis
	Guillain-Barré syndrome
	Cranial and peripheral neuropathy
	Acute psychosis
Gastrointestinal tract (14–44%)	
	Anorexia
	Nausea
	Vomiting
	Diarrhoea
	Hepatitis
	Pancreatitis
Skin (25%)	
	Macular rash
	Petechiae
	Erythema multiforme
	Stevens-Johnson syndrome
Musculo-skeletal (14–45%)	
	Myalgia
	Arthralgia
	Polyarthritis
Heart (4.5%)	
	Myocarditis
	Pericarditis
Others	
	Haemorrhagic myringitis
	Tonsillar exudates
	Cervical lymphadenopathy
	Splenomegaly
	Acute glomerulonephritis

of respiratory symptoms or only those of mild upper respiratory tract infection.[27]

CNS manifestations occur in approximately 1/1000 hospitalised cases. Aseptic meningitis and meningoencephalitis,[28] transverse myelitis,[29] brain stem dysfunction,[30] Guillain–Barré syndrome,[31] and peripheral neuropathy have all been reported. The findings in the cerebrospinal fluid in such cases are variable and may include a minimal cellular response, slightly elevated protein and low glucose. The interval between the onset of respiratory symptoms and neurological sequelae would suggest an autoimmune pathogenesis,[27] although *M. pneumoniae* has occasionally been isolated from the nasopharynx and from CSF in such patients.[31,32] While some mycoplasma elaborate a neurotoxin, this has not been described for *M. pneumoniae.* Neurological complications are usually reversible but CNS involvement is associated with increased mortality.

A wide variety of transient skin conditions have been reported in association with *M. pneumoniae* infection. Erythema multiforme or Stevens–Johnson syndrome has been reported in up to 7% of patients.[33] This complication of mycoplasma infection tends to occur in younger patients and has a male predominance (3:1). The pathogenesis is unclear. There is no clear relationship between the level of cold agglutinins and development of erythema multiforme. Although an autoimmune aetiology has been suggested,[34] *M. pneumoniae* has been isolated from skin lesions.[35]

Polyarthralgias are common in mycoplasmal pneumonia but arthritis is rare.[36] When present, arthritis may be monoarticular or migratory. Although immune mechanisms have been postulated, *M. pneumoniae* has been cultured from inflamed joint fluid.[37]

Cardiac manifestations of *M. pneumoniae* infection may occur in about 5% of patients. They become more common in older patients and can cause death.[38] The mechanism of heart damage is unknown, but the organism has been isolated from the blood and pericardial fluid of one patient who died.[39]

Haemorrhagic myringitis, tonsillar exudates, cervical lymphadenopathy and splenomegaly have all been reported in association with mycoplasma infection. Ear involvement or myringitis was associated with experimentally induced *M. pneumoniae* infection in about 20% of volunteers.[40] However, myringitis in naturally occurring infection is rare and is more often associated with bacterial and viral upper respiratory tract pathogens.[41]

Investigations and diagnosis

Examination of sputum by Gram's stain may be helpful only in the failure to identify large numbers of bacteria in purulent sputum. Lacking a cell wall, the organism is not detectable on Gram's stain and is too small to be seen on conventional light microscopy. Examination of fluid from rarely occurring pleural or joint effusion is also unrewarding.

Characteristically, the chest X-ray in mycoplasmal pneumonia shows patchy consolidation and central dense infiltrates in one or other lower lobes. Bilateral infiltrates occur in 10–40% of cases and usually extend from the hilar regions. Hilar lymphadenopathy can occur in children but is rare in adults. Chest X-ray changes usually resolve in 10–21 days but may take 4–6 weeks.[23,26,42] The white blood cell count is normal in 75–90% cases of mycoplasma pneumonia because this organism with an incomplete cell wall does not induce an neutrophil leukocytosis. Elevated cold haemagglutinins are found in 33–76%, a titre of 1:32 or greater being highly suggestive. However, these antibodies can be associated with other disorders including acute EB virus infection, adenovirus or influenza virus infection, CMV, syphilis, lymphoproliferative disorders and idiopathic chronic cold haemagglutinin disease (Table 13.3). These IgM antibodies appear after 7 days, increase to a maximum at 4 weeks and usually disappear after 4 months. Significant haemolysis and Raynaud's phenomenon are rare.[42]

Complement-fixing antibodies, although far more specific than

Table 13.3. *Causes of cold haemagglutinins*

	Infection
Common	*Mycoplasma pneumoniae*
	Acute glandular fever (EB virus)
Rare	Adenovirus
	Influenza
	Mumps
	Cytomegalovirus
	Infective endocarditis
	Syphilis
	Trypanosomiasis
	Malaria
Lymphoproliferative disorders	
	Titre usually > 1:512, monoclonal IgM
Idiopathic chronic cold haemagglutinins disease	
	Found in the elderly
	Monoclonal IgM

cold haemagglutinins, do not arise early enough in infection and, therefore, usually do not guide therapeutic decisions. They are useful in epidemiological studies to provide retrospective confirmation of the diagnosis. As previously mentioned, detection of IgM antibodies to *M. pneumoniae* may be of some value in primary infection in young children but is of much less help in adults. Culture of *M. pneumoniae* is difficult and not widely available. It requires media-containing sterols and preformed nucleic acid precursors. Colonies have a 'mulberry' appearance and confirmative tests include reduction of the dye tetrazolium from blue to yellow and detection of acid production by fermentation of glucose. Culture takes 1–2 weeks.

Management

Despite increasing understanding of the microbiology of and host response to *M. pneumoniae,* in most clinical situations the treatment is empirical, based on recognition of the clinical features. Antimicrobial therapy is not necessary for mycoplasmal upper respiratory tract infection and it is likely that the mycoplasmal aetiology of this syndrome often goes undiagnosed. Pneumonia due to *M. pneumoniae* is self-limiting and not life-threatening in most cases. However, effective treatment can shorten the illness and perhaps also reduce the spread of infection in contacts.

As would be predicted by the lack of a cell wall, *M. pneumoniae* is unaffected by β-lactam antibiotics, such as penicillins and cephalosporins. While aminoglycosides are effective *in vitro*, there is no evidence that they are effective *in vivo*. The mainstays of therapy have been tetracyclines and macrolides, particularly erythromycin. While either of these types of antimicrobial will shorten the duration of illness, organisms may continue to be culturable from sputum for several weeks after a complete course of treatment.[43] This may be because, although *M. pneumoniae* causes respiratory disease as an extracellular parasite, it also has the capacity to survive intracellularly. Although tetracyclines are very active against *M. pneumoniae,* their use is precluded in young children because of adverse effects on developing teeth and bones. On the other hand, erythromycin is often poorly tolerated due to gastrointestinal effects. These include nausea, vomiting, abdominal pain and diarrhoea. Erythromycin also raises serum theophylline levels which should be considered in patients with asthma prescribed both drugs.

Because of these adverse effects of tetracyclines and erythromycin, there is considerable increase in newer agents with affects against mycoplasma. Doxycycline is better tolerated than tetracycline and can be administered in two daily doses rather than three. The newer macrolide antibiotics, azithromycin and clarithromycin have recently become available. Azithromycin has a broader spectrum of action than erythromycin and *in vitro* has greater activity against mycoplasma pneumoniae than either erythromycin or tetracycline. It also appears to have fewer adverse effects.[44] Clarithromycin is better tolerated than erythromycin and effective against *M. pneumoniae*.[45] However, these newer macrolide antibiotics are significantly more expensive than erythromycin. Quinolone antibiotics have recently been introduced which have an action against *M. pneumoniae.* Two of these, ciprofloxacin and lomefloxacin, have been studied *in vitro* and have shown 1000 times raised activities against *M. pneumoniae* compared to erythromycin.[46] Similarly, ofloxacin has good antibacterial activity against the organism.[47] Again, however, the newer quinolone antibiotics are significantly more expensive than either tetracycline or erythromycin and this may affect the decision on which antibiotic to use.

The standard regime for mycoplasmal pneumonia would therefore be erythromycin orally 500 mg four times daily in adults and 30–40 mg/kg/day in divided doses to children weighing less than 25 kg. Tetracycline at comparable doses would be an appropriate alternative to patients older than 8 years. Although symptoms usually abate abruptly with therapy, relapses occur in up to 10% of cases unless therapy is continued for 3 weeks.

Prophylaxis

Although *M. pneumoniae* continues to be among the most common agents of community-acquired pneumonia, enthusiasm for vaccine development has waned. Initial vaccines tested on military recruits did produce specific antibody responses but protection against infection was limited to less than 50% of recipients.[48,49] Live vaccines using attenuated wild-type and temperature-sensitive mutant mycoplasma have proved no more effective.[50] Studies of the use of prophylactic antibiotics in family members exposed to mycoplasma have shown a decrease in clinical disease but serial conversion was not reported.[51]

Chlamydia spp.

Chlamydia spp. cannot synthesise ATP or GTP and are therefore, obligate intracellular pathogens. Like mycoplasmas, they are prokaryotes which have morphological and structural similarities to Gram-negative bacteria including a trilaminar cell wall. However, they lack peptidoglycan, a macromolecule that provides most prokaryotes with structural rigidity and osmotic stability. The result is an almost spore-like structure, the elementary body, that is metabolically inert.

Within the genus, *Chlamydia,* four species are currently recognised: *Chlamydia trachomatis, Chlamydia pecorum, C. psittaci* and *C. pneumoniae.* Sequence data of their RNA establishes them as a unique class of bacteria that are closely related to each other but only distantly to other eubacteria.[52] Phenotypically the four species differ antigenically, metabolically, in host cell preference, antibiotic susceptibility and inclusion morphology. *C. trachomatis* is associated with ocular trachoma and with sexually transmitted disease in humans and *C. pecorum* infects cattle. These two organisms will not be discussed further. The natural history of chlamydial infections is unknown, but it is now thought that chronic symptomatic or persistent infections are extremely frequent.

Chlamydia spp. have a unique biphasic life cycle.[52] The elementary bodies, approximately 350 nm in diameter are highly condensed and infect various host cells probably by a receptor-mediated process involving clathrin-coated pits.[53] These elementary bodies then differentiate intracellularly into the much larger replicative form, the reticulate body, which is approximately 800–1000 nm in diameter. During growth and replication, *Chlamydia* obtain high-energy phosphate compounds from the host cell and are therefore, considered ‘energy parasites’.[54] Reticulate bodies are osmotically unstable, divide by binary fission to produce enlarging cells and are incapable of infecting another cell. The organism reverts to elementary bodies before exocytosis or cell lysis and is then capable of infecting new cells.

C. psittaci

History

Psittacosis is a systemic infection that frequently causes pneumonia and its relationship to bird exposure has been known for over 100 years. Morange applied the term psittacosis (from the Greek for parrot) in 1892 after studying cases associated with sick parrots. In 1930, the organism was identified in several laboratories throughout the world; by Bedson in UK, Kromwede in USA and Levinthal in Germany.[55]

Epidemiology

Over 130 avian species of caged birds, domestic poultry and wild birds have been documented as hosts of *C. psittaci* infection which they may occasionally transmit to man.[56] The term ‘ornithosis’ is, therefore, sometimes used synonymously with psittacosis. Occupational infection can occur in pet owners, pet shop employees, poultry farmers, workers in abattoirs and processing plants and veterinarians and even handling feathers has been reported to be associated with infection.[57]

Infected birds may be asymptomatic or obviously sick. The latter may demonstrate shivering, depression, anorexia, emaciation, dyspnoea or diarrhoea. During periods of illness they excrete the largest number of organisms. Discharge from their beaks and eyes, faeces and urine and dust around their cage all become contaminated.[58] In bird populations studied, 5–8% are carriers of *C. psittaci* and this may increase to 100% when birds are subject to the stress of shipping or crowding.[56]

The infection is generally spread by the respiratory route, by direct contact or aerosolisation of infected discharges or dust. Rarely the bird may spread the infection by a bite. Strains of *C. psittaci* from turkeys and psittacine birds appear to be the most virulent for humans but in up to 25% of patients there is no history of avian exposure.[59]

Although most human infection originates from avian strains of *C. psittaci,* other animals are occasionally implicated. Disease has occurred in ranchers, exposed to infection from cows and goats[60] and abortion in sheep has been followed by abortion in women who assisted in lambing.[61] Human-to-human transmission is very rare but such cases tend to be more severe than avian-acquired disease. Environmental sanitation is important since the organism is resistant to drying and can remain viable for a week at room temperature.[56]

Microbiology

There are multiple strains of *C. psittaci* which primarily infect birds and other non-human hosts. These strains exhibit from less than 10% to 60% homology with each other and from 5% to 20% with *C. trachomatis* strains. While the reticulate bodies of all four species of chlamydia are similar, the elementary body of *C. psittaci* is indistinguishable from that of *C. trachomatis* but distinct from that of *C. pneumoniae* which is often pear shaped. *C. psittaci* form multiple small inclusions in a single infected cell with each elementary body forming its own inclusion.

Clinical features

The clinical features of pneumonia due to *C. psittaci* are summarised in Table 13.1. The illness begins after an incubation period of 5–15 days. Onset may be insidious or abrupt and the clinical presentation varies from a mild influenza-like illness to fulminant pneumonia complicated by lesions in other systems.

The most common symptom is fever occurring in 50–100% patients. Cough and breathlessness are almost as frequent but may appear after the initial presentation. Headaches, myalgias and chills are reported in 30–70% of patients. Chest soreness can occur but pleuritic chest pain is rare.[62,63] These rather non-specific symptoms make the initial diagnosis difficult. Approximately 50% of patients will be found to have pharyngeal redness, crackles on chest auscultation and hepatomegaly. There may be a relative bradycardia.

Extrapulmonary manifestations reflect the systemic nature of psittacosis (Table 13.4). Cardiac complications include pericarditis, myocarditis, and ‘culture-negative’ endocarditis. In cases of endocarditis, *Chlamydia* has been found histologically in both aortic and mitral valves and on blood culture.[64,65] Hepatitis may develop[66] and jaundice may also appear in association with haemolytic anaemia.[67] Reactive arthritis occurs 1–4 weeks after the initial illness.[68] Neurological complications include cranial nerve palsies, cerebellar signs, transverse myelitis, meningoencephalitis, and seizures. The cerebrospinal fluid may contain a few lymphocytes and a raised protein concentration. Skin lesions include Horder’s spots; a pink blanching maculopapular eruption resembling the rose spots of typhoid fever.[62,63] Erythema multiforme, erythema marginatum and erythema nodosum have all been described.[69] Other complications include acute glomerulonephritis,[70] phlebitis, pancreatitis and thyroiditis.

Table 13.4. *Extrapulmonary features of C. psittaci infection*

Haemolytic anaemia
Disseminated intravascular coagulation
Meningoencephalitis
Myocarditis
Culture negative endocarditis
Reactive arthritis
Hepatic granuloma
Rhabdomyolysis
Erythema multiforme
Erythema marginatum
Erythema nodosum

Investigations and diagnosis

The white blood cell count is usually normal or only slightly elevated. Liver function tests are mildly deranged in 50% of patients showing a cholestatic picture.

The chest X-ray is abnormal in approximately 75% of patients and, like *M. pneumoniae,* the radiological changes are far more impressive than the physical signs. The most frequent finding is consolidation in a single lower lobe but other patterns include a miliary pattern of consolidation and unilateral or bilateral hilar enlargement. These chest X-ray appearances may take up to 20 weeks to resolve, the average being 6 weeks.[62] Pleural effusions are seen in up to 50% of cases but are usually small.[71]

Culture of the organism is possible from blood in the first four days and from sputum in the first two weeks. However, culture methods are potentially dangerous and deaths have occurred in laboratory workers who have become infected.[72] Since culture is dangerous, the diagnosis of psittacosis relies on the demonstration of complement-fixing antibodies in the serum. Usually a titre of 1:64 or a four-fold increase in titre over the time course of the illness is diagnostic. However, as complement-fixing antibodies are only genus specific, they do not distinguish *C. psittaci* from *C. trachomatis* or *C. pneumoniae.* An IgM antibody to *C. psittaci* can sometimes be detected but there are cross-reactions. The serological testing for *C. psittaci* infection is at present imperfect.

Management

The treatment of choice is tetracycline 500 mg four times daily or doxycycline 100 mg twice daily for 10–21 days. Erythromycin is recommended for younger children but may be less effective than tetracycline in adults. Most patients respond within 24 hours. Untreated the mortality of psittacosis pneumonia may rise to 20% but with treatment this falls to 1%.[63] Endocarditis can be treated with rifampicin[73] but valve replacement is usually required.

Prophylaxis

There is no documented protection after infection and second infections have been seen despite elevated complement-fixing antibodies.[56] Infected birds should receive tetracycline, chlortetracycline or doxycycline for at least 45 days. Imported birds should be quarantined for at least 30 days and in the USA psittacine birds are treated with chlortetracycline during this time.

C. pneumoniae

History

C. pneumoniae is the most recently recognised of the *Chlamydiae.* The type strain of *C. pneumoniae,* isolated in 1965 from the conjunctiva of a Taiwanese child was designated TW-183 (hence the early species name, TWAR, from TaiWan, Acute Respiratory). The second strain isolated, IOL-207, came from the conjunctiva of an Iranian child with trachoma. However, an association between infection with *C. pneumoniae* and trachoma or conjunctivitis has not been reported since. *C. pneumoniae* was first identified as a respiratory pathogen in 1986 when Grayston isolated the organism from throat swabs of students with acute respiratory symptoms.[74] The name *C. pneumoniae* was chosen because pneumonia has been the most commonly recognised disease caused by infection with the organism. It is likely that some illness that had previously been attributed to *C. psittaci* were actually due to *C. pneumoniae*. This has been shown from an epidemic of 'ornithosis' in Northern Europe in the 1980s[75] and for an outbreak of respiratory illness in a school in England in 1983.[76]

Microbiology

C. pneumoniae has been characterised by restriction endonuclease and DNA hybridisation analyses. Isolates have at least 94% DNA homology with each other, but less than 5% homology with *C. trachomatis* and less than 10% with *C. psittaci.*[77] *C. pneumoniae* is more homogeneous than other *Chlamydia* spp. and only one strain or serovar has been identified. The name TWAR is therefore, synonymous with the species designated *C. pneumoniae*.

The elementary body may appear to be pear shaped unlike the round elementary bodies of other *Chlamydia* spp. The small end seems to be the site of attachment to HeLa cells in culture,[78] but this morphological characteristic is unreliable. Electron microscopy also reveals a large periplasmic space containing numerous small electron-dense 'minibodies'.[78] The major outer membrane protein (MOMP) is identical between known strains of *C. pneumoniae* and distinct from other species.

Epidemiology

Man is the only known reservoir for *C. pneumoniae*[79] and person-to-person spread is the probable mode of acquisition.[80] The symptomless carrier state[81,82] and prolonged excretion of the organism for up to one year[83] helps this type of transmission. In one study 111 (47%) of 234 healthy subjects had *C. pneumoniae* isolated from throat cultures.[82]

Antibody responses to *C. pneumoniae* are very variable which can make serological studies difficult to interpret. However, such data suggests that *C. pneumoniae* is one of the most prevalent infectious agents in both affluent and deprived communities in the western world.[83,84] Seroprevalence for *C. pneumoniae* with IgG titres of greater than 1:16 among children 2–5 years has been estimated at around 12% in both Japan[85] and Spain.[86] Seroconversion peaks among teenagers and decreases slowly thereafter. The population prevalence of antibodies to *C. pneumoniae* is 40–50% in the Northern hemisphere with a higher prevalence in men.[87] Studies of *C. pneumoniae* antibodies in adult sera from 10 areas of the world have shown a higher population prevalence in tropical countries (Panama, Taiwan) than in northerly developed countries (Canada, Denmark).[88] Asymptomatic infection is probably extremely common and it is likely that chronic carriage can occur.

There appear to be cyclical changes in incidence of *C. pneumoniae* infection. In Denmark, 2–3 years of high incidence has been followed by 3–4 years of relative low incidence[89] while serological studies in Seattle, USA., from 1963–1975 suggest a four-yearly cycle of infection.[90]

Outbreaks of *C. pneumoniae* have occurred in universities, schools, military institutions and within families.[74,87,91,92] Spread of infection is slow and case to case interval can average 30 days. The organism remains viable on a formica counter top for 30 hours and in tissue paper for 12 hours.[93] Apparent infection of *C. pneumoniae* occurred during a laboratory accident due to centrifuge malfunction, when transmission is likely to have been by aerosol inhalation.[94] Aerial transmission was also suggested by the demonstration that significant numbers of elementary bodies survive in aerosols.[95]

Experimental infection of non-human primates with *C. pneumoniae* failed to cause pneumonia but did result in conjunctival infection; the organism has been isolated from the rectal mucosa of these animals.[96,97]

Clinical features

The clinical features of *C. pneumoniae* are summarised in Table 13.1.

The illness initially described by Grayston[74] in association with *C. pneumoniae* infection was a mild pneumonia and pharyngitis with hoarseness. *C. pneumoniae* may, however, cause severe pneumonia and respiratory failure. Fever may be accompanied by confusion and a prominent headache and cough may not appear for several days, making the illness appear to be bi-phasic.[98] In a study of 593 patients with serological evidence of *C. pneumoniae* infection, many of whom were treated in general practice, 50% had a diagnosis of pneumonia, 28% bronchitis, 10% ''flu-like' illness, 4% 'upper respiratory tract infection', 4% pharyngitis, 2% sinusitis and 1% otitis media.[99] *C. pneumoniae* has also been isolated from a pleural effusion that complicated a right middle lobe pneumonia in a 19-year-old man.[100] *C. pneumoniae* has therefore been implicated in the pathogenesis of infections of variable severity at all levels within the respiratory tract. Pneumonia requiring hospital admission caused by *C. pneumoniae* appears to be milder but clinically similar to that caused by *Streptococcus pneumoniae* and mixed infections are probably common.[101] However, since most *C. pneumoniae* infections are mild or even asymptomatic, its importance as a respiratory pathogen has been neglected.[83,102]

C. pneumoniae has also been associated with exacerbations of airways disease. Seven of 74 patients with exacerbations of asthma had serological evidence of acute *C. pneumoniae* infection and in two patients the organism was identified on pharyngeal swabs.[103] In a study of 118 children with acute exacerbations of asthma, *C. pneumoniae* was isolated from 13 (11%) but only 3 had serological evidence of acute infection.[104] Asthmatic bronchitis and adult-onset asthma have also been reported occurring within 6 months of *C. pneumoniae* infection.[105] In this study, *C. pneumoniae* IgG titres of at least 1:64 were found in approximately 80% of those with adult asthma compared with 63.7% of the general population. These studies suggest that *C. pneumoniae* may have a role in exacerbations of co-existing asthma or could play a more fundamental part in the aetiology of asthma.

In contrast, *C. pneumoniae* seems to be an uncommon pathogen in patients with chronic obstructive pulmonary disease (COPD). Of 44 patients with acute exacerbations of COPD only 2 (5%) had serological evidence of acute infection with *C. pneumoniae* and in neither was the organism cultured from the nasopharynx.[106] In a similar study of 142 patients with exacerbations of COPD, only 5 had serological evidence of recent infection with *C. pneumoniae* and again the organism could not be cultured from any patient.[107]

Extrapulmonary manifestations

A wide range of extrapulmonary associations with *C. pneumoniae* has been reported (Table 13.5). In a study of 70 patients with reactive arthritis 5 (7%) had serological evidence of *C. pneumoniae* infection with specific lymphocyte proliferation in synovial fluid.[108] Lymphocytic meningoencephalitis in a patient with pneumonia was reported in which cerebrospinal fluid and throat washings both gave positive results for *C. pneumoniae* on direct immunofluorescent testing with specific monoclonal antibodies.[109] Guillain–Barré syndrome[110] and lumbosacral meningoradiculitis[111] have also both been associated with *C. pneumoniae* infections.

There are several associations between *C. pneumoniae* infection and cardiac disorders. High IgM and IgG antibodies to *C. pneumoniae* were reported in a fatal case of myocarditis in which necropsy samples of heart and lungs showed positive results by PCR.[112] A case of *C. pneumoniae* endocarditis has also been described but the organism was not detected in tissue obtained at surgery from the cardiac valve.[113]

There is considerable evidence that immunological mechanisms may have a role in the pathogenesis of acute myocardial infarction and coronary artery disease, through the production of circulating immune complexes.[114,115] There is an increasing amount of evidence base on seroepidemiological studies suggesting that *C. pneumoniae* infection may be associated with artheromatous disease of the coronary and carotid arteries.[116–118] Recently, using immunocytochemistry or PCR techniques, *C. pneumoniae* has been demonstrated in atheromatous plaques of coronary arteries at necropsy.[119] 68% of patients with an acute myocardial infarction and 50% of patients with chronic angina undergoing angiography have been shown to have IgG at a titre of $\geq$ 1:128 or IgA antibodies at a titre $\geq$ 1:32 to *C. pneumoniae* compared with 17% of control subjects.[116] While this relationship may appear causal, it has also been shown that the association is limited largely to smokers[120] who are known to be at greater risk of coronary artery disease and who may also be susceptible to *C. pneumoniae* infection. However, there is currently considerable work ongoing in this area and it may be several years before there is a full understanding of the epidemiology and consequences of *C. pneumoniae* infection.

Investigation and diagnosis

As with *M. pneumoniae,* Gram's stain of the sputum may show purulent material with no detectable bacteria. Similarly, chest radiology may show abnormalities ranging from small subsegmental lesions to

Table 13.5. *Extrapulmonary features of* C. pneumoniae *infection*

Reactive arthritis
Meningoencephalitis
Guillain-Barré syndrome
Myocarditis
Endocarditis
Coronary artery disease (?)

extensive bilateral consolidation far more widespread than clinical signs would suggest.

The diagnosis of *C. pneumoniae* infection has proved particularly difficult. Techniques used for detecting the closely related species, *C. psittaci* and *C. trachomatis,* have been less effective when applied to *C. pneumoniae,* and problems have arisen in differentiating between these three chlamydial species. Diagnosis of *C. psittaci* infection has relied upon the demonstration of complement-fixing antibodies in the serum. This test, however, uses the chlamydial genus lipopolysaccharide antigen and so cannot distinguish between chlamydia species. It, therefore, seems very likely that many patients previously diagnosed as having psittacosis were, in fact, infected with *C. pneumoniae.* In addition, this complement fixation antibody test is positive in less than one third of patients who have other evidence of *C. pneumoniae* infection.[121]

Type-specific microimmunofluorescent antibody testing allows differentiation of IgG and IgM antibodies and can distinguish *Chlamydia* spp. but it is technically difficult and currently only available in specialist laboratories.[122] A single IgM titre of ≥ 1:16 or IgG titre of ≥ 1:512 or a fourfold or greater rise in IgG or IgM antibody between acute and convalescent serum samples are usually considered diagnostic.

C. pneumoniae is difficult to isolate by culture and requires cell culture which is a specialist technique not routinely available in most hospital laboratories. Chlamydial antigen can be detected using direct fluorescent antibody staining and enzyme immunoassay.[123] Recently a PCR technique which utilises oligonucleotide primers corresponding to unique regions of the *C. pneumoniae* 16SrRNAgene has been developed. This is then combined with enzyme immunoassay (PCR-EIA).[124] Using this technique, 15 (18.8%) of 80 asymptomatic subjects had antibody levels considered to be diagnostic of acute infection but only one of these subjects had the organism identified on nasopharyngeal swabs. Similarly, 35 subjects gave positive results either by culture or by PCR-EIA, but only 8 of these had antibody titres considered diagnostic of acute infection.[124] PCR-EIA appears to have a sensitivity of 76.5% and specificity of 99.0% for identifying *C. pneumoniae.* Successful amplification of chlamydial DNA by PCR does not necessarily signify active chlamydial infection, and from the studies described above, it is clear that a single serological test may be difficult to interpret.

Treatment

As with *C. psittaci* and other 'atypical' organisms, tetracycline and macrolide antibiotics, classically erythromycin, form the basis of treatment of *C. pneumoniae. In vitro* studies suggest that clarithromycin has the lowest minimum inhibitory concentration and that tetracycline and macrolides are more active than quinolones.[125,126] However, the clinical response *in vivo* to antibiotics is often slow with persistence of symptoms and frequent clinical relapse.[74] Three of nine patients with *C. pneumoniae* infection continued to have positive cultures for the organism over an 11 month period despite treatment with tetracycline.[127] Empirical observations suggest that relapses are infrequent if erythromycin is given for less than 3 weeks.[87] Such persistence of the organism could act as a reservoir for spread of infection and may have a role in the pathogenesis of some of the chronic disorders associated with *C. pneumoniae.* Antibiotics may suppress the antibody response which could influence the value of serological tests in the diagnosis of this infection.

Prophylaxis

The search for an effective anti-chlamydial vaccine continues. Protective immunity against chlamydial ocular infection in primates is correlated with the presence of persistent serovar-specific secretory IgA antibodies in tears.[128] Putative whole-cell vaccine against *C. trachomatis* have potentiated trachoma by sensitising recipients[129] and as yet a vaccine against *C. pneumoniae* has not been developed.

Coxiella burnetti

History

In 1935, Derrick, a medical officer of health in Queensland, Australia, investigated a febrile illness that affected 20 of 800 employees of a Brisbane meat works.[130] He coined the term Q (for query) fever for this illness for which he had no diagnosis but suspected a new disease. Burnet and Freeman showed that the microorganism isolated from the blood and urine of Derrick's patients was a rickettsia.[131] Davis and Cox then isolated a microorganism from ticks (Dermacentors andersoni) collected near Nine Mile Creek, Montana.[132] Later Dyer showed that the *Rickettsia burnetti* (Burnett and Freeman's organism) was the same as *Rickettsia diaporica* (Davis and Cox's organism).[133] This organism is now known as *C. burnetti.*

Microbiology

C. burnetti is a highly pleomorphic coccobacillus with a Gram-negative cell wall. It is small, measuring 300-700 nm long and, unlike true rickettsiae, it enter host cells by a passive mechanism. *C. burnetti* functions best at a low pH and, therefore, it survives within phagolysosomes of the host cell.[134] A variety of morphological forms have been described and there is a spore stage which explains how this organism can withstand harsh environmental conditions.[135] It can survive for 7–10 months on wool at 15–20 °C, for more than 1 month on fresh meat in cold storage, and for more than 40 months in skim milk at 4–6 °C. Although it is killed by 2% formaldehyde, the organism has been isolated from infected tissues stored in formaldehyde for up to 4–5 months. It can even be cultured from fixed 'parafinised' tissues.

C. burnetti undergoes 'phase' variation. The phase I state is found in nature and in laboratory animals in which organisms can be shown to have a late reaction (45 days) to convalescent guinea pig sera.

Repeated passage of phase I organisms in embryo chicken eggs leads to conversion to the phase II avirulent form. There is no morphological difference between these two phases which do differ in sugar composition of their lipopolysaccharides.[136] Plasmids have been found in both phase I and phase II cells and there is a correlation between plasmid content and the virulence of *C. burnetti*.[135] Three different plasmid types have been isolated: the QpH1 plasmid has been found in cases of acute Q fever, while the QpRS plasmid has been reported in patients with Q fever endocarditis.[137] It is believed that there are at least six strains of *C. burnetti:*[138] Hamilton, Vacca, Rasche, Biotzere, Corazon, Dod. The first three strains contain the plasmid QpH1 and have been associated with acute Q fever. Biotzere has plasmid QpRS and Corazon has no plasmid but both strains are associated with chronic Q fever and endocarditis. The Dod strain contains the QpDG plasmid and is avirulent.

Epidemiology

C. burnetti has been identified in arthropods, fish, birds, rodents, marsupials and livestock.[139] Although the most common animal reservoirs for this organism are cattle, sheep and goats, the epidemiology of *Coxiella burnetti* seems to vary across the world. For example, collared doves have been suspected of carrying this infection from Western Europe to Ireland. In Nova Scotia, exposure to infected cats has resulted in outbreaks of Q fever.[140]

Q fever has been reported from over 51 countries on five continents.[141] It is usually an occupational disease affecting those with direct contact with infected animals such as farmers, veterinarians and abattoir workers. However, infection has been described in a wide variety of situations. For instance, 350 persons who lived along a road over which sheep travelled from mountain pastures in Switzerland, developed Q fever.[142] Similarly, exposure to contaminated straw, manure or dust from farm vehicles resulted in Q fever in those who lived near the farm.[143] Even more indirect exposure can lead to illness as in the case of laundry workers who developed Q fever after handling contaminated laundry.[144] Ingesting contaminated raw milk and skinning infected wild rabbits have also been reported as ways of contracting Q fever.[145]

Laboratory exposure to *C. burnetti*[146] and transport of infected sheep through hospitals to research laboratories have been the cause of outbreaks of Q fever.[147] Q fever can be transmitted via blood transfusion[148] or at post-mortem examination.[149] There has also been one reported person-to-person transmission of Q fever within a family,[150] one where staff in hospital were infected by a patient[142] and another where a pathologist and mortuary technician were infected during post-mortem examination.[151]

The most likely cycle of transmission of *C. burnetti* to humans is that the organism is maintained in ticks or arthropods. These insects then infect domestic and other animals. When infected these animals shed the desiccation-resistant organisms in urine, faeces, milk and particularly in birth products. The placenta of infected sheep contains up to 10^9 organisms per gram. Air samples may be positive for up to 2 weeks after parturition and viable organisms are present in the soil for periods of up to 150 days.[152,153] Humans are infected by the inhalation of contaminated aerosols and the organism then proliferates in the lungs.

Clinical features

These are illustrated in Table 13.1. Humans are the only animals known to regularly develop illness as the result of *C. burnetti* infection. After an incubation period of 20 days (range 14–39 days), patients become ill with severe headache, fever, chills, fatigue and myalgia. The severity of symptoms and variety of clinical manifestations probably depends on the dose of organism inhaled and the characteristics of the infecting strain. Several clinical syndromes are described and overall the mortality rate is 2–4%.[154]

The most common form of Q fever is a self-limiting febrile illness lasting 2–14 days in which the chest X-ray is normal. It is also likely that some cases of infection with *C. burnetti* are asymptomatic.[155] Out of 505 adults in the south of Spain who had fever of more than 1 week and less than 3 weeks duration 108 (21%) had Q fever.[156]

Pneumonia associated with Q fever can present with atypical symptoms, a rapidly progressive course or as fever with no pulmonary symptoms. The last of these is probably the most common presentation of Q fever pneumonia. The illness may be of gradual or sudden onset. Cough is a feature of only 28% of patients with radiologically confirmed Q fever pneumonia. Fever occurs in every patient and headache is characteristic occurring in 75%. Other symptoms include fatigue in 98%, chills 88%, sweats 84%, myalgia 68%, nausea 49%, vomiting 25%, pleuritic chest pain 28% and diarrhoea 21%. On occasions diarrhoea can be the presenting symptom of Q fever.[157]

The most common finding on physical examination is lung crackles,[145] but in severe cases signs of pulmonary consolidation may be present. Splenomegaly occurs in 5%. Unlike other rickettsial infections, cutaneous lesions do not occur.

Extrapulmonary manifestations

Chronic infection with *C. burnetti* can present with a variety of non-pulmonary features (Table 13.6). Five-year follow-up of 114 patients known to have Q fever in Birmingham, England, in 1989 revealed that chronic symptoms were common with 69% complaining of joint pains, 66% chronic fatigue and 65% sleep disturbance.[158]

The incidence of Q fever endocarditis may be increasing. Review of the world literature from 1968 to 1973 revealed 55 cases[159] but by 1975–1980 reviews just in England produced 79 cases.[160] Between 1975 and 1981 *C. burnetti* accounted for 3% of all cases of endocarditis reported in adults in England and Wales.[161] However, Q fever endocarditis in children appears to be rare.[162] Infection with *C. burnetti* can occur on abnormal or prosthetic cardiac valves.[163,164] Patients often have finger clubbing and hepatosplenomegaly is found in over 50%. A purpuric vasculitic rash occurs in over 20%. Features of bacterial endocarditis such as high ESR, anaemia, microscopic haematuria and hypergammaglobulinaemia can all be present. Arterial embolisation has been found in one third of patients.

In France, 61.9% of all cases of Q fever present as hepatitis.[154] In contrast, Q fever hepatitis has never been reported from Nova Scotia. Hepatitis can present as a pyrexia of uncertain origin or in association with Q fever pneumonia.[165] The classical appearance is of a 'doughnut granuloma' on liver histology with a dense fibrin ring surrounded by a central lipid vacuole.[166,167] Although *C. burnetti* has never been

Table 13.6. *Extrapulmonary manifestations of chronic Q fever*

Endocarditis
Infection of a vascular prothesis
Infection of aneurysms
Hepatitis
Meningoencephalitis
Osteomyelitis
Bone marrow aplasia
Haemolytic anaemia
Splenic rupture
Optic neuritis
Erythema nodosum
? Kawasaki disease

seen on microscopy of liver biopsy, the organism has been isolated from biopsy specimens.[159]

Aseptic meningitis and/or encephalitis appears in approximately 1% of cases of Q fever.[168] In a review of 16 cases of Q fever meningoencephalitis 8 had elevated white cells in the cerebrospinal fluid of up to 1300 cells per cubic mm.[169] The CSF protein was usually increased and glucose normal. Meningoencephalitis may be accompanied by seizures and coma.[170] Residual neurological impairment including blurred vision, sensory deficits and parasthesiae can occur.[171]

Vertebral osteomyelitis has been reported due to Q fever infection.[172] Haematological manifestations include bone marrow necrosis,[173] haemolytic anaemia,[174] transient severe hypoplastic anaemia,[175] reactive thrombocytosis and splenic rupture.[176] Bilateral optic neuritis,[177] erythema nodosum[178] and a variant of Kawasaki disease[179,180] have also all been reported. In infancy Q fever can cause pneumonia, febrile seizures, pyrexia, malaise and meningeal irritation.[181]

Serological studies have shown that 10.4% of 500 HIV positive patients had IgG antibodies in a titre of ≥ 1:25 to *Coxiella burnetti* compared to 4.1% of 925 apparently healthy blood donors[182]. Conversely, 5 (7.3%) of 68 patients hospitalised with Q fever between 1987 and 1989 were HIV antibody positive. In a review of all cases of chronic Q fever in France from 1982 –1990, 20% of 84 patients were immunocompromised in some way.[183]

Investigations and diagnosis

Patients with severe headache may undergo lumbar puncture which often produces normal cerebrospinal fluid. However, *C. burnetti* has occasionally been isolated from cerebrospinal fluid.[184] The peripheral white blood cell count is usually normal, although one-third of patients may have an elevated count. The liver enzyme levels are raised in almost all patients. Hyponatraemia due to inappropriate secretion of anti-diuretic hormone has been reported.[185]

The chest X-ray appearances of Q fever are variable.[186] Non-segmental and segmental pleural-based opacities are common and pleural effusion is found in 35% of cases.[187] Atelectasis, increased pulmonary reticular shadowing and hilar adenopathy can occur. In one series the time to clear the chest X-ray abnormalities ranged from 10–70 days with a mean of 30 days.[187] Transbronchial lung biopsy may show small coccobacilli within alveolar macrophages.[188] Lung tissue obtained at post-mortem may show severe intra-alveolar haemorrhage and focal necrotising pneumonia with necrotising bronchitis.[189] Histology of non-fatal cases of Q fever pneumonia show a mixed inflammatory cell infiltrate with bronchiolar epithelium that may be focally absent, regenerated or hypoplastic.[190]

Most hospital laboratories do not have facilities for culture of *C. burnetti.* The diagnosis of Q fever, therefore, largely depends on serological methods. The microagglutination, complement fixation, indirect microimmunofluorescence and enzyme-linked immunosorbent assay have all been used.[191,192] The diagnosis of Q fever is usually confirmed by the detection of serum antibodies to the two lipopolysaccharide antigens of *C. burnetti.* Acute infection is demonstrated by fourfold rise in phase II antibody titres between acute and convalescent serum samples at intervals of 10–14 days. Phase I antibody titres rise more slowly than phase II and a titre of ≥ 1:200 to phase I antigen is said to be diagnostic of chronic Q fever and endocarditis. Western immunoblotting of serum samples from patients with chronic Q fever show IgG antibodies to 12–15 antigens of phase I *C. burnetti,* whereas serum from patients with acute Q fever react with 7–10 *C. burnetti* antigens.[193] IgM antibody testing has been advocated in the diagnosis[194] but these antibodies may persist for up to 678 days[195] with 3% of patients having detectable IgM antibody 1 year after infection.[196]

Treatment

Antibiotic sensitivity testing using L929 fibroblast cells infected with *C. burnetti* revealed that various quinolones including ciprofloxacin and also rifampicin were highly effective.[197] Chloramphenicol, doxycycline and trimethoprim had an intermediate effect while tetracycline, gentamicin, streptomycin, erythromycin and penicillin G were less effective. There are reports of treatment failures in Q fever pneumonia using erythromycin alone with a cure produced by the addition of rifampicin.[198,199] Despite these *in vitro* results, tetracycline in a dose of 500 mg four times daily for 2–3 weeks is the treatment of choice for acute Q fever.

There is no clear consensus on antimicrobial type or duration of treatment for Q fever endocarditis[195,196] and some have advised that treatment should be continued indefinitely.[195] Combination antibiotics are recommended including doxycycline with co-trimoxazole or rifampicin for 2 years. Others have used doxycycline with pefloxacin or ofloxacin.[200] The addition of chloroquine or amantadine to doxycycline enhances the bactericidal effect by alkalinisation of the intracellular phagosome.[201] Antibody titres should be performed every 6 months during therapy and every 3 months for the first 2 years after treatment. Valve replacement is frequently necessary.

Prophylaxis

Pasteurisation of milk can eliminate some cases of Q fever and in Cyprus the incidence of *C. burnetti* infection among sheep and goats was reduced by disinfection of premises and burning of aborted material.[202] Control of ticks and other arthropods on cattle, sheep and goats is also important in control of Q fever. Vaccines[203,204] have been developed and those at risk, e.g. abattoir workers and veterinarians should be considered for this prophylaxis.

References

1. EATON MD, MEIKLEJOHN G, VAN HERICK W. Studies on the etiology of primary atypical pneumonia. II. Properties of the virus isolated and propagated in chick embryos. *J Exp Med*, 1945;82:317–21.
2. CLYDE WA. *Mycoplasma pneumoniae* infections in man. In. Tully JG, Whitcomb RF, vols. *The Mycoplasmas* v II. New York: Academic Press: 1979:275–306.
3. EATON MD, MEIKLEJOHN G, VAN HERICK W. Studies on the etiology of primary atypical pneumonia. A filterable agent transmissible to cotton rats, hamsters, and chick embryos. *J Exp Med* 1944;79:649–54.
4. EATON MD, VAN HERICK W, MEIKELJOHN G. Studies on the etiology of primary atypical pneumonia. III. Specific neutralization of the virus by human serum. *J Exp Med* 1945;82:329–433.
5. MARMION BP. Eaton-agent – science and scientific acceptance: an historical commentary. *Rev Infect Dis* 1990;12:338–41.
6. CHARNOCK RM, MUFSON MA, BLOOM HH. Eaton-agent pneumonia. *JAMA* 1961;175: 213–17.
7. CHARNOCK RM, RIFKIND D, DRAVETZ HM. Respiratory disease in volunteers infected with Eaton agent: a preliminary report. *Proc Natl Acad Sci USA* 1961;47:887–901.
8. BIBERFIELD G, GRONOWICZ E. *Mycoplasma pneumoniae* is a polyclonal B-cell activator. *Nature* 1976;261:238–43.
9. STANBRIDGE EJ, WEISS RL. *Mycoplasma* capping on lymphocytes. *Nature* 1978;276: 583–91.
10. MAHKOUL N, MERCHAV S, TATARSKY I. *Mycoplasma*-induced *in vitro* production of interleukins-2 and colony stimulating activity. *1st J Med Sci*, 1987;23:480–5.
11. CAPOBIANCHI MR, LOVINO G, LUN MT Membrane interactions involved in the induction of interferon-alpha by *Mycoplasma pneumoniae*. *Antiviral Res* 1987;8:115–17.
12. RUUTH E, PRAZ F. Interactions between *Mycoplasmas* and the immune system. *Immunol Rev* 1987;112:113–16.
13. PETERSON OL, HAN TH, FINLAND M. Cold agglutinins (auto-haemagglutinins) in primary atypical pneumonia. *Science* 1943;97:167–9.
14. FEIZI T, TAYLOR-ROBINSON D. Cold agglutinins anti-I and *Mycoplasma pneumoniae*. *Immunology* 1967;13:405–9.
15. JACOBSON LB, LONGSTRETH GF, EDINGTON TS. Clinical and immunologic features of transient cold agglutinin haemolytic anaemia. *Am J Med* 1973;54:512–16.
16. KARAYAMA Y, SHIOTA K, KOTUNI K. *Mycoplasma pneumoniae*, pneumonia associated with IgA nephropathy. *Scand J Infect Dis* 1982;14:23–6.
17. MOGABGAB WJ. *Mycoplasma pneumoniae* and adenovirus respiratory illness in military and university personnel, 1959–1966. *Am Rev Respir Dis* 1968;97:345–9.
18. NOAH ND. *Mycoplasma pneumoniae* infections in the United Kingdom, 1967–1973. *Br Med J* 1974;2:544–6.
19. TORNA S. Isolation of *Mycoplasma pneumoniae* from respiratory tract specimens in Ontario. *Can Med Assoc J*, 1987;137:48–50.
20. FOY HM, KENNY GE, COONEY MK. Longterm epidemiology of infection with *Mycoplasma pneumoniae*. *J Infect Dis* 1979;139:681–3.
21. Surveillance of *Mycoplasma* infection, 1980–1990. *Commun Dis Rep* 1990;46
22. NOAH ND. Cyclical patterns and predictability in infection. *Epidemiol Infect* 1989;102: 175–90.
23. MURRAY HW, MASUR H, SERTERFIT LB, ROBERTS RB. The manifestations of *Mycoplasma pneumoniae* infection in adults. *Am J Med* 1975;58:229–42.
24. ALI NJ, SILLIS M, ANDREWS BE. The clinical spectrum and diagnosis of *Mycoplasma pneumoniae* infection. *Quart J Med* 1986;58:241–51.
25. FINE NL, SMITH LR, SHEEDY PF. Frequency of pleural effusions in mycoplasma and viral pneumonias. *N Engl J Med* 1970;283:790–3.
26. CASSELL GH, COLE CB. *Mycoplasma* as agents of human disease. *N Engl J Med* 1981;304:80–9.
27. PONKA A. The occurrence and clinical picture of serologically verified *Mycoplasma pneumoniae* infections with emphasis on central nervous system, cardiac and joint manifestations. *Ann Clin Res* 1979;24(Suppl 11):1–60.
28. LERER RJ, KALAVSKY SM. Central nervous system disease associated with *Mycoplasma* infection. Report of five cases and review of the literature. *Pediatrics* 1973;52:658–61.
29. MILLS RW, SCHOOLFIELD L. Acute transverse myelitis associated with *Mycoplasma pneumoniae* infection: a case report and review of the literature. *Pediatr Infect Dis J* 1992;11:228–231.
30. ONG ELC, ELLIS ME, YUILL GM. Neurologic complications of *Mycoplasma pneumoniae* infection. *Resp Med* 1989;83:441–2.
31. STEELE JC, GLADSTONE RM, THORASAPHON S. *Mycoplasma pneumoniae* as a determinant of the Guillain-Barre syndrome. *Lancet* 1969;2:719–21.
32. LEVINE DP, LERNER AM. The clinical spectrum of *Mycoplasma pneumoniae* infections. *Med Clin N Am* 1978;62:961–78.
33. LEVY M, SHEAR NH. *Mycoplasma pneumoniae* infections and Stevens–Johnson syndrome. *Clin Pediatr* 1991;30:42–5.
34. KAZMIEROWSKI JA, WUEPPER KD. Erythema multiforme: clinical spectrum and immunopathogenesis. *Springer Semin Immunopathol*, 1981;4:45–9.
35. STUTMAN HR. Stevens–Johnson syndrome and *Mycoplasma pneumoniae*: evidence for cutaneous infection. *J Pediatr* 1987;111:845–8.
36. PONKA A. Arthritis associated with *Mycoplasma pneumoniae* infection. *Scand J Rheumatol* 1979;8:27–9.
37. DAVIS C.P, COCHRAN S, LISSE J. Isolation of *Mycoplasma pneumoniae* from synovial fluid samples in a patient with pneumonia and polyarthritis. *Arch Intern Med* 1988; 148:969–71.
38. SANDS MR, ROSENTHAL R. Progressive heart failure and death associated with *Mycoplasma pneumoniae*. *Chest* 1982;81:763–5.
39. NATHALIN JM, WELLISCH G, KAHANA Z. *Mycoplasma pneumoniae* septicaemia. *JAMA* 1974;228:565–7.
40. RIFKIND D, CHARNOCK R, KRAVETZ H Ear involvement (myringitis) and primary atypical pneumonia following inoculation of volunteers with Eaton agent. *Am Rev Res Dis* 1962;85:479–80.
41. KLEIN JD, TEELE DW. Isolation of viruses and mycoplasmas from middle ear effusions: a review. *Ann Otol Rhinol Laryngol* 1976;85:140–3.
42. ALI NJ, SILLIS M, ANDREWS BE. The clinical spectrum and diagnosis of *Mycoplasma pneumoniae* infections. *Quart J Med* 1986;58:241–51.
43. SMITH CB, FRIEDEWALD WT, CHARNOCK RM. Shedding of *Mycoplasma pneumoniae* after tetracycline and erythromycin therapy. *N Engl J Med* 1967;276:1172–4.
44. SCHANWALKD S, GUNJACA M, KOLANYG-BABIC L. Comparison of azithromycin and erythromycin in the treatment of atypical pneumonias. *J Antimicrob Chemother* 1990; 25:123–7.
45. CASSELL GH, DRUEC J, WAITES KB *et al.* Efficacy of clarthromycin against *Mycoplasma pneumoniae*. *J Antimicrob Chemother* 1991;27:Suppl A:47–59.
46. CASSELL GH, WAITES KB, PATE MS. Comparative susceptibility of *Mycoplasma pneumoniae* to erythromycin, ciprofloxacin and lomefloxacin. *Diag Microbiol Infect Dis* 1989;12:433–6.

47. OSADA Y, OGAWA H. Antimycoplasmal activity of ofloxacin (Dh-8280). *Antimicrob Agents Chemother* 1983;23:509–11.

48. WEIZEL RP, CRAVEN, RB, DAVIES JA. Field trial on an inactivated *Mycoplasma pneumoniae* vaccine. I. Vaccine efficacy. *J Infect Dis* 1976;134:571–4.

49. MOGABAB WJ. Protective effects of inactive *Mycoplasma pneumoniae* vaccine in military personnel. *Am Rev Resp Dis* 1968;97:359–61.

50. GREENBERG H, HELMS CM, BRUNNER H, CHANOCK RM. Asymptomatic infection of adult volunteers with a temperature-sensitive mutant of *Mycoplasma pneumoniae*. *Proc Natl Acad Sci USA* 1974;71:4015–4019.

51. JENSEN KE, SERTERFIT LB, SCULLY WE. *Mycoplasma pneumoniae* infections in children: an epidemiological approval in families treated with oxytetracycline. *Am J Epidemiol* 1967;86:419–21.

52. MOULDER JW. Looking at *Chlamydia* without looking at their hosts. *Am Soc Microbiol* News, 1984;50:353–62.

53. MOULDER JW. Interaction of *Chlamydiae* and host cells *in vivo*. *Microbiol Rev* 1991;51:143–90.

54. HATCH TP, AL-HOSSAINY E, SILVERMAN JA. Adenine nucleotide and lysine transport in *Chlamydia psittaci*. *J Bacteriol* 1982;150:662–70.

55. WEISBURG WG, HATCH TB, WOESE CR. Eubacterial origin of *Chlamydiae*. *J Bacteriol* 1986;167:570–4.

56. MACFARLANE JT, MACRAE AD. Psittacosis. *Med Bull* 1983;39:163–7.

57. PALMER SR, ANDREWS BE, MAJOR R. A common source outbraek of ornithosis in veterinary surgeons. *Lancet* 1982;ii:798–9.

58. GRIMES JE. Zoonoses acquired from pet birds. *Vet Clin* 1987;17:209–18.

59. PSITTACOSIS (editorial) *Br Med J* 1972;1:1–2.

60. BARNES MG, BRAINERD H. Pneumonitis with alveolar-capillary block in a cattle rancher exposed to epizootic bovine abortion. *N Engl J Med* 1964;271:981–5.

61. JOHN FWA, MATHESON BA, WILLIAMS H. Abortion due to infection with *Chlamydia psittaci* in a sheep farmer's wife. *Br Med J* 1985;290:592–4.

62. CROSSE B. Psittacosis : a clinical review. *J Infect* 1990;21:251–9.

63. YUNG AP, GRAYSON ML. Psittacosis – a review of 135 cases. *Med J Aust* 1988;148:228–33.

64. PAGE SR, STEWART JT, BENSTEIN JJ. A progressive pericardial effusion caused by psittacosis. *Br Heart J* 1988;60:87–9.

65. SHAPIRO DS, KENNEY SC, JOHNSON M. Brief report: *Chlamydia psittaci* endocarditis diagnosed by blood culture. *N Engl J Med* 1992;326:1192–5.

66. SAMRA Z PIK A, GUIDETTI-SHARON A. Hepatitis in a family infected by *Chlamydia psittaci*. *J Roy Soc Med* 1991;84:347–8.

67. GEDDES DM, SKEATES SJ. Ornithosis pneumonia associated with haemolysis. *Br J Dis Chest* 1977;71:135–7.

68. TSAPAS G, KLONIZAKIS I, CASAKOS K. Psittacosis and arthritis. *Chemother*, 1991;37:143–5.

69. SENEL J. Cutaneous findings in a case of psittacosis. *Arch Dermatol* 1984;120:1227–9.

70. JEFFREY RF, MORE IAR, CARRINGTON MB. Acute glomerulonephritis following infection with *Chlamydia psittaci*. *Am J Kidney Dis* 1992;1:94–6.

71. SAHN SA. Pleural effusions in the atypical pneumonias. *Semin Respir Infect* 1988; 3:322–34.

72. MEYER KF. Psittacosis-lymphogranuloma venereum agents In: Horsfall FL, Tanim I (eds). *Viral and Rickettsial Infections of Man*. 4th ed London : Pitman 1965;1006–41.

73. JARIWALLA AG, DAVIES BH, WHITE J. Infective endocarditis complicating psittacosis : response to rifampicin. *Br Med J* 1980;280:155.

74. GRAYSTON JT, KNO CC, WANG SP, ALTMAN J. A new *Chlamydia psittaci* strain, TWAR, isolated in acute respiratory tract infections. *N Engl J Med* 1986;315:161–8.

75. FRYDEN A, KIHLSTROM E, MALLER R, PERSSON K, ROMANUS V, ANSUHU S. A clinical and epidemiological study of 'ornithosis' caused by *Chlamydia psittaci* and *Chlamydia pneumoniae* (strain TWAR). *Scand J Infect Dis* 1989;21:681–91.

76. PETHER JVS, WANG SP, GRAYSTON JT. *Chlamydia pneumoniae*, strain TWAR, as the cause of an outbreak in a boys' school, previously called psittacosis. *Epidem Infect* 1989;103:395–400.

77. COX RL, KNO CC, GRAYSTON JT, CAMPBELL LA Deoxyribonucleic acid relatedness of Chlamydia species strain TWAR to *Chlamydia trachomatis* and *Chlamydia psittaci*. *Int J Syst Bacteriol* 1988;38:265–8.

78. KNO CC, CHI EY, GRAYSTON JT. Ultrastructural study of entry of *Chlamydia* strain TWAR into HeLa cells. *Infect Immunol* 1988;56:1668–72.

79. GRAYSTON JT, WANG SP, KUO CC, CAMPBELL LA. Current knowledge on *Chlamydia pneumoniae*, strain TWAR and important cause of pneumonia and other respiratory diseases. *Eur J Clin Microbiol Infect Dis* 1989;8:191–202.

80. YAMAZAKI T, NAKADA H, SAKURAI N, KUO CC, WANG SP, GRAYSTON JT. Transmission of *Chlamydia pneumoniae* in young children in a Japanese family. *J Infect Dis* 1990;162:1390–2.

81. HYMAN CL, AUGENBRAUN MH, BOLLIN PM, SCHACHTER J, HAMMERSCHLAG MR. Asymptomatic respiratory tract infection with *Chlamydia pneumoniae* TWAR. *J Clin Microbiol* 1991;29:2082–3.

82. GNARPE J, GNARPE H, SUNDERLOF B. Endemic prevalence of *Chlamydia pneumoniae* in subjectively healthy persons. *Scand J Infect Dis* 1991;23:387–8.

83. CHIRGWIN K, ROBLIN PM, GELLING M, HAMMERSCHLAG MR, SCHACHTER J. Infection with *Chlamydia pneumoniae* in Brooklyn. *J Infect Dis* 1991;163:757–61.

84. TREHARNE JD, BALLARD RC. The expanding spectrum of Chlamydia – a microbiological and clinical appraisal. *Rev Med Microbiol* 1990;1:10–18.

85. KARAMOTO Y, OUCHI K, MIZUI M, USHIO M, USUI T. Prevalence of antibody to *Chlamydia pneumoniae* TWAR in Japan. *J Clin Microbiol* 1991;29:816–18.

86. MONTES M, CILLA G, ALCORTA M, PEREZ-TRALLERO E High prevalence of *Chlamydia pneumoniae* in children and young adults in Spain. *Ped Infect Dis J* 1992;11:972–3.

87. GRAYSTON JT, *Chlamydia pneumoniae*, strain TWAR. *Chest* 1989;95:664–9.

88. WANG SP, GRAYSTON JT. Population prevalence antibody to *Chlamydia pneumoniae*, strain TWAR. In Boure WR, Caldwell HD, Jones RP, eds. *Chlamydial Infections* Cambridge, England : Cambridge University Press,1990:402–5.

89. MORDHORST CH, WANG SP, GRAYSTON JT. Epidemic 'ornithosis' and TWAR infection, Denmark 1976–1985. In Criel JD, Ridgeway GL, Schachter J, Taylor-Robinson D, Ward M. eds. *Chlamydial Infections*. Cambridge, England: Cambridge University Press, 1986;325–8.

90. GRAYSTON JT, CAMPBELL LA, KNO CC, MORDHORST CH, SAIKKU P, THOM DH. A new respiratory tract pathogen: *Chlamydia pneumoniae*, strain TWAR. *J Infect Dis* 1990;161:618–25.

91. KLEEMOLA M, SAIKKU P, VISAKOPPI R, WANG SP, GRAYSTON JT. Epidemics of pneumonia caused by TWAR, a new chlamydia organism, in military trainees in Finland. *J Infect Dis* 1988;157:230–6.

92. GHOSH K, FREW CE, CARRINGTON D. A family outbreak of *Chlamydia pneumoniae* infection. *J Infect* 1992;25(Suppl):99–103.

93. FALEY AR, WALSH EE. Transmission of *Chlamydia pneumoniae*. *J Infect Dis* 1993;168:493–6.

94. GAYDOS CA, ROBLIN PM, HAMMERSCHLAG MK, HYMAN CL, EIDEN JJ, SCHACHTER J. Diagnostic utility of PCR-enzyme immunoassay, culture and serology for

detection of *Chlamydia pneumoniae* in symptomatic and asymptomatic patients. *J Clin Microbiol* 1994;32:903–5.

95. THEURISSEN HJH, LEMMENS DEN TOOM NA, BURGGRAAF A, STOLZ E, MICHEL MF. Influence of temperative and relative humidity on the survival of *Chlamydia* pneumonia strain TWAR. *Appl Environ Med* 1993;59:2589–93.

96. BELL TA, KUO CC, WANG SP, GRAYSON JT. Experimental infection of baboons (*Paprio cynocephalus anubis*) with *Chlamydia pneumoniae* strain TWAR. *J Infect* 1989;19:47–9.

97. HOLLAND SM, TAYLOR HR, GAYDOS CA, KIAPPUS EW, QUINN TC. Experimental infection with *Chlamydia pneumoniae* in non-human primates. *Infect Immun* 1990;58:593–7.

98. FANG GD, FINE M, ORLOFF J, ARISUMI D, YU VL, KAPOOR W. New and emerging aetologies for community-acquired pneumonia with implications for therapy : a prospective multicenter study of 359 cases. *Medicine* 1990;69:307–16.

99. MYKRA W, MORDHURST CH, WANG SP, GRAYSTON JT. Clinical features of *Chlamydia pneumoniae*, strain TWAR, infection in Denmark 1975–1987. In Boure WR, Caldwell HD, Jones PP, Mardl PH, Ridgway GL, Schachter J. eds. *Chlamydial Infections.* Cambridge, England: Cambridge University Press, 1990:422–5.

100. AUGENBRAUN MH, ROBLIN PM, MANDEL L, HAMMERESCHLAG MR. *Chlamydia pneumoniae* pneumonia with pleural effusion : diagnosis by culture. *Am J Med* 1991;91:437–8.

101. KAUPPINEN MT, SAIKKU P, KIYALA P, HERVA E, SYRJALA H. Clinical picture of community-acquired *Chlamydia pneumoniae* pneumonia requiring hospital treatment : a comparison between chlamydial and pneumococcal pneumonia. *Thorax* 1996;51:185–9.

102. HAMMERSCHLAG MR. *Chlamydia pneumoniae* infections. *J Infect Dis* 1991;163:757–60.

103. ALLEGRA L, BLASI F, CERTANNI S, COSENTINI R, DENTI F, RASSENELK R. Acute exacerbation of asthma in adults: role of *Chlamydia pneumoniae* infection. *Eur Resp J* 1994;7:2165–8.

104. EMRE U, ROBLIN PM, GELLING M, DUMORNAY W, RAO M, HAMMERSCHLAG MR. The association of *Chlamydia pneumoniae* infection and reactive airways disease in children. *Arch Pediatr Adolesc Med* 1994;148:727–32.

105. HOHN DL, DODGE R, GOLUBJATRIKOV R. Association of *Chlamydia pneumoniae* (strain TWAR) infection with wheezing, asthmatic bronchitis and adult-onset asthma. *JAMA* 1991;266:225–30.

106. BEATY CD, GRAYSTON JT, WANG SP, KUO CC, RETO CS, MARTIN TR. *Chlamydia pneumoniae*, strain TWAR, infection in patients with chronic obstructive pulmonary disease. *Am Rev Resp Dis* 1991;144:1408–10.

107. BLASI F, LEGNANI D, LOMBARDO VM, NEGRETTO GG, MAGLIANO E, PAZZOLI R. *Chlamydia pneumoniae* infection in acute exacerbation of COPD. *Eur Resp J* 1993;6:19–22.

108. BRAUN J, LAITKOS S, TREHARNE J, EGGERS U, WU P, DISTLER A *Chlamydia pneumoniae* – a new causative agent of reactive arthritis and undifferentiated oligoarthritis. *Ann Rheum Dis* 1994;53:100–5.

109. SOCAN M, BEOVIC B, KESE O. *Chlamydia pneumoniae* and meningoencephalitis. *N Engl J Med* 1994;331:406.

110. HAID IS, IVARSSON S, BJERRE I, PERSSON K Guillain–Barré syndrome after *Chlamydia pneumoniae* infection. *N Engl J Med* 1992;326:576–7.

111. MICHEL D, ANTOINE JC, POZZETTO B, GAUDIN OG, LUCHT F. Lumbosacral meningoradiculitis associated with *Chlamydia pneumoniae* infection. *J Neurol Neurosurg Psychiat* 1992;55:511.

112. WESSLEN L, PAHLSON C, FRIMAN G, FOHLMAN J, LINDGUIST O, JOHANSSON C. Myocarditis caused by *Chlamydia pneumoniae* (TWAR) and sudden unexpected death in a Swedish elite orienteer. *Lancet* 1992;340:427–8.

113. MARRIE TJ, HARCZY M, MANN K, LANDYMORRE W, WANG SP, GRAYSTON JT. Culture-negative endocarditis probably due to *Chlamydia pneumoniae*. *J Infect Dis* 1990;161:127–9.

114. LOPEZ-VIRELLA MF, VIRELLA G. Immunological and microbiological factors in the pathogenesis of atherosclerosis. *Clin Immunol Immunopathol* 1985;37:377–86.

115. SMITH GW, MCARTHUR CJ, SIMPSON IJ. Circulating immune complexes in myocardial infarction. *J Clin Lab Immunol* 1983;12:197–9.

116. SAIKKU P, MATTILA K, NIEMINER MS, HUTTUNEN JK, LEINONEN M, EKMAN MR. Serological evidence of an association of a novel chlamydia, TWAR, with chronic coronary heart disease and acute myocardial infarction. *Lancet* 1988;ii:983–5.

117. MELNICK SL, SHAHAR E, FOLSOM A, GRAYSTON JT, SORLIE PD, WANG SP. Past infection by chlamydial pneumonia strain TWAR and asymptomatic carotid atherosclerosis. *Am J Med* 1993;95:499–504.

118. LINNANMAKI E, LEINONEN M, MATTILA K, NIEMINEN MS, VALTONEN V, SAIKKU P. *Chlamydia pneumoniae*–specific circulating immune complexes in patients with chronic coronary heart disease. *Circulation* 1993;87:1130–4.

119. KUO CC, SHOR A, CAMPBELL LA, FUKUSHI H, PATTON DL, GRAYSTON JT. Demonstration of *Chlamydia pneumoniae* in atherosclerotic lesions of coronary arteries. *J Infect Dis* 1993;167:841–9.

120. THOM DH, GRAYSTON JT, SISCOVOCK DS, WANG SP, WEISS NS, DALING JR Association of prior infection with *Chlamydia pneumoniae* and angiographically demonstrated coronary artery disease. *JAMA* 1992;268:68–72.

121. MARRIE TJ, GRAYSTON JT, WANG SP, KUO CC. Pneumoniae associated with the TWAR strain of *Chlamydia*. *Ann Intern Med* 1987;106:507–11.

122. WANG SP, GRAYSTON JT. Microimmunoflorescence serological studies with the TWAR organism. In Oriel JD, Ridgway G, Schachter J, Taylor-Robinson D, Ward M. *Chlamydial Infections*. Cambridge, England. Cambridge University Press, 1986:329–32.

123. SILLIS M, WHITE P, CAUL EO, PAUL ID, TRAHARNE JD. The differentiation of *Chlamydia* species by antigen detection in sputum specimens from patients with community acquired acute respiratory infections. *J Infect* 1992;25(Suppl I):77–86.

124. GAYDOS CA, ROBLIN PM, HAMMERSCHLAG MR, HYMAN CL, EIDER JJ, SCHACHTER J. Diagnostic utility of PCR-enzyme immunoassay, culture and serology for detection of *Chlamydia pneumoniae* in symptomatic and asymptomatic patients. *J Clin Microbiol* 1994;32:903–5.

125. FENELON LE, MUMTAZ G, RIDGWAY GL. The *in vitro* susceptibility of *Chlamydia pneumoniae*. *J Antimicrob Chemother* 1990;2:763–7.

126. ROBLIN PM, MONTALBAN G, HAMMERSCHLAG MR. Susceptibilities to clarithromycin and erythromycin of isolates of *Chlamydia pneumoniae* from children with pneumonia. *Antimicrob Agents Chemother* 1994;38:1588–9.

127. HAMMERSCHLAG MR, CHIRGWIN K, ROBLIN PM, GELLING M, DUNOUNAY W, MANDEL L. Persistent infection with *Chlamydia pneumoniae* infection. *Clin Infect Dis* 1992;14:178–82.

128. CALDWELL HD, STEWART S, JOHNSON S, TAYLOR H. Tear and serum antibody response to Chlamydia trachomatic antigens during acute chlamydial conjunctivitis in monkeys as determined by immunoblotting. *Infect Immun* 1987;55:93–8.

129. GRAYSTON JT, KIN KS, ALEXANDER ER, WANG SP. Protective studies in monkeys with trivalent and monovalent trachoma vaccines. In Nichols RL ed. *Trachoma and Related Disorders Caused by Chlamydial Agents*. Amsterdam: Exerpta Medica, 1971:377–85.
130. DERRICK EH. 'Q' fever, new fever entity : clinical features, diagnosis and laboratory investigations. *Med J Aust* 1937;2:281–99.
131. BURNET FM, FREEMAN M. Experimental studies on the virus of 'Q' fever. *Med J Aust* 1937;2:299–305.
132. DAVIS G, COX HR. A filter-passing infectious agent isolated from ticks: isolation from *Dermacentors andersoni*, reactions in animals and filtration experiments. *Public Health Rep* 1939;53:2259–67.
133. DYER RE. Similarity of Australian Q fever and a disease caused by an infectious agent isolated from ticks in Montana. *Public Health Rep* 1939;54:1229–37.
134. MCCAUL TF, WILLIAMS JC. Development cycle of *Coxiella burnetti*: structure and morphogenesis of vegetative and sporogenic differentiations. *J Bacteriol* 1981;147:1063–76.
135. SAWYER LA, FISHBEIN DB, MCDADE JE. Q fever : current concepts. *Rev Infect Dis* 1987;9:935–46.
136. SCHRANEK S, MAYER H. Different sugar compostions of lipopolysacchandes isolated from phase I and pure phase II cells of *Coxiella burnetti*. *Infect Immun* 1982;38:53–7.
137. MINNICK MF, HEINZEN RA, RESCHKE DK. A plasmid-encoded surface protein found in chronic disease isolates of *Coxiella burnetti*. *Infect Immun* 1991;59:4735–9.
138. MALLAVIA LP, SAMUEL JE, FRAZIER HE. The genetics of *Coxiella burnetti* : etiologic agent of Q fever and chronic endocarditis. In Williams JC, Thompson HA. eds. *Q Fever: The Biology of* Coxiella burnetti. Boca Raton, FL : CRC Press; 1991:259–84.
139. BACA OG, PARETSKY D. Q fever and *Coxiella burnetti* : a model for host–parasite interactions. *Microbiol Rev* 1983;47:127–49.
140. LANGLEY JM, MARIE TJ, COVERT A. Poker players pneumonia: an urban outbreak following exposure to a parturient cat. *N Engl J Med* 1988;319:354–6.
141. LEEDOM JM. Q fever : An update. In Remington JS, Schwartz MN. eds. *Current Clinical Topics in Infectious Diseases*. New York : McGraw-Hill, 1980:304–31.
142. CENTERS FOR DISEASE CONTROL AND PREVENTION. Q fever outbreak – Switzerland. *MMWR* 1984;33:355–61.
143. SALMON MM, HOWELLS B, GLENCROSS EJF. Q fever in an urban area. *Lancet* 1982;1:1002–4.
144. OLIPHANT JW, GORDON DA, MEIS A. Q fever in laundry workers presumably transmitted from contaminated clothing. *Am J Hyg* 1949;49:72–82.
145. BELL JA, BECK MD, HUEBNER RJ. Epidemiologic studies of Q fever in Southern California. *JAMA* 1950;142:868–72.
146. HALL CJ, RICHMOND SJ, CAUL EO. Laboratory outbreak of Q fever acquired from sheep. *Lancet* 1982;1:1004–6.
147. MEIKLEJOHN G, REINER LG, GRAVES PS, HELMICK C. Cryptic epidemic of Q fever in a medical school. *J Infect Dis* 1981;144:107–14.
148. Editorial comment on Q fever transmitted by blood transfusion. *United States Can Dis Wkly Rep* 1977;3:210.
149. HARMAN JB. Q fever in Great Britain. Clinical account of eight cases. *Lancet* 1949;ii:1028–30.
150. MANN JS, DOUGLAS JG, INGLIS JM, LEITCH AG. Q fever : person to person transmission within a family. *Thorax* 1986;41:974–5.
151. DEUTCH DL, PETERSON ET. Q fever : transmission from one human being to others. *JAMA* 1950;143:348–50.
152. WELSH HH, LENNELTE EH, ABINARTE FR. Air-borne transmission of Q fever: the role of parturition in the generation of infective aerosols. *Ann NY Acad Sci* 1958;70:528–40.
153. WELSH HH, LENNELTE EH, ABINARTE FR. Q fever studies XXI. The recovery of *Coxiella burnetti* from the soil and surface water of premises harbouring infected sheep. *Am J Hyg* 1959;70:14–20.
154. DUPONT HT, RAOULT D, BROUQUI P. Epidemiologic features and clinical presentation of acute Q fever in hospitalised patients : 323 French cases. *Am J Med* 1992;93:427–34.
155. LUOTO L, CASEY ML, PICKERS EG. Q fever studies in Montana. Detection of asymptomatic infection among residents of infected dairy premises. *Am J Epidemiol* 1965;81:356–69.
156. VICIANA P, MACHAN J, CUELLO JA. Fever of indeterminate duration in the community. A seven year study in the South of Spain. *Abstract No. 683. 32nd Interscience Conference on Antimicrobial Agents and Chemotherapy*. October 11–14, 1992. Washington DC: American Society for Microbiology.
157. LIM KC, KANG JYU. Q fever presenting with gastroenteritis. *Med J Aust* 1980;1:327.
158. FLINT N, SMITH G, AYRES JG. Five year follow up of patients involved in the 1989 Q fever outbreak. *Thorax* 1995;50:464.
159. TURCK WPG, HOWITT G, TURNBERG LA, FOX W, MATTHEWS MB, DAS GUPTA R. Chronic Q fever. *Quart J Med* 1976;45:192–217.
160. Editorial. Chronic Q fever. *J Infect* 1984;8:1–4.
161. PALMER SR, YOUNG SEJ. Q fever endocarditis in England and Wales, 1975–1981. *Lancet* 1982;2:1148–9.
162. LAU FO D, LAW PD, OBERHARSKI I. Chronic Q fever endocarditis with massive splenomegaly in childhood. *J Pediatr* 1986;108:535–9.
163. RAOULT D, PIQUET PH, GALLAIS H. *Coxiella burnetti* infection of a vascular prosthesis. *N Engl J Med* 1986;315:1358–9.
164. ROSS PJ, JACOBSON J, MUIR JR. Q fever endocarditis of porcine xenograft valves. *Am Heart J* 1983;105:151–3.
165. HOFFMAN CER, HEATON JW. Q fever hepatitis. Clinical manifestations and pathological findings. *Gastroenterology* 1982;83:474–9.
166. QIZILBASH AH. The pathology of Q fever as seen on liver biopsy. *Arch Pathol Lab Med* 1983;107:364–7.
167. TRAVIS LB, TRAVIS WD, LI C-Y. Q fever. A clinicopathological study of five cases. *Arch Pathol Lab Med* 1986;100:1017–20.
168. MARRIE TJ. Pneumonia and meningo-encephalitis due to *Coxiella burnetti*. *J Infect* 1985;11:59–61.
169. MARRIE TJ, RAOULT D. Rickettsial infections of the central nervous system. *Semin Neurol* 1992;12:213–24.
170. DRANCOURT M, RAOULT D, XERIDAT B, MARRIE TJ. Q fever meningoencephalitis in five patients. *Eur J Epidemiol* 1991;7:134–8.
171. REILLY S, NORTHWOOD JL, CAUL EO. Q fever in Plymouth, 1972–1988. A review with particular reference to neurological manifestations. *Epidemiol Infect* 1990;105:391–408.
172. ELLIS ME, SMITH CC, MOFFAT MAJ. Chronic or fatal Q fever infection. A review of 16 patients seen in the North East of Scotland (1967–1980). *Quart J Med* 1983;205:54–66.
173. BRADA M, BELLINGHAM AJ. Bone marrow necrosis and Q fever. *Br Med J* 1980;210:1108–9.
174. CARDELLACH F, FONT J, AGNST AG. Q fever and haemolytic anaemia. *J Infect Dis* 1983;148:769.
175. HITCHINS R, COBCROFT RG, HOCER G. Transient severe hypoplastic anaemia in Q fever. *Pathol* 1986;18:254–5.
176. BAUMBACH A, BREHM B, SAUER W. Spontaneous splenic rupture complicating acute Q fever. *Am J Gastroenterol* 1992;87:1651–3.
177. SCHUIL J, RICHARDHUS JH, BOARSMA GS. Q fever as a possible cause of bilateral optic neuritis. *Br J Ophthalmol* 1985;69:580–3.

178. CONGET I, MALLOLAS J, MENSA J, ROVIRA M. Erythema nodosum and Q fever. *Arch Dermatol* 1987;123:867.

179. SWABY ED, FISCHER-HOCH S, LAMBERT HP, STEM H. Is Kawasaki disease a variant of Q fever? *Lancet* 1980;2:146.

180. WEIR WRC, BOUCHET VA, MITFORD E, TAYLOR RF, SMITH H. Kwawasaki disease in European adult associated with serological response to *Coxiella burnetti*. *Lancet* 1985;2:504.

181. RICHARDHUS JH, DUNA AM, HUISMAN J. Q fever in infancy : a review of 18 cases. *Pediatr Infect Dis* 1985;4:369–73.

182. RAOULT D, LEVY P-Y, DUPONT HT. Q fever and HIV infection. *AIDS* 1993;7:81–6.

183. BROUQUI P, DUPONT HT, DRANCOURT M. Chronic Q fever : ninety-two cases from France including 27 cases without endocarditis. *Arch Intern Med* 1993;153:642–9.

184. ROBINS FC. Q fever in Mediterranean area: report of its occurrence in allied troops. *Am J Hyg* 1946;44:51–71.

185. BIGGS BA, DOUGLAS JG, GRANT IWB, CROMPTON GK. Prolonged Q fever associated with inappropriate secretion of anti-diuretic hormone. *J Infect* 1984;8:61–3.

186. GORDON JD, MACKEEN AD, MARRIE TJ. The radiographic features of epidemic and sporadic Q fever pneumonia. *J Can Assoc Radiol* 1984;35:293–6.

187. MILLAR JK. The chest film findings in Q fever – a series of 35 cases. *Clin Radiol* 1978;329:371–5.

188. PIERCE TH, YUCHT SE, GORIN AB. Q fever pneumonitis : diagnosis by transbronchial lung biopsy. *West J Med* 1979;130:453–5.

189. URSO FP. The pathologic findings in rickettsial pneumonia. *Am J Clin Pathol* 1975;64:335–42.

190. JANIGAR DT, MARRIE JT. An inflammatory pseudotumour of the lung in Q fever pneumonia. *N Engl J Med* 1983;30:86–8.

191. PETER O, DUPUIS G, BURGODAEFER W. Evaluation of the complement fixation and indirect immunofluorescence tests in the early diagnosis of primary Q fever. *Eur J Clin Microbiol* 1985;4:394–6.

192. PETER O, DUPUIS G, PEACOCK MG Comparison of enzyme-linked immunosorbent assay and complement fixation and indirect antibody tests for detection of *Coxiella burnetti* antibody. *J Clin Microbiol* 1987;25:1063–7.

193. BLANDEAU JM, WILLIAMS JC, MARRIE TJ. The immune response to phase I and phase II *Coxiella burnetti* antigens as measured by western immunoblotting. *Ann NY Acad Sci* 1990;590:187–202.

194. HUNT JG, FIELD PR, MURPHY AM. Immunoglobulin responses to *Coxiella burnetti* (Q fever): single-serum diagnosis of acute infection using an immunofluorescence technique. *Infect Immunol* 1983; 39:977–81.

195. WORSWICK D, MARMIAN BP. Antibody response in acute and chronic Q fever and in subjects vaccinated against Q fever. *J Med Microbiol* 1985;119:281–96.

196. DUPUIS G, PETER O, PEACOCK M. Immunoglobulin responses in acute Q fever. *J Clin Microbiol* 1985;22:484–7.

197. YEAMAN MR, MITSHER LA, BACA OG. *In vitro* susceptibility of *Coxiella burnetti* for antibiotics, including several quinolones. *Antimicrob Agents Chemother* 1987;31:1079–84.

198. D'ANGELO LJ, HETHERINGTON R. Q fever treated with erythromycin. *Br Med J* 1979;2:305–6.

199. ELLIS ME, DUNBAR EM. *In vivo* response of acute Q fever to erythromycin. *Thorax* 1982;37:867–8.

200. LEVY PY, DRANCOURT M, ETIENNE J. Comparison of different antibiotic regimens for therapy of 32 cases of Q fever endocarditis. *Antimicrob Agents Chemother* 1991;35:533–7.

201. MAURIN M, BEROLIEL AM, BONGRAND P. Phagolysomal alkalinisation and the bactericidal effect of antibiotics : the *Coxiella burnetti* paradigm. *J Infect Dis* 1992;166:1097–102.

202. POLYDOUROU K. Q fever in Cyprus – recent progress. *Br Vet J* 1985;141:427–30.

203. ASCHER MS, BERMAN MA, RUPPARER R. Initial clinical and immunologic evaluation of a new phase I Q fever vaccine and skin test in humans. *J Infect Dis* 1983;148:214–24.

204. MARMAN BP, ORMSBEE R, KYRKOU M. Vaccine prophylaxis of abbatoir-associated Q fever. *Lancet* 1984;2:1411–14.

14 Legionellosis

J.M. WATSON* and J.T. MACFARLANE†

*Communicable Disease Surveillance Centre, Colindale, UK; †Nottingham City Hospital, UK

Epidemiology

Legionnaires' disease was not recognised until 1976 when an outbreak of pneumonic illness occurred among American legionnaires attending a convention in a hotel in Philadelphia.[1] It was not until early the following year that the causative organism was isolated and identified.[2] Using stored sera it was subsequently possible to determine that a number of previously unexplained outbreaks of pneumonia had also been caused by *Legionnella* infections. Although the precise source of the eponymous outbreak was never identified, many other outbreaks have since been recognised and their source precisely identified.

The term 'legionellosis' encompasses any illness due to *Legionella* infection. 'Legionnaires' disease' is reserved for the pneumonic form of legionellosis whereas 'Pontiac fever' is generally used to describe the non-pneumonic form of the disease.[3] In practice *Legionella* infections may cause a spectrum of illness from an asymptomatic infection through influenza-like illness, to fulminant pneumonia. Cases of Legionnaires' disease have now been identified in patients in most industrialised countries although reports of cases from developing countries are uncommon due, at least in part, to limited diagnostic facilities.

More than 30 species of *Legionella* have been identified but only a small number have been associated with disease in man. Over three-quarters of infections are caused by *Legionella pneumophila* species most usually serogroup 1. *Legionella micdadei* is the second commonest pathogen, more often affecting immunocompromised individuals, followed by *Legionella bozemanii* and *Legionella dumoffii*.[4]

Legionella spp. are found widely in the man-made and natural environment surviving in water and soil. Although difficult to isolate in the laboratory, the organism readily colonises water systems including the domestic water systems providing hot and cold water to large buildings, as well as the water system used for cooling purposes in wet cooling systems such as air conditioning. A chain of events is required for *Legionella* to cause illness in man[1]: a virulent strain of *Legionella* must survive in a water system; environmental conditions must allow the organism to multiply to high concentrations; the water must be aerosolised into particles that permit droplet nuclei to be inhaled deep into the lungs; the aerosolised organism must be inhaled before it is inactivated by ultra-violet light or drying; the host must be susceptible to the infection. Despite the ubiquitous nature of the organism, these circumstances probably occur infrequently in situations where people will be exposed.

A comprehensive surveillance system for cases of Legionnaires' disease in England and Wales has been maintained by the Communicable Disease Surveillance Centre of the Public Health laboratory Service since 1977.[5] Cases, which must have clinical evidence of a pneumonic illness and microbiological evidence of a *Legionella* infection reaching certain minimum criteria, are reported to CDSC by hospital laboratories, clinicians and public health physicians on a voluntary basis. Ascertainment and reporting of cases of Legionnaires' disease is incomplete: many cases of pneumonia do not undergo microbiological investigation, and if they do, are not investigated for *Legionella* infection; despite appropriate investigation the timing of the collection of specimens may produce negative results; appropriately diagnosed infections may not be reported. Despite the under-ascertainment and reporting, this surveillance system, which has remained little changed for 15 years, provides useful information about the trends in the incidence of this disease and can give early warning of the occurrence of outbreaks.

Between 100 and 300 cases of Legionnaires' disease are reported each year in England and Wales although this total has been falling in the last decade (Table 14.1). The occurrence of the disease appears to increase with age but reduced opportunity for exposure may account for the slightly lower numbers in the elderly group (Fig.14.1). Men appear to be more susceptible than women even after allowing for exposure opportunities and smoking habit. About 15% of the reported cases are subsequently reported to have died.

Cases may be *sporadic*, i.e. single cases not known to be associated with any other cases of disease, or occur in *outbreaks*, i.e. clusters of two or more cases associated in time and place. Cases occur in three main settings: the community, in hospital, and in association with

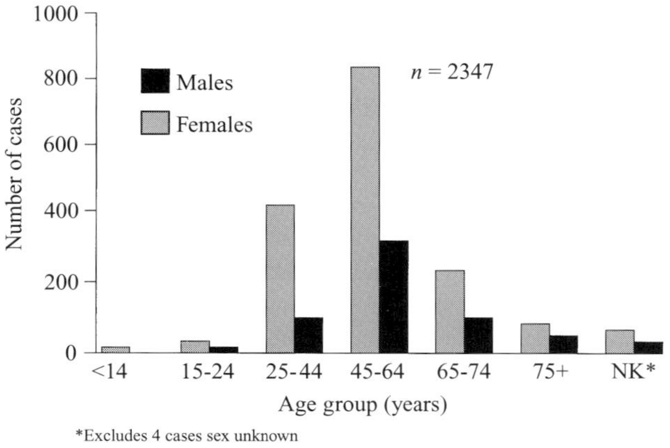

FIGURE 14.1 Age groups and sex of patients with Legionnaires' disease: residents of England and Wales, 1980–92. (Source: PHLS Communicable Disease Surveillance Centre, London.)

Table 14.1. *Legionnaires' disease in residents of England and Wales reported from 1980 to 1994*

Year	Males	Females	Total	Deaths
1980	132	50	182	23
1981	99	42	142	15
1982	96	42	138	20
1983	114	45	159	22
1984	116	34	150	15
1985	137	72	210	39
1986	136	53	190	23
1987	150	59	210	36
1988	216	62	279	17
1989	179	64	243	32
1990	147	40	187	23
1991	81	31	112	17
1992	116	33	149	25
1993	85	44	129	22
1994	121	39	160	27
Total	1926	710	2640[a]	356

[a]includes four cases with sex unknown.

Source: PHLS Communicable Disease Surveillance Centre, London.

travel. Approximately half of cases are associated with travel which, in residents of England and Wales, is most commonly associated with visits to hotels on the Mediterranean coast.[6] Hospital stay accounts for a small but important proportion of all cases as, in some of these, the infection is acquired from the hospital itself meriting urgent investigation.[7] Wet cooling systems in large buildings (cooling towers) have been associated with well-recognised large outbreaks but a greater number of outbreaks have been attributed to domestic water systems in large buildings. Little is known about the origin of sporadic cases in the community, although unrecognised transmission of infection from cooling towers within the community,[8] and possibly transmission from domestic water systems within the home,[9] have been suggested as possible sources of these infections.

A seasonal pattern in the occurrence of *Legionella* infections is apparent with cases generally being reported more frequently in the summer and autumn months (Fig.14.2). This is largely a result of the increased number of travel associated cases in the summer months but may also reflect the enhanced viability of *Legionella* spp. in warmer water and the increased use of water-cooled air-conditioning systems at this time of the year.

In view of the high proportion of cases occurring in travellers, and the potential to prevent further cases by investigation of suspected sources, a surveillance system for travel associated cases in Europe has recently been established.[5] The system permits the identification of accommodation, such as hotels, associated with two or more cases of Legionnaires' disease in travellers who may live in different European countries and whose national surveillance systems alone would be unlikely to identify the occurrence of an outbreak. Public health authorities in the countries concerned are informed so that appropriate investigations can be carried out locally.

Outbreak investigation

The essential elements of the investigation of a suspected outbreak of Legionnaires' disease include (a) confirmation of the diagnosis, (b) ascertainment of further cases, (c) application of control measures.[10]

Confirmation of the diagnosis in suspected cases of Legionnaires' disease is essential before public health action is considered. Liaison with the local microbiology laboratory, with support from the local public health laboratory and national reference centre, is important to rule out false-positive diagnoses. In particular, raised *Legionella* antibody titres are found in a small proportion of the population and recommendations have been made about the minimum levels with the standard serological tests for making a confirmed and presumptive diagnosis.[10] Additional clinical specimens should be sent as a matter of urgency if the diagnosis remains in doubt.

The occurrence of two or more cases, closely linked in time and place, strongly suggests the occurrence of a common source outbreak and the need to take action. An incident committee should be convened, usually under the chairmanship of the local consultant in communicable disease control (CCDC), but including clinicians and microbiologists as well as others dependent upon the setting of the suspected outbreak. Additional cases should be sought bearing in mind that some may be ill with pneumonia without *Legionella* infection having been suspected, and others may yet be incubating the infection. The search for further cases not only promotes the early institution of the appropriate antibiotic treatment but also provides the epidemiological information that may help to pinpoint the source of infection.

On the basis of the information available from the early cases, a geographical area or specific water system may be identified as a potential source of infection. The water systems should be examined, sampled and disinfected to prevent further possible transmission of infection. The combination of epidemiological, microbiological and environmental findings may ultimately be required to pinpoint the source of infection in an outbreak. Long-term control measures may need to take into account the findings of the detailed investigation and new

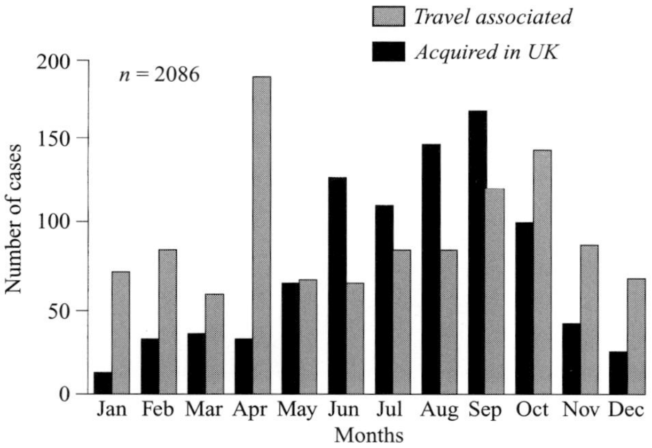

FIGURE 14.2 Seasonal distribution of cases of Legionnaires' disease: residents of England and Wales, 1980–92. (Source: PHLS Communicable Disease Surveillance Centre, London.)

information arising from the investigation should be reported to help prevent similar episodes elsewhere.[11,12]

Clinical manifestations of *Legionella* infections

Legionella infections present in the two principal forms of the disease, namely pneumonia and Pontiac fever.[3] It is not clear why people similarly exposed may develop either one or the other form of disease, although host factors and differing virulence of *Legionella* strains are likely to be relevant. It has been suggested that Pontiac fever may be a hypersensitivity reaction to *Legionella* bacteria in a previously sensitised individual or a reaction to inhaling large numbers of dead bacteria. The background prevalence of detectable *Legionella* antibodies in the community also suggests that subclinical infections resulting in seroconversion do occur.

Pontiac fever

This presents as a transient, self-limiting, influenzal-like illness and is an acute, non-pneumonic form of *Legionella* infection caused by several *Legionella* species.[13–15] The incubation period following exposure is usually 36–48 hours and the attack rate is extremely high with symptoms including high fever, headache, rigors, muscle aches and pains, malaise and dizziness. A dry cough may occur, but there are no signs of pneumonia on chest examination (Fig.14.3). The chest radiograph and white blood cell count are normal and the illness improves spontaneously, usually within 5 days. Treatment is symptomatic and the diagnosis is invariably made retrospectively by serological testing. Deaths have not been reported, although lassitude can persist following recovery.

Legionella pneumonia

Legionella infection can cause pneumonia in a number of different settings, including both community-acquired and nosocomial infections occurring sporadically or during an epidemic or on occasions due to background, endemic fever.

There is wide geographical and seasonal variation in the incidence of community-acquired *Legionella* pneumonia. Prospective clinical studies reported over recent years from Britain,[16–20] Europe,[21–26] New Zealand,[27] Australia,[28] Canada[29] and USA[30] have recorded an incidence varying from less than 1% up to 17% (Fig.14.4). Perhaps the best overall, representative figure was obtained from the multi-centre British Thoracic Society pneumonia study,[16] which identified *Legionella* pneumonia in 3% of patients who were tested. Unlike other bacterial respiratory pathogens, infection tends to lead to moderate or severe infection rather than a mild illness and *Legionella* pneumonia is the second commonest identified cause of adult community pneumonia requiring management on the Intensive Care Unit.[31]

The incubation period is usually 2–10 days and males are affected twice as often as females. The highest incidence is in the 40–70 year-old age-group (mean of 53 years) and infection at the extremes of age is rare. Risk factors include cigarette smoking, excess alcohol intake, diabetes, underlying chronic disease and those who are receiving corticosteroids or immunosuppressive therapy.

Clinical features

These are summarised in Fig.14.5. Flu-like symptoms start fairly abruptly with rigors, high fevers, severe headache and myalgia. Upper respiratory tract symptoms and skin rashes are uncommon. The cough that follows may be insignificant and dry initially, but shortness of breath is common and the illness often progresses quickly. Most patients require hospital admission within 5–7 days of developing symptoms. A story of a recent hospital or hotel stay is an important epidemiological clue for the clinician. Not infrequently, the patient will have received a β-lactam antibiotic in the community and have failed to improve.

The patient usually looks ill and toxic with a high fever of over 39 °C in the majority. Sometimes profuse diarrhoea and other non-respiratory features such as confusion and delirium can be the principle presenting complaint with the only pointer to pneumonia being localising signs detected in the chest by the alert clinician.

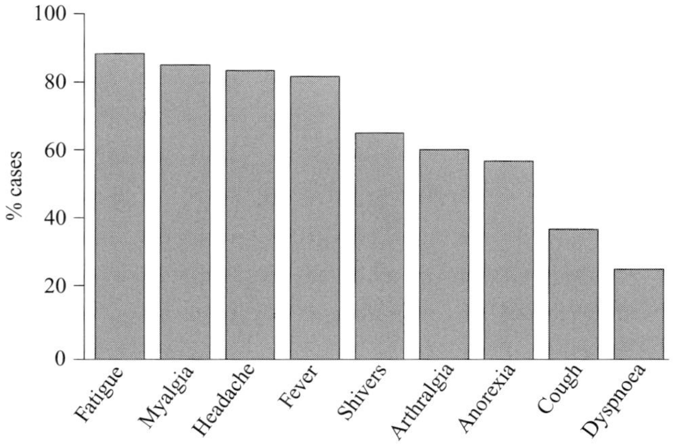

FIGURE 14.3 Clinical features of 631 patients diagnosed as having Pontiac fever. Adapted from Glick *et al.* (1978),[13] Herwaldt *et al.* (1984)[14] and Goldberg *et al.* (1989).[15]

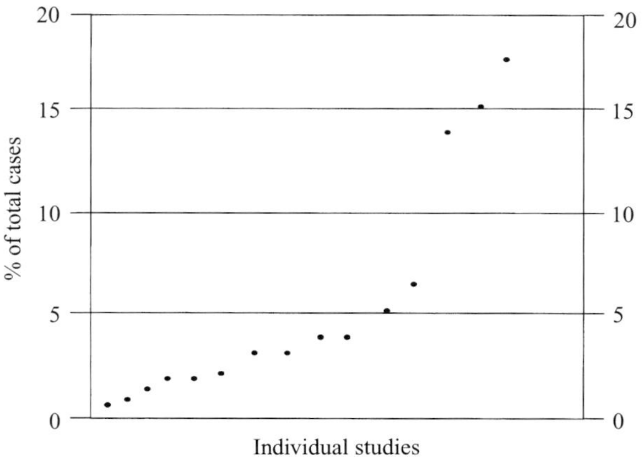

FIGURE 14.4 Incidence of *Legionella* pneumonia found in 15 recent hospital-based studies of adult community-acquired pneumonia[16–30].

Laboratory features

In contrast with other bacterial and atypical pneumonias, the total white count is usually only moderately raised up to 1000×10^6/litre in two-thirds of cases.[32] The blood film reveals a mild neutrophilia often with a lymphopenia. General disturbance of body function is common with hyponatraemia, hypoalbuminaemia and abnormal liver function tests being present in over half of cases and raised blood urea and muscle enzymes, haematuria and proteinuria and hypoxia due to advancing respiratory failure are also common.[33] Sputum may be difficult to obtain but typically Gram's stain reveals sparse pus cells and no predominant organism and initial blood and sputum cultures are negative unless dual infection is present. Dual infection is uncommon, but mostly involves added infection by *Streptococcus pneumoniae.*

Radiological features

There are no unique radiographic features of *Legionella* pneumonia.[34] The shadowing most commonly starts as segmental or lobar homogeneous consolidation, but characteristically radiographic deterioration occurs with spread of consolidation to both lungs. Some pleural fluid can be detected in a quarter of cases, although effusions are usually small. Lung cavitation is rare except in immunosuppressed patients.

The pulmonary shadows clear particularly slowly in survivors with only two-thirds of radiographs being clear within three months and some do not resolve for 6 months. It is not unusual to see persistent, irregular linear lines on the chest radiograph, presumably representing areas of fibrosis.

Complications

A wide variety of complications have been reported affecting nearly every system of the body.[35,35a] (Table 14.2) It is difficult to put these into context as most involve individual case reports. It is thought that complications occur from a multi-system toxic effect rather than from direct spread of the bacteria, by means of a bacteraemia, which appears rare.

In practical terms, the most important immediate complication is acute respiratory failure requiring assisted ventilation which occurs in up to a quarter of cases. The need for assisted ventilation may not become apparent until the second to fourth day after hospital admission and can parallel the spread of radiographic shadowing which occurs commonly in severe disease, even in spite of apparently appropriate antibiotic therapy.

Table 14.2. *Some reported complications of Legionella pneumonia*

Respiratory	Acute respiratory failure	+++
	Lung cavitation	++
	Lung fibrosis	
Cardiovascular	Pericarditis and effusion	++
	Myocarditis	++
	Endocarditis	+
	Arteriovenous fistula infection	+
Neurological	Encephalomyelitis	++
	Cerebellar involvement	+++
	Guillain–Barré syndrome	++
	Motor neuropathy	++
Musculoskeletal	Myositis	+++
	Rhabdomyolysis	++
	Arthropathy	+
Renal	Acute renal failure	++
	Interstitial nephritis	+
	Glomerulonephritis	+
Gastrointestinal	Focal gut infection	+
	Paralytic ileus	+
	Jaundice	+
	Pancreatitis	+
Others	Skin rashes	+
	Pancytopoenia	+
	Thrombocytopoenia	++
	Lymph node enlargement	+

From Macfarlane JT. Pneumonia and acute respiratory infections in adults. In Gibson CJ, Geddes DM, eds Brewis RA, *Respiratory Medicine*. London. Ballière-Tindall; 1990:907[35a].
+++ Several reports.
++ Uncommon.
+ Very rare.

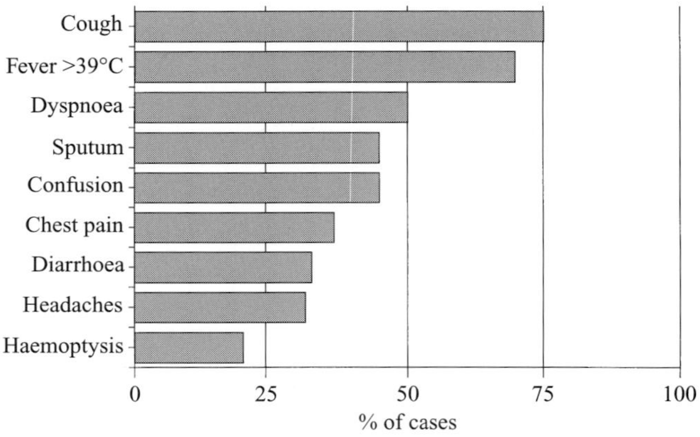

FIGURE 14.5 Clinical features of 739 patients with *Legionella* pneumonia. (Adapted from Bartlett *et al.* (1986)[3].)

Other common complications of severe disease include shock which carries a poor prognosis, and acute renal failure which may require temporary dialysis, but usually recovers completely in survivors. Other complications are summarised in Table 14.2 with further details given elsewhere.[35,35a]

Prolonged sequelae

There is unfortunately no information from properly controlled prospective follow-up studies on long-term or late sequelae of *Legionella* infection. In one review of neurological complications,[36] 20% of cases with cerebellar dysfunction had prolonged sequelae and a few had persistent memory loss. Feelings of lethargy and malaise have been reported months or even years after infection[37,38] At follow-up from a hospital-related outbreak in Stafford, England, patients who had had *Legionella* infection tended to be less active, have more feelings of breathlessness and evidence of mental impairment compared with a small number of patients with other forms of pneumonia.[39] However, lack of an appropriate control group and patients' knowledge of their disease make sensible interpretation of such observations difficult. Not infrequently, medico-legal aspects and concerns cloud the situation.

Differential diagnosis

Early suggestions that *Legionella* pneumonia could be differentiated from other pneumonias by the presence of such features as dry cough, confusion, diarrhoea, lymphopenia and hyponatraemia,[40] have not been borne out by subsequent studies.[32,41] Epidemiological clues such as recent hospital or hotel stay and infection occurring during the summer months can be valuable. High fever, confusion or delirium not explainable on obvious metabolic upsets such as hypoxia, significant biochemical abnormalities including hyponatraemia, lack of predominant pathogen on sputum Gram's stain and failure to respond to β-lactam antibiotics may act as clues.

Making the diagnosis

The diagnosis of *Legionella* infection can be made in the laboratory by a range of methods.[3,42] These include:

(a) culture of the organism,
(b) direct identification of bacteria or their nucleic acid,
(c) detection of *Legionella* antigen in the urine, and
(d) serological response.

Isolation is the method of choice, but requires specialist medium and suitable specimens such as expectorated sputum, tracheal aspirates, bronchial alveolar lavage fluid, lung tissue and pleural aspirates. Increasing numbers of microbiology laboratories can offer this service if pre-warned to culture specifically for *Legionella*, although a positive culture may take several days. A quicker diagnosis is possible by examining such samples with specific monoclonal antisera and visualising the bacteria by immunofluorescence or immunoperoxidase techniques. However, considerable experience is needed for correct interpretation. Detection of specific nucleic acid by the polymerase chain reaction is not widely available but appears promising.

Tests to detect *L. pneumophila* serogroup 1 urinary antigen, which is excreted in the urine for up to two weeks during the acute infection have a high specificity[43] and sensitivity, but are of less value for other *Legionella* serogroups and species. Detection of urinary antigen, using commercially available kits, offer the best hope of early diagnosis in many centres.

Serology is the most widely used diagnostic tool utilising either the indirect fluorescent antibody test (IFAT) or the rapid microagglutination technique (RMAT). In Britain, the serological criteria for a diagnosis of *L. pneumophila* serogroup 1 infection are either a fourfold rise in IFA titre to >64 or a single titre of >128 (or RMAT titre of >32), the single titre being presumptive evidence. Unfortunately, diagnostic seroconversion may not occur for 2–4 weeks after the beginning of the illness and is therefore of little clinical value. One study revealed that 6% of patients had diagnostic serology within one day of admission, 20% within three days and 40% within 7 days.[44] Even the presence of detectable antibodies in the early stage should alert the clinician to the possibility of *Legionella* infection. Up to a quarter of culture proven cases do not show seroconversion[45] and of those that do demonstrate seroconversion, 50% may do so only within 4 weeks and 75% within 8 weeks. The significance of antibodies to other *Legionella* species and non-serogroup 1 *L. pneumophila* is less clearly understood.

Management

Antibiotic therapy

The organism is susceptible to a wide range of antibiotics *in vitro* including macrolides, β-lactam antibiotics, co-trimoxazole, aminoglycosides, tetracyclines, chloramphenicol and rifampicin. However, these *in vitro* findings have little revelance to the treatment of human infection as, in the lung, the *Legionella* bacterium is an intracellular pathogen hiding and dividing in vacuoles within pulmonary macrophages and polymorphonuclear neutrophils in the alveolar spaces.[46] The ability of antibiotics to penetrate these pulmonary cells appears to be the major criterion for their efficacy as demonstrated in animal models. The most commonly used model is the aerosol-infected guinea pig which has supported the efficacy of rifampicin,[47] tetracycline,[48] quinolines,[47] and newer macrolides such as azithromycin and clarithromycin,[49] all producing somewhat better results than with erythromycin.

Unfortunately there are no controlled clinical trials on the efficacy of different antibiotic combinations for *Legionella* pneumonia and recommendations are empirical, based on retrospective case study and outbreak analysis as well as animal experiments. Erythromycin remains the recommended drug of choice in dosages of 500 mg–1000 mg six hourly, being given intravenously if required.[3] It is said that therapy is necessary for up to 3 weeks to prevent relapse, but in practice short courses are usually effective unless the patient is immunocompromised or has lung cavitation. Other antibiotics to consider include rifampicin, fluoroquinolone and newer macrolides.

The addition of rifampicin (600–1 200 mg daily orally or intravenously) is recommended for those patients with moderate to severe infection, although reversible hyperbilrubinaemia has been reported in 60% of individuals with severe *Legionella* pneumonia treated with rifampicin.[50] There is limited clinical experience with the use of quinolines in the treatment of legionellosis, but two reports record successful treatment of 14 severely ill patients with ciprofloxacin (200–400 mg daily intravenously) who had not improved with erythromycin with and without rifampicin.[51,52] Perfloxacin has been reported to be effective in a limited number of seriously ill patients.[53] These reports suggest that fluoroquinolines should be seriously considered as safe, additional or alternative therapy for *Legionella* infections. Of the newer macrolides, a high clinical cure rate was reported in 44 patients treated with clarithromycin (1–2 g daily by mouth).[54]

General supportive measures

Correct management of fluids, nutrition and oxygen therapy is very important, particularly in view of the frequency of both respiratory and renal failure. Patients with advancing respiratory failure should be managed on an Intensive Care Unit and many will require assisted ventilation. Severe community-acquired *Legionella* pneumonia requiring assisted ventilation has a relatively good outcome with three quarters surviving, although prolonged intermittent positive pressure ventilation may be required, sometimes for weeks. Acute renal failure requiring dialysis is common, but is reversible in survivors with only one requiring ongoing dialysis after discharge from hospital in one study.[50]

Prevention

Even a single case of *Legionella* infection requires the clinician to consider a likely source and the case should be discussed with the appropriate local consultant in communicable disease control (CCDC) or the national communicable disease surveillance centre. Two or more linked cases require an epidemiological investigation.

Prognosis

Outcome is mainly affected by the underlying state of the patients' health before the infection and effective and early use of appropriate antibiotics and supportive therapy. The mortality rate in young, previously healthy individuals is low, at around 5–15% but can approach 75% in debilitated or immunocompromised individuals.

References

1. FRASER DW, TSAI TR, ORENSTEIN W *et al.* Legionnaires' disease: description of an epidemic of pneumonia. *N Engl J Med* 1977;297:1189–97.
2. MCDADE JE, SHEPARD CC, FRASER DW, TSAI TR, REDUS MA, DOWDLE WR. Legionnaires' disease: isolation of a bacterium and demonstration of its role in other respiratory disease. *N Engl J Med* 1977;297:1197–203.
3. BARTLETT CR, MACRAE AD, MACFARLANE JT. *Legionella* infection. Edward Arnold, London, 1986.
4. REINGOLD AL, THOMASON BM, BRAKE BJ, THACKER L, WILKINSON HW, KURITSKY JN. *Legionella* pneumonia in the United States: the distribution of serogroups and species causing human illness. *J Infect Dis* 1984;149:819.
5. JOSEPH CA, HUTCHINSON EJ, DEDMAN D, BIRTLES RJ, WATSON JM, BARTLETT CL. Legionnaires' disease surveillance: England and Wales 1994. *Commun Dis Rep*, 1995;5:R180–3.
6. BARTLETT CL, WATSON JM, JOSEPH CA, BEZZANT M. Travel associated Legionnaires' disease. Proceedings of the second conference on International Travel Medicine, Atlanta, Georgia, USA. 9–12 May 1991, Atlanta. *Intern Soc Travel Med* 1992;225–7.
7. JOSEPH CA, WATSON JM, HARRISON TG, BARTLETT CL. Nosocomial Legionnaires' disease in England and Wales, 1980–1992. *Epidemiol Infect* 1994;112:329–45.
8. BHOPAL RS, FALLON RJ, BUILST EC, BLACK RJ, URQUHART JD. Proximity of the home to a cooling tower and risk of non-outbreak Legionnaires' disease. *BMJ* 1991;302:378–83.
9. STOUT JE, YU VL, MURACA P. Legionnaires' disease acquired within the home of two patients: link to the home water supply. *JAMA* 1987;257:1215–17.
10. SAUNDERS CJ, JOSEPH CA, WATSON JM. Investigating a single case of Legionnaires' disease: guidance for consultants in communicable disease control. *Commun Dis CDR Rep Rev* 1994;4:R112–14.
11. WATSON JM, MITCHELL E, GABBAY J *et al.* Piccadilly Circus Legionnaires' disease outbreak. *J Pub Health Med* 1994;16:341–7.
12. MITCHELL E, O'MAHONY M, WATSON JM *et al.* Two outbreaks of Legionnaires' disease in Bolton Health District. *Epidemiol Infect* 1990;104:159–70.
13. GLICK TH, GREGG MB, BERMAN B, MALLISON G, RHODES JR WW, KASSANOFF I. Pontiac Fever: An epidemic of unknown aetiology in a health department. 1. Clinical and epidemiological aspects. *Am J Epidemiol* 1978;107:149–60.
14. HERWALDT LA, GORMAN GW, MCGRATH T *et al.* A new *Legionella* species, *Legionella feeleii* species nova, causes Pontiac fever in an automobile plant. *Ann Intern Med* 1984;100:333–8.
15. GOLDBERG DJ, WRENCH JG, COLLIER PW *et al.* Lochgoilhead fever: Outbreak of non-pneumonic Legionellosis due to *Legionella micdadei*. *Lancet*, 1989;1:316–18.
16. BRITISH THORACIC SOCIETY AND PUBLIC HEALTH LABORATORY SERVICE. Community acquired pneumonia in adults in British hospitals in 1982–1983: a survey of aetiology, mortality, prognosis factors and outcome. *Quart J Med* 1987;239:195–220.
17. MACFARLANE JT, FINCH RG, WARD MJ, MACRAE AD. Hospital study of adult community acquired pneumonia. *Lancet* 1982:2:225–58.
18. KENNEDY DH. Respiratory infections. *Hosp Update* 1985;11(Suppl 23):11.
19. WHITE RJ, BLAINEY AD, HARRISON KJ, CLARKE SK. Causes of pneumonia presenting to a district general hospital. *Thorax* 1981;36:566–70.
20. MCNABB WR, SHANSON DC, WILLIAMS TD, LANT AF. Adult community acquired pneumonia in central London. *J Roy Soc Med* 1984;77:550–5.
21. BLANQUER J, BLANQUER R, BORRAS R *et al.* Aetiology of community acquired pneumonia in Valencia, Spain: a multicentre prospective study. *Thorax* 1991;46:508–11.
22. BEMTSSON E, BLOMBERG J, LAGERGARD T, TROLLFOSS B. Aetiology of community acquired pneumonia in patients requiring hospitalisation. *Eur J Clin Microbiol* 1985;4:268–72.
23. HOLMBERG H. Aetiology of community acquired pneumonia in hospital treatment patients. *Scand J Infect Dis* 1987;19:491–501.
24. LEVY M, DROMER F, BRION N, LETURDU F, CARBON C. Community acquired pneumonia. Importance of initial non-invasive bacteriologic and radiographic investigations. *Chest* 1988;92:43–8.
25. ORTQVIST A, HEDLUND J, GRILLNER L *et al.* Aetiology, outcome and prognostic factors in community acquired pneumonia requiring hospitalisation. *Eur Resp J* 1990;3:1105–13.
26. BURMAN LA, TROLLFORS B, ANDERSSON B *et al.* Diagnosis of pneumonia by cultures, bacterial and viral antigen detection tests, and serology with special reference to antibodies against pneumococcal antigens. *J Infect Dis* 1991;163:1087–93.
27. KARALUS NC, CURSONS RT, LENG RA *et al.* Community acquired pneumonia: aetiology and prognostic index evaluation. *Thorax* 1991;46:413–18.
28. LIM I, SHAW DR, STANLEY DP, LUMB R, MCLENNAN G. A prospective hospital study of the aetiology of community acquired pneumonia. *Med J Aust* 1989;151:87–91.
29. MARRIE TJ, DURANT H, YATES L. Community acquired pneumonia requiring hospitalisation: 5 year prospective study. *Rev Infect Dis* 1989;11:586–599.
30. FANG GD, FINE M, ORLOFF J *et al.* New and emerging aetiologies for community acquired pneumonia with implications for therapy. A prospective multicentre study of 359 cases. *Medicine* 1990;69:307–16.

31. MACFARLANE JT. Community acquired pneumonia. In Mitchell D ed. *Recent Advances in Respiratory Medicine* No 5. Churchill Livingstone; 1991.

32. WOODHEAD MA, MACFARLANE JT. Comparative clinical and laboratory features of *Legionella* with pneumococcal and mycoplasma pneumonias. *Br J Dis Chest* 1987;81:133–9.

33. WOODHEAD MA, MACFARLANE JT. Legionnaires' disease: a review of 79 community acquired cases in Nottingham. *Thorax* 1986;41:635–40.

34. MACFARLANE JT, MILLER AC, RODERICK SMITH WR, MORRIS AH, ROSE DH. Comparative radiographic features of community acquired Legionnaires' disease, pneumococcal pneumonia and psittacosis. *Thorax* 1984;39:28–33.

35. WOODHEAD MA, MACFARLANE JT. The protean manifestations of Legionnaires' disease. *J Roy Coll Phys Lond* 1985;19:224–30.

35a. MACFARLANE JT. Pneumonia and acute respiratory infections in adults. In Gibson CJ, Geddes DM, Brewis RA eds. *Respiratory Medicine*. Ballière-Tindall, London; 1990:907.

36. JOHNSON JD, RAFF MJ, VAN ARSDALL JA. Neurological manifestations of Legionnaires' disease. *Medicine* 1984;63:303–10.

37. LATTIMER GL, RHODES LV, SALVENTI JS *et al.* The Philadelphia epidemic of Legionnaires' disease: clinical, pulmonary and serological findings two years later. *Ann Intern Med* 1979;90:522–6.

38. JENKINS P, MILLER AC, OSMAN J, PEARSON SB, ROWLEY JM. Legionnaires' disease: a clinical description of 13 cases. *Br J Dis Chest* 1979;31:31–8.

39. LLOYD RS, GUEST D, FAIRFAX AJ. Long term morbidity from Legionnaires' disease. *Thorax* 1990;45:325.

40. MILLER AC. Early clinical differentiation between Legionnaires' disease and other sporadic pneumonias. *Ann Intern Med* 1979;90:526–8.

41. GRANADOS A, PODZAMCZER D, GUDIOL F, MANRESA F. Pneumonia due to *Legionella pneumophila* and pneumococcal pneumonia: similarities and differences on presentation. *Eur Resp J* 1989;2:130–4.

42. HARRISON TG, TAYLOR AG. *A Laboratory Manual for Legionella*. New York: Wiley Interscience; 1988.

43. BIRTLES RJ, HARRISON TG, SAMUEL D, TAYLOR AG. Evaluation of urinary antigen ELISA for diagnosing *Legionella pneumophila* serogroup 1 infection. *J Clin Pathol* 1990;43:685–90.

44. HARRISON TG, TAYLOR AG. Timing of seroconversion in Legionnaires' disease. *Lancet* 1988;2:795.

45. MONTFORTE R, ESTRUCH R, VIDAL J, CERVERA R, URBANO-MARQUEZ A. Delayed seroconversion in Legionnaires' disease. *Lancet* 1988;2:513.

46. KEYS TF. Therapeutic considerations in the treatment of *Legionella* infections. *Semin Resp Infect* 1987;2:270–3.

47. HAVLICHEK D, POHLOD D, SARAVOLATZ L. Comparison of ciprofloxacin and rifampicin in experimental *Legionella pneumophilia* penumonia. *J Antimicrob Chemother* 1987;20:875–81.

48. YOSHIDA S, MIZUGUCHI Y, OHTA H, OGAWA M. Effects of tetracyclines on experimental *Legionella pneumophila* infection in guinea pigs. *J Antimicrob Chemother* 1985;16:199–204.

49. FITZGEORGE RB, LEVER S, BASKERVILLE A. A comparison of the efficacy of azithromycin and clarithromycin in oral therapy of experimental airborne Legionnaires' disease. *J Antimicrob Chemother* 1993;31(Suppl E):171–6.

50. HUBBARD RB, MATHUR RM, MACFARLANE JT. Severe community-acquired *Legionella* pneumonia: Treatment, complications and outcome. *Quart J Med* 1993;86:327–32.

51. WINTER JH, MCCARTNEY C, BINGHAM J, TELFER M, WHITE LO, FALLON RJ. Ciprofloxacin in the treatment of severe Legionnaires' disease. *Rev Infect Dis* 1988;10:S218–19.

52. UNERTL KE, LENHART FP, FORST H *et al.* Ciprofloxacin in the treatment of Legionellosis in critically ill patients including those cases unresponsive to erythromycin. *Am J Med* 1989;87(Suppl 5A):128s–31s.

53. DOURNON E, MAYAUD C, WOLFF M *et al.* Comparison of the activity of three antibiotic regimens in severe Legionnaires' disease. *J Antimicrob Chemother* 1990;26(Suppl B):129–39.

54. HAMEDANI P, ALI J, HAFEEZ S *et al.* The safety and efficacy of clarithromycin in patients with *Legionella* pneumonia. *Chest* 1991;100:1503–6.

15 Tuberculosis

J.A.R. FRIEND* and J.M.WATSON†
*Aberdeen Royal Infirmary, Scotland, UK, †Communicable Disease Surveillance Centre, Colindale, London, UK

Definition

Tuberculosis is an infection caused by micro-organisms of the *Mycobacterium tuberculosis* complex, and is usually taken to include infections caused by the human and bovine strains of the organism, but not those infections caused by other 'Non–tuberculous' mycobacteria such as *Mycobacterium avium-intracellulare* and others, which are described in full detail in Chapter 11. Such non-tuberculous mycobacteria have also been described as 'atypical', 'anonymous', 'opportunistic' or '*Mycobacteria* other than tuberculosis' (MOTT), but these terms are generally discouraged.

Characteristics of *Mycobacterium tuberculosis*

The classic property of the mycobacteria in general is that of being acid fast; that is, when stained with a dye such as carbol fuchsin, as in the Ziehl–Neelsen stain, weak mineral acids do not remove the colour. The stain is also resistant to removal by alcohol, so that they are known as acid and alcohol-fast bacilli, or AAFB. This property is shared by all mycobacteria, including the non-tuberculous mycobacteria.

They are unicellular organisms, containing polysaccharides, antigenic proteins, and lipids. The cell wall has a very high lipid content and is formed in several layers, the innermost being composed of short peptide chains cross-linked with long polysaccharide chains, forming a peptidoglycan called murein. The intermediate layer of the cell wall is formed by arabinogalactan, a polysaccharide attached to long chain fatty acids called mycolic acids, and the outer layer consists of glycolipids named mycosides. Lipids comprise some 60% of the cell wall. Within this cell wall is a plasma membrane, and inside this is the cytoplasm containing a single chromosome in the nuclear body. This thick cell wall makes the live organisms resistant to acids, alkali, and detergents, so that mixed specimens of secretions such as sputum, heavily contaminated with other organisms, can be treated to leave the mycobacteria still viable for culture purposes uncontaminated by other micro-organisms. Mycobacteria as a genus are widespread in watery habitats such as streams, mud, and bogs, although the thick waxy cell wall makes them quite hydrophobic. Most are saprophytic and only a minority are parasites which require, like *M. tuberculosis*, a live host.

The *M. tuberculosis* group was formerly divided into the human and bovine strains, but further types with slightly different characteristics include a strain of human tubercle bacilli found in the Madras region of South India, which differs from the classical type originally isolated by Koch in being sensitive to an isoniazid analogue, TCH (thiophen-2-carboxylic acid hydrazide). The classical human type of *M. tuberculosis* is resistant to TCH, and also grows best under aerobic conditions. The bovine strains of *M. tuberculosis* differ from human strains both in their cultural appearance on Löwenstein–Jensen medium and in their preference for a micro-aerophilic growing atmosphere, but also in their resistance to pyrazinamide. A further type, *Mycobacterium Africanum*, is found in equatorial Africa and is somewhat intermediate between the human and bovine types, being sensitive to pyrazinamide but being micro-aerophilic [1].

The disease process

Tubercle bacilli stimulate in the host a vigorous immune response which accounts for much of the resulting disease process, rather than through any major toxic effect of the bacilli themselves. The classical lesion is a necrotising epithelioid cell granuloma, containing non-lymphoid mononuclear cells, which include blood monocytes, macrophages,epithelioid cells, and multinucleate giant cells, mainly of Langerhans type. Necrosis occurs in these granulomata, resulting in caseation. In most tuberculosis infections, the bacilli are transmitted by droplet infection, by coughing from an infected individual, though ingestion of bacilli from infected milk was an alternative method of transmission in times when infected cows' milk was common. In the case of airborne transmission, the organisms are inhaled into the lungs, usually to terminal bronchus or alveolar level and are then engulfed by macrophages. The organisms may then come to lie within a pocket of cell surface membrane, the phagosome, which fuses with lysosomes containing anti-bacterial agents such as hydrogen peroxide and superoxide radicals. In some cases this may kill the bacilli, but in other situations may merely neutralise the organism, possibly allowing a dormant state to persist for long periods. At other times, the cell may not inhibit the organism, and intracellular multiplication can occur, with eventual disruption of the cell and further dissemination of the infection.

Some macrophages with mycobacteria may migrate from the infection site to regional lymph nodes, where the foreign antigen, represented by elements of the mycobacteria, can be processed, involving active T-lymphocytes. Such T-lymphocytes become sensitised to tuberculoprotein, and a cell-mediated reaction can then develop, with sensitised T-lymphocytes and macrophages activated by lymphokines clustering around any mycobacteria, creating a granuloma as the macrophages 'mature' into epithelioid cells; some epithelioid cells will then coalesce to form multi-nucleate giant cells. The lesion consisting of the original site of infection and the associated, involved lymph node is called the primary complex.

In the course of this initial or primary infection with the mycobacterial organisms, the host will develop delayed (type IV) hypersensitivity to soluble protein antigens from mycobacteria. This hypersensitivity is cell mediated, as opposed to Type I (anaphylactic, IgE mediated), type II (Arthus, antibody dependent) and type III (immune-complex mediated). This delayed, cell-mediated hypersensitvity is evident within 6–8 weeks after the initial infection develops, and can be detected by skin testing with old tuberculin or purified protein derivative (PPD), using the so-called Mantoux test or some other form of tuberculin test, detailed further on pp. 249–250.

In most patients exposed to mycobacterial infection and developing a primary complex, the infection will be contained and all viable bacilli will be eliminated. In others, the organisms may become dormant, with a risk that in later life (and sometimes many decades later) the infection can reactivate and develop into clinical tuberculosis. In a few, the infection can progress and cause a clinical illness. If this occurs within the initial infection, it may be called primary tuberculosis; if infection develops later, once full tuberculin hypersensitivity has developed, or even by re-infection at a later stage, the disease which develops is usually called post-primary tuberculosis.

The difficulty about the host response to mycobacterial infections relates to the question of immune status, and the relationship between immunity and delayed hypersensitivity.[2] This difficulty arises from the complexity of the antigens involved, the likelihood that several different T-cell types may be involved in the cell-mediated reactions, and the technical difficulties in studying such complex interactions. There is no specific test which can measure immunity to tuberculosis infection, which can really only be assessed by epidemiological observation of groups of people with different characteristics over a period of time. It seems probable that different T-lymphocyte populations mediate immunity on the one hand, and delayed hypersensitivity on the other; these effects may arise from a combination of protective, DTH (delayed tuberculin hypersensitivity) effector, cytolytic, and memory T-cell subsets. In the case of protective immunity, evidence suggests that this is mediated mainly by CD4+ T-cells, and that these cells are class II MHC restricted in the recognition of antigen, as opposed to the class I antigens recognised by CD8+ T-cells.[3] It seems likely that class II molecules may determine both tuberculin reactivity and susceptibility to tuberculosis.[2] When immune reactions occur in tuberculous infections, they are controlled by various cytokines, which act as chemical messengers. Gamma-interferon is such a cytokine which arises from both CD4+ and CD8+ T-cells, and helps to arm macrophages for killing mycobacteria. Another cytokine, tumour necrosis factor (TNF), may contribute to tissue necrosis and pulmonary cavity formation, and therefore account for the so-called Koch phenomenon[4].

In the Koch phenomenon, the necrosis, scarring, and cavitation in tuberculosis may have some value in controlling the disease by walling off the dead tissues, and depriving them of their oxygen supply. On the other hand, when cavities open into airways, the organisms are excreted [5]. The effect of an impaired host response, as in human immunodeficiency virus-infection (HIV) is for a progressive change from a tendency to a 'normal' cavitating type of tuberculosis, to a form of tuberculosis with no cavitation, less tissue reaction, and greater dissemination to other tissues, as the T-helper cells fail. Up to a point therefore, the effects of the Koch phenomenon could be regarded as protective in the days before effective antibacterial therapy was available, but with modern anti-tuberculous therapy the Koch phenomenon may inhibit access of the drugs to more dormant organisms buried in necrotic or scar tissue. In addition to the immunological, cell-mediated responses to mycobacteria, Stanford [5] has postulated that there are other forms of protective immunity in tuberculosis which prevent the bacilli from gaining access to the interstitial lung tissues by acting within the alveoli. He suggests that modulating the cellular response during anti-tuberculous chemotherapy, using a form of immunotherapy by giving a dose of killed *Mycobacterium vaccae*, might enhance protective immunity, and reduce the Koch phenomenon, with an improved response to drug treatment. This approach is further discussed later in the chapter (page 260). But the precise relationship between the tissue reactions to mycobacteria and protective immunity remain an area of difficulty.

Epidemiology

Tuberculosis occurred in humans in prehistoric times but did not become a common disease until man lived in larger communities in later centuries[6]. The epidemic of tuberculosis in Europe only began in the seventeenth century and peaked in the eighteenth and nineteenth centuries. During this period almost the whole population became infected with *M. tuberculosis* and about a quarter of all deaths were attributed to the disease. The subsequent slow decline of tuberculosis in Europe has been attributed to the general improvement in nutrition and living standards, and probably genetic changes in the population, rendering it less susceptible to the disease. In recent decades specific therapy has also contributed to the decline. The tuberculosis epidemic in North America also peaked in the early nineteenth century, whereas in Asia it probably peaked towards the end of the nineteenth century. In Africa tuberculosis was still uncommon at the beginning of the twentieth century but its prevalence has risen considerably since then.

In 1993 the World Health Organisation declared tuberculosis a global emergency[7]. In the ten years from 1990 to 1999, the WHO estimates that 88 million new cases of tuberculosis will occur worldwide and that 30 million of these cases will die[8]. At present the WHO estimates that one in five of the world's population is infected with the tubercle bacillus and that about eight million per year progress to disease. Whilst some are cured, either spontaneously or as a result of specific therapy, nearly three million per year die and the remainder become chronic cases. The epidemic of human immunodeficiency virus (HIV) infection has contributed to the current global tuberculosis epidemic and is predicted to account for nearly one in ten of the incident cases and deaths by the end of the century[8].

While it was recognised that tubeculosis was becoming less common in the developed world during the twentieth century, and that there was a continuing probelm in developing countries, there was until about 1985 an optimism that, in due course, tuberculosis could be defeated. This led to a certain complacency, but more recent events have shown that this was misplaced. The trends in tuberculosis in

England and Wales are an example of some of the changes which have occurred in one area where the disease was thought to be in sight of eradication, and where detailed information has been collected for over 90 years.

Notification of cases of tuberculosis began in England and Wales in 1913. The clinician making the diagnosis has a statutory obligation to report cases to the local 'proper officer' who is now usually the Consultant in Communicable Disease Control (CCDC). The CCDC in turn reports the cases to the Office of Population Censuses and Surveys (OPCS). Limited information only is requested on each case including age, sex, place of residence and site of disease. The recognition of an increased occurrence of tuberculosis in recently arrived immigrants to the United Kingdom in the 1960s, and the limited amount of information available from the notification system in this group, led to the institution of a series of more detailed surveys which have examined clinical, epidemiological, microbiological and treatment aspects of the disease in greater detail.[9–12] Additional information on those cases of tuberculosis from which the organism was isolated is available through the system of laboratory reporting to the PHLS Communicable Disease Surveillance Centre in London. This system provides, in particular, the opportunity to carry out surveillance on the occurrence of drug resistance.[13] Despite the clear microbiological basis for the aetiology of tuberculosis infection, nearly 50% of the cases reported in England and Wales are not supported by microbiological evidence. In these cases the diagnosis is made on clinical grounds, supported, in some, by histopathological results and/or the results of tuberculin hypersensitivity testing.

About 100 000 cases of tuberculosis per year were reported in England and Wales in the first few years after the notification system began. Bovine tuberculosis was responsible for a substantial proportion of tuberculosis cases at the beginning of the twentieth century, especially non-pulmonary disease, but measures taken to rid milk of this infection reduced the number of cases in humans to very small numbers. Notifications fell to about 50 000 per year at the time of the second world war and continued to decline until the mid-1980s reaching a low point of 5086 notifications in 1987. Since then in England and Wales, as in some other European countries and the United States, totals of notifications have increased (Fig. 15.1). It is likely that a range of factors have contributed to this increase[14], including the possibility of an improvement in the ascertainment of cases as a result of the appointment of CCDCs to districts throughout England and Wales. Other factors contributing to the recent increase are discussed below.

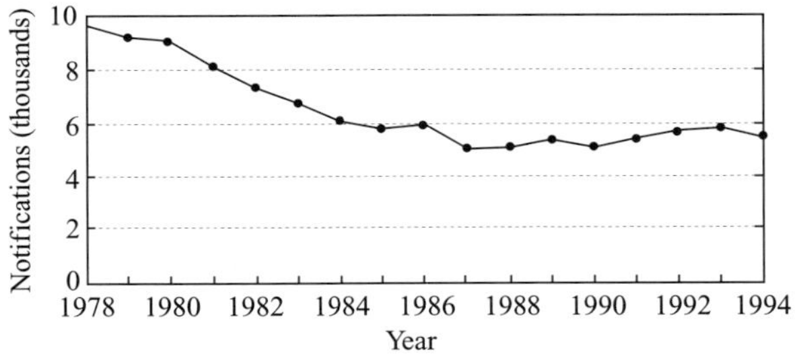

FIGURE 15.1 Tuberculosis notifications, England and Wales, 1978–94. Source: OPCS 1994 (provisional corrected).

The incidence of tuberculosis is recognised to be higher in a number of immigrant subgroups within the population. While the overall rate in England and Wales is about 10 per 100 000 per year, the rate in the population of Indian subcontinent ethnic origin has been 20 to 30 times higher than this.[12] Incidence rates in those recently arrived in this country are considerably higher than those that have been here for many years, but the rates among those immigrants born in this country remain higher than the rates in the indigenous white population. Despite the high rates, the incidence in the Indian subcontinent group in this country has been declining and the preliminary results of the 1993 National Survey of Tuberculosis Notifications suggests that this trend, after standardisation for age distribution and year of entry, continues. More recently tuberculosis is being recognised as a particular problem among immigrants, including refugees, from other parts of the world, particularly Africa. The largest increase in notifications between the 1988 and 1993 National Tuberculosis Surveys occurred in the population of black African ethnic origin[12] (PHLS unpublished data). In general, the incidence of tuberculosis increases with increasing age, with only small differences between the sexes until older age when rates in males are considerably higher (Fig. 15.2). However, the distribution by age and sex differs in different ethnic groups with a greater proportion of cases in older children and young adults occurring in populations within which substantial recent transmission of tuberculosis is occurring. Differences are also evident in the site of disease, both by age and ethnic group: in particular pulmonary disease is more common in the elderly white population and lymph node disease in younger cases and those of Indian subcontinent ethnic origin.[15,16] Large differences in the geographical distribution of tuberculosis in England and Wales are apparent but are mainly associated with demographic factors in the resident population. The rates of tuberculosis are higher in areas with a high proportion of the population within immigrant subgroups but the rates may also be increased in inner city areas in association with poverty and deprivation.[17]

The association between tuberculosis and HIV infection is well recognised and the occurrence of tuberculosis in patients with HIV infection in England and Wales was reported early in the epidemic. About 5% of AIDS patients in England and Wales are reported to contract tuberculosis[18,19] reflecting the relatively limited overlap

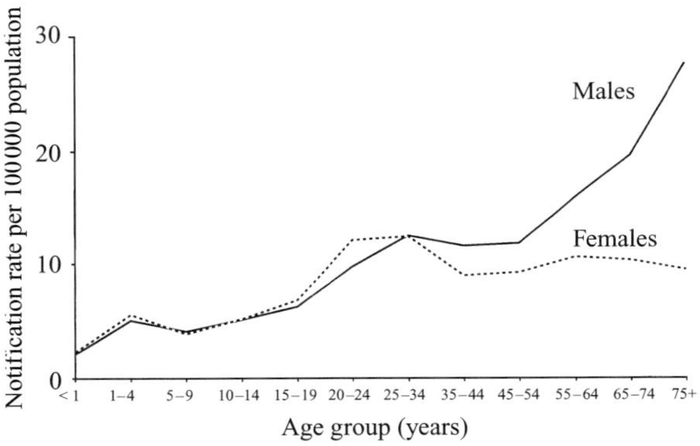

FIGURE 15.2 Aggregated notification rates of tuberculosis by age group, England and Wales, 1990–92.

between the population with HIV infection and the population with prior tuberculous infection in this country. Continued surveillance of this overlap is essential while the global epidemics of tuberculosis and HIV infection continue to develop.

Although the tubercle bacillus may infect both the rich and poor, it has long been recognised that the disease is more common in association with poverty. Overcrowding and poor nutrition may contribute to this, as well as more limited access to preventative or curative services. An association too is well recognised between tuberculosis and homelessness. A recent study in London found about 5% of a homeless population using cold weather shelters had features consistent with active tuberculosis[20] and recommendations have recently been made to improve the detection and treatment of tuberculosis in this group.[21]

Tuberculosis in other countries

In the UK the incidence of tuberculosis infection is usually assessed and recorded by the notification rate of active, treated cases; the accuracy of this depends on the identification of such active disease, and includes not only those cases which are bacteriologically confirmed, but also unconfirmed cases being treated on suspicion. In addition, some cases are undoubtedly 'missed', either because notification is omitted, or because the disease, while present, is not diagnosed. For instance, a small number of cases of tuberculosis are only detected at autopsy, and yet the autopsy rate is so low that there are probably a significant number of other undetected cases of active tuberculosis which never come to light, and the cause of death is perhaps certified as chronic bronchitis or pneumonia.

Another measure of the prevalence of tuberculosis infection is to use information from repeated mass tuberculin testing to estimate the risk of tuberculosis infection. This 'annual risk of infection', the probability that an uninfected person will become infected (but not necessarily develop clinical tuberculosis) in the course of a year, gives a measure of the extent of tuberculous infection in a community. World Health Organisation figures[22] show that the annual risk of infection is highest in the African region (1.5 to 2.5%), followed by South-east Asia and the Western Pacific (1.0 to 2.5%), Central and South America , and the Eastern Mediterranean Region (0.5 to 1.5%) .

In Africa, notifications of tuberculosis approximately doubled between 1985 and 1990, achieving levels of over 200 per 100 000 per year, compared with around 30 per 100 000 per year in Europe, North America, Japan, and the Antipodes (WHO figures), although in many of these countries notification rates are below 10 per 100 000 per year. The epidemic of HIV infection seems fundamental to this increase, not only by increasing the susceptibility to the reactivation of previous tuberculosis infection, but also by making HIV positive people vulnerable to re-infection[23]. It has been estimated that in Africa, with a total population of 750 million people, about 170 million have been infected with tuberculosis, and perhaps 6 million by the HIV virus. Around 3 million have both infections, and in some parts of Africa up to 80%of those with active clinical tuberculosis are HIV positive.

In the USA, since 1985, there has been a 16% increase in the number of cases of tuberculosis reported annually, compared with a 6% annual fall during the preceding 30 years [24]. It is estimated that this increase amounts to an additional 40 000 cases over the 8 years following 1985; most of the cases have occurred among children[25] and young adults, racial and ethnic minorities, and immigrants and refugees. In many such cases homelessness, drug abuse, and overcrowded housing was thought to be important, with additional transmission in prison and shelters for the homeless. A further possible factor in the USA has been the epidemic of HIV infection, either from reactivation of previous tuberculosis infection, or because of their greatly increased likelihood of developing tuberculous disease following a new infection. This is compounded by other problems, such as drug abuse, which make good compliance with treatment less easy to maintain, and the increasing levels of tuberculosis caused by drug-resistant organisms[26].

In Europe generally,[27] there has been a gradual decline in the risk of tuberculosis infection (as judged by tuberculin testing data) of about 10% every year, with a trend for increasing age of those who develop active disease, and a notification rate varying between 6.6 and 19.7 per 100 000 per year in different European countries in 1990. The impact of HIV infection on tuberculosis, as in England and Wales, seems small, but will require careful surveillance in the future. There is concern that increasing prevalence of tuberculosis in the Paris area of France, and in some areas of Italy and Spain, may be associated with HIV infection.

Clinical features of pulmonary tuberculosis

Primary tuberculosis

In most countries with a high prevalence of tuberculosis, the primary infection occurs in childhood, especially under the age of 5; almost all infections arise from inhalation of organisms dispersed from an infected, coughing individual, by droplet infection. Infection is usually only acquired through close and relatively prolonged contact with an infected adult. Rarely, primary infection is acquired through consumption of infected milk, which can induce infection at tonsillar level, or through the gastrointestinal tract. There is no evidence of spread through the use of cutlery, or crockery used by infected people, nor from clothing, bedding, or exposure to dust from wards in which infected patients are living.[28]

When infection develops, there may be the general symptoms of infection such as malaise and fever, or no symptoms at all. In some, the onset of the infection may be accompanied by erythema nodosum, or phlyctenular conjunctivitis, which are regarded as an aspect of the development of a hypersensitivity reaction to the mycobacteria. Some children will have a cough, but this is usually unproductive. The commonest syndrome radiologically is the presence of a visible primary complex, with a prominent lymphatic element represented by hilar lymph node enlargement, together with a peripheral lesion in lung tissue, which is usually 'soft' initially, and may be small, and situated in any zone of the lung. The size of the primary pulmonary lesion in some children may be so small as to be radiologically invisible, especially among some racial groups; those from the Indian subcontinent frequently only demonstrate enlarged hilar or paratracheal nodes. If there is substantial hilar node enlargement, this may be enough to obstruct major bronchi, leading to obstructive emphysema, or to collapse of lobes, with or without distal infection; this has been termed epituberculosis; if caseation in an infected lymph node ruptures outside the node, the material may burst into the bronchi, with development of a brisk tuberculous pneumonic reaction, or rupture may occur into other structures such as the oesophagus.

Apart from the possibility of erythema nodosum, or phlyctenular conjunctivitis, there may be no other abnormal general signs on physical examination. It is unusual to find any abnormal physical signs on examination of the chest, unless there is major airway narrowing from enlarged lymph nodes which may cause stridor, or if there is extensive consolidation, when bronchial breathing and crackles may be heard.

In most children with primary tuberculosis, the primary complex heals, often with calcification of the affected lymph nodes and the associated primary lesion. This may represent a complete cure, or there may be residual dormant organisms which can reactivate at a later date. In others, the infection can become progressive primary tuberculosis, with increasing pulmonary lesions, often productive of tubercle bacilli in sputum, and sometimes with pleural involvement and a pleural effusion. Another potentially serious consequence of the primary infection is of dissemination of bacilli via lymphatic and haematogenous routes to other organs; this can include any organ, but spread to other lymph nodes, bones, joints, and the renal tract can cause subsequent tuberculosis in these organs. If the infection spreads in the bloodstream, there is a particular risk of the development of miliary tuberculosis and tuberculous meningitis, which both carry a high mortality in children, particularly in infancy.

Post-primary pulmonary tuberculosis

This form of tuberculosis can arise either as a result of progression of the primary infection, or as a reactivation of a previously dormant primary infection, or as a result of exogenous 'new' infection from an outside source. Such reinfection is thought to be uncommon, but is difficult to investigate unless organisms or DNA from the original primary infection and the 'new' infection are available.

The symptoms of post-primary infection may be the general symptoms of any infection, including malaise, loss of appetite, and fever; weight loss will follow from reduced food intake and the catabolic effects of infection. Traditionally, the fever of tuberculosis has been associated with 'night sweats', but such a symptom is totally non-specific and can arise from any cause of protracted and recurrent fever, including other chronic infections and neoplastic diseases including lymphomas and tumours.

Other symptoms of tuberculosis arise from the local effects on lung tissue; cough is common, and as the disease progresses will be accompanied by sputum which is increasingly purulent, and also by haemoptysis. Initially, haemoptysis may only amount to slight streaking, but if there is lung destruction with cavitation, erosion of branches of the bronchial arteries may lead to substantial, and occasionally fatal, arterial haemorrhage. If the inflammatory changes in the lung occur near to the pleural surface, pleuritic pain may develop, with the possibility of pleural effusion with all the symptoms and signs which effusion causes.

The physical signs caused by pulmonary tuberculosis are very variable, and extensive tuberculosis may be present without any abnormal or localising signs on clinical examination of the chest. If the infection has been progressive over some time, there may be weight loss and general appearances suggesting chronic infection and debility. Substantial infections with consolidation of lung tissue will cause signs of consolidation with dullness on percussion, bronchial breathing, and lung crackles. Very rarely, amphoric breath sounds can be heard over large, ventilated cavities. Occasionally, bronchial narrowing can arise from bronchial infection with tuberculosis, and cause wheezing.

Investigation of possible pulmonary tuberculosis

Sputum investigation

Obtaining samples will be relatively simple where the patient is producing sputum; but if this is not the case, respiratory secretions containing bacilli may be obtained by laryngeal swabs, or by early morning gastric lavage. More recently, in cases of diagnostic difficulty, broncho-alveolar lavage (BAL) at bronchoscopy has been employed, and also sputum induction using nebulised hypertonic saline (usually 3%) has been used, as for the detection of *Pneumocystis* infections. It has been shown that sputum induction is at least as successful in diagnosing tuberculosis as BAL, and is much simpler, well tolerated, and cheaper[29].

Once the sample of sputum, or respiratory secretion, has been obtained, it is usual to undertake direct examination of the sample, and then to attempt to culture the organisms.

Direct microscopy techniques

If positive, the examination of sputum for AAFB is the single most simple way of confirming the diagnosis, and it is also the cheapest for general use world-wide. The usual procedure is to centrifuge the sample, and stain by the Ziehl–Neelsen or Kinyoun techniques, but probably best using auramin or auramin–rhodamin[30] and then to examine under the microscope. In general, there has to be a bacillary concentration of 5000–10 000 bacteria per ml. to detect infection by this method, but the technique is almost 100% specific. The sensitivity of the technique can be further increased from about 51% to almost 100% by cytocentrifugation.[31] Such direct-smear techniques do not, of course identify which species of *Mycobacterium* is present. They have the added disadvantage of identifying tuberculosis only in those patients excreting bacilli in sufficient quantities to be detected by the method; many patients with undoubted infection may be 'negative on direct smear'. It is estimated that direct smear techniques have a specificity of over 99%, and a sensitivity of over 70%.

Culture techniques

The classical culture techniques involve treatment of the sputum with chemicals such as oxalic acid, sodium hydroxide, or detergents in sufficient concentration to kill most contaminating organisms, but not so much as to destroy mycobacteria. The material is then inoculated onto solid media, such as the Löwenstein–Jensen medium, and the cultures observed for up to 12 weeks for evidence of growth. Such methods are therefore very slow, and may not provide useful diagnostic or confirmatory information for many weeks. These techniques are described in greater detail in Chapter 1.

Newer techniques

More rapid techniques have been developed[32–35] including the Bactec 460 radiometric method (Becton Dickinson Instrument Systems, Sparks, MD, USA), which uses an automated system for detecting release of $^{14}CO_2$ from bacilli during metabolism of labelled substrates. This method can identify mycobacterial infection twice as quickly as conventional culture methods, giving results in about 2 weeks. The method is relatively expensive and requires facilities for safe handling of radioactive materials.

Other newer techniques include the Septi-Chek AFB system (Becton Dickinson Microbiology Systems, Cockeysville, MD, USA) involving liquid and solid phase media, which gives results in about 3 weeks, though at lower cost than the Bactec system. Another isolation system employs detection of micro-colonies on solid media, again being quicker than traditional methods, but is labour intensive.

Identification and drug-sensitivity testing

Following culture, it is then possible to set about identifying the mycobacterial strain, normally by observing the cultural characteristics and appearances of the colonies, and their susceptibility to anti-tuberculous drugs. Such procedures can add a further 4 weeks or so of investigation before the organism is identified and the sensitivity to anti-tuberculous drugs defined. There is a possibility that new techniques involving the use of luciferase may greatly accelerate the testing of drug sensitivity. The technique consists of the treatment of mycobacteria under test with genetically engineered mycobacterial phages whose genomes contain the gene Fflux, encoding firefly luciferase. After adsorption, the phage DNA is injected into the bacterial culture, and if the organisms are still alive they will begin to glow; if they have been killed by the antibiotic, they will remain dark. This method can yield results within hours.[34]

Further new techniques include the use of nucleic acid probes, the polymerase chain reaction, and DNA fingerprinting.

Nucleic acid probes

Specific, synthesised short chain labelled oligonucleotides can hybridise specifically with heat-treated mycobacterial DNA and RNA, allowing identification of a range of mycobacteria including *M. tuberculosis* and a number of non-tuberculous mycobacteria. Although these techniques are very quick, they cannot be used on clinical samples without prior culture and preparation.

Nucleic acid amplification – polymerase chain reaction (PCR)

Using synthesised short oligonucleotides, selected DNA sequences single-stranded DNA from mycobacteria are hybridised and then copied using DNA polymerase and nucleotide building blocks , deoxyribonucleotides. This process can be repeated 40 or more times, until a large number of the specific DNA sequences has been made, and then identified by separation on gel electrophoresis, and gene probes. These techniques allow identification of some mycobacteria with a sensitivity of around 95%. False-negatives occur, however, and the test cannot distinguish between live and dead bacilli; the latter can often be excreted in sputum for months after bacilli have been killed by therapy. Also, there are still significant technical difficulties, particularly in the pre-treatment of samples to avoid contamination of the PCR process with inhibitors, and cross-contamination of the PCR process with other DNA fragments which confuse the identification process. Currently, these technical problems and major costs limit the wide application of PCR for rapid identification of mycobacteria, but automation and technical advance may well increase its value in the future.[32,33,35,36]

Fingerprinting of mycobacteria strains

Molecular genetic techniques, using restriction fragment length polymorphism, now make it possible to identify mycobacteria to subspecies level, so that it is possible to trace the spread of specific strains or clones of mycobacteria in a community; such methods can be of value in tracing the epidemiology of the spread of tuberculosis infection.[37,38]

Other techniques

Attempts have also been made to detect components of the mycobacteria in sputum and other clinical samples; for instance, by looking for cell-wall fatty acids such as tuberculostearic acid (TBSA) using gas chromatography-mass spectrometry methods. Although such techniques have value, the specificity is relatively low when applied to sputum, partly because TBSA arises from other organisms including actinomycetes and contaminant organisms. The technique is also costly, but is a valuable method for the diagnosis of tuberculous meningitis in CSF.[39]

Blood investigations for tuberculosis

Mycobacteria contain many antigens which stimulate antibody production, but so far it has not been possible to develop a test for these antibodies which has proved clinically useful. The usual approach has been to employ enzyme-linked immunosorbent assays (ELISAs),[40] using more purified antigens, but the specificity and sensitivity of these techniques falls below those of direct microscopy on sputum or other body fluids such as pleural fluid.

Skin testing in the diagnosis of pulmonary tuberculosis

Individuals infected with mycobacteria develop a range of immunological reactions, but one of the earliest is the sensitisation of lymphocytes to protein from the bacilli. This delayed hypersensitivity phenomenon, Type IV hypersensitivity, is known as tuberculin hypersensitivity, and can be detected in a variety of ways. In the past, tuberculin tests used Koch's Old Tuberculin (OT), a filtrate of a broth culture of bacilli, but now the usual material used is purified protein derivative (PPD). PPD is, however, far from pure, and 'new tuberculins' which are purer and more species specific have been developed.[41] A positive tuberculin test following injection of tuberculin consists of an area of erythema and induration, reaching a maximum at 48–72 hours. While most of this reaction is a type IV hypersensitivity response, some individuals develop an earlier reaction at 6–8 hours which has features of a 'late' phase Type I hypersensitivity in addition.

The Mantoux test

This is probably the most reliable test for clinical use in individual patients. Using a fine needle, 0.1 ml of a dilution of tuberculin is injected intradermally into the volar surface of the forearm. It is essential that the injection is given as a true intradermal injection, using an intradermal needle and raising a lump within the dermis. The reaction is examined at 48–72 hours, and the diameter of induration felt is measured. The diameter of induration should be carefully recorded in the medical notes, detailing the exact strength of tuberculin used. This induration may be most easily assessed by using a ball-point pen held perpendicular to the skin, and drawing it across the skin towards the injection site; when the pen reaches the edge of the induration, its progress will be impeded. If marks like this are made from four directions towards the lesion, then the mean diameter of the induration can be easily derived.[42] Any erythema present is disregarded – the diameter of induration is regarded as the significant reaction, and if the induration is 10 mm in diameter or more to 5 International Units (IU), then the test is positive.

The form of tuberculin used for clinical purposes is PPD-S. The strengths and dilutions differ, depending whether the USA or European dilutions are employed. They are listed in Table 15.1.

The greater dilutions of tuberculin are generally thought unreliable, because of their tendency to adhere to the glass of the storage container and the plastic of the syringe, and they are not well standardised. For general purposes it is usual in the UK to start with the 1 in 1000 strength, i.e. 0.1 ml of 1 in 1000 dilution, or 10 international units (IU). In the USA it is more usual to start with 5 IU, or to use the term TU (tuberculin units). Some fear that by using these concentrations from the outset, a vigorous reaction might result in unacceptable skin necrosis. However, if such a local reaction occurs, it can be treated effectively by the prompt application of topical corticosteroid cream. The disadvantage of starting the tuberculin testing at a greater dilution with 1 in 10 000 or first strength relates to the lack of reliability of the material and the prolongation of the procedure by having to use two strengths in sequence. The very potent preparations involving the administration of 100 or 250 IU are generally reserved for assessment of the immunological status of the patient where immunosuppression is suspected, and are again less well standardised than the intermediate strengths.

Table 15.1. *Mantoux test solutions using PPD-S*

Dilution on label	Potency on label	Potency when 0.1 ml injected
1 in 10 000 'first strength' in USA	10 IU per ml	1 IU PPD-S
1 in 2000 'intermediate strength' in USA	50 IU per ml	5 IU PPD-S
1 in 1000	100 IU per ml	10 IU PPD-S
1 in 100	1000 IU per ml	100 IU PPD-S
'second strength' in USA	25 000 IU per ml	250 IU PPD-S

Multiple puncture tuberculin tests

The Heaf test

This uses a spring-loaded 'gun' with an autoclavable, removable head with six needle points. A solution of undiluted PPD is applied to the volar surface of the forearm; the gun is then 'fired' at the stretched skin, forcing the points into the dermis usually to a depth of 2 mm. The resulting reaction can be read after an interval of 72 hours to 7 days, and is conventionally reported as in Table 15.2.

Table 15.2. *Gradings of Heaf test results*

Appearance	Grade
No reaction, or up to three papules	0
4–6 palpable papules	I
A ring of induration, linking the 6 papules	II
Centre of the ring indurated – a plaque of induration	III
Erythema extending outwith the ring of 12 mm, sometimes with blistering or necrosis	IV

A Heaf test result graded at Grades II, III, or IV is generally regarded as positive.

Another type of multiple puncture device, the Tine Test, employed a disposable unit with four tines pre-dipped in tuberculin, but is not now widely used. In general, such multiple puncture tests are of less value in patient assessment, and are of greater value for epidemiological work, or in the assessment of tuberculin hypersensitivity prior to possible BCG vaccination in large numbers of subjects.

Interpretation of tuberculin tests

In the majority of individuals, a positive tuberculin test, as defined by induration of 10 mm or more in diameter to 5 TU, indicates past or present exposure to mycobacterial infection (including past BCG vaccination). In primary tuberculosis infections, tuberculin positivity will develop in approximately 6 weeks, and even where the infection is overcome by the individual, tuberculin positivity will persist for many years and usually for life. Where the reaction is markedly stronger than 10 mm in diameter, the diagnosis of tuberculosis is more likely, but all positive tuberculin tests should be interpreted in an individual as a clinical sign, with all the variability of interpretation which that suggests, rather than as a laboratory test which provides an accurate numerical answer.

On the other hand, a negative tuberculin test to 5 or 10 TU either suggests that the subject has never been exposed to mycobacteria, or can represent suppression of previously present tuberculin hypersensitivity by any of a number of conditions where delayed hypersensitivity in general (i.e. also to such antigens as mumps antigen, candida, and DNCB) is suppressed; such conditions include severe overwhelming infections of any type (including severe tuberculosis), sarcoidosis, lymphomas, malignancy, and treatment with immunosuppressive drugs, including corticosteroid therapy. Delayed hypersensitivity is, of course, markedly impaired also in the acquired immunodeficiency syndrome.

Fuller interpretations of the tuberculin test in different circumstances have been proposed.[43]

Radiological investigation

The radiographic appearances on X-ray can be very varied, and may mimic many other conditions. More advanced tuberculosis is often bilateral, may be patchy in nature, and more commonly afflicts the upper lobes,, especially the posterior segments, and also the apical segments of the lower lobes. The presence of cavitation and of later calcification should also be seen as increasing the probability of tuberculosis. Long-standing disease may cause fibrosis, with contraction of lung tissue, and when involving the upper lobes leads to the elevation of the hilar vascular shadows. However, the diagnosis of tuberculosis in the early stages may be more difficult, as the earliest lesions are usually soft, unilateral, and have no specific features. Rarely, superficial endobronchial tuberculosis occurs with a normal chest X-ray, even when the patient may be highly infectious and shedding many bacilli from the bronchial walls. Other less common appearances seen include single rounded 'coin' lesions, which may mimic tumours; and diffuse fine nodular or reticulo-nodular changes seen in miliary tuberculosis which can mimic interstitial lung disease from other causes.

Differential diagnosis of pulmonary tuberculosis

There are four major diagnoses to be considered in any patient with respiratory symptoms and X-ray changes: (a) acute infection, such as pneumonia; (b) chronic infection, such as tuberculosis; (c) lung tumour; and finally, (d) pulmonary thrombo-embolic disease. There is , of course, a wide range of other possibilities, but to remember always these 'big four' means that none of them are overlooked; this is easily done in the case of tuberculosis, by those who do not frequently see patients with the disease; and in the case of thrombo-embolic disease, because of the very many different presentations of the disease and difficulties in validating the diagnosis. When considering the X-ray appearances seen in tuberculosis, these can resemble many other disorders, and particular patterns give rise to different differential diagnoses.

Mediastinal lymphadenopathy may also be caused by sarcoidosis, or by lymphomas, or malignant disease:

- Solitary cavities may occur in lung tumours, acute lung abscesses, and pulmonary infarcts, especially when infected.
- Multiple cavitation can arise in staphylococcal pneumonia, in *Klebsiella* pneumonia, and apparent multiple cavities are seen with severe honeycombing in the lung, as in advanced fibrotic disorders.
- Bilateral upper zone patchy opacity may be present in allergic bronchopulmonary aspergillosis, extrinsic allergic alveolitis, and in sarcoidosis, and also in pneumoconiosis.
- Unilateral shadowing may occur in any acute infection with pneumonia, or in bronchial carcinoma, whether from the tumour itself, or from infection distal to more central bronchial obstruction.

The interpretation of the X-ray will therefore depend substantially on the clinical setting of the patient, and will need in many cases to be assisted by the results of further investigations. For instance, it has been shown that there is a higher proportion of mediastinal lymphatic disease in people from the Indian subcontinent, with a higher prevalence of accompanying extra-pulmonary tuberculosis infection.[44] Also, tuberculosis among HIV positive patients demonstrates a pattern where cavitation is uncommon, and dissemination is common, both within lung and to other organs.[45]

Complications of pulmonary tuberculosis

Complications of primary tuberculosis

Most cases of primary tuberculosis cause little in the way of clinical disease, and resolve without being detected; but as detailed on pp. 247–248, local progression in lung and associated lymph node may result in symptomatic primary pulmonary tuberculosis. However, particularly where children are malnourished, or debilitated by other infections including measles, or parasitic infestation, the infection may rupture from the lung lesion into the pleural space, causing a pleural effusion, and can progress to an empyema; pleural effusions are, however, rare in children under the age of five. Lesions which progress within the lung tissue can caseate, and discharge caseous material into the bronchi and occasionally cause bronchial obstruction. The development of epituberculosis has been mentioned previously, with the obstruction of airways by enlarged hilar lymph nodes.

The most serious complications arise from haematogenous spread of bacilli from the primary complex, causing miliary tuberculosis, and tuberculous meningitis. In young children these complications usually occur early, and carry a high mortality and are further discussed later in the chapter. In addition, less overwhelming degrees of haematogenous spread may allow tubercle bacilli to reach other sites, and to initiate small tuberculous lesions in other organs, including bones and joints, kidney, lymph nodes and peritoneum; here the organisms can remain dormant; local disease can then develop in these organs many years or decades later.[46] In 1948, Wallgren proposed a 'timetable of tuberculosis',[47] in which the first stage consisted of the primary infection, taking about 6 weeks. The second stage, lasting about three months immediately after the first phase, was the vulnerable period for miliary tuberculosis and meningitis, with the third stage, lasting roughly three months, following after; during this third stage, pleural tuberculosis was more common. The fourth stage, lasting up to three years, was the time when bone tuberculosis, or post-primary tuberculosis in adolescents, was a feature. Since then, it has been pointed out that in situations where tuberculosis is less common, chemotherapy is available, and BCG vaccination has been employed, the whole timetable is altered, with most disease occurring many decades after the primary infection, often in middle-aged or elderly people.[48] Some population groups, such as those of Indian Sub-continent origin residing in the UK, are now reaching the fourth stage of Wallgren's timetable, with skeletal and post-primary lung tuberculosis in their mid-30s, with a fifth stage of genito-urinary tuberculosis 8–10 years after the fourth stage.[49]

Complications of post-primary tuberculosis

Major haemoptysis

When tuberculous disease erodes a branch of a bronchial artery, major arterial bleeding can occur into the airways, with a significant risk of causing death, either by torrential haemorrhage, or by filling the bronchial tree with blood and causing aspiration with respiratory failure. Haemoptysis was a common terminal event in the days before chemotherapy, particularly in those whose respiratory function was compromised by extensive pulmonary damage from tuberculosis or some other disease such as chronic bronchitis. In cases where the bleeding is persistent and life threatening, the patient should first undergo bronchoscopy to determine the side and, if possible, the lobar source of the bleeding; after this, selective bronchial arterial angiography using digital subtraction techniques may identify the bleeding vessel, which can then be embolised.[50] If facilities for this are not available, emergency lobectomy may be life saving, as long as the site of bleeding can be correctly identified.

Pleural complications

Pleural effusion

Pulmonary tuberculosis in adults, as a post-primary infection, usually behaves rather differently, because the host response favours a vigorous local response to the bacilli which tends to create a thick barrier of inflammatory tissue around the lesions, and may limit spread. However, spread can and will occur, and although the usual route is by rupture of lesions dispersing caseous material through the bronchi and allowing spread to other areas of lung, spread can also occur through the pleural surface causing pleuritic pain (so-called 'dry pleurisy'), which is frequently followed (sometimes after an interval of some months) by the development of pleural effusion. The pleural fluid found in tuberculosis has the characteristics of an exudate, with a protein content of 30 g/l or more, and containing a preponderance of lymphocytes. Acid-fast bacilli may be identified in the fluid on microscopy, but their numbers are usually small, the effusion often being interpreted as an exudative response to tuberculoprotein: this is likely to be the result of a delayed hypersensitivity response over the surface of the pleura, with relatively few bacilli. Pleural biopsy, using an Abram's needle or similar instrument, frequently demonstrates the presence of typical tuberculous granulomata, and acid-fast bacilli can be detected in the pleural biopsy sections with suitable staining.

Tuberculous empyema

If the pleural fluid becomes purulent from increasing numbers of inflammatory cells, which usually include neutrophil polymorphs in large numbers as well as lymphocytes, it can be defined as an empyema. Treatment will require continuing anti-tuberculous chemotherapy, and effective drainage, which may be surgical. See Chapter 20.

Pneumothorax

Spontaneous pneumothorax can occur in any healthy adult, but can also be a complication of tuberculosis, especially if a lesion near to the pleural surface ruptures. An acute pyopneumothorax can occur as a result, and should be treated by intercostal drainage and continuing anti-tuberculous therapy.

Tuberculous laryngitis

In patients with extensive tuberculosis and a large bacillary load in sputum, infection may develop on the vocal cords, causing painful hoarseness of the voice. This usually responds quickly to therapy.

Later complications

In severe tuberculosis, where significant lung damage occurs before anti-tuberculous therapy has been effective, there may be permanent damage to airways, causing airways obstruction, and to alveoli, resulting in extensive fibrosis with a restrictive defect in lung function testing. This may be particularly disabling if there is other lung disease, such as chronic bronchitis from tobacco smoking, and may become complicated after some years by chronic respiratory failure, pulmonary hypertension, and cor pulmonale.

Chronic residual cavities remaining after the successful treatment of pulmonary tuberculosis can become colonised with *Aspergillus fumigatus*, gradually building up with serum and fungus to form an aspergilloma, or mycetoma, fungus ball. The presence of aspergillus precipitins, with multiple precipitin lines, confirms the diagnosis, the mycetoma being suspected radiologically by an air crescent above a homogeneous opacity within a cavity, although such appearances are only seen if the X-ray is taken with the patient in the erect position. The presence of a mycetoma can be confirmed radiologically by antero-posterior tomography, or by computerised tomography. The main symptom is of recurrent haemoptysis, and surgical resection is sometimes required.

Carcinoma of the lung sometimes arises in patients who have been treated for tuberculosis, but there is no good evidence of an association between the two conditions other than the observation that both tuberculosis and lung cancer are more common in smokers.[51]

Non-pulmonary tuberculosis

M. tuberculosis can infect virtually any body tissue, with the commonest route of infection by inhalation of the organism from droplet infection, establishment of a focus of infection in the lung, and then by blood (or sometimes lymphatic) spread to other organs. Alternatively, organisms may be inhaled and gain access by the tonsils, or they may be swallowed from contaminated food (usually milk) or from swallowed respiratory secretions, and gain entry via the tonsils or through the gut. This chapter is not intended as an exhaustive account of extrapulmonary tuberculosis, but since pulmonary tuberculosis may occur alongside pulmonary disease, it seems appropriate to include brief details of some of the commoner manifestations of extrapulmonary tuberculosis at this point.

The prevalence of the different sites of tuberculous disease varies in different age groups, racial groups, and countries. In a UK study of all patients notified as having tuberculosis in England and Wales in 1988, demonstrated these wide variations.[52] In 1988 the notification rate for tuberculosis was 4.7 per 100 000 per year for white patients, but was about 120 per 100 000 per year for those from the Indian subcontinent (ISC) (India, Pakistan, Bangladesh). Among white UK patients, non-pulmonary tuberculosis accounted for 20% of the notifications; 4.2% of those notified had both pulmonary and non-pulmonary disease. Among those from the ISC, 46% were notified with non-pulmonary tuberculosis, and 11% of all tuberculosis notifications had both pulmonary and non-pulmonary disease. A further group of various ethnic origins including Africa showed a high rate (39%) of non-pulmonary disease, with 7% having combined pulmonary and non-pulmonary disease.

In the USA, extrapulmonary disease accounted for 17.5% of notifications in 1986.[53] Up to 70% of patients with AIDS who contract tuberculosis will have extrapulmonary tuberculous disease.

The commonest site for non-pulmonary tuberculosis is in lymph nodes, particularly in the cervical nodes. In the MRC study[52], among white patients 37% of the non-pulmonary tuberculosis was in lymph nodes, and in 52–54% of the Indian subcontinent and 'other' racial groups. Some 13% of non-pulmonary infection was in bones and joints (both white and ISC), and in white patients 28% of non-pulmonary infection was genito-urinary, with only 4% among other races. Among ISC and 'other' groups, abdominal tuberculosis contributed 14–19% of non-pulmonary TB notifications.

Life-threatening but relatively unusual forms

Miliary tuberculosis

Miliary tuberculosis, in which there is evidence of widespread dissemination of tuberculosis by lympho-haematogenous spread, has been described in two very different contexts; in children, usually in immediate continuity with the primary tuberculosis infection; and in adults, usually elderly, and as a more chronic and indolent infection.

In children, miliary tuberculosis presents with general symptoms of fever, malaise, and weight loss; later, dyspnoea and cyanosis can occur as lung parenchymal involvement extends, and up to 30% will develop tuberculous meningitis. Most organs including liver and spleen are involved. Sometimes, careful examination of the retinae at fundoscopy will show choroidal tubercles. Chest X-rays show extensive miliary (fine nodular) changes throughout the lung fields, and mycobacteria may be identified in urine or gastric secretions; biopsy of bone marrow, lymph node, or liver can demonstrate tubercles or acid-fast bacilli. With prompt anti-tuberculous therapy, recovery is usual, but this requires the diagnosis to be considered in the first place.

In older people, a more chronic form of miliary tuberculosis has been described.[54] This may be characterised by fever; in patients who have a pyrexia of unknown origin, still not explained after 3 weeks of investigation, chronic cryptic miliary tuberculosis is one of the more likely causes; or it may present in a variety of unexplained haematological disorders, with pancytopenia, neutropenia, or lymphocytosis. Patients with chronic cryptic miliary tuberculosis may have a completely normal chest X-ray, but the diagnosis can be made from bone marrow aspiration and culture for mycobacteria; but as this may take several weeks, a therapeutic trial using anti-tuberculous drugs which are specific for *M. tuberculosis*, such as isoniazid and ethambutol, may support the diagnosis. If a previously unremitting fever settles within two weeks or so of such therapy, the diagnosis of tuberculosis is virtually confirmed In addition to the chronic cryptic form of miliary tuberculosis, cases of more classical miliary tuberculosis still occur among adults, where the presenting symptoms include cough and dyspnoea, with classical miliary changes on chest X-ray.

The incidence of miliary tuberculosis in adults is difficult to define; some cases are only diagnosed at autopsy, and with the relatively low autopsy rates among elderly people, it is likely that some cases never come to light. Two reports from the UK give some idea of the pattern and prognosis of miliary tuberculosis in a 'developed' country; in Edinburgh,[55] among a mainly Caucasian population, 40% of the adult cases were of the cryptic type, and the mortality overall was 50% The mean age of the 29 patients studied was 73 years. In Blackburn[56] with a much higher proportion of people of Indian subcontinent origin, the average age of the 10 Caucasian patients was 52 years, whereas that of the 28 Indian Sub-continent origin patients was 38 years; the overall mortality was 10%. In this series, nearly 70% of the cases were of the chronic cryptic type.

Tuberculous meningitis

This remains the most serious form of *M. tuberculosis* infection, with high mortality and in survivors, significant disability. In addition, patients with AIDS are vulnerable to meningitis from both *M. tuberculosis* and non-tuberculous mycobacteria.

The organisms usually reach the meninges as a result of blood spread, but occasionally from direct spread from vertebral infection. Clinical findings can be very non-specific initially, with general ill-health for a few weeks, and classical signs of meningitis may not be obvious until quite late in the disease progression. There may, or may not, be varying degrees of meningism, with neck stiffness, headaches, and vomiting; other signs can include involvement of cranial nerves where they leave the base of the brain; the development of blocks to the flow of cerebrospinal fluid, causing hydrocephalus and impaired consciousness; and sometimes, by causing arteritis as the arteries enter the brain, epileptic fits, or even brain infarcts with loss of function[57,58].

The diagnosis is usually confirmed by examination of the cerebrospinal fluid, which commonly shows the classical changes of increased numbers of lymphocytes, raised protein estimation, and low glucose levels. Acid fast bacilli may be seen in at least 40% of patients, or detected by subsequent culture; some of the newer identification techniques discussed on p. 249 are of particular value in the speedy diagnosis of tuberculous meningitis, in view of the relative purity of the sample being examined compared to sputum.

Treatment is often difficult, because not all anti-tuberculous drugs penetrate the meninges effectively. In a detailed review of this problem, isoniazid and pyrazinamide cross the meninges well, achieving levels of up to 100% of blood levels even when the meninges are not inflamed. Rifampicin and ethambutol cross poorly, but reach about 20% of blood levels when the meninges are inflamed[59]. Streptomycin achieves about 20% of blood levels, and second line drugs such as ethionamide, cycloserine and kanamycin have all been used in difficult cases with drug-resistant organisms. The information available suggests that isoniazid, pyrazinamide, and rifampicin should all be given as initial treatment, with ethambutol and streptomycin in addition for acute meningeal inflammation. Where a good response occurs, ethambutol, streptomycin and pyrazinamide can be stopped after 8 weeks and isoniazid and rifampicin continued for a further 4 to 10 months, depending on progress.

More common forms of non-pulmonary tuberculosis

Lymph-node tuberculosis

In the past, much lymph node tuberculosis was caused by *M. bovis*, but *M. tuberculosis* is now the commonest strain isolated. The disease can develop at almost any age after primary infection, by progressive infection or by reactivation of dormant disease after many years or decades. Characteristically, around 70% of the infections become apparent in cervical nodes, with a gradual enlargement which later may become painful and red. Usually a group of nodes is involved which may coalesce, and without therapy lead to abscess formation and sometimes progress to discharge of pus and sinus formation. Particularly in patients from Asia and Africa, paratracheal and mediastinal lymph nodes are involved, and may progress to abscesses which cause pressure effects on mediastinal structures.

The diagnosis may be suspected by other evidence of tuberculosis on X-ray, including calcification in the neck from previous chronic lymph node infection. The Mantoux test is usually strongly positive. Biopsy or aspiration of pus from a node, and microscopy and culture for AFB will commonly confirm the diagnosis.

Treatment consists of conventional anti-tuberculous therapy, but there may well be a recurrent need for aspiration of pus or even surgical resection during treatment,[60] and even up to the completion of therapy. This may arise because of the continuing delayed hypersensitivity response to tuberculoprotein within the node even when the mycobacteria have been killed.[61]

However, the final outcome of therapy using conventional 'short course' treatment seems satisfactory and curative.[62] Grzybowski and Allen have written an interesting account of the history of tuberculous lymphadenopathy[63] ('scrofula').

Bone and joint tuberculosis

Bone and joint involvement takes some time to develop after the primary infection, even in children, where it does not usually appear for 3 years or more. The commonest bones to be affected are the spinal vertebrae and the vertebral discs, but any bone or synovial joint may be infected, by haematogenous spread. In the case of spinal tuberculosis, back pain is usual, and if untreated, patients develop collapse of vertebrae with wedging and the development of the angulated 'gibbus', frequently in the dorsal vertebrae, which accounted for the hunchbacks of history. Involvement of the lumbar vertebrae may be complicated by paravertebral abscess formation, and pus may accumulate in the psoas muscle (a psoas abscess), track down within the ilio-psoas, and emerge at the groin. When bones are infected by tuberculosis, the characteristic radiological feature is the presence of simultaneous osteolysis and osteosclerosis, with areas of both bone destruction and new bone formation. In the spine, disc spaces are often involved.

The treatment of orthopaedic tuberculosis should follow the same principles as with pulmonary disease, with short-course regimens being effective. Surgical treatment is rarely required unless evidence of spinal cord compression becomes evident and decompression is required. For the majority, ambulatory chemotherapy seems to give excellent results.[64]

Genitourinary tuberculosis

Renal tuberculosis is usually a late event after primary infection, 5–15 years or more later. The infection can attack any part of the renal tract, but most frequently involves the kidney itself, the lower end of the ureter (causing obstruction) and the bladder itself. When the bladder is affected the symptoms consist of frequency of micturition, haematuria, dysuria, and 'sterile' pyuria, where pus cells abound in urine but conventional culture is negative.[65]

In men, the seminal vesicles, prostate and epididymes may become infected with tuberculosis; in women, the Fallopian tubes and endometrium are possible sites of infection. In both sexes, infertility may result, either from obstruction to epididymis, or to the Fallopian tube.[66]

Treatment consists of conventional multiple drug chemotherapy, although it has been suggested that adding corticosteroid treatment may help to prevent late stricture, as for instance at the lower end of the ureter.[67]

Other sites for non-pulmonary tuberculosis

Other tissues where tuberculosis can develop include:

- the pericardium, causing pericardial effusion and later constrictive pericarditis;
- the gastrointestinal tract, at any point but particularly terminal ileum (in the past infection was mainly from *M. bovis*, from infected milk; now more often by ingestion of bacilli from pulmonary disease). Ulceration of the mucosa, and fistulae can occur;
- the peritoneum, causing ascites;
- the adrenal glands, causing Addison's disease;
- skin, causing lupus vulgaris;
- mouth, tonsil, tongue.

In all cases the proper treatment consists of a full course of multidrug anti-tuberculous therapy, plus any other measures to remedy the effects of the disease, such as the surgical release of constrictive pericarditis.

Treatment of tuberculosis

Prior to the introduction of the first true anti-tuberculous drugs, treatment was based on rest, good nutrition, and fresh air; the sanatorium regimes of the first 50 years of the twentieth century relied substantially on such measures, supplemented by surgical techniques which by the early 1950s included artificial pneumothorax, phrenic nerve crush, pneumoperitoneum, thoracoplasty, plombage, and resection of diseased lung. During this period the prognosis for those with more advanced disease remained poor – the 5-year survival for those with pulmonary disease demonstrating cavity formation was about 25%. Many of the surgical approaches listed above were aimed at 'collapsing' the affected lung and closing cavities, to prevent further spread of the disease. The discovery and introduction for general use of streptomycin in 1948, followed by para-aminosalicylic acid (PAS) and then isoniazid, transformed the outlook for patients with tuberculosis. Following the crucial and innovative multi-centre controlled clinical trials by the Medical Research Council in the UK, it was then possible to offer patients a cure for tuberculosis. During the second half of the twentieth century tuberculosis treatment has advanced further with the development of new agents, but it is a tragedy that improper use of the drugs by both doctors and patients has led to increasing problems with strains of *M. tuberculosis* which are resistant to some or most of the available anti-tuberculous drugs. At the same time, many of the lessons learnt during the early days of effective drug treatment have been ignored; the vital importance of community control measures in tuberculosis and the proper supervision of treatment have been neglected, and in many countries throughout the world tuberculosis is resurgent, and represents a major health challenge.

The essential components of a programme for the modern treatment of tuberculosis include:

- Effective diagnosis, with ability to determine drug sensitivity of the organisms
- Good drug treatment regimens, starting with at least three effective anti-tuberculous agents, and continuing for a proper duration under supervision to ensure compliance
- A comprehensive community tuberculosis control programme.

Drugs used in the treatment of tuberculosis

The principal drugs are shown in Table 15.3. Some of the relevant clinical pharmacological properties of the three first-line drugs are discussed below. For reviews of the pharmacokinetics and adverse effects of these and other-antituberculosis drugs, see Holdiness[68–71] and Girling.[72] For a fuller review of the treatment of tuberculosis, see Davidson and Le,[73] and WHO Guidelines.[74]

Major anti-tuberculosis drugs

Isoniazid (INH, or H)

Isoniazid is the hydrazide of isonicotinic acid, and is bactericidal to growing tubercle bacilli, by interfering with cell wall synthesis. It is invaluable as a first-line drug in combination therapy with rifampicin and pyrazinamide. It is also used as a single agent in chemoprophylaxis to prevent tuberculosis infection in susceptible people in contact with tuberculosis (primary chemoprophylaxis), and also to prevent activation in individuals with dormant, inactive infection (secondary chemoprophylaxis). As with all other antituberculosis drugs, isoniazid should *never* be used as a single agent to treat active tuberculosis, because of the high risk of inducing drug-resistant organisms; if in doubt, secondary chemoprophylaxis should be given with two or more effective drugs.

Isoniazid is well and rapidly absorbed after oral dosing on an empty stomach (peak concentration attained in 1 to 2 hours), more slowly with food. The distribution of isoniazid is extensive, including cerebrospinal fluid, with negligible protein binding, and it persists in caseous material. Metabolism is by acetylation (at a rate which is genetically determined) and hydroxylation. Patients who are 'slow' acetylators have higher concentrations of active isoniazid and this appears to increase the frequency of some adverse reactions (see below). On the other hand, 'rapid' acetylators are less likely to be effectively treated with some of the intermittent regimens which involve once weekly doses, though they respond equally as well as slow acetylators to a twice weekly, bactericidal and sterilising regimen. The elimination half life of isoniazid (normally 0.75 to 1.8 hours in rapid acetylators or 2 to 4.5 hours in slow acetylators) is prolonged in acute or chronic liver disease and also in neonates (up to 19.8 hours), but does not appear to be significantly altered in renal dysfunction.[68]

The recommended dose of isoniazid is 3 to 5 mg/kg/day but children tolerate much higher doses (up to 20 mg/kg/day). Twice weekly (and in slow acetylators, once weekly) regimens (usually combined with pyridoxine to reduce or reverse neurological and haematological adverse reactions) are also used (Table 15.3). The dose should be reduced or therapy stopped in hepatic insufficiency because the rate of elimination of isoniazid is prolonged. In severe renal insufficiency, monitoring of serum concentrations is indicated, particularly in patients who are slow acetylators.

Adverse reactions to isoniazid are infrequent if the above recommendations are followed and the benefits outweigh the risks of therapy. However, at higher dose levels (more than 6 mg/kg/day) peripheral neuropathy, particularly in slow acetylators, occurs. This can usually be prevented and treated with the use of pyridoxine supplements. In addition, isoniazid-induced hepatic injury is now well recognised. This reaction appears to be associated with one of the metabolites of isoniazid, monoacetylhydrazine, via the formation of a reactive intermediate. Increasing age, slow acetylation and alcohol consumption appear to be risk factors for isoniazid-induced hepatotoxicity.

The onset of the hepatotoxic reaction is variable (1 week to many months) and the severity varies from a mild reversible reaction (elevation of transaminases in 10 to 20% of patients) to severe hepatitis with considerable morbidity and some mortality.

In the treatment of active pulmonary tuberculosis, initial therapy should include a minimum of three of the above drugs, because of the ready development of resistance to a single drug. If resistance is suspected, then four or more drugs should be used as initial therapy.

Rifampicin(R) (rifampin)

Rifampicin is a potent first-line bactericidal antituberculosis agent, probably effective through inhibition of RNA-polymerase. It is a semisynthetic antibiotic, obtainable in both oral and intravenous formulations, which, along with pyrazinamide, has the ability to kill so-called 'persisters' – mycobacteria that lie dormant, often within cells or caseous material.

Absorption of rifampicin is practically complete and rapid (peak levels attained within 2 to 4 hours) after dosage on an empty stomach. The presence of food causes marked variations in serum concentrations. Concurrent isoniazid (as in combined formulations) does not affect its absorption. Rifampicin and rifabutin are subject to hepatic 'first-pass' metabolism and transferred to bile. At rifampicin doses above 300 to 450 mg the excretory capacity of the liver is saturated. Increases in the dose of rifampicin above these levels lead to relatively higher serum concentrations. Protein binding of rifampicin is to albumin (weak, reversible, approximately 80%). Distribution is extensive and patients should be warned about probable red–brown colouration of body fluids (e.g. urine, sweat, tears, faeces, etc). The metabolism of rifampicin is principally by desacetylation. The desacetylated metabolite is active and accounts for most of the biliary antibacterial activity. Rifampicin also stimulates its own metabolism as well as being a potent inducer of hepatic drug metabolising enzymes of certain

Table 15.3. *Principal antituberculosis drugs*

Drug	Dose (daily)	Notes	Main adverse effects
Isoniazid	300 mg, 5 mg/Kg Child 10 mg/kg	Take 30 min before food for peak levels Bactericidal in high doses Penetrates to CSF Active against intracellular organisms Reduce in slow acetylators Dosage in twice weekly intermittent therapy 15 mg/kg plus10 mg pyridoxine	*Side-effects:* few at less than 350 mg/day *Hypersensitivity reactions:* rare – fever, rash, lymphadenopathy. Slow acetylators have greater incidence of some side effects, esp. peripheral neuropathy (pyridoxine responsive) Optic neuritis is rare, Occasional liver disturbance also ataxia, euphoria,convulsions, tinnitus, insomnia and muscle twitching. Occasional hyperglycaemia, gynaecomastia, pellagra-like state, dryness of mouth, epigastric discomfort, urinary retention. *Caution:* in convulsive disorders, renal and hepatic dysfunction, alcoholism, breast-feeding. Contraindicated: in manic states, porphyria, drug-induced liver disease. *Interaction:* with diazepam, also with carbamazepine, ethosuximide and phenytoin in slow acetylators. Antacids (e.g. aluminium hydroxide) reduce absorption.
Rifampicin	450 to 600 mg Child 10 mg/kg	Take 30 mins before food Bactericidal Penetrates to CSF only partly via inflamed meninges Reduce dose in hepatobiliary disease Dose in twice weekly intermittent therapy should be less than 15mg/kg	*Side effects:* gastrointestinal disturbance, modest elevations of bilirubin and hepatic enzymes, not precluding continuation of therapy – usually transient. All patients pass orange-red urine, may have staining of saliva, tears (and hence soft contact lenses), sweat, and bowel mucus. Jaundice, skin rashes can occur. In those on intermittent therapy, an influenza-like syndrome with chills, fever, and aches may occur. Rarely shock, breathlessness, haemolytic anaemia, acute renal failure, thrombocytopenic purpura, eosinophilia, leukopenia. *Contraindications:* porphyria, hepatic disease. *Interactions:* rifampicin induces liver enzymes, hastens metabolism of oral contraceptives, so patients must use additional means of contraception. Other important interactions with anticonvulsant drugs, anticoagulants and oral hypoglycaemic drugs, diazepam, Beta-blockers, cyclosporin, calcium-channel blockers, anti-dysrhythmics such as diisopyramide, mexilitine, tricyclic antidepressants, cimetidine, thyroxine, theophyllines – all may have action reduced as a result of accelerated metabolism. Absorption reduced by antacids..
Pyrazinamide	1.5–2 g Child 35 mg/kg	Bactericidal, especially in acid pH Penetrates to CSF	*Side-effects:* Gastrointestinal disturbance, hepatotoxicity; fever, nausea, vomiting, jaundice, liver failure; liver function should be monitored during therapy. Also can precipitate gout, arthralgia, urticaria, sideroblastic anaemia *Contraindications:* porphyria, liver disease; *Caution:* diabetes, gout, impaired renal function *Interactions:* antagonises uricosuric effect of sulphinpyrazone and probenecid
Ethambutol:	15 mg/kg– 25 mg/kg	Bacteriostatic Partial penetration to CSF via inflamed meninges Reduce dose in renal failure; avoid in severe renal failure unless no alternative Absorption not reduced by food In intermittent therapy, 30 mg/kg three times weekly, 45 mg/kg twice weekly	*Side effects:* Optic neuropathy, red/green colour blindness, peripheral neuropathy; optic effects more common in higher doses. all patients should have visual acuity recorded before therapy starts, and be rechecked regularly; should also be warned to report any visual change. *Contraindications:* poor vision, young children under 6 years. Reduce dose in renal impairment
Streptomycin	1g , dose. reduced in patients over 40 years and under 50kg	Intramuscular injection, an amino glycoside Bactericidal in combination with pyrazinamide Partial penetration to CSF Useful in some fully supervised intermittent regimens	*Side effects:* as for aminoglycosides; ototoxicity (especially disorders of balance), renal damage, skin rashes, fevers, paraesthesiae around mouth. *Caution:* in renal disease, reduce dose and watch blood levels to prevent ototoxicity.

Adapted from *Avery's Drug Treatment*, 4th edn by permission of the editor and publisher.

other drugs, leading to clinically important adverse drug interactions (Table 15.3). Rifampicin does not affect isoniazid acetylation. Its elimination half-life ranges between 2.3 and 5.1 hours following initial doses, but this decreases to 2 to 3 hours following repeated administration due to increased hepatic metabolism.[68] The excretion of rifampicin is both biliary and renal, and modifications in dosage are required in patients with hepatobiliary or hepato-renal insufficiency.

Adverse reactions to rifampicin are infrequent particularly if attention is paid to recommended dosage levels, dosage intervals, associated disease and concurrent drug therapy;[72] (Table 15.3). Interpretation of cause and effect relationships (e.g. hepatic dysfunction) is complicated by the fact that rifampicin is usually combined with isoniazid, which has important adverse reactions of its own.

Other rifamycins

Rifapentin is a rifamycin with a longer (20 hours) half-life than rifampicin, so it can be used in one-dose a week regimens, but shares the same pattern of effectiveness with rifampicin, so is of no value in rifampicin resistant infections. Rifabutin is, on the other hand, effective against 30% of rifampicin-resistant strains, and is more active against *M. avium–intracellulare.*[75,76] The usual dosage is 150 mg daily, but with more resistant organisms and *M. avium–intracellulare* infections, 300–600 mg daily is recommended.

Pyrazinamide (Z)

This drug is especially bactericidal to mycobacteria multiplying intracellularly at low pH levels, and it has been clearly shown in several studies that inclusion of pyrazinamide in the first 2 months of a treatment regimen can reduce the later relapse rate and allow a shorter duration of continuation therapy.

Pyrazinamide is well absorbed after oral administration and is eliminated principally by hepatic metabolism (half-life 9 to 10 hours); only about 3% of an oral dose is excreted unchanged in the urine in the first 24 hours. As an with isoniazid, pyrazinamide penetrates well into cerebrospinal fluid, and is therefore especially useful in tuberculous meningitis. The drug is not always well tolerated and commonly causes nausea, flushing and arthralgia. Hepatotoxic reactions have also occurred (see Table 15.3) and may limit the duration of therapy.

Important supportive drugs

Ethambutol (E)

Ethambutol is an essentially bacteriostatic drug, which seems to inhibit mycobacterial cell wall synthesis. It is well absorbed after oral administration (75 to 80%), with peak levels at 2 hours. Though distributed to most body fluids and with 40% protein binding, it does not cross the blood–brain barrier, and even in meningitis transmission is variable. Hepatic metabolism is less than with isoniazid or rifampicin and the drug is mainly excreted unchanged in the urine, so the drug can be used safely in liver disease, but in renal insufficiency the dose must be modified (Table 15.3). Adverse reactions with ethambutol are infrequent at recommended doses. The most important reaction is the occurrence of a dose-related retrobulbar neuritis (see also Table 15.3) and the drug should be immediately withdrawn if visual symptoms occur. Fortunately most patients with retrobulbar neuritis recover normal vision if the ethambutol is stopped with the first symptoms, but it is recommended that all patients started on ethambutol should have regular checks of visual acuity, and be firmly warned of the possibility of, and the need to report promptly, any visual impairment.

Streptomycin (S)

Streptomycin is an aminoglycoside which must be given by injection, usually intramuscularly. It is well distributed in the tissues, but does not cross particularly well to the cerebrospinal fluid. As with other aminoglycosides, high blood levels of streptomycin cause eighth cranial nerve damage, particularly vestibular, and drug rashes are common. As the drug is 90% excreted in the urine, particular care is required in patients with renal impairment.

Standard courses of antituberculosis treatment in situations where drug resistance is not anticipated

Detailed recommendations for the treatment of tuberculosis have been published by the Joint Tuberculosis Committee of the British Thoracic Society,[77] World Health Organisation[74] and the American Thoracic Society,[78] and are regularly updated. There is wide agreement that treatment should consist of an initial intensive phase, usually of 2 months, followed by a longer continuation phase of 4 to 16 months depending on the drugs used.

Initial intensive treatment

Once specimens of sputum have been obtained for culture, treatment should be started with at least three drugs to which the organism is likely to be sensitive. Multiple drug therapy is more effective and reduces infectivity and the development of resistant strains of *M. tuberculosis*. The three drugs of first choice are isoniazid, rifampicin, and pyrazinamide and should be taken before food (Table 15.2). The choice of initial therapy may however be influenced by other factors such as cost, availability, convenience and toxicity, and also by preexisting liver disease, renal disease, or pregnancy. In such circumstances alternative drugs may be required, but the requirement to treat with a minimum of three drugs must be adhered to. The initial three-drug regimen should be continued for at least 8 weeks and ideally until the sensitivities of the organism have been established (usually 8 to 12 weeks, though new techniques sometimes allow earlier results). The importance of adequate instruction and surveillance in tablet taking cannot be over-emphasised. In areas where drug-resistant organisms are prevalent, it may be essential to give more that three drugs as initial therapy, until the drug sensitivities of the infecting organism are known.

All three of the main anti-tuberculous drugs have a potential to cause hepatotoxicity in about 3–4% of treated patients. It is now recommended,[79] as an additional recommendation to the Joint Tuberculosis Committee Guidelines of 1990[77] that:

1. All patients should have pretreatment measurements of liver function.
2. Standard treatment should be given under the supervision of a respiratory or other suitably qualified physician.

Table 15.4. *Other anti-tuberculosis drugs*

Drug	Dose (daily)	Notes	Main adverse effects
Thiacetazone	150 mg	Bacteriostatic Well absorbed Cheap	Nausea, vomiting and diarrhoea in up to 20% of patients. Bone marrow depression, vertigo, ataxia, occasional liver toxicity, exfoliative dermatitis
Ethionamide (and prothionamide)	500–750 mg 7.5–15 mg/kg	Chemically related to isoniazid, but usually highly effective in isoniazid-resistant infections Bactericidal Crosses to CSF and placenta?	Frequent gastrointestinal side-effects, liver toxicity; rarely, hypotension, hypoglycaemia, alopecia, convulsions, neuropathy. Prothionamide may be better tolerated than ethionamide.
Cycloserine	10 mg/kg/day (adults) 10–20 mg/kg/day (children)	Bactericidal Well absorbed, crosses CSF and placenta	Frequent CNS effects; drowsiness, vertigo, disorientation, confusion, coma, psychosis, personality changes in up to 50%.
Capreomycin (also kanamycin, amikacin)	1 g, reduced if aged over 40 years, and if renal impairment intramuscular injection	Aminoglycosides, similar activity to streptomycin, but may be effective in streptomycin resistant infections.	As for aminoglycosides, but may have higher incidence of eighth nerve toxicity than streptomycin.
Clofazimine	100–200 mg	Riminophenazine compound, mainly used in leprosy, but now used in drug-resistant tuberculosis and atypical mycobacterial infections. Half-life 70 days. Crystallises in many organs, including fatty tissues. Not found in CSF or brain.	Brown discolouration of the skin
Fluoroquinolones (Including ciprofloxacin and ofloxacin)	Ciprofloxacin; 1–1.5 g Ofloxacin; 400–600 mg/day parfloxacin	Value in drug-resistant tuberculosis and in infections with mycobacteria other than tuberculosis being explored	Generally well tolerated, apart from some gastrointestinal upset in about 5%
β-lactams	Clavulanic acid and amoxycillin	Some activity against mycobacteria; clinical activity unclear so far	
Macrolides	Azithromycin Clarithromycin Roxithromycin	Some evidence of anti-mycobacterial activity, including *M. avium–intracellulare*	

Adapted from *Avery's Drug Treatment*, 4th edn by permission of the editor and publisher.

3. All patients (and their general practitioners) should be warned of the possible side-effects and action to take if they arise, preferably in writing.
4. Regular monitoring of liver function is required for those with any known chronic liver disease.

The application of these recommendations in developing countries where resources are limited could prove particularly difficult or impossible, and in such circumstances the balance of benefit and risk will have to be carefully considered.

Continuation treatment

Once the sensitivities of the organism have been established, or the initial 8-week period completed, therapy is continued with the two most appropriate drugs until the completion of the recommended course.[80,81] The usual drugs included in the continuation regimen are rifampicin and isoniazid, and using these drugs, only a further 4 months of treatment is required. These 6-month regimens of isoniazid and rifampicin, supplemented for the first two months by pyrazinamide (the so-called 2HRZ/4HR regimen) has been shown to be as effective as the previously favoured 9-month regimen of isoniazid and rifampicin supplemented for the first two months by ethambutol

(2EHR/7HR regimen).[82] If for reason of cost or toxicity one of these first-line drugs cannot be used, a reserve drug (Table 15.3) should be substituted and the course of therapy extended to 18 months, especially if rifampicin is not included. In African countries, an 8-month regimen is employed with 2 months of isoniazid, rifampicin, and pyrazinamide followed by 6 months of isoniazid and thiacetazone, 150mg daily, though for those with HIV infection there are particular problems in the tolerance of thiacetazone in this group.

During continuation therapy, patients should be reviewed at regular intervals to monitor clinical and bacteriological progress and to assess compliance with drug therapy. In patients who are suspected of irregular tablet taking a supervised daily or intermittent (twice weekly) regimen should be introduced, where a clinic or practice nurse watches while the medication is administered. This is usually called directly observed therapy, or DOT. In extreme situations, where patients cannot be relied upon to attend and take therapy, the rights of their contacts at risk and the community as a whole may have to take precedence, and rarely treatment may be administered in a compulsory, court-ordered secure facility.

Intermittent regimens of antituberculosis therapy

Intermittent therapy, given twice or thrice weekly, permits greater supervision of treatment, and may be more convenient and cheaper, particularly in developing countries. A wide variety of effective intermittent regimens have been devised, with a daily initial phase followed by twice or thrice weekly continuation therapy, and some thrice-weekly regimens have proved to be effective even without an initial daily phase of treatment. To be effective, the individual doses may need to be higher than those used in daily therapy, at the risk of inducing side-effects. For a thrice weekly regimen, the dose of rifampicin can be similar to the daily dose; isoniazid can be given in doses of 200–400 mg thrice weekly according to body weight, along with rifampicin. After an 8-week daily initial therapy with isoniazid, rifampicin, and pyrazinamide, 4 months of thrice weekly rifampicin and isoniazid is an effective continuation regimen. An alternative regimen consists of twice weekly streptomycin, 0.75 g or 1 g according to weight, plus isoniazid, 14 mg/kg twice weekly, along with pyridoxine 10 mg, to prevent isoniazid induced peripheral neuropathy with the higher isoniazid doses, but with this regimen, the continuation phase must be continued for 16 months after the initial phase of daily treatment. Rifampicin can be used in twice weekly regimens, but there is a higher risk of adverse reactions (especially 'chills' and 'flu'-like symptoms) which may be reduced by reducing the dose to below 15 mg/kg twice weekly. For details of other regimens, including intermittent regimens, see Crofton, Horne, and Miller,[46] and Davies.[84]

Particular treatment problems in tuberculosis

Treatment of tuberculosis during pregnancy

The transplacental pharmacokinetics of antituberculosis drugs have been reviewed by Holdiness.[71] In general, active tuberculosis in pregnancy should be treated employing the usual principles of treating with at least three drugs, and giving a course for the full effective duration. In general, isoniazid, ethambutol, and rifampicin seem to reasonably safe in pregnancy, even though placental transmission occurs. There is no clear evidence of a teratogenic effect of these three antituberculosis drugs, although caution is advised in using rifampicin in the first trimester. Streptomycin also crosses the placenta, but carries the risk of ototoxicity in up to one in six of the foetuses exposed, so is best avoided. Little is known about the other drugs in pregnancy, though some, such as thiocetazone and pyrazinamide are poorly tolerated. Ethionamide is teratogenic and is contraindicated. A standard regimen with isoniazid, pyrazinamide, and rifampicin can be used in pregnancy, substituting ethambutol if any of the first three drugs prove unsuitable or are poorly tolerated.

Therapy of tuberculosis in patients with renal disease

Ethambutol is largely excreted by the kidney, whereas most isoniazid, rifampicin and pyrazinamide is either metabolised or excreted through the biliary system. Consequently, rifampicin can be given in normal doses to patients with renal failure, but the other drugs may have to be given in reduced dosage, particularly in severe renal failure, and pyridoxine should be given to prevent isoniazid neuropathy. Ethambutol is best avoided in severe renal failure, particularly if the glomerular filtration rate is less than 50 ml/min, because of the increased risks of visual field defects and colour-blindness. With pyrazinamide, caution is required because of the tendency to precipitate gout. Streptomycin should only be given if essential, and at reduced dosage with blood level monitoring. For patients on renal dialysis, ethambutol and streptomycin can be given immediately after each dialysis treatment.

Therapy of patients with tuberculosis who have pre-existing liver disease

Isoniazid, rifampicin, ethionamide and pyrazinamide can all be hepatotoxic, although not necessarily all of them together in the same patient. Patients with hepatic failure can be treated with ethambutol, streptomycin, and isoniazid, with careful monitoring of liver function tests, though if the patient can tolerate rifampicin, there are considerable advantages in shortening the treatment course; clearly, great caution and regular liver function monitoring are required.

Treatment of tuberculosis in children

Children with active tuberculosis can be treated with the standard initial regime of isoniazid, rifampicin, and pyrazinamide; ethambutol is best avoided because they may not be able to report any visual side-effects. In most children the bacillary load in the tuberculous lesions may be quite small, and pyrazinamide can be omitted if there is no likelihood of drug-resistant organisms, but it will in that case be necessary to continue therapy with isoniazid and rifampicin for 9 months. The recommended doses of anti-tuberculous drugs for children are detailed in Tables 15.3 and 15.4.

Treatment of drug-resistant tuberculosis

Tubercle bacilli have a spontaneous tendency to mutations which are resistant to antimicrobial drugs; it has been estimated that spontaneous mutations could account for one in every 10^6 organisms becoming resistant to isoniazid, and one in every 10^8 being resistant to rifampicin.[85] As a result of this, patients treated with a single anti-tuberculous drug can rapidly develop strains resistant to that drug, hence the essential principle that *all patients should be treated with a minimum of two drugs to which the organisms are known or likely to be sensitive*. Unfortunately, through improperly prescribed therapy, erratic drug ingestion, inadequate dosage or incomplete therapy, or a combination of these defects in therapy, there have been steep increases in the frequency of tubercle bacilli resistant to multiple anti-tuberculous drugs in many areas of the world, both in developing countries and also in major cities such as New York. It is usual to classify drug resistance as being primary, if the organisms are isolated from an individual who has never previously received TB drug therapy, or secondary resistance, where previous therapy has been taken, though such information is not always easy to verify. In New York, organisms resistant to two or more drugs accounted for 33% of all isolates, though half of these came from patients who had previous TB treatment, so could not be classed as primary drug resistant cases. Among previously untreated patients, 7% showed resistance to both isoniazid and rifampicin.[86] In another New York study, the rates of combined isoniazid and rifampicin resistant organisms rose from 2.5% in 1971 to 16% in 1991.[87] Rates of primary multiple drug resistance may be as high as 20–30% in China, India, Pakistan and the Philippines.[88] This compares with the UK, where current rates of primary resistance run at 6% resistant to isoniazid, and 0.6% resistant to both isoniazid and rifampicin.

HIV-positive individuals seem particularly susceptible to such infections, and transmission of the infection by exogenous infection, rather than reactivation of previously dormant disease, seems particularly likely. Such a pattern of transmission was seen when DNA fingerprinting techniques were used to trace the transmission of the infection.[89]

Patients with multidrug-resistant tuberculosis infection present a serious global problem for the future of tuberculosis control, particularly with the ease of rapid world travel. It is, however, possible to regain control by a disciplined and obsessional approach to tuberculosis control and therapy, such as was demonstrated in Korea, where the prevalence of drug resistance fell from 48% overall in 1980 to 2% in 1990 through a rigorous programme of management which reduced the numbers of 'failed' TB treatment cases.[90] To begin to deal with drug resistance problems, it is essential to have a community control programme which can identify new cases, determine the drug sensitivity of the organisms, and treat the affected patients with a fully effective regimen, usually fully supervised, ensuring cure wherever possible.

A variety of regimens have been suggested for treating patients with multiple resistance to such drugs as isoniazid, rifampicin, and pyrazinamide, employing multiple (even up to six or seven) second-line drugs in prolonged treatment regimens continuing for 2 years or more. Such patients should only be treated by experts; segregation, especially from vulnerable contacts such as those with AIDS, is essential; and treatment must be given in a fully supervised manner to achieve the best possible outcome both for the individual and the community at large. Iseman has written a detailed review.[91] Surgical resection of affected parts of lung may be necessary.

The treatment of patients with infection with non-tuberculous mycobacteria, which are usually resistant to many of the standard anti-tuberculous agents, is also exceptionally difficult, and such patients are also properly treated by experts. For further details, see Chapter 11.

Mycobacterial infections associated with AIDS are discussed further in Chapter 22.

Other therapies for tuberculosis

Immunotherapy

While the relationship between tuberculin hypersensitivity and protective immunity in tuberculosis remains puzzling, there is increasing interest in the development of vaccines which may improve the host response to mycobacterial infections. The particular vaccine of promise currently is prepared from *M. vaccae*, a fast-growing saprophytic organism derived from mud samples found on the shores of Lake Kyoga in Uganda. Work with vaccines prepared from a strain entitled R877R, using a dose containing 10^9 irradiation killed organisms, suggested that there was benefit in terms of improved survival, reduced mycobacterial excretion, and greater weight gain even where patients had drug-resistant organisms, or failed to receive an adequate course of anti-tuberculous drug therapy.[92] A further study with the same vaccine in Kuwait showed increased weight gain, and reduced skin test responses to tuberculin in those given the vaccine when compared with placebo.[93] There is also a suggestion that *M. vaccae* immunisation can improve survival and sputum clearance of organisms in HIV-related tuberculosis.[94]

A further report of the use of such a vaccine in Africa has suggested benefits from this approach, even when drugs are hard to obtain, and where tuberculosis occurs alongside human immunodeficiency virus infection[95]. A single dose of an autoclaved suspension of *M. vaccae* or placebo was given in the first 3 weeks of a course of anti-tuberculous drug therapy. After 10 to 14 months, against the background of the difficulties of TB treatment in Africa, of those receiving the active preparation, 11% were still excreting bacilli, compared with 84.6% of those given placebo: the mean weight gain was almost 8 kg in the active group, and only 2 kg in the placebo group. These results from a simple single-dose therapy in difficult conditions suggest the need for further study in view of the possibility that such treatment could be applied widely and cheaply. The studies so far reported have been relatively small and there is a need for large, well-controlled and well-designed studies before reliable conclusions can be drawn about the place of *M. vaccae* immunotherapy. However, if the results were to be confirmed under fully controlled conditions, immunotherapy could provide an important additional treatment in tuberculosis generally, but especially in 'hard-to treat' mycobacterial infections with multi-drug resistant organisms or infections with non-tuberculous *Mycobacteria*.

The method of action of such therapy remains unclear, but it has been suggested that the injected preparation contains a molecule which induces long-term production of a substance in the host which secondarily regulates cellular immunity, perhaps a regulatory antibody, to diminish the Koch phenomenon.[96]

Steroid therapy

Since the development of anti-tuberculous chemotherapy, corticosteroid therapy has sometimes been used at the same time, on the basis that some of the more harmful effects of tuberculosis infection were the result of the inflammatory process. The field is fully reviewed by Sendorowitz and Viskum.[97] It is known, of course, that corticosteroid therapy suppresses the tuberculin reaction. In pulmonary tuberculosis, corticosteroid therapy can hasten the resolution of fever, and results in more rapid weight gain and X-ray resolution, especially in those with more fulminant disease. However, the dangers of dissemination of tuberculosis infection if the anti-tuberculosis drugs are not taken, or if the organisms are drug resistant, are real so such therapy is not generally advised unless the patients are well supervised and ill enough to justify adding corticosteroid treatment. However, there is a better case for using corticosteroids alongside anti-tuberculous therapy where there is a brisk inflammatory reaction, as with rapidly re-accumulating tuberculous pleural effusions, or where inflammatory changes cause obstruction to a viscus; examples of the latter include tuberculosis of the renal tract with developing stricture of the lower end of the ureter, or where enlarged mediastinal lymph nodes cause bronchial obstruction in tuberculosis in children. The value of corticosteroids in tuberculous meningitis is much more controversial; it has been suggested that corticosteroids might reduce the risk of spinal block and subsequent hydrocephalus by inhibiting the development of exudate, but there are no adequate fully controlled trials to help make a decision. However, in those with very severe disease, particularly with altered consciousness and neurological deficit, corticosteroid therapy may well be justified. A placebo-controlled trial of corticosteroids in tuberculous pericarditis showed significant benefit in terms of survival and rate of improvement.[98]

The current place of surgery for tuberculosis

In the past, and particularly from 1930 until about 1955, surgical techniques were frequently employed in an attempt to treat pulmonary tuberculosis. At this time, and before anti-tuberculous drugs had been full developed and their potential realised, the prognosis for pulmonary tuberculosis was serious: in those with established cavitating disease, the 5-year survival was about 25%. Attempts were therefore made to close cavities, because they were seen as the means of disseminating bacilli to other areas of the lung. Techniques included 'collapse' therapy by phrenic nerve crush and artificial pneumothorax, or pneumoperitoneum, often maintained by regular refills for months or years. More permanent methods of achieving the same effect included thoracoplasty, and plombage. Occasionally, infected areas of lung were resected.

Such surgical methods of treatment were rendered almost totally redundant by the advent of anti-tuberculous drugs, but with the advent of multi-drug resistant strains of *M. tuberculosis*, it seems possible that some of these techniques may need to be reconsidered for such hard-to treat disease.[99]

Drug therapy for tuberculosis in developing countries, and the economics of tuberculosis treatment

Developing countries are handicapped by shortages of funds, not only for the purchase of antituberculosis drugs, but for the essential measures to control tuberculosis in a community, and for training of medical personnel. Excellent handbooks for tuberculosis treatment and control are available at low cost.[46,100]

The cost of antituberculosis drugs clearly has a major influence on the effectiveness of a tuberculosis control programme, and is detailed in the *WHO Guidelines*[74] published in 1993. Tables 15.5 and 15.6 indicate the comparative costs of the individual antituberculosis drugs, together with the costs of complete courses of combined drug therapy.

General conclusions on the treatment of tuberculosis

The effective treatment of tuberculosis in a world with an increasing prevalence of drug-resistant organisms, and a population which includes some very susceptible people with inadequate housing, poor nutrition, and risk factors such as HIV infection, requires a committed and obsessional approach to detail. Part of this includes an ability to communicate with patients – to have an understanding of their lives and the constraints upon them, and to help them to understand the wider aspects of the problem, to gain trust, and co-operation. At times this may bring conflicts between the rights of the patient to decide whether to take advice and treatment, and the wider needs of the community where there is a need to prevent the spread of infection, and sanctions may sometimes be needed, such as the use of local legislation to insist on segregation and treatment of infectious people, or at least the threat of such sanctions, in particularly difficult patients.

At the same time, the requirements of good treatment vary widely; it may be a relatively simple matter to treat a fully compliant patient in a country with a low rate of tuberculosis, caused by drug-sensitive organisms. Different clinical situations require a different approach, depending whether early treatment of ordinary patients, or delayed diagnosis in deprived, difficult situations.[101]

But to treat an outbreak of tuberculosis in an environment where there is poverty, drug resistance, high levels of HIV infection, and a lack of basic medical care is one of the most daunting challenges to the health care services, and will not be soluble without a political commitment in that country to a comprehensive tuberculosis control programme, as described in the following section.

Control and prevention of tuberculosis

Tuberculosis cannot be controlled without a comprehensive programme which includes the expeditious diagnosis and effective treatment of all active cases, checking of close contacts, and preventive measures in the community. In 1990, a Subcommittee of the Joint Tuberculosis Committee of the British Thoracic Society[102] made recommendations, which were updated in 1994.[103] These recommendations covered the issue of necessary segregation of tuberculosis patients, contact and hospital staff procedures, and the use of BCG vaccination in defined circumstances. The American Thoracic Society also made detailed recommendations in 1992,[78] as has the World Health Organisation.[74] The International Union against Tuberculosis and Lung Disease has also published valuable Guides to the management of tuberculosis in low income countries[100] and high prevalence countries,[104] and Crofton, Horne and Millar's book[46] represents a particularly helpful guide to tuberculosis management for those working in developing countries.

Table 15.5. *Costs of drug for 2 months treatment at average adult doses in US dollars (derived from WHO Guidelines (1993), using UNICEF prices)*

Drug	Daily dose	Cost, US Dollars
Isoniazid	300 mg	0.426
Rifampicin	600 mg	11.0
Pyrazinamide	1500 mg	6.44
Streptomycin	1 g	16.3 (plus injection costs)
Ethambutol	1 g	3.5

Table 15.6. *Costs of commonly used regimens of antituberculosis therapy in US dollars (derived from WHO Guidelines (1993) using UNICEF prices)*

Initial phase	Cost, US $
2HRZ	25
2HRZS	44
2HRZE	29
$2H_3R_3Z_3$	11
Continuation phase	US $
4HR	31
6HT	2
$4H_3R_3$	13
6HE	11

H= isoniazid, R=rifampicin, Z=Pyrazinamide, S=Streptomycin, E=Ethambutol, T=Thiacetazone.
Large numerals indicate duration of therapy in months; Small subscript numerals indicate doses of therapy per week, but where no subscript, daily therapy is indicated.

In general, the recommended approach to tuberculosis control has been similar worldwide except for a differing view on the value and place of BCG vaccination, which has not been previously regarded as generally valuable by medical opinion in the United States, and this area will be discussed further below.

Tuberculosis is an infectious disease, usually spread by droplet infection, but with a widely variable period of latency between the primary infection (which may be sub-clinical and undetected, and is rarely infectious), and the possible subsequent development of a clinical and usually post-primary infection where the affected person can become infectious to others. It therefore follows that any person with tuberculosis must have contracted the disease from another individual, and could, if excreting the bacilli, infect others in turn. Tracing of the contacts of the 'index case', both to find a source for infection and to detect any people who may have been infected by the index case or others in the circle of contacts, is therefore an important part of tuberculosis control policies.

The effectiveness of a tuberculosis control programme will depend on the available resources, but decision-makers must be made aware that financial economies in TB control programmes lead to very expensive problems in the future if the numbers of active cases increases, and drug-resistant organisms become a problem.

For the best control of tuberculosis in a community, the following components are necessary:

1. Detection of people with clinically active disease. This will require the education of health staff to consider TB as a cause of disease, good diagnostic facilities, and a willingness to seek disease in vulnerable groups, such as the elderly, and recent immigrants from areas of high tuberculosis prevalence.
   All diagnosed cases should be notified, both to allow epidemiological trends to be measured, and to trigger contact procedures.
2. Tracing of contacts of diagnosed cases, both to find sources of infection and secondary cases. Procedures to check contacts will vary in different countries, particularly depending on the attitude to BCG vaccination. A discussion of contact procedures follows below.
3. Treatment of active cases to the highest standards, usually to an agreed protocol, should be supervised by a respiratory physician; treatment should be monitored at least monthly. In patients known to be sputum positive on direct smear, segregation from vulnerable contacts is necessary until therapy has been in progress for 2 weeks. Many less infectious patients can be treated without segregation.
4. Protection of health care workers, prison staff, and other groups at higher risk of exposure to tuberculosis.
5. Pre-employment screening of prospective health care staff, school staff, and others, who could, if infected, pass tuberculosis to vulnerable groups such as children and the immunosuppressed.

Tuberculosis surveillance procedures, including contact checking

The USA approach[78] relies substantially on the value of tuberculin testing as evidence of past or present infection with tuberculosis, and the giving of preventive therapy with isoniazid to those with positive tuberculin tests but no evidence of active clinical tuberculosis or old fibrotic lesions on X-ray (such patients are treated with full multi-drug anti-tuberculous therapy). Thus tuberculin tests are applied to all possible cases of tuberculosis, to all recent TB contacts, and to those who are vulnerable to TB, such as those with diabetes, chronic renal disease, immunosuppression, or known or suspected HIV infection. Some HIV positive people should be considered for preventive isoniazid therapy even when tuberculin negative, because the test is a poor indicator of exposure in the HIV positive person, and they are especially vulnerable to tuberculosis infection if they are living in a high prevalence environment. In addition, people under the age of 35, with positive tuberculin tests who are recent immigrants from high incidence countries, or residents of long-term care institutions such as nursing homes, mental institutions, and correctional institutions are recommended to have tuberculin tests.

If tuberculin testing in these people is positive, or becomes positive after an interval after known TB contact, this is regarded as evidence of tuberculosis infection, and chest X-ray is performed. if there is no clinical or radiological evidence of active tuberculosis, the person is then advised to have chemoprophylaxis, or prophylactic treatment, with isoniazid. The dosage recommended is 10 mg/kg daily for children, and up to 300 mg daily for adults, continuing for 6 to 12 months, with the longer duration for those who are immunosuppressed. There is a small but real risk of hepatic side-effects, with clinical hepatitis in 0.5–3%, and raised transaminases in 10–15%[105,106] and compliance with therapy taken over many months in an asymptomatic group may not be high. Such treatment has been estimated to reduce the subsequent incidence of active disease by 54–88%.

BCG vaccination is now being recommended in the USA for the protection of infants and children in particularly vulnerable positions, such as continuing exposure to sputum positive cases, and in groups where there is a high incidence of tuberculosis (greater than 1% new infections per year). Selective BCG vaccination of other groups at risk in the USA has now being proposed, particularly because the groups most vulnerable to tuberculosis infection are those very individuals where it is difficult to supervise a satisfactory programme of isoniazid preventive therapy.[107] BCG is however, contra-indicated in HIV-positive people, as the BCG organism may give rise to disseminated BCG infection in such immunosuppressed subjects.

The UK approach (see JTC, 1994)

Much greater reliance is placed on increasing the immunity of individuals, and hence the population, using BCG vaccination[103] (see the following paragraph). The majority of people in the UK are offered BCG vaccination at the age of 13–14 years, giving a perceived 80% protection against tuberculosis. After BCG vaccination, most people develop low-level tuberculin hypersensitivity, giving a Heaf test at Grade I or up to grade II. As an a result, the value of tuberculin testing as evidence of tuberculosis infection in people after BCG vaccination is reduced, and tuberculosis contact procedures have to take account of this.

Tuberculosis contact procedures for the UK

The latest recommendations suggest that all tuberculosis contacts should have a Heaf test. For those with previous BCG vaccination (as evidenced by a vaccination record, or a typical BCG vaccination scar, usually over the insertion of the left deltoid muscle insertion on the lateral aspect of the upper arm), a Grade 0, 1 or 2 reaction is regarded as reassuring, and the contact can generally be advised to report the development of any new symptoms, such as a persistent cough or malaise, to a doctor, reminding the doctor of previous TB contact and the possible need for a chest X-ray. If, on the other hand, the Heaf test is Grade 3 or 4 positive, then an X-ray should be taken; if this is normal, and the contact is aged over 16, but the index case was highly infectious (sputum positive), then the contact should be kept under observation and a further X-ray performed after 3 months and probably again at 12 months. Any contacts with Grade 3 or 4 Heaf tests aged under 16 who have a normal X-ray should be given chemoprophylaxis under supervision. Clearly, any contacts who have an abnormal X-ray should be treated as having active tuberculosis unless proved otherwise.

In the cases of contacts who have *not* had BCG, the Heaf test result is also used to determine management. Those with Heaf grade 2, 3, or 4, are X-rayed, and dealt with in the same way as those detailed above who have had BCG and who have Grade 3 and 4 positive Heaf tests. Those with Heaf grade 0 or 1, must be considered vulnerable to the development of tuberculosis, depending on the infectiousness of the index case; if the index case is sputum positive, then it is usual to repeat the Heaf test after 6 weeks, to see whether 'conversion' to grade 2, 3, or 4 has occurred. If so, then those with a normal X-ray should receive chemoprophylaxis, and those with an abnormal film should be considered as having tuberculosis and treated accordingly. Those whose second Heaf test remains Grade 0 or 1 should, if children or young adults, be given BCG vaccination; older adults should be warned to report the symptoms which might suggest the later development of tuberculous infection.

Children under the age of 2 are at particular risk of tuberculosis infection, since they are vulnerable to dissemination of tuberculosis and to miliary disease and tuberculous meningitis. If such a child has never had BCG vaccination and has been in close contact with a sputum positive case of tuberculosis, they should receive immediate chemoprophylaxis whatever their Heaf test result; many will give chemoprophylaxis to all child contacts under the age of 5 years. If it is considered important not only to treat possible developing tuberculosis infection in such children, but also simultaneously to achieve future protective immunity, it was in the past possible to obtain isoniazid-resistant strains of BCG vaccination which could be effective, even while children were receiving chemoprophylaxis, but isoniazid-resistant BCG vaccine is no longer available. It is now reccommended, therefore, that standard BCG vaccination is given after an effective period of chemoprophylaxis.

There is a clear need to examine in this way the close contacts of people with infectious tuberculosis, but judgements need to be made as to both 'closeness' and the 'infectiousness' of the index case. Close family contacts are clearly not in doubt for full contact procedures, but there may be more occasional or remoter contacts, usually at work but sometimes at home, who are at less risk of infection. Such more casual contacts need only be examined if they are unusually susceptible, for instance, young children, or the immunosuppressed. Other less immediate contacts need only be told of the very low risk of infection, and advised to report any persistent symptoms which develop in the future which should suggest the need for investigation.

Special procedures will be required in schools where a teacher has been found to be smear or culture positive.

Case finding

Elderly people in long-stay institutions are vulnerable to reactivation of previous tuberculous infection, so evidence of previous tuberculosis should be noted on admission, and the development of any chronic respiratory symptoms such as chronic cough need to be investigated.

New immigrants from areas of high tuberculosis incidence should be checked for evidence of infection, as though they were TB contacts, with X-rays of those with symptoms, chemoprophylaxis where appropriate, and BCG vaccination of uninfected people, particularly among infants and children in view of the much higher levels of tuberculosis among such communities; tuberculosis is up to 28 times more common in some immigrant groups than in the lifelong indigenous population of the UK.[52]

Protection of vulnerable groups

Health care workers, including those who handle specimens and work in mortuaries, and those who work in prisons, are recommended to undergo pre-employment screening; this involves getting details of previous BCG vaccination. In those who have no evidence of previous BCG vaccination, a Heaf test is undertaken, and those with a negative or grade 1 Heaf reaction should be given BCG. For those with a most strongly positive Heaf reaction, only those with symptoms need to be X-rayed; and all such people should be advised to seek an X-ray if symptoms develop in the future. Regular X-rays of asymptomatic health workers exposed to tuberculosis are not required.

Bacille Calmette–Guérin (BCG)

In 1924, Calmette produced an attenuated strain of bovine *M. tuberculosis* which could not cause disease in laboratory animals, and by 1950 BCG vaccination, by intradermal injection, was recommended for use in Europe by the World Health Organisation. Trials in Europe, such as a UK trial in British school leavers, showed a 77% reduction in vaccinated subjects compared with controls over a 20-year follow-up.[108] However, trials in other countries, and particularly in Georgia and Alabama[109] in the USA, and Puerto Rico,[110] and also in South India,[111] where no protective effect could be demonstrated. Since these studies, there have been up to 40 reports of BCG trials, giving widely varying results in different situations, which have been reviewed.[112,113] While the protective effects of BCG in preventing pulmonary tuberculosis were very variable, there does seem to be a consistent effect in reducing the rates and fatality from tuberculous meningitis and miliary tuberculosis.

A variety of explanations has been proposed for the variations between 0% and 80% effectiveness, including differences in the vaccines used, and also the impact of non-specific hypersensitivity and immunity resulting from exposure to environmental non-tuberculous mycobacteria in the warmer latitudes of the world.[114] There are also suggestions that BCG is more effective in urban than in rural populations. It has been proposed that infections with such environmental organisms may in themselves give some protective immunity against *M. tuberculosis* infection, so that the impact of BCG would be much less in countries where such mycobacteria are common, as in Puerto Rico, compared to the UK, where they are rare. On the other hand, the effect of BCG in Puerto Rico appeared to be similar whether the initial tuberculin tests were completely negative, or where they were weakly positive suggesting previous non-specific mycobacterial infection, so a simple protective effect of non-tuberculous mycobacterial infection may not be the complete explanation for the lack of BCG effect in this study. There is much clearer evidence of the benefit of BCG in the prevention of leprosy, which is, of course, also a mycobacterial infection.[115] Fine[112] proposes that there is a need to develop and test other vaccines, in view of the apparently selective value of BCG in differing environments.

Current practice for BCG in the UK and elsewhere

BCG vaccination may be given as an intradermal injection, over the humeral insertion of the left deltoid muscle (0.05 ml for those under 1 year old, 0.1 ml for all others), or by the more recently approved percutaneous method, using a multiple puncture head.[116]

BCG vaccination is recommended in the UK[103] for:

1. Infants and children of immigrants from high-tuberculosis areas of the world. BCG may be given to such children under the age of 3 months without prior tuberculin testing if there is no known prior contact with TB.
2. All schoolchildren aged 10–14 years who are tuberculin negative. It had been suggested that this was becoming unnecessary in view of the cost of the programme in relation to the number of TB cases prevented, but the rise in tuberculosis notifications has delayed such a decision meantime,[117] and the Joint Committee on Vaccination and Immunisation has decided in 1996 that the BCG programme for 10–14 year-olds should continue in the UK.

Even if the general programme of BCG vaccination were to be abandoned, there would remain some high-risk groups for whom BCG will be appropriate. These groups include health care workers at risk, infants in high prevalence ethnic groups, and tuberculin-negative immigrants from countries where tuberculosis is common.

The vaccination is usually trouble-free, with a small red papule developing at the injection site after 3 weeks or so, gradually fading over the ensuing weeks, and leaving a small white scar about 5 mm in diameter. There is no systemic effect. In some subjects, a pustule may develop with the discharge of pus, but again spontaneous healing is usual. Occasionally, and especially if the injection is given subcutaneously rather than intradermally, a larger reaction can develop with inflammation of draining axillary nodes; if this occurs, the reaction can be controlled by giving a short course of isoniazid or erythromycin, to which the BCG organism is sensitive.

The decision as to which countries might employ a policy of universal BCG vaccination is a difficult one which depends on the prevalence of tuberculosis in that country, and economic factors. Current recommendations for countries with a high prevalence of tuberculosis advise BCG vaccination for all at birth, with probable re-vaccination at school entry age.[104] The IUATLD has also issued a statement as to when universal BCG programmes may be discontinued in countries with a low prevalence of tuberculosis,[118] in which the criteria for low prevalence are as follows: either the notification rate for smear-positive tuberculosis should be below 5 cases per 100 000 per year for three consecutive years, *or* the average annual notification rate of tuberculous meningitis in children under 5 should be less than one case per ten million of the general population for the previous five years, or the average risk of tuberculous infection should be 0.1% or less.

General conclusions

Despite the fact that effective drug treatment for tuberculosis has been available for over 40 years, the disease remains a global health problem for both the developed and developing world. Much of this can be blamed on the medical profession and global economics; the simple rules of appropriate, well-designed and supervised therapy have been neglected, and community control measures have been widely abandoned or never applied, either through poverty, ignorance or complacency. The resulting increasing incidence of the infection, assisted in some countries by the HIV epidemic, has been complicated by the emergence of drug-resistant organisms. This is a challenge to politicians, physicians, and health workers, if tuberculosis is not to become a world disaster from which no country is immune.[119]

References

1. GRANGE JM. *Mycobacteria and Human Disease*. London: Edward Arnold. 1988.
2. BOTHAMLEY GH, GRANGE JM. The Koch phenomenon and delayed hypersensitivity. *Tubercle* 1991;72: 7–11.
3. ORME I. Processing and presentation of mycobacterial antigens: implications for the development of a new improved vaccine for tuberculosis control. *Tubercle* 1991; 72: 250–2.
4. ROOK GAW, AL ATTIYAH R. Cytokines and the Koch phenomenon. *Tubercle*; 1991; 72: 13–20.
5. STANFORD JL. Koch's phenomenon: can it be corrected? *Tubercle* 1991; 241–9.
6. DANIEL TM, BATES JH, DOWNES KA. History of tuberculosis. In Bloom BR, ed. *Tuberculosis: Pathogenesis, Protection and Control*. Washington DC 20005: American Society for Microbiology, 1994;13-23.
7. NAKAJIMA H. *Tuberculosis: A Global Emergency* (editorial). World Health 1993; 46: 3.
8. DOLIN PJ, RAVIGLIONE MC, KOCHI A. Global tuberculosis incidence and mortality during 1990–2000. *Bull WHO* 1994; 72: 213–20.
9. BRITISH TUBERCULOSIS ASSOCIATION. Tuberculosis among immigrants to England and Wales: A National Survey in 1965. *Tubercle* 1966; 47: 145–56.
10. MEDICAL RESEARCH COUNCIL TUBERCULOSIS AND CHEST DISEASES UNIT. National survey of tuberculosis notifications in England and Wales 1978–9. *Br Med J* 1980; 281: 895–8.
11. MEDICAL RESEARCH COUNCIL TUBERCULOSIS AND CHEST DISEASES UNIT. National survey of notifications of tuberculosis in England and Wales in 1983. *Br Med J* 1985; 291: 658–61.
12. MEDICAL RESEARCH COUNCIL CARDIOTHORACIC EPIDEMIOLOGY GROUP. National survey of notifications of tuberculosis in England and Wales in 1988. *Thorax* 1992; 47: 770–5.
13. WARBURTON ARE, JENKINS PA, WAIGHT PA, WATSON JM. Drug resistance in initial isolates of *Mycobacterium* tuberculosis in England and Wales, 1981–1991. *Communicable Disease Report* 1993; 3: R175–9.
14. WATSON JM. Tuberculosis in Britain today (editorial). *Br Med J* 1993; 306: 221–2.
15. MEDICAL RESEARCH COUNCIL TUBERCULOSIS AND CHEST DISEASES UNIT. National survey of tuberculosis notifications in England and Wales in 1983: characteristics of disease. *Tubercle* 1987; 68: 19–32.
16. GRANGE JM, YATES MD, ORMEROD LP. Factors determining ethnic differences in the incidence of bacteriologically confirmed genitourinary tuberculosis in south east England. *J Infect* 1995; 30: 37–40.
17. SPENCE DPS, HOTCHKISS J, WILLIAMS CSD, DAVIES PDO. Tuberculosis and poverty. *Br Med J* 1993; 307: 759–61.
18. HELBERT M, ROBINSON D, BUCHANAN D, HELLYER T, MCCARTHY M, BROWN I *et al*. Mycobacterial infection in patients infected with the human immunodeficiency virus. *Thorax* 1990; 45: 907–8.
19. WATSON JM, MEREDITH SK, WHITMORE–OVERTON E, BANNISTER B, DARBYSHIRE JH. Tuberculosis and HIV: estimates of the overlap in England and Wales. *Thorax* 1993; 48: 199–203.
20. KUMAR D, LEESE J, CITRON K, WATSON J. Tuberculosis among the homeless in London. *J Epidemiol Community Health* 1993; 47: 401.
21. CITRON KM, SOUTHERN A, DIXON M. *Out of the Shadow: Detecting and Treating Tuberculosis Amongst Single Homeless People*. London: Crisis, 1995
22. SUDRE P, TEN DAM G, KOCHI A. Tuberculosis: a global overview of the situation today. *Bull WHO* 1992; 70(2): 149–59.
23. STEEL M. Tuberculosis recurrence in Africa: true relapse or re-infection? *Lancet*, 1993; 342: 756–7.
24. COMMUNICABLE DISEASES CENTER. Tuberculosis morbidity in the United States: final data, 1990. *MMWR CDC Surveill Sum* 1991; 40(SS-3): 23–7.
25. DRUCKER, E, ALCABES, P, BOSWORTH, W, SCKELL, B. Childhood tuberculosis in the Bronx, New York. *Lancet* 1994; 343: 1482–5.
26. SNIDER, DE, ROPER, WM. The new tuberculosis. *N Engl J Med* 1992; 326: 703–5
27. REIDER, HL. Epidemiology of tuberculosis in Europe. *Eur Resp J* 1995; 8: 620s– 32s
28. RILEY RL, MILLS CC, O'GRADY F *et al.* Infectiousness of air from a tuberculosis ward. *Am Rev Resp Dis* 1974; 85: 511–25.
29. ANDERSON C, INHABER N, MENZIES D. Comparison of sputum induction with fiber-optic bronchoscopy in the diagnosis of tuberculosis. *Am J. Resp Crit Care Med* 1995: 152: 1570–4
30. HUEBNER RE, GOOD RC, TOKARS JI. Current practices in mycobacteriology: results of a survey of state public health laboratories. *J Clin Microbiol* 1993; 31: 771–5
31. SACEANU CA, PFEIFFER NC, MCLEAN T. Evaluation of sputum smears concentrated by cytocentrifugation for detection of acid-fast bacilli. *J Clin Microbiol*. 1993; 31: 2371–4.
32. KÄLLENIUS G, HOFFENR SE, MIÖRNER H, SVENSON SB. Novel approaches to the diagnosis of *Mycobacterial* infections. *Eur Resp J* 1994; 7: 1921–4.
33. KOX LFF. Tests for detection and identification of *Mycobacteria*: how should they be used? *Resp Med* 1995; 89: 399–408.
34. JACOBS WR, BARLETTA RG, UDANI R *et al.* Rapid assessment of drug susceptibilities of *Mycobacterium tuberculosis* by means of luciferase reporter phages. *Science* 1993; 260: 819–22.
35. GROSSET J, MOUTON Y. Is PCR a useful tool for the diagnosis of tuberculosis in 1995? *Tubercle and Lung Dis* 1995; 76: 183–4
36. GODFREY-FAUSSETT P. Molecular diagnosis of tuberculosis: the need for new diagnostic tools. *Thorax* 1995; 50: 709–11.
37. EDLIN BR, TOKARS JI, GRIECO MH *et al.* An outbreak of multi-drug resistant tuberculosis among hospitalised patients with the acquired immunodeficiency syndrome. *N Engl J Med* 1992; 326: 1514–22.
38. SMALL PM, HOPEWELL PC, SINGH SP *et al.* The epidemiology of tuberculosis in San Francisco – a population-based study using conventional and molecular methods. *N Engl J Med* 1994; 330: 1703–9.
39. FRENCH GL, TEOH R, CHAN CY *et al.* Diagnosis of tuberculous meningitis by detection of tuberculostearic acid in cerebrospinal fluid. *Lancet* 1987; ii: 117– 9.
40. BOTHAMLEY GH, RUDD R, FESTENSTEIN F, IVANI J. Clinical value of the measurement of *Mycobacterium tuberculosis* specific antibody in pulmonary tuberculosis. *Thorax* 1992; 47: 270–5.
41. ANONYMOUS EDITORIAL. New tuberculins. *Lancet* 1984; i: 199–200.
42. SOKAL JE. Measurement of delayed skin test responses. *N Engl J Med* 1975; 293: 501–2.
43. MURTHY NK, DUTT AK. Tuberculin skin testing: present status. *Sem Resp Infect* 1994; 9: 78–83.
44. MEDICAL RESEARCH COUNCIL TUBERCULOSIS AND CHEST DISEASES UNIT. National Survey of tuberculosis notifications in England and Wales 1983: characteristics of disease. *Tubercle* 1987; 68: 19–32.
45. SORIANO E, MALLOLAS J, GATELL JM *et al.* Characteristics of tuberculosis in HIV-infected patients; a case-control study. *AIDS* 1988; 2: 429–32.
46. CROFTON J., HORNE N., MILLER F. *Clinical Tuberculosis*. London: Macmillan Education Ltd.; 1992.
47. WALLGREN A. The timetable of tuberculosis. *Tubercle* 1948; 29: 245–51.
48. RUBILAR M., SIME PJ., MOUGDIL H *et al.*

Time to extend the 'timetable of tuberculosis'? *Res Med* 1994; 88: 481–2.

49. GRANGE JM, YATES MD. The time-table of tuberculosis. *Resp Med* 1995; 89: 313–14.

50. BOOKSTEIN JJ, MOSER KM, KALFER ME *et al.* The role of bronchial arteriography and therapeutic embolisation in haemoptysis. *Chest* 1977; 72: 658–61.

51. STERNITZ R. Pulmonary tuberculosis and carcinoma of the lung: a survey from two population-baased disease registers. *Am Rev Resp Dis* 1965; 92: 758–66

52. MEDICAL RESEARCH COUNCIL CARDIOTHORACIC EPIDEMIOLOGY GROUP. National survey of notifications of tuberculosis in England and Wales in 1988. *Thorax* 1992; 47: 770–5.

53. PITCHENIK AE, FERTEL D, BLOCH AB. Pulmonary effects of AIDS: mycobacterial disease – epidemiology, diagnosis, treatment and prevention. *Clin Chest Med* 1988; 9: 425–41.

54. PROUDFOOT AT, AKHTAR AJ, DOUGLAS AC *et al.* Miliary tuberculosis in adults. *BMJ* 1969; ii: 273–6.

55. SIME PJ, CHILVERS ER, LEITCH AG. Miliary tuberculosis in Edinburgh – a comparison between 1984–1992 and 1954–1967. *Resp Med* 1994; 88: 609–11.

56. ORMEROD LP, HORSFIELD N. Miliary tuberculosis in a high prevalence area of the UK: Blackburn 1978–1993. *Resp Med* 1995; 89: 555–7.

57. PARSONS M. *Tuberculous Meningitis*. Oxford: Oxford University Press; 1979.

58. PARSONS M. Tuberculous meningitis. *Br J Hosp Med* 1982; 27: 682–4.

59. HOLDINESS MR. Management of tuberculous meningitis. *Drugs* 1990; 39: 224–33.

60. NEWCOMBE J. Tuberculous glands in the neck. *Br J Hosp Med* 1979; 22: 553–5.

61. BRITISH THORACIC SOCIETY RESEARCH COMMITTEE. Short-course chemotherapy for tuberculosis of the lymph nodes: a controlled trial. *Br Med J* 1985; 290: 1106–8.

62. BRITISH THORACIC SOCEITY RESEARCH COMMITTEE. Short-course chemotherapy for lymph node tuberculosis: final report at 5 years. *Br J Dis Chest* 1988; 82: 282–4.

63. GRZYBOWSKI S, ALLEN, EA. History and importance of scrofula. *Lancet* 1995; 346: 1472–4.

64. MEDICAL RESEARCH COUNCIL WORKING PARTY ON TUBERCULOSIS OF THE SPINE. A controlled trial of six-month and nine-month regimens of chemotherapy in patients undergoing radical surgey for tuberculosis of the spine in Hong Kong. *Tubercle* 1986; 67: 243–59.

65. GOW J. Genitourinary tuberculosis. *Br J Hosp Med.* 1979; 22: 556–68.

66. SUTHERLAND AM. Gynaecological tuberculosis. *Br J Hosp Med.* 1979; 22: 569–76.

67. GOW JG, BARBOSA S. Genitourinary tuberculosis. A study of 1117 cases over a period of 35 years. *Br J Urol* 1984; 56: 449–55.

68. HOLDINESS MR. Clinical pharmacokinetics of the antituberculosis drugs. Clin Pharmacokinetics 1984; 9:511.

69. HOLDINESS MR. Cerebrospinal fluid pharmacokinetics of the antituberculosis drugs. *Clin Pharmacokinetics* 1985; 10: 532.

70. HOLDINESS M.R. Neurological manifestations and toxicities of the antituberculosis drugs. *Med Toxicol* 1987; 2:33.

71. HOLDINESS M.R. Transplacental pharmacokinetics of the antituberculosis drugs. *Clin Pharmacokinetics* 1987; 13: 125.

72. GIRLING DJ. Adverse effects of antituberculosis drugs. *Drugs* 1982; 23: 56.

73. DAVIDSON PT, LE HQ. Drug treatment of tuberculosis. *Drugs* 1992; 43: 651.

74. WORLD HEALTH ORGANISATION. *Treatment of Tuberculosis; Guidelines for National Programmes*. Geneva: WHO; 1993.

75. DAVIES PDO. The clincal efficacy of rifabutin in the treatment of pulmonary tuberculosis. *Rev Contemp Pharmacother* 1995; 6: 121–7.

76. NARANG PK. Clinical pharmacology of rifabutin: a new antimycobacterial. *Rev Contemp Pharmacother* 1995; 6: 129–51

77. JOINT TUBERCULOSIS COMMITTEE OF THE BRITISH THORACIC SOCIETY. Chemotherapy and management of tuberculosis in the United Kingdom: recommendations. *Thorax* 1990; 45: 403.

78. AMERICAN THORACIC SOCIETY; control of tuberculosis in the United States. *Am Rev Resp Dis* 1992; 146: 1623.

79. ORMEROD LP, SKINNER C, WALES J. Hepatotoxicity of anti-tuberculous drugs. *Thorax* 1996; 51: 111–13.

80. BRITISH THORACIC ASSOCIATION. A controlled trial of six months chemotherapy in pulmonary tuberculosis: first report: results during chemotherapy. *Br J Dis Chest* 1981; 75: 141–53.

81. BRITISH THORACIC ASSOCIATION. A controlled trial of six months chemotherapy in pulmonary tuberculosis: 2nd report. *Am Rev Resp Dis* 1982; 126: 460–2

82. BRITISH THORACIC SOCIETY. A controlled trial of six months chemotherapy in pulmonary tuberculosis: results during the 36 months after the end of chemotherapy and beyond. *Br J Dis Chest* 1984; 78: 330–6.

84. DAVIES PDO ed. *Clinical Tuberculosis*. London: Chapman and Hall Medical; 1994

85. HAYWARD CMM, HERRMAN J-L, GRIFFIN GE. Drug-resistant tuberculosis: mechanisms and management. *Br J Hosp Med* 1995; 54: 494–500.

86. FRIEDEN TR, STERLING T., PABLOS MENDEZ A., KILBURN JO., CAUTHEN G.M., DOLLEY SW. The emergence of drug-resistant tuberculosis in New York City. *N Eng J Med* 1993; 328: 521–6.

87. NEVILLE K, BROMBERG A, BROMBERG R *et al.* The third epidemic – multidrug-resistant tuberculosis. *Chest* 1994; 105: 45–8.

88. VEEN J. Drug resistant tuberculosis: back to sanatoria, surgery, and cod-liver oil? *Eur Resp J* 1995; 8: 1073–5.

89. FRIEDMAN CR, STOEKLE MY, KREISWIRTH BN *et al.* Transmission of multidrug-resistant tuberculosis in a large urban setting. *Am J Resp Crit Care Med* 1995; 152: 355–9.

90. KIM, SJ, HONG, YP. Drug resistance of *Mycobacterium* tuberculosis in Korea. *Tuberc Lung Dis* 1992; 73: 219–24.

91. ISEMAN MD. Treatment of multidrug-resistant tuberculosis. *New Engl J Med* 1993; 329: 784.

92. STANFORD JL, BAHR GM, BYASS P *et al.* A modern approach to the immunotherapy of tuberculosis. *Bull Int Union Tub Lung Dis* 1990; 65: 27–9.

93. STANFORD JL, BAHR GM, ROOK GAW *et al.* Immunotherapy with *Mycobacterium vaccae* as an adjunct to chemotherapy in the treatment of pulmonary tuberculosis. *Tubercle* 1990; 71: 87–93.

94. STANFORD JL, GRANGE JM. The promise of immunotherapy for tuberculosis. *Resp Med* 1994; 88: 3–7.

95. ONYEBUJOH PC, ABDULMUMINI T, ROBINSON S *et al.* Immunotherapy with *Mycobacterium vaccae* as an addition to chemotherapy for the treatment of pulmonary tuberculosis under difficult conditions in Africa. *Resp Med* 1995; 89: 199–207.

96. STANFORD JL. Koch's phenomenon: can it be corrected? *Tubercle* 1991; 72: 241–9.

97. SENDOROWITZ T, VISKUM K. Corticosteroids and tuberculosis. *Resp Med* 1994; 88: 561–5.

98. STRANG JIG, KAKAZA HHS, GIBSON DG *et al.* Controlled trial of prednisolone as adjuvant in treatment of tuberculous constrictive pericarditis in Traskei. *Lancet* 1987; 2: 1418–22.

99. ISEMAN MD, MADSEN L, GOBLE M *et al.* Surgical intervention in the treatment of pulmonary disease caused by drug-resistant *Mycobacterium* tuberculosis. *Am Rev Resp Dis* 1990; 141: 623–5.

100. INTERNATIONAL UNION AGAINST TUBERCULOSIS AND LUNG DISEASE. *Tuberculosis Guide for Low Income Countries.*

3rd ed. 68 boulevard Saint-Michel, 75006, Paris, France: IUATLD; 1994.

101. NARDELL EA. Beyond four drugs; Public Health policy and the treatment of the individual patient with tuberculosis. *Am Rev Resp Dis* 1993; 148: 2–5.

102. SUBCOMMITTEE OF THE JOINT TUBERCULOSIS COMMITTEE OF THE BRITISH THORACIC SOCIETY. Control and prevention of tuberculosis in Britain: an updated code of practice. *Br Med J* 1990; 300: 995–9.

103. JOINT TUBERCULOSIS COMMITTEE OF THE BRITISH THORACIC SOCIETY. Control and prevention of tuberculosis in the United Kingdom: Code of Practice 1994. *Thorax* 1994: 49: 1193–200.

104. INTERNATIONAL UNION AGAINST TUBERCULOSIS AND LUNG DISEASE. *Tuberculosis Guide for High Prevalence Countries*. 2nd ed. 68 boulevard Saint-Michel, 75006, Paris, France: IUATLD.

105. JORDAN TJ, LEWITT EM, REICHAMN IB. Isoniazid preventive therapy for tuberculosis. *Am Rev Resp Dis* 1991; 144: 1357–60.

106. STEELE MA, BURK RF, DESPREZ RM. Toxic hepatitis with isoniazid and rifampin. *Chest* 1991; 99: 465–71.

107. KOCH-WESER D. BCG vaccination: can it contribute to tuberculosis control? *Chest* 1993; 103: 1641.

108. MEDICAL RESEARCH COUNCIL STATISTICAL RESEARCH AND SERVICES UNIT. BCG and Vole vaccines in the prevention of tuberculosis in adolescence and early adult life. Final Report. *BMJ* 1977; 2: 293–5.

109. COMSTOCK GW, WOOPERT SF, LIVESAY VT. Tuberculosis studies in Muscogee County, Georgia. Twenty-year evaluation of a community trial of BCG vaccination. *Publ Health Rep* 1976; 91: 276–80.

110. COMSTOCK GW, LIVESY VT, WOOLPERT SF. Evaluation of BCG vaccination among Puerto Rican children. *Am J Publ Health* 1974; 64: 283–91.

111. TUBERCULOSIS PREVENTION TRIAL MADRAS. Trial of BCG vaccines in South India for tuberculosis prevention. *Ind J Med Res* 1980; 72:(suppl) 1–74.

112. FINE PEM. Variation in protection by BCG: implications of and for heterologous immunity. *Lancet* 1995; 346: 1339–45.

113. SMITH, PG. BCG vaccination. In Davies PDO, ed. *Clinical Tuberculosis*, London: Chapman and Hall, 1994; 297–310.

114. COLDITZ GA, BREWER TF, BERKEY CS *et al.* Efficacy of BCG vaccination in the prevention of tuberculosis. *JAMA* 1994; 271: 698–702.

115. FINE PEM, RODRIGUES LC. Mycobacterial vaccines. *Lancet* 1990: 335: 1016–20.

116. DEPARTMENTS OF HEALTH, JOINT COMMITTEE ON VACCINATION AND IMMUNISATION. *Immunisation Against Infectious Disease*. London: HMSO; 1992.

117. ORMEROD LP, SHAW RJ, MITCHELL DM. Tuberculosis in the UK.; current issues and future trends. *Thorax* 1994; 49: 1085–9.

118. INTERNATIONAL UNION AGAINST TUBERCULOSIS AND LUNG DISEASE. Criteria for the discontinuation of vaccination programmes using Bacille Calmette Guerin (BCG) in countries with a low prevalence of tuberculosis. *News IUATLD* 1994; 20–2.

119. ENARSON DA, GROSSET J, MWINGA A *et al.* The challenge of tuberculosis: statements on global control and prevention. *Lancet* 1995; 346: 809–19.

16 Fungal respiratory disease

MICHAEL E. ELLIS

King Faisal Specialist Hospital and Rsearch Centre, Riyadh, Saudi Arabia

Introduction

This chapter describes the major fungal respiratory tract infections which are usually acquired in hospital or in individuals who are substantially immunocompromised.

Aspergillosis

Aspergillus moulds are highly ubiquitous, being found in soil, dust and water, often present in food stuffs, flowers and tobacco and commonly in decaying organic material. Therefore, the scene for human infection is easily set. Yet of the 300 or so species only approximately 20 are pathogenic to man of which *Aspergillus fumigatus* is the most frequently encountered. *Aspergillus niger*, *Aspergillus flavus*, and *Aspergillus clavatus* are seen less often. Appropriate settings of exposure, virulence factors and host response interact to produce several disease entities often distinctive but occasionally overlapping. This section will describe the pulmonary manifestations both in the normal host, namely, those due to colonisation phenomena, hypersensitivity reactions, chronic invasive pulmonary aspergillosis and in the immunocompromised host – acute invasive disease.

Microbiology

Aspergillus spp. grow well on organic substrates and best at 37 °C though they will grow at temperatures up to 45 °C. On laboratory media and in tissue fluffy powdery (Fig. 16.1) or velvety colonies of different colours are produced, which darken with sporulation. Mycelia are composed of the asexual reproductive conidiophores which bear conidia (Fig. 16.2). Specimens from the airways reflecting colonisation are characterised by the presence of these conidiophores. Hyphae are thick (not always uniformly) septate approximately 4 μ in diameter and branching at 45° angles. Tissue specimens of patients with invasive aspergillosis usually show these hyphae (Fig. 16.3). The organism may be identified by haematoxylin and eosin but PAS and silver stains are better. Colonial morphology will differentiate the *Aspergillus* spp. However, expertise is required for confident histological diagnosis and other fungi such as *Fusarium* spp. can be easily mistaken. In addition atypical morphological features, for example, due to degenerative hyphae may pose a problem for diagnosis.

Pathogenesis/host defence overview

The portal of entry is normally the respiratory tract; inhalation of the < 3 μ conidia spores results in their proximal and distal (including alveolar) deposition. Therefore, outbreaks of aspergillosis have been well documented in association with high atmospheric spore levels[1], and during hospital construction alterations[2]. Atmospheric spore levels partly depend on geographical location and time of the year. A rare pulmonary source is cannabis smoking. Although primary skin inoculation is well described, it is not clear whether this can act as a focus for haematogenous dissemination. Secondary infection of intravenous lines has been reported. Right-sided *Aspergillus* endocarditis can sometimes be the origin of multiple pulmonary lesions.

The first host defence is the mucociliary escalator of the respiratory tree. Abnormal inflammatory responses of the larger airways to

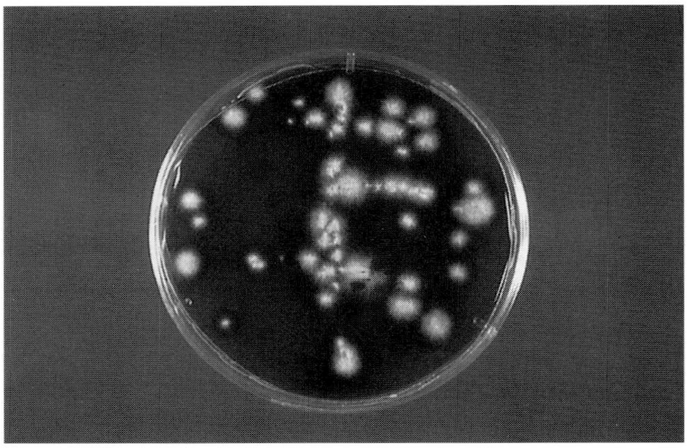

FIGURE 16.1 *Aspergillus*: white powdery colonies. (Courtesy of Dr Fouad Al Dayel.)

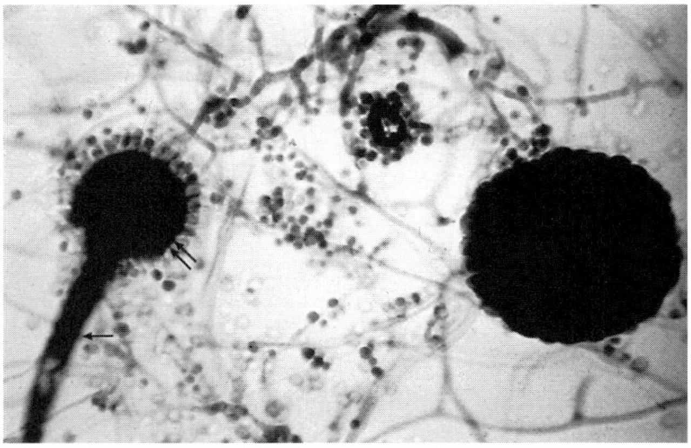

FIGURE 16.2 *Aspergillus*: conidiophore (arrow); phialide (arrows). (Courtesy of Dr Fouad Al Dayel.)

Aspergillus spores and the biochemical composition of mucus may allow colonisation. Should spores escape this line of defence, impaction occurs onto respiratory epithelium. Defective lung clearance mechanisms found in cavitary lung disease and bronchiectasis permit *Aspergillus* colonisation.

Further defence is largely dependent on the degree of intactness of, and response by, the host immune system. Of prime importance are the phagocytic neutrophils, monocytes and macrophages. Bronchoalveolar macrophages phagocytose and kill inhaled spores. A prerequisite to phagocytosis is the attachment of conidia to resident bronchoalveolar macrophages. This depends on fungal–polysaccharide cell wall component interaction with β-glucan receptors on the macrophages. Neutrophils also attach and damage fungal hyphae, e.g. via lysozyme. Ingested conidia are then killed by macrophage-generated oxygen radicals. Should spores fail to be phagocytosed or macrophages fail to kill, the conidia germinate and form hyphae, resulting in tissue invasion and triggering further immune responses. The larger neutrophils and monocytes kill by various means, including interactive oxidant mechanisms and production of defensins [3].

Prolonged qualitative and quantitative neutrophil defects, e.g. secondary to immunosuppressive and steroid therapy are the most critical factors predisposing to invasive aspergillosis[4,5]. Macrophage function, particularly chemotaxis, may also be impaired after cytotoxic chemotherapy. Eosinophils contribute little to host defence but produce important inflammatory responses in subjects prone to *Aspergillus* hypersensitivity reactions. The role of antibodies is not clear, despite the demonstration by immune electronmicroscopy of binding of monoclonal antibodies to *Aspergillus* antigen[6]. Patients with immunoglobulin deficiency syndromes are not at risk from severe fungal disease. However, surface deposition of opsonic C3b and chemoattractant C5a complement onto *Aspergillus* appears to be important in attracting inflammatory cells and for subsequent internalisation of the spores. Some species can inhibit the activation of the alternative complement pathway and decrease binding of C3b to fungi, which may prove advantageous to the fungus by reducing optimal association of *Aspergillus* conidia and polymorphonuclear cells[7]. Lymphocyte-mediated cellular activity is not a major defence mechanism against *Aspergillus*; hence, invasive aspergillosis is rare in such immunodeficiency states, e.g. in AIDS[8]. Finally, normal iron homeostasis may play a role in limiting *Aspergillus* infection. This fungus secretes essential nutrient iron attracting siderophores, and certain patients with iron overload states are at increased risk from fungus infections, though mucormycosis is usually the most commonly described[9].

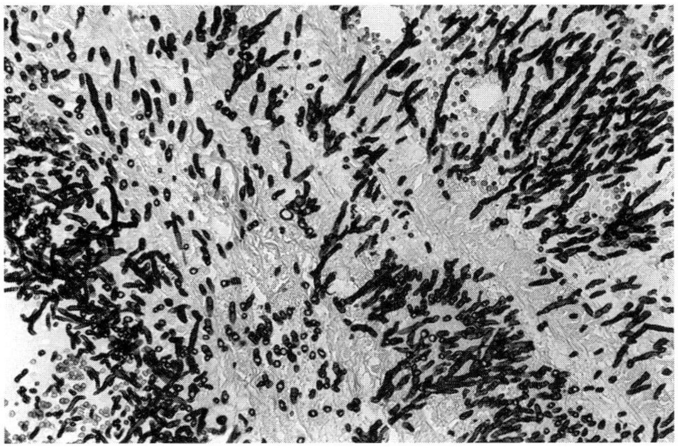

FIGURE 16.3 Septated hyphae of aspergillus stained GMS. Some of them show dichotomous branching. (Courtesy of Dr S. M. Hussein Qadri.)

Tissue invasion by *Aspergillus* is generally thought to be facilitated by the production of elastases, proteases and toxins and their presence has been found to correlate with tissue destruction, at least in animal models[10,11] but some doubt has been cast on their role as important virulence determinants[12]. *A. flavus* can inhibit the fusion of phagocytic liposomal granules to the ingested fungi within phagocytic vacuoles, thus, preventing intracellular killing of the fungus. The cell walls of both *A. fumigatus* and *A. flavus* have mild endotoxin-like activity. This can induce fever, a degree of shock and participate in haemorrhage and necrosis in animals which typifies certain manifestations of *Aspergillus* infection. The exact role in humans, however, remains unclear. Other defined fungal virulence factors include gliotoxin production which inhibits phagocytosis, diffusible compounds which inhibit neutrophil-induced toxic oxygen radical production and enzymes which produce fibrinolysis, coagulopathy and proteolysis.

In addition, *Aspergillus* conidia are relatively resistant to oxidant killing. *Aspergillus* spp. are capable of crossing tissue barriers which include bone and blood vessels.

Disease spectrum

Pulmonary infection caused by *Aspergillus* is either (i) hypersensitivity type, e.g. asthma; extrinsic allergic alveolitis; allergic bronchopulmonary aspergillosis (ii) non-invasive, e.g. colonisation; aspergilloma; bronchitis; or (iii) invasive, e.g. chronic necrotising aspergillosis; acute invasive pulmonary aspergillosis; acute tracheobronchitis.

Host defence/background profile and nature of exposure determine the particular expression of *Aspergillus* lung disease. Overlap and dynamic interchange of the three categories occurs.

Hypersensitivity reactions

Allergic asthma is a hyper-reactive type IgE-mediated response to *Aspergillus* antigens, resulting in episodic bronchospasm, the usual features of asthma and response to bronchodilators. Löffler's syndrome characterised by fleeting pulmonary infiltrates, eosinophilia, fever and cough is another manifestation (see Chapter 28).

Extrinisc allergic alveolitis (EAA) occurs in individuals who become sensitised by repeated exposure to *Aspergillus* antigens (conidia) and *Aspergillus* associated chemicals, e.g. the amylase from *Aspergillus oryzae* which results in Baker's asthma. Type III and IV reactions are the most frequent seen. Inhaled particulate matter is postulated to provoke an initial acute inflammatory reaction. This leads to a lymphocyte-histiocytic predominant response with granuloma formation. The coining of such descriptions as malt worker's lung, farmer's lung[13] and baker's asthma underscores the occupational aetiology sometimes found. In EAA associated with *Aspergillus* spp., *A. fumigatus* and *A. clavatus* are the usual causative agents. Many other fungi including *Penicillium* spp., *Aureobasidium* spp.

as well as thermophilic bacteria, animal proteins and amoeba are capable of eliciting a hypersensitivity pneumonitis. Among farmer's lung one of the commonest forms of EAA, *Micropolyspora faenia* is, in fact, implicated more often than *Aspergillus* spp[14].

Cough, dyspnoea, fever, chills, fatigue and myalgia develop characteristically a few hours after exposure. Bilateral crepitations are auscultatible. These symptoms resolve after a few days. If unrecognised and in the face of continued exposure a chronic alveolar and distal airways granulomatous reaction occurs resulting in pulmonary fibrosis and cor-pulmonale. Chronic cough, weight loss, fatiguability and shortness of breath then are the usual features which eventually become dominated by right ventricular failure and cyanotic signs and symptoms. The diagnosis strongly depends on the occupational history supported by the presence of serum *Aspergillus* precipitating antibodies. Pulmonary function testing in the acute stage reveals a diminished DLCO and lung capacity. Features of bronchospasm have been described but are unusual. In the chronic situation gross reduction in lung volumes and DLCO are found. Alveolar-arterial gradients are widened with resulting hypoxemia. A chest radiograph may be normal or show non-specific infiltrates. Features of lung fibrosis may develop. Aerosol challenge to purified specific antigen may be necessary for establishing the diagnosis in uncertain cases. BAL and lung biopsy may also be helpful. Treatment involves removal from the source and systemic steroids if necessary.

Allergic broncho-pulmonary aspergillosis (ABPA) (and allergic broncho-pulmonary fungosis) develops in some patients with asthma or cystic fibrosis who mount a highly host damaging immunological response to *Aspergillus*[15] usually *A. fumigatus*. This was first described by Hinson *et al.* in 1952[16]. The diagnosis is made[17] in established atopic asthmatics who have a variety of allergic symptomatologies, including eczema and rhinitis, who in addition have a combination of features, mainly (i) eosinophilia $> 1 \times 10^9/l$; (ii) high serum IgG or IgE titres to *Aspergillus* with elevated total IgE in excess of 15 000 ng/ml; (iii) transient pulmonary infiltrates often affecting the upper lobes; (iv) central bronchiectasis with normal distal bronchi tapering preserved; (v) positive serum *Aspergillus* precipitins; (vi) documented type I skin reaction. Some of these features also occur in regular asthma patients but the presence of all six serves to differentiate. High level serum IgE and eosinophils are usually notable, and increase further during acute exacerbations.

Allergic *Aspergillus* sinusitis (see Chapter 25) is a newly recognised similar entity and thought to be of similar aetiology to ABPA[18]. This comprises one part of the spectrum of aspergillosis of the sino-nasal tract namely aspergilloma, chronic indolent sinusitis, invasive fulminant sinusitis and allergic sinusitis[19].

The diagnostic criteria for ABPA alluded to above also serve to differentiate ABPA from other pulmonary eosinophilic syndromes, namely: tropical and parasitic eosinophilia (due to *Wuchereria, Ascaris, Brugia, Toxocara, Ancylostoma, Necator,* and *Strongyloides*), chronic eosinophilic pneumonia, Churg–Strauss allergic granulomatosis/angiitis, Löffler's syndrome and hypereosinophilic syndrome. Furthermore, fibrinous bronchitis, allergic bronchopneumonia, mucoid impaction of the bronchus and bronchocentric granulomatosis have considerable clinical and radiological similarities and have to be considered in the differential diagnosis[20]. In addition, although ABPA is generally considered a non-invasive entity, limited tissue invasion has been described which includes some of the aforementioned features namely bronchocentric mycosis/granulomatosis and mucoid impaction. This highlights the fact that overlap can occasionally be seen in the different forms of aspergillosis[21,22].

The pathophysiology is not clearly understood but there may be abnormal airways secretion properties which predispose patients to exhibit inappropriate immune hyper-responsiveness to *Aspergillus*. It is postulated that virulent protease-producing fungi colonise the mucus-epithelial surface and elicit intense immunological reactions and eosinophilic airways infiltration[23]. This results in damage to the epithelium and lung matrix proteins. Inefficient clearing of fungi from the airways leads to permanent bronchial mucosal damage and bronchiectasis. Types I (broncho-spasmic, associated with excessively high levels of histamine release), Type III (inflammatory lesions leading to bronchial plugs and bronchiectasis) and Type IV (producing bronchocentric granulomatous reactions, leading to irreversible fibrotic lung disease) reactions are found. Recently, concanavalin A nonbinding *A. fumigatus* antigens have been identified in the cellular immunoresponse[24]. Histopathologically most often there is mucosal infiltration by eosinophils, plasma cells and histiocytes. Intraluminal bronchial plugs contain *Aspergillus* hyphae. There may be proximal saccular bronchiectasis, atelectasis and an eosinophilic pneumonitis. A bronchocentric granulomatous reaction may also be present[25].

Patients may expectorate brown mucus plugs and *Aspergillus* can occasionally and sometimes repeatedly be cultured from the sputum. Other associated features[26,27] include recurrent episodes of dyspnea, fatiguability, fever, haemoptysis and pleuritic or non-specific chest pain. The chest radiograph[28] may be normal or show features of fleeting infiltrates or thickened bronchial walls and mucus impaction manifest by ring shadows (= cystic bronchiectasis) and parallel line shadows (= dilated bronchi). Changes of proximal cystic bronchiectasis and other features are best visualized by bronchography or thin section/high resolution CT scanning[29,30]. Lobar consolidation and generalised hyperinflation may also be found. Pulmonary function tests indicate initial obstruction with less reversibility compared to that usually found in asthmatics. Eventually a restrictive pattern may emerge. The DLCO is diminished. Finally respiratory failure may occur characterised by finger clubbing, cyanosis and cor-pulmonale.

Occasionally, patients with a syndrome resembling ABPA present with unusual clinical and pathological features. These include the presence of fungal species other than *Aspergillus* (for example, *Candida*, *Mucor*, *Curvularia*, *Drechslera*) and *Pseudallescheria boydii* when the syndrome is called allergic broncho-pulmonary fungal disease (ABPF)[31–34] and maybe associated with Churg–Strauss angiitis and allergic fungal sinusitis[32]. There may be histological features such as follicular and xanthomatous bronchiolitis[31]. In other patients, including children, ABPA may be present at an early stage without fulfilling all diagnostic criteria, e.g. there may be negative serology[17,35]. The CT scan may have low sensitivity for diagnosing central bronchiectasis compared to bronchography. Some patients may be labelled 'ABPA sero-positive' only, to distinguish from those who also have positive radiological features[36]. A high index of suspicion is thus required in what appears to be a broader disease spectrum than previously recognised – so much so that it is suggested that ABPA should be positively excluded in all patients with chronic asthma[37]. Thus, at least 10% of patients with asthma in one series had ABPA[38].

ABPA evolves from the acute episode (Stage I) through remissions (Stage II) and exacerbations (Stage III), corticosteroid dependence (Stage IV) and finally fibrosis (Stage V). While approximately one-fifth patients not on treatment progress to end stage pulmonary fibrosis by the age of 40[25], others remit to asthma which may be steroid dependent or non-dependent. Exacerbations are known to occur during periods of high ambient spore counts.

The mainstay of management is intermittent or prolonged use of systemic steroids to resolve infiltrates, improve the IgE levels and eosinophilia, and to decrease dyspnoea and sputum production. Steroids also reduce the number of exacerbations and reduce pulmonary fibrosis. Serial IgE monitoring may be a useful guide to disease activity in the presence of asymptomatic infiltrates. The usual dose of prednisone in Stage I or III is 0.5 mg/kg daily for at least 2 weeks followed by alternate daily administration for 3 months, then tapering or discontinuation[39]. However, the clinical response and serum IgE levels should determine the fine tuning of the steroid dose programme. Only 10% of patients achieve prolonged remission over a long-term follow-up period and may remain steroid dependent[39]. Additional important adjunctive therapies include bronchodilators, postural drainage and removal of the patient from the source of high spore counts, e.g. prohibiting farmers from working with compost piles. Antifungal therapy has not been extensively studied but reports suggest, at best, a transient clinical improvement. This is possibly related to poor drug delivery and recolonisation during discontinuation of treatment[40–42].

Colonisation and aspergillomas

The lower respiratory tract of as many as 10% of hospitalised patients is colonised by *Aspergillus*. In patients with normal mechanical/humoral/cellular immunity mechanisms, this situation is asymptomatic and non-progressive.

Patients who have long-standing mechanical host defence deficiencies, particularly cavitary lung disease are at risk from the development of aspergilloma due to *Aspergillus* colonisation. Such patients include those with cavities secondary to previous TB and non-tuberculous mycobacteriosis, idiopathic bronchiectasis, sarcoidosis, malignancy, emphysema, ankylosing spondylitis, pulmonary sequestration, bronchogenic cysts and post-operative stumps. Aspergilloma, fungus ball or mycetoma are interchangeable descriptive terms for this manifestation. Occasionally, aspergillomas develop at the site of scar tissue. Such aspergillomas are termed secondary. Old tuberculous cavities are the commonest disposition to the development of aspergilloma. Approximately 15% of patients with inactive tuberculous cavitary lung disease and 10% of patients with sarcoidosis develop aspergillomas by 3 years[43].

Recently, aspergillomas have been documented in patients with cystic fibrosis. This had not been previously described despite up to 60% of patients with cystic fibrosis being colonised with *Aspergillus* spp. Increased longevity of these patients may have resulted in the switch over from colonisation of the cystic fibrosis patients necrotic tissue/cyst to aspergilloma[44].

Although aspergilloma usually develops in a pre-existing cavity of some duration, it occasionally arises concomitant with the evolution of the cavity, particularly in association with lung abscess or lung neoplasia. These acute, primary, aspergillomas can occur in patients with aspiration pneumonia or other conditions, for example, pulmonary infarction which predisposes to lung necrosis. Occasionally primary aspergilloma occurs following invasive *Aspergillus* lung disease in neutropenic patients[46] or in patients with allergic bronchopulmonary aspergillosis. The term mycotic lung sequestrum has been proposed to differentiate this from a fungus ball arising in a preformed cavity[45]. Other fungi such as *Mucor* spp. rarely give rise to mycetomas.

Intracavitary aspergilloma appears to be a dynamic process of host–fungus interactions as evidenced by positive serum precipitins, a type III skin reaction and the production of certain *Aspergillus* metabolites[46]. Within the cavities are masses of hyphae, host debris and inflammatory tissue lying free or attached to the wall but without evidence of lung parenchymal invasion. The cavity is composed of a surrounding fibrous wall within which may be lining epithelium. Unless the host defences are impaired, fungal invasion of the wall is unusual.

The natural history of secondary aspergillomas is variable but most patients have stable disease and occasionally spontaneous regression occurs[47,48] (up to 10% particularly in those arising from abscesses). Very rarely invasive aspergillosis may arise from the mycetoma. This could occur as a result of increased immunosuppression, e.g. high dose steroid therapy or in patients having lung transplants. Massive haemoptysis and death is unusual.

Secondary aspergillomas may be asymptomatic being an incidental finding on chest radiographic examination. However, three-quarters of all patients will eventually develop symptoms – usually cough with a variable degree of haemoptysis. Haemoptysis may range from trivial to severe/fatal. The aetiology may be related to rupture of a bronchial or pulmonary blood vessel in the cavity wall or due to direct frictional trauma of the aspergilloma or *Aspergillus* derived haemolytic endotoxin or anticoagulant. It is unusual to have systemic symptoms unless the aspergilloma is due to chronic necrotising pulmonary aspergillosis or the patient develops secondary bacterial infection, e.g. from bronchial obstruction by the mycetoma. Dyspnoea from pleural environment is unusual. Fistula formation, e.g. broncho-pleural is rare.

Examination may reveal features of chronic fibrosis, cavitary lung disease or of the predisposing condition.

A plain chest radiograph may show a cavity with a variable thickness wall containing an ovoid round mass usually in the upper lobes which may be somewhat mobile, surrounded by a crescent of air (Fig. 16.4 (*a*)). CT/MRI may provide further radiological information (Fig. 16.4 (*b*))[49]. However, these classical features may not always be present[49], particularly in cavities due to carcinoma[50].

Serum *Aspergillus* precipitins are usually present in patients with aspergillomas. Recently IgG-ELISA serology, IgG-binding to 32 kD serine protease and other proteins have been shown to correlate with disease progression and treatment response[51]. Sputum examination reveals *Aspergillus* in a half of all cases. Skin testing is not helpful. Occasionally, bronchoscopy with brushing, washings or biopsy, transthoracic fine needle aspiration or pleural biopsy may be necessary to establish the diagnosis. FNA may produce tangled mats of fungal hyphae to provide the diagnosis in patients with cavities[52].

Aspergillomas arising *de novo*, so-called 'primary aspergilloma' or 'apparent mycetoma' or 'mycotic lung sequestrum' to distinguish from secondary forms behave differently[53]. These are formed from normal lung which has become invaded with *Aspergillus* usually as the result of severe immunocompromisation and consists of necrotic pulmonary tissue infiltrated with fungus. Patients with mycotic lung sequestra are at significant risk from fatal haemoptysis in about 50% of cases[53].

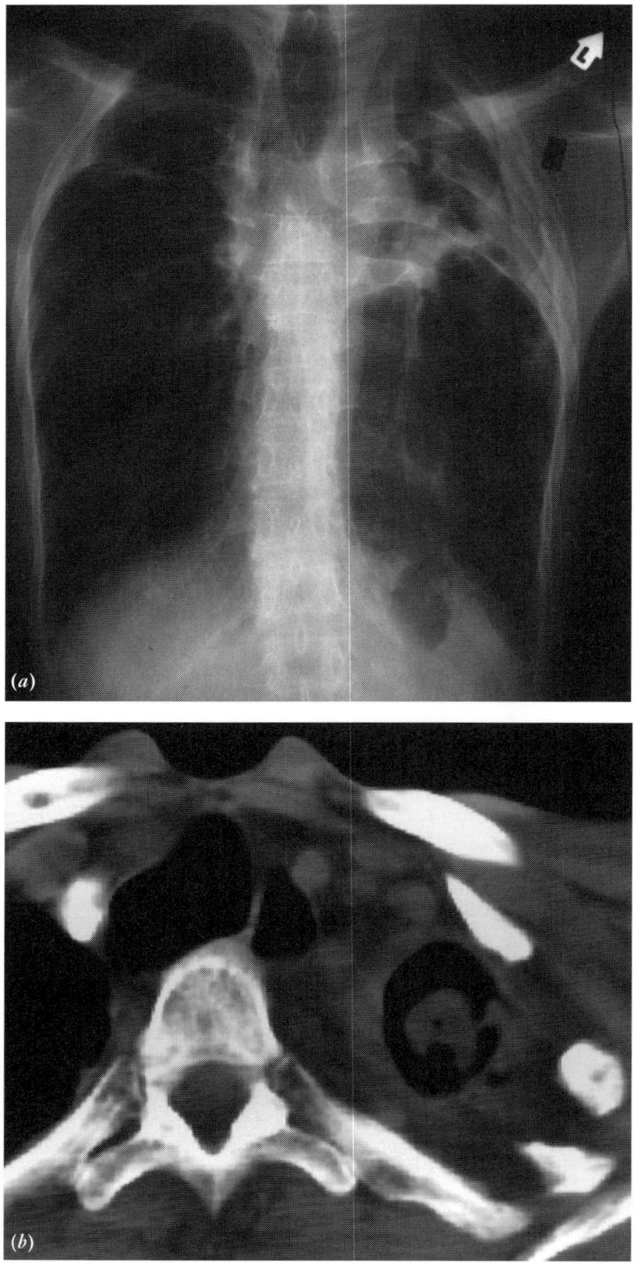

FIGURE 16.4 (*a*) 33-year-old male with previous TB, now haemoptysis, CXR shows collapse of left upper lobe, cavity and fungus ball. (*b*) CT scan of same patient. (Courtesy of Dr W. von Sinner.)

Apart from patients with mycotic lung sequestra when surgical intervention is strongly advised[53], the management of most patients with aspergilloma is conservative. Should haemoptysis become recurrent or severe, then active intervention is indicated. Resective surgery is curative though hazardous due to the poor underlying pulmonary status which is present in many patients. Complications of surgery include bronchopleural fistula, empyema, and therefore perioperative administration of amphotericin B is usually advocated[54]. Complications are more common with pleural aspergillosis and in multicavitary aspergillomas. Systemic amphotericin B with or without 5-flucytosine has little effect in the majority of patients because of the extremely poor penetration of the antifungals into the site of infection. Intracavitary installation has been attempted occasionally with some success but wide experience with this technique is lacking[55,56]. However, this may be a feasible alternative in selected patients who present a poor operative risk. Embolisation of the feeding artery is an alternative approach. The source of bleeding is often the pulmonary artery in aspergillomas arising from bronchiectatic cavities and the bronchial artery in other cases. Late recurrences may be observed.

Aspergillus bronchitis

This is an unusual entity occurring either as a primary event or secondary to ongoing chronic suppurative lung disease, e.g. chronic bronchitis/bronchiectasis or following thoracic surgery (local bronchial stump remnant *Aspergillus* infection). Pseudomembranous necrotising bronchial aspergillosis is usually a limited version of invasive aspergillosis and is described later.

Invasive aspergillosis

Extension of *Aspergillus* into tissue is termed invasive aspergillosis. This may be locally and moderately invasive (tracheobronchitis), acutely and dramatically invasive (acute invasive pulmonary aspergillosis), or chronically invasive (chronic necrotising aspergillosis).

Aspergillus tracheobronchitis

In this manifestation[22,57–59] (see also Chapter 25) the infection is largely limited to the tracheobronchial tree. Less than 10% of all cases of intrathoracic aspergillosis affects the airways solely. It has several morphological presentations. Single or multiple segmental circumferential intraluminal growth without tissue invasion of the bronchial tree is one form. This may lead to mucoid impaction consisting of bronchial casts of mucus and mycelia. Another is typified by the formation of discrete plaques which often invade the adjacent bronchial/tracheal mucosa and cartilage in lung tissue. Pseudomembranous tracheobronchitis describes an extensive pantracheobronchial involvement by a membranous slough which contains *Aspergillus* hyphae. A form of aspergillosis of the smaller bronchi/bronchioles in which bronchocentric granulomatosis and mucosal necrosis is also described. Occasionally, pulmonary parenchymal involvement or dissemination occurs, particular in patients with severe immunocompromisation, for example, HIV infection[59].

The host risk setting for these unusual forms varies throughout the spectrum from the immunocompetent or mildly immunocompromised host (e.g. patients on steroids, antibiotics or who are diabetic) to the severely immunocompromised (e.g. patients with leukaemia, HIV disease, lung transplantation)[22,57–60]. In general, though, there is less neutropenia, less exposure to steroids and cytotoxins than patients with invasive pulmonary parenchymal involvement[57]. In addition, intrinsic airways disease may predispose to *Aspergillus* tracheobronchitis, for example, increased mucus production, decreased mucociliary clearance, mucosal carcinoma or endotracheal intubation damage[57].

Presentation is highly variable. Some patients are initially asymptomatic although many have a degree of dyspnoea, cough and haemoptysis. Significant intraluminal growth can cause obstruction with localised wheeze, distal lung collapse, perhaps with secondary bacterial infection or life-threatening major airways respiratory obstruction. If invasion occurs, for example, in the plaque forming variety, then pneumonia, lung abscess may occur or lung haemorrhage/infarction with haemoptysis which may be fatal[61]. Intrathoracic fistula formation can occur as a result of invasion. Examination of expectorated plugs of purulent sputum in these conditions will reveal *Aspergillus*. Chest radiographical appearances are likewise variable from normal to atelectasis with infiltrates, and other features appropriate to the particular pathology. Diagnosis can be made on bronchoscopy with histological/microbiological examination of respiratory secretions or biopsy material. Unrecognised and untreated the disease carries a high mortality though progression may be either slow or rapid. Preferred treatment is with systemic amphotericin B; itraconazole may be a useful alternative[57]. Airways debris may be removed using rigid bronchoscopy[61]. Surgical resection of a lung may be indicated.

Acute invasive pulmonary aspergillosis

The increasing population of the iatrogenic immunocompromised host secondary to increasing complex and sophisticated medical care has carried with it a tremendous increase in the risk for, and disease from, nosocomial acute invasive aspergillosis (Chapter 21). In some bone marrow transplantation centres it is the most common cause of death[62]. Invasive pulmonary aspergillosis (IPA) presents a challenging diagnostic and therapeutic dilemma. *A. fumigatus* is most commonly involved; *A. flavus* and rarely *Aspergillus terreus* have been incriminated[63].

Granulocytopoenia, particularly if severe ($< 0.1 \times 10^9$/l) and prolonged, is the single most important risk factor as this removes the host defence against germinated stages of *Aspergillus*[4,64]. Thus, patients with acute leukaemia or bone marrow transplantation have a much higher incidence of IPA compared to those with reticuloendothelial malignancies or recipients of solid organ transplants. By 3 to 5 weeks of neutropenia, between 4.5% and 14% of patients with leukaemia receiving chemotherapy/radiotherapy or bone marrow transplant recipients may develop IPA[65–67]. However, the incidence varies widely from centre to centre. An international autopsy study has shown that 25% of patients dying with leukaemia or organ transplantation, 12% of patients with lymphoma and 5% with solid tumours had fungal infections of which two-thirds were due to *Candida* and one-third *Aspergillus*[68]. Recurrent pulmonary aspergillosis is well recognised in patients with haematological malignancy[69] and these patients require prophylactic amphotericin B in subsequent granulocytopenic episodes, despite apparent clinical and radiological resolution of previous IPA.

Conditions which produce neutrophil dysfunction also predispose to invasive aspergillosis, such as chronic granulomatous disease[70]. The overriding importance of the defensive neutrophils is reflected by the paucity of IPA reported in patients with AIDS[8,71].

Another important factor is high dose corticosteroid use which down-modulates polymorphonuclear and bronchoalveolar macrophage function, and fails to arrest the germination of ingested *Aspergillus* spores, since the fusion of lysosomes to vacuoles is inhibited. This is exemplified by the occurrence of IPA in patients with Cushing's syndrome[72].

Other predisposing host factors include the use of broad spectrum antibiotics, immunosuppressant drugs, organ transplantation, intravascular devices, total parenteral nutrition, breaches of the mucosal barrier, treatment for graft vs. host disease, malignancies and concomitant cytomegalovirus disease[73–76].

Occasionally, invasive aspergillosis can occur in patients with less severe immunocompromisation, such as chronic lung disease, bronchial carcinoma, hepatic failure, uraemia and steroid administration[77].

IPA has also been described rarely in patients with a normal host defence system[78]. However, many of these patients have a background history of COAD or alcoholism. Inhalation of extremely high concentrations of spores in children with no apparent underlying disease can produce self-limiting acute respiratory distress syndrome typified by miliary radiological changes and fever.

The source for the majority of cases of IPA is the hospital environment, in association with inadequate or defective air ventilation systems. The evidence for this comes from the documented increase in cases during periods of maintenance of ventilatory systems and other hospital fixtures or of hospital construction/building renovations, and their decrease once the source of *Aspergillus* has been corrected[2,79–81]. However, not all instances of hospital building activities have been shown to produce excess cases of IPA.

The fungus–host interactive mechanisms have already been described. Following hyphae formation in the endobronchial tree, *Aspergillus* invades lung parenchyma and blood vessels to produce thrombosis and haemorrhagic pulmonary infarction. Fungal proliferation occurs in a centrifugal fashion from respiratory bronchioles into the lung parenchyma, causing well-defined whitish areas of consolidation which may contain cavities or hyphae containing necrotic areas, as well as producing a bronchopneumonia. Vascular infiltration also features prominently. The vessel's wall becomes invaded and nodular necrosis of the supplied tissue follows. The distribution and histological description of the nodular lesions appears to favour coagulative necrosis rather than an ischaemic necrosis mechanism. Some of the lesions are blood filled. Other lesions are caused primarily by the ischaemia resulting from vascular occlusion resulting in wedge/triangular shaped lesions. Haematogenous dissemination to distant organs occurs, particularly the brain, kidneys and heart[68].

The cardinal clinical presenting feature of IPA is unremittent and persistent fever in the appropriate setting of a granulocytopenic patient – usually with a background of leukaemia or bone marrow transplantation, who has been receiving antimicrobials directed towards a broad spectrum of Gram-positive and Gram-negative organisms (antibiotic resistant neutropenic fever)[82]. Onset is typically subacute, though a few cases are acute with a fulminant course. Other findings include cough, often unproductive, pleuritic chest pain and tachypnoea which are common early features, though may not appear until later[83,84]. Crepitations and a pleural rub may be auscultated. Hypoxia initially is not a major feature. As the disease becomes more established, haemoptysis may ensue due either to pulmonary infarction, bleeding from mycetoma or from mycotic aneurysm rupture (which may prove catastrophic). Sometimes haemoptysis is sudden, unexpected and occurs shortly after the recovery from chemotherapy induced aplasia[85]. Respiratory failure may also occur. Clinical and radiological features appear or become prominent sometimes only at the time of marrow recovery. Superior vena caval obstruction is an unusual presentation.

It is not uncommon for the paranasal sinuses to be involved, sometimes with intracranial extension. Features include headache, sinus pain, rhinitis (which may involve blood stained and necrotic discharge), facial swelling, proptosis and focal cranial nerve or other neurological features. There may be associated intraoral spread, for example, palatal necrosis and sloughing. This presentation characterises tissue invasive and angioinvasive sino-nasal aspergilloses to distinguish them from the saprophytic forms of sinus aspergillomas and *Aspergillus* sinusitis[19].

From the lung, direct spread to the pleura, chest wall and myopericardium may occur as well as haematogenous dissemination to other organs, including the central nervous system (most commonly), skin (Fig. 16.5), bone, eye, GI tract, kidneys, and thyroid. Features of pleural effusion, pericarditis or myocardial infarction, seizures, with focal long tract and cranial nerve palsies and skin lesions typified by central necrosis, may then present.

Pleural aspergillosis can also occur as a result of spread from a bronchial plaque or other form of tracheobronchitis, from an aspergilloma and rarely post-operatively in patients operated on for pulmonary aspergillosis. Widespread haematogenous dissemination from an initial focus can sometimes lead to miliary aspergillosis[86].

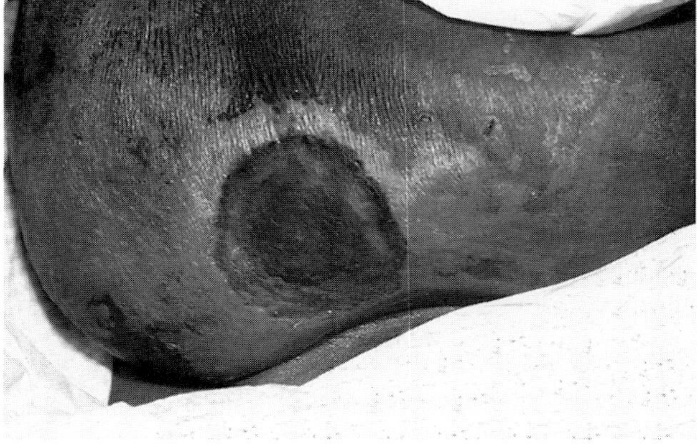

FIGURE 16.5 Pulmonary aspergillosis: massive skin necrosis of thigh.

The diagnosis of IPA may be either presumptive or definitive, but often is missed ante-mortem. A plain chest radiograph initially is often clear, or shows subtle features (Fig. 16.6 (*a*)) which is not surprising in the face of an ineffectual host response. Later, non-specific diffuse infiltrates, or well-defined single or multiple nodules appear[75] (Fig. 16.6 (*b*)). The infiltrates may increase rapidly to produce consolidation in a broncho-pneumonic or lobar pattern[75]. Cavitation secondary to necrosis may occur[75]. Primary lung aspergilloma may develop (Fig. 16.6 (*c*)). It is the presence of cavitation, particularly with crescent formation, which is the radiological appearance most suggestive of IPA[87]. Triangular infiltrates commensurate with pulmonary infarction may be mistaken for pulmonary embolism and infarction may also be found[87,88]. However, no radiological pattern is diagnostic of IPA or other fungi. Microorganisms and noninfective processes can present a similar picture. Computerised tomography has been shown to be more sensitive than plain radiology in demonstrating cavitation/air crescent formation and this may prove useful in early diagnosis and management (Fig. 16.7, Fig. 16.8)[89–91]. The air-crescent sign, however, is not pathognomonic of IPA – mucor, TB, bacterial sepsis and *Nocardia* can also produce this[90–93].

The halo sign – a distinctive zone or halo surrounding a round pulmonary mass, having an attenuation lower than the mass centre, but higher than that of the surrounding lung parenchyma appears before crescent formation and is highly suggestive of IPA[91,94].

MRI is even more sensitive than CT scanning. Rim enhancement post gadolinium, intranodular blood and increased number of nodules visualized compared to CT have been demonstrated[95].

In many cases the diagnosis of IPA is presumptive, i.e. based upon clinical and radiological features in an appropriate granulocytopenic host. An attempt to quantify the likelihood of a diagnosis of IPA, based upon 11 clinical and radiological variables and without microbiological support, was presented as a discriminate score card. This gave a sensitivity and specificity of between 63% and 93% and 88% and 98% respectively and, in addition, identified patients with IPA 4 days prior to clinical recognition of disease and initiation of amphotericin B treatment[82].

Since many of these patients are critically ill and some have uncorrectable coagulopathies, a tissue diagnosis may not always be feasible. A fully expressed clinical picture, i.e. a febrile granulocytopenic patient with pulmonary infiltrates unresponsive to antibiotics associated with sinusitis with bony destruction is highly suggestive of IPA. However, other fungi can (less often) produce an indistinguishable clinical picture. Since *Aspergillus* can colonise the respiratory tract, care has to be taken in the interpretation of the finding of this fungus in specimens other than tissue. Nevertheless, the presence of *Aspergillus* spp. in sputum, nasal swab, sinus aspirate, respiratory secretions or from bronchoalveolar lavage specimens is in general predictive of IPA in neutropenic patients who have appropriate clinical and radiological signs and should not necessarily be dismissed as contaminants or colonisers[96–98]. On the other hand, their absence does not exclude the diagnosis[99]. The positive predictive value of *Aspergillus* in BAL is highest with diffuse rather than focal lesions[100–103]. Nevertheless, up to 40% of neutropenic patients with *Aspergillus* isolated from respiratory secretions may have no evidence of IPA[97]. The presence of *Aspergillus* in other extrapulmonary sites such as the skin, pericardium, nasal eschars or brain will also strongly support the diagnosis of IPA.

Clearly then the finding of *Aspergillus* in respiratory specimens is suggestive but by no means conclusive of IPA. Positive identification of *Aspergillus* within lung tissue will establish the diagnosis without doubt. Transbronchial biopsy may be subject to sampling error and may have a high incidence of bleeding complications in such compromised patients. Open lung biopsy provides a controlled means of obtaining substantial diseased lung tissue for examination and bleeding can generally be successfully controlled[104]. Open lung biopsy provides much more diagnostic information and is generally safe[104,105]. However, fungal disease can still be missed even on an open lung biopsy sample. Definitive impact on patient outcome has yet to be conclusively demonstrated by resorting to open lung biopsy and it is a moderately invasive procedure.

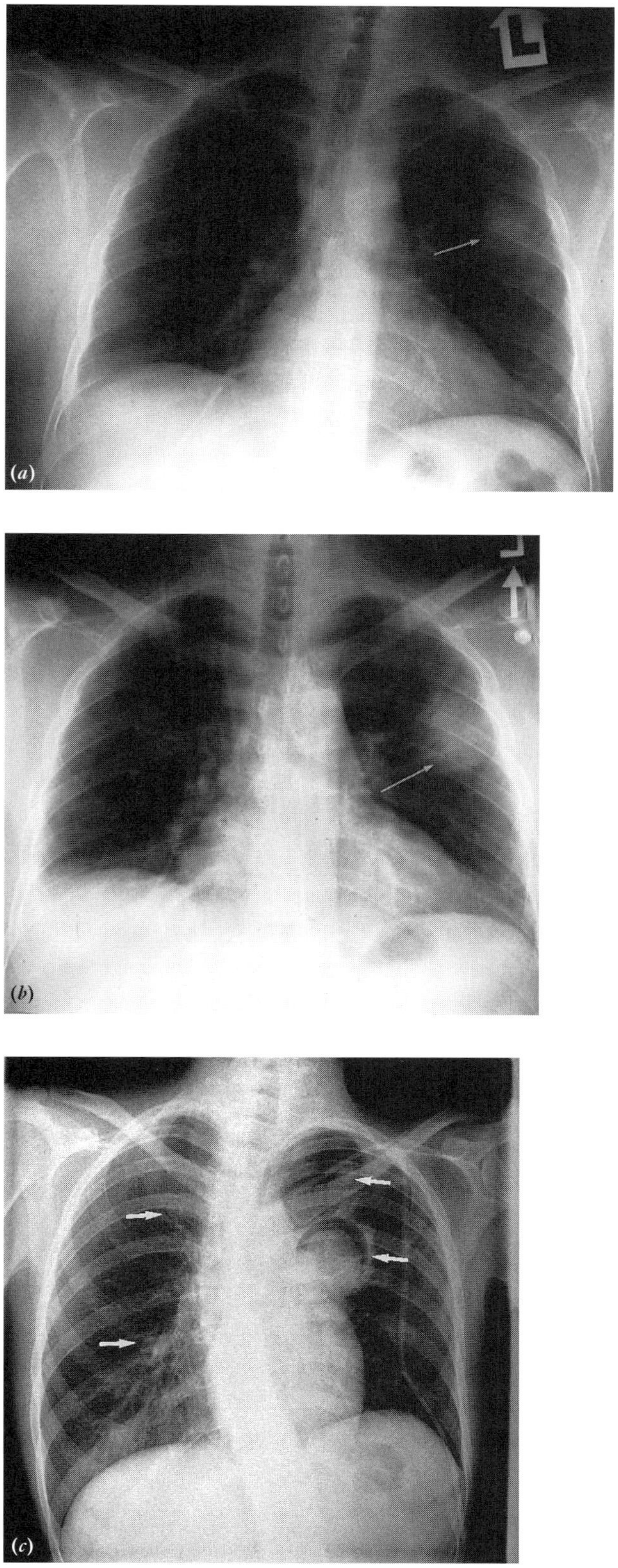

FIGURE 16.6 (*a*) Circumscribed rounded lesion of pulmonary aspergillosis left mid zone barely visible. (*b*) Same patient as in Fig. 16.5 (*a*), 2 days later obvious large lesion. (*c*) Multiple fungal balls (arrowed) in a patient with prolonged severe neutropoenia.

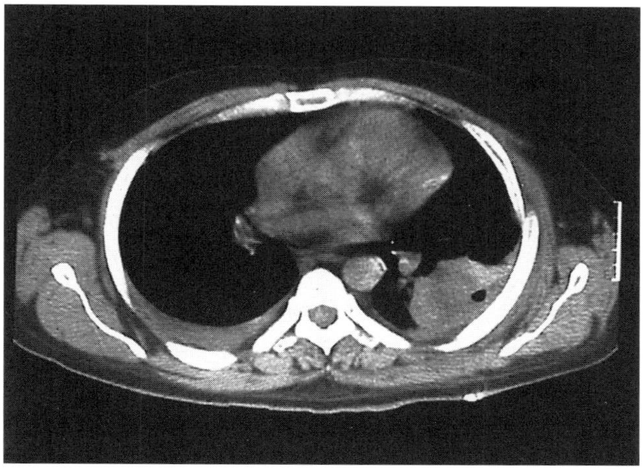

FIGURE 16.7 CT scan of same patient as in Fig. 16.5 (*a*): large pleural based lesion with early cavitation.

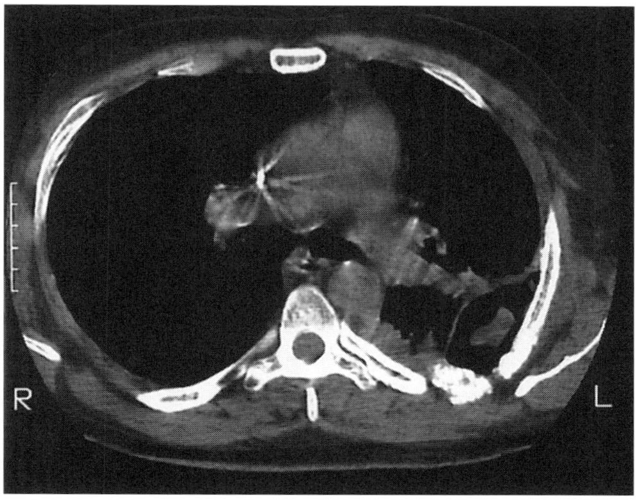

FIGURE 16.8 CT scan of same patient as in Fig. 16.5 (*a*) 4 weeks later: lesion has now cavitated. Note rib periosteal reaction.

The presence of wide septated 45° branching hyphae on microscopical examination is highly suggestive of invasive aspergillosis – (Fig. 16.1, 16.9) however, other fungi including *Fusarium* spp. and *Pseudallescheria* spp. can be mistaken. Cultures are mandatory to provide distinction, since not all fungi are uniformly sensitive to antifungal agents. Blood cultures are rarely positive in IPA, possibly as a result of the intermittent fungaemia.

The serological diagnosis of IPA focused on antibody and antigen detection has received a great deal of attention in recent years, since specimens can be obtained relatively non-invasively. However, most tests are still not widely applied in clinical practice. Previous experience aimed at looking for antibodies to *Aspergillus* has proved neither particularly sensitive nor specific[106]. The development of primary binding enzyme immunoassays with increased sensitivity to detect low concentration of specific antibodies, however, is promising.

The identification of immunodominant protein antigens, e.g. 41, 54, and 71 kD antigens has permitted development of antibody detection assays[107]. Animal studies have demonstrated that antibody seroconversion to the 41 kD antigen occurs during experimental animal IPA. Techniques to increase the sensitivity of assays are being investigated. To date such tests are unsatisfactory for routine diagnostic clinical use although some studies indicate that up to 70% of patients develop an antibody response to infection[108]. Generally speaking, antibody detection is less sensitive than antigen detection in invasive aspergillosis[109].

A number of antigen detection methods also have been developed at an investigational level. Foremost has been galactomannan polysaccharide detection by countercurrent immunoelectrophoresis, radioimmunoassay, enzyme-linked immunoassay or latex agglutination tests. The sensitivities of these tests when applied to serum samples approximate 75%, and specificities 90%[110]. Recent studies using latex agglutination have returned figures of 95% and 99%, respectively[108]. Some studies have indicated that a positive test can pre-date standard clinical/laboratory diagnosis of IPA in about one-third of patients[110] – a finding crucial to the institution of early antifungal therapy. The limitations of these tests may be related to fluctuating serum levels (due to hepatic removal of *Aspergillus* antigens), immune complex formation (which requires dissociation to free up detectable antigen), and complex structures of the antigens. Serial serum sampling, BAL specimens and 24-hour urine collection may increase the detection rate. Several other ill-defined antigens have been detected and are undergoing evaluation. Further laboratory and clinical data are urgently required to clarify the role of such serodiagnosis tests.

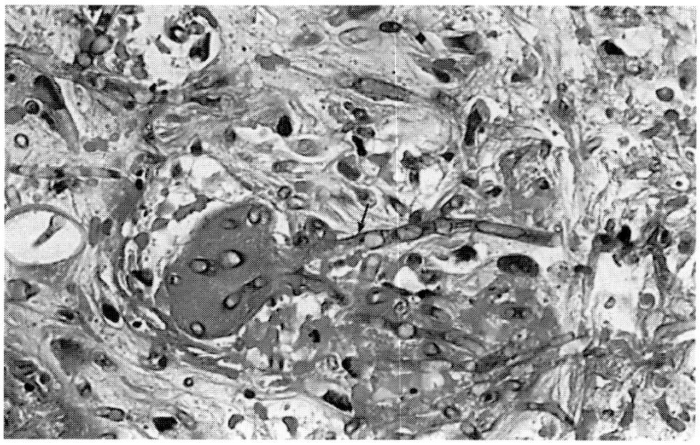

FIGURE 16.9 *Aspergillus* invading blood vessel (arrow).

Other diagnostic tests not generally in use include detection of oxalate crystals and mannitol production, unique to some strains of *Aspergillus*.

The place of the PCR is currently undergoing evaluation. Using the PCR to amplify fragments of genes encoding alkaline proteases from *A. fumigatus* and *A. flavus* to detect these organisms in BAL, sensitivity was found to be 100% and specificity 94% for immunocompromised patients with proven/probable IPA[111]. In non-immunocompromised patients, however, without IPA a PCR positive rate of almost 20% was found, and this was thought to represent colonisation. Others have also confirmed a similarly high false positive rate for invasive aspergillosis when using the PCR to predict for this[112]. This situation may reflect the ubiquitous nature of the organism in terms of colonisation of the patient or contamination of reagents and samples. Occasionally, negative PCRs are seen in patients with characteristic radiological and clinical features of IPA, but with negative microbiological culture. Whether this represents true false negatives or the presence of fungal pathogens other than *Aspergillus* spp. cannot be determined at this time[113]. Clearly, the PCR in general can easily identify fungal nucleic acid sequences but cannot as yet provide the clinician with the significance of the result, i.e. cannot differentiate IPA from *Aspergillus* colonisation.

Chronic necrotising pulmonary aspergillosis

This is a slowly progressive (over several months) destructive pulmonary infection due to *A. fumigatus*[114] and occasionally to *A. flavus*[114] or *A. niger*[115] that occurs against the background of mild immunosuppression (or none), or in the presence of diabetes mellitus, alcoholism, general debility or in patients with chronic lung disease. However, no specific immune disturbance has been documented, although an association with preceding viral infections has been mooted[116]. Superinfection with *Mycobacterium tuberculosis* may also occur rarely. The fungus grows slowly and invades locally, and does not appear to extend beyond pleural boundaries or spread to distant extrapulmonary sites. Histologically, examination of adequate biopsies reveals fungal elements within a milieu of fibrotic avascularity (Fig. 16.10)[116]. Necrotising granulomatous inflammation resembling chronic fibrocaseous TB is found. Nevertheless, severe cavitating lung disease may occur. Invasion of major local structures may be present (Fig. 16.11). Secondary aspergillomas may result. The chronicity and propensity for upper lobe involvement often leads to an initial mistaken diagnosis of TB or carcinoma particularly when patients have systemic features of fever, weight loss and cough.

Fever, cough and sputum production over several months is the characteristic presentation[114–117]. Treatment has to be individualised and is often difficult. Local disease can sometimes be resected. Successful systemic antifungal administration is limited by the dense avascular nature of the inflammatory tissue surrounding the fungi which presumably limits adequate drug delivery to the infected tissue. The role of high dose regular amphotericin B, liposome-encapsulated amphotericin B, or itraconazole – all these alone or in combination with rifampicin/flucytosine – has yet to be properly evaluated though successes have been reported with intravenous, inhaled and intracavity routes of regular amphotericin B[37,118,119]. The outcome is generally poor with many patients developing respiratory failure and cor-pulmonale.

Management of invasive aspergillosis

Medical management with amphotericin B (AB) is the key therapeutic manipulation, supported as appropriate by surgery and immunomodulation. The consensus of opinion is that early administration of high dose (1–1.5 mg/kg/day) AB should be administered for IPA in neutropenic patients[120]. This is based on circumstancial reports of higher clinical failure rates with lower dosages, necessity to achieve adequate tissue levels (some patients, for example, with chronic necrotising aspergillosis have a notable avascular milieu, Fig. 16.10), and relatively high MICs for some *Aspergillus* isolates. A cumulative dosage of 2–4 g is generally administered. However, AB should be given until the neutrophil count has recovered, clinical signs have disappeared and radiological improvement has been substantial. In most cases clinical and radiological response in established IPA is slow with strong dependence on recovery of the neutrophil count (Fig. 16.12). Dose-limiting toxicity is a serious consideration which often precludes the administration of high doses. However, the availability of lipid preparations such as liposomal amphotericin B, e.g. Ambisome[121] enables doses as high as 4–5 mg/kg/day to be given with little toxicity. Whether these very high doses will prove to be more beneficial than the usual maximum dose of 1.5 mg/kg/day of regular AB remains to be proven in a scientific-controlled trial setting. In the meantime, there is accumulating evidence that liposomal amphotericin B may prove successful in the face of failure on regular amphotericin B and be at least as effective[122–125]. A controlled study of Ambisome vs regular AB in children with haematological malignancy and cryptic fungal infections (antibiotic resistant neutropenic fever) has demonstrated statistically significant improved efficacy of Ambisome[126].

In general, the outcome for IPA treated with AB in other groups of patients, e.g. bone marrow transplant recipients, solid organ transplant recipients and those with a lesser degree of immunosuppression is better than for those with neutropenia, with survival rates of 50–82%[127]. In these it is often possible to use lower (0.5 mg/kg/day) dosages of AB. In renal transplant patients, nephrotoxicity of AB may be compounded by the use of cyclosporin, whilst graft loss may be significant if immunosuppressive therapy is reduced to lessen the immunosuppressive drive[128].

The concomitant use of other antifungals such as 5-flucytosine or rifampicin is controversial. Despite the demonstration of *in vitro* synergy between AB and 5- flucytosine or AB and rifampicin, animal models have not proved a consistent additive or synergistic effect[127], but none has proved antagonistic. There have been no prospective human studies addressing this issue. If flucytosine is used, its

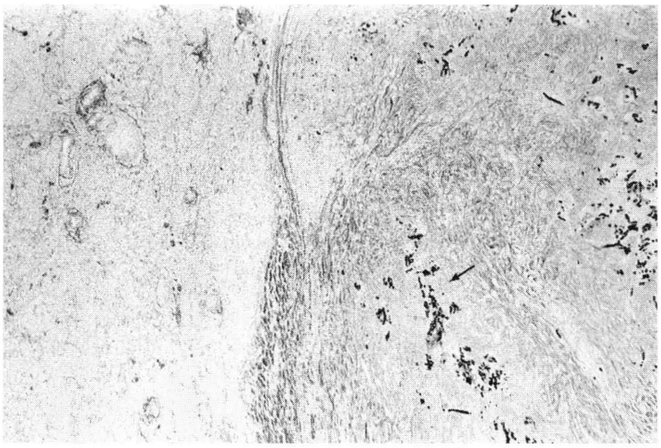

FIGURE 16.10 Lymph node biopsy: numerous fungi (arrow) engulfed in dense fibrous avascular tissue.

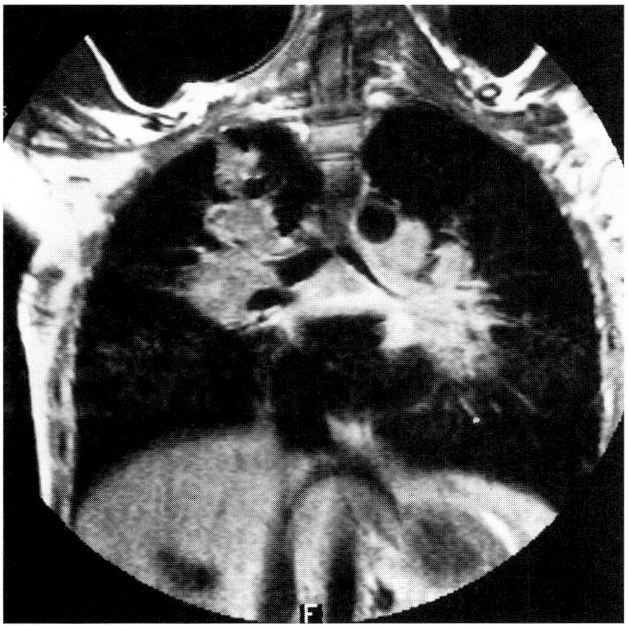

FIGURE 16.11 MRI of chronic necrotising pulmonary aspergillosis: bilateral hilar, subcarinal, right apex and aorto-pulmonary region invasion.

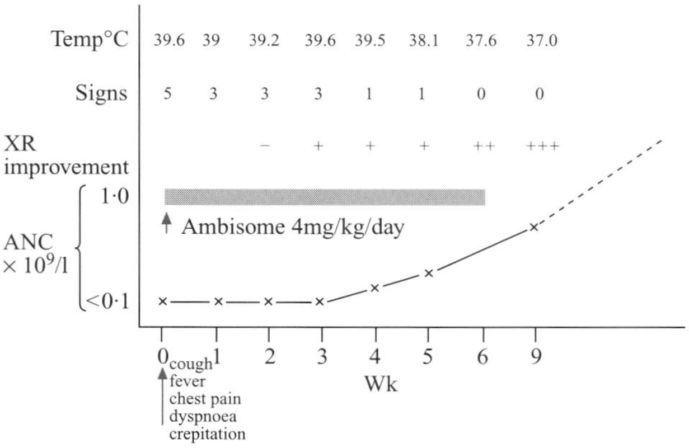

FIGURE 16.12 Clinical and radiological response not apparent until the white count recovers.

myelosuppressive action may cause concern, particularly in patients already neutropenic. However, serum level monitoring is easily accomplished to reduce this risk.

Miconazole, ketoconazole and fluconazole have rarely been used to treat IPA[127] and cannot be recommended. Itraconazole, on the other hand, has been used with some success in patients with IPA who were not neutropenic[129]. However, approximately 20% of patients experience low serum levels. The liquid formulation of itraconazole may produce more reliable and constant levels. Interaction with rifampicin, phenytoin, cyclosporin and other drugs may be a problem with itraconazole. Some reports indicate that combinations of AB with azoles may be antagonistic[130], but clear clinical evidence of this is lacking.

Surgery in IPA may be useful in appropriate circumstances. Certainly in patients who develop life-threatening haemoptysis secondary to mycetoma formation recourse to early surgical resection may prove life saving[131]. Pulmonary resection has also been recommended for fungal infection in bone marrow transplant patients[132]. This may reduce fungal load and chance of recurrence of dissemination especially during relapse of leukaemia. Comparative data of surgery + AB vs AB alone is not available and major thoracic surgery in patients with granulocytopenia is potentially hazardous. Patients with post-operative bronchial stump, pleural or laryngeal aspergillosis are further indications for surgery[127]. Therapeutic embolisation of feeder arteries is an alternative approach in patients with uncontrolled haemoptysis but who are high operative risks.

The restoration of adequate granulocytes can be assisted with granulocyte infusions or with the use of growth factors and this would theoretically seem a reasonable objective given the central role that the neutrophil has in IPA. This has not been studied extensively and there have been mixed efficacy results[87,133]. Pulmonary toxicity due to AB-granulocyte interaction[134], inability to maintain a sufficient donor supply and mismatch reactions limit this approach. Recently, Enaissie *et al.* reported that neutropenic patients with refractory mycoses appear to have an initial favourable response when infused leukopherised white cells from healthy matched donors given growth factors[135]. The use of white cell colony stimulating factors shortens neutropenia, improves their function, reduces febrile and bacterial infections[136] but there is no evidence to date of any impact on established invasive fungal infections[137].

AB used at doses of between 0.15 and 0.5 mg/kg/day administered empirically to leukaemic patients with refractory fever compromised by severe therapy-induced neutropenia has been shown to reduce the incidence of deep fungal infections[138]. In patients with previous IPA, the risk of recurrence in subsequent episodes of neutropenia is high, of the order of 50%[69]. However, the rate can be significantly reduced in these patients by the prophylactic administration of AB (1 mg/kg/day) combined with 5-flucytosine[141,142]. The use of AB as a primary prophylactic given to neutropenic patients at risk from invasive fungal infections has been recently studied in prospective randomised comparative studies, following retrospective reports that the incidence of invasive mycoses might be reduced with AB. Results were conflicting: reduction in oropharyngeal *Candida* colonisation, reduction in systemic fungal-infections, mainly *Candida*, increased survival (not necessarily due to reduction in fungal-related mortality) and incidence of AB toxicity being variably demonstrated[143,144]. Few control patients developed IPA to be able to comment on the efficacy against this fungus.

The administration of fluconazole as a primary prophylactic in high risk leukaemic and bone marrow transplant patients has also been tested in several studies[145,146,147,148,149]. In general, results indicate a reduction in colonisation, reduction in the incidence of invasive fungal infections (mainly *Candida* though a trend towards reduction in moulds including *Aspergillus* spp. has been shown by some studies) and improved survival in some studies have been shown. Advantages of fluconazole over amphotericin B are reduced toxicity, increased compliance and efficacy which is at least equivalent[150]. Other less commonly used agents include itraconazole which has also been shown to reduce the incidence of invasive fungal diseases, mainly candidiasis, but not to a significant level[151].

Of paramount importance in the prevention of IPA is limiting the environmental exposure of patients at risk. Prohibition of building works and repairs of ventilatory systems in the vicinity of neutropenic patients are probably the most important measures. Simple barriers and positive pressure ventilated rooms should be employed in the nursing of such patients. The use of laminar air flow and HEPA filters are additional measures for particular at risk environments[152].

Amphotericin B (AB), flucytosine, azoles and rifampicin

AB is a polyene macrolide first isolated from *Streptomyces nodosus* in the 1950s. Most strains of *Aspergillus* remain sensitive. Being virtually water insoluble, it is administered as a deoxycholate micellar formation, intravenously. By an unknown mechanism, the drug penetrates fungal cell walls and binds to the cell membrane sterol nodosus; ergosterol more avidly than cholesterol[153], when it induces lethal permeability effects. Other modes of action may include oxygen radical-dependent macrophage stimulation[154]. Its action is fungistatic/cidal depending on tissue concentration and organism susceptibility.

The side-effects of AB are formidable and are related in part to the binding to cholesterol in mammalian cell membranes. These include systemic effects of headache, chills, rigors, myalgia, nausea and vomiting. The frequency and severity of these side-effects may be unrelated to time of infusions[155], although others have suggested that rapid infusions are more toxic[156]. Established chills and rigors may be caused by tumour necrosis factor and interleukin release and can be alleviated with corticosteroids and pethidine. Nephrotoxicity, mainly self-limiting, occurs in most patients. In addition, tubular cell permeability changes, arteriolar spasm, calcium deposition and tumour necrosis factor α have all been implicated as mechanisms. Changes in tubular permeability can cause a fall in a glomerular filtration rate (GFR) via a tubulo-glomerular feedback mechanism. In many patients, the GFR falls to 60% of normal. Pyuria, albuminuria, urinary casts, hypokalaemia, hypomagnesaemia, renal tubular acidosis, and nephrocalcinosis can all occur. Since AB is commonly administered to very ill patients who are often hypotensive and septic and receiving other nephrotoxic drugs or who are hyperuricaemic, the role for amphotericin B-related nephrotoxicity in any particular patient is often unclear. There is some evidence that co-administering normal saline can reduce the incidence of renal dysfunction. Potassium and magnesium supplements are usually required. Should renal toxicity be severe, for example, the GFR fall exceeding 50% of baseline, then the drug can be temporarily discontinued.

Normochromic-normocytic anaemia may also occur after some weeks of prolonged treatment due to inhibition of red blood cell production or secondary to renal toxicity. Leukopenia and thrombocytopenia are rare; but at a concentration in excess of 5 mg/l neutrophil function may be compromised. Thrombophlebitis is common and may be prevented by administering AB via a central line. Heparin will lower concentrations of the drug.

Occasionally, acute allergic reactions with bronchospasm and hypotension occur. Liver toxicity has been described but is not clearly related to administration of the drug. Rare side-effects include peripheral neuropathy and cardiac arrest (possibly related to hypo/hyperkalaemic states).

AB appears to have immunomodulatory activity on lymphocytes, phagocytes, and macrophages, but the clinical significance of this is unknown.

Another potential problem with AB is adverse drug interactions. These include enhanced aminoglycoside, cyclosporin and antineoplastic nephrotoxicity, enhanced action of digoxin, and possibly acute pulmonary distress during simultaneous transfusion of granulocytes. The concomitant use of colony-stimulating factors such as GMCSF may also interact in the same way.

AB is usually given, first as a test dose of 1 mg intravenously over 30 minutes to rule out an adverse drug reaction and this is followed with definitive treatment. The usual dosage is then 0.25 mg/kg in 5% dextrose given over 4–6 hours and the dosage subsequently increased daily, depending on clinical response, severity of illness and drug toxicity, up to a maximum daily dosage of 1.5 mg/kg. There is some debate over optimal daily dosage and patients' total dosage requirements. In most cases of less serious infections, 1–2 g cumulative dosage suffices, but in severe infections 2–4 g may be necessary to effect cure. High dosage (1–1.5 mg/kg/day) of AB administered early and escalated rapidly over a few days from the starting dose and continued until neutrophil recovery occurs, is most likely to be associated with a successful outcome in IPA[67] possibly due in part to better tissue penetration of the drug.

Should significant toxicity, particularly renal, occur, AB dosage and frequency of dosing will have to be reduced. No modification of dosage is necessary in patients with renal/hepatic toxicity unattributable to the drug. Relatively higher dosages should be used in children since they have a smaller volume of distribution and a higher clearance than adults.

Combination therapy with rifampicin and/or 5-flucytosine is often used in particularly sick patients. Some studies show synergistic activity, others indifferent but non-antagonistic[157–159]. However, clinical experience is limited. Rifampicin or flucytosine should not be used as single agents because of the rapid selection of fungal resistance.

Alternative fungal therapy includes lipid preparations of AB, azoles and several experimental drugs. By combining AB with lipid vehicles, it is hoped to greatly improve the therapeutic index as a result of diminished toxicity. Liposomes, phospholipid bilayers, have been used to encapsulate amphotericin B. One of these is called Ambisome, in which AB is encapsulated within phosphatidylcholine/cholesterol/distearoylphosphatidylglycerol[160]. This lyophilised, stable preparation is avidly taken up by reticuloendothelial cells to produce substantially higher concentrations in such organs as liver, spleen and brain when compared to regular AB. There is large accrued uncontrolled data to indicate remarkable reduction of toxicity even when used in patients who had severe nephrotoxicity on regular AB[161,162]. In addition, circumstantial evidence of improved success rates have been claimed[121–6,161,163,164], though large controlled studies are needed to determine if the liposomal preparations are superior in efficacy to regular AB. Several other lipid preparations are available[121]. However, their structure, pharmacokinetics and toxicity vary with the particular preparation.

Several systemic antifungal agents are available, whose mechanism of action involves inhibition of cytochrome P450 mediated 14α demethylase activity, thereby reducing formation of membrane ergosterol from lanosterol. However, of the presently available drugs, only itraconazole has substantial activity against *Aspergillus*. It is a triazole, administered orally only, absorbed well after meals, has a long half-life of approximately 18 hours and produces concentrations in most tissues at least twice those in serum. The drug is metabolised by the liver but liver toxicity is low. No alteration in dosage is required in patients with renal dysfunction. Unlike ketoconazole, no effect on testicular or adrenal steroid synthesis has been documented. Drug interactions are uncommon, but data on cyclosporin interaction is conflicting. Although its role in IPA has not been extensively studied, reports do suggest efficacy comparable to AB[165,166], making itraconazole a possible alternative and therapeutic choice in patients unable to tolerate AB. In view of reports of antagonism[167], the role of combination treatment with AB remains to be clarified. Other investigation/experimental azoles with anti-*Aspergillus* activity include saperconazole, the cyclic lipopeptides which inhibit the crucial cell wall enzyme 1,3,β glucan synthetase such as cilofungin (but causes metabolic acidosis), allylamines, which inhibit squalene epoxidase dependent sterol synthesis and pentaene macrolides such as faerifungin[168].

5-flucytosine is a fluorinated pyrimidine, initially developed as a cytotoxic drug for leukaemia whose antifungal mechanism is due to inhibition of DNA synthesis (via the 5-fluorouracil and 5-fluorodeoxyuridine intermediates). It can be given orally or intravenously at a daily dosage of 150–200 mg/kg in four divided doses. Dose reduction is necessary in patients with renal dysfunction. It has high bioavailability. Gastrointestinal side-effects of nausea, vomiting and diarrhoea, occur in up to 18% of patients particularly with the oral form and which may be prevented by giving each dosage of the drug in divided aliquots at 5-minute intervals. Haematological side-effects, particularly dose-dependent bone marrow suppression due to the toxic intermediary fluorouracil, are particularly worrying, since many patients already have bone marrow suppression. Ideally serum level monitoring should be done to maintain the levels within a therapeutic range of 25–100 μg/ml and thereby decrease the incidence of toxicity. Other side effects include dose-dependent hepatotoxicity (liver cell necrosis has been described). The use of flucytosine in aspergillosis may be rather limited by the resistance of the organism, though combination therapy with other antifungals has sometimes shown synergism[158,159,169].

Rifampicin is often used in patients failing to respond to AB, this antibiotic used alone has no antifungal activity. AB permits rifampicin to cross the damaged fungal cytoplasmic membrane. *In vitro* and a few *in vivo* studies suggests synergism[159].

Candidal respiratory tract infection

Candidal lung disease is rare but of increasing importance because of a rising incidence and challenges for diagnosis and management.

Candida organisms are Gram-positive, round/oval unicellular fungi, approximately 5μ in diameter which grow by budding. The buds or blastoconidia do not separate but produce a cell chain called a pseudohypha. These pseudophypae can be differentiated from true hyphae by 'nipping' of the walls at the cell interfaces in comparison with the strictly parallel walls in true hyphae. They are usually identified by microscopy of KOH treated (to disrupt epithelium) material. *Candida albicans*, the commonest in human disease, can be differentiated by the formation of tubular projections called germ tubes (Fig. 16.13). Various fermentation requirements and products characterise different *Candida* spp. In addition to *C. albicans* only nine of well over a hundred *Candida* spp. are important human pathogens: *Candida krusei*, *Candida parapsilosis*, *Candida tropicalis*, *Candida pseudotropicalis*, *Candida stellatoidea*, *Candida lusitaniae*, *Candida rugosa*, *Candida guilliermondii* and *Torulopsis* (*Candida*) *glabrata*.

Candida spp. are found in soil, food, colonising the gastrointestinal tract, skin and the hospital environment. Evidence has accrued that candidal infections are playing an increasing role in the nosocomial infectious arena of high risk patients, particularly those in intensive care and those with host immune defects, particularly granulocytopenia. Thus, over 50% of patients dying with invasive mycoses have *Candida* spp. isolated[68]. In addition, there is an increasing contribution of the non-albicans spp. to disease[170,171], for example, *C. tropicalis*[172], *T. glabrata*[145], *C. parapsilosis*[173], and *C. krusei*[174]. In a large centre in the USA in 1992, *C. parapsilosis*, *C. tropicalis* and *T. glabrata* accounted for 70% of all *Candida* isolates compared to 13% in 1987[175]. Importance of the non-*albicans* spp. includes resistance to amphotericin B, e.g. with *C. lusitaniae*, resistance to fluconazole, e.g. *T. glabrata* and variable pathogenecity, for example, *C. parasilopsis* is less and *C. tropicalis* is more virulent than *C. albicans*.

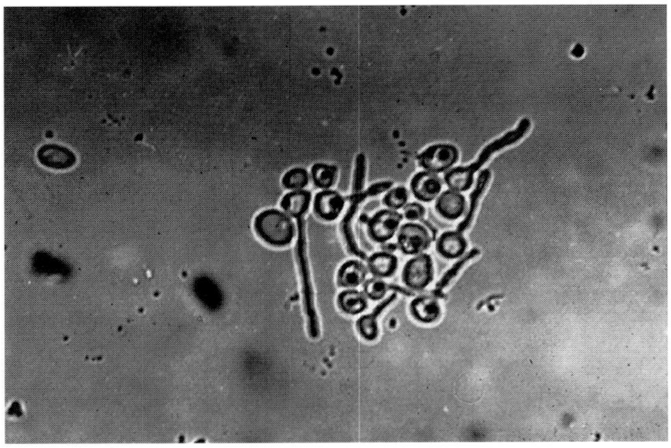

FIGURE 16.13 *Candida albicans*: germ tubes. (Courtesy of Dr S. M. Hussein Qadri.)

In the context of the clinical spectrum of *Candida* infection, pathological involvement of the respiratory tract is one of the least common, despite the high incidence (approximately 25%) colonisation of the respiratory tract. Among autopsies from cancer centres the incidence of primary candidal pneumonia is of the order of 0.2% to 1%[176].

There is considerable controversy concerning the role that azoles have to play in selecting out species of *Candida* other than *C. albicans*. Some countries have reported an increased incidence of non-*albicans* spp. following widespread institutional usage of azoles[175], whilst others have not demonstrated such a phenomenon[177].

Host factors which predispose to severe candidal infections include (i) disruption of the mechanical skin or mucosal barrier. This occurs in in burns patients, those with extensive abdominal surgery, in patients with intravenous lines (hyperalimentation is an additional risk factor)[178], bladder catheterisation, intravenous drug abuse and in haematological patients with critically damaged gastrointestinal tract mucosal surfaces; (ii) disturbance of normal gastrointestinal tract flora by broad spectrum antibiotics; (iii) neutropenia induced by chemotherapy or secondary to leukaemia – since phagocytosis by engulfing and killing organisms is a major line of defence against tissue invasion and dissemination; (iv) qualitative neutrophil dysfunction – either severe such as occurs in chronic granulomatous disease or mild such as antimicrobial mediated neutrophil dysfunction as occurs with aminoglycosides, tetracyclines, sulphonamides or secondary to corticosteroid therapy and diabetes mellitus; (v) impaired cell-mediated immunity, responsible for preventing severe mucocutaneous infections, such as occurs in patients on steroids, HIV disease and those taking cyclosporin A; (vi) humoral defects including complement deficiencies and hypoimmunoglobulinaemia. In a few patients, however, no obvious predisposing factors can be identified[179].

A number of key virulence factors operate in antagonism to the host defence system. These include (i) germ tube formation which permits the organism to resist polymorph killing; (ii) production of enzymes including proteases which have lytic activity against keratinocytes and permit invasion and phospholipases which have epithelial penetrating properties; (iii) enhanced adhesion in a hyperglycaemic milieu such as diabetes mellitus.

In an appropriate situation therefore, entry of *Candida* spp. is facilitated from the skin, oropharynx and gastrointestinal tract. The more heavily these sites are colonised, the more likely the chance of invasive *Candida* infection[180]. It is particularly the hyphal phase of *Candida* which invades mucosal cells. Candidaemia then occurs which may culminate in spontaneous resolution (aided by removal of an accessible primary focus such as an intravenous line), multiorgan dissemination (including the skin, retina, central nervous system, endocardium, joints, kidneys, liver, spleen and the lung), or the patient may develop overwhelming fungal sepsis.

The major portal of entry for pulmonary candidal infection is therefore the skin or gastrointestinal tract from which haematogenous dissemination to the lungs occurs[181]. The respiratory tract is in general not usually a source for candidal invasion either of the lung *per se* or as a focus of haematogenous dissemination, despite the high frequency with which respiratory tract colonisation occurs. However, patients with a major risk for lung aspiration who are prone to vomiting and aspiration may then develop primary or bronchogenic candidal pneumonia[176,182]. These include neonates or the foetus which may acquire candidal pneumonia perinatally as a result of maternal vaginal candidiasis or even intrauterine from chorioamniitis, patients with malignancy or debilitation or chronic disease, the aged, or recipients of lung transplant.

Candida can either colonise the respiratory tract without tissue invasion or produce infection involving the larynx, epiglottis, bronchial tree and pulmonary tree[182]. Histologically, candidal pneumonia shows a spectrum of changes[176]. Thus, bronchopneumonia, intra-alveolar haemorrhage and exudates, focal lung abscesses associated with small limited adjacent areas of lung destruction and haemorrhage (in contrast to more extensive and severe involvement in *Aspergillus* lung disease), are the commonest. The inflammatory response is also diverse with polymorph, histiocytic or granulomatous lesions. Occasionally there may be no inflammatory response to the organism particularly in the immunocompromised[176,182].

High risk patients are therefore mainly those with cancer, haematological malignancy transplant recipients, those with long-term indwelling intravenous lines, burns patients, those having major and repeated abdominal surgery and others with reduced host defence factors as described. Among patients undergoing marrow transplantation, increased age, acute graft vs. host disease and donor mismatch are particular risk factors for invasive candidal infection[183]. In a neutropenic setting patients with haematological malignancies who are also receiving prophylactic antibiotics, the risk of invasive candidiasis is five-fold higher in patients with multiple colonised non-contiguous body sites compared to non-colonised patients[184]. Among neonates, particularly preterm infants, a high index of suspicion for candidal pneumonia is required[185,186].

The more common manifestations[176,187] of *Candida* respiratory infections include bronchitis, laryngitis, epiglottitis, mycetoma, lung abscesses and pneumonia. Pneumonia may present with non-specific features including fever, cough, chest pain, tachypnoea and altered mental status. Often, the presence of extrapulmonary features overshadows the respiratory tract presentation. Candidaemia may persist for several days prior to pulmonary seeding in the haematogenous aetiological situation[181]. Chest radiographic appearances may be normal initially[181]. When established disease is present, fine bilateral nodular infiltrates and/or interstitial/alveolar infiltrates will be seen. Lobar/non-lobar, segmental/non-segmental, distribution can also be found (Fig. 16.14)[187]. Although cavitation may be present, it occurs less commonly compared to other invasive fungi particularly aspergillosis[187]. The radiological pattern, however, is not specific. In addition, there may be features to suggest disseminated candidiasis, e.g. red nodular skin lesions with central necrosis, unilateral retinal exudates, meningoencephalitis/focal brain abscesses, endocarditis, septic arthritis and hepatosplenomegaly.

The diagnosis of *Candida* pneumonia should ideally be confirmed by lung biopsy (open, transbronchial or transthoracic), to demonstrate tissue invasion. However, many patients are too ill to undergo this procedure and diagnosis must depend upon the appropriate clinical setting, absence of other causes for the pneumonia and demonstration of hyphal forms obtained from the distal bronchial tree by protected specimen techniques. The presence of multiple body site colonisation in a high risk patient with appropriate clinical signs may provide good circumstancial evidence for invasive candidiasis[188]. Blood cultures are positive in approximately 50% of cases of disseminated candidiasis. The yield may be increased with improved laboratory techniques which include lysis centrifugation[189], use of vented systems, quantitative colony counting, prolonged incubation and the use of different markers for microbial growth, e.g. carbon dioxide production, gas consumption, fluorescent pH and redox probes. Rapid identification of *Candida* spp. at colonial level has been possible using differential colour media.

The usefulness of serological diagnosis is severely limited particularly with respect to antibody production, in terms of poor sensitivity and delayed sero-conversion. Detection of antibodies towards major cytoplasmic antigens, mannan, the pseudohyphae and germling protoplasts have all had variable or unvalidated results. The epitope LKVIRKIV has been found to be immunodominant in patients recovering from systemic candidiasis[190] and could be used as a prognostic marker. Detection of specific antigens namely mannan[191] cytoplasmic protein and heat labile glycoprotein antigens by EIA, RIA and latex agglutination are showing some promise[192]. Production of antibodies to candidal enolase[193] and heat shock protein 90[194] has made it possible to explore the usefulness of detection of these antigens, but sensitivity and specificity can be low. High level molecular biological techniques such as the use of PCR for detecting *Candida* DNA and BAL are proving exquisitely sensitive. For example, detection of the portion of the gene encoding lanosterol 14α demethylase at a sensitivity of 100 organisms/ml can now be accomplished[195]. Others include the detection of fungus specific metabolites such as D arabinitol[196]. Detection of virulence molecular markers such as aspartyl-proteinase might serve to differentiate colonising from invasive strains. Electrophoretic karyotype patterns, pulse field electrophoresis, DNA fingerprinting and restriction length polymorphism analysis allows biotyping of *C. albicans*.

However, these techniques are not generally available and need to

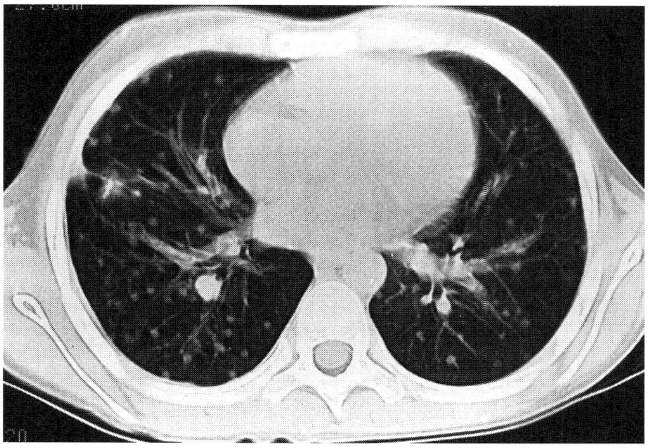

FIGURE 16.14 11 year-old with AML in relapse and neutropenic fever. Multiple round lesions of *Candida* spp. throughout most lung segments.

be validated in clinical practice. Therefore, the diagnosis is often one of probable candidal pneumonia in at-risk patients, and as such is often overdiagnosed, although disseminated candidiasis, on the other hand, is often only diagnosed postmortem[68,197].

Treatment of candidal pneumonia involves removal of any source such as infected intravascular lines, improvement of neutropenia, optimisation of nutritional status and systemic antifungals. The outcome of candidal pneumonia is generally poor particularly in patients with underlying malignancies[198]. Patients with lesser degrees of immunodeficiency fare relatively better[199]. Overall, the mortality of disseminated candidiasis is of the order of 25–40%. Amphotericin B is the mainstay and first choice treatment. Approximately 2–3 g are administered over 2–3 weeks. This may be combined with 5-flucytosine or rifampicin particularly in patients who are severely ill, in patients with complicated disease such as lung abscess[178,200] or in patients with disseminated candidiasis, since *in vitro* synergy may translate into increased survival[201,202]. Itraconazole or fluconazole are alternative therapies. In general, the older azole ketoconazole is inferior to amphotericin B and probably to the newer azoles, has a high toxic profile and inconstant bioavailability. Fluconazole alone has been demonstrated to be successful in the treatment of hepatosplenic candidiasis[169]. Experience of its use in candidal pneumonia is somewhat limited. Therefore, fluconazole or itraconazole should be used only in specific circumstances, for example, those patients in which amphotericin B resistant *Candida* spp. have been isolated, in patients in whom clinical deterioration occurs despite the use of other antifungals or in which there is unacceptable toxicity with other antifungals. Severe infections due to tolerant *C. parapsilosis* have been treated with the newer azoles including fluconazole[203]. An alternative approach in difficult cases with resistant organisms is to combine amphotericin B with flucytosine and this may be effective, for example in abating recalcitrant *C. albicans* fungaemia in which the organism is resistant to amphotericin B[204]. *T. glabrata* associated with pneumonia in the immunocompromised host[205] may prove problematical for effective treatment even with the combination of amphotericin B and flucytosine. The increasing number of systemic infections with fluconazole resistant *C. krusei* poses a problem for effective antifungal treatment[176]. Novel antifungal agents including lipid preparations of amphotericin B[206], the echinocandins and others[168] are being tested. Clinical studies of innovative dosing regimes such as sequential administration of antifungals are in their infancy.

Immunomodulatory therapy with growth factors does reduce the duration of neutropenia and improves the quality of function of neutrophils but to date there has been no demonstrable clinical impact on established candidal infections.

There is considerable debate surrounding the issue of susceptibility testing for *Candida* spp. In general, laboratory standards are improving in this area and this is now technically feasible[207]. Most physicians involved in the management of patients with deep candidal infection would support species identification and susceptibility testing particularly since the number of species of *Candida* having increased MICs has increased in recent years[175].

In recent years, emphasis has been given to the prophylaxis of candidal and other fungal infections particularly with fluconazole, itraconazole and parenteral amphotericin B. In patients undergoing bone marrow transplantation, Goodman *et al.* in a key paper established that fluconazole significantly reduced systemic fungal infections compared to a placebo group and that there were statistically fewer deaths ascribed to acute fungal infections in the group receiving fluconazole[145]. Broadly similar results for fluconazole have also been shown by other investigators[146,147]. However, not all studies have shown uniformly similar results. This probably reflects differences in the patient population studied, intra-study variation in fluconazole dosages and different methodologies. There have been several other controlled and non-controlled studies which have been reviewed[208]. Only two prospective controlled studies have been performed with amphotericin B in at-risk patients[143,144]. One study[144] did show a reduction in early systemic fungal infections in bone marrow transplant recipients but was not confirmed by the other[143].

A change in the distribution of *Candida* spp. following the widespread use of antifungal prophylaxis is being extensively discussed. Thus *C. albicans* was the predominant (87%) species in 1987 but accounted for only 31% of isolates after 5 years of fluconazole use[175]. Use of fluconazole has been associated with an increase in *C. krusei* isolates. However, this experience has not been universally confirmed. For example, from a large Eastern European Cancer Centre the distribution of species has remained unchanged over a similar 5-year period despite widespread fluconazole use[177]. Even in those centres reporting an increased detection of non-albicans *Candida* spp., invasive disease due to these species does not appear to have increased[209,210]. Clearly, there are unknown local factors which strongly influence the colonisation and disease profile. Long-term fluconazole treatment has led to resistant *C. albicans*. This phenomenon is largely confined to AIDS patients[211].

Mucormycosis

Mucormycosis is a general term used to describe the diseases produced by fungi of the Mucorales order. The commonest pathogens are *Rhizopus arrhizus*, *Rhizomucor* spp., *Absidia corymbifera*. Less commonly *Cunninghamella*, *Mortierella*, *Saksenaea*, *Apophysomyces* and *Mucor* spp. are the causative agents. These fungi are ubiquitous, found in decaying organic material, fruit, bread, soil and the hospital environment. Nosocomial outbreaks of mucormycosis sometimes linked to hospital reconstructions have been described[212]. Although they are not fastidious and can grow over an extremely wide temperature range of between 25 °C and 55 °C, they grow best at around 29 °C and in an acid medium. Wide irregular aseptate right angle branching hyphae approximately 15 μ in diameter characterise their appearance in tissue specimens, following KOH treatment and staining with PAS or Grocott-Gomori methenamine silver stains. Culture is more difficult to achieve compared with *Aspergillus* spp. Formation of sporangia spores leads to airbone dissemination.

Inhalation of mucorales spores permits their impaction onto nasal epithelium or pulmonary alveoli. Rarely direct inoculation into the skin in the situations of trauma, burns or contaminated dressings or of the respiratory tract surgery or via the gastrointestinal tract are alternative modes of acquisition. In a suitably susceptible host, rapid tissue invasion occurs.

Effective host defence against Mucorales hinges primarily around the presence of adequate numbers of and functional integrity of bronchoalveolar macrophages and polymorphonuclear leukocytes. Bronchoalveolar macrophages block spore germination perhaps through production of toxic oxygen radicals[213] and defensins, whilst polymorphonuclear leukocytes cover and damage hyphae. Diabetes mellitus results in reduced phagocytic properties of polymorphonuclear leukocytes as well as failure of bronchoalveolar macrophages to prevent spore germination[214,215]. Acidosis but not only the ketocoacidosis associated with uncontrolled diabetes mellitus, but that secondary to other metabolic causes, e.g. methylmalonicaciduria[216] and renal failure, appears to be an important factor. Acidosis may lead to an increase in unbound freely circulating iron which the fungus utilises. Furthermore, patients who receive desferrioxamine treatment are at risk from mucormycosis[217]. Other polymorphonuclear leukocyte deficiency states particularly those induced by corticosteroids, as well as neutropenia contribute towards the pathogenesis of mucormycosis. On occasions no immunological or host defence defect can be recognised[218].

As with invasive aspergillosis, Mucorales have a propensity for direct invasion of major blood vessels resulting in thrombosis, ischaemic necrosis of tissue, adjacent lung infarction and pulmonary haemorrhage which may be severe in thrombocytopenic patients. Pus is often black in colour. Transversing anatomical boundaries may lead to chest wall, pleural or mediastinal involvement.

Clinical presentation

Mucormycosis manifests most often as an upper respiratory tract infection: sinusitis, rhinocerebral mucormycosis (see Chapter 25). Pulmonary disease, cutaneous, gastrointestinal/pelvic, disseminated and miscellaneous forms, e.g. heart involvement are less common. Whereas rhinocerebral mucormycosis/sinusitis usually involves diabetic patients, pulmonary mucormycosis is usually confined to patients who are highly immunocompromised as a result of neutropenia and corticosteroid use. Patients at greatest risk for pulmonary mucormycosis are those with leukaemia or recipients of bone marrow transplantation[219,220]. Patients with solid tumours are at less risk unless they have also received corticosteroids[221]. Pulmonary mucormycosis has also been described in HIV disease[222] and in recipients of renal, heart and other solid organ transplants[223,224]. Occasionally, patients who have lesser degrees of immunosuppression, for example, those who are malnourished particularly patients in the ICU setting[225], those on steroids alone, diabetics or even patients without apparent immunodeficiency[218] may also develop pulmonary disease. This category of patients, however, tends to develop less severe disease[226] and the course is usually more indolent than the usual fulminant course which occurs in leukaemics[227].

Cases of pulmonary mucormycosis may be primary or occur secondary to rhinocerebral mucormycosis or as part of the disseminated picture. The presentation of pulmonary mucormycosis is indistinguishable from aspergillosis – a patient profoundly neutropenic receiving broad spectrum antibiotics develops fever followed by dyspnoea, pleuritic chest pain and haemoptysis as a result of pulmonary infarction or erosion of blood vessels. Haemoptysis may be massive and fatal[228]. Airways obstruction may occur[229]. Respiratory failure may develop. Fistulae connecting bronchi to the chest wall, pleural cavity and other signs may be evident. The course is usually rapid and the final outcome is generally poor with death occurring within a few weeks of diagnosis. Occasionally, indolent or subclinical disease occurs and some cases may only be discovered at autopsy.

Chest radiography may show scattered infiltrates, areas of well-defined consolidation, rounded lesions, cavities resembling primary mycetoma, pleural effusion or changes consistent with pulmonary infarction (Fig. 16.15). In the less severe forms, solitary pulmonary nodules and subacute infiltrates may be found. CT and MRI scanning have been evaluated in the setting of rhinocerebral mucormycosis but its role in pulmonary disease has yet to be delineated.

The specific diagnosis of pulmonary mucormycosis is not easy since the clinical and radiological presentation mimics aspergillosis and other invasive mycoses and no serological tests are clinically available. However, there are a few reports describing the production of antibodies[230]. Cultures of airways secretion are often negative. Positive cultures, whilst not known to be predictive for disease, should not be dismissed as contaminants or colonisation in an appropriate clinical setting. Lung tissue obtained by invasive techniques such as open lung biopsy is the only way of making a firm diagnosis. At bronchoscopy the occasional unusual presentation of endobronchial mucormycosis may be seen.

The mainstay of treatment of mucormycosis involves aggressive surgery and antifungal agents. Removal of pulmonary necrotic tissue is the goal. Residual disease[231] and extrapulmonary lesions should also be resected. Amphotericin B at doses of 1–1.5 mg/kg/day intravenously to provide a total dosage of between 2 and 4 g should be administered. Occasionally, patients with limited disease will respond

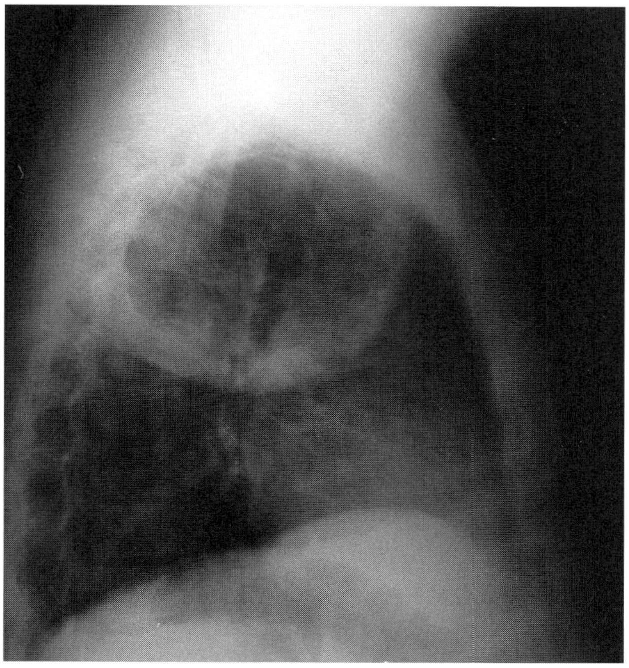

FIGURE 16.15 Renal transplantation. Mucormycosis of right upper lobe: cavitating lesion with surrounding parenchymal compression.

to amphotericin B therapy alone[232] but this approach is not favoured unless the patient has a major contraindication to surgery. The role of higher dose amphotericin B in lipid formulations, e.g. ambisome has not yet been evaluated. Addition of rifampicin, 5-flucytosine or other antifungal agents is an unproven approach[233]. The clinical efficacy of the older azoles such as ketoconazole or miconazole as well as the newer ones such as itraconazole and fluconazole is unknown.

Hyperbaric oxygen is known to be fungistatic and this has been used in rare instances with apparent effect, for example, in one small non-randomised study[234] and as reported in anecdotal case reports[235]. If HBO therapy is available, then it should be employed as adjunctive therapy. Ideally a multicentre prospective study is required to assess efficacy.

Correction of the underlying predisposition is important and this involves reduction of the dosage of immunosuppressant drugs and steroids, correction of neutropenia and restoration of a normal pH.

The outcome is generally guarded with an overall mortality rate approaching 90%. The prognosis, however, is better in patients without neutropenia. Approximately 50% of these patients would be expected to respond. The poor prognosis is possibly related to delay in diagnosis as well as to the underlying disease process.

Pseudallescheriasis

Pseudallescheria boydii grows easily on regular laboratory media and best at 30 °C to 37 °C. There are different morphological forms: the perfect or sexual form is *P. boydii* and the imperfect or asexual form is called *Scedosporium* (or *Monosporium*) *apiospermum*. Hyphae are thin, septated and may display dichotomous branching. In general, histopathological examination fails to differentiate *P. boydii* from *Aspergillus* spp. and other similar fungi. However, *P. boydii* produces asexual conidia. Culture of clinical specimen is necessary for definitive diagnosis.

P. boydii is found widely in soil, sewage, manure and polluted water. Although most infections are traumatically acquired in temperate regions and manifest as subcutaneous mycetomas often associated with sinus tracts, the respiratory tract is the next common site. Infection is usually acquired through the inhalational route. In this regard, *P. boydii* infections imitate *Aspergillus* spp. infections. Being of low virulence thoracic disease expression for the main part is entirely dependent on predisposing host factors and are virtually identical to those described for pulmonary aspergillosis. Disseminated disease is also part of the clinical spectrum. One well-established mode of acquisition occurs in patients who have aspirated polluted water. Near drowning scenarios have led to pulmonary and disseminated infection even in normal individuals because of the large inoculum[236].

In patients who are immunocompetent but have a background history of chronic lung disease or a past history of lung disease such as sarcoid or cancer who may or may not be treated with steroid therapy[237] or who have lung cavities[238], colonisation is the most frequent pulmonary infection described[239]. Invasive pneumonia is described but is exceptional in these types of patients. Fungus ball formation, indistinguishable radiographically and clinically from that due to *Aspergillus* spp. is well described[240]. Invasive pulmonary disease with consolidation, solitary nodules, necrotising pneumonia and abscess formation occurs almost exclusively in highly immunocompromised patients particularly those with haematological malignancy, neutropenia, steroid treatment and organ transplantation[239,241]. Dissemination to the central nervous system, heart, eyes, kidneys, bones and joints may occur. *P. boydii* sinusitis also occurs[242] sometimes in normal individuals or else in patients with some degree of immunocompromisation, for example, diabetes and leukaemia. Bony erosion with extension to the central nervous system may ensue.

Diagnosis depends on culture. Serology has not been extensively studied but precipitating antibodies may be detected[243]. Treatment involves resectional surgery as the main approach[237,244] supported by systemic antifungal therapy. Surgery is particularly useful in localised or cavitary lung disease. Amphotericin B and 5-flucytosine display limited efficacy, possibly due to the high MICs. However, ongoing problems of standardising and interpreting laboratory data for such moulds may well cloud this issue. Most reports appear to suggest that miconazole[245] or perhaps ketoconazole[237] are antifungals of choice. Experience with the other azoles including fluconazole and itraconazole is extremely limited.

Sporotrichosis

Sporothrix schenckii is a dimorphic fungus growing at 25 °C on Sabouraud's medium producing branching hyphae 2 μ in diameter, septated with conidiophore bearing conidia. However, at 37 °C in carbon dioxide 4 μ ovoid yeast like cells are produced that may be confused with *Candida* spp.

S. schenckii is found globally in soil, wood, plants and sphagnum moss. Exposure to these sources or to infected cats presents a risk for acquisition. Localised nodular subcutaneous or ulcerated skin lesions following trauma is the most common presentation. Lymphangitis leading to multiple cutaneous lesions may occur. Haematogenous spread to deeper organs, bones, joints, kidneys, central nervous system, muscles, etc. including widespread disseminated disease occurs uncommonly. Inhalation of spores is thought to lead to primary pulmonary disease[246,247]. Alternatively, haematogenous dissemination from an extrapulmonary source can seed the lungs. The lungs can themselves act as a focus leading to haematogenous dissemination.

Pulmonary disease usually occurs in normal individuals though a history of alcoholism is frequent[248]. Underlying malignancy, immunosuppressive therapy, organ transplantation or HIV has also been described in patients with disseminated disease[249–251].

Pulmonary disease may be asymptomatic but usually presents as a TB-like picture with chronic productive cough, slight fever, weight loss, anorexia, malaise and a chest radiograph usually showing unilateral or bilateral nodules or cavities in the apical upper lobes[246,247]. Other radiographical findings include hilar lymphadenopathy, pulmonary infiltrates, pleural effusion and fungus ball formation. There may be associated features of extrapulmonary involvement particularly the skin.

Diagnosis is based initially on clinical suspicion, for example, in a patient with a provisional diagnosis of pulmonary tuberculosis who fails to respond to anti-tuberculous therapy. The organism may be visualised with some difficulty in sputum or lung tissue using a variety of stains including Gram's, methenamine silver or fluorescent antibody techniques. Culture is the sure way of diagnosis. Sporotrichosis agglutination and complement fixation tests are available but there is a significant rate of false-negativity. Skin testing is not commonly available and lacks specificity.

The optimal management involves a combination of resectional surgery with amphotericin B (total dosage 2–2.5 g). Cure rates of the order of 80% are possible with such a combined approach compared to only 50% with medical treatment alone[246,252]. Potassium iodide as a saturated solution has been used for skin sporotrichosis but has no effect in pulmonary disease[246]. The experience with ketoconazole, miconazole or itraconazole is rather limited in pulmonary disease. Failure in cutaneous forms have been reported using these azoles.

Fusariosis

Previously *Fusarium* spp. caused mainly nail, corneal and cutaneous infections and also gastrointestinal symptomatology associated with aplastic anaemia (toxic alimentary aleukia). Over the last 20 years, however, disseminated deep tissue infections occurring almost exclusively in profoundly and protracted granulocytopenic immunocompromised hosts testifies to its role as an emergent pathogen[253]. Of the 60 species in this genus, *F. solani*, *F. oxysporum*, and *F. verticilloides* are the commonest found in human disseminated clinical disease.

Acquisition is by the inhalational or subcutaneous routes (Fig. 16.16). Occasionally immunocompetent patients develop disseminated fusarial infections, e.g. secondary to burns[254].

Angioinvasion and subcutaneous tissue necrosis is similar to that found in infections due to *Aspergillus* spp. and in mucormycosis. Blood cultures are often positive. Rapidly progressive erythematous maculopapular skin lesions which evolve to necrosis are found in 75% of patients. These two last features are points of contrasts with infections due to *Aspergillus* spp. Dissemination to other organs is common. The fungal elements on biopsy are often mistaken for *Aspergillus*.

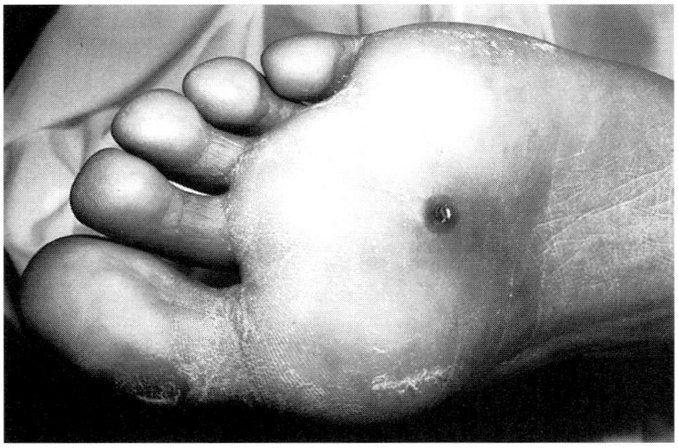

FIGURE 16.16 Source of *Fusarium* infection (plantar needle stick) in neutropenic patient.

The lungs are involved in about 20% of cases and the sinuses in 6%[253]. Treatment is with high dose amphotericin B, although there is variable susceptibility and failure in murine models has been documented[255]. In addition, fusarial infections have developed even in patients receiving prophylactic amphotericin B[256]. Liposomal amphotericin B may be successful as salvage treatment[257]. Addition of rifampicin is synergistic. Despite this, the mortality of fusarial infections in the immunocompromised host is at least of the order of 60% to 70%. It is higher in patients with persistent neutropenia and correction of the neutropenia is mandatory for cure. Excision of early accessible foci is strongly advised to prevent dissemination[258,259].

Trichosporon beigelii

T. beigelii, which usually produces hair infection in the immunocompetent together with *Trichosporon capitatum* have been described as producing pulmonary lesions in the immunocompromised[260,261]. Radiographical appearances are similar to aspergillosis (Fig. 16.17). Maculopapular skin lesions or evidence of widespread organ dissemination may be present. This infection is often unrecognised premortem unless tissue is obtained for histology and culture. The cross reaction which occurs in the *Cryptococcus neoformans* antigen agglutination test producing a false positive result for *Cryptococcus* infection may be a useful diagnostic tool. Treatment is with amphotericin B but a mortality rate of the order of 80% is usual for the disseminated form.

Malassezia infections

Fungaemia due to *Malassezia furfur* and *Malassezia pachydermatis*, associated with lipid/TPN infusions and related to intravenous catheter infection has been described in preterm, malnourished infants and also in adults[262–264].

This has been associated with interstitial pneumonitis in several instances and sometimes associated with concurrent infection with *pneumocystis* or *Pseudomonas*.

The organism's growth is dependent on lipids. The organism can

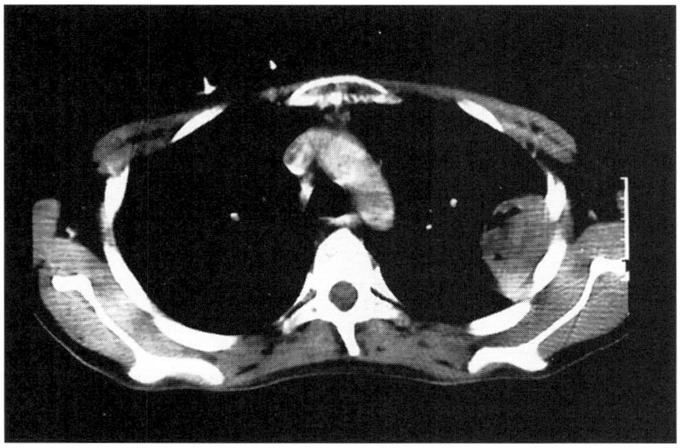

FIGURE 16.17 Pleural-based lesion of *Trichosporon beigelii*.

be cultured from (catheter) blood. Management involves discontinuation of lipids, catheter removal and amphotericin B or fluconazole. The mortality rate is high for patients with pulmonary infection.

Penicillium infections

P. marneffii appears to occur in patients who are residents of Southeast Asia or in non-Asian visitors to those endemic areas. It can produce disseminated, pulmonary or endocardial disease in the immunocompetent including HIV-positive individuals, intravenous drug abusers, patients with lymphoma and acute lymphoblastic leukaemia. It can also occur after cardiac valve replacement. Molluscum contagiosum-like skin lesions may accompany the picture[265,266].

Rare fungi

Other rare opportunistic fungi which have produced disseminated or deeply invasive infections which have included documentation of lung involvement in the immunocompromised host include *Acremonium* spp.[267], *Paecilomyces* spp.[268], *Scopulariopsis*[269], *Alternaria* spp.[270], *Cladosporum* spp.[271], *Bipolaris* spp.[272], *Curvularia* spp.[273], and *Chaetomium* spp.[274].

References

1. RHAME FS. Prevention of nosocomial aspergillosis. *J Hosp Infect* 1991;18:466–72.
2. ARNOW PM, ANDERSON RL, MAINOUS PD *et al.* Pulmonary aspergillosis during hospital renovation. *Am Rev Resp Dis* 1978;118:49–53.
3. WALDORF AR Pulmonary defence mechanisms against opportunistic fungal pathogens. *Immunol Ser* 1989;47:243–71.
4. GERSON SL, TALBOT GH, HURWITZ S, STROM BL, LUSK EJ, CASSILETH PA. Prolonged granulocytopenia: the major risk factor for invasive pulmonary aspergillosis in patients with acute leukaemia. *Ann Intern Med* 1984;100:345–51.
5. PALMER LB, GREENBERG HE, SCHIFF MJ. Corticosteroid treatment as a risk factor for invasive aspergillosis in patients with lung disease. *Thorax* 1991;46:15–20.
6. REIJULA KE, KURUP VP, KUMAR A, FINK JN. Monoclonal antibodies bind identically to both spores and hyphae of *Aspergillus fumigatus*. *Clin Exp Allerg* 1992;22:547–53.
7. STURTEVANT J, LATGE JP. Participation of complement in the phagocytosis of the conidia of *Aspergillus fumigatus* by human polymorphonuclear cells. *J Infect Dis* 1992; 166:580–6.
8. SINGH N, YU VL, RIHS JD. Invasive aspergillosis in AIDS. *South Med J* 1991;84:822–7.
9. DALY AL, VELAZQUEZ LA, BRADLEY LA, KAUFMAN CA. Mucormycosis: association with desferoxamine therapy. *Am J Med* 1989;87:468–71.
10. RHODES JC, AMLUNG TW, MILLER MS. Isolation and characteristic of an elastinolytic proteinase from *Aspergillus flavus*. *Infect Immun* 1990;58:2529–34.
11. KOTHARY MH, CHASE T JR, MACMILLAN JD. Correlation of elastase production by some strains of *Aspergillus fumigatus* with ability to cause pulmonary invasive aspergillosis in mice. *Infect Immun* 1984;43:320–5.
12. HOLDEN DW, TANG CM, SMITH JM. Molecular genetics of *Aspergillus* pathogenicity. *Antonie van Leeuwenhoek* 1994;65:251–5.
13. FULLER CJ. Farmer's lung. *Dis Chest* 1962;42:176–80.
14. ROBERTS RC, WENZEL FJ, EMANUEL DA. Precipitating antibodies in the Midwest dairy farming population toward antigens associated with farmer's lung disease. *J Allergy Clin Immunol* 1976;57:518–24.
15. GREENBERGER PA, PATTERSON R. Diagnosis and management of allergic bronchopulmonary aspergillosis. *Ann Allerg* 1986;56:444.
16. HINSON KFW, MOON AJ, PLUMMER NS. Bronchopulmonary aspergillosis. A review and a report of eight new cases. *Thorax* 1952;7:317–33.
17. ROSENBERG M, PATTERSON, R, MINTZER R, COOPER BJ, ROBERTS M, HARRIS KE. Clinical immunologic criteria for the diagnosis of allergic bronchopulmonary aspergillosis. *Ann Intern Med* 1977;86:405–14.
18. WAXMAN JE, SPECTOR JG, SALE SR, KATZENSTEIN A. Allergic-*Aspergillus* sinusitis: concepts in diagnosis and treatment of a new clinical entity. *Laryngoscope* 1987;97:261–6.
19. HARTWICK RW, BATSAKIS JG. Sinus aspergillosis and allergic fungal sinusitis. *Ann Otol Rhinol Laryngol* 1991;100:427–30.
20. SULAVIK SB. Bronchocentric granulomatosis and allergic bronchopulmonary aspergillosis. *Clin Chest Med* 1988;9:609–21.
21. RILEY DJ, MACKENZIE JW, UHLMAN WE, EDELMAN NH. Allergic bronchopulmonary aspergillosis: evidence of limited tissue invasion. *Am Rev Resp Dis* 1975;111:232–6.
22. KEMPER CA, HOSTETLER JS, FOLLANSBEE SE *et al.* Ulcerative and plaque-like tracheobronchitis due to infection with *Aspergillus* in patients with AIDS. *Clin Infect Dis* 1993;17:344–52.
23. KAUFFMAN HF, TOMEE JF, VAN DER WERF TS, DE MONCHY JF, KOETER GK Review of fungus-induced asthmatic reactions. *Am J Resp Crit Care Med* 1995;151:2109–15.
24. MURALI PS, KRUP VP, GREENBERGER PA, FINK JN. Concanavalin a non-binding *Aspergillus fumigatus* antigen: a major immunogen in allergic bronchopulmonary aspergillosis. *J Lab Clin Med* 1992;119:377–84.
25. PATTERSON R, GREENBERGER PA, HALMO JM *et al.* Allergic bronchopulmonary aspergillosis. Natural history and classification of early disease by serologic and roentgenographic studies. *Arch Intern Med* 1973;54:16–21.
26. MCCARTHY D, PEPYS J. Allergic bronchopulmonary aspergillosis. Clinical immunology: clinical features. *Clin Allergy* 1971;1:261–86.
27. SAFIRSTEIN BH, DISOUZA MF, SIMON G *et al.* Five year follow-up of allergic bronchopulmonary aspergillosis. *Am Rev Resp Dis* 1973;108:450–9.
28. MALO J, PEPYS J, SIMON G Studies in chronic allergic bronchopulmonary aspergillosis. 2. Radiological findings. *Thorax* 1977;36:262–8.
29. CURRIE DC, GOLDMAN JM, COLE PF, STRICKLAND B. Comparison of narrow section computed tomography and plain chest radiography in chronic allergic bronchopulmonary aspergillosis. *Clin Rad* 1987;38:593–6.
30. NEELD DA, GOODMAN LR, GURNEY JW, GREENBERGER PA, FINK JN. Computerized tomography in the evaluation of allergic bronchopulmonary aspergillosis. *Am Rev Resp Dis* 1990;142:1200–5.
31. TRAVIS WD, KWON-CHUNG KJ, KLEINER DE *et al.* Unusual aspects of allergic bronchopulmonary fungal disease: report of two cases due to *Curvularia* organisms associated with allergic fungal sinusitis. *Hum Pathol* 1991;22:1240–8.

32. LAKE FR, FROUDIST JH, MCALEER R *et al.* Allergic bronchopulmonary fungal disease caused by bipolaris and curvularia. *Aust NZ J Med* 1991;21:871–4.

33. MILLER MA, GREENBERGER PA, AMERICAN R *et al.* Allergic bronchopulmonary mycosis caused by *Pseudallescheria boydii Am Rev Resp Dis* 1993;148:810–2.

34. TRAVIS WD, KWON-CHUNG KJ, KLEINER DE *et al.* Unusual aspects of allergic bronchopulmonary fungal disease: report of two cases due to *Curvularia* organisms associated with allergic fungal sinusitis. *Human Path* 1991;22:1240–8.

35. TURNER ES, GREENBERGER PA, SIDER L. Complexities of establishing an early diagnosis of allergic bronchopulmonary aspergillosis in children. *Allergy Proc* 1989;10:63–9.

36. PATTERSON R, GREENBERGER PA, HALWIG JM *et al.* Allergic bronchopulmonary aspergillosis: natural history and classification of early disease by serologic and radiographic studies. *Arch Intern Med* 1986;146:916–21.

37. GREENBERGER PA, PATTERSON R. Allergic bronchopulmonary aspergillosis and the evaluation of the patient with asthma. *J Allerg Clin Immunol* 1988;81:646–53.

38. HENDERSON AH, ENGLISH MP, VECHT RJ. Pulmonary aspergillosis: a survey of its occurrence in patients with chronic lung disease and a discussion of the significance of diagnostic tests. *Thorax* 1968;23:513–23.

39. PATTERSON R, GREENBERGER PA, RADIN RC, ROBERTS M. Allergic bronchopulmonary aspergillosis: staging as an aid to management. *Ann Intern Med* 1982;96:286–91.

40. CURRIE DC, LUECK C, MILBURN HJ *et al.* Controlled trial of natamycin in the treatment of allergic bronchopulmonary aspergillosis. *Thorax* 1990;45:447–50.

41. FOURNIER EC Trial of ketoconazole in allergic bronchopulmonary aspergillosis. *Thorax* 1987;42:831.

42. SHALE DJ, FAUX JA, LANE DJ. Trial of ketoconazole in non-invasive pulmonary aspergillosis. *Thorax* 1987;42:26–31.

43. BRITISH THORACIC AND TUBERCULOSIS ASSOCIATION. Aspergilloma and residual tuberculous cavities – the results of a resurvey. *Tubercle* 1970;51:227–45.

44. MAGUIRE CP, HAYES JP, HAYES M, MASTERSON J, FITZGERALD MX. Three cases of pulmonary aspergilloma in adult patients with cystic fibrosis. *Thorax* 1995;50:805–6.

45. KIBBLER CC, MILKINS SR, BHAMRA A, SPITERI MA, NOONE P, PRENTICE HG. Apparent pulmonary mycetoma following invasive aspergillosis in neutropenic patients. *Thorax* 1988;43:108–12.

46. SEVERO LC, GEYER GR, PORTO NS. Pulmonary aspergillus intracavitary colonisation. *Mycopathologia* 1990;112:93–104.

47. HAMMERMAN KJ, CHRISTIANSON CS, HUNTINGTON I *et al.* Spontaneous lysis of aspergillomata. *Chest* 1973;64:697–9.

48. RAFFERTY P, BIGGS BA, CROMPTON GK, GRANT IWB. What happens to patients with pulmonary aspergilloma? Analysis of 23 cases. *Thorax* 1983;38:579–83.

49. ROBERTS CM, CITRON KM, STRICKLAND B. Intrathoracic aspergilloma: role of CT in diagnosis and treatment. *Radiology* 1987;165:123–28.

50. SMITH FB, BENECK D. Localised aspergillus infestation in primary lung carcinoma. Clinical and pathological contrasts with post TB intracavitary aspergilloma. *Chest* 1991;100:554–6.

51. TOMEE JF, VAN DER WERF TS, LATGE JP, KOETER GH, DUBOIS AE, KAUFFMAN HF. Serologic monitoring of disease and treatment in a patient with pulmonary aspergilloma. *Am J Resp Crit Care Med* 1995;151:199–204.

52. STANLEY MW, DEIKE M, KNOEDLER J, IBER C. Pulmonary mycetomas in immunocompetent patients: diagnosis by fine–needle aspiration. *Diag Cytopath* 1992;8:577–9.

53. KIBBLER CC, MILKINS SR, BHAMRA A *et al.* Apparent pulmonary mycetoma following invasive aspergillosis in neutropenic patients. *Thorax* 1988;43:108–12.

54. DALY RC, PAIROLERO PC, PIEHLER JM *et al.* Pulmonary aspergilloma: results of surgical treatment. *F Thorac Cardiovasc Surg* 1986;92:981–8.

55. HENZE G, ALDENHOFF P, STEPHANI U *et al.* Successful treatment of pulmonary and cerebral aspergillosis in an immunosuppressed child. *Eur J Pediatr* 1982;138:263–65.

56. RYAN PJ, STABLEFORTH DE, REYNOLDS J, MUHDI KM. Treatment of pulmonary aspergilloma in cystic fibrosis by percutaneous instillation of amphotericin B via indwelling catheter. *Thorax* 1995;50:809–10.

57. CLARKE A, SKELTON J, FRASER RS. Fungal tracheobronchitis. Report of 9 cases and review of the literature. *Medicine* 1991;70:1–14.

58. KRAMER MR, DENNING DW, MARSHALL SE *et al.* Ulcerative tracheobronchitis following lung transplantation: a new form of invasive aspergillosis. *Am Rev Resp Dis* 1991;144:552–6.

59. PERVEZ NK, KLEINERMAN J, KATTAN M *et al.* Pseudomembranous necrotising bronchial aspergillosis: a variant of invasive aspergillosis in a patient with hemophilia and acquired immune deficiency syndrome. *Am Rev Resp Dis* 1985;131:961–3.

60. NICHOLSON AG, SIM KM, KEOGH BF, CORRIN B Pseudomembranous necrotising bronchial aspergillosis complicating chronic airways limitation. *Thorax* 1995;50:807–8.

61. PUTNAM JB, DIGNANI MC, MEHRA RC, ANAISSE EJ, MORICE RC, LIBSHITZ HI. Acute airway obstruction and necrotising tracheobronchitis from invasive mycosis. *Chest* 1994;106:1265–7.

62. PETERSEN PK, MCGLAVE P, RAMSAY NKC *et al.* A prospective study of infectious diseases following bone marrow transplantation: emergence of aspergillus and cytomegalovirus as the major causes of mortality. *Infect Control* 1983;4:81–9.

63. TRITZ DM, WOODS GL. Fatal disseminated infection with *Aspergillus terreus* in immunocompromised hosts. *Clin Infect Dis* 1993;16:118–22.

64. ANDRIOLE VT. Invasive aspergillosis: serologic diagnosis. In Schimpff SC, Klastersky J, eds. *Infectious Complications in Bone Marrow Transplantation: Recent Results in Cancer Research*. Heidelberg: Springer-Verlag; 1993.

65. GERSON SL, TALBOT GH, HURWITZ S *et al.* Prolonged granulocytopoenia: the major risk factor for invasive pulmonary aspergillosis in patients with acute leukaemia. *Ann Intern Med* 1984;100:345–51.

66. WINGARD JR, BEALS SU, SANTOS GW, MERZ WG, SARAL R. *Aspergillus* infections in bone marrow transplant recipients. *Bone Marrow Transpl* 1987;2:175–81.

67. BURCH PA, KARP JE, MERZ WG, KUHLMAN JE, FISHMAN EK. Favourable outcome of invasive aspergillosis in patients with acute leukaemia. *J Clin Oncol* 1987;5:1985–93.

68. BODEY G, BUELTMANN B, DUGUID W *et al.* Fungal infections in cancer patients. An international autopsy survey. *Eur J Clin Microbiol Infec Dis* 1992;11:99–109.

69. ARTIS WM, FOUNTAIN JA, DELCHER HK *et al.* A mechanism of susceptibility to mucormycosis in diabetic ketoacidosis. Transferrin and iron availability. *Diabetes* 1982;31:1109–14.

70. COHEN MS, ISTURICH RE, MALECH HL *et al.* Fungal infection in chronic granulomatous disease. The importance of the phagocyte in defence against fungi. *Am J Med* 1981;71:59–66.

71. DENNING DW, FOLLANSBEE SE, SCOLARO M *et al.* Pulmonary aspergillosis in the acquired immunodeficiency syndrome. *N Engl J Med* 1991;324:654.

72. WALSH TJ, MENDELSOHN G. Invasive aspergillosis complicating Cushing's syndrome. *Arch Intern Med* 1981;141:1227–8.

73. FISHER BD, ARMSTRONG D, YU B, GOLD JWM. Invasive aspergillosis. Progress in early diagnosis and treatment. *Am J Med* 1981;71:571–7.

74. WEILAND D, FERGUSON RM, PETERSON PK *et al.* Aspergillosis in 25 renal transplant patients: epidemiology, clinical presentation, diagnosis and management. *Ann Surg* 1983;198:622.

75. ORR DP, MYEROWITZ RL, DUBOIS PJ. Patho-radiologic correlation of invasive pulmonary aspergillosis in the compromised host. *Cancer* 1978;41:2028–39.

76. MAYER JM, NIMER L, CARROLL K. Isolated pulmonary aspergillar infection in cardiac transplant recipients: case report and review. *Clin Infect Dis* 1992;15:698–700.

77. PALMER LB, GREENBERG HE, SCHIFF MJ. Corticosteroid treatment as a risk factor for invasive aspergillosis in patients with lung disease. *Thorax* 1991;46:15–20.

78. THOMMI G, BELL G, LIU J, NUGENT K. Spectrum of invasive pulmonary aspergillosis in immunocompetent patients with chronic obstructive pulmonary disease. *South Med J* 1991;84:828–31.

79. LENTINO JR, ROSENKRANZ MA, MICHAELS JA *et al.* Nosocomial aspergillosis. A retrospective review of airborne disease secondary to road construction and contaminated air conditioners. *Am J Epidemiol* 1982;116:430–5.

80. OPAL SM, ASP AA, CANNADY PB *et al.* Effect of infection control measures during a nosocomial outbreak of aspergillosis associated with hospital construction. *J Infect Dis* 1986;153:634–7.

81. SARUBBI FA, KOPF HB, WILSON MB *et al.* Increased recovery of *Aspergillus fluvus* from respiratory specimens during hospital construction. *Am Rev Resp Dis* 1982;125:33–8.

82. GERSON SL, TALBOT GH, HURWITZ S, LUSK EJ, STROM BL, CASSILETH PA Discriminant scorecard for diagnosis of invasive pulmonary aspergillosis in patients with acute leukaemia. *Am J Med* 1985;79:57–64.

83. YOUNG RC, BENNETT JE, VOGEL CL, CARBONE PP, DEVITA VT. Aspergillosis: the spectrum of the disease in 98 patients. *Medicine* 1970;49:147–73.

84. SPEARING RL, PAMPHILON DH, PRENTICE AG. Pulmonary aspergillosis in immunosuppressed patients with haematological malignancies. *Quart J Med* 1986;59:611–25.

85. PAGANO L, RICCI P, NOSARI A *et al.* Fatal haemoptysis in pulmonary filamentous mycosis: an underevaluated cause of death in patients with acute leukaemia in haematological complete remission. A retrospective study and review of the literature. Gimema Infection Program (Gruppo Italiano Malattie Ematologiche dell'Adulto). *Br J Haematol* 1995;89:500–5.

86. PENNINGTON JE, FELDMAN NT. Pulmonary infiltrates and fever in patients with hematologic malignancy. *Am J Med* 1977;62:581–7.

87. SINCLAIR AJ, ROSOFF AH, COLTMAN CA. Recognition and successful management in pulmonary aspergillosis in leukaemia. *Cancer* 1978;42:2019–24.

88. KUHLMAN JE, FISHMAN EK, BURCH PA, KARP JE, ZERHOUNI EA, SIEGELMAN SS. Invasive pulmonary aspergillosis in acute leukaemia. *Chest* 1987;92:95–9.

89. KUHLMAN JE, FISHMAN EK, BURGH PA *et al.* Invasive pulmonary aspergillosis in acute leukaemia – the contribution of CT to early diagnosis and aggressive management. *Chest* 1987;92:95–9.

90. KUHLMAN JE, FISHMAN EK, SIEGELMAN SS. Invasive pulmonary aspergillosis in acute leukaemia: characteristic findings on CT, the CT halo sign, and the role of CT in early diagnosis. *Radiology* 1985;157:611–14.

91. KUHLMAN JE, FISHMAN EK, BURCH PA, KARP JE, ZERHOUNI EA, SIEGELMAN SS. CT of invasive pulmonary aspergillosis. *AJR* 1988;150:1015–20.

92. LIBSHITZ HI, PAGANI JJ. Aspergillosis and mucormycosis: two types of opportunistic fungal pneumonia. *Radiology* 1981;140:301–6.

93. DYKHUIZEN RS, KERR KN, SOUTAR RL. Air crescent sign and fatal haemoptysis in pulmonary mucormycosis. Scand *J Infect Dis* 1994;26:498–501.

94. HRUBAN RH, MEZIANE MA, ZERHOUNI EA, WHEELER PS, DUMLER JS, HUTCHINS GM. Radiologic–pathologic correlation of the CT halo sign in invasive pulmonary aspergillosis. *J Comp Ass Tomog* 1987;11:534–6.

95. HEROLD CJ, KRAMER J, SERTL K *et al.* Invasive pulmonary aspergillosis: evaluation with MR imaging. *Radiology* 1989;173:717–21.

96. YU VL, MUDER RR, POORSATTAR A. Significance of isolation of aspergillus from the respiratory tract in diagnosis of invasive pulmonary aspergillosis. Results of a three-year prospective study. *Am J Med* 1986;81:249–54.

97. FISHER BD, ARMSTRONG D, YU B *et al.* Invasive aspergillosis : progress in early diagnosis and treatment. *Am J Med* 1981;71:571–7.

98. NALESNIK MA, MYEROWITZ RL, JENKINS R, LENKEY J, HERBERT D. Significance of *Aspergillus* species isolated from respiratory secretions in the diagnosis of invasive pulmonary aspergillosis. *J Clin Microbiol* 1980;11:370–6.

99. TREGER TR, VISSCHER DW, BARTLETT MS *et al.* Diagnosis of pulmonary infection caused by *Aspergillus* Usefulness of respiratory cultures. *J Infect Dis* 1985;152:572–6.

100. ALBELDA SM, TALBOT GH, GERSON SL, MILLER WT, CASSILETH PA. Role of fiberoptic bronchoscopy in the diagnosis of invasive pulmonary aspergillosis in patients with acute leukaemia. *Am J Med* 1984;76:1027–34.

101. SAITO H, ANAISSIE EJ, MORICE RC, DEKMEZIAN R, BODEY GP. Bronchoalveolar lavage in the diagnosis of pulmonary infiltrates in patients with acute leukaemia. *Chest* 1988;94:745–9.

102. CORDONNIER C, BEMAUDIN JF, BIERLING P, HUET Y, VERNANT JP. Pulmonary complications occurring after allogeneic bone marrow transplantation: a study of 130 consecutive transplanted patients. *Cancer* 1986;58:1047–54.

103. MCWHINNEY PHM, KIBBLER CC, HAMON MD *et al.* Progress in the diagnosis and management of aspergillosis in bone marrow transplantation: 13 years' experience. *Clin Infect Dis* 1993;17:397–404.

104. ELLIS ME, SPENCE D, BOUCHAMA A *et al.* Open lung biopsy provides a higher and more specific diagnostic yield compared to bronchoalveolar lavage in immunocompromised patients. *Scand J Infect Dis* 1995;27:157–62.

105. WONG K, WATERS CM, WALESBY RK. Surgical management of invasive pulmonary aspergillosis in immunocompromised patients. *Eur J Cardiothorac Surg* 1992;6:138–42.

106. YOUNG RC, BENNETT JC. Invasive aspergillosis: absence of detectable antibody response. *Am Rev Resp Dis* 1971;104:710–15.

107. DE REPENTIGNY L, KILANOWSKI E, PEDNEAULT L, BOUSHIRA M Immunoblot analyses of the serological response to *Aspergillus fumigatus* antigens in experimental invasive aspergillosis. *J Infect Dis* 1991;163:1305–11.

108. ROGERS TR, HAYNES KA, BARNES RA. Value of antigen detection in predicting invasive pulmonary aspergillosis. *Lancet* 1990;336:1210–13.

109. WEINER MH, TALBOT GH, STANTON L *et al.* Antigen detection in the diagnosis of invasive aspergillosis. Utility in controlled, blinded trials. *Ann Intern Med* 1983;99:777–82.

110. TALBOT GH, WEINER MH, GERSON SL, PROVENCHER M, HURWITZ S. Serodiagnosis of invasive aspergillosis in patients with hematologic malignancy: validation of the *Aspergillus fumigatus* antigen radioimmunoassay. *J Infect Dis* 1988;152:946–53.

111. TANG CM, HOLDEN DW, AUFAUVRE-BROWN A, COHEN J. The detection of aspergillus spp. by the polymerase chain reaction and its evaluation in bronchoalveolar lavage fluid. *Am Rev Resp Dis* 1993;148:1313–17.

112. BRETAGNE S, COSTA JM, MARMORAT-

KHUONG A *et al.* Detection of aspergillus species DNA in bronchoalveolar lavage samples by competitive PCR. *J Clin Microbiol* 1995;33:1164–8.

113. VERWEIJ PE, LATGE JP, RIJS AJ *et al.* *J Clin Microbiol* 1995; 33:3150–3.

114. BINDER RE, FALING J, PUGATCH RD, MAHASSEN C, SNIDER SL. Chronic necrotising pulmonary aspergillosis: a discrete clinical entity. *Medicine* 1982;61:109–24.

115. WIGGINS J, CLARK TJH, CORRIN B. Chronic necrotising pneumonia caused by *Aspergillus niger*. *Thorax* 1989;44:440–1.

116. ELLIS ME, DOSSING M, AL-HOKAIL A, QADRI SH, HAINAU B, BURNIE J. Progressive chronic pulmonary aspergillosis: a diagnostic and therapeutic challenge. *J Roy Soc Med* 1991;763–4.

117. GEFTER WB, WEINGRAD TR, EPSTEIN DM, OCHS RH, MILLER WT. Semi-invasive pulmonary aspergillosis. *Radiology* 1981;140:313–21.

118. HARGIS JL, BONE, RC, STEWART J *et al.* Intracavitary amphotericin B in the treatment of symptomatic pulmonary aspergillomas. *Am J Med* 1980;68:389–92.

119. RODENHAUS S, BEAUMONT F, KAUFFMAN HF, SLUITER HJ. Invasive pulmonary aspergillosis in a non-immunosuppressed patient: successful management with systemic amphotericin and flucytosine and inhaled amphotericin. *Thorax* 1984;39:78–9.

120. BURCH PA, KARP JE, MERZ WG, KHULMAN JE, FISHMAN EK. Favorable outcome of invasive aspergillosis in patients with acute leukaemia. *J Clin Oncol* 1987;5:1985–93.

121. DE MARIE S, JANKNEGT R, BAKKER-WOUDENBERG IAJM. Clinical use of liposomal and lipid-complexed amphotericin B. *J Antimicrob Chemother* 1994;33:907–16.

122. NG TTC, DENNING DW. Liposomal amphotericin B (AmBisome) therapy in invasive fungal infections. *Arch Intern Med* 1995;155:1093–8.

123. BERENGUER J, MUNOZ P, PARRAS F, FERNANDEZ-BACA V, HERNANDEZ-SAMPELAYO T, BOUZA E. Treatment of deep mycoses with liposomal amphotericin B. *Eur J Clin Microbiol Infect Dis* 1994;13:504–7.

124. TOLLEMAR J, ANDERSSON S, RINGDEN O, TYDEN G. A retrospective clinical comparison between antifungal treatment with liposomal amphotericin B (AmBisome) and conventional amphotericin B in transplant recipients. *Mycoses* 1992;35:215–20.

125. MILLS W, CHOPRA R, LINCH DC, GOLDSTONE AH. Liposomal amphotericin B in the treatment of fungal infections in neutropenic patients: a single-centre experience of 133 episodes in 116 patients. *Br J Haematol* 1994;86:754–60.

126. GRANT-PRENTICE H. New information on AmBisome. Presentation at session VIII. Trends in invasive fungal infection 3. Brussels 1995.

127. DENNING DW, STEVENS DA. Antifungal and surgical treatment to invasive aspergillosis: review of 2,121 published cases. *Rev Infect Dis* 1990;12:1147–1201.

128. BURTON JR, ZACHERY JB, BESSIN R *et al.* Aspergillosis in four renal transplant recipients. Diagnosis and effective treatment with amphotericin B. *Ann Intern Med* 1972;77:383–8.

129. DENNING DW, TUCKER RM, HANSON LH, STEVENS DA. Treatment of invasive aspergillosis with itraconazole. *Am J Med* 1989;86:791–800.

130. SHAFFNER A, FRICK PG. The effect of ketoconazole on amphotericin B in a model of disseminated aspergillosis. *J Infect Dis* 1985;151:902–10.

131. ALBELDA SM, TALBOT GM, GERSON SL, MILLER WT, CASSILETH PA. Pulmonary cavitation and massive haemoptysis in invasive pulmonary aspergillosis. Influence of bone marrow recovery in patients with acute leukaemia. *Am Rev Resp Dis* 1985;131:115–20.

132. LUPINETTI FM, BEHRENDT DM, GILLER RH, TRIGG ME, DE ALARCON P. Pulmonary resection for fungal infection in children undergoing bone marrow transplantation. *J Thorac Cardiovasc Surg* 1992;104:684–7.

133. VOGLER WR, WINTON EF. A controlled study of the efficacy of granulocyte transfusions in patients with neutropoenia. *Am J Med* 1977;63:548–55.

134. HABER RH, ODDONE EZ, GURBEL PA, STEAD WW. Acute pulmonary decompensation due to amphotericin B in the absence of granulocyte transfusions. *N Engl J Med* 1986;315:836–9.

135. ENAISSIE E. Role of colony stimulating factors either as adjuvant treatment with antifungal therapy or to stimulate donors for white cell transfusion. Presentation session VII: trends in invasive fungal infections 3. Brussels 1995.

136. DALE DC. Potential role of colony-stimulating factors in the prevention and treatment of infectious diseases. *Clin Infect Dis* 1994;18:S180–8.

137. OFFNER F. The use of hematopoietic growth factors in cancer patients: indications and impact on invasive fungal infections. Presentation session VII: Trends in invasive fungal infections 3. Brussels 1995.

138. KARP JE, MERZ WG, CHARACHE P. Response to empiric amphotericin B during antileukaemic therapy-induced granulocytopenia. *Rev Infect Dis* 1991;13:592–9.

139. WALSH TJ, RUBIN M, HATHORN J *et al.* Amphotericin B vs high-dose ketoconazole for empirical antifungal therapy among febrile, granulocytopenic cancer patients. *Arch Intern Med* 1991;151:765–70.

140. ROUSEY SR, RUSSLER S, GOTTLIEB M, ASH RC. Low-dose amphotericin B prophylaxis against invasive *Aspergillus* infections in allogeneic marrow transplantation. *Am J Med* 1991;91:484–92.

141. KARP JE, BURCH PA, MERZ WG. An approach to intensive antileukaemia therapy in patients with previous invasive aspergillosis. *Am J Med* 1988;85:203–6.

142. RICHARD C, ROMON I, BARO J *et al.* Invasive pulmonary aspergillosis prior to BMT in acute leukaemia patients does not predict a poor outcome. *Bone Marrow Transpl* 1993;12:237–41.

143. PERFECT JR, KLOTMAN ME, GILBERT CC *et al.* Prophylactic intravenous amphotericin B in neutropenic autologous bone marrow transplant recipients. *J Infect Dis* 1992;165:891–7.

144. RILEY DK, PAVIA AT, BEATTY PG *et al.* The prophylactic use of low-dose amphotericin B in bone marrow transplant patients. *Am J Med* 1994;97:509–14.

145. GOODMAN J, WINSTON DJ, GREENFIELD RA *et al.* A controlled trial of fluconazole to prevent fungal infections in patients undergoing bone marrow transplantation. *N Engl J Med* 1992;326:845–51.

146. WINSTON DJ, CHANDRASEKAR PH, LAZARUS HM *et al.* Fluconazole prophylaxis of fungal infections in patients with acute leukaemia. Results of a randomized placebo-controlled, double-blind, multicenter trial. *Ann Intern Med* 1993;118:495–503.

147. ELLIS ME, CLINK H, ERNST P *et al.* Controlled study of fluconazole in the prevention of fungal infections in neutropenic patients with hematologic malignancies and bone marrow transplant recipients. *Eur J Clin Microbiol Infect Dis* 1994;13:3–11.

148. BODEY GP, ANAISSIE EJ, ELTING LS, ESTEY E, O'BRIEN S, KANTARJIAN H. Antifungal prophylaxis during remission induction therapy for acute leukaemia fluconazole versus intravenous amphotericin B. *Cancer* 1994;73:2099–106.

149. PHILIPOTT-HOWAR JN, WADE JJ, MULTI GJ, BRAMMER KW, EHNINGER G. Randomized comparison of oral fluconazole versus oral polyenes for the prevention of fungal infection in patients at risk of

neutropoenia. *J Antimicrob Chemother* 1993;31:973–84.

150. BODEY GP, ANAISSIE EJ, ELTING LS, ESTEY E, O'BRIEN S, KANTARJIAN H. Antifungal prophylaxis during remission induction therapy for acute leukaemia fluconazole versus intravenous amphotericin B. *Cancer* 1994;73:2099–106.
151. VREUGDENHIL G, VAN DIJKE BJ, DONNELLY JP *et al.* Efficacy of itraconazole in the prevention of fungal infections among neutropenic patients with hematologic malignancies and intensive chemotherapy. A double blind, placebo controlled study. *Leukaemia Lymphoma* 1993;11:353–8.
152. ANDRIOLE VT. Infections with *Aspergillus* species. *Clin Infect Dis* 1993;17:S481–6.
153. KINSKY SC. Antibiotic interaction with model membranes. *Ann Rev Pharmacol* 1970;10:119–42.
154. WILSON E, THARSON L, SPEERT DP. Enhancement of macrophage superoxide anion production by amphotericin B. *Antimicrob Agents Chemother* 1991;35:796–800.
155. OLDFIELD EC 3D., GARST PD, HOSTETTLE RM, WHITE M, SAMUELSON D. Randomised, double-blind trial of 1 versus 4 hr amphotericin B infusion duration. *Antimicrob Agents Chemother* 1990;34:1402–6.
156. ELLIS ME, AL-HOKAIL A, CLINK HM *et al.* Double-blind randomised study of the effect of infusion rates on toxicity of amphotericin B. *Antimicrob Agents Chemother* 1992;36:172–9.
157. LAVER BH, RELLER LB, SCHROTER GPJ. Susceptibility of aspergillus to 5 fluorocytosine and amphotericin B alone and in combination. *J Antimicrob Chemother* 1978;4:375.
158. PARK GR, DRUMMOND GB, LAMB D *et al.* Disseminated aspergillosis occurring in patients with respiratory, renal and hepatic failure. *Lancet* 1982;2:179–84.
159. ARROYO J, MEDOFF G, KOBAYASHI GS. Therapy of invasive aspergillosis with amphotericin B in combination with rifampicin or 5 fluorocytosine. *Antimicrob Agents Chemother* 1977;11:21–5.
160. ADLER-MOORE J. Ambisome targeting to fungal infections. *Bone Marrow Transpl* 1994;14:S3–7.
161. RINGDEN O, MEUNIER F, TOLLEMAR J *et al.* Efficacy of amphotericin B encapsulated in liposomes (Ambisome) in the treatment of invasive fungal infections in immunocompromised patients. *J Antimicrob Chemother* 1991;28:73–82.
162. MEUNIER F, PRENTICE HG, RINGDEN O. Liposomal amphotericin B (Ambisome): safety data from a phase II/III clinical trial. *J Antimicrob Chemother* 1991;28:83–91.
163. SCULIER JP, COUNE A, MEUNIER F *et al.* Pilot study of amphotericin B entrapped in sonicated liposomes in cancer patients with fungal infections. *Eur J Cancer Clin Oncol* 1988;24:527–38.
164. CHOPRA R, BLAIR S, STRANG J *et al.* Liposomal amphotericin B (Ambisome) in the treatment of fungal infections in neutropoenic patients. *J Antimicrob Chemother* 1991;28:93–104.
165. DENNING DW, TUCKER RM, HANSON LH, STEVENS DA. Treatment of invasive aspergillosis with itraconazole. *Am J Med* 1989;86:791–800.
166. VAN'T WOUT JW. Itraconazole in neutropoenic patients. *Chemotherapy* 1992;38:23–6.
167. POLAK A. Combination therapy of experimental candidiasis, cryptococcosis, aspergillosis and wangiellosis in mice. *Chemotherapy* 1987;33:381–95.
168. GEORGOPAPADAKOU NH, WALSH TJ. Human mycoses: drugs and targets for emerging pathogens. *Science* 1994;264:371–3.
169. ANAISSIE K, BODEY GP, KANTARJIAN H *et al.* Fluconazole therapy for chronic disseminated candidiasis in patients with leukaemia and prior amphotericin B therapy. *Am J Med* 1991;91:142–50.
170. HORN R, WONG B, KIEHN TE, ARMSTRONG D. Fungemia in a cancer hospital: changing frequency, earlier onset, and results of therapy. *Rev Infect Dis* 1985;7:645–55.
171. KOMSHIAN SV, UWAYDAH AK, SOBEL JD *et al.* Fungemia caused by *Candida* species and *Torulopsis glabrata* in hospitalised patients. Frequency, characteristics and evaluation of factors influencing outcome. *Rev Infec Dis* 1989:3:379–90.
172. KOMSHIAN SV, UWAYDAH AK, SOBEL JD *et al.* Fungemia caused by *Candida* species and *Torulopsis glabrata* in hospitalised patients. Frequency, characteristics and evaluation of factors influencing outcome. *Rev Infec Dis* 1989:3:379–90.
173. SALO J, RIBERA JM, BLADE J *et al.* Sepsis caused by candida parapsilosis. Joint and lung involvement in 2 patients with acute leukaemia. *Med Clin* 1990;94:58–60.
174. MERZ WG, KARP JE, SCHRON D, SARAL R. Increased incidence of fungaemia caused by *Candida krusei J Clin Microbiol* 1986;24:581–4.
175. PRICE MF, LAROCCO MT, GENTRY LO. Fluconazole susceptibilities of *Candida* species and distribution of species recovered from blood cultures over a 5-year period. *Antimicrob Agents Chemother* 1994;38:1422–24.
176. HARON E, VARTIVARIAN S, ANAISSIE E, DEKMEZIAN R, BODEY GP. Primary candida pneumonia. Experience at a large cancer center and review of the literature. *Medicine* 1993;72:137–42.
177. KUNOVA A, TRUPL J, SPANIK S *et al. Candida glabrata, Candida krusei*, non-*albicans Candida* spp., and other fungal organisms in a sixty-bed National Cancer Center in 1989–1993: no association with the use of fluconazole. *Chemotherapy* 1995;41:39–44.
178. O'DRISCOLL BRC, COOKE RDP, MAMTORA H, HIRVING M, BERNSTEIN A. *Candida* lung abscesses complicating parenteral nutrition. *Thorax* 1988;43:418–9.
179. GERBERDING KM, EISENHUT CC, ENGLE WA, COHEN MD. Congenital candida pneumonia and sepsis: a case report and review of the literature. *J Perinat* 1989;9:159–61.
180. THALER M, PASTAKIA B, SHAWKER TH *et al.* Hepatic candidiasis in cancer patients: the evolving picture of the syndrome. *Ann Int Med* 1988;108:88–100.
181. ROSE HD, SHETH NK. Pulmonary candidiasis. A clinical and pathological correlation. *Arch Intern Med* 1978;138:964–5.
182. MASUR H, ROSEN PP, ARMSTRONG D. Pulmonary disease caused by *Candida* species. *Am J Med* 1977;63:914–25.
183. GOODRICH JM, REED EC, MORI M. Clinical features and analysis of risk factors for invasive candida infection after marrow transplantation. *J Infect Dis* 1991;164:731–40.
184. MARTINO P, GIRMENIA C, MICOZZI A, DE BERNARDIS F, BOCCANERA M, CASSONE A. Prospective study of candida colonisation, use of empiric amphotericin B and development of invasive mycosis in neutropenic patients. *Eur J Clin Microbiol Infec Dis* 1994;13:797–804.
185. LOKE HL, VERBER I, SZYMONOWICZW W, YU VY. Systemic candidiasis and pneumonia in preterm infants. *Aust Ped J* 1988;24:138–42.
186. GERBERDING KM, EISENHUT CC, ENGLE WA, COHEN MD. Congenital *Candida* pneumonia and sepsis: a case report and review of the literature. *J Perinatol* 1989;9:159–61.
187. BUFF SJ, MCLELLAND R, GALLIS HA, MATTHAY R, PUTMAN CE. *Candida albicans* pneumonia: radiographic appearance. *Am J Roentgenol* 1982;138:645–8.
188. BODEY GP. Fungal infections complicating acute leukaemia. *J Chron Dis* 1966;19:667–87.
189. BILLE J, STOCKMAN L, ROBERTS JD *et al.* Evaluation of a lysis – centrifugation system for recovery of yeasts and filamentous fungi from the blood. *J Clin Microbiol* 1983;18:469–74.
190. AL-DUGHAYM AM, MATTHEWS RC, BURNIE JP. Epitope mapping human heat-shock protein 90 with sera from infected patients. FEMS *Immunol Med Microbiol* 1994;8:43–8.
191. WEINER MH, COATS-STEPHEN M. Immunodiagnosis of systemic candidiasis:

mannan antigenemia detected by radioimmunoassay in experimental and human infection. *J Infect Dis* 1979;140:989–93.

192. WALSH TJ, HATHORN JW, SOBEL JD *et al.* Detection of circulating *candida* enolase by immunoassay in patients with cancer and invasive candidiasis. *NEJM* 1991;324:1026–31.

193. WALSH TJ, HEYTHORNE JW, SEVILLE JD. Detection of circulating *Candida* enolase by immunoassay in patients with cancer and invasive candidiasis. *N Engl J Med* 1991;324:1026–31.

194. MATTHEWS RC, BURNIE JP, LEE W. The application of epitope mapping in the development of a new serological tests for systemic candidosis. *J Immunol Meth* 1991;143:73–9.

195. BURGENER-KAIRUZ P, ZUBER JP, JAUNIN P, BUCHMAN TG, BILLE J, ROSSIER. Rapid detection and identification of *Candida albicans and Torulopsis (candida) glabrata* in clinical specimens by species-specific nested PCR amplification of a cytochrome P-450 lanosterol-α-demethylase (L1A1) gene fragment. *J Clin Microbiol* 1994;32:1902–7.

196. REISS E, MORRISON CJ. Nonculture methods for diagnosis of disseminated candidiasis. *Clin Microbiol Rev* 1993;6:311–23.

197. MAARTENS G, WOOD MJ. The clinical presentation and diagnosis of invasive fungal infections. *J Antimicrob Chemother* 1991;28:13–22.

198. MEUNIER-CARPENTIER F, KIEHN TE, ARMSTRONG D. Fungemia in the immunocompromised host: changing patterns, antigenemia, high mortality. *Am J Med* 1981;71:363–70.

199. ROSENBAUM RB, BARBER JV, STEVENS DA. *Candida albicans* pneumonia. Diagnosis by pulmonary aspiration, recovery without treatment. *Am Rev Resp Dis* 1974;109:373–8.

200. SCHIFFMAN RL, JOHNSON TS, WEINBERGER SE, WEISS ST, SCHWARTZ A. *Candida* lung abscess: successful treatment with amphotericin B and 5-flucytosine. *Am Rev Resp Dis* 1982;125:766–8.

201. HORN R, WONG B, KIEINTE, ARMSTRONG D. Fungemia in a cancer hospital: changing frequency, earlier onset and results of therapy. *Rev Infect Dis* 1985;7:646–55.

202. EDWARDS JE, MORRUON J, HENDERSON DK *et al.* Combined effort of amphotericin B and rifampin on *Candida* species. *Antimicrob Agents Chemother* 1980;14:484–8.

203. WEEMS JJ. Candida parapsillosis: epidemiology, pathogenicity, clinical manifestations and antimicrobial susceptibility. *Clin Infect Dis* 1992;14:756–66.

204. CONLY J, RENNIE R, JOHNSON J, FARAH S, HELLMAN L. Disseminated candidiasis due to amphotericin B resistant *Candida albicans J Inf Dis* 1992;165:761–4.

205. AISNER J, SICKLES SC, SCHIMPFF SC *et al.* Torulopsis glabrata pneumonitis in patients with cancer. Report of 3 cases. *JAMA* 1974;230:584–5.

206. MEUNIER F. Alternative modalities of administering amphotericin B: current issues. *J Infect* 1994;28:51–6.

207. NATIONAL COMMITTEE FOR CLINICAL LABORATORY STANDARDS. 1992. Reference method for broth dilution antifungal susceptibility testing of yeasts. Proposed guideline M27-P. National Committee for Clinical Laboratory Standards, Villanova, Pa.

208. BEYER J, SCHWARTZ S, HIENEMANN V, SIEGERT W. Strategies in prevention of invasive pulmonary aspergillosis in immunosuppressed or neutropenic patients. *Antimicrob Agents Chemother* 1994;38:911–17.

209. ELLIS ME, QADRI SMH, SPENCE D *et al.* The effect of fluconazole as prophylaxis for neutropenic patients on the isolation of *Candida* spp. from surveillance cultures. *J Antimicrob Chemother* 1994;33:1223–8.

210. CHANDRASEKAR PH, GATNY CM, BONE MARROW TRANSPLANTATION TEAM. The effect of fluconazole prophylaxis on fungal colonisation in neutropenic cancer patients. *J Antimicrob Chemother* 1994;33:309–18.

211. SANGUINETI A, CARMICHAEL JK, CAMPBELL K. Fluconazole-resistant *Candida albicans* after long-term suppressive therapy. *Arch Intern Med* 1993;153:1122–4.

212. WALSH TJ, DIXON DM. Nosocomial aspergillosis: environmental microbiology, hospital epidemiology, diagnosis, and treatment. *Eur J Epidemiol* 1989;5:131–42.

213. DIAMOND RD, HAUDENSCHILD CC, EIKSON NF III. Monocyte-mediated damage to *Rhizopus oryzae* hyphae *in vitro*. *Infect Immun* 1982;38:292–7.

214. CHINN RYW, DIAMOND RD. Generation of chemotactic factors by *Rhizopus oryzae* in the presence and absence of serum; relationship to hyphal damage mediated by human neutrophils and effects of hyperglycemia and ketoacidosis. *Infect Immun* 1982;38:1123–9.

215. WALDORF AR, RUDERMAN N, DIAMOND RD. Specific susceptibility to mucormycosis in murine diabetes and bronchoalveolar macrophage defence against *Rhizopus*. *J Clin Invest* 1984;74:150–60.

216. LEWIS LL, HAWKINS HK, EDWARDS MS. Disseminated mucormycosis in an infant with methylmalonicaciduria. *Pediatr Infect Dis J* 1990;9:851–4.

217. WINDUS DW, STOKES TJ, JULIAN BA *et al.* Fatal *Rhizopus* infections in hemodialysis patients receiving deferoxamine. *Ann Intern Med* 1987;107:678–80.

218. MAJID AA, YII NW. Granulomatous pulmonary zygomycosis in a patient without underlying illness. Computed tomographic appearances and treatment by pneumonectomy. *Chest* 1991;100:560–1.

219. PARFREY NA. Improved diagnosis and prognosis of mucormycosis. A clinico-pathologic study of 33 cases. *Medicine* 1986;65:113–8.

220. VENTURA GJ, KANTARJIAN HM, ANAISSIE E, HOPFER RL, FAINSTEIN V. Pneumonia with Cunninghamella species in patients with hematologic malignancies. A case report and review of the literature. *Cancer* 1986;58:1534–6.

221. MEYER RD, ROSEN P, ARMSTONG D. Phycomycosis complicating leukaemia and lymphoma. *Ann Intern Med* 1972;77:871.

222. REED AE, BODY BA, AUSTIN MB, FRIERSON HF JR. *Cunninghamella bertholletiae* and *Pneumocystis carinii* pneumonia as a fatal complication of chronic lymphocytic leukaemia. *Hum Pathol* 1988;19:1470–2.

223. STUDEMEISTER AE, KOZAK K, GARRITY E, VENEZIO FR. Survival of a heart transplant recipient after pulmonary cavitary mucormycosis. *J Heart Transpl* 1988;7:159–61.

224. MORDUCHOWICZ G, PITLIK SD, SHAPIRA Z *et al.* Infections in renal transplant recipients in Israel. *Israel J Med Sci* 1985;21:791–7.

225. AGGER WA, MAKI DG. Mucormycosis. A complication of critical case. *Arch Intern Med* 1978;138:925–7.

226. BIGBY TD, SEROTA ML, TIERVEY LM *et al.* Clinical spectrum of mucormycosis. *Chest* 1986;89:435–9.

227. BAUM JL. Rhino-orbital mucormycosis, occurring in an otherwise apparently healthy individual. *Am J Ophthalmol* 1967;63:335.

228. WATTS WJ. Bronchopleural fistural followed by massive fatal haemoptysis in a patient with pulmonary mucormycosis. A case report. *Arch Intern Med* 1983;143:1029–30.

229. SCHWARTZ JRL, NAGLE MG, ELKINS RC *et al.* Mucormycosis of the trachea. An unusual case of upper airway obstruction. *Chest* 1982;81:653–4.

230. JONES KW, KAUFMAN L. Development and evaluation of an immunodiffusion test for diagnosis of systemic zygomycosis (mucormycosis): preliminary report. *J Clin Microbiol* 1978;7:97.

231. SMITH JL, STEVENS DA. Survival in cerebro-rhino-orbital zygomycosis and cavernous sinus thrombosis with combined therapy. *South Med J* 1986;79:501–4.

232. GALE AM, KLEITSCH WP. Solitary

pulmonary nodule due to phycomycosis (mucormycosis). *Chest* 1972;62:752–4.

233. CHRISTENSON JC, SHALIT I, WELCH DF, GURUSWAMY A, MARKS MI. Synergistic action of amphotericin B and rifampin against *Rhizopus* species. *Antimicrob Agents Chemother* 1987;31:1175–8.

234. FERGUSON BJ, MITCHELL TG, MOON R *et al.* Adjunctive hyperbaric oxygen for the treatment of rhinocerebral mucormycosis. *Rev Infect Dis* 1988;10:551–9.

235. COUCH L, THEILEN F, MADER JT. Rhinocerebral mucormycosis with cerebral extension successfully treated with adjunctive hyperbaric oxygen therapy. *Arch Otolaryngol Head Neck Surg* 1988;114:791–4.

236. HACHIMI-INDRISSI S, WILLEMSEN M, DESPRECHINS B *et al. Pseudallescheria boydii* and brain abscesses. *Pediatr Infect Dis J* 1990;9:737–41.

237. GALGIANI J, STEVENS D, GRAYBILL J *et al. Pseudallescheria boydii* infections treated with ketoconazole. *Chest* 1984;86:219–24.

238. KATHURIA S, RIPPON J. Non-*Aspergillus* aspergilloma. *Am J Clin Pathol* 1982;78:870–3.

239. TRAVIS L, ROBERTS G, WILSON W. Clinical significance of *Pseudallescheria boydii*: a review of 10 years' experience. *Mayo Clin Proc* 1985;60:531–7.

240. SEVERO L, LONDERO A, PICON P *et al. Petriellidium boydii* fungus ball in a patient with active tuberculosis. *Mycopathologia* 1982;77:13–17.

241. COOPER DKC, LANZA RP, OLIVER S *et al.* Infections complications after heart transplantation. *Thorax* 1983;38:822–8.

242. MORGAN M, WILSON W, NEEL H, ROBERTS G. Fungal sinusitis in healthy and immunocompromised individuals. *Am J Clin Pathol* 1984;82:597–601.

243. HAINER JW, OSTROW HJ, MACKENZIE DWR. Pulmonary monosporosis: report of a case with precipitating antibody. *Chest* 1974;66:601–3.

244. JUNG J, SALAS R, ALMOND C *et al.* The role of surgery in the management of pulmonary monosporosis. *J Thorac Cardiovasc Surg* 1977;73:139–45.

245. DWORZACH D, CLARK R, BORKOWSKI W *et al. Pseudallescheria boydii* brain abscess: association with near drowning and efficacy of high-dose, prolonged miconazole therapy in patients with multiple abscesses. *Medicine (Baltimore)* 1989;68:218–24.

246. ROHATGI PK. Pulmonary sporotrichosis. *South Med J* 1980;73:1611–18.

247. PLUSS JL, OPAL SM. Pulmonary sporotrichosis: review of treatment and outcome. *Medicine (Baltimore)* 1986;65:143–53.

248. MOHR JA, GRIFFITHS W, LONG H. Pulmonary sporotrichosis in Oklahoma and susceptibilities *in vitro*. *Am Rev Resp Dis* 1979;119:961–4.

249. EWING GE, BOSL GJ, PETERSON PK. *Sporothrix schenckii* meningitis in a farmer with Hodgkin's disease. *Am J Med* 1980;68:455–7.

250. KUROSAWA A, POLLOCK SC, COLLINS MP, KRAFF CR, TSO MOM. *Sporothrix schenckii* endophthalmitis in a patient with human immunodeficiency virus infection. *Arch Ophthal* 1988;106:376–80.

251. GULLBERG RM, QUINTANILLA A, LEVIN ML, WILLIAMS J, PHAIR JP. Sporotrichiosis: recurrent cutaneous, articular and central nervous system infection in a renal transplant recipient. *Rev Infect Dis* 1987;9:369–75.

252. GERDING DN. Treatment of pulmonary sporotrichosis. *Semin Respir Infect* 1986;1:61–5.

253. RABODONIRINA M, PIENS MA, MONIER MF, GUEHO E, FIERE D, MOJON M. *Fusarium* infections in immunocompromised patients: case reports and literature review. *Eur J Clin Microbiol Infect Dis* 1994;13:152–61.

254. WHEELER MS, MCGINMS MR, SCHELL WA, WALKER DH. Fusarium infection in burned patients. *Am J Clin Path* 1981;75:304–11.

255. ANAISSIE EJ, HACHEM R, LEGRAND C, LEGENNE P, NELSON P, BODEY GP. Lack of activity of amphotericin B in systemic murine fusarial infection. *J Infect Dis* 1992;165:1155–7.

256. BLAZAR BR, HURD DD, SNOVER DC, ALEXANDER JW, MCGLAVE PB. Invasive fusarial infections in bone marrow transplant recipients. *Am J Med* 1984;77:645–51.

257. COFRANCESCO E, BOSCHETTI C, VIVIANI MA *et al.* Efficacy of liposomal amphotericin B (AmBisome) in the eradication of *fusarium* infection in a leukaemic patient. *Haematologica* 1992;77:280–3.

258. ELLIS ME, CLINK H, YOUNGE D, HAINAU B. Successful combined surgical and medical treatment of fusarium infection after bone marrow transplantation. *Scand J Infect Dis* 1994;26:225–8.

259. LUPINETTI FM, GILLER RG, TRIGG ME. Operative treatment of *Fusarium* fungal infection of the lung. *Ann Thoracic Surg* 1990;49:991–2.

260. ANAISSIE EJ, BODEY GP, KANTARJIAN H *et al.* Non spectrum of fungal infections in patients with cancer. *Rev Infect Dis* 1989;11:369–78.

261. QADRI S, ELLIS ME. Localised pulmonary disease to trichosporon beigelie. *J Nat Med Assoc* 1992;84:449–52.

262. MARCON MJ, POWELL DA. Epidemiology, diagnosis and management of *Malassezia furfur* systemic infection. *Diag Microbiol Infect Dis* 1987;7:161–75.

263. DANKNER WM, SPECTOR SA, FIERER J, DAVIS CE. *Malassezia* fungemia in neonates and adults: complications of hyperalimentation. *Rev Infect Dis* 1987;9:743–53.

264. MICKELSEN PA, VIANO-PAULSON MC, STEVENS DH, DIAZ PS. Clinical and microbiological features of infection with *Malassezia pachydermatis* in high risk infants. *J Infect Dis* 1988;157:1163–8.

265. DENG Z, RIBAS JL, GIBSON DW, CONNOR DH. Infections caused by *Penicillium marneffei* in China and Southeast Asia. Review of eighteen published cases and report of four non-Chinese cases. *Rev Infect Dis* 1988;10:640–52.

266. SUPPARATPINYO K, CHIEWCHANVIT S, HIRUNSRI P, UTHAMMACHAI C, NELSON KE, SIRISANTHANA T. *Penicillium marneffei* infection in patients infected with human immunodeficiency virus. *Clin Infect Dis* 1992;14:871–4.

267. BOLTANSKY H, KWON-CHUNG KJ, MACHER AM, GALLIN JI. *Acremonium strictum*-related pulmonary infection in a patient with chronic granulomatous disease. *J Infect Dis* 1984;149:653–5.

268. DHARMASENA FMC, DAVIES GSR, CATOVSKY D. *Paecilomyces variotii* pneumonia complicating hairy cell leukaemia. *Br Med J* 1985;290:967–8.

269. WHEAT LJ, BARTLETT M, CICCARELLI M, SMITH JW. Opportunistic scopulariopsis pneumonia in an immunocompromised host. *South Med J* 1984;77:1608–9.

270. LOBRITZ RW, ROBERTS TH, MARRARO RV, CARLTON PK, THORP DJ. Granulomatous pulmonary disease secondary to alternaria. *J Am Med Assoc* 1979;241:596–7.

271. DIXON DM, WALSH TJ, MERZ WG, MCGINNIS MR. Infections due to *Xylohypha bantiana (Cladosporium trichoides)*. *Rev Infect Dis* 1989;11:515–25.

272. ADAM RD, PAQUIN ML, PETERSEN EA *et al.* Phaeohyphomycosis caused by the fungal genera *Bipolaris* and *Exserohilum*: a report of 9 cases and review of the literature. *Medicine* 1986;65:203–17.

273. LAMPERT RP, HULTO JH, DONNELLY WH, SHULMAN ST. Pulmonary and cerebral mycetoma caused by *Curvularia pallescens*. *J Pediat* 1977;91:603–5.

274. HOPPIN EC, MCCOY EL, RINALDI MG. Opportunistic mycotic infection caused by chaetomium in a patient with acute leukaemia. *Cancer* 1983;52:555–6.

Part 3: Major respiratory syndromes

17 Community-acquired pneumonias

J.A.R. FRIEND
Aberdeen Royal Infirmary, Scotland, UK

Definition

The term pneumonia is rarely defined as a clinical entity in the literature, although it can be more clearly defined as a pathological term. However, it is generally agreed to be a lung infection with micro-organisms in which the alveoli are involved, with resulting consolidation of the alveolar air spaces. Such a definition distinguishes pneumonia from bronchitis, which involves the airway mucosa and walls. Pneumonia results in impairment of the function of the affected lung tissue in its task of gas exchange, and the consolidation usually also causes shadowing of the affected lung tissue as seen on chest X-ray, so that some element of X-ray opacity is usually a requirement for the clinical diagnosis of pneumonia. In one study,[1] the definition of X-ray opacity sufficient to define pneumonia required 'either opacity at least involving a segment, or present in more than one lobe, which was neither pre-existing nor of other known cause'.

Some organisms can affect either the airways alone, causing bronchitis, or can involve primarily the alveoli causing pneumonia, but the distinction between bronchitis and pneumonia is not clear-cut, and in some infections there may be a combination of bronchitis and pneumonia in different degrees in different parts of the lungs in the same subject. Examples of such infections include those caused by organisms such as *Streptococcus pneumoniae* or *Haemophilus influenzae*.

The term community-acquired pneumonia (CAP) describes pneumonia arising in people of any age who have no obvious pathological impairment of host defences, and where the infection has been acquired while living in the normal environment outside hospital. This is in contrast to nosocomial, or hospital-acquired pneumonia, which is caused by the more unusual range of organisms found in hospitals, and pneumonias arising in immunocompromised individuals, often with organisms which are not pathogenic in fully healthy people. This chapter intends to describe the clinical approach to adults developing pneumonia in the community, in whom there is no particular predisposing disease, and where the causative organism is not known at the time of diagnosis of the pneumonia.

Epidemiology

Incidence

It is difficult to determine the true incidence of pneumonia in a given population, because CAP may range from a mild infection which goes unreported by the patient to a severe, life-threatening illness requiring intensive therapy. Indeed, many cases of pneumonia may be so mild as to be virtually symptomless, and an unknown number of milder cases may consist of simple febrile illnesses, often not reported to a doctor. In addition, there will be milder illnesses labelled by doctors as being influenza or 'chest infections', without further investigation, which may also amount to pneumonia, but which are not diagnosed as such. Reports of incidence will therefore depend on whether the diagnosis is made in the family doctor's or physician's consulting room, whether an X-ray is taken, whether the data derives from hospital attendances (at an emergency room, and from admissions to hospital wards) or only from those ill enough to need hospital admission. Studies of CAP have therefore varied in their inclusion and exclusion criteria. For instance, there is a divergence of definition as to whether elderly people developing pneumonia in nursing homes should be defined as having CAP (as is usually taken to be the case in US studies) or whether nursing homes should be regarded as institutions which are not part of the wider community, as has been the case in UK studies.

Respiratory tract infections are very common, and one of the commonest reasons for consulting a family doctor. In a single family practice in England, the incidence of lower respiratory tract infections in adults requiring antibiotic therapy was 44 per 1000 per year.[2] In an earlier study in family practice in the UK,[3] patients with lower respiratory infections with new focal signs on clinical examination, all had a subsequent X-ray to determine whether pneumonia was present or not; in this study, the incidence of community-acquired pneumonia in adults aged 15 to 79 was 4.7 per 1000 population per year, with an incidence of 3.6 per 1000 per year if all ages were included. Most of these patients (78%) were treated at home, so that from this study, only about one case per 1000 population per year required hospitalisation. Cases of radiologically confirmed pneumonia comprised only 5.6% of all the lower respiratory tract infections in this study for which antibiotics were prescribed, so that pneumonia represents a small proportion of all lower respiratory infections. In a study in Finland[4] involving all ages, and where 97% of the subjects had the diagnosis confirmed by chest X-ray, Jokinen *et al.* found a higher annual incidence of pneumonia for all ages of 11.6 per 1000. In 19% of all the patients, there was an underlying chronic condition, such as chronic heart or lung disease, cancer, diabetes, or alcoholism. Of all the patients 42% were admitted to hospital with their pneumonia. The overall incidence of CAP in the USA has also been estimated to be about 10 to 12 cases per 1000 people a year.[5,6]

The effect of age on the incidence of pneumonia

The Finnish study,[4] which included 546 patients, showed that the highest incidence of CAP was in young children and the elderly: the incidence for those aged under 5 was 36 per 1000 population per year, and for adults over 75 was 34 per 1000. The incidence at other ages was as follows: aged 5–14, 16.2, aged 15–59, 6.0, and aged 60–74, 15.4 cases per 1000 of the population per year. In an earlier study in Seattle, USA, rates for pneumonia in the under-5s were 12 to 18 cases per 1000 per year, with over 30 per year for the over 75 age-group.[5]

Incidence of pneumonia in different sexes

In the Finnish Study,[4] 59% of the CAP patients were males, with a particularly striking preponderance of males among the very young (under 5 years), where 73% were male, and the very old (over 75 years) where 61% were male. The sex ratio was equal (51%) in those aged 5 to 44 years.

Incidence in different countries

Even in developed countries, it is difficult to estimate the true incidence of pneumonia, because of the varied methods of definition, case finding, and diagnosis. However, in industrialised countries an incidence of about 10 per 1000 per year for all ages seems likely from the many and varied studies. In developing countries a true measure of the incidence of CAP is harder to achieve if X-ray changes are considered to be a necessary part of the diagnosis, though respiratory tract infections are common, particularly in children, with a high mortality rate. For instance, a study of nearly 9000 children under 15 from poor areas of Colombia[7] yielded an incidence of 70 cases of lower respiratory tract infection per 1000 per year, of whom over a quarter were diagnosed as having pneumonia, particularly in the under two age-group. The mortality in the pneumonia group was less than 1%. In an undeveloped area of India, the attack rate for pneumonia in children under the age of 5 was estimated at 130 per 1000 per year, with mortality as high as 13.5% in areas where there was no access to medical care.[8]

Predisposition–vulnerable groups

It is usual to exclude from the diagnosis of CAP those who have an obvious condition with immunosuppression, such as those with acquired immune deficiency syndrome (AIDS), those on chemotherapy for haematological or other malignancy, or on immunosuppression for organ transplantation. While such immunosuppressed patients are relatively simple to define, there are others who seem to be at increased risk for reasons other than age alone, including, in Jokinen *et al.*'s study,[4] those with severe chronic lung disease, chronic heart disease (7.5% of the study group overall), severe chronic heart disease (6.6% of the group) diabetes (4%) and a smaller number with cancer, connective tissue disorder, and alcoholism (4%). The majority of these patients were in the over 60 age-group, 46% of whom had one of these underlying risk factors.

A further study of people aged over 60 in Finland[9] also showed the importance of previous heart and lung disease, including asthma, and also the greater likelihood of pneumonia in those on immunosuppressive therapy, and with alcoholism. All these risk factors except alcoholism also increased the need for hospitalisation for pneumonia. A Spanish study also highlighted the importance of alcoholism as a risk factor for pneumonia in middle-aged people.[10] However, in 45% of the elderly subjects in the Finnish study[9] there was no obvious risk factor for the development of pneumonia, confirming that pneumonia can, and does occur in previously fit individuals.

Mortality

Pneumonia is the sixth most common cause of death in the USA.[11] There is, however, a tendency for physicians to certify pneumonia as a cause of death in many people dying of other underlying conditions, so that it is more reliable to look at the mortality in formal prospective studies of community-acquired pneumonia. The mortality of CAP varies, however, in different reports, depending on the selection of patients included. In Jokinen *et al.*s' study,[4] the overall mortality within 2 weeks of onset was 4%, but inevitably varied with age, with no deaths under age 5, but 11% over 60, and 17% over 75. In a survey of CAP treated in hospital among adults aged 15 to 74 in the UK,[1] the mortality was 5.7%, but this study excluded older patients, those from nursing homes, those where pneumonia was not the main reason for admission, and those where the pneumonia was seen as being 'an expected terminal event'. A number of very high risk patients were therefore excluded from this study, but who contributed to the mortality in other studies. It has been estimated that mortality rates for CAP in developed countries are probably less than 5% for pneumonia treated as an out-patient, but up to 25% for all those admitted as in-patients, and even higher for those requiring treatment in an intensive care unit.[11] In several studies the factors evident on admission which were associated with mortality have been assessed by multi-variate analysis, and these are considered later in this chapter in relation to the identification of patients with particularly severe CAP. In a meta-analysis of 127 studies of CAP, including over 33 000 patients, *S. pneumoniae* accounted for 86% of the deaths occurring in patients where the pathogen was clearly identified.[12]

Aetiology of community-acquired pneumonia

A number of large studies have been undertaken to estimate the relative importance of different infecting organisms in the aetiology of CAP, but all differ in their method of case selection, and in the diagnostic methods used to determine the cause. Much of the data has been summarised in the consensus papers from the Canadian, American, and British organisations, which have been published in recent years from the Canadian CAP Consensus Conference Group in 1993,.[13] the American Thoracic Society, USA 1993,[14] and the British Thoracic Society, 1993.[15] Some of the largest studies of CAP have been undertaken in Canada:[16] the United States of America,[17] the United Kingdom,[1] Spain,[18] and Sweden.[19] The spectrum of infecting agents will vary depending on whether the patients derived from an out-patient group, from hospitalised patients, and on their age and sex characteristics, and the presence of underlying disease. In addition, the prevalence of particular infecting organisms may vary with time and place, so that there may be higher levels of, for instance, *Mycoplasma pneumoniae* infections some years,[20] and variations in the frequency of *Legionella* infections in others. In addition to this, 32% to 47% of the causative organisms are never identified despite careful investigation. Possible reasons for this may include the previous use antibiotic therapy, the transient presence of the organism, or the inadequacy of the diagnostic procedures.

In most studies, the commonest cause of CAP in adult patients is *S. pneumoniae* (see Chapter 5) which is detected in 8–46% of CAP patients in the larger studies listed above. The chances of isolating pneumococci from patients with pneumonia are greatly reduced by prior antibiotic therapy–in one study,[1] pneumococcal infection was diagnosed in 47% of those who had not had prior antibiotics, and in only 18% of those who had; in patients with subsequent good evidence of pneumococcal infection (either by sputum culture, blood culture, or pneumococcal antigen in sputum, blood, or urine) sputum cultures were positive in 14% of those who had not had prior antibiotics, but in only 2% of those who had prior antibiotic therapy.

H. influenzae (see Chapter 7) accounts for 2–11%, of CAP, and *Legionella* for 2–14%, this latter organism being variable and occurring in epidemics; *Staphylococcus aureus* is isolated in 1–4%, and Gram-negative enteric bacilli (such as *Klebsiella pneumoniae, Escherischia coli, Pseudomonas aeruginosa,* and others) are found as the causative organism in 1–6% of CAP (see Chapter 8). The place of Gram-negative enteric bacilli as a cause of pneumonia has been a matter of some difficulty.[21] Because of prior antibiotic therapy, and contamination of sputum samples by oral secretions, it is harder to judge whether Gram-negative infections are, in individual cases, the major pathogen. Certainly, the proportion of pneumonias caused by Gram-negative organisms is higher in those studies which include the more elderly patients and those from nursing homes.[22, 23]

Non-bacterial pneumonias are attributed to *M. pneumoniae* in 2–18%, this being particularly variable because of epidemics, to *Chlamydia* in 2–6%, and to viral infections in up to 20%.[1,16–19] For further details, the reader should consult the specific chapters relating to infections by these micro-organisms.

Rarely, community-acquired pneumonia may arise from less usual organisms: pneumonia may be acquired by transmission from animals; examples include Q fever (caused by *Coxiella burnetii*), usually passed from animals such as sheep and deer, especially to those who work in abattoirs or in contact with animal blood, such as shepherds; pneumonic plague, caused by *Yersinia pestis* carried to man from rodents by fleas, and subsequently by human-to-human transmission; anthrax, caused by *Bacillus anthracis* from infected animal materials, and tularaemia (*Francisella tularensis* from tick bites); but these are rare causes of pneumonia, probably accounting together for less than 1% of all CAP. Despite their rarity, a knowledge of the patient's environment and workplace, and of the current prevalence of specific infections causing pneumonia, may help to increase the chances of defining the aetiology of pneumonia in an individual patient. Where such hints in the clinical history towards a possible aetiology exist, then the antibiotic therapy should take account of such an infection until the aetiology is determined.

The clinical approach

Symptoms

The symptoms arising from pneumonia depend on the causative organism, and the severity of the infection. Some of the symptoms will be *the general symptoms of any infection*, such as malaise and fever, which is present in about 78%,[16] and in severe pneumonia, there may be more demanding symptoms of clinical shock and prostration. In addition, there may be *local symptoms* such as *pleuritic pain*, occurring where the lung inflammation extends to the visceral pleura, and spreads across the pleural space to stimulate the pain endings present in the branches of the intercostal nerves serving the parietal pleura. Generally, pain experienced from stimulation of the intercostal sensory nerves is felt in the area the nerves serve, but pleurisy affecting the more central parts of the diaphragmatic parietal pleura causes referred pain experienced in the shoulder tip on the affected side, via phrenic nerve afferents. Pleuritic pain is characteristically felt during coughing and deep breathing, as the inflamed visceral and parietal layers of the pleura rub against each other. However, pleuritic pain is only present in about 40% of patients with pneumonia,[16] presumably because not all pneumonias extend to the visceral pleural surface with such severity as to cause inflammation and pain in the parietal pleura.

Cough is common, occurring in some 82%[16] and in some infections (and particularly in *M. pneumoniae*) may be paroxysmal, persistent, and cause retching and vomiting. Depending on the pathogen, the cough may be productive of *sputum* which is *purulent or blood-stained*–this is particularly common in bacterial pneumonias. Acute pneumococcal pneumonia may cause the expectoration of rust-coloured sputum, in which the purulent sputum is uniformly mixed with red blood cells and haemosiderin from the consolidated lung tissue.

Consolidation of lung tissue inevitably results in impaired ventilation of the affected area, whether this be lobule, segment, lobe or more; perfusion may continue, so that there will be shunting of less oxygenated blood through the area and consequent relative arterial hypoxaemia. If an extensive area of lung is consolidated, the hypoxaemia may cause *breathlessness*; this may be out of proportion to the hypoxia and can be interpreted as a result of the reduced compliance of the consolidated lung and stimulation of stretch receptors. The sensation of breathlessness may be increased by the difficulty in breathing resulting from pleuritic pain.

Clinical signs

The general signs of infection will include fever, with rigors, sweating, and obvious illness depending on the severity of the infection. In severe infection the patient may be prostrated with hypotension and septic shock with bacteraemia, which may, in turn, lead to renal failure.

If substantial areas of lung are consolidated, blood perfusing the consolidated lung will effectively be shunted from the pulmonary arterial circulation through pulmonary capillaries to the pulmonary veins without uptake of oxygen or release of carbon dioxide, resulting in signs of hypoxia such as cyanosis, and where there is severe hypoxia, confusion. The reduced compliance of stiff lung and the need to excrete carbon dioxide will lead to increased ventilation with tachypnoea, unless the patient has pre-existing chronic lung disease, especially chronic airways obstruction, in which case ventilation may not be adequate to maintain a normal arterial carbon dioxide level and hypoventilation with arterial hypercapnia may develop.

On examination of the chest, substantial areas of consolidation at the pleural surface will be detected as areas of dullness to percussion (29%), and if the main airways remain patent, the better transmission of the sound frequencies of turbulent air flow in the large airways will lead to the transmission of bronchial breath sounds to the stethoscope, accompanied by increased vocal resonance. Accompaniments will consist most commonly of coarse crackles over the affected areas (78%), if these are large enough and near to the auscultation site. Wheezes are less common, being recorded in 34% in Marrie's series.[16] If pleurisy is present, a pleural rub may be felt with the hand or heard through a stethoscope. It is not uncommon for a pleural friction rub to be heard even where the patient has not experienced pleuritic pain. However, such classical signs of pneumonia and consolidation occur mainly in lobar pneumonia, where a large enough volume of lung is involved at the pleural surface of the lung – many patients with more patchy, central, or limited pneumonia have few if any abnormal physical signs.

Investigations

Investigations are aimed at (a) confirming or establishing the clinical diagnosis, and then (b) attempting to detect and identify the causative organism, so that the most appropriate antibiotic therapy can be given. Some of the investigations will also be aimed at (c) defining the severity of the infection, so that those who are severely ill and at the most risk can be assigned to intensive care. At the same time, the physician will attempt (d) to detect any underlying conditions such as diabetes, cardiac or lung disease, or other predisposing conditions such as bronchial obstruction or immunosuppression.

For those ill enough to be admitted to hospital, Table 17.1 lists the *immediate* initial investigations which are regarded by most authorities as being important and valuable to fulfil the objectives detailed above.

Table 17.1. *Important immediate investigations in patients admitted to hospital with possible CAP*

Full blood count, biochemical profile including renal and liver function tests
Gram staining and culture of sputum[a];
Blood culture
Arterial blood gas analysis
Chest X-ray
HIV testing (especially for patients aged 15 to 54)
Initial blood sampling for antibody studies

Consider aspiration of pleural fluid, if present; analysis, microbiology including aerobic and anaerobic bacteria, mycobacteria.
Where a more detailed assessment of the pathogen is required, options include: 1 nasopharyngeal aspirate for virus antigen detection studies (see Chapter 1); sputum antigen detection for *S. pneumoniae, Legionella, Pneumocystis;* urine antigen detection for *S. pneumoniae, Legionella.*
[a] See Chapter 1 for further details.
(After Bartlett and Mundy 1995,[24] Ortqvist, 1994.[25])

The place of more invasive investigations

Other more invasive diagnostic procedures, such as transtracheal aspiration, bronchoscopy and broncho-alveolar lavage, percutaneous fine needle lung aspiration, and sampling by a protected specimen brush in the airways, have been advocated: the merits of such techniques in the intensive care unit are a matter for debate.[26,27] All such investigations carry a variable level of risk to the patient, which must be carefully balanced against the potential benefits. While such techniques may be particularly appropriate, and simpler to perform, in patients who have started ventilator treatment for CAP, or who have developed pneumonia while on ventilator treatment for another condition, their place in the investigation of less severe CAP is much less certain. The place of such investigations in the Intensive Care Unit is discussed in Chapter 27. One of the listed techniques, i.e. trans-tracheal aspiration, has, however, been employed in less severely ill patients with CAP. Even in this situation, it has been the subject of debate.

Trans-tracheal aspiration

In this technique, the crico-thyroid membrane is punctured by a needle after infiltration with local anaesthetic, and a catheter passed through the needle into the trachea. About 4 ml of 0.9% saline is instilled into the trachea, and then suction applied to the catheter, and sputum aspirated.[28] The advantage of this technique is the avoidance of contamination of the sample by upper respiratory organisms. In Østergaard's series of 119 patients only one procedure was complicated,[28] and this by prolonged bleeding from the puncture site, but a further 135 patients with community-acquired pneumonia were not subjected to the procedure because they were thought to be high risk by virtue of respiratory insufficiency or cardiac disease, haemorrhagic risk, or poor general condition. Another study[29] dating from 1972, reported a 15% complication rate from the procedure, ranging from subcutaneous emphysema to death, and the technique is rejected as unacceptable by some.[6] However, in Østergaard's series[28] it was possible to make an aetiological diagnosis in 71 of the 119 patients (59.6%) investigated by trans-tracheal aspiration by immediate microscopic examination and Gram's and methylene blue stains, and in 54% by subsequent culture of the sample aspirated.

Additional laboratory studies

So far, there have been few studies of the value of the polymerase chain reaction (PCR) in making a rapid diagnosis of the cause of infection in a patient with community acquired pneumonia; although there is evidence of possible future value of PCR techniques in the diagnosis of *Pneumocystis carinii* pneumonia, and possibly also in Cytomegalovirus and *Mycobacterium tuberculosis*; in the case of community-acquired pneumonia only a few preliminary results are available for infection with *M. pneumoniae,* and *Legionella pneumophila*.[30]

Differential diagnosis

The combination of fever, respiratory symptoms, and X-ray shadowing is used by most doctors to suggest the diagnosis of pneumonia; in this chapter the more acute infections have been discussed, but it is essential to remember that infections which are sometimes regarded as more chronic can nevertheless mimic acute community-acquired pneumonia, and the most important of these is tuberculosis (see Chapter 15).

There is, in addition, a wide variety of non-infectious disorders which can cause the same clinical combination of fever, respiratory symptoms, and X-ray opacity. These are discussed in much greater detail in Chapter 28, but the important other causes of such a clinical picture are listed in Table 17.2.

Identifying the dangerously ill

Several studies have undertaken univariate and multi-variate analysis to attempt to identify those findings evident on admission which are associated with a higher risk of death during the episode.[31] For instance, the British Thoracic Society study of community-acquired pneumonia in adults admitted to hospital[1] concluded that, in addition to death being more likely in those over 60 years, the risk of death was increased at any age in patients with any of the following signs on admission:

- high respiratory rate (330 per minute)[a]
- low diastolic blood pressure (≤ 60 mm Hg)[a]
- confusion
- raised blood urea (>7 mmol/l)[a]
- low arterial oxygen tension (<8 kPa {60 mmHg}) on admission
- very low or very high white cell count (<4 or >30 $\times 10^9$/l)
- low serum albumin (<35 g/l)

[a]The risk of death in this study was increased 21-fold in any patient with two of these three factors.

It was interesting to note that the *absence* of chest pain was also a worse prognostic sign in this study. The absence of chest pain was also noted as an adverse sign in the study by Fine and colleagues,[32] along with increasing age, mental status change, and abnormal vital signs. The presence of neoplasm, bronchial obstruction, or evidence of aspiration were also more likely to be associated with a fatal outcome. A further study by Marrie *et al.*[33] found that age, residence in a nursing home, and the number of lobes involved were factors associated with an increased risk of death, and the importance of a low serum albumin was confirmed as an important factor in another study.[19]

The detection of any of the major adverse signs detailed above should immediately raise the issue of transfer of the patient to an intensive care unit (ICU), with facilities for full respiratory, circulatory and metabolic support should this become necessary.

Pneumonia requiring ICU treatment can be defined as severe pneumonia. Because of the risk to life, and the great importance of appropriate treatment, it is necessary to augment the diagnostic procedures if a causative organism has not been identified, with an early resort to more invasive techniques if the simpler investigations of sputum, blood culture, etc, are unproductive.

Table 17.2. *Non-infectious conditions which may cause fever, respiratory symptoms, and lung infiltrates*

Lung tumours:	primary tumours, sometimes with pneumonia distal to bronchial obstruction	
	primary tumours causing shadowing *per se:*	
	e.g. bronchial carcinoma	
	broncho-alveolar carcinoma	
	lymphoma, leukaemic infiltrates	
	Kaposi's sarcoma	
Pulmonary embolism		
Bronchiolitis obliterans organising pneumonia (BOOP)		
Collagen vascular diseases:	Systemic lupus erythematosus	
	Polyarteritis nodosa	
	Rheumatoid arthritis	
	Polymyositis/ dermatomyositis	
	Systemic sclerosis	
	Mixed connective tissue disorders	
Drug-induced lung diseases		
Hypersensitivity pneumonitis (allergic alveolitis)		
Granulomatous vasculitides	Wegener's granulomatosis	
	Churg–Strauss disease	
	Lymphomatoid granulomatosis	
	and various other rare forms of vasculitis	
Pulmonary haemorrhage		
Pulmonary oedema		
Sarcoidosis		
Acute forms of cryptogenic fibrosing alveolitis		
Pulmonary eosinophilia		
Toxic lung syndromes, e.g. paraquat pneumonitis		
Radiation pneumonitis		
Adult respiratory distress syndrome		

Adapted from *Avery's Drug Treatment*, 4th edn by permission of editor and publisher.

Complications

Pleural effusion, empyema

Pleural effusions, usually transudates, are a common accompaniment to pneumonia, and are apparent in the plain chest X-ray in up to 25% of CAP, though decubitus views may demonstrate small effusions in up to 57%[34] of patients with pneumococcal pneumonia. Such effusions usually contain polymorphonuclear leukocytes, but it is relatively rare to be able to culture *S. pneumoniae* from the fluid. Pleural effusions accompany about 25–40% of Staphylococcal pneumonias, about the same proportion of Gram-negative pneumonias, and about 30% of *Legionella* infections. When the numbers of leukocytes in the fluid increase to the point that the aspirated fluid is cloudy and no longer translucent, the condition is usually termed an empyema: at this point the fluid may become thicker and frankly purulent, with a tendency to loculation. For full details, the reader should consult Chapter 20.

Other complications

In the majority of pneumonias there will be a degree of respiratory failure, resulting from 'shunting' of blood from the pulmonary circulation through perfused but unventilated areas of pneumonic consolidation. If there is underlying chronic lung disease, such as chronic bronchitis, there will also be a tendency to carbon dioxide retention, and a resulting need for ventilatory support. Further complications include septicaemia and septic shock, with the consequent risk of renal failure and diffuse intravascular coagulation, and the development of the adult respiratory distress syndrome (ARDS). The development of these complications usually results in the definition of the pneumonia as 'severe', and requires intensive care unit management; these complications are further discussed in Chapter 27.

Prevention

Those most susceptible to CAP include the very young, the elderly, those with underlying diseases of the heart and lungs particularly, and those with a history of smoking and considerable alcohol consumption. Clearly, the achievement and maintenance of good general health through adequate nutrition, prevention of infectious diseases (especially among young children) and the avoidance of adverse factors such as tobacco smoking and excessive alcohol consumption can play a major part in reducing the prevalence and mortality from CAP. More specific preventative measures against CAP also include the use of influenza and pneumococcal vaccines.

Influenza vaccine

Influenza infection can cause viral pneumonia, but is more often a precursor of bacterial pneumonia with *S. pneumoniae, H. influenzae*, and *Staphylococcus aureus.* Vulnerable groups should therefore be offered and advised to have influenza vaccination annually, and those usually included in the 'vulnerable' category usually include:

- those with chronic cardiopulmonary disease, including chronic bronchitis, bronchiectasis, cystic fibrosis, and cardiac failure;
- those needing regular care for chronic diseases such as diabetes mellitus, renal failure, haemoglobinopathies, immunosuppression (including HIV positive people);
- people over 65 years living in nursing homes, long-stay hospitals, to prevent epidemics of influenza.
- In addition, influenza vaccination has been recommended for health care workers including doctors, nurses, and care workers who might, by transmitting influenza to those in their care, put elderly or infirm people at risk.

Influenza vaccination usually has few and minor side-effects, but should not be given to those with known hypersensitivity to eggs, in which the vaccine is prepared: they should be considered for chemoprophylaxis instead, using anti-viral drugs. The rationale for, and use of, influenza vaccine, and the occasional prophylactic use of anti-viral drugs such as amantadine and rimantadine is fully detailed in Chapter 19.

Prophylaxis against pneumococcal infection

A multi-valent pneumococcal vaccine was developed in 1983 containing capsular polysaccharides to 23 strains of *S. pneumoniae*, covering about 85% of the invasive strains usually found. Young people have a good antibody reaction to the vaccine with protective levels of antibody persisting for 7–10 years after a single inoculation. In older people, lower antibody levels are achieved, and the value of routine vaccination of the elderly is not clearly proven.[35] In this study, the overall protection given by vaccination was 57%; the protection was best among those with diabetes mellitus (84%), and chronic heart and lung disease (65%), but was least among those with chronic renal disease (27%) with no obvious efficacy in cirrhosis and alcoholism. Those for whom pneumococcal vaccination should be considered mandatory include those who have had an actual or functional splenectomy, whether after trauma, or through a haematological disorder. The case for wholesale vaccination of other population groups, such as the elderly, is still not entirely clear, although in USA pneumococcal vaccination is recommended for those aged over 65 years, those with chronic cardiac and respiratory disease, diabetes mellitus, alcoholism, and cirrhosis. It is suggested that pneumococcal vaccination should also be considered for those with chronic renal disease, Hodgkin's disease, myeloma, chronic lymphocytic leukaemia, and HIV infection.[36] For a fuller discussion of pneumococcal vaccine, see Chapter 5.

Therapy

Antibiotic therapy

Detailed guidelines for the management of community-acquired pneumonia have been published in the USA by the American Thoracic Society (1993),[14] in Canada by the Canadian Community Acquired Pneumonia Consensus Conference Group (1993),[13] and in the UK by the British Thoracic Society (1993).[15] Predictably, and as with all Guidelines, there has been a variety of views as to the appropriateness of the antibiotic therapy recommended, and the wisdom of Guidelines in general,[37] and some surprise as to the widely differing recommendations for the UK and USA[24, 38]

Much of the debate centres on the importance of investigation to determine the pathogen; a simple approach, with basic investigation and empirical 'best guess' therapy is generally suggested by the American and Canadian guidelines.[39]

On the other hand, a more active approach to diagnostic testing, with at the very least Gram's staining of sputum, and tests to detect capsular polysaccharide or cell-wall antigen for *S. pneumoniae* in sputum and pleural fluid has been advocated. This allows early specific treatment in many cases, which has advantages with the current increasing trend towards antibiotic resistance among pneumococcal infections[24]. Some of the argument revolves around the cost of investigation, and all those involved in the debate recognise the need for more research and careful validation of the guidelines in terms of patient outcome.

Despite these reservations, the practical issue is that, in most cases of community-acquired pneumonia, the pathogen cannot be identified at the moment the diagnosis of pneumonia is made; and even when the results of investigations are available, the causative organism cannot be identified in up to 47% of cases. Occasionally, special clinical features can suggest a particular pathogen; for instance, a patient with pleuritic pain, a lobar shadow on X-ray, and rusty sputum, is more likely to have pneumococcal pneumonia; and a younger patient, with the protracted, insidious onset of a harsh cough, in an epidemic year for *M. pneumoniae* infection may well have *M. pneumoniae*; initial therapy can therefore take account of such clinical hints. The value of such clinical hints, is, however, very limited; in a multivariate analysis of patients in the BTS pneumonia study,[40] using five admission variables (age, number of days ill before admission, presence or absence of bloody sputum, lobar infiltration on X-ray, and leukocytosis) the analysis could only predict whether the organism was *S. pneumoniae*, *M. pneumoniae,* 'other', or 'undetermined' in 42% of the cases. A further study of 359 patients with CAP confirmed how much overlap there was in the clinical syndromes, chest X-rays, and laboratory data accompanying pneumonias of different aetiology, that they could not be used to predict a cause.[17] Yet another study confirms the difficulty of using X-rays to attempt to differentiate between pathogens in CAP.[41] While investigations can provide important epidemiological information, and in cases where progress is unsatisfactory, important guidance for changes in antibiotic therapy, it is clear that for the broad mass of patients with pneumonia, treatment must be started on an empirical basis.

Table 17.3 and Table 17.4 show the anti-microbial therapy recommended in the available published Guidelines from the USA and UK. For *hospitalised patients*, the ATS recommends:

> second or third generation cephalosporins (e.g. cefotaxime, ceftriaxone);
> *or*
> β-lactam/β-lactamase inhibitor, with a macrolide if *Legionella* is suspected.

In the case of more *severe pneumonias*, demonstrating the features associated with a poorer prognosis noted above, antibiotic therapy recommended is shown in Table 17.4.

Why should the recommendations be so different, when there is little evidence to suggest that CAP on opposite sides of the Atlantic Ocean differs clinically, or in the range and proportion of causative organisms? Both guideline groups recognised the need to 'cover' the possibility of *Mycoplasma* and *Legionella* infections with a macrolide, but in the UK it was felt that this did not have to be an invariable maxim, since the most common pathogen was the pneumococcus. Only when *Legionella* or *Mycoplasma* is suspected need a macrolide be given. This may be good advice in the UK, where very few pneumococci are resistant to penicillin. Elsewhere, there are reports of an increasing prevalence of penicillin-resistant *S. pneumoniae* organisms in different countries; a recent report in the USA states that over 25% of isolates are penicillin resistant, and up to 80% show intermediate resistance.[42] The proportion of penicillin-resistant strains approaches 50% in several countries, including South Africa, Hungary, Spain, and Israel.[43] Despite such findings, one Spanish study,[44] while confirming high levels of penicillin-resistant pneumococci (29%), showed that the mortality from pneumonia with penicillin-resistant strains of *S. pneumoniae*, treated with penicillin G or ampicillin, did not differ from the mortality in patients where the organisms were penicillin sensitive. The same report noted that 6% of the organisms were also resistant to second generation cephalosporins such as cefotaxime and ceftriaxone. There is also an increasing level of resistance to other antibiotics in some countries: in Uruguay, 31% of strains of *S. pneumoniae* are resistant to erythromycin; and some resistance to cephalosporins has also been reported.[45] A knowledge of local resistance patterns is therefore essential, and all isolates should be tested for resistance so that antibiotic therapy is appropriate, particularly if pneumococcal infection is suspected. On the other hand, it is important to recognise that, although macrolides remain the mainstay of treatment for pneumonia caused by *S. pneumoniae* where there is penicillin hypersensitivity or in countries where there are significant levels of penicillin-resistant *S. pneumoniae* strains, there is nevertheless a trend towards increasing macrolide resistance, as discussed in greater detail in Chapter 5. The use of quinolones in the treatment of respiratory infections is also increasing, yet there is evidence that they are less effective in pneumococcal infections than other antibiotics.[46]

Table 17.3. *Recommended therapy for non-severe community-acquired pneumonia*

	BTS Guidelines	ATS Guidelines
Tolerant of penicillin	amoxycillin 500 mg 8-hourly orally *or* ampicillin 500 mg 6-hourly i/v *or*	aged 60 years or less; out-patient therapy erythromycin or other macrolide; possible tetracycline
	benzylpenicillin 1.2 g 6-hourly i/v *but* Erythromycin if *Legionella* or *Mycoplasma* suspected; in epidemics of influenza, add anti-staphylococcal agent	aged over 60 years, out-patient: second-generation cephalosporin *or* TMP/SMX *or* β-lactam/β-lactamase inhibitor, with or without a macrolide
Penicillin hypersensitivity	Erythromycin 500 mg 6-hourly orally *or* i/v cefuroxime *or* i/v cefotaxime	See above

Adapted from *Avery's Drug Treatment*, 4th edn by permission of editor and publisher.

Table 17.4. *Recommended therapy for severe pneumonias*

BTS Guidelines	ATS Guidelines
Erythromycin, 1 g. 6-hourly, *plus* second or third generation cephalosporin, e.g. cefuroxime, 1.5 g or cefotaxime, 2 g, 8-hourly, i/v *or* ampicillin, 1 g *and* flucloxacillin, 2 g *and* erythromycin, 1 g all in combination, 6-hourly, i/v	Macrolide *plus* third-generation cephalosporin with anti-*pseudomonas* activity *or* other antibiotic with similar activity, e.g. imipenem, or ciprofloxacin

Adapted from *Avery's Drug Treatment*, 4th edn by permission of editor and publisher.

Antibiotic therapy after the causative organism is identified–therapy for specific pneumonias

The reader is directed to the infection-specific chapters, but a summary of the usual recommendations is given herewith.

Pneumococcal pneumonia: *Streptococcus pneumoniae*

This organism remains the commonest cause of community-acquired pneumonia in the general population, and further details of the increased susceptibility of patients after splenectomy, or people with sickle-cell anaemia, are detailed in Chapter 5. Other people vulnerable to Streptococcal infection include those with hepatic cirrhosis, and those with hypogammaglobulinaemia, particularly of IgG2 and IgG4.

Until recently, *S. pneumoniae* was sensitive to almost all antibiotics except aminoglycosides, and could be effectively treated with penicillin G intramuscularly or intravenously, or penicillin V by mouth; the effective dose is 1–3 G daily, in four or more divided doses. For those with hypersensitivity to penicillin, macrolides or cephalosporins are the usual alternative. The emergence of increasing numbers of strains of *S. pneumoniae* showing resistance to β-lactams, macrolides, tetracyclines, and co-trimoxazole has meant that it is necessary to be aware of the antibiotic sensitivity pattern for pneumococci for the country where the infection has arisen, and treat accordingly; antibiotics such as cefotaxime, imipenem, or even rifampicin may be required in the more multiply-resistant varieties of *S. pneumoniae* infection.

In most cases treatment brings about a rapid fall in fever, followed by a gradual resolution of the physical signs over a few days. Radiological clearing of the pneumonia usually takes about 2 weeks, but may take up to 10 weeks, especially in the elderly or in those with underlying lung disease, such as chronic bronchitis. If clinical improvement does not occur, it will be important to consider the presence of antibiotic-resistant strains, but also the possibility of other diagnoses, accompanying the pneumonia, such as, for example, an obstructing bronchial tumour or pulmonary embolism.

Staphylococcal pneumonia: *Staphylococcus aureus*

Staphylococcal pneumonia may be a primary infection, or may occur as a complication of influenza, particularly in major epidemics of influenza; it is a severe pneumonia, with a mortality rate of about 30%. The appearance of penicillinase-producing strains requires that Staphylococcal pneumonia must be treated with penicillins resistant to β-lactamases, such as flucloxacillin. Doses of up to 2 g flucloxacillin four times daily intravenously may be required in severe cases; the addition of fusidic acid, 0.5–1 g three times daily, or an aminoglycoside, may bring added benefits. More recently, methicillin-resistant strains of *S. aureus* have posed particular problems in some hospitals, and for such organisms vancomycin is the treatment of choice.

Gram-negative pneumonias

H. influenzae, a common pathogen in infective exacerbations of chronic bronchitis, is also increasingly recognised as a cause of adult community-acquired pneumonia. More than 10% of strains are now capable of producing β-lactamase, so ampicillin is no longer the antibiotic of choice in many areas; recommended antibiotics include the amoxycillin and clavulanic acid combination (co-amoxyclav), or a second-generation cephalosporin such as cefotaxime; or ciprofloxacin, or co-trimoxazole.

Infections with organisms such as *P. aeruginosa*, *Acinetobacter*, *K. pneumoniae*, *Enterobacter*, *Proteus* species, *Serratia marcescens*, and *E.coli* are rarely found as community-acquired infections, being almost always associated with hospital nosocomial infections or occurring in immunosuppressed patients. They are best treated following careful assessment of the antibiotic sensitivities, but treatment may be started with a third-generation cephalosporin such as ceftazidime in combination with an aminoglycoside such as gentamicin, tobramycin, or netilmicin. Subsequent therapy, once antibiotic sensitivities are known, may include other agents such as the quinalones (e.g. ciprofloxacin), monobactams (e.g. aztreonam) and carbapenems (e.g. imipenem).

Legionnaire's disease *Legionella pneumophila* (see Chapter 14)

This is a severe pneumonia with many potential complications and a mortality rate of around 15%. Sporadic community–acquired cases may account for 2% of all community-acquired pneumonias, but outbreaks have also occurred, often being attributed to contamination of water in air conditioning systems with evaporative condensers, or water fittings in showers and sinks; a number of these outbreaks have occurred in hospitals, and from other public buildings. Erythromycin administered in high doses (1 g 6-hourly intravenously or orally) is the antibiotic of choice. In severe cases, and in those not responding adequately to erythromycin alone, the addition of rifampicin is recommended, and ciprofloxacin is a further option.

Other bacterial pneumonias–zoonoses

Pneumonic plague (*Y. pestis*) responds to tetracyclines and chloramphenicol, also to streptomycin. *B. anthracis* (anthrax pneumonia) responds to penicillin, and tularaemia to gentamicin and streptomycin.

Mycoplasmal, chlamydial and rickettsial pneumonias (see Chapter 13)

The so-called atypical pneumonias due to *M. pneumoniae*, *Chlamydia psittaci* and *Coxiella burnetii* (the causative agent of Q fever) differ from common bacterial pneumonias in having an influenza-like presentation, often with generalised symptoms, and in responding to tetracyclines and macrolides rather than penicillins. *M. pneumoniae* may be suspected in epidemic years, which occur every 4–5 years, and by the very persistent cough which often induces retching. Infection with *C. psittaci* is usually contracted from infected birds, though person-to person transmission has been suggested in the TWAR strain. *C. burnetii* infection is usually contracted by those such as abattoir workers or shepherds who are exposed to the blood of infected animals.

M. pneumoniae infection responds to erythromycin or the tetracyclines, though even with therapy the course of the illness may be prolonged for up to 6 or 8 weeks. Tetracyclines are the drugs of choice for *C. psittaci* and *C. burnetii* infection.

Supportive therapy

Oxygen therapy

If a substantial area of lung is consolidated in pneumonia, arterial hypoxaemia is likely because some of the pulmonary blood flow will take place through unventilated lung tissue. The aim should therefore be to restore arterial oxygen tension (P_aO_2) and saturation (S_aO_2) to levels which allow the oxygen content of arterial blood to be adequate for tissue oxygenation. Although the normal P_aO_2 is usually defined as being between 12 and 13.3 kPa (90–100 mm Hg), which means that, for a haemoglobin level of 15 g/dl of blood, the oxygen content is 200 ml of oxygen per litre, the content of oxygen in hypoxia does not usually fall significantly until the P_aO_2 has fallen to 8 kPa or 60 mm Hg, so the aim of therapy should always be to give sufficient oxygen to exceed this level with a margin to spare. If there is a large 'shunt' across the pulmonary circulation as a result of a large consolidated, perfused area of lung, it may be necessary to give high concentration oxygen; this increases the amount of *dissolved* oxygen in plasma (up to 20 ml per litre) and thus increases the oxygen content even when a proportion of the pulmonary blood flow does not take part in the gas-exchanging process. Therefore, in many cases, oxygen can, and should, be given through a mask which allows the delivery of 40–60% oxygen. Rarely, even higher levels may be required, delivered by a system with valves which can deliver concentrations of 80% oxygen or more. However, patients who have such severe hypoxaemia should properly be considered for intensive care management and assisted ventilation. As with all patients requiring oxygen therapy, and particularly those with pre-existing chronic lung disease such as chronic bronchitis, there is a risk of the development of hypoventilation with hypercapnia, and any hint of this should raise the immediate question of ventilatory support.

Other supportive measures

Patients with pneumonia should also receive good nursing care, including attention to good hydration, if necessary intravenously. Physiotherapy will be required to assist the patient who has much sputum to expectorate.

References

1. BRITISH THORACIC SOCIETY AND PUBLIC HEALTH LABORATORY SERVICE. Community acquired pneumonia in adults in British Hospitals in 1982–1983: a survey of aetiology, mortality, prognostic factors and outcome. *Quart J Med* 1987;239:195–220.
2. MACFARLANE JT, COLVILLE A, GUION A, *et al.* Prospective study of aetiology and outcome of adult lower-respiratory-tract infections in the community. *Lancet* 1993;341:511–14.
3. WOODHEAD MA, MACFARLANE JT, MCCRACKEN JS *et al.* Prospective study of the aetiology and outcome of pneumonia in the community. *Lancet* 1987;i:671–4.
4. JOKINEN C, HEISKANEN L, JUVONEN H *et al.* Incidence of community acquired pneumonia in the population of four municipalities in Eastern Finland. *Am J Epidemiol* 1993;137: 977–88.
5. FOY HM, COONEY MK, ALLAN I *et al.* Rates of Pneumonia during influenza epidemics in Seattle, 1964 to 1975. *JAMA* 1979;241:253–8.
6. MARRIE TJ. Community acquired pneumonia. *Clin Infect Dis* 1994;18:501–15.
7. BERMAN S, DUENAS A, BEDOYA A *et al.* Acute lower respiratory tract illnesses in Cali, Colombia: a two-year ambulatory study. *Pediatrics* 1983;71:210–18.
8. BANG AB, BANG RA, TALE O *et al.* Reduction in pneumonia mortality and total child mortality by means of community-based intervention trial in Gadchiroli, India. *Lancet* 1990;336:201–6.
9. KOIVULA I, STEN M, MAKELÄ PH. Risk factors for pneumonia in the elderly. *Am J Med* 1994;96:313–20.
10. FERNANDEZ-SOLA J, JUNQUE A, ESTRUCH R *et al.* High alcohol intake as a risk and prognostic factor for community-acquired pneumonia. *Arch Int Med* 1995;155:1649–54.
11. NIEDERMAN MS. Respiratory infections in the 1990s. *Curr Opin Pulm Med* 1995;1:155–62.
12. FINE MJ, SMITH MA, CARSON CA *et al.* Prognosis and outcomes of patients with community-acquired pneumonia: a meta-analysis. *JAMA* 1996;275:134–41.
13. MANDELL LA, NIEDERMAN M. Canadian Community Acquired Pneumonia Consensus Conference Group. Antimicrobial treatment of community acquired pneumonia in adults: a conference report. *Can J Infect Dis* 1993;4:25–8.
14. AMERICAN THORACIC SOCIETY. Guidelines for the initial management of adults with community-acquired pneumonia: diagnosis, assessment of severity, and initial antimicrobial therapy. *Am Rev Resp Dis* 1993;148:141.
15. BRITISH THORACIC SOCIETY. Guidelines for the management of community-acquired pneumonia in adults admitted to hospital. *Br J Hosp Med* 1993;49.346.
16. MARRIE TJ, DURRANT H, YATES L. Community acquired pneumonia requiring hospitalisation: 5-year prospective study. *Rev Infect Dis* 1989;11:586–99.
17. FANG G, FINE M, ORLOFF J *et al.* New and emerging aetiologies for community acquired pneumonia with implications for therapy. *Medincine (Baltimore)* 1990;69:307–16.
18. BLANQUER J, BLANQUER R, BORRAS R *et al.* Aetiology of community acquired pneumonia in Valencia, Spain: a multicentre prospective study. *Thorax* 1991;46:508–11.
19. ÖRTQVIST A, HEDLUND J, GRILLNER L *et al.* Aetiology, outcome, and prognostic factors in community acquired pneumonia requiring hospitalisation. *Eur Resp J* 1990;3:1105–13.
20. LIND K, BENTZAN MW. Changes in the epidemiological pattern of *Mycoplasma pneumoniae* infections in Denmark. *Epidemiol Inf* 1988;101:377–86.
21. MACFARLANE J. An overview of community acquired pneumonia with lessons learned from the British Thoracic Society study. *Semin Resp Infect* 1994;9:153–65.
22. KARALUS NC, CURSONS RT, LENG RA, *et al.* Community acquired pneumonia: etiology and prognostic index evaluation. *Thorax* 1991;46:413–18.
23. LIM I, SHAW DR, STANLEY DP *et al.* A prospective hospital study of the aetiology of community acquired pneumonia. *Med J Aust* 1989;151:87–91.
24. BARTLETT JG, MUNDY LM. Community-acquired pneumonia. *New Engl J Med* 1995;333:1618–24.
25. ÖRTQVIST A. Initial investigation and treatment of the patient with severe community acquired pneumonia. *Semin Resp Infect* 1994;9:166–79.
26. NIEDERMAN MS, TORRES A, SUMMER W. Invasive diagnostic testing is not needed routinely to manage ventilator-associated pneumonia *Am J Resp Crit Care Med* 1994;150:565–9.
27. CHASTRE J, FAGON JY. Invasive Diagnostic Testing should be routinely used to manage ventilated patients with suspected pneumonia *Am J Resp Crit Care Med* 1994;150: 570–4.
28. ØSTERGAARD L, ANDERSEN PL. Etiology of community acquired pneumonia: evaluation by transtracheal aspiration, blood culture or serology. *Chest* 1993;104:1400–7.

29. SPENCER CD, BEATY HN. Complications of transtracheal aspiration. *N Engl J Med* 1972;286:304–6.

30. SCHLUGER NW, ROM WN. The Polymerase Chain Reaction in the diagnosis and evaluation of pulmonary infections. *Am J Resp Crit Care Med* 1995;152:11–16.

31. GILBERT K, FINE MJ. Assessing prognosis and predicting outcomes in community acquired pneumonia. *Semin Resp Infect* 1994;9:140–52.

32. FINE MJ, ORLOFF JJ, ARISUMI D *et al.* Prognosis of patients hospitalised with community acquired pneumonia. *Am J Med* 1990;88:5-1N–8N.

33. MARRIE TJ, DURANT H, YATES L. Community-acquired pneumonia requiring hospitalisation: 5-year prospective study. *Rev Infect Dis* 1989;11:586–99.

34. TARYLE DA, POTTS DE, SAHN SA. The incidence and clinical correlates of parapneumonic effusions. *Chest* 1978;74: 170–3.

35. BUTLER JC, BREIMANN RF, CAMPBELL JF *et al.* Pneumococcal polysaccharide vaccine efficacy: an evaluation of current recommendations. *J Am Med Assoc* 1993;270:1826–31.

36. ORTIZ CR, LA FORCE FM. Prevention of community-acquired pneumonia. *Med Clin N Am* 1994;78:1173–83.

37. FEIN AM, NIEDERMAN MS. Guidelines for the initial management of Community-acquired pneumonia: Savory recipe or cookbook for disaster? *Am J Resp Crit Care Med* 1995; 152:1149–53.

38. MANDELL LA. Community acquired pneumonia; aetiology, epidemiology, and treatment. *Chest* 1995;108:35S–42S.

39. MANDELL LA, NIEDERMAN MS. Community-acquired pneumonia. *N Engl J Med* 1996; 334: 861. (letter)

40. FARR BM, KAISER DL, HARRISON BDW, CONNOLLY CK. Prediction of microbial aetiology at admission to hospital for pneumonia from the presenting clinical features. *Thorax* 1989;44:1031–5.

41. MACFARLANE JT, MILLAR AC, SMITH WHR, MORRIS AH, ROSE DH. Comparative radiographic features of acquired legionnaires' disease, pneumococcal pneumonia, and psittacosis *Thorax* 1984;39:28–33.

42. HOFMAN J, CETRON MS, FARLEY MM *et al.* The prevalence of drug-resistant *Streptococcus pneumococci* in Atlanta. *N Engl J Med* 1995;333:481–6.

43. FRIEDLAND IR, MCCRACKEN GH. Management of infections caused by antibiotic-resistant *Streptococcus pneumoniae*. *New Engl J Med* 1994;331:377–82.

44. PALLARES R, LINARES J, VADILLO M *et al.* Resistance to penicillin and cephalosporin and mortality from severe pneumococcal pneumonia in Barcelona, Spain. *N Engl J Med* 1995;333:474–80.

45. FRIEDLAND IR, MCCRACKEN GH. Management of infections caused by anti-biotic-resistant *Streptococcus pneumoniae N Eng J Med* 1992;331:377–82.

46. THYS JP, JACOBS F, BYL B. Role of quinolones in the treatment of bronchopulmonary infections, particularly pneumococcal and community-acquired pneumonia. *Eur J Clin Microbiol Infect Dis* 1991;10:304–15.

18 Community-acquired fungal pneumonias

DAVID S. MCKINSEY
Research Medical Center, Kansas City, USA

Introduction

Community-acquired fungal pneumonias are uncommon diseases but can cause substantial morbidity and even mortality. The endemic fungi *Histoplasma capsulatum*, *Blastomyces dermatitidis*, *Coccidioides immitis* and *Paracoccidioides brasiliensis* cause disease primarily in localised areas in North, Central, and South America, but the geographical distribution of these pathogens is actually quite widespread and cases are occasionally seen outside of the traditional endemic areas. Moreover, the global population is now so mobile that many individuals who reside in non-endemic areas come into contact with the endemic fungi while traveling for business or leisure activities. Other fungal respiratory tract pathogens including *Cryptococcus neoformans* and *Sporothrix schenkii* have worldwide distributions.

The patient with community-acquired fungal pneumonia often poses a significant diagnostic challenge because the clinical manifestations of the endemic and non-endemic pulmonary mycoses are varied and non-specific. The presentations of these forms of pneumonia often mimic bacterial pneumonia, tuberculosis, or malignancy. Thus, it is important for the clinician to have a high index of suspicion for fungal pneumonias in a variety of settings.

The diagnostic approach to the patient with suspected fungal pneumonia depends upon the specific aetiology under consideration in an individual case. Available diagnostic techniques include smears and cultures of clinical specimens and various serological tests. Although some forms of fungal pneumonia are self-limited, treatment is indicated in many cases. Treatment options for fungal pneumonia have expanded substantially with the availability of the azole antifungal compounds ketoconazole, fluconazole, and itraconazole.

This chapter will review features of six community-acquired fungal pneumonias. Particular attention will be focused on the epidemiology, clinical manifestations, diagnosis, and treatment of these infections. Fungal respiratory infections acquired in hospital are described in Chapter 16.

Histoplasmosis

History

The first case of histoplasmosis, reported by Darling in 1906, was a young Panamanian man who died from a subacute febrile illness and was noted to have an unusual microorganism scattered throughout the organs of the reticuloendothelial system[1]. Darling named the organism *Histoplasma capsulatum* because he believed that it infected histiocytes (macrophages), was a parasite *(plasmas* = parasite), and possessed a capsule. The latter two counts later were proven incorrect when it was shown that the organism is a fungus that is not encapsulated, but the original name has been maintained.

In 1932, Dodd and Tompkins made the first ante-mortem diagnosis of histoplasmosis in a child who subsequently died from the disease[2]. DeMonbreun cultured *H. capsulatum* from tissue specimens from this child and demonstrated that *H. capsulatum* is a thermal dimorphic fungus. *H. capsulatum* infection was considered invariably fatal until the 1940s when Christie, Peterson, and Palmer showed that histoplasmosis was a common cause of asymptomatic pulmonary calcifications in the midwestern and southern United States[3–6].

Emmons cultivated the organism from soil in 1948[7]. Later it was shown that *H. capsulatum* thrives in soil contaminated with bird or bat guano[8] and that aerosolisation of organisms is its route of transmission. A number of point-source epidemics were reported in association with activities such as cleaning chicken coops or spelunking[9].

Since the early 1980s, attention has focused on the epidemiology and clinical manifestations of histoplasmosis in immunocompromised individuals including patients with AIDS.

Mycology

Three pathogenic varieties of *H. capsulatum* have been identified: *H. capsulatum var. capsulatum, H. capsulatum var. dubosii,* and *H. capsulatum var. farciminosum. H. capsulatum var. dubosii* causes African histoplasmosis, a disease manifested primarily by bone and skin lesions; pulmonary disease is extremely uncommon[10]. *H. capsulatum var. farciminosum* is a cause of lymphangitis in mules and horses but is not pathogenic in humans. The remainder of this discussion will address *H. capsulatum var. capsulatum,* which shall be referred to as *H. capsulatum* for the sake of convenience.

H. capsulatum is a dimorphic fungus. At temperatures less than 37 °C, the organism exists as a mycelium. This saprophytic form consists of vegetative hyphae associated with two types of conidia: macroconidia, which measure up to 15 μM in diameter and have characteristic finger-like tuberculate surfaces, and microconidia, which are 2 to 4 μM in diameter and have smooth surfaces. The mycelial form of *H. capsulatum* has an extensive natural reservoir in soil and decaying vegetation. It grows best in warm, humid areas contaminated by chicken, starling, or bat guano. Organisms live primarily in the top 15 cm of soil and are not found more than 22.5 cm below the ground surface[11]. At 37 °C, *H. capsulatum* converts to an oval yeast which reproduces by budding and measures 3 to 4 μM in diameter.

Epidemiology

Cases of histoplasmosis have been reported from all five continents[12]. However, the primary endemic areas are in North and South America, particularly in the Ohio and Mississippi River valleys in the United States (Fig. 18.1). Within the endemic area the distribution of organisms in the soil is patchy, with highest concentrations occurring in such microfoci as blackbird roosts, chicken coops, decaying trees, and caves contaminated with bat guano[13]. Skin test surveys have been useful in mapping endemic areas by identifying individuals with prior subclinical infection. Such surveys have shown that 20% of the population of the continental United States, i.e. approximately 50 million people as of the mid-1990s, have been infected with *H. capsulatum*[14]. In highly endemic areas, asymptomatic infection occurs in approximately 3% of the population per year[15].

Most symptomatic cases of histoplasmosis are sporadic and are acquired by inhalation of airborne organisms from environmental foci. Rare cases of laboratory-acquired disease have occurred due to mishandling of culture plates[16]. Human-to-human transmission due to renal transplantation has been documented[17]. There have been numerous epidemics of histoplasmosis, which have been traced to activities associated with exposure to avian droppings or contaminated soil, e.g. exploring caves or cleaning bird roosts, chicken coops, or old parks[18,19]. An urban epidemic in Indianapolis, Indiana, during which more than 100 000 persons were infected, occurred in the late 1970s following the demolition of an amusement park[20,21]. Specific high-risk exposures which have been associated with histoplasmosis and with other forms of fungal pneumonia are shown in Table 18.1.

Future studies of the epidemiology of histoplasmosis will be aided by the development of new molecular biology techniques. Restriction frequent length polymorphism (RFLP) studies have been used to identify five distinct classes of *H. capsulatum*[22]. Genetic diversity has been documented within isolates in the same classes[22].

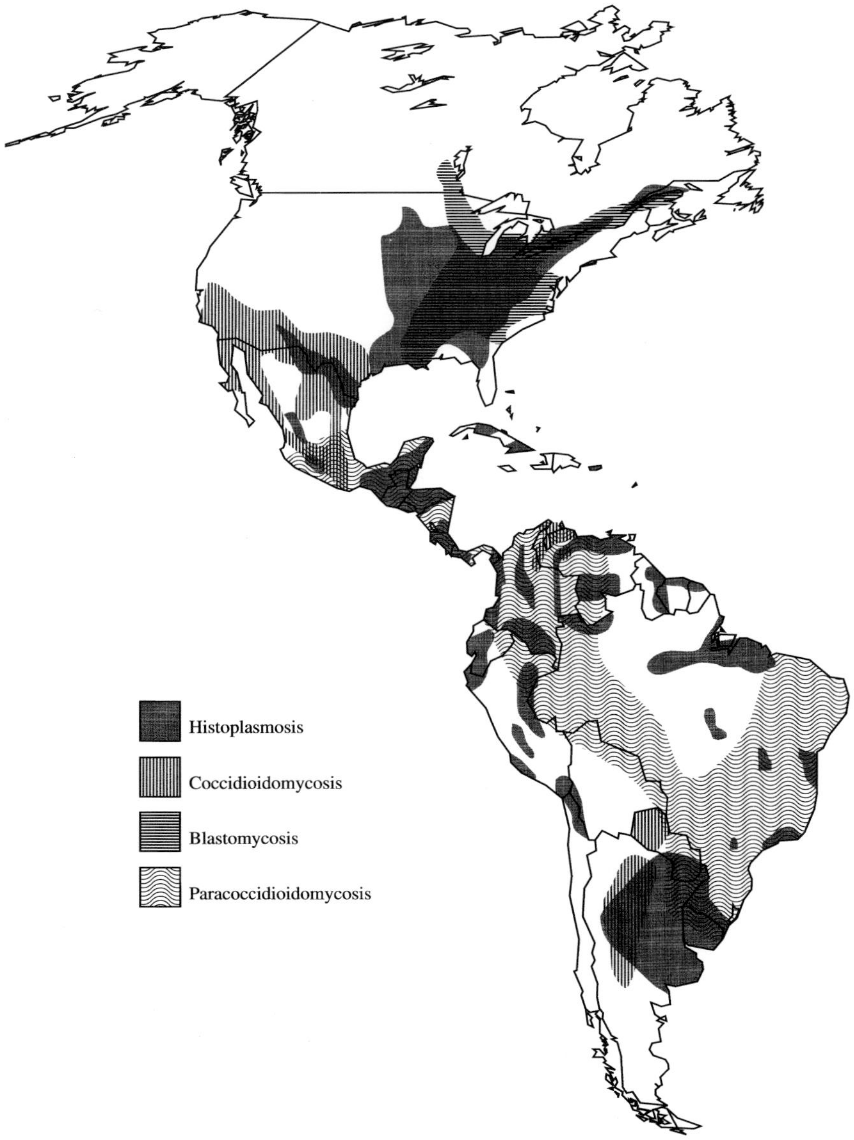

FIGURE 18.1 Primary endemic areas for histoplasmosis, coccidioidomycosis, blastomycosis, and paracoccidioidomycosis.

Table 18.1. *High-risk exposures for fungal pneumonias*

Disease	Exposure
Histoplasmosis	Residence in Mississippi or Ohio River Valleys Spelunking Woodcutting through logs contaminated with avian excrement Construction work Chicken coop exposure Bird roost exposure
Blastomycosis	Residence in upper midwestern or southeastern US or southern Canada Hunting, fishing, or camping in wooded areas along streams or lakes Construction work
Coccidioidomycosis	Residence in Sonoran Life Zone in southwestern US and northwestern Mexico or in endemic areas in Argentina Agricultural work Construction work Archeological exploration Laboratory exposure Fomite exposure from endemic area
Cryptococcosis	None known
Sporotrichosis	Exposure to contaminated sphagnum moss, straw, or wood
Paracoccidioidomycosis	Residence in endemic areas in Mexico, Central America, or South America Agricultural work

Use of genetic fingerprinting techniques during future epidemics may enable more accurate analysis of the epidemiology and pathogenesis of histoplasmosis.

Pathophysiology

Infection is initiated by inhalation of airborne *H. capsulatum* microconidia into the alveoli. A large inoculum of organisms is required to establish an infection. After 3 to 5 days, microconidia convert to yeast which replicate by budding and then spread to contiguous alveoli. Neutrophils have potent antifungal activity *in vitro* against mycelial and yeast forms of *H. capsulatum* and probably play a role in limiting spread of infection[23,24]. Macrophages ingest *H. capsulatum* yeast forms, but in non-immune individuals organisms are able to replicate within macrophages[25,26]. Infected macrophages enter pulmonary lymphatic channels and drain to hilar lymph nodes, which often become enlarged during primary infection. Subsequently, widespread haematogenous dissemination occurs in many cases, as indicated by the common occurrence of splenic calcifications among individuals residing in endemic areas[27]. Organisms can spread to the liver, spleen, bone marrow, lymph nodes, adrenal glands, central nervous system, and other sites.

After 1 to 2 weeks, a cellular immune response develops. Activated macrophages are fungistatic and participate in formation of caseating granulomas[26]. Granulocyte-macrophage colony-stimulating factor (CSF), macrophage CSF, and interleukin 3 all increase the fungistatic capability of activated macrophages *in vitro*[25,28]. The crucial role of the CD4+ T lymphocyte in the cellular immune response against *H. capsulatum* has been emphasised by the markedly increased risk of severe histoplasmosis in patients with AIDS who have diminished CD4+ T-cell counts[29,30].

In individuals with healed histoplasmosis, granulomas become calcified approximately 6 months after resolution of infection. *H. capsulatum* organisms can be detected within calcified granulomas for many years[27]. It is unclear whether or not such foci of infection can reactivate in a manner analogous to reactivation tuberculosis. The occurrence of disseminated histoplasmosis in non-endemic areas such as New York City[31] and Europe[32] among individuals who previously visited endemic areas suggests that reactivation of latent foci of infection can occur.

Clinical manifestations

The majority of *H. capsulatum* infections are asymptomatic and self-limited. Symptomatic disease develops in individuals who have been exposed to a large inoculum of organisms or in persons with impaired cellular immune function. Clinical manifestations of histoplasmosis vary based upon the inoculum of organisms inhaled, the underlying health status of the patient, and the immunological response of the host to the pathogen (Table 18.2).

Acute pulmonary histoplasmosis

Approximately 1% of persons exposed to *H. capsulatum* develop acute pulmonary histoplasmosis[33]. The median incubation period is 2 weeks (range 4 to 30 days)[34,35]. Clinical manifestations of this disease have been well characterised in studies of epidemics, as summarised by Bullock[36]. Among 450 patients reported in four epidemics, the following symptoms occurred: fever, 92%; headache, 89%; malaise, 64%; substernal chest pain (thought to be secondary to sudden enlargement of hilar lymph nodes), 62%; chills, 61%; non-productive cough, 56%; myalgias, 40%[19,34,35,37]. Other common symptoms included anorexia and weight loss. Symptoms of acute histoplasmosis resolve spontaneously within 2 weeks in most cases, although a few patients develop a severe infection complicated by acute respiratory distress syndrome (Fig. 16.2).[38]

There are a variety of uncommon clinical manifestations of acute pulmonary histoplasmosis. Pericarditis occurs in approximately 6% of cases[39]. Pericardial tamponade has been reported rarely[40]. Small, self-limited pleural effusions are seen in a few cases. Six percent of patients develop a rheumatological syndrome which closely resembles sarcoidosis. These individuals have monoarthritis or polyarthritis and erythema nodosum for approximately 2 weeks in most cases, although occasionally symptoms persist for up to a year[41].

Physical findings in acute pulmonary histoplasmosis are nonspecific. Fever and tachypnea occur frequently. Lung examination is generally normal. In rare cases hepatosplenomegaly is observed; this finding suggests a high likelihood of progression to disseminated histoplasmosis. Chest radiographs generally demonstrate patchy

Table 18.2. *Histoplasmosis: clinical manifestations*

Asymptomatic infection
Acute symptomatic infection
Pulmonary histoplasmosis
Pericarditis
Arthralgias or arthritis with erythema nodosum
Chronic pulmonary histoplasmosis
Mediastinal fibrosis
Disseminated histoplasmosis

pulmonary infiltrates that are unilateral or bilateral (Fig. 18.3)[42]. Infiltrates occur in any location in the lungs but primarily affect the lower lobes. Hilar and/or mediastinal lymphadenopathy is often seen[42]. Cavitation has been reported rarely (Fig. 18.4)[43,44].

Mediastinal granulomatosis and fibrosis

During acute pulmonary histoplasmosis, an intense inflammatory response can occur in mediastinal lymph nodes. Enlarged mediastinal nodes sometimes coalesce to form a cystic structure in the mediastinum called a mediastinal granuloma, which can compress the oesophagus[45], trachea, bronchi, or great vessels[46]. Occasionally calcified debris from a granuloma erodes into a bronchus, causing broncholithiasis[47].

In approximately 1 in 5000 cases of pulmonary histoplasmosis an excessive host inflammatory response to *H. capsulatum* antigens causes an exuberant fibrotic reaction[46]. Fibrosis usually occurs in the mediastinum but also can involve the pericardium or pleura[48]. Clinical manifestations of this life-threatening condition include superior vena cava syndrome, oesophageal compression, constrictive pericarditis, and trapping of a lung (Fig. 18.5)[46].

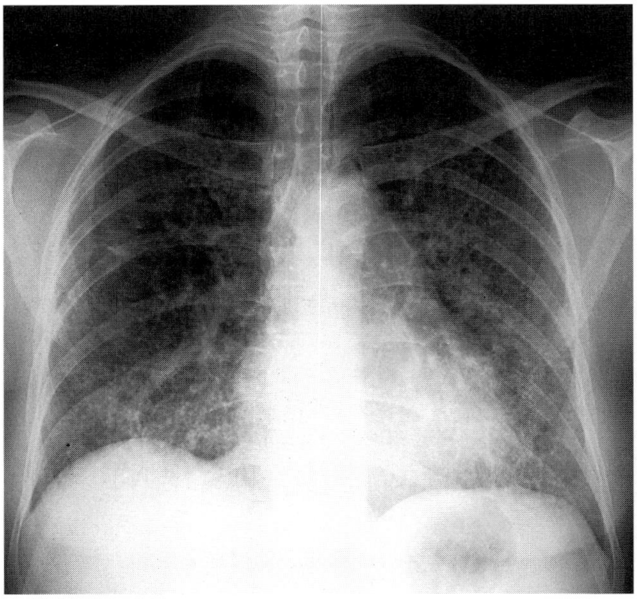

FIGURE 18.2 Acute pulmonary histoplasmosis. Diffuse, bilateral interstitial pulmonary infiltrates in a woman exposed to starling guano while cleaning window sills at an old home in rural Missouri.

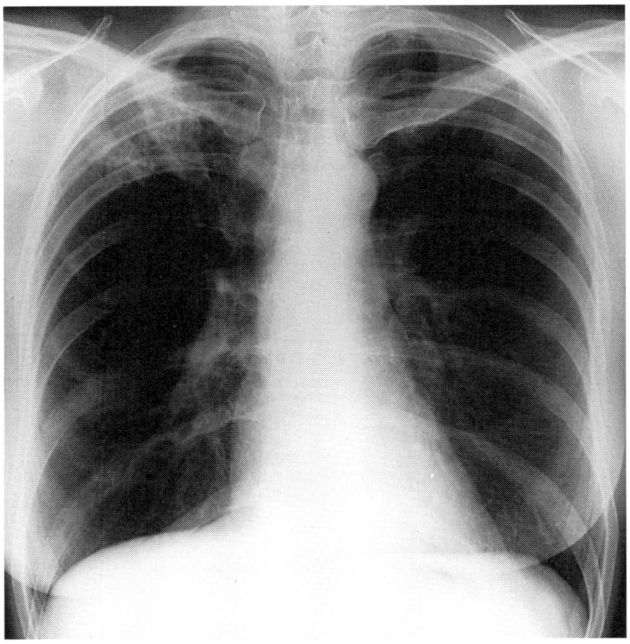

FIGURE 18.3 Acute pulmonary histoplasmosis. Focal alveolar infiltrate is present in right upper lobe. (Courtesy of J. Bower, MD.)

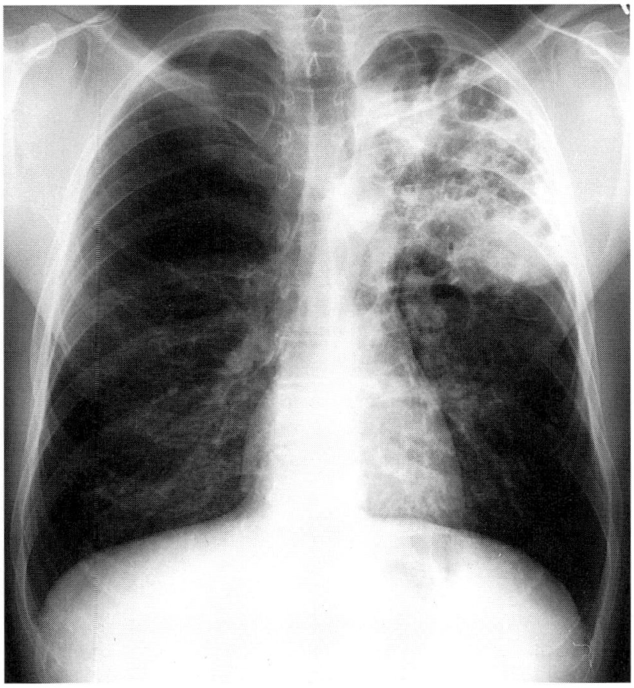

FIGURE 18.4 Acute cavitary pulmonary histoplasmosis. Numerous cavities are present within an alveolar infiltrate in the left upper lobe.

Histoplasmoma

Healed pulmonary foci of histoplasmosis occasionally create coin lesions called histoplasmomas. A histoplasmoma consists of a calcified granuloma containing yeast phase organisms surrounded by a circumferential fibrotic reaction. Histoplasmomas are usually located in subpleural areas. They are asymptomatic but are clinically significant in that their radiographical appearance can be identical to that of bronchogenic neoplasms.

Chronic pulmonary histoplasmosis

Persons with pulmonary emphysema or chronic bronchitis are at risk for chronic pulmonary histoplasmosis. This disease closely mimics pulmonary tuberculosis; indeed, prior to the 1950s, many patients hospitalised in American tuberculosis sanitariums actually had chronic pulmonary histoplasmosis[49].

Risk factors for chronic pulmonary histoplasmosis include male sex, white race, age above 40 years, chronic obstructive pulmonary disease, and immunosuppression[43]. Most patients have been ill for several weeks to months before seeking medical attention. Clinical manifestations include weight loss, fatigue, productive cough, chest pain, dyspnoea, or hemoptysis. Fever occurs in only one-quarter of cases. Physical examination is generally unremarkable aside from the typical stigmata of chronic obstructive pulmonary disease[50].

Infiltrates occur in the apical and posterior segments of both upper lobes, are located peripherally[50], and are associated with pulmonary cavities in 80 to 90% of cases (Fig. 18.6, 7, 8)[43,50]. One-quarter of patients have bilateral cavities; in the remaining three-fourths, the right upper lobe is affected more frequently than the left upper lobe[43]. The cavities tend to enlarge over time and eventually lead to fibrosis and retraction of surrounding lung tissue[50].

Disseminated histoplasmosis

Symptomatic disseminated histoplasmosis occurs in approximately 1 in 2000 patients infected with *H. capsulatum*[20]. Disseminated histoplasmosis is a life-threatening infection which has protean clinical manifestations. Extra-pulmonary disease dominates the clinical presentation, although one-quarter of patients present with non-productive cough and dyspnoea[51]. In these cases miliary pulmonary infiltrates (identical to those seen in miliary tuberculosis) are present. For a detailed description of the clinical manifestations of disseminated histoplasmosis the reader is referred to an excellent review of the subject[51].

Histoplasmosis in the acquired immunodeficiency syndrome (AIDS)

In certain communities in the endemic area for *H. capsulatum*, disseminated histoplasmosis has been diagnosed in up to 30% of patients with AIDS[30,52,53]. Cases also have occurred in locations outside the

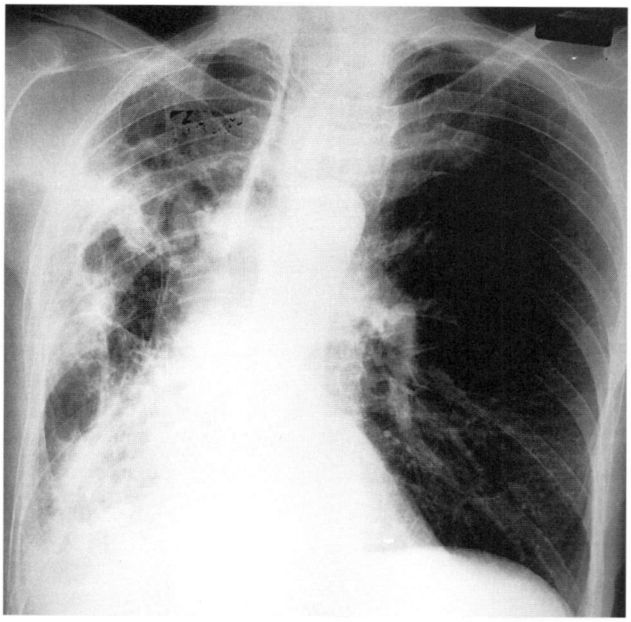

FIGURE 18.6 Chronic pulmonary histoplasmosis. Extensive infiltrate in right lung is associated with cavitation and volume loss. (Courtesy of M. Driks, MD.)

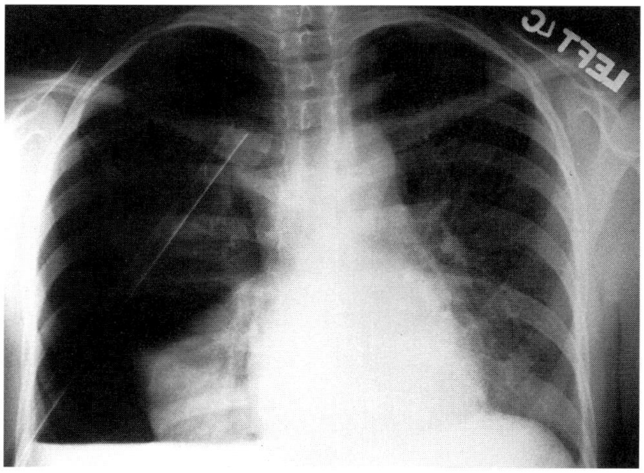

FIGURE 18.5 Trapped right lung in patient with pleural fibrosis secondary to histoplasmosis.

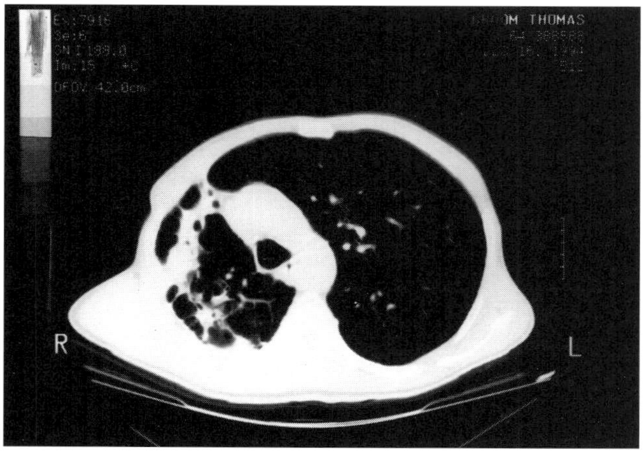

FIGURE 18.7 Chronic pulmonary histoplasmosis. Computerized tomography scan shows destruction of lung parenchyma, cavity formation, and fibrosis. (Courtesy of M. Driks, MD.)

endemic area (e.g. California, New York, France)[31,32] among individuals who previously visited endemic regions.

Histoplasmosis in AIDS occurs most commonly in individuals with CD4+ lymphocyte counts ≤ 150/l[54]. The disease generally presents as a subacute febrile wasting illness although in up to 10% of cases the presentation is fulminant and multiple organ system failure occurs[53]. Virtually all infections are disseminated; however, rare cases of pneumonia without dissemination have been reported[53].

Symptoms of respiratory tract infection, e.g. cough and dyspnoea, occur in about half of patients with AIDS and disseminated histoplasmosis[55]. Pulmonary infiltrates are seen in two-thirds of cases[55,56]. Bilateral interstitial or interstitial-alveolar infiltrates are the typical finding[56] (Fig. 18.9). This radiographic pattern can be indistinguishable from that of *Pneumocystis carinii* pneumonia, the most common form of AIDS-associated opportunistic pneumonia[56]. In the endemic area, therefore, disseminated histoplasmosis should be included in the differential diagnosis of all cases of opportunistic pneumonia in AIDS.

Diagnosis

Direct examination

H. capsulatum organisms can be observed directly in blood smears, sputum, cerebrospinal fluid, or biopsy specimens (Fig. 18.10). Wright's stains of peripheral blood smears demonstrate *H. capsulatum* yeast forms within neutrophils in about one-third of patients with AIDS and disseminated histoplasmosis[52] but far less frequently in HIV-seronegative patients. Preparation of Buffy coat smears from peripheral blood may facilitate diagnosis. Giemsa or Wright's stains of sputum or bronchial washings are positive in 10–16% of cases of acute or chronic pulmonary histoplasmosis[57,58]. In tissue biopsy specimens, Periodic Acid Schiff stain and Gomori Methenamine Silver stain are useful for visualising *H. capsulatum* organisms, although the latter stain is not specific. Other yeasts, *P. carinii* cysts, or staining artefacts may be confused with *H. capsulatum*.

Culture

Fungal cultures of sputum or bronchial washings are usually negative in acute pulmonary histoplasmosis but are positive in 30–60% of cases of chronic pulmonary histoplasmosis. Cultures of lung or lymph node tissue specimens are often positive. In patients with suspected disseminated histoplasmosis, blood and bone marrow

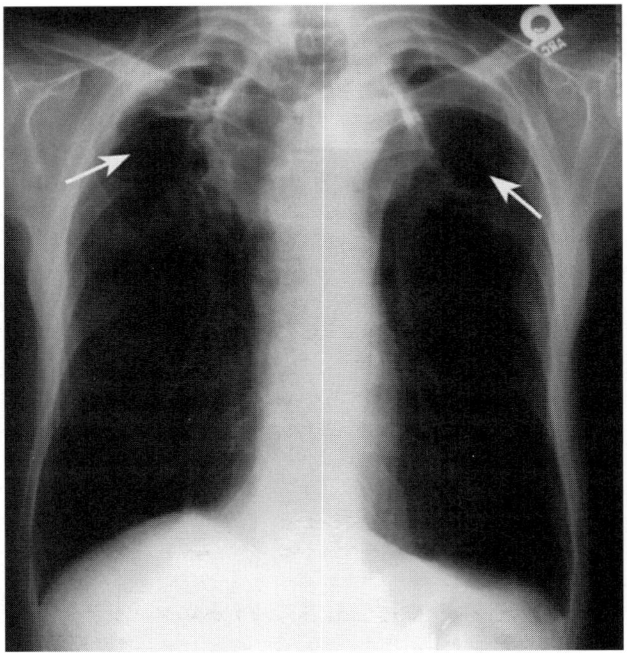

FIGURE 18.8 Chronic pulmonary histoplasmosis. There are bilateral apical cavities (arrows) without associated infiltrates. Patient presented with severe hemoptysis.

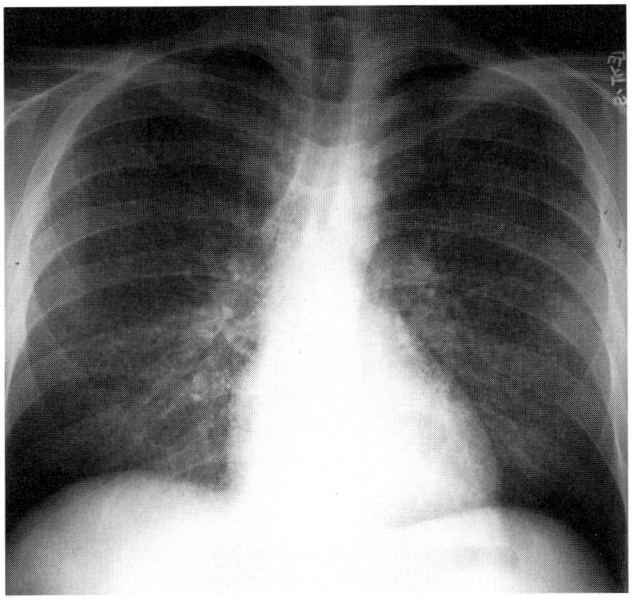

FIGURE 18.9 Disseminated histoplasmosis in AIDS. Diffuse bilateral miliary interstitial pulmonary infiltrates are present.

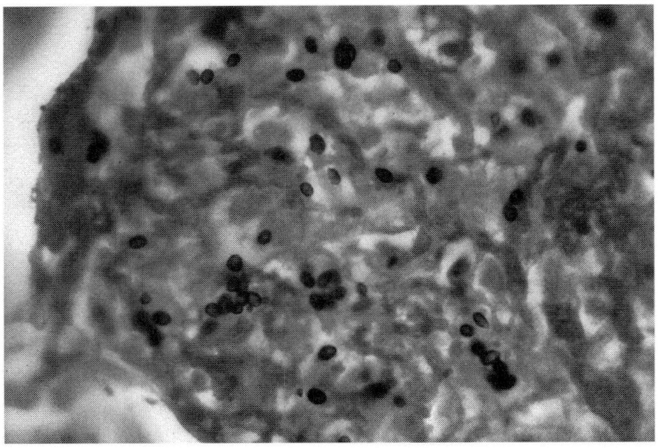

FIGURE 18.10 *Histoplasma capsulatum.* Gomori Methenamine Silver stain of open lung biopsy specimen from patient with acute pulmonary histoplasmosis (× 1000). (Courtesy of R. Givler, MD.)

cultures have the highest diagnostic yield, particularly when the lysis-centrifugation technique is utilised[59]. Traditionally, confirmation of the identity of *H. capsulatum* has been contingent upon establishing the dimorphic nature of the fungus by converting it to the yeast phase at 37 °C. The use of an RNA genetic probe specific for Histoplasma, however, has enabled confirmation to be obtained much more rapidly, i.e. within a few hours after colony growth is first noted[60].

Serology

Complement fixation (CF) antibodies against the yeast or mycelial antigens are positive in 85% of patients with acute pulmonary histoplasmosis[58], 93% of patients with chronic pulmonary histoplasmosis[43], and 70% of cases of disseminated histoplasmosis[57]. Although a CF titre of 1:8 is considered positive, in most cases the titre is ≥ 1:32 in patients with documented infection, and titres of 1:8 or 1:16 should be considered equivocal. In acute histoplasmosis CF titers may not become positive until up to 6 weeks after onset of symptoms; therefore, the CF test is primarily useful in confirming the diagnosis retrospectively[61]. As many as 16% of the population in endemic areas have detectable CF antibodies due to prior exposure[62], limiting the specificity of a positive test result in an endemic region. False-positive reactions can occur in patients with blastomycosis or coccidioidomycosis.

Immunodiffusion antibodies to the h and m bands become detectable 1–4 weeks later than CF antibodies and persist for several years after resolution of histoplasmosis. Sensitivity of immunodiffusion for acute or chronic pulmonary histoplasmosis varies from 50–75%[61,63]. Because positive CF results can be obtained in patients with negative immunodiffusion tests and vice versa, both studies should be done in patients with suspected histoplasmosis.

Histoplasma polysaccharide antigen

Histoplasma polysaccharide antigen (HPA) is a glycoprotein antigen that can be detected in serum, urine, bronchial washings, or cerebrospinal fluid from patients with histoplasmosis[64–66]. The sensitivity of this test is highest in patients with disseminated infection and lowest in those with acute or chronic pulmonary histoplasmosis[33,64]. Specificity is excellent: false-positive results have been observed only in patients with blastomycosis or paracoccidioidomycosis. (J. Wheat, personal communication)

HPA is useful in following the clinical course of patients undergoing treatment for disseminated histoplasmosis, because patients with relapse of infection develop increasing HPA levels[67]. The major role of HPA testing in pulmonary histoplasmosis is for patients with severe acute pneumonia, in whom the sensitivity of the test exceeds 50%.

Skin Testing

Histoplasmin skin testing is useful in epidemiological studies but not for diagnostic purposes[68]. Skin tests become reactive following initial infection and remain positive for life in about 90% of cases[69]; thus, a positive result cannot differentiate between remote and active infection. Moreover, skin tests are negative in 20% of patients with documented chronic pulmonary histoplasmosis[50] and in two-thirds of patients with disseminated histoplasmosis[51].

Histopathology

Biopsy or necropsy specimens from infected tissues show characteristic inflammatory reactions. In acute pneumonia, large numbers of macrophages are seen and epithelioid cells and multinucleated giant cells are present. In later stages of infection, caseating granulomas which are often indistinguishable from those found in tuberculosis are observed.

Diagnostic approach

The suggested diagnostic evaluation for histoplasmosis is shown in Table 18.3.

Treatment

Acute pulmonary histoplasmosis

Asymptomatic or mildly symptomatic cases require no specific treatment. In patients with persistent or progressive pulmonary histoplasmosis, itraconazole appears to be the most effective of the three available azole drugs. When administered at daily doses of 200 mg, 300 mg, or 400 mg, itraconazole was effective in all seven patients studied who had mediastinal or pulmonary infection[70]. Experience with ketoconazole and fluconazole has been limited. A few patients have been treated successfully but efficacy rates have not been determined. Ketoconazole has the least favourable toxicity profile of the 3 available azole drugs and thus has a limited role. Because of lower efficacy with fluconazole than with itraconazole in patients with AIDS and disseminated histoplasmosis[71], fluconazole therapy should be reserved for those situations in which intolerance, poor absorption, or drug interactions prevent the use of itraconazole. Severe cases of histoplasmosis associated with respiratory failure respond to a 10- to 14-day course of amphotericin B, 0.5–0.6 mg/kg/day[38].

Chronic pulmonary histoplasmosis

Although self-limited cases of chronic histoplasmosis have been reported, untreated infection usually causes progressive destruction of lung parenchyma, so antifungal treatment is recommended for all patients with this disease. Amphotericin B, at cumulative doses of 35–40 mg/kg, was effective in 59–100% of patients reported in 3 series but relapses occurred in 10–15% of these cases[63, 72, 73]. Clinical experience with the azole drugs has been limited. Ketoconazole, 400 mg or 800 mg daily, was effective in 19 of 23 cases (84%) in one series[74]. Itraconazole at doses of 200 mg, 300 mg, or 400 mg daily was effective initially in 16 of 20 cases (80%) studied by Dismukes, *et al.*, but 15% of patients relapsed[70]. Five of eleven patients (45%) with chronic pulmonary histoplasmosis responded to fluconazole, 200–800 mg daily in a Mycoses Study Group protocol[75].

Disseminated histoplasmosis

The treatment of disseminated histoplasmosis varies according to the patient's HIV seropositivity status. In HIV-seronegative patients, untreated disseminated histoplasmosis is fatal in 90% of cases[76,77] so treatment is always indicated. Amphotericin B, in cumulative doses of 35–40 mg/kg, has been effective in 68–91% of cases, but post-treatment relapses have occurred in 7–20% of cases[76]. Ketoconazole in doses of at least 400 mg/day was effective in 70% of cases in a prospective study; however, less than half of patients with underlying

Table 18.3. *Histoplasmosis: diagnostic approach*

Acute pulmonary
Acute and convalescent CF[a] and ID[b] serology
Urine HPA[c] (severe cases only)
Sputum or bronchial washing fungal cultures
Lung biopsy and culture (severe, progressive cases only)
Chronic pulmonary
Acute and convalescent CF and ID serology
Sputum fungal culture
Disseminated
Urine and sputum HPA
Peripheral blood smear review for intracellular organisms
Acute and convalescent CF and ID serology
Blood cultures (lysis–centrifugation technique)
Bone marrow biopsy, fungal culture
Consider biopsy/culture of other potentially involved tissues (oral ulcers, skin lesions, lymph nodes, adrenal glands)

[a]CF = complement fixation.
[b]ID = immunodiffusion.
[c]HPA = Histoplasma polysaccharide antigen.

Table 18.4. *Histoplasmosis: treatment*

Acute pulmonary
None
Amphotericin B, 0.5–0.6 mg/kg/d for 10–14 days
Itraconazole 200–400 mg QD for 2 to 6 weeks
Fluconazole 400–800 mg QD for 2 to 6 weeks
Ketoconazole 400 mg QD for 2 to 6 weeks
Chronic pulmonary
Itraconazole 200–400 mg QD for at least 6 months
Fluconazole 400–800 μg QD for at least 6 months
Ketoconazole 400 mg QD for at least 6 months
Pericarditis or rheumatological syndrome
Non-steroidal anti-inflammatory drug
Disseminated
Amphotericin B, 35–40 mg/kg cumulative dose (life-threatening cases or inability to absorb oral medications)
Itraconazole, 200–400 mg QD for at least 6 months
Fluconazole 400–800 mg QD for at least 6 months
Ketoconazole, 400 mg QD for at least 6 months

immunosuppression responded to treatment[74]. Itraconazole, 200 mg to 400 mg QD, was effective in all ten patients studied and post-treatment relapses did not occur[70]. Itraconazole is considered the drug of choice except in life-threatening cases, in which amphotericin should be used.

Disseminated histoplasmosis in AIDS is invariably fatal if not treated. Severe cases should be treated initially with amphotericin B, until a cumulative dose of approximately 500 mg is attained; in mild to moderately severe cases, itraconazole should be administered at a dose of 400 mg daily[78]. Because at least 60% of patients have a relapse of infection, long-term maintenance therapy should be given routinely[79]. Amphotericin B, 50 mg weekly or bi-weekly, has been effective maintenance therapy in 82–97% of cases,[53,79,80] and itraconazole 200 mg QD has prevented relapse in 97%[81]. Fluconazole, 100–400 mg QD, has prevented relapse in 91% of patients who received prior antifungal therapy[82]. However, relapse occurred in one-third of patients who received fluconazole for both induction and maintenance therapy[71]. Ketoconazole maintenance therapy prevented relapse in just 9% of cases[53] and is not recommended.

Other forms of histoplasmosis

Histoplasma pericarditis and the rheumatologic syndrome are immunologically mediated processes which should be treated with anti-inflammatory drugs but not antifungal therapy. Mediastinal fibrosis does not respond to medical treatment, but symptoms of obstruction can be alleviated by surgery in some cases.

Treatment recommendations

Specific guidelines for treatment of histoplasmosis are shown in Table 18.4.

Prevention

Treatment of soil with 3% formalin solution is effective for decontamination prior to cleaning or construction activities. Because of concerns about the ecological impact of this practice, such treatment should be administered only under the auspices of the local or state health department. Education about high-risk work practices and leisure activities is important for persons who reside in endemic areas. An effective vaccine against *H. capsulatum* has not been developed. A placebo-controlled trial of itraconazole prophylaxis against histoplasmosis in HIV-infected patients showed that treatment with itraconazole capsules 200 mg QD prevents histoplasmosis in patients with CD4 counts < $100/mm^3$ [82a].

Blastomycosis

History

Gilchrist reported the first case of blastomycosis in 1894[83]. The causative organism was isolated from a second patient with cutaneous blastomycosis by Gilchrist and Stokes in 1898, and was named *Blastomyces dermatitidis* (*blastomycete,* any fungus; *dermatitidis*, cutaneous disease)[84]. During the next two decades numerous additional patients with cutaneous blastomycosis were reported, and cases of systemic infection, primarily involving the lungs, were described[85,86]. Initially, it was believed that systemic disease was a distinct entity from cutaneous infection, which was thought to occur due to direct inoculation of the fungus into the skin. However, the studies of Schwartz and Baum, published in 1951, showed that cutaneous disease occurs after dissemination of infection from a pulmonary source, indicating that inhalation of organisms is the primary route of acquisition of infection[87]. Studies of the epidemiology and ecology of *B. dermatitidis* have been hampered by lack of availability of an accurate skin test and by great difficulty in culturing the organism from environmental sources. Despite these limitations, the endemic area of blastomycosis has been identified to include the southeastern and upper midwestern United States, and sporadic cases of blastomycosis have been reported elsewhere. Environmental foci of *B.dermatitidis* have been found in soil and decaying vegetation in association with freshwater lakes and streams.

Mycology

Blastomyces dermatitidis is a dimorphic organism which exists as a mycelium at temperatures below 37 °C. Single terminal conidiophores, which grow on branching hyphae, are the infectious forms of the organism. Conidiophores measure 2–10 μM in diameter and are oval or spherical in shape. Conversion to the yeast form occurs at temperatures of 37 °C or higher. Yeast cells measure 8–15 μM in diameter, have highly refractile cell walls, and produce characteristic broad-based buds between parent and daughter cells (Fig. 18.11). Growth of *B.dermatitidis in vitro* typically requires 1 to 3 weeks' incubation.

Epidemiology

The absence of an accurate skin test for blastomycosis has hampered efforts to define the endemic area. Current concepts about the epidemiology of blastomycosis are based on published case reports and case series and analyses of several small epidemics.

The endemic area for blastomycosis in North America is shown in Fig. 18.1 and includes several states in the southern and upper midwestern United States as well as an area along the St Lawrence River. Cases have also been reported from the Canadian provinces of Manitoba, Alberta, Saskatchewan, Ontario, and Quebec. Within the endemic area the incidence of disease varies substantially. For example, in Wisconsin the average annual incidence was 0.48/100 000 population between 1973 and 1982[88] compared to 6.8/100 000 in Washington Parish, Louisiana, between 1976 and 1985[89] and 40.4/100 000 in Vilas County, Wisconsin, between 1979 and 1990[90]. Although most cases have been reported from the endemic area in the United States, the geographical distribution of blastomycosis is quite widespread. The disease is endemic in Africa, and autochthonous cases also have been reported from Poland[91], Saudi Arabia[92], Israel[93], Lebanon[94], and India[95].

The ecological niche of *B.dermatitidis* remains poorly characterised. The primary environmental reservoir is thought to be in soil, although most attempts to isolate *B.dermatitidis* from soil have been unsuccessful. Indeed, the organism survives for less than 6 weeks when experimentally inoculated into soil specimens[96,97]. Until 1984 *B.dermatitidis* had been cultured from soil only rarely and never in association with human disease. In that year Klein and associates studied an epidemic of blastomycosis among school children and adults who visited a beaver dam in a remote area in northern Wisconsin. *B.dermatitidis* was successfully cultivated from decomposed wood along the shoreline of the beaver pond and from two soil specimens obtained from the beaver lodge[98]. Klein and co-workers also cultivated *B.dermatitidis* from soil and organic debris from a river bank in 1985 while investigating two additional outbreaks[99]. Thus, the organism does exist in the soil, which is its probable environmental reservoir. The presence of decaying organic debris and high humidity probably favours the growth of *B.dermatitidis*[100].

Epidemiologic studies have demonstrated that cases occur most often in individuals with intimate exposure to soil in endemic areas. Although early reports suggested that persons with outdoor occupations (e.g. loggers, farmers, construction workers) were at greater risk[101,102], most recent epidemics have occurred in individuals from urban areas who pursued recreational activities such as hunting, fishing, or camping in wooded areas along streams or lakes[90,98,99,103–107]. The incidence of blastomycosis is highest in the winter months[100].

Analysis of the reported epidemics of blastomycosis has shown no consistent differences in risk based on age, sex, race, or occupation[90]. There are no apparent risk factors aside from residential, recreational, or occupational exposures to the outdoors. Indeed, most persons who develop this disease have been in excellent health beforehand[90].

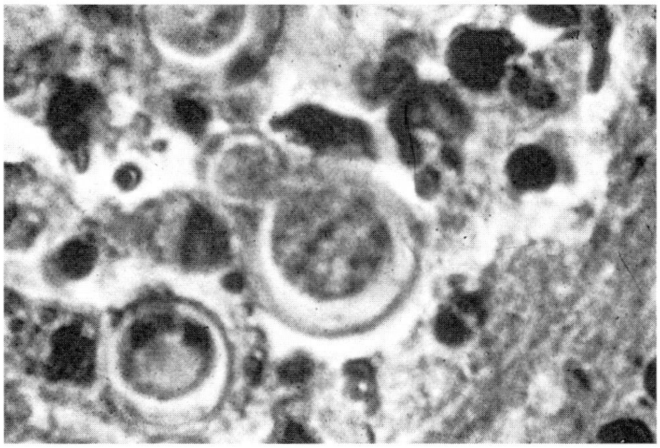

FIGURE 18.11 *Blastomyces dermatitidis.* Haematoxylin and Eosin stain of skin biopsy specimen from patient with cutaneous blastomycosis. (Courtesy of R. Gunnoe, MD.)

Pathophysiology

Blastomycosis can be acquired by inhalation of organisms from an environmental source or by sexual transmission from men with genitourinary infection to their partners[108–110]. Laboratory-acquired infection has occurred due to subcutaneous inoculation of organisms during necropsy[111] or inhalation of organisms from culture plates[87].

Following inhalation of *B. dermatitidis* organisms, a focal pulmonary infiltrate develops. Drainage of organisms via lymphatics then leads to development of hilar lymphadenopathy in some cases. Disseminated infection can occur due to haematogenous spread of organisms to other sites such as skin, bones, genitourinary tract, central nervous system, adrenals, or oropharynx. Disease can progress at one or more of these sites even in the face of resolution or regression of pulmonary lesions.

The host immune response to *B. dermatitidis* is incompletely understood. Neutrophils and macrophages both kill conidia more efficiently than yeast *in vitro*, and phagocytes play a limited role in initial control of infection[112,113]. Although antibodies can be detected in the majority of persons with blastomycosis, humoral immunity does not appear to be important in eradication of the infection. Cellular immunity is the major defence mechanism against *B.dermatitidis;* the cellular immune response is manifested by development of non-caseating granulomas. Immunodeficiency is not a major risk factor for blastomycosis.

Clinical manifestations

Acute blastomycosis

Since the lungs are the portal of entry of the organism, acute blastomycosis is almost always manifested by pneumonia, which is the only clinical finding in half to three-quarters of cases[90]. The incubation period varies from 21 to 105 days, with a median of 45 days[98,99,100]. The onset of symptoms is usually subacute and the clinical presentation is non-specific; typical symptoms include fever, chills, myalgias, and productive cough.[90] Pleuritic chest pain is present in more than half of cases[90]. Rarely, acute pulmonary blastomycosis causes acute respiratory distress syndrome[114,115].

Chest radiographical findings are variable. Four patterns of involvement have been described: airspace consolidation, nodular mass lesions, interstitial infiltrates, and cavitation[116,117]. Upper lobe consolidation and mass lesions are the most common findings[116,118,119]; cavitation occurs within approximately one-third of infiltrates (Fig. 18.12)[117,120]. Other radiographic findings include focal patchy pulmonary infiltrates[121], miliary infiltrates[122], hilar lymphadenopathy, and pleural effusion[120]. Typical chest radiographic findings in blastomycosis and other forms of fungal pneumonia are shown in Table 18.5.

Chronic blastomycosis

Patients with chronic pulmonary blastomycosis generally have been ill for weeks to months prior to presentation. Common symptoms include fever, weight loss, cough, purulent sputum production, or haemoptysis. In chronic pulmonary blastomycosis, spontaneous resolution of infection is uncommon and progression of disease is the rule. Various findings have been noted on chest radiography, including lobar pulmonary infiltrates, mass lesions mimicking malignancy, miliary infiltrates, diffuse infiltrates, and pleural thickening[102,118,119,121,122]. There is no predilection for a particular lobe. Cavitation occurs in less than 10% of cases[119]. Hilar lymphadenopathy and pleural effusion are extremely uncommon. Pulmonary calcifications do not occur in healed lymph nodes or parenchymal lesions[117,118,121].

There are numerous extrapulmonary manifestations of chronic blastomycosis[102,120]. Extrapulmonary lesions can occur concomitantly with pulmonary blastomycosis although in some cases infiltrates have resolved by the time extra-thoracic disease becomes apparent. The most commonly involved site is the skin[102,120,123,124]. Single or multiple verrucous lesions with well-circumscribed margins (Fig. 18.13) can be noted anywhere on the skin surface. Such lesions contain microabscesses, and purulent material can be easily expressed from their margins. Ulcerative skin lesions with erythematous, friable bases are present in some cases.

Other extra-pulmonary manifestations include the following: bone and joint lesions, primarily involving the extremities, vertebrae, or ribs, and often associated with contiguous soft-tissue abscesses[125,126]; genitourinary tract disease, with involvement of the prostate or epididymis[127]; central nervous system infection, manifested by chronic meningitis or intracranial mass lesions[128]; or involvement of mucosal surfaces, liver, spleen, lymph nodes, pericardium, adrenal glands, or eyes.

Immunocompromised hosts

Blastomycosis does not have a predilection for immunocompromised patients. However, when a compromised host does develop blastomycosis, clinical manifestations tend to be severe[129,130].

Despite the frequency of HIV infection in the endemic area for blastomycosis, only 24 cases of blastomycosis in AIDS had been reported as of July 1994[131]. Two patterns of infection have been

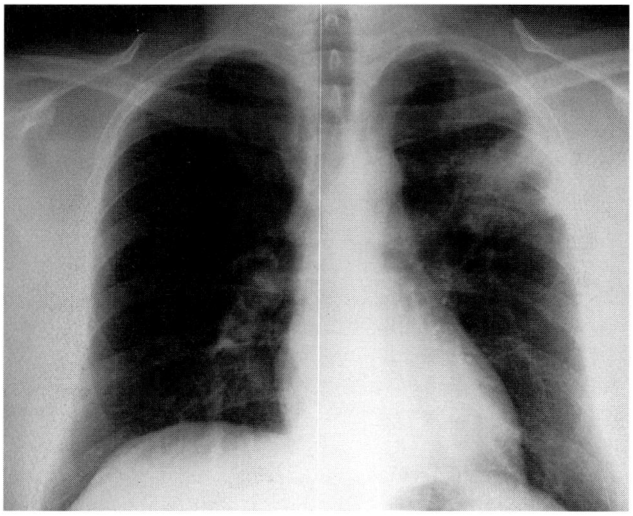

FIGURE 18.12 Acute pulmonary blastomycosis. An alveolar pulmonary infiltrate containing an area of cavitation is present in the left upper lobe. (Courtesy of R. Bradsher, MD.)

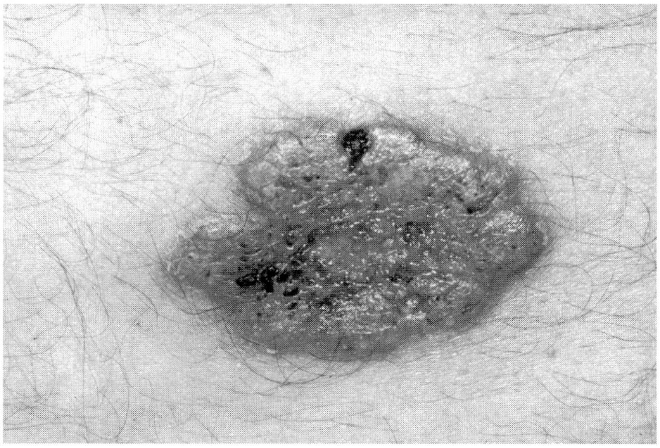

FIGURE 18.13 Cutaneous blastomycosis. Verrucous skin lesion on right thigh. Purulent material was easily expressed from the margins of this lesion. (Courtesy of R. Gunnoe, MD.)

Table 18.5. *Chest radiographical findings in fungal pneumonia*

Disease	Parenchymal infiltrate	Interstitial infiltrate	Mass lesion	Coin lesion	Cavitation	Hilar lymphadenopathy	Pleural effusions	Calcification
Histoplasmosis	X	X		X	X	X		X
Blastomycosis	X	X	X		X	X		
Coccidioidomycosis	X	X		X	X	X	X	
Cryptococcosis	X	X	X		X			
Sporotrichosis	X	X			X			
Paracoccidioidomycosis	X				X			

described: localised pulmonary involvement and disseminated infection. The latter occurs in two-thirds of cases[132]. The majority of reported patients with disseminated disease have had widespread, rapidly progressive, fatal disease[132]. Central nervous system involvement has occurred up to ten times more frequently in patients with AIDS than in HIV-seronegative patients[131].

In a series of 34 HIV-seronegative immunocompromised hosts with blastomycosis, 26 patients had pulmonary infiltrates and 15 had extra-pulmonary disease. Respiratory failure occurred in four cases and two patients had involvement of multiple visceral organs[129]. Mortality from blastomycosis in this group of patients approached 25%[129].

Diagnosis

The diagnosis of blastomycosis can be confirmed by observing organisms in a clinical specimen or by obtaining a positive culture. *B. dermatitidis* is usually easy to identify by direct observation. Sputum, purulent material aspirated from the periphery of a skin lesion, or centrifuged specimens of pleural fluid, cerebrospinal fluid, or urine should be placed on a glass slide and covered with a coverslip. Under the high dry objective, *B. dermatitidis* yeasts measure 8 to 15 μM in diameter, have a globose configuration, possess a highly refractile cell wall, and often have daughter cells which are attached to the mother cells by broad-based buds. Atypical forms of the yeast occasionally may be confused with other fungi such as *Cryptococcus neoformans*, *Histoplasma capsulatum*, or *Paracoccidioides brasiliensis*, but atypical yeasts are generally outnumbered by organisms with the typical appearance described above, so misdiagnosis is unlikely.

Organisms can be visualised by cytology preparation using the Papanicolaou smear[109,133]. Cytology studies of sputum or bronchial washings are particularly helpful in making the diagnosis. In tissue specimens, Gomori Methenamine Silver (GMS) stain is useful for identifying organisms, although it does not provide information about the host inflammatory response. In that regard, Periodic Acid-Schiff (PAS) stain is helpful because it stains the yeast form of *B. dermatitidis* and also demonstrates the pyogranulomatous reaction which is typically seen in blastomycosis.

Culture is the gold standard for diagnosis. The specimen should be inoculated onto brain–heart infusion (BHI) agar or Sabouraud's agar and incubated at 30 °C. The mycelial form of the organism grows within 2 weeks in most cases. Confirmation of the diagnosis requires conversion of the mycelium to the yeast phase by incubation at 37 °C. Exoantigen analyses[134] and DNA probe assays[135] can also be used to confirm the presence of *B. dermatitidis*.

Unfortunately, serological studies and skin tests are of limited value. The sensitivity of complement fixation antibody testing varies from 9–43%[136,137] and that of immunodiffusion ranges from 28–79%[134,136–139]. Specificity of the two tests has been reported as 30–100% and 100%, respectively[136,140]. An ELISA test is more sensitive (83%) but less specific[134,136,141]. Radioimmunoassay and indirect fluorescent antibody tests have been developed[142,143] but are not available in clinical laboratories. The ELISA is the only commercially available test with adequate sensitivity to be used in clinical practice, but its major role is in epidemiological studies rather than in evaluation of individual patients with blastomycosis. Currently, no serological tests are recommended for routine use.

Blastomycin skin test reactivity occurs in only 41% of patients with active blastomycosis[98]. Cross-reactions to blastomycin have occurred in individuals with histoplasmosis. Because of the poor sensitivity and specificity of the blastomycin skin test, no commercially marketed forms of blastomycin are available. Although lymphocyte transformation tests using the ASWS antigen are positive in 81% of cases[98], results do not become positive until at least two weeks after the onset of symptoms, limiting the usefulness of this test during initial diagnostic evaluation.

Treatment

In the era prior to the availability of effective antifungal therapy, blastomycosis was typically a progressive disease: mortality was 78% in one large series[85]. Even in patients who appear to have recovered, extra-pulmonary infection can become apparent months to years later. Based on the unfavourable natural history of blastomycosis all documented cases should be treated with a systemic antifungal drug. Because asymptomatic colonisation does not occur, any patient with a positive smear or culture for *B. dermatitidis* should be considered to have active infection and should be treated accordingly.

Amphotericin B was the first systemic drug which was clinically effective[144]. Efficacy rates have varied from 75–90% in patients who received cumulative doses of at least 1500 mg[144]; lower doses have been associated with a high risk of post-treatment relapse of infection[123]. Controlled clinical trials of amphotericin therapy have not been done, so the optimal dosage and duration of treatment are unknown. It is recommended that patients receive 0.4–0.6 mg/kg/day until a cumulative dose of 1.5–2.0 grams is attained.

The oral azole drugs ketoconazole and itraconazole are effective in the treatment of blastomycosis and have largely supplanted amphotericin B except for the most severe cases. Ketoconazole therapy was assessed in two clinical trials. In one study, efficacy was 79% in patients treated with 400 mg daily and 100% in those who received 800 mg daily; patients treated with the higher dose experienced much more toxicity[75]. Another study reported efficacy of 80% in patients who received 400 mg daily for at least two weeks[145].

Itraconazole was studied at daily doses of 200 mg, 300 mg, or 400 mg in a prospective trial in which 48 patients were evaluated. Overall efficacy was 90%, and in those patients who were compliant with therapy, efficacy was 95%. Toxicity occurred less frequently than had been reported with ketoconazole[71].

Fluconazole therapy was evaluated in a pilot study which assessed daily doses of 200 mg and 400 mg. Treatment was successful in 62% of patients who received 200 mg QD and in 70% of those treated with 400 mg QD. The median duration of therapy for successfully treated patients was 6.7 months[146].

Based on its excellent clinical efficacy and favourable toxicity profile, itraconazole is considered the drug of choice for mild to moderately severe cases of blastomycosis. It is unclear whether a daily dose of 400 mg is superior to 200 mg, so most authorities recommend starting with 200 mg daily and then increasing the dose up to 400 mg daily if there is an incomplete clinical response. For the immunocompromised patient, or the patient with diffuse pulmonary infiltrates and respiratory failure, amphotericin B should be used rather than itraconazole.

Patients with meningeal or genitourinary blastomycosis pose special treatment problems. Neither itraconazole nor ketoconazole penetrate the blood-brain barrier well, and neither drug is excreted into the urine in appreciable concentrations[147]. Patients with central nervous system disease should be treated with amphotericin. If genitourinary infection is treated with an oral drug, it is recommended that a high dose be used and that the patient be monitored closely during and after treatment for evidence of relapse. Fluconazole attains much higher concentrations in the urinary tract than ketoconazole or itraconazole[147], but its role in treatment of genitourinary blastomycosis remains to be defined.

Surgery has an extremely limited role in the management of blastomycosis. Surgical resection of pulmonary disease is not curative since there is a high likelihood of extra-pulmonary dissemination of infection. The only substantial role for surgery is in the drainage of empyemas or soft-tissue abscesses.

Prevention

A vaccine for blastomycosis does not exist. Because of the sporadic nature of this disease and our current inability to identify high-risk patients, antifungal prophylaxis has not been studied and is not recommended.

Coccidioidomycosis

History

An Argentinian soldier who developed an ulcerative skin lesion in 1891 was the first reported case of coccidioidomycosis[148]. During the next 5 years, two additional cases were diagnosed in California. Rixford and Gilchrist isolated the causative organism from one of these patients in 1896 and concluded incorrectly that it was a protozoan: hence the pathogen was named *Coccidioides* (resembling *Coccidia*, a protozoan) *immitis* (not mild)[149]. Orphüls and Moffitt cultured *C. immitis* from clinical specimens in 1900, determined that the organism is a dimorphic fungus rather than a protozoan, and identified the lung as its portal of entry[150].

The recognised clinical spectrum of coccidioidomycosis was expanded in 1929 when a self-limited case of pulmonary coccidioidomycosis occurred in a medical student who accidentally inhaled *C. immitis* spores from a culture plate[151]. Subsequently it was determined that Valley Fever, a well-known syndrome associated with acute pneumonia and erythema nodosum, is caused by *C. immitis* infection[152].

In 1932, the organism was isolated from the soil of a farm in the San Joaquin Valley of California where four migrant workers had developed severe cases of coccidioidomycosis. In the 1940s and 1950s it was determined that the disease is endemic in certain areas in the southwestern United States and Central and South America. The association between exposure to dust clouds and development of coccidioidomycosis led to dust control efforts during construction activities in southern California. In the 1990s there has been a marked increase in the incidence of coccidioidomycosis because of two large epidemics in California, and many cases have been reported among persons with AIDS in the endemic area.

Mycology

Coccidioides immitis is a dimorphic fungus. In the environment *C. immitis* exists as a mycelium, which reproduces through the so-called saprophytic cycle. Hyphae produce branches that then become septated, culminating in the formation of several barrel-shaped arthroconidia within individual hyphae. Arthroconidia can become airborne and travel to new environmental sites to start other saprophytic cycles or they can be inhaled, in which case the parasitic cycle begins. Once within human tissue, arthroconidia swell to become spherules, which then become progressively larger and eventually attain sizes of 30 μM to 60 μM in diameter. Internal cleavage of spherules leads to formation of endospores which typically measure 3 μM to 5 μM in diameter. A fully mature spherule can contain up to 800 endospores. Eventually the spherule ruptures and releases its endospores, each of which can begin a new parasitic cycle.

Ecology and epidemiology

Coccidioides immitis lives in soil in areas with arid or semiarid climates. Factors favourable to the growth of the fungus include low altitude, low rainfall, soil alkalinity, high summer temperatures, and mild winters. The endemic area, which generally correlates with the Lower Sonoran Life Zone[153], includes portions of seven states in the southwestern United States, as well as localised areas in Guatemala, Honduras, Colombia, Venezuela, Paraguay, and Argentina (Fig. 18.1). Within the endemic region the distribution of organisms is patchy. *C. immitis* is recovered particularly frequently from the vicinity of rodent burrows[154,155]. Some investigators have noted an association between soil contamination with *C. immitis* and growth of the creosote bush[154,155].

Skin test surveys have demonstrated that more than half of the population in endemic areas such as Kern County, California, have reactive coccidioidin skin tests indicative of prior subclinical infection[156]. Susceptibility to asymptomatic coccidioidomycosis is not influenced by age, sex, or race. However, disseminated disease develops much more frequently in dark-skinned races. African–Americans and Filipinos develop disseminated disease 10 to 15 times more frequently than Caucasians[157,158], and dissemination is more common in Mexicans, Native Americans and Asians. Disseminated disease also occurs more often in transplant recipients[159], other patients receiving immunosuppressive therapy[160], and patients with AIDS[161,162].

Coccidioidomycosis is generally not contagious from person to person. One exceptional case involved a patient with a fracture and a draining wound who had a plaster cast that became contaminated with *C. immitis* arthrospores. During manipulation of the cast, six health care personnel inhaled arthrospores and subsequently developed pulmonary coccidioidomycosis[163].

Disease transmission through exposure to contaminated fomites has been well documented. Cases have been described among textile workers in the southeastern United States who were exposed to contaminated cotton from California[164,165]. An imported case has also been reported from Great Britain[166]. *C. immitis* is highly contagious to laboratory workers. Numerous laboratory-acquired cases have been reported[151,167] and at least one fatal case has occurred[151]. Occupational exposure is a risk to individuals with extensive exposure to soil dust in the endemic area, including archaeologists[168], construction workers, and agricultural workers[169].

The incidence of coccidioidomycosis is influenced by climatic factors and therefore exhibits seasonal variability. The fungus grows upward into the surface layers of the soil during the rainy season[170]; after the soil becomes dry, arthrospores are dispersed by the wind[171]. The major peaks in incidence are in the summer and the late autumn[172]. A large epidemic in Southern California occurred in the late 1970s due to a severe windstorm[173]. An epidemic in Kern County, California during 1991–1993 affected approximately 7000 people and was associated with a period of heavy rainfall following a prolonged drought[171,173]. In 1994, an epidemic occurred following an earthquake in the Los Angeles area. Persons who were exposed to dust clouds immediately after the earthquake had a markedly increased risk of infection[174].

Coccidioidomycosis has been a particularly important opportunistic infection among patients with AIDS who reside in the endemic area[161,162]. In a prospective study by Ampel, *et al.*, the cumulative incidence of coccidioidomycosis was 25% in HIV-infected patients in Tucson, Arizona. No specific exposures were associated with increased risk for coccidioidomycosis among patients with AIDS; the major risk factor was a CD4+ lymphocyte count below 250/μl[175].

Pathophysiology

Infection is generally initiated by inhalation of arthroconidia into the lungs although in rare cases percutaneous inoculation of organisms can be the portal of entry[176]. The arthroconidia then convert to spherules and begin the parasitic cycle of multiplication. A brisk inflammatory response manifested by infiltration of alveolar macrophages and neutrophils occurs within 24 hours after infection, with a peak response developing after 4 days[177]. Although neutrophils are unable to kill *C. immitis* spherules, the inflammatory response can lead to abscess formation[177]. Subsequently killer T cells limit fungal replication; this process is enhanced by interferon[178]. Granulomas, which can contain areas of caseous necrosis, are the typical pathological lesions. Most cases of coccidioidomycosis are confined to the lungs, but haematogenous dissemination of organisms can occur, and virtually any organ system can be infected.

Clinical manifestations

Primary coccidioidomycosis

Primary coccidioidomycosis is asymptomatic in 60% of cases[179]. The incubation period for symptomatic disease varies from 1 to 4 weeks[180]. The clinical presentation of primary pulmonary coccidioidomycosis is usually non-specific. Patients typically have fever, malaise, anorexia, diffuse myalgias, cough, or chest pain[172,180]. The cough is generally non-productive although clear or purulent sputum may be produced. Self-limited haemoptysis occurs in some cases.

Typical radiographical manifestations include one or more patchy pulmonary infiltrates (Fig. 18.14) or frank consolidation[181,182]. Hilar lymphadenopathy is seen in 20% of cases[182]. In approximately 5% of cases, resolution of a pulmonary infiltrate is accompanied by development of a focal nodule, the appearance of which mimics a neoplasm (Fig. 18.15)[182]. Such coccidioidal nodules cavitate in about half of cases (Fig. 18.16)[183]. After 2 years, half of these cavitary lesions close spontaneously[184]. Cavities can cause haemoptysis or can extend into contiguous bronchi, resulting in bronchopleural fistula or empyema. Small unilateral pleural effusions are present in approximately 20% of cases; rarely, large effusions are observed[181]. In cases

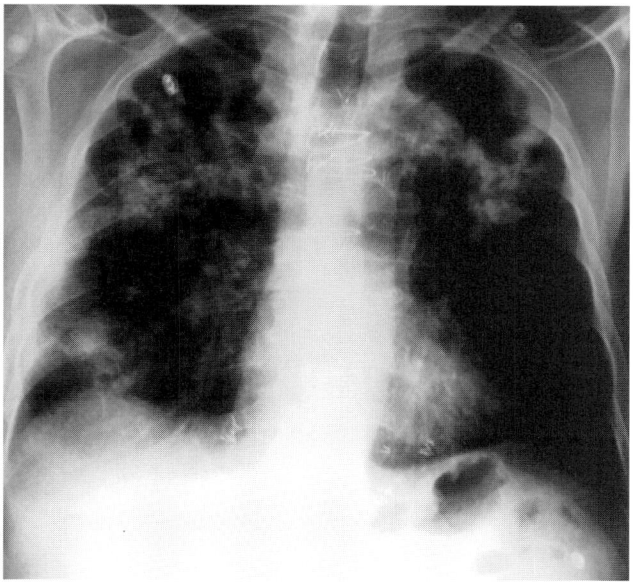

FIGURE 18.14 Acute pulmonary coccidioidomycosis. Bilateral upper lobe nodular alveolar infiltrates present. (Courtesy of J. Weems, MD.)

of disseminated coccidioidomycosis, miliary pulmonary infiltrates are seen frequently[178].

Skin lesions can be important clues to the diagnosis of coccidioidomycosis. An erythematous macular rash is often present during the first few days of illness[168]. Erythema nodosum occurs in 20% of cases and is particularly common in Caucasian women[178]. Erythema multiforme lesions may be present on the trunk and upper extremities. Skin lesions, which are thought to be due to excessive delayed-type hypersensitivity reactions, are associated with a good prognosis.

Chronic coccidioidomycosis

A small subset of patients develop chronic, progressive pulmonary coccidioidomycosis[185]. This disease is associated with apical fibronodular infiltrates (Fig. 18.17) which sometimes cause fibrosis and retraction of lung parenchyma. Clinical findings mimic pulmonary tuberculosis or chronic pulmonary histoplasmosis[185].

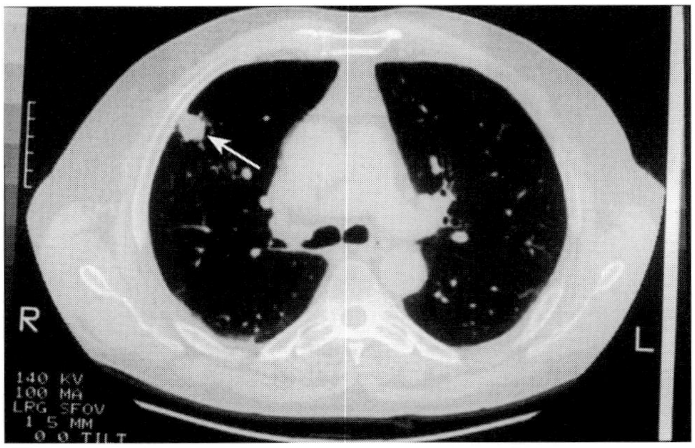

FIGURE 18.15 Coccidioidal pulmonary nodule. Computerised tomography scan shows subpleural coin lesion in right upper lobe (arrow). (Courtesy of M. Driks, MD.)

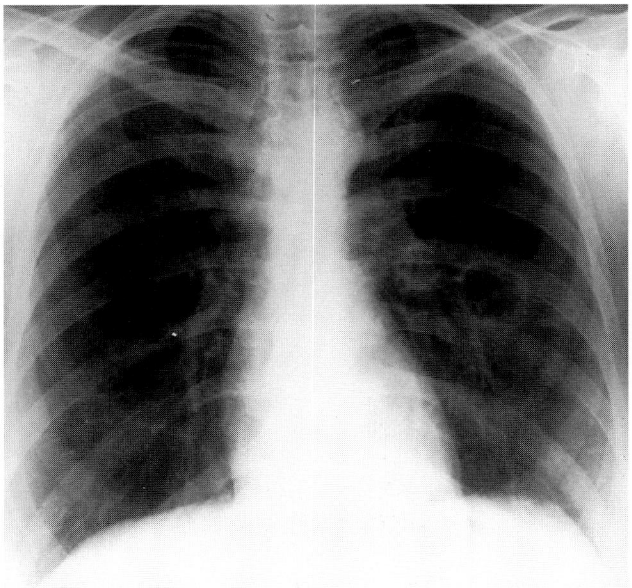

FIGURE 18.16 Coccidioidal cavity in left mid-lung zone. (Courtesy of M. Waxman, MD.)

Disseminated coccidioidomycosis

Haematogenous dissemination of coccidioidomycosis occurs in a small percentage of Caucasian patients (approximately 0.5%) but is much more common in dark-skinned races[156,157]. Disseminated coccidioidomycosis carries an unfavourable prognosis. Numerous organ systems can be involved, and in many cases concomitant disease is noted in two or more systems. A variety of skin lesions can occur due to haematogenous dissemination, including subcutaneous abscesses, ulcers, nodules, verrucous papules, draining sinuses, or large proliferative lesions. Approximately 20% of disseminated cases are associated with bone lesions, usually involving the skull, vertebrae, or long bones[186]. Septic arthritis of the knees or ankles can occur due to contiguous spread from a bony lesion[187]. Coccidioidal meningitis occurs in up to half of cases of disseminated coccidioidomycosis. Clinical findings include headache, confusion, diplopia, ataxia, or focal neurological deficits[188]. Other sites which can be involved include lymph nodes, liver, spleen, adrenals, kidneys, eyes, ears, larynx, or genitourinary tract.

Coccidioidomycosis in AIDS

Six patterns of disease have been reported in patients with AIDS: focal pulmonary infection, diffuse pulmonary disease, cutaneous disease, meningitis, liver or extrathoracic lymph node involvement, or positive serology without evidence of localised infection[161]. Three-quarters of patients have pulmonary infiltrates, of whom 60% have

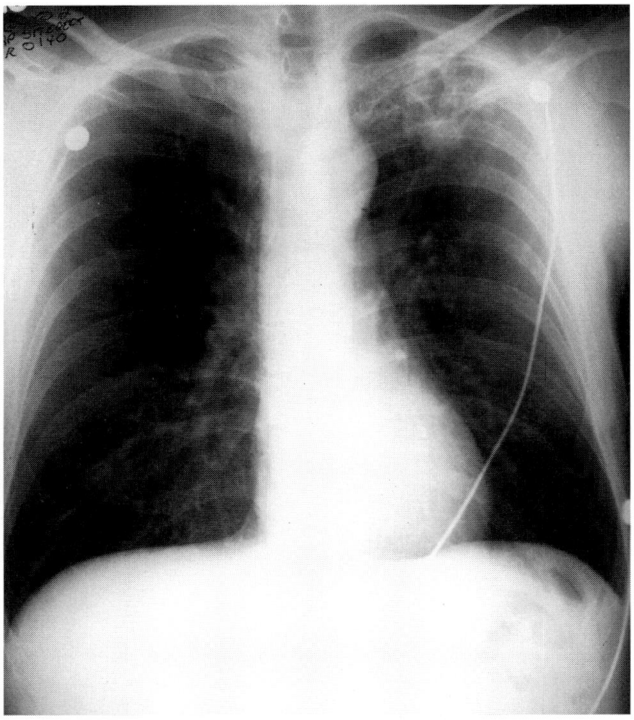

FIGURE 18.17 Chronic pulmonary coccidioidomycosis. Alveolar infiltrate is present in left upper lobe. (Courtesy of M. Waxman, MD.)

diffuse bilateral infiltrates and 40% have focal infiltrates, nodules, hilar adenopathy, or pleural effusions[161]. The clinical presentation of pulmonary coccidioidomycosis in AIDS closely mimics *Pneumocystis carinii* pneumonia and other forms of opportunistic pneumonia.

Diagnosis

C. immitis spherules are so unique in appearance that observation of a spherule is diagnostic for coccidioidomycosis. Spherules are found easily in purulent drainage and are seen occasionally in sputum, bronchial washings, joint fluid, and tissue specimens. Organisms are visualised rarely in pleural fluid, cerebrospinal fluid, blood, or urine. Potassium hydroxide preparations can be utilised, but Gomori Methenamine Silver stain is more sensitive. Other stains that demonstrate coccidioidal spherules include Periodic Acid Schiff and the Gridley fungus stain.

Coccidioides immitis can be cultured from clinical specimens on Sabouraud's agar, brain–heart infusion (BHI) agar, or blood agar. Culturing *C. immitis* poses a significant hazard to laboratory workers[166], and appropriate biohazard precautions should be followed. The organism typically grows after 3 to 5 days' incubation. The identity of *C. immitis* can be confirmed by conversion of the mycelial form to the spherule form. This procedure has been largely supplanted by the exoantigen test[189] and by a DNA probe which has sensitivity of 98.8% and specificity of 100%[190].

Serology has been a time-honoured method for diagnosing coccidioidomycosis. Complement fixation (CF) antibody titres are negative in 98% of patients with solitary pulmonary nodules or cavities, but are positive in 92% of cases of severe primary infection and in 99% of cases of disseminated coccidioidomycosis in HIV-seronegative patients[191]. However, one-third of patients with AIDS and disseminated coccidioidomycosis have non-reactive CF tests[161]. In the past, elevated titres were said to correlate with disseminated disease; in one study a titre greater than 1:32 was present in 61% of patients with disseminated disease but in less than 5% of those without evidence of dissemination[192]. Because of inter-laboratory variability, however, the significance of an individual titre elevation of greater than 1:32 is unclear. Serial CF titres are useful in assessing response to therapy: falling titres denote a good clinical response whereas rising titres often correlate with treatment failure[193]. False-positive CF tests can occur in patients with histoplasmosis.

A variety of immunodiffusion antibody tests for coccidioidomycosis are available. Immunodiffusion has excellent sensitivity and specificity[194,195] although false-positive results can be seen in patients with histoplasmosis or blastomycosis. A quantitative immunodiffusion test which correlates well with CF titres is available[196]. Other serology tests include the tube-precipitin test[196], which is not currently being done by most laboratories, and the latex agglutination test. False-positive latex agglutination reactions occur in 6–10% of cases[197]. Radioimmunoassay and enzyme immunoassay tests have been developed to detect coccidioidal antigen in serum[198,199]; the clinical utility of these tests is unclear.

Skin testing is primarily of value in epidemiological studies. There are two commercially available skin test antigens: coccidioidin, prepared from mycelial phase organisms, and spherulin, made from coccidioidal spherules[200]. Although the two antigens have not been directly compared in the same patient population, their sensitivity and specificity are probably similar, and there is no apparent advantage of one antigen over the other[201]. Skin test results can be negative in patients with active coccidioidomycosis[68] but are positive in one-third to half of healthy persons who reside in endemic areas[202,203]. Thus, skin testing is of less value than serology in establishing the diagnosis and should not be done routinely. Skin testing is perhaps most useful in assessing prognosis, i.e. a negative test in a patient with disseminated infection is an unfavourable prognostic finding.

Diagnostic approach

The suggested diagnostic approach for coccidioidomycosis is shown in Table 18.6.

Treatment

Primary coccidioidomycosis

Primary pulmonary coccidioidomycosis is often a self-limited disease, and antifungal therapy is warranted only in severe cases. Indications for treatment include persistence of symptoms for more than 6 weeks, progression of pulmonary infiltrates, suspected dissemination of infection (i.e. markedly elevated CF titre, presence of paratracheal lymphadenopathy), or underlying conditions associated with increased risk for dissemination (dark-skinned race, HIV seropositivity, immunosuppression, or late stages of pregnancy).

Amphotericin B has been the mainstay of therapy since 1959 when the drug was first used for treatment of coccidioidomycosis[204,205]. The typical daily dose is in the range of 30 to 35 mg for adults. The duration of treatment should be based on clinical response; a cumulative dose of 500 mg to 1000 mg is generally warranted[205]. The role of ketoconazole, itraconazole, and fluconazole for treatment of primary pulmonary coccidioidomycosis has not been defined.

Cavitary pulmonary lesions do not respond to antifungal therapy. Because many coccidioidal cavities close spontaneously and dissemination of infection from cavitary lesions does not occur, conservative management is warranted in almost all cases[182]. Surgical resection of cavities is indicated in certain uncommon situations, including recurrent or severe haemoptysis, bronchopleural fistula, or recurrent bacterial superinfections[183,206,207]. Surgical resection carries the risk of inducing bronchopleural fistulae or coccidioidal empyema[207]. Since concomitant small cavities may not be noted at the time of surgery, adjunctive antifungal therapy is warranted during the perioperative period. Typically, amphotericin B has been administered for 2 weeks before and after surgery[206,207], although the use of an oral antifungal drug could be considered.

Chronic coccidioidomycosis

Chronic coccidioidal pneumonia poses a difficult management problem. In untreated cases, apical infiltrates progress over a span of several months, leading to pulmonary cavitation and fibrosis. Amphotericin B therapy is effective, although there is a high risk of relapse unless a cumulative dose of at least 30 mg/kg is administered[205]. Ketoconazole was effective in 43% of cases treated with either 400 mg or 800 mg daily in a Mycoses Study Group study; there was no improvement in efficacy with the higher dose[208]. In another clinical trial fluconazole was effective in 28% of patients who received

Table 18.6. *Coccidioidomycosis: diagnosis*

Smear and fungal culture of sputum, bronchial washings, pus, or other clinical specimens
Complement fixation and immunodiffusion serology
Coccidioidin or spherulin skin testing

Table 18.7. *Coccidioidomycosis: treatment*

Primary infection
None
Amphotericin B, cumulative dose of 500–1000 mg (severe cases)
Fluconazole, 200–400 mg QD
Itraconazole, 200–400 mg QD
Ketoconazole, 400 mg QD
Surgical resection of cavitary lesion (for recurrent haemoptysis or superinfections)
Chronic pulmonary infection
Amphotericin B, cumulative dose ≥ 30 mg/kg
Itraconazole, 200–400 mg QD
Ketoconazole, 400 mg QD
Disseminated infection
Amphotericin B, cumulative dose ≥ 2000 mg
Itraconazole, 200–400 mg QD
Fluconazole, 200–400 mg QD

200 mg daily and in 46% of those who received 400 mg daily. Although the median duration of therapy was close to 2 years, 39% of patients experienced relapse of infection after discontinuation of fluconazole[209]. Itraconazole, 200 mg to 400 mg daily, was effective in 12 of 22 patients (54%) with chronic pulmonary coccidioidomycosis in another Mycoses Study Group protocol[210]. In a pilot study of itraconazole therapy at doses of 50 mg to 400 mg daily, clinical response was seen in 57% of 37 patients reported by Tucker, *et al.*[211]. Of patients studied by Diaz and colleagues who were treated with itraconazole 400 mg QD, 93% had partial or complete responses[212]. Prognosis for complete recovery is poor regardless of the form of treatment. Treatment with an oral azole drug should be continued for at least 12 months and perhaps indefinitely. Currently it is unclear whether itraconazole is superior to fluconazole or vice-versa[213]. An ongoing clinical trial is comparing the two drugs for treatment of coccidioidomycosis.

Disseminated coccidioidomycosis

Disseminated coccidioidomycosis is a life-threatening infection which should always be treated. This is a particularly challenging infection to manage because of the high risk of persistent or recurrent infection despite prolonged treatment. Amphotericin B is often effective when cumulative doses of 2000 to 4000 mg are administered but relapse can occur after discontinuation of treatment[205]. In an open study of fluconazole 50 mg to 100 mg daily, 12 of 14 patients with pulmonary, osteoarticular, genitourinary, or soft tissue infection responded to treatment initially but only 4 had complete resolution of infection[214]. Clinical response rates were improved when doses of 200 mg to 400 mg daily were used[209].

Objective parameters which can be followed to assess response to treatment include defervescence, improvement in pulmonary infiltrates, declining CF serology titre, decreasing erythrocyte sedimentation rate, and development of coccidioidin skin test reactivity. In cases of chronic coccidioidal pneumonia or disseminated coccidioidomycosis, improvement may occur very slowly, over a span of months to years. Treatment should not be discontinued until several months after normalisation of these clinical parameters.

Coccidioidomycosis in AIDS

Treatment regimens for coccidioidomycosis in AIDS have not been standardised. Initial treatment should consist of amphotericin B in doses of 0.5–0.6 mg/kg/day. Lifelong oral maintenance therapy should be given after a brief course of amphotericin B[215]. Because cases of coccidioidomycosis have occurred in HIV-infected patients being treated with ketoconazole for other reasons[215], ketoconazole generally is not recommended. Itraconazole and fluconazole appear to be effective as maintenance therapy, but controlled clinical trials have not been done[216].

Treatment recommendations

Specific treatment recommendations are reviewed in Table 18.7.

Prevention

A vaccine developed from killed *C. immitis* spherules has been protective in several animal species but not in humans[217]. A placebo-controlled trial of fluconazole prophylaxis against coccidioidomycosis in patients with AIDS is under way in Arizona. Currently, no forms of immunoprophylaxis or chemoprophylaxis have been shown to be effective.

Cryptococcosis

History

The first case of cryptococcosis, reported by Busse and Buschke in 1894, was a young German woman who presented with a tibial lesion and eventually died from disseminated disease[218]. The causative organism was cultured from the bone lesion. During the first half of the twentieth century, the organism was named *Torula histolytica* based on the mistaken impression that it caused lysis of tissues; the term 'torulosis' was used to refer to cryptococcal infection. In 1950 the organism's name was changed to *Cryptococcus neoformans* and the term cryptococcosis was coined to refer to the infection caused by this pathogen[219]. In the 1950s, the fungus was cultivated from soil and its growth was shown to be enhanced by the presence of pigeon excrement. In the early 1980s cryptococcosis was recognised as a common opportunistic infection in AIDS. Subsequently the incidence of cryptococcal disease has increased dramatically as the result of the AIDS epidemic.

Mycology

Cryptococcus neoformans exists only in yeast form in its pathogenic stage. Based on antigenic specificity of the cryptococcal polysaccharide capsule, four serotypes have been identified, designated A, B, C, and D. There are two varieties of *C. neoformans: C. neoformans var. neoformans,* which includes serotypes A and D, and *C. neoformans var. gattii*, which includes serotypes B and C. The environmental reservoirs of these two varieties differ, as will be discussed below.

Cryptococci measure 5 to 10 μM in diameter and reproduce by budding (Fig. 18.18). Most organisms are encapsulated, although non-encapsulated isolates have been reported. Capsules may attain sizes as large as 20 μM in diameter. *C. neoformans* can be differentiated in the laboratory from various non-pathogenic species of cryptococcus by its growth at 37 °C and its abilities to hydrolyse urea and to assimilate various sugars.

Ecology and epidemiology

C. neoformans has a worldwide distribution and there are no localised endemic areas. The distribution of the two varieties varies considerably, however, based on the defined ecological niches of the organisms.

C. neoformans var. neoformans has been isolated from soil repeatedly. In particular, soil contaminated by pigeon droppings often contains large quantities of the fungus[220]. *C. neoformans* can metabolise creatinine into a nitrogen source[221], and avian droppings contain large amounts of creatinine. Pigeon roosting sites such as barns, window ledges, and towers often are heavily contaminated with *C. neoformans*. The organism also grows in sites contaminated with droppings of other avian species.

Conversely, *C. neoformans var. gattii* is not found in areas contaminated with avian droppings, despite the fact that it can metabolise creatinine[222]. Rather, this organism lives in the bark of *Eucalyptus camaldulensis* (red river gum) and *Eucalyptus tereticornis* (forest red gum) trees. Particularly high levels of *C. neoformans var. gattii* can be detected in the air during periods when these trees are flowering[220,222]. In tropical and subtropical areas where eucalyptus trees live, the *gattii* variety predominates, whereas in other areas the *neoformans* variety is the predominant pathogen[220]. In regions such as Brazil where both varieties are present *C. neoformans* is more likely to cause disease in immunocompromised hosts than *C. gattii* which tends to infect nonimmunosuppressed patients[223].

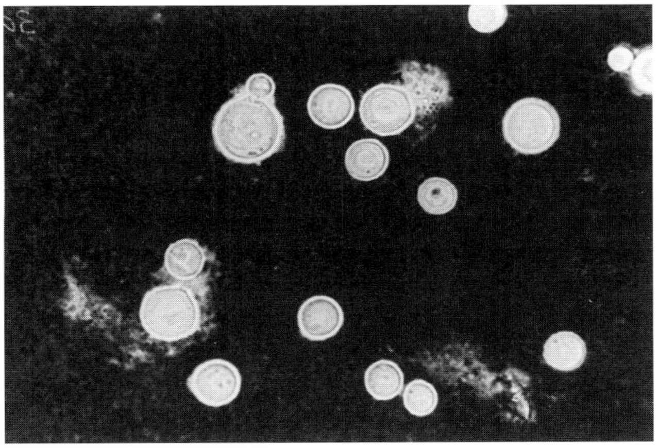

FIGURE 18.18 *Cryptococcus neoformans var neoformans.* India ink preparation shows minimally encapsulated cells, some of which are budding. (Courtesy of M. Dykstra, PhD.)

Infection occurs due to aerosolisation of cryptococci from environmental sources and inhalation into the alveoli. Interestingly, persons with intense exposure to known environmental sources do not appear to be at increased risk for development of cryptococcal disease[220,224], although skin test surveys have demonstrated that subclinical infection occurs more commonly in these individuals[220,225,226]. In most cases, a specific high-risk exposure cannot be identified in a patient with active cryptococcal disease. Epidemics of cryptococcal infection have not occurred among groups of people exposed to contaminated areas.

Cryptococcal infections are not contagious from person to person except in the rare case of organ transplantation from a donor with active infection[227]. Animal-to-human spread does not occur even after exposure to large quantities of the organism.

The availability of molecular epidemiological techniques such as restriction fragment-length polymorphisms and DNA probes will be useful in future epidemiological studies of cryptococcosis[228]. Widespread genetic variability in this fungus has been noted within individual geographical areas[228].

Pathophysiology and risk factors

A cryptococcal infection is initiated when *C. neoformans* is inhaled from an environmental source into the lower respiratory tract. There is a high level of natural immunity, and most infections are asymptomatic. Cryptococci do not produce toxins and do not induce tissue necrosis or haemorrhage; manifestations of infection occur due to mechanical pressure from the organisms.

The host immune response to cryptococci is complex. Neutrophils and alveolar macrophages ingest and kill cryptococci within 2 hours in an *in vitro* model[229] and are the host's first line of defense. However, the cryptococcal polysaccharide capsule can inhibit chemotaxis and block phagocyte recognition of the organism resulting in incomplete phagocytosis, especially following exposure to a large inoculum of organisms[230,231]. Cell-mediated immunity plays an important role in control of cryptococcal infection. CD8 cells are required for development of effective cell-mediated immunity[232]. Macrophages and killer T cells can kill cryptococci[233], and the fungicidal activity of these cells is enhanced by granulocyte-macrophage colony-stimulating factor, interleukin-2, and interferon[234]. The histopathologic manifestations of infection vary from absence of inflammatory response to presence of well-formed non-caseating granulomas. Pulmonary calcifications and fibrosis do not develop following resolution of cryptococcosis.

Cryptococcal disease can occur in normal persons or in immunocompromised hosts; clinical manifestations vary depending on the patient's underlying health status. Normal hosts generally develop self-limited pneumonia without extra-pulmonary manifestations of disease, although cryptococcal meningitis can occur due to haematogenous seeding of the meninges even in previously healthy patients[235]. A variety of conditions associated with impaired cellular immunity increase the risk of cryptococcal infection. AIDS is the most important predisposing condition; indeed, approximately 90% of new cryptococcal infections occur in patients with AIDS, and 5–10% of American AIDS patients develop cryptococcal disease[236,237].

Other risk factors include prolonged systemic corticosteroid therapy, sarcoidosis, malignancies of the reticuloendothelial system (chronic lymphocytic leukaemia, Hodgkin's disease, reticulum cell sarcoma, hairy cell leukaemia), or organ transplantation[235,238]. The incidence of cryptococcosis in transplant recipients, however, has declined since the advent of cyclosporin, which has anticryptococcal activity *in vitro*[239].

In patients with impaired cellular immunity, haematogenous dissemination of cryptococcosis to extra-pulmonary sites occurs frequently and host response to infection may be blunted. Cryptococci have a particular predilection for the central nervous system: cerebrospinal fluid serves as an excellent growth medium for *C. neoformans*[240], perhaps owing to its lack of complement or soluble anticryptococcal factors[241].

Clinical manifestations

The clinical manifestations of pulmonary cryptococcosis are protean and non-specific. Cryptococcal pneumonia is a subacute or chronic process. Approximately half of cases are asymptomatic. Among symptomatic patients, presenting complaints include dry cough, dyspnoea, and chest pain. Rarely, severe pneumonia causes respiratory failure. An important clue to the diagnosis is the presence of extra-pulmonary disease, although in many cases extra-pulmonary manifestations occur after spontaneous resolution of pneumonia. The most common and serious extra-pulmonary form of cryptococcosis is meningitis, which is manifested by chronic headache, fever, cranial nerve palsies, blindness, or mental status changes[236]. Virtually any other organ system can be affected. Cryptococcal skin lesions may present as papules, pustules, or ulcers, often involving the face and scalp[242]. Osteolytic bone lesions involving the extremities, ribs, or vertebrae are noted in approximately 5% of cases[243]. Asymptomatic prostatitis is a particularly common manifestation in patients with AIDS[244].

Chest radiographic findings of cryptococcal pneumonia are non-specific. Single or multiple well-circumscribed pulmonary infiltrates or discrete nodules are the most common findings (Fig. 18.19, 18.20); cavitation can occur. Pleural effusions and hilar lymphadenopathy occur only rarely[245]. Other radiographical patterns include patchy alveolar infiltrates (Fig. 18.21), or diffuse bilateral interstitial infiltrates.

In individuals with AIDS who develop cryptococcosis, the infection is almost always disseminated. Approximately one-quarter of such patients have pulmonary involvement[246]. A wide variety of pulmonary manifestations have been reported including focal nodules, lobar consolidation, interstitial infiltrates, pleural effusions, and hilar or mediastinal adenopathy[247].

Diagnosis

Asymptomatic colonisation of the airway with *C. neoformans* can occur so it is important to correlate laboratory data with the patient's clinical status to determine that the patient has invasive cryptococcal infection. Confirmation of the diagnosis of pulmonary cryptococcosis requires a positive culture of sputum, bronchial washings, or lung tissue for *C. neoformans* in the appropriate clinical setting. The yield of culture is increased with the use of birdseed agar[248]. Although *C. neoformans* can grow at 37 °C, growth occurs more rapidly at 30 °C so culture media should be incubated at the lower temperature if the diagnosis is suspected. *C. neoformans* is a rapidly growing fungus and organisms are generally observed within 3–4 days, though cultures should be held for 4 weeks to detect more slowly growing organisms. The relative sensitivity of sputum culture as compared to bronchial

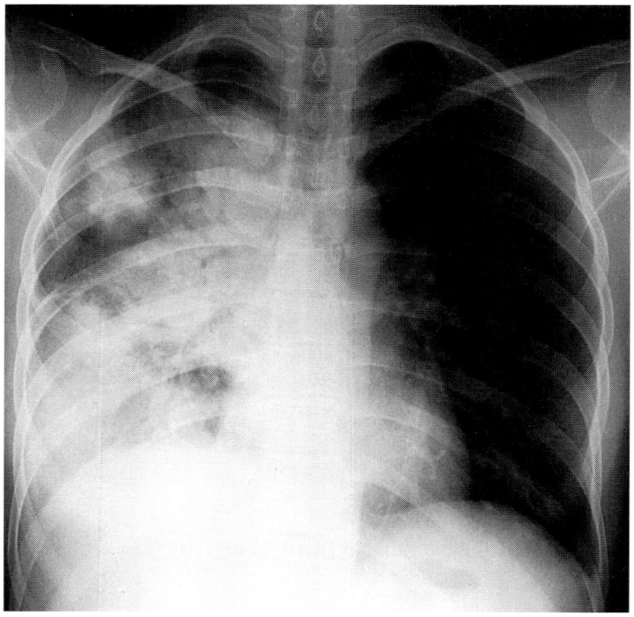

FIGURE 18.19 Pulmonary cryptococcosis. Extensive alveolar infiltrate in right lung of woman with steroid-dependent ulcerative colitis.

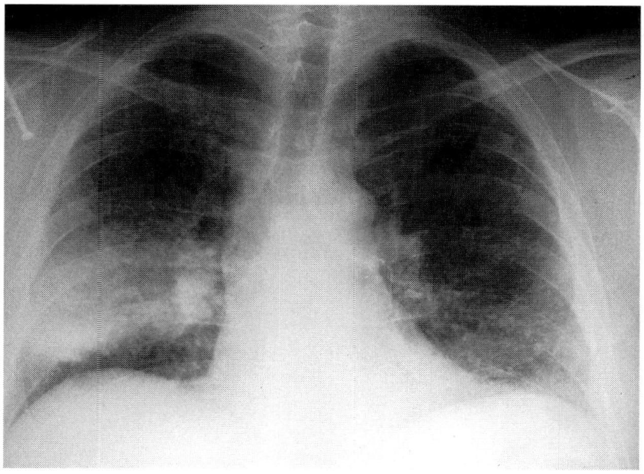

FIGURE 18.20 Pulmonary cryptococcosis in patient with pre-existing eosinophilic granuloma. Dense alveolar infiltrate in right lower lobe is due to cryptococcosis, bilateral pulmonary interstitial infiltrates are secondary to eosinophilic granuloma.

washing culture has not been determined, although in the author's experience the latter is more likely to be positive. Cultures should be obtained not only from sputum and bronchial washings but also from other potentially involved sites such as blood, skin lesions, cerebrospinal fluid, or bone lesions. A commercially available DNA probe for *C. neoformans* has 100% sensitivity and specificity and enables rapid confirmation of the identity of clinical isolates[60].

Direct visualisation of organisms is useful but not diagnostic, since non-pathogenic yeasts or various artefacts may be confused with *C. neoformans*. Organisms are most likely to be visualised in cerebrospinal fluid by India ink preparation, although this technique has been largely supplanted by antigen testing (see below). Sputum, bronchial washings, or tissue specimens should be stained with Gomori Methenamine Silver, Periodic Acid Schiff, or Mayer's mucicarmine. The latter is particularly useful because it stains the cryptococcal polysaccharide capsule a rose colour but does not stain other fungi.

The cryptococcal antigen test is remarkably accurate in diagnosing cryptococcal meningitis but is of limited value in diagnosing respiratory tract infections. Although the sensitivity of serum and cerebrospinal fluid cryptococcal antigen testing exceeds 90% in patients with cryptococcal meningitis, the test is positive in cryptococcal pneumonia only in the setting of extensive infiltrates or extra-pulmonary disease[249]. False-positive results can occur in the presence of rheumatoid factor[250]. Treatment of serum or cerebrospinal fluid with pronase has been shown to increase the sensitivity of the cryptococcal antigen test by eliminating false-negative tests due to the prozone effect[251]. The value of cryptococcal antigen testing of bronchoalveolar lavage fluid or pleural fluid has not been determined. Serial cerebrospinal fluid cryptococcal antigen values do not correlate with response to therapy in AIDS patients with cryptococcal meningitis[252]; whether or not serial serum antigen titres correlate with outcome of cryptococcal pneumonia remains unknown.

Although some patients who have recovered from cryptococcal pneumonia have detectable antibodies in serum, cryptococcal serology is not useful diagnostically. A cryptococcin skin test has been developed, but it has no role in diagnosis and is not commercially available[225].

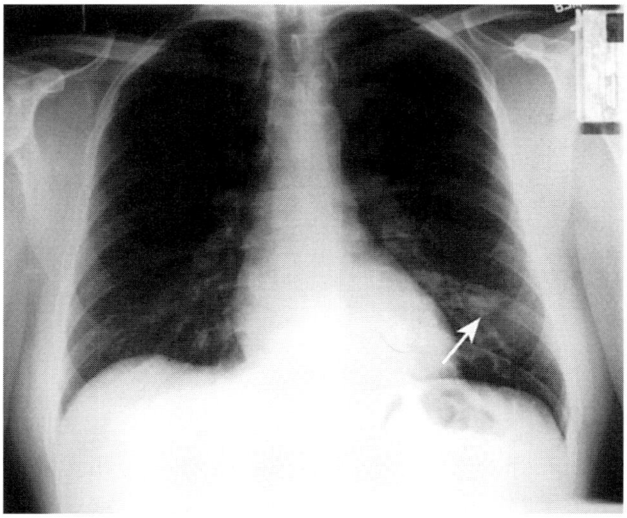

FIGURE 18.21 Pulmonary cryptococcosis. Faint focal infiltrate in left lower lobe (arrow). (Courtesy of M. Hagan, MD.)

Treatment

The decision about whether or not to treat a patient with cryptococcal pneumonia depends primarily upon two factors: the presence or absence of extra-pulmonary disease, and the underlying health status of the patient. Any patient with documented or suspected extra-pulmonary infection clearly requires systemic antifungal therapy. If disease is confined to the respiratory tract, the decision to treat is based upon the severity of pneumonia and the presence or absence of immunosuppression. Patients with extensive infiltrates or with cavitary lesions should be treated. Individuals who are HIV-seropositive or who have histories of haematological malignancies, chronic corticosteroid therapy, or other conditions associated with cellular immunodeficiency are at markedly increased risk for extra-pulmonary dissemination and require systemic antifungal therapy. Whether or not to treat the non-immunosuppressed patient with localised pulmonary disease remains an unresolved issue. Because many such cases are self-limited, most authorities recommend withholding antifungal therapy and monitoring the patient's clinical status closely. Unless the pneumonia progresses or extra-pulmonary disease develops, treatment is unnecessary. Others argue that all patients should be treated, because of the availability of relatively non-toxic drugs with excellent anticryptococcal activity *in vitro*, e.g. fluconazole.

No controlled clinical trials assessing the treatment of cryptococcal pneumonia have been done, so treatment recommendations are empirical and are extrapolated from the large body of clinical experience with treatment of cryptococcal meningitis. Available treatment options include intravenous amphotericin B, oral flucytosine, intravenous or oral fluconazole, and oral itraconazole.

A prospective clinical trial showed that amphotericin B, with or without concomitant flucytosine, is effective therapy for cryptococcal meningitis[253]. A 6-week course of amphotericin B, 0.3 mg/kg/day, plus flucytosine 150 mg/kg/day was more effective and less toxic than a 10-week course of amphotericin monotherapy, 0.4 mg/kg/day[253]. Clinical experience with fluconazole and itraconazole has been limited primarily to treatment of cryptococcal meningitis in patients with AIDS. A prospective study comparing amphotericin to fluconazole, 400 mg daily, found no significant difference in outcome between the two drugs, but deaths within the first 2 weeks were more common with fluconazole and cerebrospinal fluid sterilisation occurred more slowly[254]. In a comparative study of the two drugs for maintenance therapy, fluconazole 200 mg daily was superior to amphotericin B 1 mg/kg weekly[255]. Another trial of maintenance therapy found that fluconazole 200 mg daily was significantly more effective than itraconazole 200 mg daily (M. Saag, personal communication).

For the patient with cryptococcal pneumonia who does not have concomitant meningitis, both the dose and the duration of amphotericin therapy are arbitrary and should be based on clinical response. Most authorities recommend a dose of 0.5–0.6 mg/kg/day, continued until a cumulative dose of 500 mg to 1000 mg is attained. Because of the risk of flucytosine toxicity (bone marrow suppression, gastrointestinal side-effects)[256], concomitant flucytosine therapy generally is not given in the absence of meningitis. Flucytosine can be used only in combination with another antifungal drug, typically amphotericin, because of the risk of rapid development of resistance during flucytosine monotherapy. Less severe cases of cryptococcal pneumonia can be treated with fluconazole, administered orally or intravenously. The optimal dose of fluconazole is unknown, but given the high therapeutic index of this drug a daily dose of at least 400 mg seems preferable. Therapy should be continued until at least 2 weeks after resolution of pulmonary infiltrates. The efficacy of itraconazole for cryptococcal pneumonia is unknown, although treatment with this drug could be considered if the patient is unable to tolerate both amphotericin B and fluconazole.

A murine monoclonal anti-cryptococcal antibody has been studied in a mouse model of disseminated cryptococcal infection. Survival was significantly prolonged in treated mice compared to controls[257]. Subsequent studies showed that lung fungal burden and brain and lung weight were significantly reduced in mice who received monoclonal antibody[258].

Prevention

A cryptococcal vaccine has been developed but has not been tested in humans. Antifungal drug prophylaxis in patients with AIDS has been assessed in three studies. Nightingale *et al.* studied the incidence of cryptococcosis in HIV-infected patients with CD4+ lymphocyte counts below 68/μl who were treated with fluconazole 200 mg daily. As compared to untreated historical control patients from the previous year, there was a significant reduction in disease: less than 1% of treated patients developed cryptococcal infections, compared to 4% of control patients[259]. Powderly and associates performed a double-blinded trial comparing fluconazole, 200 mg daily, to clotrimazole troches in the prevention of fungal infection in HIV-infected patients with CD4+ lymphocyte counts below 200. Cryptococcal infection occurred in 0.9% of treated patients and in 7.1% of untreated patients[260]. A third study showed that itraconazole prophylaxis, 200 mg daily, prevented cryptococcosis in patients with CD4+ counts below 150/mm^3. Despite the clear-cut efficacy of fluconazole and itraconazole prophylaxis, such prophylaxis is not routinely recommended given the low incidence of cryptococcal infection in western countries and the risks of drug toxicity, drug interactions, or emergence of fluconazole-resistant yeast.

Miscellaneous forms of fungal pneumonia

Sporotrichosis

Sporotrichosis is caused by the dimorphic fungus *Sporothrix schenckii*. This organism is found worldwide, although most cases of sporotrichosis have been reported from North and South America. *S. schenckii* lives in sphagnum moss, straw, and wood. Exposure to these substances increases the risk of developing disease. The most common form of sporotrichosis is lymphocutaneous infection which occurs after inoculation of *S. schenckii* into the skin or subcutaneous tissues. A variety of extracutaneous manifestations have been reported, including osteoarticular disease, meningitis, and pneumonia.

Pulmonary sporotrichosis is quite uncommon but has been well described. In a series of 51 cases reported by Pluss and Opal, there was a six-fold higher incidence in males. Three-quarters of patients were Caucasian; average age was 46 years (range, 30 to 60 years). More than one-third of patients had underlying chronic medical illnesses including alcoholism, diabetes mellitus, sarcoidosis, or tuberculosis[261].

Pulmonary sporotrichosis is a chronic infection which does not cause significant systemic toxicity. Typical symptoms include low-grade fever, weight loss, and dry cough. Haemoptysis occurred in 18% of cases reported by Pluss and Opal[261]; massive, fatal haemoptysis has been described. Chest radiographs typically demonstrate unilateral or bilateral cavitary lesions, often associated with surrounding pulmonary infiltrates. The upper lobes are the predominant sites of involvement. Hilar lymphadenopathy and pleural effusions are seen infrequently[261]. Diagnosis is made by culturing the organism from sputum, bronchial washings, or lung tissue. Serology studies and skin tests for sporotrichosis are available but are considered inaccurate and are not recommended for routine use.

Saturated solution of potassium iodide (SSKI) has been used for treatment of lymphocutaneous sporotrichosis but is ineffective for pneumonia. Treatment options for pulmonary sporotrichosis include amphotericin B, the azole antifungal compounds, and surgical resection. Treatment failures are common with amphotericin B therapy even when cumulative doses in excess of 2 g are used[261]. Of the azole drugs, itraconazole has been the most effective for treatment of lymphocutaneous disease[262]. Only four patients with pulmonary sporotrichosis treated with itraconazole have been reported in the literature, three of whom responded[262,263]; however, one of the responders still had a positive sputum culture for *S. schenkii* after 12 months of treatment. Ketoconazole therapy has been ineffective[264,265]. Fluconazole appears less effective than itraconazole for extracutaneous sporotrichosis but has not been assessed for the treatment of pneumonia[266]. Based on currently available data, the treatment of choice for pulmonary sporotrichosis is itraconazole 400 mg daily. Treatment should be continued for at least a year in most cases. After completion of therapy, patients should be monitored closely for evidence of relapse of infection.

Paracoccidioidomycosis

Paracoccidioides brasiliensis is the aetiological agent of paracoccidioidomycosis, also named South American blastomycosis. Paracoccidioidomycosis is an endemic mycosis which occurs in the southern half of Mexico, all of Central America, and portions of South America[267] (Fig. 18.1). Disease is thought to result from inhalation of the organism from an environmental source. Epidemiological studies have failed to demonstrate the environmental niche of *P. brasiliensis*, although in a few cases the organism has been isolated from soil. Person-to-person transmission does not occur. Paracoccidioidomycosis occurs most frequently in persons over 30 years of age. In one series, males were affected 39 times more frequently than females[268]. Alcoholism is a risk factor for this infection[269].

Primary paracoccidioidomycosis is asymptomatic in most cases. After a variable latency period following exposure (up to 30 years), chronic pneumonia occurs in approximately 90% of patients who develop symptomatic infection[268]. Systemic toxicity is uncommon. Cough and sputum production occur in almost all cases, and approximately one-quarter of patients have haemoptysis or chest pain[270]. Half of patients with pneumonia also have extra-pulmonary disease, such as skin lesions, mucosal ulcerations in the nose and mouth, or diffuse lymphadenopathy[268,270–272]. Chest radiographs generally demonstrate bilateral nodular or alveolar pulmonary infiltrates which are often symmetrical. Cavitation occurs in 20% of cases[268]. Hilar lymphadenopathy and pleural effusion are uncommon findings[267,268].

Diagnosis can be made by direct observation, culture, or serology tests. In more than 90% of cases, KOH preparations of sputum or purulent drainage demonstrate round to oval budding yeasts measuring up to 40 μM in diameter[267]. The so-called 'pilot wheel' cell is a typical finding (Fig. 18.22). Cultures usually do not become positive for at least 2 to 3 weeks, and should be held for a minimum of 4 weeks. Serology tests for paracoccidioidomycosis are quite accurate. Immunodiffusion antibodies can be detected in 95% of cases; specificity approaches 100%[273]. Sensitivity of the complement fixation test is approximately 80% and specificity exceeds 95%[273], although false-positive reactions can occur in patients with histoplasmosis. Declining CF titres correlate with clinical response to treatment, so serial CF titres should be monitored in all cases[267,274,275]. Antigenaemia has been detected in patients with paracoccidioidomycosis but antigen measurement is not useful diagnostically[267]. Paracoccidioidin skin tests are positive in 70% of cases[268] but generally are non-reactive in persons with severe infection; skin testing is not of diagnostic value.

All patients with documented paracoccidioidomycosis should be treated. The oral azole drugs are the agents of choice for non-life-threatening cases. Ketoconazole, at a dose of 400 mg daily for 1 to 3 months followed by 200 mg daily for at least 3 months, was effective in approximately 90% of cases in two clinical trials, and relapse occurred in only about 10% of patients[276,277]. Itraconazole, 100 mg daily, appears to be as effective as ketoconazole and is less toxic[278,279]. Fluconazole therapy, 200 mg to 400 mg daily, was effective in all five cases assessed in a pilot study[280]. Of the three available azole drugs, itraconazole is considered the drug of choice.

Amphotericin B should be used in patients with life-threatening infection[267], and in those unable to receive oral medications. Among 250 patients who received 6 to 8 weeks of amphotericin treatment, 84% responded[267]. Because of a high risk of relapse, all patients treated with amphotericin should receive maintenance therapy with ketoconazole or itraconazole for 1 to 2 years[267]. Relapse occurs in 5–10% of cases; risk of relapse is greater with ketoconazole[267].

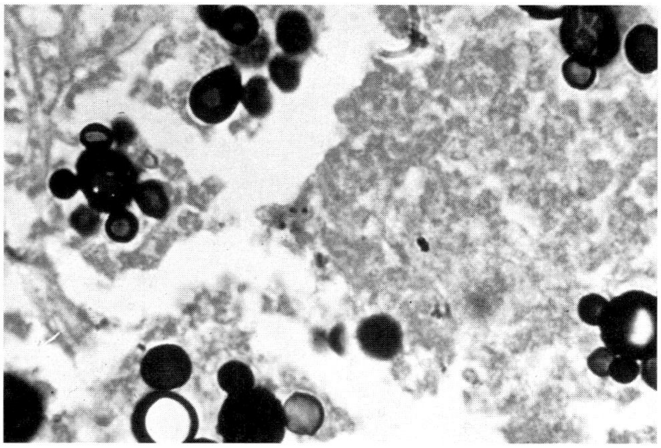

FIGURE 18.22 *Paracoccidioides brasiliensis*. Periodic Acid Schiff stain shows typical 'pilot wheel' cells. (Courtesy of M. Dykstra, PhD.)

In contrast to the other systemic mycoses, paracoccidioidomycosis responds to sulphadiazine. Sulpha maintenance therapy is reserved for those patients who are not candidates for oral azole therapy because of poor toleration or potential for drug interactions. Typical daily sulphadiazine dosage is 6 g for adults or 60–100 mg/kg for children[267]. Sulpha maintenance therapy is continued for 3 to 5 years[267]. In approximately 35% of sulphadiazine-treated patients, relapse of infection occurs, often due to development of fungal resistance to the drug[267]. Trimethoprim and sulphamethoxazole are synergistic *in vitro* against *P. brasiliensis*, even in strains resistant to sulphamethoxazole[281], but clinical experience with the combination of the two drugs is limited.

Conclusions

Histoplasma capsulatum is ubiquitous in the midwestern and southern United States and is also found in many areas in the Caribbean and Latin America. This fungus can cause asymptomatic infection, acute pneumonia, pericarditis, a rheumatological syndrome that mimics sarcoidosis, chronic pneumonia, pulmonary coin lesions, pulmonary calcifications, mediastinal or pleural fibrosis, or disseminated infection that can involve numerous organ systems. The diagnostic approach varies depending on the clinical manifestations in an individual case. Smears and cultures of clinical specimens, serology tests, and *Histoplasma* polysaccharide antigen are useful diagnostic tests. Treatment options include intravenous amphotericin B, oral itraconazole, intravenous ketoconazole or oral fluconazole or oral ketoconazole. The role of fluconazole in the treatment of histoplasmosis has not been defined fully. No forms of chemoprophylaxis or immunoprophylaxis have been shown to be effective.

Blastomyces dermatitidis is encountered in the southern and upper midwestern United States and in southern Canada. Clinical manifestations include acute or chronic pneumonia and extra-pulmonary disease involving the skin, mucosal surfaces, musculoskeletal system, genitourinary tract, or central nervous system. Diagnosis is made by direct observation of organisms in clinical specimens or by culture of body fluids or tissues. Serological tests are of limited value. Amphotericin B is the drug of choice for severe cases whereas itraconazole should be used for non-life-threatening disease. Ketoconazole and fluconazole also are effective in some cases. Since it is not possible to identify high-risk patients, prophylaxis against blastomycosis is not feasible.

Coccidioides immitis is found in arid climates in the lower Sonoran Life Zone in the United States and Mexico and in some areas in South America. Clinical manifestations include asymptomatic infection, acute pneumonia which sometimes is associated with skin lesions, chronic pulmonary nodules which occasionally cavitate, chronic pneumonia, or disseminated infection involving the skin, meninges, musculoskeletal system, or various other sites. Diagnosis can be established by visualisation and culture of organisms or by complement fixation and immunodiffusion serology studies. Amphotericin therapy is effective in severe cases; fluconazole, itraconazole, or ketoconazole are recommended for non-life-threatening infection. Treatment for chronic coccidioidomycosis should be quite prolonged and perhaps should be continued indefinitely. Although a vaccine has been developed, it has not been shown to be effective.

Cryptococcus neoformans has a widespread geographic distribution. The incidence of cryptococcosis has increased dramatically as a result of the AIDS epidemic. Cryptococcal pneumonia is frequently associated with extra-pulmonary manifestations of infection such as meningitis, cutaneous disease, or musculoskeletal lesions. Diagnosis is made by culture of sputum, bronchial washings, or tissue specimens; serum cryptococcal antigen is positive in severe cases. Treatment recommendations are hampered by the lack of controlled clinical trials assessing therapy of this infection. Amphotericin B is considered the drug of choice for severe cases, and fluconazole can be used for milder infections.

Sporothrix schenkii is best known as a cause of lymphocutaneous infection, but this fungus also can cause chronic pneumonia, particularly in persons with underlying serious medical illnesses. Diagnosis is made by culturing the organism from respiratory tract secretions. The low efficacy of antifungal therapy has been disappointing. Itraconazole and amphotericin B are preferred for treatment of this uncommon infection.

Paracoccidioides brasiliensis is prevalent in some areas of Mexico, Central America, and South America. The most common presentation of paracoccidioidomycosis is chronic pneumonia, which is associated with extra-pulmonary lesions in approximately half of cases. The diagnosis can be confirmed by smear, culture, or serology studies. Amphotericin B, itraconazole, ketoconazole, or fluconazole can be used to treat paracoccidioidomycosis. Because the risk of relapse of infection is high, long-term maintenance therapy with an azole drug should be administered.

References

1. DARLING ST. A protozoan general infection producing pseudotubercles in the lungs and focal necroses in the liver, spleen, and lymph nodes. *JAMA* 1906; 46: 1283–5.
2. DODD K, TOMPKINS EH. Case of histoplasmosis of Darling in an infant. *Am J Trop Med* 1934; 14: 127–37.
3. CHRISTIE A, PETERSON JC. Pulmonary calcification in negative reactors to tuberculin. *Am J Public Health* 1945; 35: 1131–47.
4. CHRISTIE A, PETERSON JC. Histoplasmin sensitivity. *J Pediatr* 1946; 29: 417–32.
5. CHRISTIE A. Histoplasmosis and pulmonary calcification – geographic distribution. *Am J Trop Med* 1951; 31: 742–9,
6. PALMER CE. Geographic differences in sensitivity to histoplasmin among student nurses. *Public Health Rep* 1946; 61: 475–87.
7. EMMONS CW. Isolation of *Histoplasma capsulatum* from soil. *Public Health Rep* 1949; 64: 892–6.
8. ZEIDBERG LD. Isolation of *Histoplasma capsulatum* from soil. *Am J Public Health* 1952; 12: 930–5.
9. FURCULOW ML, GRAYSTON JT. Occurrence of histoplasmosis in epidemics. *Am Rev Tuberc* 1953; 68: 307–20.
10. DUPONT B, DROUHET E, LAPRESLE G. Histoplasmose généralisée à *Histoplasma duboisii*. *Nouv. Presse Med* 1974; 3: 1005–7.
11. BRANDESBERG JW. Fungi found in association with *Histoplasma capsulatum* in a naturally contaminated site in Clarksburg, Maryland. *Sabouraudia* 1968; 6: 246–54.
12. AJELLO L. Histoplasmosis – a dual entity: *Histoplasmosis capsulati* and *Histoplasmosis duboisii*. *Hyg Mod* 1983; 79: 3–30.
13. FURCULOW ML, NEY PE. Epidemiologic aspects of histoplasmosis. *Am J Hyg* 1957; 65: 264–70.
14. US NATIONAL COMMUNICABLE DISEASE CENTER. Annual Supplement, summary 1968, *MMWR* 1969; 17.
15. FURCULOW ML, WILLIS MJ, WOOD LE, MANTZ HL. Tuberculin-histoplasmin conversion rates in Kansas City as an indication of the prevalence of infection. *Am Rev Tuberc* 1954; 69: 234–40.
16. MURRAY JF, HOWARD DH. Laboratory-acquired histoplasmosis. *Am Rev Resp Dis* 1964; 89: 631–40.
17. HOOD AB, INGLIS FG. Histoplasmosis and thrombocytopenic purpura: transmission by renal homotransplantation. *Can Med Assoc J* 1965; 93: 587–92.
18. MCKINSEY D, SMITH D, DRIKS M, O'CONNOR M. Histoplasmosis in Missouri: historical review and current clinical concepts. *Mo Med* 1994; 91: 27–32.
19. BRODSKY AL, GREGG MB, LOEWENSTEIN MS *et al.* Outbreak of histoplasmosis associated with the 1970 Earth Day activities. *Am J Med* 1973; 54: 333–42.
20. WHEAT LJ, SLAMA TG, EITZEN HE, KOHLER RB, FRENCH MLV, BIESECKER JL. A large outbreak of histoplasmosis: clinical features. *Ann Intern Med* 1981; 94: 331–7.
21. SCHLECH WF, WHEAT LJ, HO JL *et al.* Recurrent urban histoplasmosis, Indianapolis, Indiana, 1980–81. *Am J Epidemiol* 1983; 118: 301–12.
22. KEATH EJ, KOBAYASHI GS, MEDOFF G. Typing of *Histoplasma capsulatum* by restriction fragment length polymorphisms in a nuclear gene. *J Clin Microbiol* 1992; 30: 2104–7.
23. BAUGHMAN RP, KIM CK, VINEGAR A *et al.* The pathogenesis of experimental pulmonary histoplasmosis. Correlative studies of histopathology, bronchoalveolar lavage, and respiratory function. *Am Rev Resp Dis* 1986; 134: 771–4.
24. NEWMAN SL, GOOTE L, GABAY J. Human neutrophil-mediated fungistasis against *Histoplasma capsulatum*. Localization of fungistatic activity to the azurophil granules. J Clin Invest 1993; 92: 624–31.
25. NEWMAN SL, GOOTEE L, BUCHER C *et al.* Inhibition of intracellular *Histoplasma capsulatum* yeast cells by cytokine-activated human monocytes and macrophages. *Infect Immun* 1991; 59: 737–41.
26. SANCHEZ SB, CARBONELL LM. Immunological studies on *Histoplasma capsulatum*. *Infect Immun* 1975; 11: 387–94.
27. STRAUB M, SCHWARZ J. The healed primary complex in histoplasmosis. *Am J Clin Pathol* 1955; 25: 727–41.
28. NEWMAN SL, GOOTEE L. Colony stimulating factors activate human macrophages to inhibit intracellular growth of *Histoplasma capsulatum* yeasts. *Infect Immun* 1992; 60: 4593–7.
29. MCKINSEY D. Histoplasmosis and aspergillosis: clinical manifestations, diagnosis, and treatment. *Postgrad Med* 1995; Special Report: 35–41.
30. MCKINSEY D, DRIKS M. Histoplasmosis in HIV disease. *AIDS Reader* November 1993: 203–9.
31. SALZMAN SH, SMITH RL, ARANDO CP. Histoplasmosis in patients at risk for AIDS in a

non-endemic setting. *Chest* 1988; 93: 916–21.

32. BRIVET F, ROULOT D, NAVEAU D *et al.* The acquired immunodeficiency syndrome: B-cell lymphoma, histoplasmosis, and ethics and economics. *Ann Intern Med* 1986; 104: 447.
33. WHEAT LJ. Histoplasmosis – diagnosis and management. *Infect Dis Clin Pract* 1992; 1: 287–90.
34. LARRABEE WF, AJELLO L, KAUFMAN L. An epidemic of histoplasmosis on the isthmus of Panama. *Am J Trop Med Hyg* 1977; 27: 281–5.
35. WARD JI, WEEKS M, ALLEN D *et al.* Acute histoplasmosis: clinical, epidemiologic and serologic findings of an outbreak associated with exposure to a fallen tree. *Am J Med* 1977; 66: 587–95.
36. BULLOCK WE. *Histoplasma capsulatum.* In Mandell G, Bennett JE, Dolin R. *Principles and Practice of Infection Diseases.* 4th ed. New York: Churchill Livingston; 1995: 2340–53.
37. BARTLETT PC, VONBEHREN LA, TEWARI RP *et al.* Bats in the belfry: an outbreak of histoplasmosis. *Am J Public Health* 1982; 72: 1369–72.
38. KATARIA YP, CAMPBELL PB, BURLINGTON BT. Acute pulmonary histoplasmosis presenting as adult respiratory distress syndrome: effect of therapy on clinical and laboratory features. *South Med J* 1981; 74: 534–7.
39. WHEAT LF, STEIN L, CORYA BC *et al.* Pericarditis as a manifestation of histoplasmosis during two large urban outbreaks. *Medicine* 1983; 62: 110–19.
40. FREDRICKSON RT, COHEN LS, MULLINS CB. Pericardial windows or pericardiocentesis for pericardial effusions. *Am Heart J* 1971; 82: 158–62.
41. ROSENTHAL J, BRANDT KD, WHEAT LJ *et al.* Rheumatologic manifestations of histoplasmosis in the recent Indianapolis epidemic. *Arthritis Rheum* 1983; 26: 1065–70.
42. RUBIN SA, WINER-MURAM HT. Thoracic histoplasmosis. *J Thorac Imaging* 1992; 7: 39–50.
43. WHEAT LJ, WASS J, NORTON J, KOHLER RB, FRENCH MLV. Cavitary histoplasmosis occurring during two large urban outbreaks: analysis of clinical, epidemiologic, roentgenographic, and laboratory features. *Medicine* 1984; 63: 201–9.
44. BENNISH M, RADKOWSKI MA, RIPPON JW. Cavitation in acute histoplasmosis. *Chest* 1983; 84: 496–7.
45. JENKINS DW, FISK DE, BYRD RB. Mediastinal histoplasmosis with esophageal abscess. *Gastroenterology* 1976; 70: 109–11.
46. GOODWIN RA, NICKELL JA, DES PREZ RM. Mediastinal fibrosis complicating healed primary histoplasmosis and tuberculosis. *Medicine* 1972; 51: 227–46.
47. FELSON B. Thoracic calcifications. *Dis Chest* 1969; 56: 330–43.
48. KILBURN C, MCKINSEY D. Recurrent massive pleural effusion due to pleural, pericardial, and epicardial fibrosis in histoplasmosis. *Chest* 1991; 100: 1715–17.
49. FURULOW ML, BRASHER CA. Chronic progressive (cavitary) histoplasmosis as a problem at tuberculosis sanitariums. *Am Rev Tuberc Pulm Dis* 1956; 73: 609–19.
50. GOODWIN RA, OWENS FT, SNELL JD *et al.* Chronic pulmonary histoplasmosis. *Medicine* 1976; 55: 413–52.
51. GOODWIN RA, SHAPIRO JL, THURMAN GH. *et al.* Disseminated histoplasmosis: clinical and pathologic correlations. *Medicine* 1980; 59: 1–32.
52. KURTIN PK, MCKINSEY DS, GUPTA MR, DRIKS M. Histoplasmosis in patients with AIDS: hematologic and bone marrow manifestations. *Am J Clin Pathol* 1990; 93: 367–72.
53. WHEAT LJ, CONNOLLY-STRINGFIELD P, BAKER RL *et al.* Disseminated histoplasmosis in the acquired immune deficiency syndrome: clinical findings, diagnosis and treatment, and review of the literature. *Medicine* 1990; 69: 361–74.
54. MCKINSEY D, SPIEGEL R, HUTWAGNER L *et al.* Prospective study of histoplasmosis in patients with human immunodeficiency virus infection. Incidence, risk factors and pathophysiology. *Clin Infect Dis* 1997 (in press)
55. JOHNSON PC, KHARDORI N, NAJJAR A *et al.* Progressive disseminated histoplasmosis in patients with AIDS. *Am J Med* 1988; 85: 152–8.
56. MCKINSEY D, WAXMAN M, IDSTROM M. Differentiation of disseminated histoplasmosis from *Pneumocystis carinii* pneumonia in AIDS. *Infect Med* 1993; 10: 30–8.
57. WHEAT LJ, FRENCH MLV, KOHLER RB *et al.* The diagnostic laboratory tests for histoplasmosis: analysis of experience in a large urban outbreak. *Am Intern Med* 1982; 97: 680–5.
58. SATHAPATAYVONGS B, BATTEIGER BE, WHEAT J, SLAMA TG, WASS JL. Clinical and laboratory features of disseminated histoplasmosis during two large urban outbreaks. *Medicine* 1983; 62: 264–70.
59. BILLE J, STOCKMAN L, ROBERTS GD *et al.* Evaluation of a lysis-centrifugation system for recovery of yeasts and filamentous fungi from blood. *J Clin Microbiol* 1983; 18: 469–71.
60. HUFFNAGLE KE, GANSER RM. Evaluation of Gen-probe's *Histoplasma capsulatum* and *Cryptococcus neoformas* accuprobes. *J Clin Microbiol* 1993; 31: 419–21.
61. DAVIES SF. Serodiagnosis of histoplasmosis. *Semin Resp Infect* 1986; 1: 9–15.
62. GEORGE RB, LAMBERT RS. Significance of serum antibodies to *Histoplasma capsulatum* in endemic areas. *South Med J* 1984; 77: 161–3.
63. PARKER JD, SAROSI GA, DOTA IL, BAILEY RE, TOSH FE. Treatment of chronic pulmonary histoplasmosis. *N Engl J Med* 1970; 238: 225–9.
64. WHEAT LJ, KOHLER RB, TEWARI RP. Diagnosis of disseminated histoplasmosis by detection of *Histoplasma capsulatum* antigen in serum and urine specimens. *N Engl J Med* 1986; 314: 83–8.
65. WHEAT LJ, KOHLER RB, TEWARI RP, GARTEN ML, FRENCH MLV. Significance of *Histoplasma* antigen in the cerebrospinal fluid of patients with meningitis. *Arch Intern Med* 1989; 149: 302–4.
66. WHEAT LJ, CONNOLLY-STRINGFIELD P, WILLIAMS B, CONNOLLY K, BLAIR R, BARTLETT M, DURKIN M. Diagnosis of histoplasmosis in patients with the acquired immunodeficiency syndrome by detection of *Histoplasma capsulatum* polysaccharide antigen in bronchoalveolar lavage fluid. *Am Rev Resp Dis* 1992; 145: 1421–4.
67. WHEAT LJ, CONNOLLY-STRINGFIELD P, BLAIR R *et al.* Histoplasmosis relapse in patients with AIDS: detection using *Histoplasma capsulatum* variety capsulatum antigen levels. *Ann Intern Med* 1991; 115: 936–41.
68. SAROSI GA, CATANZARO A, DANIEL TM, DAVIES, SF. Clinical usefulness of skin testing in histoplasmosis, coccidioidomycosis, and blastomycosis. *Am Rev Resp Dis* 1988; 138: 1081–2.
69. FURCULOW, ML. Tests of immunity in histoplasmosis. *N Engl J Med* 1963; 268: 357–61.
70. DISMUKES WE, BRADSHER RW, CLOUD GC *et al.* Itraconazole therapy for blastomycosis and histoplasmosis. *Am J Med* 1992; 489–97.
71. WHEAT L, MAWHINNEY S, HAFNER R, MCKINSEY D. Fluconazole treatment for histoplasmosis in AIDS: prospective multicenter noncomparative trial (abstract 1233) In *Program and Abstracts of the 34th Interscience Conference on Antimicrobial Agents and Chemotherapy*. Washington, DC: American Society for Microbiology, 1994: 214.
72. BAUM GL, LARKIN JL, SUTLIFF WD. Follow up of patients with chronic pulmonary histoplasmosis treated with amphotericin B. *Chest* 1970; 8: 562–5.
73. VETERANS ADMINISTRATION – ARMED

FORCES COOPERATIVE STUDY ON HISTOPLASMOSIS. Histoplasmosis cooperative study, II. Chronic pulmonary histoplasmosis treated with and without amphotericin B. *Am Rev Resp Dis* 1964; 89: 641–50.

74. DISMUKES WE, CLOUD G, BOWLES C *et al.* Treatment of blastomycosis and histoplasmosis with ketoconazole. *Ann Intern Med* 1985; 103: 861–72.

75. MCKINSEY D, PAPPAS P, KAUFMAN C, *et al.* Fluconazole therapy for histoplasmosis. *Clin Infect Dis* 1996; 23: 996–1001.

76. SAROSI GA, VOTH DW DAHL BA, DOTO IL, TOSH FE. Disseminated histoplasmosis: results of long-term follow-up. *Ann Intern Med* 1971; 75: 511–16.

77. RUBIN H. The course and prognosis of histoplasmosis. *Am J Med* 1959; 27: 278–87.

78. WHEAT LJ, HAFNER R, KORZUN AH *et al.* Itraconazole treatment of disseminated histoplasmosis in patients with AIDS. *Am J Med* 1995; 98: 336–42.

79. MCKINSEY D, GUPTA M, RIDDLER S *et al.* Long-term amphotericin B therapy for disseminated histoplasmosis in patients with AIDS. *Ann Intern Med* 1989; 11: 655–9.

80. MCKINSEY DS, GUPTA MR, DRIKS MR *et al.* Histoplasmosis in patients with AIDS: efficacy of maintenance amphotericin B therapy. *Am J Med* 1992; 92: 225–7.

81. WHEAT LJ, HAFNER RE, WULFSOHN M *et al.* Prevention of relapse of histoplasmosis with itraconazole in patients with AIDS. *Am Intern Med* 1993; 118: 610–16.

82. NORRIS J, WHEAT J, MCKINSEY D *et al.* Prevention of relapse of histoplasmosis with fluconazole in patients with AIDS. *Am J Med* 1994; 96: 504–8.

82a. MCKINSEY D, WHEAT J, CLOUD G *et al.* Itraconazole is effective primary prophylaxis against systemic fungal infections in patients with advanced human immunodeficiency virus infection (abstract LB9). In: Addendum to program and abstracts of the 36th interscience conference on antimicrobial agents and chemotherapy. Washington DC American Society for Microbiology, 1996.

83. GILCHRIST TC. Protozoan dermatitidis. *J Cutan Genitourin Dis* 1894; 12: 496–9.

84. GILCHRIST TC, STOKES WR. A case of pseudolupus caused by blastomyces. *J Exp Med* 1898; 3: 53–78.

85. MARTIN DS, SMITH DT. Blastomycosis I: a review of the literature. *Am Rev Tuberc* 1939; 39: 275–304.

86. MARTIN DS, SMITH DT. Blastomycosis II: a report of thirteen new cases. *Am Rev Tuberc* 1939; 39: 488–515.

87. SCHWARTZ J, BAUM GL. Blastomycosis. *Am J Clin Pathol* 1951; 21: 999–1029.

88. KLEIN BS, DAVIS JP. A laboratory-based surveillance of human blastomycosis in Wisconsin between 1973 and 1982. *Am J Epidemiol* 1985; 122: 897–903.

89. LOWRY PW, KELSO KY, MCFARLAND LM. Blastomycosis in Washington Parish, Louisiana, 1976–1985. *Am J Epidemiol* 1989; 130: 151–9.

90. BAUMGARDNER DS, BUGGY BP, MOTTSON BJ, BURDICK JS, LUDWIG D. Epidemiology of blastomycosis in a region of high endemicity in north central Wisconsin. *Clin Infect Dis* 1992; 15: 629–35.

91. KOWALSKI M. North American blastomycosis and possibilities of its occurrence in Poland. *Przegl Dermatol* 1976; 63: 641–7.

92. KINGSTON M, EL-MISHAD MM, ALI MA. Blastomycosis in Saudi Arabia. *Am J Trop Med Hyg* 1980; 29: 464–6.

93. KUTTIN ES. Occurrence of *Blastomyces dermatitidis* in Israel: first autochthonous Middle Eastern case. *Am J Trop Med Hyg* 1978; 27: 1203–5.

94. HASAN FM. The association of adenocarcinoma of the lung and blastomycosis from an unusual geographical location. *Br J Dis Chest* 1978; 72: 242–6.

95. RANDHAWA HS, KHAN ZU, GAUR SN. *Blastomyces dermatidis* in India: first report of its isolation from clinical material. *Sabouraudia* 1983; 21: 215–21.

96. MCDONOUGH ES. Studies on the growth and survival of *Blastomyces dermatitidis* in soil. In Gibbons NE, ed. *Recent Progress in Microbiology.* Toronto: University of Toronto Press: 1963.

97. MCDONOUGH ES, VAN PROOIEN R, LEWIS AL. Lysis of *Blastomyces dermatitidis* yeast-phase cells in natural soil. *Am J Epidemiol* 1965; 81: 86–94.

98. KLEIN BS, VERGERONT JM, WEEKS RJ *et al.* Isolation of *Blastomyces dermatitidis* in soil associated with a large outbreak of blastomycosis in Wisconsin. *N Engl J Med* 1985; 314: 529–34.

99. KLEIN BS, VERGERONT JM, DISALVO AF *et al.* Two outbreaks of blastomycosis along rivers in Wisconsin: isolation of *Blastomyces dermatitidis* from river-bank soil and evidence of its transmission along waterways. *Am Rev Resp Dis* 1987; 136: 1333–8.

100. KLEIN BS, VERGERONT JM, DAVID JP. Epidemiologic aspects of blastomycosis, the enigmatic systemic mycosis. *Semin Resp Infect* 1986; 1: 29–39.

101. MENGES RW, DOTO IL, WEEKS RJ. Epidemiologic studies of blastomycosis in Arkansas. *Arch Environ Health* 1969; 18: 956–71.

102. WITORSCH P, UTZ JP. North American blastomycosis: a study of 40 patients. *Medicine* 1968; 47: 169–200.

103. KITCHEN MS, REIBER CD, EASTIN GB. An urban epidemic of North American blastomycosis. *Am Rev Resp Dis* 1977; 115: 1063–6.

104. SMITH JG, HARRIS JS, CONANT NF *et al.* An epidemic of North American blastomycosis. *JAMA* 1955; 158: 641–6.

105. TOSH FE, HAMMERMAN KJ, WEEKS RJ *et al.* A common source epidemic of North American blastomycosis. *Am Rev Resp Dis* 1974; 109: 525–9.

106. COCKERILL FR, ROBERTS GD, ROSENBLATT JE *et al.* Epidemic of pulmonary blastomycosis (Nanekagan fever) in Wisconsin canoeists. *Chest* 1984; 86: 688–92.

107. ARMSTRONG CW, JENKINS SR, KAUFMAN L *et al.* Common source outbreak of blastomycosis in hunters and their dogs. *J Infect Dis* 1987; 155: 568–70.

108. CRAIG MW, DAVEY WN, GREEN RA. Conjugal blastomycosis. *Am Rev Resp Dis* 1970: 86–90.

109. DYER ML, YOUNG TL, KATTINE AA, WILSON D. Blastomycosis in a Papanicolau smear: report of a case with possible venereal transmission. *Acta Cytol* 1983; 27: 285–7.

110. FARBER ER, LEAHY MS, MEADOWS TR. Endometrial blastomycosis acquired by sexual contact. *Obst gyn* 1968; 32: 195–9.

111. LARSON DM, ECKMAN MR, ALBER RL *et al.* Primary cutaneous (inoculation) blastomycosis: an occupational hazard to pathologists. *Am J Clin Pathol* 1983; 79: 253–5.

112. DRUTZ DJ, FREY CL. Intracellular and extracellular defenses against *Blastomyces dermatitidis* conidia and yeasts. *J Lab Clin Med* 1985; 105: 737–50.

113. SCHAFFNER A, DAVIS CE, SCHAFFNER T *et al. In vitro* susceptibility of fungi to killing by neutrophil granulocytes discriminates between primary pathogenicity and opportunism. *J Clin Invest* 1986; 78: 511–24.

114. EVANS ME, HAYNES JB, ATKINSON JB *et al. Blastomyces dermatitidis* and the adult respiratory distress syndrome. *Am Rev Resp Dis* 1982; 126: 1099–102.

115. MEYER KC, MCMANUS EJ, MAKI DG. Overwhelming pulmonary blastomycosis associated with the adult respiratory distress syndrome. *N Engl J Med* 1993; 329: 1231–6.

116. WINER-MURAM HT, RUBIN SA. Pulmonary blastomycosis. *J Thoracic Imaging* 1992; 7: 23–8.

117. SHEFLIN JR, CAMPBELL JA, THOMPSON GP. Pulmonary blastomycosis: findings on chest radiographs in 63 patients. *AJR* 1990; 154: 1177–80.

118. BROWN LR, SWENSEN SJ, VAN SCOY RE, PRAKASH UBS, COLES D, COLBY TV. Roentgenologic features of pulmonary blastomycosis. *Mayo Clin Proc* 1991; 66: 29–38.

119. WINER-MURAM HT, BEALS DH, COLE FH. Blastomycosis of the lungs: CT features. *Radiology* 1992; 182: 829–32.

120. BLASTOMYCOSIS COOPERATIVE STUDY OF THE VETERANS ADMINISTRATION: Blastomycosis I: a review of 198 collected cases in Veterans Administration Hospitals. *Am Rev Resp Dis* 1964; 89: 659–72.

121. BROWN LR, SWEASEN SJ, VANSCOY RE *et al.* Roentgenologic features of pulmonary blastomycosis. *Mayo Clin Proc* 1991; 66: 29–38.

122. STELLING CB, WOODWRING JH, REHM SR *et al.* Miliary pulmonary blastomycosis. *Radiology* 1984; 150: 7–13.

123. LOCKWOOD WR, ALLISON F, BATSON BE *et al.* The treatment of North American blastomycosis: Ten years experience. *Am Rev Resp Dis* 1969; 100: 314–20.

124. DUTTERA MJ, OSTERHOUT S. North American blastomycosis: a survey of 63 cases. *South Med J* 1969; 62: 295–301.

125. MACDONALD PB, BLACK GB, MACKENZIE R. Orthopaedic manifestations of blastomycosis. *J Bone Joint Surg* 1990; 72: 860–4.

126. PRICHARD DJ. Granulomatous infections of bones and joints. *Orthop Clin N Am* 1975; 6: 1029–47.

127. EIKENBERG HA, AMIN M, LICH RI. Blastomycosis of the genitourinary tract. *J Urol* 1975; 113: 650–2.

128. GONYEA EF. The spectrum of primary blastomycotic meningitis. A review of central nervous system blastomycosis. *Ann Neurol* 1978; 3: 26–39.

129. PAPPAS PG, THRELKELD MG, BEDSOLE GD *et al.* Blastomycosis in immunocompromised patients. *Medicine* 1993; 72: 311–25.

130. SERODY JS, MILL MR, DETTERBECK FC, HARRIS DT, COHEN MS. Blastomycosis in transplant recipients: report of a case and review. *Clin Infect Dis* 1993; 16: 54–8.

131. WITIG RS, HOADLEY DJ, GREER DL, ABRIOLA KP, HERNANDEZ RL. Blastomycosis and human immunodeficiency virus: three new cases and review. *South Med J* 1994; 85: 715–19.

132. PAPPAS PG, POTTAGE JC, POWDERLY WG *et al.* Blastomycosis in patients with acquired immunodeficiency syndrome. *Ann Intern Med* 1992; 116: 857–63.

133. TRUMBULL ML, CHESNEY T. The cytological diagnosis of pulmonary blastomycosis. *JAMA* 1981; 245: 836–8.

134. TURNER S, KAUFMAN I. Immunodiagnosis of blastomycosis. *Semin Resp Infect* 1986; 122–8.

135. STOCKMAN L, MURPHY-CLARK K, ROBERTS G. Evaluation of commercially available acridium ester-labeled chemiluminescent DNA probes for culture identification of *Blastomyces dermatitidis, Coccidioides immitis, Cryptococcus neoformans* and *Histoplasma capsulatum. J Clin Microbiol* 1993; 31: 845–50.

136. KLEIN BS, KURITSKY WAC, KAUFMAN L *et al.* Comparison of enzyme immunoassay, immunodiffusion and complement fixation in detecting antibody in human serum to the A antigen in *B. dermatitidis. Am Rev Resp Dis* 1986; 133: 144–8.

137. KLEIN BS, VERGERONT JM, KAUFMAN L *et al.* Serological tests for blastomycosis: assessments during a large point-source outbreak in Wisconsin. *J Infect Dis* 1987; 155: 262–8.

138. KAUFMAN L, MCLAUGHLIN DW, CLARK MJ *et al.* Specific immunodiffusion tests for blastomycosis. *Appl Microbiol* 1973; 26: 244–7.

139. WILLIAMS JE, MURPHY R, STANDARD PG *et al.* Serologic response in blastomycosis: Diagnostic value of double immunodiffusion assay. *Am Rev Resp Dis* 1981; 123: 209–12.

140. KAUFMAN L, MCLAUGHLIN O, CLARK M *et al.* Specific immunodiffusion tests for blastomycosis. *Appl Microbiol* 1973; 26: 244–7.

141. LAMBERT RS, GEORGE RB. Evaluation of enzyme immunoassay as a rapid screening test for histoplasmosis and blastomycosis. *Am Rev Resp Dis* 1987; 136: 316–19.

142. GEORGE RB, LAMBERT RS, BRUCE MJ *et al.* Radioimmunoassay: a sensitive screening test for histoplasmosis and blastomycosis. *Am Rev Resp Dis* 1981; 124: 407–10.

143. GREEN JH, HARRELL WK, JOHNSON J *et al.* Preparation of reference antisera for laboratory diagnosis of blastomycosis. *J Clin Microbiol* 1979; 10: 1–7.

144. PARKER JD, DOTO IL, TOSH FE. A decade of experience with blastomycosis and its treatment with amphotericin B. *Am Rev Resp Dis* 1969; 99: 895–902.

145. BRADHSER RW, RICE DC, ABERNATHY RS. Ketoconazole therapy for endemic blastomycosis. *Ann Intern Med* 1985; 103: 872–9.

146. PAPPAS PG, BRADSHER RW, CHAPMAN SW *et al.* Treatment of blastomycosis with flucconazole: a pilot study. *Clin Infect Dis* 1995; 20: 267–271.

147. COMO JA, DISMUKES WE. Oral azole drugs as systemic antifungal therapy. *N Engl J Med* 1994; 330: 263–72.

148. POSADAS A. Un nuevo case de micosis fungoidea con psorospermias. *Ann Circ Med Argent* 1892; 15: 585–97.

149. RIXFORD E, GILCHRIST TC. Two cases of protozoan (coccidioidal) infection of the skin and other organs. *Johns Hopkins Hosp Rep* 1896; 1: 209–69.

150. OPHÜLS W, MOFFITT HC. A new pathogenic mould (formerly described as a protozoan: *Coccidioides immitis* pyogenes): preliminary report. *Phil Med J* 1900; 5: 1471–72.

151. KRUSE RH. Potential aerogenic laboratory hazards of *Coccidioides immitis. Am J Clin Pathol* 1962; 37: 150–5.

152. DICKSON EG. 'Valley fever' of the San Joaquin Valley and fungus *Coccidioides. California West Med* 1937; 47: 151–5.

153. EGEBERG RO, ELY AI. *Coccidioides immitis* in the soil of southern San Joaquin Valley. *Am J Med Sci* 1956; 231: 151–4.

154. MADDY KT. Observations on *Coccidioides immitis* found growing naturally in soil. *Ariz Med* 1965; 22: 281–8.

155. MADDY KT. Ecological factors possibly relating to the geographic distribution of *Coccidioides immitis.* In *Proceedings of a Symposium on Coccidioidomycosis.* Public Health Service Publ. No. 575. Atlanta: Centers for Disease Control; 1957: 144–57.

156. EDWARDS LB, PALMER C. Prevalence of sensitivity to coccidioidin, with special reference to specific and non-specific reactions to coccidioidin and histoplasmin. *Dis Chest* 1957; 31: 35–60.

157. PAPPAGIANIS D. Ethnic background and the clinical course of coccidioidomycosis. *Am Rev Resp Dis* 1979; 120: 959–61.

158. HUNTINGTON RW. Morphology and racial distribution of fatal Coccidioidomycosis: report of a ten-year autopsy series in an endemic area. *JAMA* 1959: 115–18.

159. CALHOUN DL. Coccidioidomycosis in recent renal or cardiac transplant recipients. In Einstein HE, Catanzaro A, eds. *Proceedings of the 4th International Conference on Coccidioidomycosis.* Washington, DC, National Foundation for Infectious Diseases; 1985; 312–18.

160. RUTALA PJ, SMITH JW. Coccidioidomycosis in potentially compromised hosts: the effects of immunosuppresive therapy in dissemination. *Am J Med Sci* 1978; 275: 283–95.

161. BRONNIMANN DA, ADAM RD, GALGIANI JN *et al.* Coccidioidomycosis in the acquired immunodeficiency syndrome. *Ann. Intern Med* 1987; 106: 372–9.

162. FISH DG, AMPEL NM, GALGIANI JN *et al.* Coccidioidomycosis during human immunodeficiency virus infection: a review of 77 patients. *Medicine* 1990; 6: 384–91.

163. ECKMANN BH, SCHAEFER GL, HUPPERT M. Bedside interhuman transmission of coccidioidomycosis via growth on fomites: an epidemic involving six persons. *Am Rev Resp Dis* 1964; 89: 175–85.

164. ALBERT BL, SELLERS TF. Coccidioidomycosis from fomites. *Arch Intern. Med* 1963; 112: 253–61.

165. GEHLBACH SH, HAMILTON JD, CONANT NF. Coccidioidomycosis: an occupational disease in cotton mill workers. *Arch Intern Med* 1973; 131: 254–5.

166. SYMMERS W, ST C. Case of coccidioidomycosis seen in Britain. In Ajello L, ed. *Coccidioidomycosis.* Tucson: University of Arizona Press: 1978: 301–5.

167. JOHNSON JE, PERRY JE, FEKETY FR *et al.* Laboratory-acquired coccidioidomycosis. A report of 210 cases. *Ann Intern Med* 1964; 60: 941.

168. WERNER SB. An epidemic of coccidioidomycosis among archeology students in northern California. *N Engl J Med* 1972; 286: 507–12.

169. FIESE MJ. *Coccidioidomycosis.* Springfield, II: Charles C. Thomas; 1958.

170. EGEBERG RO, ELCOVIN A. Effect of salinity and temperature on *Coccidioides immitis* and three antagonistic soil saprophytes. *J Bacteriol* 1964; 88: 473–6.

171. EINSTEIN HE, JOHNSON RH. Coccidioidomycosis: new aspects of epidemiology and therapy. *Clin Infect Dis* 1993; 16: 349–56.

172. KERRICK SS, LUNDERGAN LL, GALGIANI JN. Coccidioidomycosis at a university health service. *Am Rev Resp Dis* 1985; 131: 100–2.

173. PAGGAGIANIS D, EINSTEIN H. Tempest from Tehachapi takes toll, or *coccidioides* conveyed aloft and afar. *West J Med* 1978; 129: 527–30.

174. CDC. Coccidioidomycosis following the Northridge earthquake–California. 1994. *MMWR* 1994; 43: 194–5.

175. AMPEL NM, DOLS CL, GALGIANI JN. Coccidioidomycosis during human immunodeficiency virus infection: results of a prospective study in a coccidioidal endemic area. *Am J Med* 1993; 94: 235–40.

176. WILSON J, SMITH C, PLUNKETT O. Primary cutaneous coccidioidomycosis, the criteria for diagnosis and report of a case. *Calif Med* 1953; 79: 233–9.

177. SAVAGE DC, MADIN SH. Cellular responses in lungs of immunized mice to intranasal infection with *Coccidioides immitis. Sabouraudia* 1968; 6: 94–101.

178. PETKUS AF, BAUM LL. Natural killer cell inhibition of young spherules and endospores of *Coccidioides immitis. J Immunol* 1987; 139: 3107–11.

179. SMITH CE, BEARD RR, WHITING EG *et al.* Varieties of coccidioidal infection in relation to the epidemiology and control of the disease. *Am J Public Health* 1946; 36: 1394–401.

180. TOM PF, LONG TJ, FITZPATRICK SB. Coccidioidomycosis in adolescents presenting as chest pain. *J Adolesc. Health Care* 1987; 8: 365–71.

181. BATRA P. Pulmonary coccidioidomycosis. *J Thorac Imaging* 1992; 7: 29–38.

182. CASTELLINO RA, BLANK N. Pulmonary coccidioidomycosis: the wide spectrum of roentgenographic manifestations. *Calif Med* 1968; 109: 41–8.

183. HYDE L. Coccidioidal pulmonary cavitation. *Dis Chest* 1968; 54 (Suppl 1): 273–7.

184. WINN WA. A long term study of 300 patients with cavity-abscess lesions of the lung of coccidioidal origin. *Dis Chest* 1968; 54 (Suppl. 1): 268–72.

185. SAROSI GA, PARKER JD, DOTO IL, TOSH FE. Chronic pulmonary coccidioidomycosis. *N Engl J Med* 1970; 283: 325–9.

186. IGER M. Coccidioidal osteomyelitis. In: Ajello L, ed. *Coccidioidomycosis. Current Clinical and Diagnostic Status.* Miami: Symposia Specialists: 177, 1977.

187. POLLOCK SF, MORRIS JM, MURRAY WR. Coccidioidal synovitis of the knee. *J Bone Joint Surg* 1967; 49A: 1397–9.

188. BOUZA, E, DRYER JS, HEWITT WL *et al.* Coccidioidal meningitis: an analysis of thirty-one cases and review of the literature. *Medicine* 1981; 60: 139–72.

189. KAUFMAN L, STANDARD P. Improved version of the exoantigen test for identification of *Coccidioides immitis* and *Histoplasma capsulatum* cultures. *J Clin Microbiol* 1978; 8: 42–5.

190. BEARD JS, BENSON PM, SKILLMAN L. Rapid diagnosis of coccidioidomycosis with a DNA probe to ribosomal RNA. *Arch Dermatol* 1993; 129: 1589–93.

191. SMITH CE, SAITO MT, SIMONS SA. Pattern of 39,500 serologic tests in coccidioiomycosis. *JAMA* 1956; 160: 546–552.

192. SMITH CE, SAITO MT. Serologic reactions in coccidioiomycosis. *J Chronic Dis* 1957; 5: 571–7.

193. SMITH CE. Serological tests in the diagnosis and prognosis of coccidioidomycosis. *Am J Hyg* 1950; 52: 1–21.

194. HUPPERT M, BAILEY JW. The use of immunodiffusion tests in coccidioidomycosis. *Am J Clin Pathol* 1965; 44: 364–8.

195. PAPPAGIANIS D, ZIMMER BL. Serology of coccidioidomycosis. *Clin Microbiol Rev* 1990; 3: 247–68.

196. KAUFMAN L, CLARK MJ. Value of the concomitant use of complement fixation and immunodiffusion tests in the diagnosis of coccidioidomycosis. *Appl Microbiol* 1974; 28: 641–3.

197. HUPPERT M. Evaluation of a latex particle agglutination test for coccidioidomycosis. *Am J Clin Pathol* 1968; 49: 96–102.

198. GALGIANI JN, DUGGER KO, ITO JJ, WIEDEN MA. Antigenemia in primary coccidioidomycosis. *Am J Trop Med Hyg* 1984; 33 645–9.

199. WEINER MH. Antigenemia detected in human coccidioidomycosis. *J Clin Microbiol* 1983; 18: 136–42.

200. STEVENS DA, LEVINE HB, DERESINSKI SC *et al.* Epidemiological and clinical skin testing studies with spherulin. In Ajello L, ed. *Coccidioidomycosis. Current Clinical and Diagnostic Status.* Miami: Symposia Specialists; 1977; 107.

201. GIFFORD J, CATANZARO A. A comparison of coccidioidin and spherulin skin testing in the diagnosis of coccidioidomycosis. *Am Rev Resp Dis* 1981; 124: 440–4.

202. LEBOWITZ MD, JOHNSON WM, KALTENBORN W. Coccidioidin skin test reactivity and cross-reactivity with histoplasmin in a Tucson population. In Ajello L, ed. *Coccidioidomycosis: Current Clinical and Diagnostic Status.* Miami: Symposia Specialists; 1977; 45–61.

203. EMMETT J. Coccidioidin sensitivity among school children in Phoenix (skin test and X-ray survey). *Am J Public Health* 1952; 42: 241–5.

204. WINN WA. The use of amphotericin B in the treatment of coccidioidal disease. *Am J Med* 1959; 26: 617–35.

205. DRUTZ DJ. Amphotericin B in the treatment of coccidioidomycosis. *Drugs* 1983; 26: 337–46.

206. SALOMON NW, OSBORNE R, COPELAND JG. Surgical manifestations and results of treatment of pulmonary coccidioidomycosis. *Ann Thorac Surg* 1980; 30: 433–8.

207. GRANT AR, STEINFOFF NG, MELICK DW. Resectional surgery in pulmonary coccidioidomycosis: a review of 263 cases. In Ajello L, ed *Coccididioidomycosis: Current Clinical and Diagnostic Status.* Miami: Symposia Specialists; 1977: 209–21.

208. GALGIANI JN, STEVENS DA, GRAYBILL JR *et al.* Ketoconazole therapy of progressive coccidioidomycosis. *Am J Med* 1988; 84: 603–10.

209. CATANZARO A, GALGIANI JN, LEVINE BE *et al.* Fluconazole in the treatment of chronic pulmonary and nonmeningeal coccidioidomycosis. *Am J Med* 1995; 98: 249–56.

210. GRAYBILL JR, STEVENS DA, GALGIANI JN *et al.* Itraconazole treatment of coccidioidomycosis. *Am J Med* 1990; 89: 282–90.

211. TUCKER RM, DENNING DW, ARATHOON EG *et al.* Itraconazole therapy of nonmeningeal coccidioidomycosis: clinical and laboratory observations. *J Am Acad Dermatol* 1990; 23: 593–601.

212. DIAZ M, PUENTE R, DE HOYES LA, CRUZ S. Itraconazole in the treatment of coccidioidomycosis. *Chest* 1991; 100: 682–4.

213. GALGIANI JN. Coccidioidomycosis. *Inf Dis Clin Pract* 1992; 1: 357–62.

214. CATANZARO A, FIERER J, FRIEDMAN PJ. Fluconazole in the treatment of persistent coccidioidomycosis. *Chest* 1990; 97: 666–9.

215. GALGIANI JN, AMPEL NM. Coccidioidomycosis in human immunodeficiency virus-infected patients. *J Infect Dis* 1990; 162: 1165–9.

216. GALGIANI JN. Coccidioidomycosis: changes in clinical expression, serological diagnosis, and therapeutic options. *Clin Infect Dis* 1992; 14 (Suppl 1): 100–5.

217. PAPPAGIANIS D AND THE VALLEY FEVER VACCINE STUDY GROUP. Evaluation of the protective efficacy of the killed *Coccidioides immits* spherule vaccine in man. *Am Rev Resp Dis* 1993; 148: 656–60.

218. BUSSE O. Über parasitäre Zelleinschlüsse und irhe Züchtung *Zentralb Bacteriol* 1894; 16: 175–80.

219. BENHAM RW. Cryptococcosis and blastomycosis. *Ann NY Acad Sci* 1950; 50: 1299–14.

220. LEVITZ SM. The ecology of *Cryptococcus neoformans* and the epidemiology of cryptococcosis. *Rev Infect Dis* 1991; 13: 1163–9.

221. POLACHECK I, KWON-CHUNG KJ. Creatinine metabolism in *Cryptococcus neoformans. J Bacteriol* 1980; 142: 15–20.

222. ELLIS DH, PFEIFFER TJ. Natural habitat of *Cryptococcus neoformans var. gattii. J Clin Microbiol* 1990; 28: 1642–4.

223. ROZENBAUM R, CONCLAVES AJR, WANKE B *et al. Cryptococcus neoformans* varieties as agents of cryptococcosis in Brazil. *Mycopathologia* 1992; 119: 133–6.

224. FINK JN, BARBORIAK JJ, KAUFMAN L. Cryptococcal antibodies in pigeon breeder's disease. *J Allergy* 1968; 41: 297–301.

225. NEWBERRY WM, WALTER JE, CHANDLER JW *et al.* Epidemiologic study of *Cryptococcus neoformans. Ann Intern Med* 1967; 67: 724–32.

226. ATKINSON AJ, BENNETT JE. Experience with a new skin test antigen prepared from *Cryptococcus neoformans. Am Rev Resp Dis* 1968; 97: 637–43.

227. GOTTESDIENER KM. Transplanted infections: donor to host transmission of the allograft. *Ann Intern Med* 1989; 110: 1001–16.

228. CURRIE BP, FREUNDLICH LF, CASADEVALL A. Restriction fragment length polymorphism analysis of *Cryptococcus neoformans* isolates from environmental (pigeon excreta) and clinical sources in New York City. *J Clin Microbiol* 1994; 32: 1188–92.

229. DIAMOND RD, ROOT RK, BENNETT JE. Factors influencing killing of *Cryptococcus neoformans* by human leukocytes *in vitro. J Infect Dis* 1972; 25: 367–76.

230. KOZEL TR, HERMERATH CA. Binding of cryptococcal polysaccharide to *Cryptococcus neoformans. Infect Immun* 1984; 43: 879–86.

231. DROUHET E, SEGRETAIN G. Inhibition de la migration leucocytaire *in vitro* par un polyoside capsulaire de *Torulopsis (Cryptococcus) neoformans. Ann Inst Pasteur* 1951; 81: 674–6.

232. MODY CH, PAINE R, JACKSON C, CHEN G-H, TOEWS GB. CD8 cells play a critical role in delayed type hypersensitivity to intact *Cryptococcus neoformans. J Immunol* 1994; 152: 3970–9.

233. LEVITZ SM, FARRELL TP, MAZIARZ RT. Killing of *Cryptococcus neoformans* by human peripheral blood mononuclear cells in culture. *J Infect Dis* 1991; 163: 1108–13.

234. MODY CH, TYLER CL, SITRIN RG *et al.* Interferon-γ activates rat alveolar macrophages for anticryptococcal activity. *Am J Resp Cell Mol Biol* 1991; 5: 19–26.

235. DIAMOND RD, BENNETT JE. Prognostic factors in cryptococcal meningitis: a study of 111 cases. *Ann Intern Med* 1974; 80: 176–81.

236. DISMUKES WE. Cryptococcal meningitis in patients with AIDS. *J Infect Dis* 1988; 157: 624–8.

237. CURRIE BP, CASADAVALL A. Estimation of the prevalence of cryptococcal infection among patients infected with the human immunodeficiency virus in New York City. *Clin Infect Dis* 1994; 19: 1029–33.

238. KAPLAN MH, ROSE PP, ARMSTRONG D. Cryptococcosis in a cancer hospital. *Cancer* 1977; 39: 2265–74.

239. MODY CH, TOEWS GB, LIPSCOMB MF. Cyclosporin A inhibits the growth of *Cryptococcus neoformans* in a murine model. *Infect Immun* 1988; 56: 7–12.

240. IGEL JH, BOLANDE RP. Humoral defense mechanisms in cryptococcosis: substances in normal human serum, saliva and cerebrospinal fluid affecting the growth of *Cryptococcus neoformans. J Infect Dis* 1966; 116: 75–83.

241. DIAMOND RD, MAY JE, KANE MA *et al.* The role of the classical and alternate complement pathways in host defenses against *Cryptococcus neoformans* infection. *J Immunol* 1974; 112: 2260–70.

242. HERNANDEZ AD. Cutaneous cryptococcosis. *Dermatol Clin* 1989; 7: 269–74.

243. BEHRMAN RE, MASCI JR, NICHOLAS P. Cryptococcal skeletal infections: case report and review. *Rev Infect Dis* 1990; 12: 181–90.

244. LARSON RA, BOZZETTE S, MCCUTCHAN JA *et al.* Persistent *Cryptococcus neoformans* infection of the prostate after successful treatment of meningitis. *Ann Intern Med* 1989; 111: 125–8.

245. CONCES DJ, VIX VV, TARVER RD. Pleural cryptococcosis. *J Thorac Imaging* 1990; 5: 84–6.

246. ZUGER A, LOUIS E, HOLZMAN RS, SIMBERKOFF MS, RAHAL SS. Cryptococcal disease in patients with AIDS: diagnostic features and outcome of treatment. *Ann Intern Med* 1986; 104: 234–40.

247. CHECHANI V, KAMHOLZ SL. Pulmonary manifestations of disseminated cryptococcosis in AIDS. *Chest* 1990; 98: 1060–6.

248. DENNING DW, STEVENS DA, HAMILTON JR. Comparison of *Guizotia abyssinica* seed extract (birdseed agar) with conventional media for selective identification of *Cryptococcus neoformans* in patients with the acquired immunodeficiency syndrome. *J Clin Microbiol* 1990; 28: 2565–7.

249. TAELMAN H, BOGAERTS J, BATUNGWANAYO J, VAN DE PERRE P, LUCAS S, ALLEN S. Failure of the cryptococcal serum antigen test to detect primary pulmonary cryptococcosis in patients infected with human immunodeficiency virus [letter]. *Clin Infect Dis* 1994; 18: 119–20.

250. POWDERLY WG, CLOUD GA, DISMUKES WE, SAAG MS. Measurement of cryptococcal antigen in serum and cerebrospinal fluid: value in the management of AIDS-associated cryptococcal meningitis. *Clin Infect Dis* 1994; 18: 789–92.

251. BENNETT JE, BAILEY JW. Control for rheumatoid factor in the latex test for cryptococcosis. *Am J Clin Pathol* 1971; 56: 360–5.

252. HAMILTON JR, NOBLE A, DENNING DW, STEVENS DA. Performance of Cryptococcus antigen latex agglutination kits on serum and cerebrospinal fluid specimens of AIDS patients before and after pronase treatment. *J CLin Microbiol* 1991; 29: 333–9.

253. BENNETT JE, DISMUKES WE, DUMA RJ *et al.* A comparison of amphotericin B alone and combined with flucytosine in the treatment of cryptococcal meningitis. *N Engl J Med* 1979; 301: 126–31.

254. SAAG MS, POWDERLY WG, CLOUD GA *et al.* Comparison of amphotericin B with fluconazole in the treatment of acute AIDS-

associated cryptococcal meningitis. *N Engl J Med* 1992; 326: 83–9.

255. POWDERLY WG, SAAG MS, CLOUD GA *et al.* A controlled trial of fluconazole or amphotericin B to prevent relapse of cryptococcal meningitis in patients with the acquired immunodeficiency syndrome. *N Engl J Med* 1992; 326: 793–8.

256. FRANCIS P, WALSH TJ. Evolving role of flucytosine in immunocompromised patients: new insights into safety, pharmacokinetics, and antifungal therapy. *Clin Infect Dis* 1992; 15: 1003–8.

257. MUKHERJEE J, SCHARF MD, CASADEVALL A. Protective murine monoclonal antibodies to *Cryptococcus neoformans*. *Infect Immun* 1993; 60: 4534–41.

258. MUKHERJEE S, LEE S, MUKHERJEE J, SCHART MD, CASADAVALL A. Monoclonal antibodies to *Cryptococcus neoformans* capsular polysaccharide modify the course of intravenous infection in mice. *Infect Immun* 1994; 62: 1079–88.

259. NIGHTINGALE SD, CAL SX, PETERSON DM *et al.* Primary prophylaxis with fluconazole against systemic fungal infections in HIV-positive patients. *AIDS* 1992; 6: 191–4.

260. POWDERLY WG, FINKELSTEIN DM, FEINBERG J *et al.* A randomized trial comparing fluconazole with clotrimazole troches for the prevention of fungal infections in patients with advanced human immunodeficiency virus infection. *N Engl J Med* 1995; 332: 700–5.

261. PLUSS JL, OPAL SM. Pulmonary sporotrichosis: review of treatment and outcome. *Medicine* 1986; 65: 143–53.

262. SHARKEY-MATHIS PK, KAUFFMAN CA, GRAYBILL JR *et al.* Treatment of sporotrichosis with itraconazole. *Am J Med* 1993; 95: 279–85.

263. BREELING J, WEINSTEIN L. Pulmonary sporotrichosis treated with itraconazole. *Chest* 1993; 103: 313–14.

264. CALHOUN DL, WASHKIN H, WHITE MP *et al.* Treatment of systemic sporotrichosis with ketoconazole. *Rev Infect Dis* 1991; 13: 47–51.

265. DALL L, SALZMAN G. Treatment of pulmonary sporotrichosis with ketoconazole. *Rev Infect Dis* 1987; 9: 795–8.

266. KAUFFMAN C, PAPPAS P, MCKINSEY D *et al.* Treatment of lymphocutaneous and visceral sporotrichosis with fluconazole. *Clin Infect Dis* 1996; 22: 46–50.

267. BRUMMER E, CASTAÑEDA E, RESTREPO A. Paracoccidioidomycosis: an update. *Clin Microbiol Rev* 1993; 6: 89–117.

268. RESTREPO MA. Paracoccidioidomycosis (Southern American blastomycosis): a study of 39 cases observed in Medellin, Colombia. *Am J Trop Med Hyg* 1970; 19: 68–76.

269. MARTINEZ R, MOYA MJ. Associacao entre paracoccidioidomycosis e alcoholism. *Rev Saude Publ Sao Paulo* 1992; 26: 12–16.

270. LONDERO AT, RAMOS CD, LOPES JOS. Progressive pulmonary paracoccidioidomycosis: a study of 34 cases observed in Rio Grande do Sul (Brazil). *Mycopathologia* 1978; 63: 53–6.

271. LONDERO AT, RAMOS CD. Paracoccidioidomycosis: a clinical and mycologic study in forty-one cases observed in Santa Maria, RS, Brazil. *Am J Med* 1972; 52: 771–5.

272. RESTREPO A, GREER DL, VASCONCELLOS M. Paracoccidioidomycosis: a review. *Rev Med Vet Mycol* 1973; 8: 97–123.

273. DEL NEGRO GMB, GARCIA NM, RODRIGUES EG *et al.* The sensitivity, specificity and efficiency values of some serological tests used in the diagnosis of paracoccidioidomycosis. *Rev Inst Med Trop Sao Paulo* 1991; 33: 277–80.

274. FERREIRA-DA CRUZ MF, FRANCESCONE-DO VALLE AC, ESPINERA MCD *et al.* Study of antibodies in paracoccidioidomycosis: follow-up of patients during and after treatment. *J Med Vet Mycol* 1990; 28: 151–7.

275. MARQUES SA *et al.* Paracoccidioidomycosis: a comparative study of the evolutionary serologic, clinical and radiologic results for patients treated with ketoconazole or amphotericin B plus sulfonamides. *Mycopathologia* 1985; 89: 19–23.

276. NEGRONI R. Ketoconazole in the treatment of paracoccidioidomycosis and histoplasmosis. *Rev Infect Dis* 1980; 2: 643–9.

277. RESPREPT, A. Paracoccidioidomycosis (South American Blastomycosis). In Jacobs PH, Hall L, eds. *Antifungal Drug Therapy: A Complete Guide for the Practitioner.* New York: Marcel Dekker; 1990: 181–205.

278. NARANJO MS, TRUJILLO M, MUNERA MI *et al.* Treatment of paracoccidioidomycosis with itraconazole. *J Med Vet Mycol* 1990; 28: 67–76.

279. MENDES R, NEGRONI R, ARECHAVALA A. Treatment and control of cure. In Franco M, Lacaz CS, Restrepo A, eds. *Paracoccidioidomycosis*. Boca Raton, FL: CRC Press; 1994: 373–92.

280. DIAZ M, NEGRONI R, MONTERO-GEI F *et al.* A Pan American five-year study of fluconazole therapy for deep mycoses in the immunocompetent host. *Clin Infec Dis* 1992; 14 (Suppl 1): S68–76.

281. STEVENS DA, VO PT. Synergistic interaction of trimethoprim and sulfamethoxazole on *Paracoccidioides brasiliensis*. *Antimicrob Agents Chemother* 1982; 21: 852–4.

19 Hospital-acquired pneumonia

GARY MILLER and MICHAEL E. ELLIS
King Faisal Specialist Hospital and Research Centre, Riyadh, Saudi Arabia

Introduction

Pneumonia occurring after admission to hospital is a major contribution to all hospital acquired infections. In a UK Public Health Laboratory Service study of 43 hospitals involving 18 186 patients in 1980, lower respiratory tract infection accounted for 16.8% of all hospital infections (the third most frequent after urinary tract infection at 30.3% and wound infections at 18.9%)[1]. In the USA, hospital-acquired pneumonia (HAP) ranks second only to urinary tract infection and accounts for 6 in 1000 hospitalised patients according to the National Nosocomial Infections Study[2]. In addition to substantial patient morbidity and mortality, there are considerable financial burdens on health care. The increasing incidence of HAP is complicated by the emergence of resistant pathogens. This disease poses dynamic challenges for management and prevention.

In this chapter, we review the aetiological highlights, pathogenesis, diagnosis, antimicrobial management and aspects of prevention. Special emphasis is given to the patient who is critically ill since complex pathological events interact to profoundly alter the normal haemodynamic ventilatory and host immune responses. The patient's baseline health status, severity of underlying illness, coupled with invasive intravascular monitoring, mechanical ventilation and possible cytotoxic effects of drug therapy contribute to the increased frequency of nosocomial infection. Hence we will include the particular problems encountered by the patient in this exceptional environment including limitations and discussion of diagnostic techniques and differential diagnosis. Aspects of ventilatory management and problems posed by extra-pulmonary multi-organ system failure are covered in Chapter 27.

Epidemiological highlights

Differences in definitions of pneumonia preclude a precise description of the global presence of HAP. Until recently, most investigators adopted or modified the criteria of Johanson *et al.*[3] to define pneumonia; namely, purulent tracheobronchial secretions, fever, leukocytosis and new or progressive pulmonary infiltrates. Other investigators[4] added to these criteria a sputum Gram's stain associated with greater than 25 leukocytes and less than 10 squamous cells per low-power field with recovery of a specific pathogen on Gram's stain or culture. In a UK survey, HAP was defined as an active infection not present on admission, requiring the presence of sputum *de novo* or increase in the amount of purulent sputum, with chest signs and/or X-ray changes not attributable to embolus, heart failure or aspiration, which were not present during any recent previous admission[1]. This, however, includes patients not only with pneumonia but other lower respiratory tract infections. Furthermore, critically ill ventilated and other patients may have additional problems which obscure or mimic the clinical picture of pneumonia such as tracheobronchitis, non-pneumonic infiltrates on chest radiography and fever from causes such as pulmonary embolism, atelectasis or drug reactions (Table 19.1). CDC definitions for nosocomial pneumonia in patients > 12 months of age include an infection which develops ≥ 72 hours after admission, characterised by either (i) chest signs and either new purulent or change in the character of sputum, or a positive blood culture, or isolation of pathogens from transtracheal aspiration, or bronchial biopsy, or brush biopsy or (ii) new chest radiographical signs and either new purulent or change in the character of sputum, or a positive blood culture, or isolation of the pathogen from transtracheal aspiration, brush biopsy or bronchial biopsy, or isolation of virus, or detection of viral antigens in respiratory secretions, or a diagnostic IgM titre, or biopsy evidence[5].

Table 19.1. *Non-infectious pulmonary infiltrates*

Atelectasis	Vasculitis
Aspiration	Pulmonary embolism
ARDS	Cardiogenic pulmonary oedema
Pulmonary haemorrhage	Pleural effusion
Drug-induced pneumonitis	Neoplasm
Lung contusion	Transfusion reaction

Studies using histopathology as a reference standard have demonstrated that the clinical diagnosis of lung infections in patients receiving mechanical ventilation is inaccurate. In a study by Andrews *et al.*[6] clinical diagnoses were in error in approximately 30% of patients. Similarly, Bell *et al.*[7] demonstrated that 38% of the cases of pneumonia were misdiagnosed. Several recent prospective studies by Fagon and associates[8,9] have failed to identify clinical features that permit accurate diagnosis of nosocomial pneumonia in ventilated patients which often results in inappropriate or suboptimal antibiotic therapy for these patients.

At a recent International Consensus Conference on Ventilator-Associated Pneumonia, the participants recommended adoption of standardised terminology for the following categories: definite pneumonia, probable pneumonia, definite absence of pneumonia, probable absence of pneumonia[10]. These are summarised in Table 19.2.

Despite the previous wide-ranging definitions with their limitations, it is possible to make some general inferences on the frequency and occurrence of HAP. HAP occurs in between 0.5 to 5.0 per thousand

Table 19.2. *Definitions of (ventilator associated) pneumonia*

Definite pneumonia. New (progressive) or persistent infiltrate and purulent tracheal secretions and one of the following:

1. Radiographical (preferably CT) evidence of pulmonary abscess and positive needle aspirate culture.
2. Histological evidence of pneumonia, open lung biopsy or post-mortem examination immediately after death demonstrating abscess formation or an area of consolidation with intense PMN leukocyte accumulation plus a positive quantitative culture of lung parenchyma ($>10^4$ microorganisms per gram of lung tissue).

Probable pneumonia. New (progressive) or persistent infiltrate and purulent tracheal secretions plus one of the following:

1. Positive quantitative culture of a sample of secretions from the lower respiratory tract obtained by a technique minimising contamination with upper respiratory tract flora (protected specimen brush, bronchoalveolar lavage).
2. Positive blood culture unrelated to another source and obtained within 48 hours of respiratory sampling which is identical to the organism cultured from lower respiratory tract secretions.
3. Positive pleural fluid culture in the absence of previous pleural instrumentation which is identical to the organism cultured from lower respiratory tract secretions.
4. Histologic evidence of pneumonia from open-lung biopsy or post-mortem examination immediately after death demonstrating abscess formation or an area of consolidation with intense PMN leukocyte accumulation plus a negative quantitative culture ($<10^4$ microorganism per gram of lung tissue)

Definite absence of pneumonia. In patients not meeting the criteria for definite pneumonia, the absence of pneumonia is definitive if one of the following criteria is met.

1. Post-mortem exam within 3 days of clinical suspicion of pneumonia demonstrating no histologic of lung infection.
2. Definite alternative aetiology with no bacterial growth on a reliable respiratory specimen.
3. Cytologic identification of a process other than pneumonia without significant bacterial growth on the reliable respiratory specimen.

Probable absence of pneumonia. Probable absence of pneumonia is indicated by the lack of significant growth on the reliable respiratory specimen with one of the following:

1. Resolution without antibiotic therapy of one of the following: fever, radiographical infiltrate, or radiographical infiltrate and a definitive alternative diagnosis.
2. Persistent fever and radiographical infiltrate with a definite alternative diagnosis.

Adapted from Cook D, Brun-Buisson C, Guyatt GH, Sibbald WJ. Evaluation of new diagnostic technologies: bronchoalveolar lavage and the diagnosis of ventilator-associated pneumonia. *Crit Care Med* 1994; 22:1314–22[10a].

patients admitted to hospital[1,2,11,12]. Its prominence has increased and it is now the second most common nosocomial infection in the USA and the third most common in the UK[1,2]. The European Prevalence of Infection in Intensive Care (EPIC) Study examined the prevalence of infection in 1417 intensive care units in Western Europe on a single day in 1992 and of the 10 000 patients surveyed, 45% had at least one infection[13]. The most common ICU infections were pneumonia followed by urinary tract and bloodstream infections. The annual infection rate is twofold greater in patients admitted to large teaching hospitals compared to non-teaching hospitals[14]. Within any one centre, the incidence varies depending on particular identifiable factors. For example, post-operatively, almost 20% of patients develop pneumonia[15]. Approximately one in ten patients admitted to a respiratory/surgical ICU had HAP as the primary diagnosis for admission[16]. Of 178 patients with severe pneumonia requiring ICU support, 31 had HAP[17].

It appears that, as the complexity of the patient's medical and surgical problems and their intensivity of care increase (including exposure to invasive devices), particularly in intubated and mechanically ventilated patients on critical care units, or those with severe trauma[18–21] the risk for acquisition of pneumonia also rises substantially. ICU units themselves pose a considerable risk for acquiring pneumonia – approximately 10% in one study[16]. In the NNIS study, 1986–1990, the median number of ventilator-associated pneumonias was 13/1000 ventilator days for coronary and medical ICUs and 18/1000 ventilator–days for medical and surgical ICUs[22]. Ventilator-associated pneumonia remains a frequent and serious complication in critically ill mechanically ventilated patients, and is associated with increased mortality, deterioration in pulmonary haemodynamics and function, increased cost and length of ICU stay, and development of multi-system organ failure. To differentiate early pneumonia (present at or developing soon after intubation), from late pneumonia (not present or incubating at time of intubation) a time span of 48 hours should have elapsed. Increased duration of stay, which may also reflect the complex environment of critically ill patients, is another factor.

Mortality associated with HAP is substantial although multiple risk factors such as multi-organ failure, sepsis syndrome and underlying disease interplay to make attribution of mortality directly due to HAP *per se*, a complex issue to delineate. Certain organisms particularly *Pseudomonas* spp., carry a higher mortality rate over and above that of the underlying disease[8,23]. Pneumonia in patients on medical ICUs or community ICUs carry relatively lower death rates at around 5–10%[3,24,25] whilst in respiratory/surgical ICU's the rate is between 35% and 60%[21,26,27]. Crude mortality associated with ventilated associated pneumonia varies between 50% and 70% depending on whether ARDS is present[7,9,28,29]. More sophisticated statistical methods are needed to assess the impact of pneumonia *per se* as well as survival in these patients. In some such studies, pneumonia has been established as an independent significant factor contributing to mortality[8,30]. This underscores the need for earlier recognition, treatment and if possible, prevention. This is of particular importance since two studies have demonstrated that in those patients without a terminal illness, appropriate antibiotic treatment significantly affects survival[19,28]. Others, however, although demonstrating a gross mortality rate in ventilated patients who had pneumonia being twofold that of ventilated patients without pneumonia, when stepwise logistical regression analysis was employed, pneumonia *per se* was not found to give an additional mortality hazard[26].

Direct economic implications of acquiring pneumonia in hospital are staggering in terms of costs for increased duration of hospitalization, antimicrobial treatment and loss of life[31]. It is estimated that nosocomial pneumonia prolongs hospital stay up to 10 days resulting in at least US$3000 – $8000 in extra charges per infection equivalent to an annual cost of US$4 532 million[32,33].

Microbial aetiology

Knowledge of the most likely organisms responsible for HAP is important for initial empirical antimicrobial selection. Diagnostic methodology varies considerably from study to study ranging from simple sputum examination through bronchoalveolar lavage (BAL) to tissue biopsy. These methods vary in diagnostic sensitivity and specificity and this may limit the validity of comparing published data. *Streptococcus pneumoniae*, *Haemophilus influenzae* or *Mycoplasma* account for roughly more than 50% of identifiable agents associated with community-acquired pneumonia whereas *Pseudomonas* spp., *Klebsiella* spp. and other Gram-negatives are responsible for more than 75% of cases of HAP[2,6,9,34,35]. *Pseudomonas aeruginosa* is the single most common agent responsible for nosocomial pneumonia (Figs 19.1 and 19.2), followed by *Staphylococcus aureus*, *Klebsiella* spp. and *Enterobacter* spp.[2,36] (Table 19.3). A polymicrobial aetiology is found in approximately 40% of infections[9,35]. However, variations from this overall pattern are found. For example, in a non-tertiary care setting such as community hospitals, the frequency of organisms may closely resemble those found in community-acquired pneumonia, namely, *S. pneumoniae* or *H. influenzae* being the main players[24], with only 15% being due to Gram-negative bacilli. In the elderly patient often with a background of lung disease, *S. pneumoniae*, *H. influenzae* or *Moraxella* spp. may predominate[24]. Even in such hospitals, Gram-negative bacilli assume relatively more important roles within those wards with a higher acumen of medical or surgical care, i.e. Gram-negative bacilli accounted for a quarter of cases of pneumonia on acute medical and surgical wards compared with only 10% on the intermediate medical or nursing home wards[24]. A certain seasonal variance has been described for Gram-negative bacilli associated with HAP, for example, *Klebsiella* spp. and *Pseudomonas* spp. assume an increase during summer months[14].

Major changes in the distribution and antimicrobial susceptibility of pathogens responsible for nosocomial pneumonia have been observed recently[14,34]. Through the 1980s there has been a substantial increase in HAP due to *P. aeruginosa* (from 12% to 17%), *S. aureus* (from 13% to 17%), *Enterobacter* spp. (from 9% to 11%), *Candida albicans* (from 3% to 5%), coagulase negative *Staphylococcus* (from 1% to 2%), and accompanied by a decrease in cases due to *Escherischia coli* (from 9% to 6%), *Klebsiella* spp. (from 11% to 8%) and *Proteus* spp. (from 7% to 3%). Cases due to *Enterococci* have not changed in incidence (2%). It is speculative whether these have arisen as a direct result of a change in antimicrobial and infection control policies (for example, antibiotic prophylaxis for surgical procedures) or the increasing sophistication of supportive care (for example, the increased use of invasive devices). An accompanying phenomenon has been the emergence of pathogens showing a decreased susceptibility to antimicrobial agents particularly *Pseudomonas* spp. and *Enterococcus* spp.. This aspect of increased antimicrobial resistance in Gram-negative bacteria has been covered in Chapter 8.

Table 19.3. *Most frequently isolated pathogens from lower respiratory infections in the United States, 1984*

Pathogen	Frequency (%)
Pseudomonas aeruginosa	16.9
Staphylococcus aureus	12.9
Klebsiella species	11.6
Enterobacter species	9.4
Escherichia coli	6.4
Serratia species	5.8
Proteas species	4.2
Candida species	4.0
Enterococci	1.5
Coagulase-negative staphylococci	1.5

[a]Data from Horan TC, White JW, Jarvis WR *et al.*: *MMWR* 1986; 35:SS17–29[2].

The exact role and contribution of anaerobic bacteria in the setting of HAP is surprisingly unclear. In large national studies both from the UK[1] and from the USA[14], anaerobes were either noted as not identified or infrequently (about 2%) found. Yet other reports implicate anaerobes as contributory pathogens in up to one-third of patients with HAP[37,38] whereas as a sole pathogen, they are found in only 7%. The reason for their absence in larger surveillance reports may be due to the fastidious techniques required for their identification (See Chapter 1). *Peptococcus, Peptostreptococcus, Fusobacterium* and *Bacteroides* spp. are the most common. Antibiotic regimes chosen for the management of HAP may provide scant anaerobic cover – a matter of some concern which should direct attention towards clarifying this issue.

Organisms other than Gram-negative bacteria and *S. aureus* are implicated in specific risk groups such as the chronically ill, debilitated or the severely immunocompromised host. Enterococcal pneumonia has been observed especially in patients receiving broad spectrum cephalosporins and enteral feeding[7], and more recently in patients given topical antimicrobials for selective decontamination of the digestive tract[39]. Outbreaks of *Acinetobacter* spp. associated nosocomial pneumonia have been increasing and are associated with a poor prognosis[8]. Less frequently isolated bacterial pathogens include *Citrobacter* and *Aeromonas* spp., *Xanthomonas maltophilia, Moraxella catarrhalis* and *Flavobacterium* spp..

Bone marrow transplant patients, those undergoing intensive induction or consolidation therapy for leukaemia, and experiencing severe and prolonged neutropenia are vulnerable to pulmonary opportunistic fungal infections. Renal transplant, liver transplant and burn patients are also at risk for *Aspergillus, Fusarium, Candida albicans* and *Candida* non-*albicans* spp. (see Chapters 16 and 21). In some centres, *Aspergillus* is the major cause of nosocomial pneumonia and carries a crude mortality of the order of at least 75% and an attributable mortality of about 62%[40]. Nosocomial outbreaks of aspergillosis including both colonisation and invasion have also been documented in non-immunocompromised hosts[41].

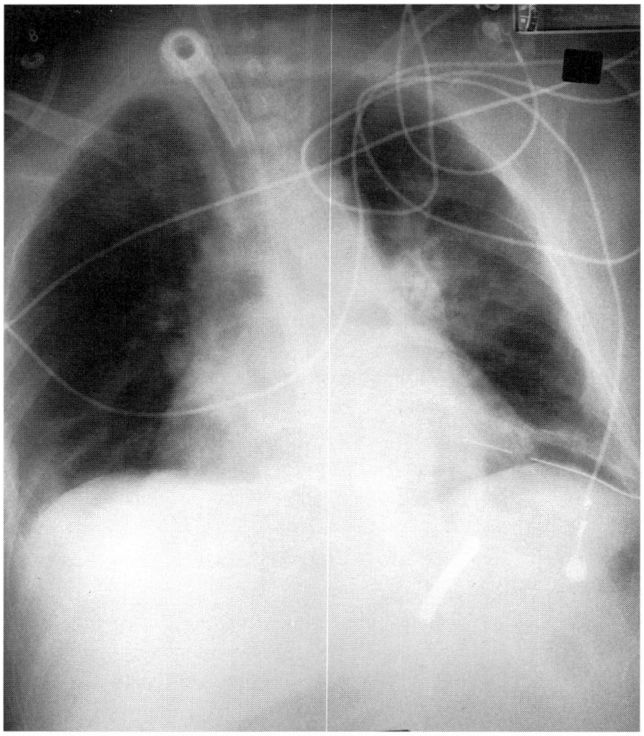

FIGURE 19.1 *Pseudomonas aeruginosa* nosocomial pneumonia involving the left lung in a 42-year-old patient following multiple trauma and chest contusion.

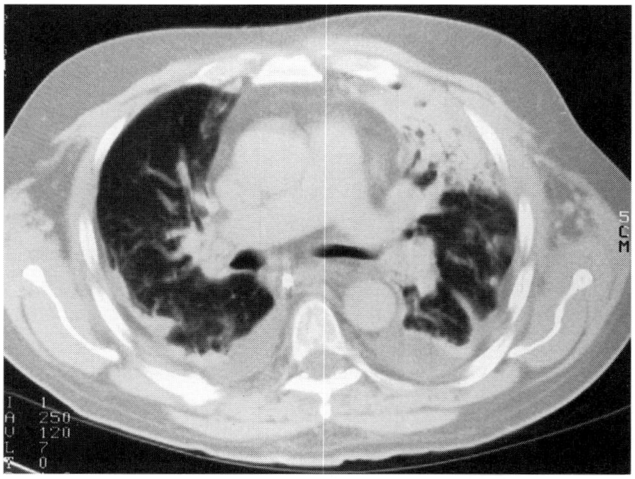

FIGURE 19.2 CT-scan of a patient with multiple trauma showing extensive pneumonia changes. PSB cultures grew >10^3 cfu/ml of *Pseudomonas aeruginosa*.

Respiratory syncytial virus (*RSV*) is another pathogen which has on occasions produced nosocomial pneumonia, particularly in children, but is less commonly recognised in adults. RSV nosocomial pneumonia especially in the setting of outbreaks is described in the elderly, those with immunocompromised states or in intensive care units[42–45]. The respiratory secretions of both healthy personnel and of index patients admitted are sources for spread[44]. The mortality rate may be particularly high (78%) in patients who are severely immunocompromised such as bone marrow transplant patients[45]. The possibility of such a viral infection should be borne in mind during recognised community outbreaks since specific antiviral therapy with ribavirin is available and effective particularly if administered early[45] (Chapter 9).

Herpes simplex and *Cytomegalovirus (CMV)* pneumonia characterises other immunocompromised patients particularly those with bone marrow and solid organ transplants, and CMV is often associated with graft rejection (Chapter 10). *Nocardia, Pneumocystis carinii, Mycobacterium tuberculosis*, non-tuberculous mycobacteria and *Toxoplasma gondii* occasionally occur in the setting of polymicrobial aetiology, and are other important opportunists that should be considered in such patients (Chapters 11, 12, 15, 21, 22 and 30).

Nosocomial-acquired legionellosis should always be included in the differential diagnosis of HAP though the frequency of occurrence is highly variable – between 0% and 30%[46,47]. Patients at greatest risk are post-operative, transplant and other immunocompromised patients, who become infected by aerosols generated from tap water and showerheads, humidifiers and respiratory equipment. Details of the epidemiology, clinical presentation, management and prevention are discussed in Chapter 14.

Finally, patients with HIV are highly susceptible not only to Gram-negative and Gram-positive bacterial pneumonia but to *Pneumocystis* and mycobacterial infections as well as other more commonly recognised pathogens. Spread of tuberculosis with rapid clinical progression among HIV-infected persons in a communal setting is a recently described phenomenon[48]. Of particular concern is the spread to health care workers of multi-drug resistant tuberculosis[49] and highlights the need for protection of patients and staff by appropriate respiratory precautions. BCG vaccination is recommended for protection of staff in many parts of the world, such as New Zealand and the United Kingdom. Reconsideration of its reintroduction in the US by some authorities in the wake of the increased risk for tuberculosis is of some interest[50]. Despite advances in diagnostic techniques and microbiological methods, the agents responsible for nosocomial pneumonia remain unknown in about 38% of cases.

Details of the particular pulmonary problems in the immunocompromised host are covered in Chapter 21.

Colonisation of airways and relation to HAP

Bacterial colonisation of the upper respiratory tract is a normal and well-recognised phenomenon. In the late 1960's, Johansen showed that, during illness and hospitalisation, individuals experience a continuing and increasing dramatic change in their normal bacterial oral flora from a largely anaerobic Gram-positive profile (in 90% of healthy people, with only 10% having transient and low numbers of Gram-negative organisms) to aerobic Gram-negative bacteria. This occurs in 40% of patients within 4 days of admission to the intensive care unit (ICU), and in 75% within 21 days of stay in the ICU. The degree of change parallels the severity or chronicity of the underlying illness. Colonisation switch to Gram-negative aerobes is found in up to 73% of the very ill[3,51].

Table 19.4. *Major risk factors associated with the development of airways colonisation and HAP*

Tracheal intubation	Thoracoabdominal surgery
Advanced age	Reintubation
Pre-existing lung disease	Gastric aspiration
H_2 receptor blockers	Frequent manipulation of ventilator circuits
Duration of mechanical ventilation	

Risk factors

Increased Gram-negative bacterial colonisation of the oral pharynx is enhanced with intubation, the elderly, antibiotic use, corticosteroid use, surgery, prolonged hospitalisation, severity of illness, major surgery, pulmonary disease, smoking, malnourishment, and renal disease[52] (Table 19.4). Others include prior respiratory viral illness, malnourishment, malignancy, antibiotics, cardiac disease, neurological disorders, chronic lung disease such as chronic bronchitis, cystic fibrosis, bronchiectasis, and acute lung injury.

The use of H_2 receptor antagonist/antacids is associated with increased oropharyngeal colonisation but less so if sucralfate is used to protect the stomach[27]. Systemic antibiotics may remove 'colonising protective' bacteria, leaving a microbial niche to be filled by more pathogenic (including Gram-negative) bacteria.

A nasogastric feeding tube is one factor which could facilitate oropharyngeal colonisation (OPC) through increased risk of regurgitation and through bypassing the mechanical defence barrier of the nose and the oesophageal sphincter. Furthermore, foodstuffs themselves may be a source of bacterial contamination. Posture of the patient is also important since an erect position will be less likely than a supine one to induce aspiration.

More distally the tracheobronchial tree is usually totally sterile in non-smoker. Smokers tend to be colonised, but not always, with enteric Gram-negative bacteria – streptococci are frequently found.

The introduction of an endotracheal tube readily and rapidly induces enteric Gram-negative bacterial colonisation particularly with *Pseudomonas* spp.[53]. The same holds true for patients with tracheostomies[54]. Polymicrobial colonisation is usual. The upper airways (with the mucus ciliary escalator, intact surface epithelial cells and secretions, cough reflex, maintenance of normal air temperature and humidity, swallowing mechanisms, etc.) present an effective first line of defence to bacterial pathogens. Construction of an artificial airway by the placement of a naso/orotracheal tube circumvents these barriers. An excess of pathogenic bacteria from the oropharynx, respiratory ventilatory equipment, pooled secretions around the cuff, and from the hands of personnel can then directly enter the lower airways. In addition, the foreign body nature of the tube induces excessive mucus secretion which promotes Gram-negative bacterial binding. Local trauma induced particularly by the cuff leads to increased bacterial colonisation[55]. A tracheostomy will have similar adverse effects on the normal protective mechanisms against pathogenic bacteria. The risk for HAP in one study appeared to increase with the increasing complexity involved in providing an airway and maintenance of respiration, i.e. endotracheal intubation (1.3%), tracheostomy (25%), tracheostomy and mechanical ventilation (66%), compared to 0.3% for patients hospitalised with none of these procedures[56]. Intubation and ventilation in multivariate analysis were associated with a sevenfold increase in pneumonia[19]. Approximately one in five who required at least 48 hours of continual mechanical ventilation developed pneumonia[26]. The longer the duration of intubation and ventilation among severely injured patients, the greater the probability of HAP – rising from 0.05% to 0.15% on day 1 to over 90% by day 7[20]. This effect has also been noted in other series, the risk increasing from 1% to 6% of day 1 to approximately 70% at 30 days or more[9,57]. A recent study from Denmark also indicated that the risk of nosocomial pneumonia significantly increased with increased intubation time[21]. Another analysis by Joshi *et al.*[58] has, to some extent, modified the conclusion that endotracheal intubation carries the highest risk for HAP. They showed that intubation was a risk factor during day 4 to 10 of ICU stay only – it was not present during the first 3 or after day 9. These discrepancies are not easy to explain but reflect the complexities of interacting factors in such patients.

A provocative finding from the Joshi study was that bronchoscopy performed for respiratory toilet in ICU ventilated patients was identified as a risk factor for pneumonia[58]. Although evidence for a clear causal relationship was not forthcoming from that study (the patients who had the procedure might have been at high risk for HAP anyway) the authors stated that it might be an avoidable risk procedure.

Malnutrition is an important factor in promoting airways colonisation through increased bacterial adherence to upper respiratory cells and by direct adverse effects on both humoral and cell mediate immune mechanisms. Thus, local IgA production is diminished, chemotaxis is blunted and reduced numbers of alveolar macrophages are found.

The elderly (over 65 years of age) is an important group in the context of HAP since they represent an increasing proportion of the hospital population in general. Thus, the incidence of nosocomial pneumonia is twice as common compared to younger (25–50 years) patients and the elderly tend to have higher rates of malnutrition, neuromuscular disease and prior aspiration[31]. Low albumin, neuromuscular disease and tracheal intubation are strong independent predictors for nosocomial pneumonia in this group.

Protection of the lower airways to some extent is dependent upon intact normally mechanical functioning pharyngeal, oesophageal and tracheobronchial passages. Diseases which adversely affect these mechanisms predispose the patient to aspiration of oropharyngeal or oro-oesophageal gastric contents and therefore pneumonia. Thus, an acute cerebral vascular incident, Parkinson's disease, cerebral dementia, intracranial trauma, motor neurone disease, depressed consciousness, Guillain–Barré syndrome, muscular dystrophy, myasthenia gravis, tracheoesophageal fistula, hiatus hernia, epilepsy, multiple sclerosis and achalasia of the oesophagus are examples. Many of these are more commonly present in the elderly population compared to younger patients[31]. In long-term care facilities the nosocomial pneumonia rate varies between 0.6 and 4.7 per 1000 patient days and two-thirds of all patients in one study had a history of chronic aspiration and neurogenic oropharyngeal dysphagia[59].

Some of the biological mechanisms for colonisation in the ill, hospitalised patient includes increased bacterial adherence mechanisms, removal of surface fibronectin by elaboration of neutrophil elastase in the salivary secretions[60], which therefore destroys this glycoprotein's blocking of epithelial Gram-negative receptors and removal of respiratory IgA. In fact, bacterial adherence may be the major pathogenic mechanism unifying the many risk factors for airway colonisation. Thus, surgery, malnutrition, endotracheal intubation and smoking stimulate oropharyngeal epithelial cells to express more binding sites for Gram-negative bacteria[61]. Some species of *Pseudomonas* attach directly to oropharyngeal epithelial cells via their pili [62].

Studies, in general, indicate a close association between airway colonisation and pneumonia. For example, pneumonia is seven times more likely to occur in prior colonised compared to non-colonised patients[3]. This is perhaps not surprising as the organisms found colonising the oropharynx and tracheobronchial tree are similar and the risk factors for HAP are similar to those for colonisation. Progression of bacteria from proximal to more distal airways occurs. For example, oropharyngeal colonisation (OPC) may lead to tracheal colonisation[53] and tracheobronchitis leads to recurrent pneumonia[63]. This progression of airways colonisation is particularly true for the enterobacteriaceae. However, in the case of *Pseudomonas* spp., colonisation of the trachea via adherence to tracheal epithelial cells appears to occur independently of, and prior to, OPC[64]. Presence or absence of a capsule, surface appendages and exoproducts may also play a role. Most studies indicate that patients with HAP had been previously colonised by Gram-negative bacteria[3,65]. It has therefore been postulated that aspiration of oropharyngeal microbes directly leads to HAP[66], a process facilitated by the impaired host defence status in seriously ill patients. However, despite such a close association of colonisation with pneumonia, it is not always clear how colonisation of the upper or lower airways relates exactly to the development of pneumonia. For example, the idea that the oropharynx is an intermediate station on the gastropulmonary route was not supported in a recent study which showed that no Gram-negative oropharyngeal isolate was identical to that found in the lower respiratory tract[66]. Other studies indicate that the trachea can be colonised by *P. aeruginosa* without prior oropharyngeal colonisation[64]. These findings have led some to suggest that colonisation in some cases may be a surrogate marker of the very ill patient. Nevertheless, not only does the presence of airways bacteria correlate with the development of pneumonia but the *specific* bacteria identified from distal airways by more sensitive and specific techniques, namely, BAL and PSB correspond well with the histological diagnosis of pneumonia caused by the same bacteria – providing strong evidence for a causal relationship (see pp. 342–344 this chapter).

Sources of airways colonisation

Hospital personnel

Health care workers may be colonised with Gram-negative bacteria and *S. aureus*. The use of gloves and gowns has been shown to significantly reduce nosocomial infections and pneumonia in the paediatric ICU[67]. In addition, hospitals with effective infection control and surveillance programmes have significantly lower rates of pneumonia compared to those without such programmes. Hence, identification of high risk patients, staff education and appropriate infection control policies are essential to reduce and hopefully prevent nosocomial infections.

Respiratory therapy equipment

Respiratory therapy equipment *per se* has long been recognised as an important exogenous source of nosocomial pulmonary pathogens for the patient on whom the equipment is used. In addition, patients in the same vicinity are at risk (through atmospheric contamination and inhalation within the range of patients up to many feet away) or who are nursed by the same personnel, via the hands of attendant health care workers. Patients who require intubation alone have a 60-fold less risk for HAP than those who are ventilated with a tracheostomy[56]. Nebulisers generate extremely small water particles containing particulate microorganisms and these can easily reach the distal trachea, terminal bronchioles and alveoli, and cause necrotising Gram-negative pneumonia[68]. Equipment with redundant tubings[69] have the potential for collecting stagnant water at temperatures < 50 °C thereby permitting rapid (within a few hours) growth of pathogenic organisms – a source of tracheal inoculation and subsequent pneumonia. Interestingly, the risk is higher if the ventilatory breathing circuits are changed too frequently, i.e. 24-hourly rather than 48-hourly[26]. Over-manipulation of these circuits leads to increased circuit contamination and direct propulsion of infected liquid into the respiratory tree with the subsequent development of pneumonia. Recently, it has been shown that there is no difference in the incidence of pneumonia irrespective of whether the ventilatory tube is left unchanged or changed every 48 hours throughout the period of ventilation[70]. Modification of ventilatory equipment with heated circuits (to reduce the amount of condensate and to destroy thermolabile microorganisms) and one-way water valves (to prevent aspiration) condensate eliminators, exercising care when interrupting inspiratory circuits, for example, on delivering medications (to reduce exogenous contamination), use of expiratory filters (to reduce patient to patient spread), and bubble through rather than aerosol generating equipment (to reduce aerosolisation of bacteria) have all reduced the risk of pneumonia. Use of heat moisture exchanges (to recycle the patient's heat and moisture and obviate the requirement for an humidifier) may also reduce the risk of pneumonia. Other equipment with potential for introducing microbes responsible for HAP include diagnostic and therapeutic spirometers, resuscitation bags, mist tents, and nasotracheal/nasogastric suctioning devices. Appropriate and regular use of disposable gloves by personnel, and sterilisation of, or use of, disposable equipment as appropriate is crucial to reduce the incidence of HAP.

Current practical recommendations regarding respiratory therapy equipment to reduce the frequency of nosocomial pneumonia in ventilated patients are summarised as follows: ventilator circuits should be changed every 48 hours as opposed to 24 hours to reduce the rate of pneumonia, appropriate elimination of tubing condensate, and avoidance of accidental contamination of patient's trachea, avoidance of transfer of equipment between patients, ongoing review and care of in-line medication nebulisers, appropriate disinfection of respiratory therapy devices such as ventilator tubing, spirometers and resuscitation bags.

Gastric colonisation

It has been known for over of 20 years that the normally sterile stomach and small bowel become rapidly colonised with Gram-negative aerobic bacteria in patients admitted to an ICU[71] and that colonisation appears to be linked to rises in the stomach pH values, above normal bactericidal levels, particular to above 3.5[72,73]. Patients admitted to an ICU who are ventilated, rapidly develop a high gastric pH[27]. Patients who are at risk from such gastric colonisation are those with achlorhydria, malnourished, elderly, abnormalities of GI tract function, for example, gastrointestinal stasis which may lead to retrograde gastric colonisation, and recipients of antacids or H_2 receptor antagonists[27,74–76]. Earlier observations suggested a link between such colonisation and the development of pneumonia[77–79].

The organisms that colonise gastric juice are typically Gram-negative aerobic bacteria and their source appears not to be swallowed oropharyngeal secretions but small intestinal contents which have moved in a retrograde fashion to the stomach[79–81]. The use of oral selective decontaminating agents, in conjunction with systemic parentally administered antibiotics has been shown to reduce Gram-negative bacterial colonisation of the stomach and is associated with a reduced incidence of pneumonia. The confounding effect of the systemic antimicrobials used has been eliminated in more recent series and an independent effect of decreased colonisation and an associated decrease in pneumonia by the selective oral agents has been shown by some studies[82], but not by others[83]. Direct intragastric administration of antibiotics has also been shown to be associated with a reduced incidence of HAP[84]. In addition to Gram-negative bacilli, Gram-positive bacteria and fungi have also been identified.

Critically ill patients and others admitted to the ICU are at substantial risk for stress ulceration and upper gastrointestinal bleeding. It has become common practice to prophylactically administer antacids, H_2 receptor antagonists, or cytoprotective drugs although the evidence that they have an impact on the reduction of haemorrhage is debatable[85,86]. Substantial evidence has accrued that the use of H_2 blockers has a direct effect on the development of gastric colonisation and hence, a possible role in the aetiology of HAP[26,76,78,87]. For example, at 24 hours of cimetidine administration to patients in an ICU, the gastric contents of all patients became colonised[79]. It appears probably the H_2 receptor blockers are risk factors for pneumonia as a direct result of the increased gastric pH and hence increased gastric colonisation[78] rather than by another unknown inherent effect.

The association of H_2 blockers with pneumonia has been demonstrated in several placebo controlled studies, for example, the two-fold increase in pneumonia in surgical patients given pre-operative cimetidine and a fourfold incidence in pneumonia in major abdominal surgery[87,88]. Similar findings have been found in retrospective studies[26]. Studies in homogenous patient populations have documented a gastric pH rise to a value of > 4 associated with an increased gastric colonisation. Others, however, with different population groups such as neurosurgical patients (which are not nursed in a supine position) or patients with a low overall frequency of pneumonia or a short period of follow-up, or in which gastric pH is not different between the two groups may show a weaker relationship between H_2 blockers and pneumonia[89–91]. A recent randomised controlled trial of ranitidine versus placebo in intubated medically critically ill patients demonstrated at least 90% rate of gastric colonisation by 48 days of intubation in both groups but pneumonia occurred significantly more frequently (81% vs. 50%) and earlier in the ranitidine arm[86].

Over the past 10 years there has been a significant reduction in the incidence of stress ulcer bleeding. Cook and colleagues in a recent multi-centre Canadian study[92] reported the incidence of clinically important GI bleeding (with associated haemodynamic compromise or the need for blood transfusion) as 1.5% in 2252 patients. Respiratory failure and coagulopathy were the two independent risk factors for developing clinically significant bleeding. Of the 1400 patients without these risk factors only 0.1% developed GI bleeding. It was the contention of that group that in patients without either risk factor, namely, no coagulopathy or mechanical ventilation for less than 48 hours, prophylaxis against stress ulcer bleeding could safely be withheld. One can speculate that the factors for reducing the incidence of GI bleeding may be improved and earlier institution of nutritional support especially enteral feeding, improvements in mechanical ventilation and possibly earlier management of shock, although there is no data to substantiate this. A recent trial by Ben-Menachem[93] reported that routine prophylaxis with sucralfate or cimetidine in patients entering the medical ICU was not warranted, given that the incidence and severity of haemorrhage from stress-related gastritis were not significant when compared to no treatment.

Sucralfate is a complex salt of sucrose sulphate and aluminium hydroxide which acts as a cytoprotective antiulcer medication whose mechanism is other than reduction in gastric acidity. It acts by adhesion to the gastric mucosa and increasing PGE_2 in the gastric lumen. Several studies have documented that gastric colonisation is less frequent and of lesser magnitude in mechanically ventilated patients treated with sucralfate than with antacids or histamine type 2 blockers[27,94,95]. Driks *et al.*[27] showed that 24% of patients receiving sucralfate were found to have sterile gastric juice as compared to only 4% in patients receiving acid-suppressing medications. In the sucralfate group, 19% of patients showed bacterial colonisation in contrast to 58% of specimens in the antacid H_2 antagonist group which showed Gram-negative bacterial colonisation. Tryba's study[96] corroborated the findings, i.e. in sucralfate treated patients there was significantly less gastric pharyngeal and tracheal colonisation with Gram-negative bacilli.

The rate of nosocomial pneumonia is also lower by at least 1.5 to threefold compared to patients receiving H_2 antagonists or antacids[94,95–97]. The complexity of analysing such studies is again highlighted by Driks[27] in which several other different risk factors interoperate, for example, whether the patient is a surgical or a medical patient, different durations of intubation, whether combinations of antacids have been used, previous antibiotics used, enteral feeds, and so on. In fact, in one small subgroup in this study the pneumonia rate was the same irrespective of sucralfate or H_2 antagonists. This phenomenon may not be related to an effect of sucralfate on gastric pH *per se* but an intrinsic antibacterial action of sucralfate and preservation of gut mucosal integrity[78,98]. In two studies comparing sucralfate to H_2 antagonists, using a different patient profile and design from others, for example, post-resuscitation, and a high incidence of alkaline gastric juice in both study arms, a short-term follow-up and lower dosages of cimetidine, the incidence of pneumonia was the same in each arm[99,100]. In a more recent randomised controlled trial comparing nosocomial pneumonia in mechanically ventilated patients receiving antacids, ranitidine or sucralfate as stress ulcer prophylaxis, Prod'hom[101] found the risk of bleeding was no less effective with sucralfate than antacids or H_2 blockers. However, the risk of late onset pneumonia (> 4 days) was significantly reduced in the sucralfate-treated group compared with antacid or ranitidine. Of note, was that mortality did not differ among the treatment groups and patients receiving sucralfate had a lower median gastric pH and less frequent gastric colonisation.

How exactly do these gastrointestinal Gram-negative organisms produce HAP? One theory is that gastric colonisation places the oropharynx and upper airways under threat of direct colonisation by gastric organisms and through retrograde movement leads to aspiration into the patient's trachea and the subsequent development of pneumonia. Evidence in support of this has been published in a paper from Manchester. This claimed retrograde colonisation was increased in ranitidine rather than sucralfate patients and linked to an increase in pneumonia[94]. Direct aspiration of the patient's stomach contents is an alternative mechanism, for example, by vomiting secondary to gastric stasis in patients in a supine position or from enteral tube feedings, into the trachea (even bypassing cuffed endotracheal tubes). Clinical and radiotracer studies have clearly shown that gastric aspiration occurs[102]. The species of organisms identified in the stomach appear to be similar to those colonising the trachea and causing pneumonia[86]. Nevertheless, pneumonia also occurs even in the absence of prior gastric colonisation[86]. The gastric bacteria similar to those found in the tracheobronchial tree usually appear in the respiratory tract after at least 2 days[71,75,78,94]. Meticulous microbial typing techniques (plasmid typing, genomic DNA finger printing) has shown identical organisms in the stomach and the lower respiratory tract[66], which provides strong evidence that the organisms responsible for ventilator-associated pneumonia aspirate from the intestine. The presence of bile both in the gastric and tracheal aspirates supports a direct duodeno-gastro-pulmonary route, with the original key event being disordered intestinal motility, leading to duodenogastric reflux. In that study, the organisms in the oropharynx were not the same as in the lower respiratory tree – upper airways colonisation and subsequent pneumonia may not always be linked[66].

Aspiration of nasogastric feeds is particularly common in critically ill patients. Enteral feeds have a pH ranging from 6–7. There appears to be a high incidence of gastric colonisation and nosocomial pneumonia associated with continuous intragastric enteral feeding. Jacobs *et al.*[103] corroborated that 54% of mechanically ventilated patients on continuous intragastric enteral feeding for more than 72 hours developed pneumonia. In their study, an elevated gastric pH was noted in 12 of 13 patients who developed pneumonia. The same group in a separate study showed that intermittent intragastric feeding of critically ill ventilated patients significantly reduced the incidence of pneumonia. Bonten and colleagues[104] studied the influence of different stress ulcer prophylactic agents and enteral feeding on gastric pH and colonisation in ICU patients. Although this was an open prospective trial and pH measurements were done via a litmus paper method, their observations were in keeping with the Jacobs study showing that continuous enteral feeding increased gastric pH and colonisation. Whether additional strategies to lower gastric pH of enteral feeds will modify the risk of nosocomial pneumonia has yet to be demonstrated.

An alternative theory is that bacteria do not reach the lungs via a direct aspiration route but through the process of translocation. It is proposed that, as a result of a breach in the mucosal integrity, gut bacteria bypass the regional lymph nodes, enter the portal venous system, pass through the liver and ultimately arrive in the lung. It has been shown, for example, that gut wall ischaemia which occurs in the setting of hypovolemic shock, cytotoxic chemotherapy, heat injury, intestinal obstruction and inflammatory bowel disease, leads to an increase in microorganisms recoverable from the regional lymph nodes[105]. The presence of bowel ischaemia is a strong determinant of post-operative pneumonia[106]. Animal models using radiolabelled bacteria demonstrate bowel bacteria targeting the lung following experimental gut ischaemia.

Diagnosis of HAP

Both accurate and specific diagnosis of HAP are demanding goals often not achieved in everyday clinical practice. Thus, in patients with ARDS, pneumonia may be under-diagnosed in one-third and over diagnosed in one-fifth[6]. Criteria for pneumonia vary and this poses limitations when comparing published data. For example, in both the CDC and UK criteria for HAP[1,5] it is possible to accept a case as one of HAP on the basis of chest rales and change in the character of sputum alone. However, these findings are also commonly found in exacerbations of chronic bronchitis or in tracheobronchitis without pneumonia and are therefore clearly imprecise. Reasonable minimal clinical requirements for the diagnosis of hospital-acquired bacterial pneumonia would appear to be the presence of new pulmonary infiltrates, increasing FIO_2 and/or ventilatory requirements, leukocytosis, fever, and increase in the purulence of respiratory secretions. A definitive diagnosis is only possible when lung tissue shows the characteristic histopathological changes and bacteria are seen or grown (Table 19.2). In many patients this is a pinnacle of perfection rarely achieved in everyday practice. Furthermore, HAP in a ventilated patient may be difficult to differentiate from left ventricular failure, ARDS, pulmonary drug toxicity, pulmonary embolism and indeed two or more of these events may be concurrent particularly ARDS with HAP (Table 19.1). In these situations, HAP may be both over-diagnosed and under-diagnosed[6,107,108].

The ideal diagnostic study to identify the presence or absence of nosocomial lung infection and identify the aetiologic agent if present should fulfil the following criteria: (i) only uncontaminated lower airway secretions would be sampled thus providing a sample representative of the alveolar space and not transbronchial contamination; (ii) minimally invasive; (iii) easily repeatable; (iv) low cost; and (v) have significant positive impact on physician practice and patient outcome. Unfortunately, there is much controversy amongst the leading researchers in this field as to what is the most appropriate technique to obtain this information. There are the proponents who advocate invasive diagnostic studies as a routine in the workup for suspected pneumonia in mechanically ventilated patients[109] and those who take the opposing view[110]. There is consensus that nosocomial pneumonia in critically ill patients has major implications regarding morbidity, mortality and ICU length of stay and hospital cost; however, as yet a unifying scheme to obtain a definitive diagnosis is not available. This is not surprising given that one cannot rely on clinical criteria and that treatment with unnecessary antibiotics can lead to highly resistant pathogens and poor patient outcome. More importantly perhaps is that other causes of fever or potential sites of infection may not be scrutinised and again may lead to higher mortality rates.

Table 19.5. *Diagnostic pulmonary procedures*

Non-invasive
Tracheal aspirate
Mini bronchoalveolar lavage
Protected bronchoalveolar lavage
Telescoped plugged catheter
Invasive
Protected specimen brush (PSB)
Bronchoalveolar lavage (BAL)
Protected bronchoalveolar lavage
Transthoracic needle aspiration
Transbronchial biopsy
Open lung biopsy

Diagnostic methods

This section describes the diagnostic approach from a clinician's perspective. Chapter 1 emphasises the microbiologist's perspective.

Non-invasive diagnostic methods

These are described in Table 19.5. Sputum and tracheal samples are often unreliable as they may be contaminated by oropharyngeal flora as indicated by a relatively high squamous epithelial to polymorphonuclear cell ratio. The relation, particularly between upper airway colonising bacteria and the bacterial agents actually causing pneumonia has still not been clearly defined. Some studies show poor correlation between the upper and lower respiratory tract flora and the causative agent of pneumonia as identified by open lung biopsy or protected specimen brush[23,35,66,111]. Therefore, the presence of, for example, *Staphylococcus* or Gram-negative bacteria in a sputum or tracheal aspirate is usually difficult to interpret. Recent clinical studies have again confirmed a high false-positive rate for pneumonia using such specimens[35,112,113].

Papazian[114] was able to improve specificity through the use of quantitative cultures at a 10^5 cfu/ml or greater cut-off for blind bronchial suctioning. Marquette[115] found that 10^6 cfu/ml was the most accurate diagnostic threshold where a high level of agreement exists between endotracheal aspirates and protected specimen brush using 10^3 cfu/ml to establish the diagnosis of nosocomial pneumonia. Unfortunately, open lung biopsies for histological analyses were not performed thus precluding a definite conclusion regarding the diagnostic yield of endotracheal quantitative cultures in the diagnosis of nosocomial pneumonia. Other methods to improve diagnostic accuracy tracheal aspirates include grading of Gram's stains, presence of elastin fibres and presence of antibody-coated bacteria (ACB).

By grading of Gram's stains according to the number of organisms and polymorphs and analysing endotracheal aspirates for elastin fibres, a specific indicator for necrotising pneumonia, the diagnostic accuracy was markedly improved in the detection of nosocomial pneumonitis[4,116]. It should be noted, however, that in the presence of the adult respiratory distress syndrome in which non-infectious lung necrosis occurs, recovery of elastin fibres is less specific (50%) for the diagnosis of pneumonia.

To date, the presence of ACB in sputum or tracheal aspirates has yielded conflicting results with sensitivities ranging from 48% to 73% and specificities ranging from 50% to 100%[117–119].

Positive blood or pleural fluid cultures are highly specific but have a low yield (of the order of 5–10%).

Non-bronchoscopic semi-invasive techniques

A number of non-invasive techniques to obtain specimens from the distal airways offer several advantages including less risk to the patient, lower cost and greater availability to those ICUs without a 24-h bronchoscopy service. Although these procedures are done without knowing the exact location from where the specimen was obtained, there is evidence to suggest that the pneumonic process is frequently widespread but especially in the posterior segments of the lower lobes[120,121]. Recent studies have demonstrated a close association between cultures obtained from different sites via non-bronchoscopic techniques and those obtained by protected specimen brush via the bronchoscope[122,123]. This, however, has not been universally accepted[124,125]. Sensitivities of quantitative cultures using $> 10^3$ cfu/ml for threshold of infection was 64% vs 71% with a predictive value of 100% for both[112]. The use of a plugged telescoping catheter (PTC) was studied by Pham[122] and colleagues who reported that blinded or directed PTC sampling had similar results to those of protected specimen brush samples obtained by bronchoscopy with a sensitivity of 100% and specificity of 82%.

Similarly, non-bronchoscopic techniques for bronchoalveolar lavage have recently been investigated in critically ill ventilated patients, which avoid aspiration of material through a non-sterile bronchoscopic channel. After one sterile catheter with a polyethylene glycol plug is inserted into the endotracheal tube and blindly advanced to the distal airways, the plug is expelled and the second catheter is passed through the first one beyond its distal tip. Twenty mls of saline are injected and the aspirate collected for Gram's stain, cell count and culture[123]. Other investigators[126] have developed curve-tipped catheters which can be used for selective left-sided bronchial catheterisation. In one study[123], minibronchoalveolar lavages performed 24–48 hours prior to death were compared to the culture results of lung tissue at post-mortem. On the basis of cell criteria (to differentiate lung infection from colonisation) and semi-quantitative cultures there was a sensitivity of 80% and specificity of 66% for diagnosing nosocomial pneumonia in patients receiving antimicrobial therapy. Of the organisms cultured from the lung tissue, 75% were found in the bronchoalveolar lavage specimen. Another trial[121] of this technique to diagnose nosocomial pneumonia (histologically proven) in patients with ARDS revealed the sensitivity to be 70% and specificity 69% with a 77% concordance of the organism cultured. Other studies[127,128] using non-bronchoscopic bronchoalveolar lavage report equal or better sensitivities and correlations for the type of organisms grown.

Bronchoscopic techniques

BAL via fibre-optic bronchoscopy (FOB) is now readily available for sampling of the distal airways. The safety of fiberoptic bronchoscopy critically ill patients includes those with the adult respiratory distress syndrome[129,130]. Despite the possible occurrence of arrhythmias, transient hypoxaemia, bronchospasm, bleeding and fever, the use of appropriate sedation plus short-acting neuromuscular blockers and close monitoring during the procedure has limited any major complications. Relative contraindications for bronchoscopy[130,131] include: P_aO_2 < 10 kPa on F_iO_2 of 1.0, positive and expiratory pressure ≥ 15 cm H_2O, severe bronchospasm, acute ischaemic heart disease (acute myocardial infarction, unstable angina), severe hypotension (mean arterial pressure < 65 mm Hg on vasopressors), increased intracranial pressure, and severe bleeding diathesis. The differential cell count, cytological examination, and search for haemosiderin laden macrophages can be performed. This has been utilised as a diagnostic tool in a number of non-infectious conditions including sarcoidosis, cancer, alveolar proteinosis and pulmonary haemorrhage. Identification of a microbiological organism by BAL which is not normally present in the airways is diagnostic of disease due to this organism, for example, *Pneumocystis, Toxoplasma, Legionella, Mycoplasma,* Influenza and RSV. The presence of CMV is somewhat more conjectural[132–134], unless accompanied by the characteristic intranuclear and intracytoplasmic cytological changes[135]. The diagnosis of fungal parenchymal lung disease carries a low sensitivity[136] but the presence of *Aspergillus* in an appropriate clinical and radiological setting is highly suggestive of invasive fungal disease[137]. Similarly, the finding of non-tuberculous mycobacteria, *Candida,* Herpes simplex, and *Cryptococcus* has to be interpreted in the context of the patient's signs and symptoms. It is in the area of bacterial pneumonia that BAL and PSB has generated the most interest since the majority of patients with HAP will have a bacterial aetiology. In order to obtain meaningful and comparative information, standard guidelines should be maintained for performing the procedure, choosing an appropriate sampling site, optimising sampling technique, processing the microbiological specimens and establishing appropriate microscopic criteria and diagnostic thresholds[131,138].

A number of specific questions remain to be answered: what is the evidence supporting bronchoscopically obtained specimens, which technique namely BAL or PSB or both has the highest diagnostic yield, how useful is microscopic analysis of specimens for intracellular organisms, cell count, differential and elastin fibres, what is the appropriate semi-quantitative culture cut off threshold for the diagnosis of pneumonia from PSB and BAL, and what is the role of bronchoscopy in patients previously on antibiotics?

Sampling area

Currently, there is conflicting data in the literature on where to obtain samples for analysis. Post-mortem studies have demonstrated that nosocomial pneumonia is frequently widespread involving predominantly the gravity-dependent regions of the lower lobes[120,123]. Recent studies[122,128] have demonstrated a good correlation between culture results of blindly advanced PSB and bronchoscopically directed PSB and between PSB obtained from radiographically involved areas and those in the contralateral lung without radiographic abnormality[115]. However, two other investigators[124,139] reported significant differences between culturing the involved versus the contralateral side. Meduri[140] has advocated bilateral sampling in patients with ARDS and in the immunocompromised patient with diffuse infiltrates. The Consensus Conference[131] recommends that sampling be directed to lung segments with new or progressive radiologic infiltrates or from purulent secretions observed in distal airways during bronchoscopy.

Sampling technique

To avoid contamination of lower airway secretions, Wimberley and colleagues[141] described the use of a PSB technique which is introduced through the inner channel of the fibre-optic bronchoscope and advanced under direct vision to the specified lung segments to be brushed. The polyethylene glycol plug is displaced and the specimen collected by advancing the brush into secretions under direct vision. As the volume of respiratory secretions collected by PSB is 0.001 ml, a quantitative culture of 10^3 cfu/ml corresponds to 10^5–10^6 cfu/ml at the site of collection, and this has been accepted as the diagnostic threshold for lower respiratory tract infection[107,142].

Several excellent studies in animals and humans have demonstrated the usefulness of the PSB technique in the diagnosis of nosocomial pneumonia in critically ill patients who are not receiving antibiotics[107,120,143] and see Table 19.6. Chastre and colleagues performed bronchoscopy with the PSB on 26 patients immediately after death while still being ventilated. This lung segment was then removed by thoracotomy and subjected to histological analysis and quantitative bacterial culture. Using the diagnostic threshold of $\geq 10^3$ cfu/ml, PSB culture yielded 15 of 19 species present in the lung culture with no false-negatives for a sensitivity of 100% but a lower specificity of 60%. Subsequent reports by other investigators[124], have shown high sensitivities and specificities using the bronchoscopically guided PSB technique and a diagnostic cut off of $\geq 10^3$ cfu/ml to diagnose nosocomial pneumonia. A recent meta analysis[144] evaluated many prospective clinical trials comprising 524 critically ill patients suspected of having ventilator-associated pneumonia who were not receiving antibiotics, and concluded that the PSB technique had a sensitivity of 90% and specificity of 94.5%. Unfortunately, the use

Table 19.6. *Frequency of organisms recovered from protected brush specimens in significant concentrations (>10^3 colony-forming units per millilitre) in 52 episodes of ventilator-associated pneumonia*

Organism	Frequency (%)
Gram-negative bacteria	75
Pseudomonas aeruginosa	31
Acinetobacter species	15
Proteus species	15
Moraxella (Branhamella) catarrhalis	10
Haemophilus species	10
Escherichia coli	8
Klebsiella species	4
Enterobacter cloacae	2
Citrobacter freundii	2
Legionella pneumophila	2
Gram-positive bacteria	52
Staphylococcus aureus	33
Streptococcus pneumoniae	6
Other streptococci	15
Corynebacterium species	8
Anaerobes	2

[a]Data from Rouby JJ, Rossingnon MD, Nicolas MH *et al. Anesthesiology* 1989; 71:679–85[123].

of antimicrobial therapy prior to PSB sampling produces a high incidence of false-positives and false-negatives. Follow-up culture of PSB specimens obtained 24 and 48 hours after initiation of antibiotics in established cases of nosocomial pneumonia were negative in 40% after 24 hours, and 65% after 48 hours[145]. The sensitivity of the PSB technique has been found to be low in critically ill patients on antimicrobial therapy[146,147] and causes individual variability in repeated quantitative culture thresholds in those suspected of nosocomial pneumonia[115,148].

A number of limitations of the PSB technique deserve mention. Not withstanding that bronchoscopy is regarded as safe for most patients, the cumulative cost of the catheter, procedure, and cultures have been found to be less than those projected to empirically treat all critically ill patients on clinical grounds alone[149]. Availability of cultures may take up to 48 hours and thus there is a delay in obtaining useful data on which to guide therapy. Moreover, due to the limited sampling area, false-negative results may occur if the specimen is not taken from an affected segment and places these critically ill patients at significant risk if therapy is withheld. The diagnostic threshold of 10^3 cfu/ml may increase the number of false-positives and hence patients with bronchiolitis may be inappropriately treated. Conversely, patients with borderline PSB culture results ($\geq 10^2$ cfu/ml but $< 10^3$ cfu/ml) with underlying pneumonia may be missed. A recent study of patients with suspected HAP who had a PSB of $\geq 10^2$ but $< 10^3$ cfu/ml indicated that approximately one-half of these patients at a second interval PSB specimen gave $\geq 10^3$ cfu/ml of the original organism whilst the remainder were repeat negative. These findings suggests that follow-up PSBs are needed in such borderline cases to identify those patients who require treatment[150]. Therefore, close monitoring and repeated PSB cultures are indicated in those patients in whom clinical suspicion of pneumonia remains and who have initial PSB cultures which do not reach the diagnostic threshold. Lastly, in those patients who have received antibiotics prior to PSB culture there is considerable variability[147] rendering PSB an unreliable predictor of nosocomial pneumonia.

BAL is a technique used to sample lower airway secretions from a larger area of lung (approximately 1 million alveoli) and the material recovered can be immediately examined microscopically for cell count, differential cytology, intracellular organisms, elastin fibres, and Gram's stain as well as being quantitatively cultured. The tip of the fibre-optic bronchoscope is wedged into a third or fourth-generation bronchus under visual guidance and 20–30 ml aliquots of saline are instilled and aspirated until 120–140 ml has been injected. Given the larger amount of lung tissue sampled it is estimated than in patients with pneumonia the BAL may recover five–tenfold more organisms than with PSB[140].

As the dilution of alveolar secretions is 10 to 100 fold, a colony count of 10^4 cfu/ml represents 10^5 to 10^6 bacteria/ml in the original specimen. Unfortunately, to date, there is no standardised diagnostic technique nor threshold for quantitative culture in BAL samples. Culture thresholds of 10^3 cfu/ml to 10^5 cfu/ml have provided sensitivities of 53–97% and specificities of 60–100%[35,120,123,142].

Another disadvantage is the possible contamination of the sample from the upper respiratory tract in heavily colonised patients or those with bronchitis, and occurs in up to 30% of specimens[35,142]. Attempts to enhance the diagnostic accuracy have included routine assessment of squamous epithelial cell count, avoidance of topical anaesthetic agents due to their potential bacteriostatic properties, and discarding the initial aspirate[131].

A number of studies employing the use of BAL in diagnosing pneumonia in non-ventilated patients used a threshold of greater than 10^5 cfu/ml[151,152]. In Thorpe's study, Gram's stain of centrifuged BAL fluid was positive only in the patients with active bacterial pneumonia. In the study by Kahn and Jones they attempted to exclude upper airway contamination by evaluating only cultures with less than 1% squamous epithelial cells in a differential cell count. Organisms were cultured in concentrations of $>10^5$ cfu/ml in 16 of 18 patients with pneumonia yet no patients without pneumonia and less than 1% squamous epithelial cells grew $>10^5$ cfu/ml in BAL cultures. Unfortunately, in this and other studies[153], contamination of lavage fluid by upper airway secretions was reported to be high and the 10^5 cfu/ml threshold could lead to withholding treatment in patients with pneumonia. Johanson[120] has proposed a bronchoalveolar lavage bacterial index (the sum of the logarithmic concentrations of any species recovered) to diagnose nosocomial pneumonia based on a baboon model which yielded a sensitivity of 100% and specificity of 92%. Given that nosocomial pneumonia is polymicrobial in up to 30% of cases, this may be a reasonable approach which requires further validation. Although the current recommended threshold for BAL specimens is $>10^4$ cfu/ml, Torres[154] found a 35% false-positive result using a cut off of 10^4 cfu/ml and 15% false-positive rate at 10^5 cfu/ml in mechanically ventilated patients without pulmonary infiltrates.

To reduce the likelihood of BAL fluid contamination from upper airways Meduri[140] introduced a protected BAL technique which yielded a sensitivity of 97% and specificity of 92%. Two important clinically observations were that protected BAL specimens decreased sample contamination (<1% squamous epithelial cells) and withholding antimicrobial therapy in stable patients with negative protected BAL findings had no adverse effects on patient outcome. Other non-bronchoscopic techniques of BAL and protected BAL have recently been studied and the results compared favourably (sensitivity 73%, specificity 96%) to bronchoscopically obtained PSB specimens (93% and 100%, respectively)[112,122,128]. There is no general consensus as to which technique provides superior diagnostic information with conflicting results being dependent to an extent on methodology, microbial scoring system, diagnostic criteria, antibiotic usage and types of patients investigated[35,120,142]. However, it is generally acknowledged that BAL is a less hazardous procedure.

Similar problems regarding the diagnostic accuracy of BAL in patients receiving antibiotics prior to the procedure have been raised by a number of investigators[140,147,154]. Studies comparing quantitative BAL cultures to PSB cultures in ventilated patients suspected of pneumonia have provided conflicting results[35,142,155] ranging from 50%–100% (sensitivity and specificity). Contributing factors to the wide variability include assessment of different patient populations, prior use of antibiotics, and the lack of a gold standard reference, namely, histology and culture of lung tissue.

Microscopic analysis

Recently several investigators have confirmed the diagnostic value of microscopic examination of BAL fluid for cell count and differential, presence or absence of intracellular organisms, Gram's stain, elastin fibres and cytology, particularly in light of the prompt availability of critical information on which to base therapeutic decisions. There is some evidence showing an increase in the neutrophil count in BAL specimens of patients with nosocomial pneumonia. However, in ARDS patients, non-infectious causes can produce similar findings. There seems to be a growing consensus that the microscopic identification of intracellular organisms with Giemsa or Gram's stained cytocentrifuged bronchoalveolar lavage fluid of critically ill patients is a good predictor of pneumonia. However, various thresholds for significance have ranged from 2% to 25%[128,140,142,156,157]. These investigators found that the presence of intracellular organisms corresponded extremely well with protected specimen brush cultures in patients without prior antimicrobial therapy and a close correlation between BAL and Gram's stain findings for the diagnosis of ventilator associated pneumonia has ranged from 73–100% and 88–100%, respectively[128,131,157]. Some of the differences are probably due to variations in the technique which has yet to be standardised, and whether percentage of total cells or percentage of only neutrophils is used as the denominator. As many encapsulated bacteria exist primarily extracellularly, it is important to assess these as well, at least semi-quantitatively. Limitations of this technique merit cautious interpretation of results in immunocompromised patients and especially in patients on antibiotic therapy[158].

Elastin fibres have been found to be a marker for necrotising pneumonia caused by Gram-negative infections[4]. However, its usefulness in the diagnosis of nosocomial pneumonia is probably limited because of the frequent occurrence in ARDS patients.

Cytological analysis of BAL fluid is useful in ventilated patients suspected of pneumonia to establish alternative diagnoses including opportunistic infections, pulmonary haemorrhage and carcinoma.

Other invasive procedures

Transtracheal aspiration (TTA), transthoracic needle aspiration and transbronchial biopsy are invasive techniques with particular disadvantages including unpleasantness for the alert patient, risk of haemorrhage, sampling discrepancies, pneumothoraces and secondary infections[136,159–161]. TTA was originally advocated to obviate oropharyngeal colonisation but still has a low specificity (high false-positive rate) although sensitivity is high. It is difficult to perform in critically ill or ventilated patients (who may have a coagulopathy) and carries an increased risk of pneumothorax. Transthoracic needle aspiration likewise is a hazardous procedure with a similar profile to TTA. It does, however, carry a high specificity[162], but low sensitivity due to the difficulties in localising the affected lung region, small sampling area, and limited specimen volume for microbiological assessment. Thoracoscopic biopsy under direct visualisation has been shown to be beneficial in immunocompromised patients[163,164] and clinical trials may prove this to be a useful technique in nosocomial pneumonia despite being somewhat more invasive.

Transbronchial needle aspiration has been shown to have a low sensitivity and specificity in a canine model[165] and in a subsequent study[166] was not found to have any advantage over protected specimen brush technique in the diagnosis of pneumonia.

Transbronchial biopsy although more risky in critically ill ventilated patients particularly from haemorrhage, (especially in those with uncontrolled coagulopathy), might help to differentiate between colonisation and tissue invasion particularly with fungal diseases such as those due to *Aspergillus* spp. Papin and co-workers[167] retrospectively studied 15 patients in which transbronchial biopsy was done during mechanical ventilation. Diagnostic information was obtained in 30% of cases and therapeutic decisions were altered in approximately 50% of patients. The major complications were transient hypoxaemia, bleeding and pneumothorax. A recent retrospective study supported the use of transbronchial biopsy in a large group of immunocompromised patients, where the combined yield of transbronchial biopsy plus BAL increased the yield by 33%. However, only a small number of ventilated patients underwent this modality of investigation[168].

Open lung biopsy (OLB) is relatively safe in mechanically ventilated patients[111,169,170] and produces a high diagnostic yield. Its place, however, is best in the setting of the severely immunocompromised patient at risk for opportunistic infections such as invasive pulmonary aspergillosis, CMV, or *P. carinii* or in whom a non-infective aetiology such as pulmonary haemorrhage, drug toxicity, or non-specific interstitial pneumonitis (NSIP) is part of the differential diagnosis. It is also useful for patients in whom a significant bleeding dyscrasia is present which would not be controlled at transbronchial biopsy. Radiographical findings in such patients are usually non-specific. Sputum and tracheal aspirates are unreliable to make a diagnosis. Hence resort is made to OLB. A number of studies[169,171] in primarily immunocompromised patients with or without mechanical ventilation reported that a specific aetiologic diagnosis was found in 66% of patients, and a change in therapeutic strategy was initiated in 70% of the study group. However, survival rates did not improve. Several investigators[136,172] have suggested that transbronchial lung biopsy and BAL provide a diagnostic yield of 85% for infections compared to 88% for OLB in AIDS patients. However, OLB was the only procedure to diagnose Kaposi's sarcoma in lung. Meduri[173] referred eight patients with ARDS and worsening respiratory function and no clinical evidence of infection to OLB and all were found to have lung changes consistent with the proliferative phase of ARDS; no infection was found. In these patients, institution of corticosteroids was associated with an improvement in lung injury score and patient survival. What little data is available comparing concurrent diagnostic yields of OLB with BAL[174,175] suggest a much higher yield from OLB. This is also supported by retrospective and other comparative studies[176–178]. Fear over excessive technique generated morbidity and mortality associated with OLB appears largely unfounded[175,176,179–181]. A recent study performed in our hospital[175] on 13 bone marrow transplant and leukaemic patients all of whom had diffuse pulmonary infiltrates (presumed non-bacterial aaetiology) who underwent synchronous BAL and OLB produced 16 distinct diagnoses on OLB. These were: seven infections – CMV, PCP, bacterial pneumonia and nine non-infectious – pulmonary haemorrhage, pulmonary embolism. In comparison BAL produced only six diagnoses: 5 infections, one pulmonary haemorrhage. In no patient was BAL able to yield the exact same specific diagnoses as the OLB. However, even OLB may fail to detect some cases of lung pathology particularly fungal infection[132,175,177,182] and on that account caution should be exercised if down-modulating existing antimicrobial therapy is contemplated, based on the OLB findings. Information gained from the knowledge of specific, histological and cultural diagnoses from the OLB, however, may rationalise antimicrobial use, introduce other appropriate treatment for non-infectious processes and is probably cost-effective. Whether the ultimate outcome of these very sick patients is modified as a result of such intervention is controversial[177,179,182,183] and can only be assessed by studies involving a larger number of patients. Undoubtedly, the approach to any particular patient needs to be individualised.

Clinical and radiological features of nosocomial pneumonia

It is clear from the preceding discussions that clinical judgement based on the presence of new pulmonary infiltrates, purulent tracheal secretions, fever or leukocytosis are not helpful in the diagnosis of nosocomial pneumonia particularly in intubated patients. In other studies evaluating the accuracy of clinical diagnosis[184] the presence of pneumonia was accurately diagnosed in only 62% of the patients with nosocomial pneumonitis and appropriate antimicrobial treatment was initiated in 33% of cases. Meduri and colleagues[185] prospectively studied 50 patients with fever, pulmonary infiltrates and clinical features of ventilator-associated pneumonia to determine their aetiology, and to evaluate the diagnostic yield of a protocol based on a series of investigations. In 45 of 50 patients a cause for fever was established with infection as the major source and in many patients more than one infection was identified. Pneumonia was identified in only 42% of these patients, with sinusitis, catheter related and urinary tract infection comprising most of the others. Infection was the cause of radiological changes in less than half of these patients, and in those without ARDS, congestive heart failure and atelectasis were responsible for producing the X-ray findings. In patients with ARDS, non-infectious causes of fever were more likely, and in 25% of patients pulmonary fibroproliferation was the only source.

Pugin[128] analysed the diagnostic accuracy of combining a number of clinical features and expanded it to include radiological variables, oxygen parameters and semiquantitative cultures of tracheal aspirates to produce a clinical pulmonary infection score (CPIS). Although a good correlation was found between the CPIS score and the quantitative bacteriology, further studies are needed to validate it.

Physical examination may provide valuable clues regarding the aetiological agent such as as skin lesions characteristic of disseminated bacterial or fungal infections. In addition, positive blood, pleural, CSF, and joint fluid culture may be useful in selected cases in identifying the infecting organisms. However, two studies[23,149] have demonstrated the importance of searching for other sources of bacteraemia especially in patients with respiratory failure, new pulmonary infiltrates and tracheal secretions. Bacteraemia associated with nosocomial pneumonia was found in 24%–36%.

There are a number of technical problems limiting the use of radiological diagnosis of pneumonia in critically ill mechanically ventilated patients. Variability of technique, absence of lateral X-rays, difficulties in positioning patients and lack of standard formats in interpretation are some of the major factors[186].

The usual radiological signs of pneumonia in non-intubated patients such as air bronchograms, interstitial and alveolar infiltrates, or the silhouette sign are not helpful in distinguishing pneumonia from other processes in the lungs of mechanically ventilated patients. This is especially true in patients with adult respiratory distress syndrome as many of them develop bilateral diffuse pulmonary infiltrates prior to nosocomial pneumonia. In a study of 60 suspected cases of pneumonia[187] whose clinical and chest X-rays were reviewed only 30% were correctly diagnosed. There are limited studies in the use of CT scanning in patients with acute lung injury mainly from Gattiononi[188] and colleagues who reported compression atelectasis in the gravity-dependent lung regions with sparing of the non-gravity-dependent zones. An expanded role for CT scanning may be useful in revealing previously undiagnosed lung cavities, empyemas, pneumothoraces or pleural effusions and further studies are likely to be performed to evaluate its role in the diagnosis of nosocomial pneumonia. Of the roentgenographic signs, only the presence of air bronchograms correlated with pneumonia in 64% of patients, however, in intubated patients with diffuse bilateral infiltrates no single or combination of signs were useful[189]. Non-infectious causes of pulmonary infiltrates in ventilated patients include alveolar haemorrhage, lung contusion, atelectasis, pulmonary edema, pleural effusions, pulmonary emboli and tumours.

Sinusitis

Although sinusitis resulting from predominantly nasotracheal intubation and nasogastric tubes has been documented in recent years[190–193], specific criteria for diagnosis including radiological assessment and microbiological diagnosis without contamination of the nasopharynx have not been uniform. The diagnosis of sinusitis on CT scan has included opacification or presence of air fluid levels and the microbiological criteria include the presence of pus with proliferation of organisms in high concentrations from the sinus cavity after extensive disinfection of the nares. Westergren[194] recently reported a method to reduce potential contamination when culturing the maxillary antrum.

Two recent prospective research studies have brought to light the risk factors and clinical relevance of nosocomial maxillary sinusitis in critically ill ventilated patients[195,196]. In the first study[195] 300 patients were randomised to oral versus nasotracheal intubation. Gastric intubation followed the same route as endotracheal intubation. Sinus CT scans were performed every 7 days or earlier if a patient developed purulent nasal discharge or fever and if radiographical features of sinusitis were present, sinus puncture for quantitative culture was obtained. If pneumonia was suspected, a PSB culture was obtained from the affected lung segment. Although nosocomial pneumonia and septicaemia were more frequent in the nasotracheal group than the orotracheal group, the difference was not statistically significant. Similar organisms were cultured from the sinuses and lungs in 9 of 16 patients who had pneumonia and sinusitis. The second study by Rouby[196] and co-workers randomised those patients with negative maxillary sinus CT scans to receive oral or nasotracheal intubation. Repeat CT scans on the seventh day revealed a 96% incidence of radiological maxillary sinusitis in the nasotracheal group versus 22.5% in the orotracheal intubated group. Of those patients with radiographical changes, 38% had confirmed sinus infections following maxillary sinus aspiration. Those investigations confirmed the increased incidence of nosocomial pneumonia in patients with sinusitis and in 38% of cases pathogens identified from sinus aspiration and bronchoalveolar lavage were identical. Often the organisms were polymicrobial and were predominantly Gram-negative in 47%, Gram-positive in 35% and yeasts were present in 18%. Of patients with microbiologically confirmed sinusitis, 47% had resolution of fever and signs of sepsis following surgical drainage of the infected sinus. It is also important to treat sphenoid or ethmoid sinusitis with appropriate drainage measures as often pansinusitis may be present[197]. Given the association between infected maxillary sinusitis and pneumonia, it is conceivable that the nasopharynx acts as a reservoir for high concentrations of bacteria and, given the right conditions, pneumonia or sinusitis may develop. Alternatively, sinusitis may be the source of bacterial contamination leading to bronchitis or pneumonia. One recent study[195] reported a reduction in sinusitis and nosocomial pneumonia with the placement of orotracheal and orogastric tubes. Appropriate treatment measures for sinusitis include removal of nasotracheal and nasogastric tubes, surgical drainage and appropriate antimicrobials.

Antimicrobial prophylaxis of nosocomial pneumonia

The apparent association between airway colonisation with enteric Gram-negative bacteria and HAP, with its attendant high mortality, has prompted an approach whereby through reducing colonisation of the respiratory tree, the incidence of pneumonia and mortality might be reduced. Two major thrusts on this front have been tested: local installation of antibiotics and selective decontamination of the digestive system (SDD). In addition, systemically administered antibiotics have been tested on a number of occasions and appear to offer no advantage in terms of decreased colonisation, pneumonia or mortality[198,199]. Furthermore, there is concern of Gram-negative bacterial overgrowth and increased rates of bacteraemia. In fact, selective pressure of perioperative antimicrobial prophylaxis is well known to increase the risk of gastrointestinal colonisation and subsequent pneumonia.

A few studies have addressed the issue of decontaminating the respiratory tree with topical antibiotics administered endotracheally or by nebulisation. These antimicrobials have included gentamicin and polymyxin B. Although both Gram-negative oropharyngeal colonisation and HAP appear to be reduced, there is a serious risk of emergence of resistant organisms, and overall mortality is unchanged. In fact, heightened mortality may occur in those patients who subsequently develop pneumonia[200–202]. This approach is therefore not indicated at this time. Further investigations into the mechanism and distribution of antimicrobials administered in this fashion might provide a lead for more effective regimens.

SDD (with or without systemic antibiotics) to attempt to reduce the risk of HAP has been used extensively in recent years. Antimicrobial regimens have included one or two component arms[203,204]. A topical arm of orally administered nonabsorbable antibiotics produces high concentrations of lethal antimicrobials within the gut, which targets aerobic pathogenic Gram-negative bacilli, and at the same time, preserves the anaerobic microflora, affording protection against colonisation with other more pathogenic organisms[205]. A common combination is polymyxin (active against Gram-negatives other than *Proteus*, *Morganella* and *Serratia* spp.) with tobramycin (with polymyxin is synergistically active against *Pseudomonas, Proteus, Morganella* and *Serratia* spp.). Amphotericin B (active against *Candida* spp.), is sometimes added, although its use has been questioned as fungal disease is not common in most patients at risk from HAP, apart from those with prolonged neutropenia or other specific risk factors. The regimen is usually administered both in a mucosal adherent paste which coats the oropharynx and also via a nasogastric tube to the stomach. Alternative or additional antimicrobials have included vancomycin, norfloxacin or ofloxacin, gentamicin and nalidixic acid. A short course (usually for 72 hours) of a systemically administered third generation cephalosporin – usually cefotaxime – is sometimes given to cover the possibility of subclinical infection and to cover certain organisms which would otherwise not be treated by topical antimicrobials – such as pneumococci[203].

The first study reported was by Stoutenbeck *et al.* in 1984[204] which showed a significant reduction in infection among multiple trauma patients. A considerable number of studies over the next decade were published with conflicting results. However, two independent meta-analyses have been performed[206,207]. Inclusion criteria for both studies were similar -namely the trials were prospective, randomised and controlled, and were performed in patients admitted to intensive care units. The European study reviewed the results among 4142 patients. Selective decontamination was found to significantly reduce the odds of developing a respiratory tract infection by 64%. Analysis of a subgroup of patients who had received systemic antibiotics initially and orotopical therapy indicated that six patients would need to be treated to prevent one respiratory tract infection. However, although there was a definite trend towards an improved overall survival, this did not achieve statistical significance when all patient groups were included in the analysis. Analysis of patients who had been treated with both oral and systemic antibiotics did show a significant reduction (24%) in the odds of death occurring. It is a moot point, however, whether this effect had been achieved entirely due to use of systemic antibiotics. The US study was based on 2270 patients. Confirmation of the significant reduction in pneumonia ($p < 0.0001$) was forthcoming and appeared to be due to a reduction in Gram-negative pneumonia only – the incidence of Gram-positive bacterial pneumonia remained unchanged. However, the cumulative mortality rate was virtually unchanged by prophylaxis. Both studies therefore agree that the incidence of pneumonia can be reduced but they differ in the conclusions over mortality. Despite the impressive reduction in the rate of pneumonia, cost benefits were not analysed. Of some concern is that, whilst a significant association between the presence of respiratory tract infection and mortality had been confirmed[207] no association was found between the reduction of pneumonia and reduction in mortality[206,207]. ICU patients may therefore be dying because of infection related (e.g. multi-organ failure) or infection of unrelated causes rather than from pneumonia *per se*.

A number of variables may be responsible for these findings. These include a high degree of heterogeneity of the patients and their background illnesses, variability in antimicrobial regimes used and whether systemic antibiotics were included, whether H_2 antagonist blockers were prescribed, non-uniform criteria for diagnosis of pneumonia and variable compliance with the entry criteria of the study, e.g. randomisation. In order to clarify these important issues, a more homogenous population group, filtered by stringent inclusion criteria, and adhering strictly to randomised protocols which include uniform active treatment arms is necessary. Another approach to clarifying the issue of selective decontamination would be to analyse results of various trials based on an individual patient data basis and this may provide more conclusive information[207].

Three recent randomised, double-blind studies[208–210] failed to demonstrate reduction in the incidence of nosocomial pneumonia, mortality, length of stay, or the duration of mechanical ventilation. Discrepancies from earlier studies may partly be attributable to the recent use of protected specimen brush samples or bronchoalveolar lavage specimens rather than clinical, radiographical, or tracheal secretions, for establishing the diagnosis of pneumonia.

An important homogenous group of patients at particular risk for sepsis (including pneumonia) is granulocytopenic patients, for example, those receiving bone marrow transplantation or who have acute leukaemia[211]. Selective decontamination regimens, mainly using co-trimoxazole, have been in widespread use for some time[212]. However, as for studies in other patient groups the results have tended to be inconclusive. Unique problems in this group of patients have included undue myelosuppressive toxicity from co-trimoxazole. Selection of resistant organisms has also posed a problem[213]. An interesting study recently suggested that the efficacy of co-trimoxazole may be more related to serum and tissue concentrations of co-trimoxazole rather than gut activity[212].

Selection of microorganisms with resistance to the particular antibiotic prophylaxis being used may be another reason for the failure to demonstrate a reduction in infection-related mortality. In addition, it generates concern for the spread of clinically important resistant strains. Indeed some of the studies reviewed provide evidence of, for example, an increase in colonisation and clinical infection due to enterococci, resistant coagulase negative staphylococci, methicillin resistant *S. aureus*, and other resistant Gram-positive bacteria[206,214].

Until, and if, unequivocal conclusions and guidelines are forthcoming, the general use of SDD appears unjustified. However, until then there may be indications for limited use of SDD regimens in certain circumstances[203,214], for example, in certain centres with homogenous populations of patients known to be at significant risk for increased morbidity and mortality, and in which a significant effect on mortality has been clearly shown in some studies, for example, trauma patients. Another indication would be to control outbreaks of infection associated with multiresistant bacteria by interrupting patient to patient transmission, for example, *Klebsiella* infections[215]. Recently, it was found that the use of erythromycin reduced *K. pneumoniae* carriage but had no effect on other multiresistant enterobacteriaceae[216]. In the meantime, continued implementation of good infection control practices including handwashing, appropriate respiratory isolation procedures, education, proper use and care of ventilatory equipment and appropriate use of antibiotics should remain the mainstay of prophylaxis of respiratory infections in hospital.

Treatment of HAP

Treatment of critically patients with nosocomial pneumonia requires a multi-faceted approach. Unfortunately, failure of therapy is common with mortality rates ranging from 25–60% in selected high risk patients. However, early and effective antibiotic therapy has been shown to improve survival[19]. Therefore, appropriate antimicrobials, optimal oxygenation and ventilation, endotracheal suctioning, use of bronchodilators where necessary, cardiovascular, nutritional and nursing support are all essential components of therapy.

Antimicrobial treatment

The principles of antimicrobial treatment in pneumonia in detail has been covered in Chapter 4 and for specific microorganisms in other appropriate chapters. A few key points will be reiterated here. Selection of an antimicrobial regimen has to encompass the following requirements.

Prediction of the most likely pathogen

If the patient is severely immunocompromised, organisms apart from those producing bacterial pneumonia should be suspected. For example, *Nocardia* (renal transplantation), cytomegalovirus (bone marrow transplantation patients with graft vs. host disease). If pneumonia develops in a patient who has been discharged from hospital within the last 10 days then the pneumonia is likely to be hospital-acquired rather than community-acquired. This will make the *Pneumococcus* a less viable aetiological candidate compared to a Gram-negative organism. Associated extra-pulmonary features might provide a clue, for example, the development of renal failure, diarrhoea and confusion may suggest legionellosis. A recent history of aspiration may suggest anaerobic infection. Viral respiratory tract infection makes the patient vulnerable to staphylococcal disease and patients having received previous extensive antibiotic therapy may be at risk from the emergence of resistant organisms. Radiologicalal features may occasionally be useful, for example, localised consolidation with cavitation would suggest *Klebsiella*, *Staphylococcus* or tuberculosis, whilst diffuse perihilar infiltrates would favour *Legionella*, viral respiratory infection or *Pneumocystis carinii*.

Knowledge of the local hospital and community epidemiology can be useful. A high incidence of pneumonia due to *Legionella* in the hospital, community outbreaks of RSV and hence the likelihood of carriage by health care personnel, contamination of respiratory equipment with *Pseudomonas* spp., as well as the antibiogram of known organisms is further useful information.

Diagnosis

Every effort should be made to try to achieve a specific microbial diagnosis by high quality techniques, e.g. good sputum production and if possible by quantitative PSB/BAL. This will allow for the tailoring of directed antimicrobial therapy.

Knowledge of antimicrobial kinetics and toxicity

Antibiotics should be chosen for their superior penetration into respiratory secretions and lung tissue. It is important to remember that the inflammatory response in the lungs can affect antibiotic kinetics. For example, clindamycin and clarithromycin penetrate lung tissue far more efficiently than third-generation cephalosporins or ticarcillin.

The toxicity of antimicrobials is generally enhanced in a HAP/ICU setting. For example, many patients have renal impairment secondary to sepsis or hypotensive injury and in this setting, dosing of antibiotics such as imipenem, aminoglycosides and amphotericin B may increase the risk of convulsions and nephrotoxicity, respectively. Revision of traditional dosing regimes, for example, once daily aminoglycoside rather than divided doses may offset some of these toxic events. Careful dosing of aminoglycosides is essential for optimum therapeutic success whilst minimising toxicity. This will involve regular monitoring of the serum peak and trough levels and individualisation of dosing, using tables or computers. The input of a clinical pharmacokineticist should be obtained. Alternative agents with a higher therapeutic/toxicity ratio should be used as far as possible or careful frequent serum monitoring performed as outlined above. Similarly, it is important to avoid drugs which increase nephrotoxicity in a patient already renally impaired, for example, using liposomal amphotericin B rather than regular amphotericin B.

Appropriate use of antibiotics

Inappropriate prolonged antimicrobial use leads to emergence of resistant organisms with the propensity for patient to patient spread. Close monitoring of the duration of antimicrobial therapy will reduce this risk. Details of prior/current antibiotic therapy in patients with ongoing pneumonia may suggest modification of an antibiotic regimen. Inappropriate choices of antibiotics may be a feature in many hospitals. For example, the use of metronidazole alone in treating anaerobic infection of the lung may not be effective.

Initial antibiotic choice

This is shown in Table 19.7. For patients with HAP in whom no epidemiological/clinical clues are present to direct therapy, broad spectrum antibiotics with Gram-negative cover (including *Pseudomonas*) together with an antibiotic with antistaphylococcal cover are indicated. Suitable combinations include ceftazidime or ticarcillin or piperacillin or aztreonam together with nafcillin. Controversy exists over the use of aminoglycosides in the treatment of HAP-associated Gram-negative pneumonia. The rationale for their inclusion (synergistic effect, rapid rate of bacterial killing, prolonged post-antibiotic effect, diminution of resistant organisms, possible reduction in mortality rate) has already been discussed elsewhere. However, some physicians believe that they have little impact on the clinical outcome. Thus, there may be a narrow therapeutic–toxic ratio and poor penetration into respiratory secretions and infected lung. Studies which have compared β-lactam monotherapy to combination therapy of a β-lactam with an aminoglycoside have not shown significant differences in outcome. However, non-uniformity of study design, e.g. different β-lactams may have been used in the two arms[217] poses problems for precise evaluation. Nevertheless, in highly septic patients or those with neutropenia, addition of an aminoglycoside is wise. Many authorities would also routinely recommend this approach for any patient with pseudomonal pneumonia since the mortality rate is high. Moore and co-workers[218] reported that improved patient outcome from Gram-negative pneumonia was associated with gentamicin or tobramycin levels > 6 μg/ml and > 24 kg/ml for amikacin. Trials of large single daily dosing of aminoglycosides are ongoing. Penicillin-allergic patients could receive vancomycin in place of nafcillin and should be given aztreonam rather than other β-lactam antimicrobials as the cross-hypersensitivity of aztreonam with other β-lactams is extremely small. Alternatively, a quinolone could be used. It is important to remember that some monotherapy regimes whilst providing excellent Gram-negative coverage will cover *S. aureus* rather poorly, for example, third-generation cephalosporins when compared to second-generation cephalosporins.

If there is a background of chronic lung disease, *H. influenzae* will have to be covered. A third-generation cephalosporin such as ceftazidime would provide good therapy for both *Haemophilus* and *Pseudomonas* spp. If aspiration pneumonia is suspected then clindamycin or cefoxitin or imipenem (or meropenem) or metronidazole

Table 19.7. *Empirical antimicrobial therapy for HAP*

Acute HAP	Third-generation cephalosporin or anti-pseudomonal penicillin (± gentamicin) plus Nafcillin	(Aztreonam or ciprofloxacin for penicillin allergy) (vancomycin for penicillin allergy)
Aspiration pneumonia	Clindamycin or Cefoxitin or third-generation cephalosporin plus Metronidazole	
MRSA pneumonia	Vancomycin ± Rifampicin	

HAP = hospital-acquired pneumonia.
MRSA = methicillin resistant *S. aureus*.

in combination with another broader spectrum antimicrobial are reasonable first choices. For patients at high risk of MRSA pneumonia, then vancomycin ± rifampicin is indicated. In certain immunocompromised patients who may be at risk for nosocomial Legionellosis, intravenous erythromycin or ciprofloxacin should be used. For the treatment of patients at risk from fungal, viral, protozoal or tuberculosis see relevant chapters on these agents, and in the risk settings.

Inhaled antimicrobials

The outcome of pneumonia treated with aminoglycosides may be related to the attainment of adequate peak levels, which in turn may reflect the importance of achieving optimum bronchial secretion levels[218]. This issue and the relatively high incidence of aminoglycoside related toxicity has led to the exploration of the use of inhaled aminoglycosides.

This approach has been used particularly in cystic fibrosis patients in whom modest improvement in parameters such as pulmonary function tests, sputum volume, and general well-being has been noted in some studies[219]. Antipseudomonal penicillins and cephalosporins have also been used in these patients with some benefit (see Chapter 24).

In patients other than those with cystic fibrosis who have Gram-negative pneumonia, there has been some success in terms of a significant reduction in mortality rate in patients receiving endotracheal sisomicin with carbenicillin when compared to carbenicillin and endotracheal saline[200], but in another study comparing endotracheal tobramycin or saline + systemic tobramycin + ceftazidime/piperacillin, there was no reduction in mortality or impact on clinical improvement, although there was a increased eradication of pathogens from tracheal secretions[220]. Instillation of antimicrobials directly into the endotracheal tree is therefore not routinely advocated at this time but may have a place in individual complex cases.

As with the prophylactic role of locally administered antibiotics, detailed pharmacokinetic studies need to be performed to describe the amount and anatomical distribution of antibiotics as well as its absorption in order to rationalise the mode of administration – as has been done for aerosolised pentamidine in the treatment and prophylaxis of *P. carinii* pneumonia. Once this has been completed, carefully designed prospective studies can be performed to investigate this potentially important therapeutic option.

Immunotherapy

In the light of the high mortality associated with nosocomial pneumonia, new therapeutic strategies for prevention or therapy are currently being studied. Serotype specific vaccines, hyperimmune globulins and monoclonal antibodies against Gram-negative pathogens such as *P. aeruginosa* are some of the immunological approaches being investigated. In addition, anticytokine antibody therapy to down-modulate infection-initiated inflammatory lung damage has been another approach of investigation but, to date, there has been no clinical evidence supporting immunotherapy related treatment for patients with nosocomial pneumonia.

Antimicrobial use and abuse in nosocomial pneumonia

Antimicrobial prescribing in hospitals, in general, is inappropriate in between 11% and 87% of patients[221–224]. Although data specifically relating to HAP is sparse, there is no reason to believe that the inappropriate use of antibiotics is any less of a feature. In fact, the frequency of usage of antibiotics among patients admitted to ICUs, many of whom have pneumonia, is usually well in excess of 50%[225,226] and in these more ill patients one might expect a tendency to a high frequency of usage. In a study of patients with community- and hospital-acquired pneumonia, it is common practice to treat sicker patients with multiple or extreme broad spectrum antibiotics whilst errors towards undertreating appear to be rather uncommon[227]. An unsatisfactory clinical outcome including a high mortality rate is often associated with a larger number of antibiotics per patient[227] – which may reflect diagnostic uncertainty. HAP may be over-diagnosed in as many as a fifth of patients[6] – for example, colonisation may be confused with infection, non-infectious processes confused with infectious processes, for example, pulmonary haemorrhage or ARDS – and may lead to unnecessary use of antimicrobials. In a recent report of pneumococcal bacteraemia (of which 85% had pneumonia) an unnecessarily broad spectrum antibiotic was given, despite a specific microbiological diagnosis, in more than one-third of patients[228]. Other reports have focused on the poor quality of prescribing of antibiotics, for example, incorrect timing of administration of intravenous antibiotics which could result in subtherapeutic levels or inappropriately high prescribing of parenteral antibiotics when oral preparations would be as effective[229].

A reliable method requires to be established in this complex field of evaluating antimicrobial drug use[230], on which to base approaches to assess and improve this aspect of patient care. In the case of HAP, an organised approach to the diagnosis is necessary. This involves obtaining a specific microbial aetiology by appropriate investigations wherever possible and extrapolating from the patient's clinical profile and local hospital epidemiology and hence selecting and correctly

Table 19.8. *Patients off antibiotics, haemodynamically stable*

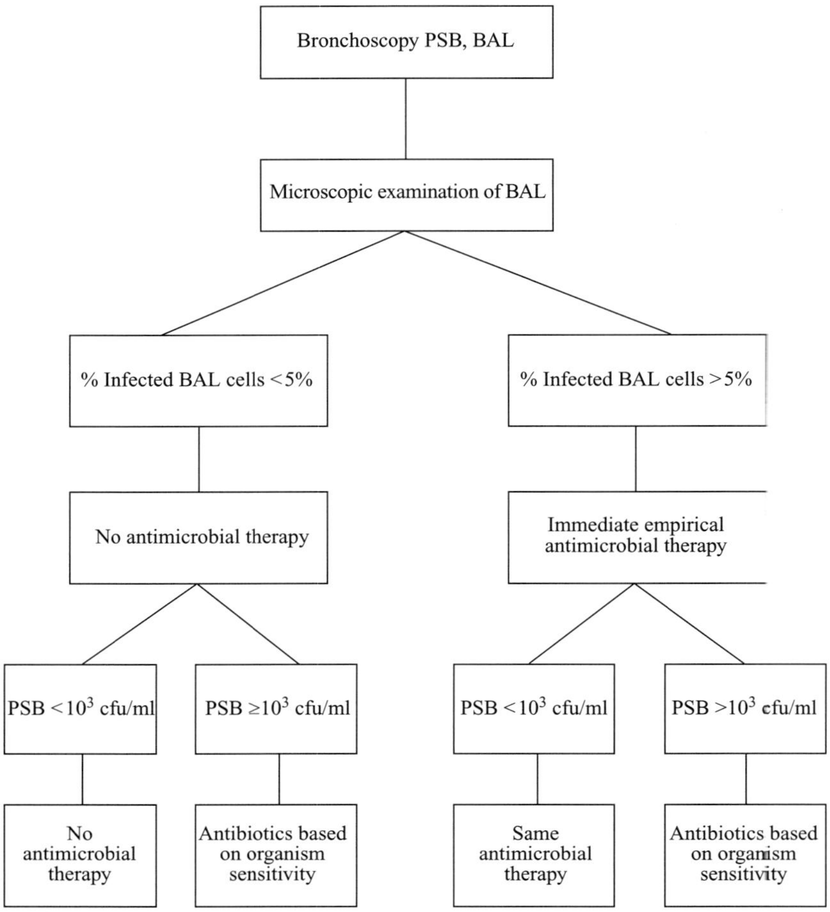

utilising antimicrobial therapy. Attempts at optimising antibiotic use have included an up-to-date local formulary, restriction of antibiotics, educational lectures and audits[231]. The success of these various methods in improving the use of antibiotics have, at best, been variable. Probably non-confrontational clinical interaction between the primary physician, an infectious diseases physician and a clinical pharmacologist would be the most acceptable and fruitful way to improve the use of antibiotics[226,231]. Some such studies have already suggested that benefits can be achieved – for example, considerable cost savings[232], but further good studies are needed to assess other outcomes including emergence of antibiotic resistance and ultimate patient outcome.

Recommendations for diagnosis and management of HAP in ventilated patients

For critically ill mechanically ventilated patients not receiving antibiotics who develop clinical features suggestive of pneumonia and have no contraindications to bronchoscopy (haemodynamically stable) then protected specimen brush and bronchoalveolar lavage is recommended as part of the diagnostic workup (Table 19.8). Nonbronchoscopically obtained bronchoalveolar lavage or plugged telescoped catheter are alternative methods to obtain lung secretions for analysis[185]. Microscopic examination BAL fluid for intracellular organisms >5%[109] is suggestive of pneumonia and Gram's stain can guide antimicrobial therapy pending results of quantitative cultures. If the results prove negative for lung infection, other potential sources for fever and pulmonary infiltrates should be sought out. In cases where borderline quantitative culture results are obtained or no alternative cause for fever can be found, a follow-up bronchoscopy may yield positive results. In those patients with evidence of systemic sepsis and hypotension, initiation of broad spectrum antibiotics should not be delayed. Exclusion of extra-pulmonary sources of infection which may exist in addition to pneumonia require full investigation from common sites such as vascular lines, urinary catheters, sinuses and intra-abdominal sources[185].

For those patients receiving antimicrobial therapy for a specified infection, a full course should be completed. However, if nosocomial pneumonia develops while on antibiotics, the likelihood of resistant organisms to the current antibiotic regimen is high. The options (Table 19.9) then are to empirically change antibiotics or perform bronchoscopy with PSB and BAL knowing the results may be difficult to interpret. In patients who do not have evidence of systemic inflammatory response syndrome or worsening multi-system organ failure, withholding antibiotics for 24–48 hours and obtaining respiratory secretions by invasive or non-invasive techniques may be the most appropriate strategy.

Table 19.9. *Patients on antimicrobial therapy*

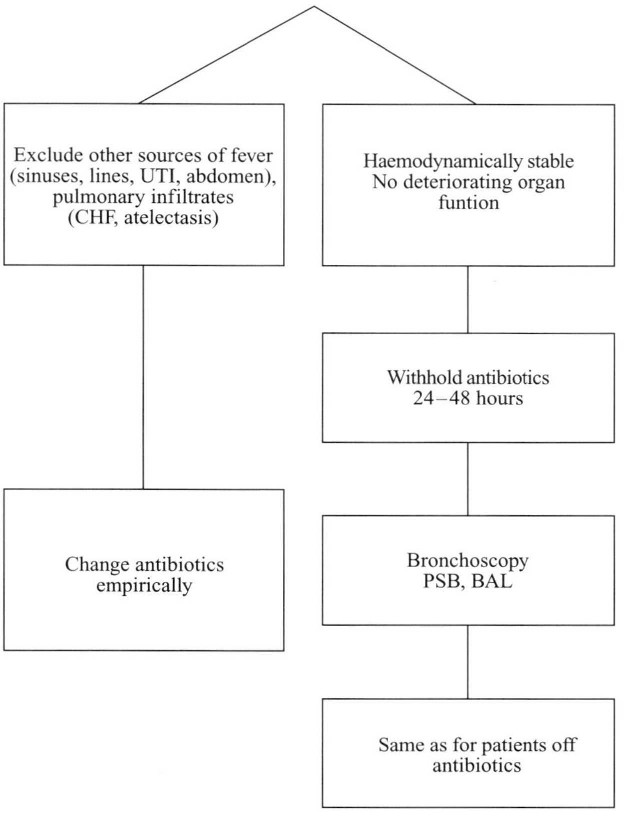

References

1. MEERS PD, AYLIFFE GAJ, EMMERSON AM *et al.* Survey of infection in hospitals. *J Hosp Infect* 1981; 2:1–11.
2. HORAN TC, WHITE JW, JARVIS WR *et al.* Nosocomial infection surveillance 1984. MMWR CDC *Surveillance Summaries* 1986; 35:SS17–29.
3. JOHANSON WG JR, PIERCE AK, SANFORD JP, THOMAS GD Nosocomial respiratory infections with gram-negative bacilli: the significance of colonisation of the respiratory tract. *Ann Intern Med* 1972; 77:701–6.
4. SALATA RA, LEDERMAN MM, SHLAES DM *et al.* Diagnosis of nosocomial pneumonia in intubated intensive care patients. *Am Rev Resp Dis* 1987; 135(2):426–32.
5. GARNER JS, JARVIS WR, EMORI TG, HORAN TC. CDC definitions for nosocomial infections. *Am J Infect Control* 1988; 16:128–40.
6. ANDREWS CP, COALSON JJ, SMITH JD, JOHANSON WG JR. Diagnosis of nosocomial bacterial pneumonia in acute diffuse lung injury. *Chest* 1981; 80:254–8.
7. BELL RC, COALSON JJ, SMITH JD, JOHANSON WG JR. Multiple organ system failure and infection in adult respiratory distress syndrome. *Ann Intern Med* 1983; 99:293–8.
8. FAGON JY, CHASTRE J, HANCE AJ, MONTRAVERS P, NOVORA A, GIBERT C. Nosocomial pneumonia in ventilated patients: a cohort study evaluating attributable mortality and hospital stay. *Am J Med* 1993; 94:281–8.
9. FAGON JY, CHASTRE J, DOMART Y *et al.* Nosocomial pneumonia in patients receiving continuous mechanical ventilation: prospective analysis of 52 episodes with use of a protected specimen brush and quantitative culture technique. *Am Rev Resp Dis* 1989; 139:877–84.
10. PINGLETON SK, FAGON JY, LEEPER KU. Patient selection for clinical investigation of ventilator-associated pneumonia. Criteria for evaluating diagnostic techniques. International Consensus Conference on the Clinical Investigation of Ventilator Associated Pneumonia. *Chest* 1992; 102(5):553S–6S.

10a. COOK D, BRUN-BUISSON C, GUYATT GH, SIBBALD WJ. Evaluation of new diagnostic technologies: bronchoalveolar lavage and the diagnosis of ventilator-associated pneumonia. *Crit Care Med* 1994; 22:1314–22.

11. HALEY RW, HOOTEN TM, CULVER DH *et al.* Nosocomial infections in US hospitals 1975–1976; estimated frequency by selected characteristics of patients. *Am J Med* 1981; 70:947–59.
12. PUGLIESE G, LICHTENBERG DA. Nosocomial bacterial pneumonia: an overview. *Am J Infect Control* 1987; 15:249–65.
13. VERBIST L, for the International Study Group. Epidemiology of ICU and hematology/oncology bacterial isolates in Europe. *18th International Congress of Chemotherapy*, Stockholm, Sweden, 1993. Abstract No 5031.
14. HUGHES JM, CULVER DH, WHITE JW *et al.* Nosocomial Infection Surveillance 1980–82. *MMWR CDC Surveillance Summaries* 1983; 32:1SS–16SS.
15. GARIBALDI RA, BRITT MR, COLEMAN

ML, READING JC, PACE NL. Risk factors for postoperative pneumonia. *Am J Med* 1981; 70:677–80.

16. STEVENS RM, TERES D, SKILLMAN JJ, FEINGOLD DS. Pneumonia in an intensive care unit: a thirty-month experience. *Arch Intern Med* 1974; 134:106–11.
17. POTGEITER PD, HAMMOND JMJ. Aetiology and diagnosis of pneumonia requiring ICU admission. *Chest* 1992; 101:199–203.
18. RELLO J, AUSINA V, CASTELLA J, NET A, PRATS G. Nosocomial respiratory tract infections in multiple trauma patients. Influence of level of consciousness with implications for therapy. *Chest* 1992; 102:525–9.
19. CELIS R, TORRES A, GATELL JM, ALMEDA M, RODRIGUEZ RR, AGUSTI VA. Nosocomial pneumonia. A multivariate analysis of risk and prognosis. *Chest* 1988; 93:318–24.
20. RODRIGUEZ JL. Hospital-acquired gram-negative pneumonia in critically ill, injured patients. *Am J Surg* 1993; 165:34–42.
21. NIELSEN SL, RODER B, MAGNUSSEN P, ENGQUIST A, FRIMODT-MOLLER N. Nosocomial pneumonia in an intensive care unit in a Danish University Hospital: incidence, mortality and aetiology. *Scand J Infect Dis* 1992; 24:65–70.
22. JARVIS WR, EDWARDS JR, CULVER DH *et al.* The National Nosocomial Infections Surveillance System. *Am J Med* 1991; 91:185–91.
23. BRYAN CS, REYNOLDS KL. Bacteremic nosocomial pneumonia: analysis of 172 episodes from a single metropolitan area. *Am Rev Resp Dis* 1984; 129:668–71.
24. SCHLEUPNER CJ, COBB DK. A study of the etiologies and treatment of nosocomial pneumonia in a community based teaching hospital. *Infect Control Hosp Epidemiol* 1992; 13:515–25.
25. CRAIG CP, CONNELLY S. Effect of intensive care unit nosocomial pneumonia on duration of stay and mortality. *Am J Infect Control* 1984; 12:233–8.
26. CRAVEN DE, KUNCHES LM, KILINSKY V, LICHTENBERG DA, MAKE BJ, MCCABE WR. Risk factors for pneumonia and fatality in patients receiving continuous mechanical ventilation. *Am Rev Resp Dis* 1986; 133:792–6.
27. DRIKS MR, CRAVEN DE, CELLI BR *et al.* Nosocomial pneumonia in intubated patients given sucralfate as compared with antacids or histamine type 2 blockers: the role of gastric colonisation. *N Engl J Med* 1987; 317:1376–82.
28. TORRES A, AZNAR R, GATELL JM *et al.* Incidence, risk, and prognosis factors of nosocomial pneumonia in mechanically ventilated patients. *Am Rev Resp Dis* 1990; 142:523–8.
29. SEIDENFELD JJ, POHL DF, BELL RC, HARRIS GD, JOHANSON WG JR. Incidence, site, and outcome of infections in patients with the adult respiratory distress syndrome. *Am Rev Resp Dis* 1986; 134:12–16.
30. MOSCONI P, LANGER M, CIGADA M, MANDELLI M. Epidemiology and risk factors of pneumonia in critically ill patients. Intensive Care Group for Infection Control. *Eur J Epidemiol* 1991; 7:320–7.
31. HANSON LC, WEBER DJ, RUTALA WA. Risk factors for nosocomial pneumonia in the elderly. *Am J Med* 1992; 92:161–6.
32. KAPPSTEIN I, SCHULGEN G, BEYER U, GEIGER K, SCHUMACHER M, DASHNER FD. Prolongation of hospital stay and extra costs due to ventilator-associated pneumonia in an intensive care unit. *Eur J Clin Microbiol Infect Dis* 1992; 11:504–8.
33. SPENCER RC. Nosocomial infection in the intensive care unit: a question of surveillance. *Intens Care World* 1993; 10(4):173–6.
34. SCHABERG DR, CULVER DH, GAYNES RP. Major trends in the microbial aetiology of nosocomial infection. *Am J Med* 1991; 91:72–5.
35. TORRES A, PUIG DE LA BELLACASSA J, XAUBERT A *et al.* Diagnostic value of quantitative cultures of bronchoalveolar lavage and telescoping plugged catheters in mechanically ventilated patients with bacterial pneumonia. *Am Rev Resp Dis* 1989; 140:306–10.
36. CRAVEN DE, BARBER TW, STEGER KA, MONTECALVO MA. Nosocomial pneumonia in the 90's: update of epidemiology and risk factors. *Semin Resp Infect* 1990; 5:157–72.
37. HESSEN MT, KAYE D. Nosocomial pneumonia. *Crit Care Clin* 1988; 4:245–57.
38. BARTLET JG, O'KEEFE P, TALLY FP, LOUIE TJ, GORBACH SL. Bacteriology of hospital acquired pneumonia. *Arch Int Med* 1986; 146:868–71.
39. BONTEN MJM, VAN TIEL FH, VAN DER GEEST S *et al.* Enterococcus faecalis pneumonia complicating topical antimicrobial prophylaxis. *N Engl J Med* 1993; 328:209–10.
40. PANNUTI C, GINGRICH R, PFALLER MA, KAO C, WENZEL RP. Nosocomial pneumonia in patients having bone marrow transplant. *Cancer* 1992; 69:2653–62.
41. HUMPHREYS H, JOHNSON EM, WARNOCK DW, WILLATTS SM, WINTER RJ, SPELLER DCE. An outbreak of aspergillosis in a general ITU. *J Hosp Infect* 1991; 18:167–77.
42. KIMBALL AM, FOY HM, COONEY MK, ALLAN ID, MATLOCK M, PLORDE JJ. Isolation of respiratory syncytial virus and influenza viruses from the sputum of patients hospitalised with pneumonia. *J Infect Dis* 1983; 147:181–4.
43. ENGLUND JA, ANDERSON LJ, RHAME FS. Nosocomial transmission of respiratory syncytial virus in immunocompromised adults. *J Clin Microbiol* 1991; 29:115–19.
44. GUIDRY GG, BLACK-PAYNE CA, PAYNE DK, JAMISON RM, GEORGE RB, BOCCHINI JA JR. Respiratory syncytial virus infection among intubated adults in a university medical intensive care unit. *Chest* 1991; 99:1377–84.
45. HARRINGTON RD, HOOTON TM, HACKMAN RC *et al.* An outbreak of respiratory syncytial virus in a bone marrow transplant centre. *J Infect Dis* 1992; 165:987–93.
46. RHAME FS, STREIFEL AJ, KERSEY JH JR, MCGLAVE PB. Extrinsic risk factors for pneumonia in the patient at high risk for infection. *Am J Med* 1984; 76(5A):42–52.
47. JOHNSON JT, YU VL, BEST MG *et al.* Nosocomial legionellosis in surgical patients with head and neck cancer: implications for epidemiologic reservoir and mode of transmission. *Lancet* 1985; 2:298–300.
48. CENTERS FOR DISEASE CONTROL. Tuberculosis outbreak among HIV infected persons. *MMWR* 1991; 40:649–52.
49. CENTERS FOR DISEASE CONTROL. Nosocomial transmission of multidrug resistant tuberculosis to health care workers and HIV infected patients in an urban hospital in Florida. *MMWR* 1990; 39:718–22.
50. GREENBERG PD, LAX KG, SCHECTER CB. Tuberculosis in house staff. A decision analysis comparing the tuberculin screening strategy with the BCG vaccination. *Am Rev Resp Dis* 1991; 143:490–5.
51. JOHANSON WG JR, PIERCE AK, SANFORD JP. Changing pharyngeal bacterial flora of hospitalised patients: emergence of Gram-negative bacilli. *N Engl J Med* 1969; 281:1137–40.
52. NIEDERMAN MS, CRAVEN DE, FEIN AM, SCHULTZ DE. Pneumonia in the critically ill hospitalised patient. *Chest* 1990; 97:170–81.
53. SCHWARTZ SN, DOWLING JN, BENKOVIC C, DEQUITTNER-BUCHANAN M, PROSTKO T, YEE RB. Sources of Gram-negative bacilli colonizing the trachea of intubated patients. *J Infect Dis* 1978; 138:227–31.
54. BARTLETT JG, FALING LJ, WILLEY S. Quantitative tracheal bacteriologic and cytologic studies in patients with long term tracheostomies. *Chest* 1978; 74:635–9.
55. SOTTILE FD, MARRIE TJ, PROUGH *et al.* Nosocomial pulmonary infection: possible etiologic significance of bacterial adhesion to endotracheal tubes. *Crit Care Med* 1986; 14:265–70.
56. CROSS AS, ROUP B. Role of respiratory assistance devices in endemic nosocomial pneumonia. *Am J Med* 1981; 70:681–5.

57. LANGER M, MOSCONI P, CIGADA M, MANDELLI M. Long-term respiratory support and risk of pneumonia in critically ill patients. Intensive Care Unit Group of Infection Control. *Am Rev Resp Dis* 1989; 140:302–5.
58. JOSHI N, LOCALIO AR, HAMORY BH. A predictive risk index for nosocomial pneumonia in the intensive care unit. *Am J Med* 1992; 93:135–42.
59. MCDONALD AM, DIETSCHE L, LITSCHE M *et al.* A retrospective study of nosocomial pneumonia at a long-term care facility. *Am J Infect Control* 1992; 20:234–8.
60. WOODS DE. Role of fibronectin in the pathogenesis of gram-negative bacillary pneumonia. *Rev Infect Dis* 1987; 9:5386–90.
61. JOHANSON WG JR, HIGUCHI JH, CHAUDHURI T, WOODS DE. Bacterial adherence to epithelial cells in bacillary colonisation of the respiratory tract. *Am Rev Resp Dis* 1980; 121:55–63.
62. WOODS DE, STRAUS DC, JOHNSON WG JR, BERRY UK, BASS JA. Role of pili in adherence of pseudomonas aeruginosa to mammalian buccal epithelial cells. *Infect Immunol* 1980; 29:1146–51.
63. BROOK I. Bacterial colonisation, tracheostomy and long-term intubation in pediatric patients. *Chest* 1978; 74:635–9.
64. NIEDERMAN MS, MANTOVANNI R, SCHOCH P, PAPAS J, FEIN AM. Patterns and routes of tracheobronchial colonisation in mechanically ventilated patients: the role of nutritional status in colonisation of the lower airway by *Pseudomonas* species. *Chest* 1989; 95:155–61.
65. BRYANT LR, TRINKLE JK, MOBIN-UDDIN K, BAKER J, GRIFFEN WO JR. Bacterial colonisation profile with tracheal intubation and mechanical ventilation. *Arch Surg* 1972; 104:647–51.
66. INGLIS TJJ, SHERRATT MJ, SPROAT LJ, GIBSON JS, HAWKEY PM. Gastroduodenal dysfunction and bacterial colonisation of the ventilated lung. *Lancet* 1993; 341:911–13.
67. KLEIN BS, PERLOFF WH, MAKI DG. Reduction of nosocomial infection during pediatric intensive care protective isolation. *N Engl J Med* 1989; 26:1714–21.
68. REINARZ JA, PIERCE AK, MAYS BB *et al.* The potential role of inhalation therapy equipment in nosocomial pulmonary infection. *J Clin Invest* 1965; 44:831–9.
69. CRAVEN DE, GOULARTE TA, MAKE BJ. Contaminated condensate in mechanical ventilator circuits. A risk factor for nosocomial pneumonia? *Am Rev Resp Dis* 1984; 129:625–8.
70. DREYFUSS D, DJEDAINI K, WEBER P *et al.* Prospective study of nosocomial pneumonia and of patient and circuit colonisation during mechanical ventilation with circuit changes every 48 hours vs no change. *Am Rev Resp Dis* 1991; 143:738–43.
71. ATHERTON ST, WHITE DJ. Stomach as source of bacteria colonizing the respiratory tract during artificial ventilation. *Lancet* 1978; 2:968–9.
72. GORBACH SL. Population control in the small gut. *Gut* 1976; 8:530–2.
73. GIANELLA RA, BROITMAN SA, ZAMCHECK N. Influence of gastric acidity on bacterial and parasitic enteric infections. A perspective. *Ann Intern Med* 1973; 78:271–6.
74. REED PJ, SMITH PL, HAINES K, HOUSE FR, WALTERS CL. Gastric juice *N*-nitrosamines in health and gastrointestinal disease. *Lancet* 1980; 2:550.
75. DONOWITZ LG, PAGE MC, MILEUR BL, GUENTHNER SH. Alteration of normal gastric flora in critical care patients receiving antacid and cimetidine therapy. *Infect Control* 1986; 7:23–6.
76. RUDDELL WSJ, AXON ATR, FINDLAY JM. Effect of cimetidine on the gastric bacterial flora. *Lancet* 1980; 1:672–4.
77. DU MOULIN GC, PATERSON DG, HEDLEY-WHYTER J, LISBON A. Aspiration of gastric bacteria in antacid treated patients: a frequent cause of postoperative colonisation of the airway. *Lancet* 1982; 1:242–5.
78. DASCHNER F, KAPPSTEIN I, ENGELS I *et al.* Stress ulcer prophylaxis and ventilation pneumonias: prevention by antibacterial cytoprotective agents. *Infect Control Hosp Epidemiol* 1988; 9:59–65.
79. FORSTER A, NIETHAMER T, SUTER P *et al.* Influence de la cimetidine sur la croissance baterienne dans le liquide gastrique. *Nouv Press Med* 1982; 11:2281–83.
80. SJOSTEDT S, KAGER L, HEIMDAHL A, NORD CE Microbial colonisation of tumours in relation to the upper gastrointestinal tract in patients with gastric carcinoma. *Ann Surg* 1988; 207:341–6.
81. SCHINDLBECK NE, LIPPERT M, HEINRICH C, MULLER-LISSNER SA. Intragastric bile acid concentrations in critically ill artificially ventilated patients. *Am J Gastroenterol* 1989; 84:624–8.
82. UNERTL K, RUCKDESCHEL G, SELBMANN HK *et al.* Prevention of colonisation and respiratory infections in long-term ventilated patients by local antimicrobial prophylaxis. *Intens Care Med* 1987; 13:106–13.
83. BRUN-BUISSON C, LEGRAND P, RAUSS A *et al.* Intestinal decontamination for control of nosocomial multiresistant Gram-negative bacilli. *Ann Intern Med* 1989; 110:873–81.
84. GODARD J, GUILLAUME C, REVERDY ME *et al.* Intestinal decontamination in a polyvalent ICU: A double blind study. *Intens Care Med* 1990; 16:307–11.
85. BROWN C, REES WDW. Drug treatment for acute gastrointestinal bleeding. *Br Med J* 1992; 304:135–6.
86. APTE NM, KARNAD DR, MEDHEKAR TP, TILVE GH, MORYE S, BHAVE GG. Gastric colonisation and pneumonia in intubated critically ill patients receiving stress ulcer prophylaxis. A randomised control trial. *Crit Care Med* 1992; 20:590–3.
87. CHEADLE WG, VITALE GC, MACKIE CR, CUSCHIERI A. Prophylactic postoperative nasogastric decompression. A prospective study of its requirement and the influence of cimetidine in 200 patients. *Ann Surg*ery 1985; 202:361–6.
88. LUNDELL L, PERSSON G. Does preoperative treatment with cimetidine increase the risk of postoperative infection. *Ann Chirug et Gynecol* 1983; 72:312–16.
89. REUSSER P, ZIMMERLI W, SCHEIDEGGER D, MARBET GA, BUSER M, GYR K. Role of gastric colonisation in nosocomial infections and endotoxemia: a prospective study in neurosurgical patients on mechanical ventilation. *J Infect Dis* 1989; 160:414–21.
90. HOLZAPFEL L, DAVEAU L, COUPRY A *et al.* Prophylaxis against stress induced bleeding and nosocomial pneumonia in patients on mechanical ventilation (Abstract). *Intensive Care Med* 1990; 16(1):54.
91. KARISTADT R, HERSON J, PALMER R, FRANK W, YOUNG M. Cimetidine reduces upper GI bleeding and nosocomial pneumonia in intensive care unit patients (Abstract). *Am J Gastroenterol* 1989; 84:1162.
92. COOK DJ, FULLER HD, GUYATT *et al.* Risk factors for gastrointestinal bleeding in critically ill patients. *N Engl J Med* 1994; 330:377–81.
93. BEN-MENACHEM T, FOGEL R, PATEL R *et al.* Prophylaxis for stress induced gastric haemorrhage in the medical intensive care unit. *Ann Intern Med* 1994; 121:568–75.
94. EDDLESTON JM, VOHRA A, SCOTT *et al.* A comparison of the frequency of stress ulceration and secondary pneumonia in sucralfate or ranitidine treated intensive care unit patients. *Crit Care Med* 1991; 19:1491–6.
95. KAPPSTEIN I, SCHULGEN G, FRIEDRICH T *et al.* Incidence of pneumonia in mechanically ventilated patients treated with sucralfate or cimetidine as prophylaxis for stress bleeding, bacterial colonisation of the stomach. *Am J Med* 1991; 91(Suppl2A):125S–31S.
96. TRYBA M. Risk of acute stress bleeding and nosocomial pnemonia in ventilated intensive care unit patients: sucralfate versus antacids. *Am J Med* 1987; 83(3B):125–7.
97. GARCIA-LABATTUT A, RODRIGUEZ-MUNOZ S, GOBERNADO-SERRANO M.

Sucralfate versus cimetidine in stress bleeding prophylaxis (Abstract). *Intens Care Med* 1990; 16(1):S19.

98. TRYBA M. Stress bleeding prophylaxis with sucralfate. Pathophysiological basis and clinical use. *Scan J Gastroenterol* 1990; 25:22–33.

99. VOGELAERS D, COLARDYN F, VERSCHRAEGEN G *et al.* A comparison of cimetidine and sucralfate for stress ulcer prophylaxis in medical patients in the ICU. *Am J Med* (in press).

100. RYAN P, DAWSON J, TERES D, NAVAB F Continuous infusion of cimetidine versus sucralfate: incidence of pneumonia and bleeding compared (Abstract). *Crit Care Med* 1990; 18:S253.

101. PROD'HOM G, LEVENBERGER P, KOERFER J *et al.* Nosocomial pneumonia in mechanically ventilated patients receiving antacid, ranitidine or sucralfate as prophylaxis for stress ulcer. a randomized control trial. *Ann Intern Med* 1994; 120:653–62.

102. TREOLAR DM, STECHMILLER J. Pulmonary aspiration in tube-fed patients with artificial airways. *Heart Lung* 1984; 13:667–71.

103. JACOBS S, CHANG RWS, LEE B *et al.* Continuous enteral feeding: a major cause of pneumonia among ventilated intensive care unit patients. *J Parenter Enteral Nut* 1990; 14:353–6.

104. BONTEN MJM, GAILLARD CA, VAN TIEL FH, VAN DER GEEST S, STROBBERINGH EE. Continous enteral feeding counteracts preventive measures for gastric colonisation in intensive care unit patients. *Crit Care Med* 1994; 22:939–44.

105. REDAN JA, RUSH BF, LYSZ TW, SMITH S, MACHIEDO GW. Organ distribution of gut derived bacteria caused by bowel manipulation or ischemia. *J Trauma* 1990; 159:85–90.

106. FIDDIAN-GREEN RG, BAKER S. Nosocomial pneumonia in the critically ill: product of aspiration or translocation? *Crit Care Med* 1991; 19:763–9.

107. CHASTRE J, VIAU F, BRUN P *et al.* Prospective evaluation of the protected specimen brush for the diagnosis of pulmonary infections in ventilated patients. *Am Rev Resp Dis* 1984; 130:924–9.

108. WUNDERINK RG, WOLDENBERG LS, ZEISS J, DAY CM, CLEMINS LACHER DA. The radiological diagnosis of autopsy-proven ventilator-associated pneumonia. *Chest* 1992; 101:458–63.

109. CHASTRE J, FAGON JY. Invasive diagnostic testing should be routinely used to manage ventilated patients with suspected pneumonia. *Am J Resp Crit Care Med* 1994; 150:570–4.

110. NIEDERMAN MS, TORRES A, SUMMER W. Invasive diagnostic testing is not needed routinely to manage suspected ventilator-associated pneumonia. *Am J Resp Crit Care Med* 1994; 150:565–9.

111. HILL J, RATLIFF JL, PARROT JCW *et al.* Pulmonary pathology in acute respiratory insufficiency: lung biopsy as a diagnostic tool. *J Thorac Cardiovasc Surg* 1976; 71:64–71.

112. TORRES A, PUIG DE LA BELLACASSA, RODRIGUEZ-ROISON R, JIMINEZ DE, ANTA MT, AGUSTI-VIDAL A. Diagnostic value of telescoping plugged catheters in mechanically ventilated patients with bacterial pneumonia using the Metras catheter. *Am Rev Resp Dis* 1988; 138:117–20.

113. EL-EBIARY M, TORRES A, GONZALES J *et al.* Diagnosis of ventilator associated pneumonia: diagnostic value of quantitative cultures of endotracheal aspirates (Abstract). *Am Rev Resp Dis* 1991; 143:A104.

114. PAPAZIAN L, MARTIN C, ALBANESE J *et al.* Comparison of two methods of bacteriologic sampling of the lower respiratory tract: a study in ventilated patients with nosocomial bronchopneumonia. *Crit Care Med* 1989; 17:461–4.

115. MARQUETTE CH, GEORGES H, WALLET F *et al.* Diagnostic efficiency of endotracheal aspirates with quantitative bacterial cultures in intubated patients with suspected pneumonia: comparison with the protected specimen brush. *Am Rev Resp Dis* 1993; 148:138–44.

116. EL-EBIARY M, TORRES A, GONZALES J *et al.* Use of elastin fibre detection in the diagnosis of ventilator associated pneumonia. *Thorax* 1995; 50:14–17.

117. WINTERBAUER RH, HUTCHINSON JF, REINHARAT GW *et al.* The use of quantitative cultures and antibody coating of bacteria to diagnose bacterial pneumonia by fiberoptic bronchoscopy. *Am Rev Resp Dis* 1983; 17:255–9.

118. LAMBERT RS, VEREEN LE, GEORGE RB Comparison of tracheal aspirate and protected specimen brush catheter specimens for identifying pathogenic bacteria in mechanically ventilated patients. *Am J Med Sci* 1989; 297:377–82.

119. WUNDERINK RG, RUSSELL GB, MEZGER E *et al.* The diagnostic utility of the antibody coated bacteria test in intubated patients. *Chest* 1991; 99:84–88.

120. JOHANSON WG JR, SIEDENTELD JJ, GOMEZ P, DELOS SANTOS R, COALSON JJ. Bacteriologic diagnosis of nosocomial pneumonia following prolonged mechanical ventilation. *Am Rev Resp Dis* 1988; 137:259–64.

121. ROUBY JJ, MARTIN DE LA SALLE E, POETE P *et al.* Nosocomial pneumonia in the critically ill. Histologic and bacteriologic aspects. *Am Rev Resp Dis* 1992; 146:1059–66.

122. PHAM LH, BRUN-BUISSON P, LEGRAND P *et al.* Diagnosis of nosocomial pneumonia inmechanically ventilated patients. Comparison of a plugged telescoping catheter with the protected specimen brush. *Am Rev Resp Dis* 1991; 143:1055–61.

123. ROUBY JJ, ROSSIGNON MD, NICOLAS MH *et al.* A prospective study of protected bronchoalveolar lavage in the diagnosis of nosocomial pneumonia. *Anesthesiology* 1989; 71:679–85.

124. BAUGHMAN RP, THORPE JE, STANECK J, RASHKIN M, FRAME PT. Use of the protected specimen brush in patients with endotracheal or tracheostomy tubes. *Chest* 1987; 91:233–6.

125. BRONSON M, MEDURI GU, LEEPER KV *et al.* Pneumonia in ARDS: Diagnostic value of bilateral sampling (abstract). *Am Rev Resp Dis* 1993; 147:A355.

126. KUBOTA Y, MAGARIBUCHI T, TOYODA Y *et al.* Selective bronchial suctioning in the adult using a curve-tipped catheter with a guide mark. *Crit Care Med* 1982; 10:767–9.

127. GASSORGUES P, PIPERNO D, BACHMAN P *et al.* Comparison of non-bronchoscopic broncheolar lavage to open lung biopsy for bacteriologic diagnosis of pulmonary infections in mechanically ventilated patients. *Intens Care Med* 1989; 15:94–8.

128. PUGIN J, AUCKENTHALER R, MILI N, JANSSENS JP, LEW PD, SUTER PM. Diagnosis of ventilator associated pneumonia by bacteriologic analysis of bronchoscopic and nonbronchoscopic 'blind' broncheolar lavage fluid. *Am Rev Resp Dis* 1991; 143:1121–9.

129. MONTRAVERS P, GAUZIT R, DOMBRET MC, BLANCHET F, DESMONTS JM. Cardiopulmonary effects of bronchoalveolar lavage in critically ill patients. *Chest* 1993; 104:1541–7.

130. STEINBERG KP, MITCHELL DR, MAUNDER RJ, MULBERG JA, WHITCOMB ME, HUDSON LD. Safety of bronchoalveolar lavage in patients with adult respiratory distress syndrome. *Am Rev Resp Dis* 1993; 148:556–61.

131. MEDURI GU, CHASTRE J. The standardisation of bronchoscopic techniques for ventilator associated pneumonia. *Chest* 1992; 102 (suppl 1):557S–64S.

132. CRAWFORD SW, BOWDEN RA, HACKMAN RC, GLEAVES CA, MEYERS JD, CLARK JG. Rapid detection of cytomegalovirus pulmonary infection by bronchoalveolar lavage and centrifugation culture. *Ann Intern Med* 1988; 108:180–5.

133. RUUTU P, RUUTU R, VOLIN L, TUKIAINEN P, UKKONEN P, HOVI T. Cytomegalovirus is frequently isolated in bronchoalveolar lavage fluid of bone marrow transplant recipients without pneumonia. *Ann Intern Med* 1990; 112:913–6.

134. SCHMIDT GM, HORAK DA, NILAND JC, DUNCAN SR, FORMAN SJ, ZAIA J, AND THE CITY OF HOPE-STANDARD-SYNTEX CMV STUDY GROUP. A randomized controlled trial of prophylactic ganciclovir for cytomegalovirus pulmonary infection in recipients of allogenic bone marrow transplants. *New Engl J Med* 1991; 324:1005–11.

135. CHANEZ P, AUBAS P, SEGONDY G *et al.* Approaches to the diagnosis of viral pneumonias in the immunocompromised host: importance of assaying cytopathic viral effects in bronchoalveolar lavage cells. *Eur Resp J* 1988; 1:553–7.

136. STOVER DE, ZAMAN MB, HAJDU SI, LANGE M, GOLD J, ARMSTRONG D. Bronchoalveolar lavage in the diagnosis of pulmonary infiltrates in the immunosuppressed host. *Ann Intern Med* 1984; 101:1–7.

137. KHAN FW, JONES JM, ENGLAND DM. The role of bronchoalveolar lavage in the diagnosis of invasive aspergillosis. *Am J Clin Path* 1986; 86:518–23.

138. BASLESKI VS, EL-TORKY M, COALSON J, GRIFFIN J. The standardisation of criteria for processing and interpreting laboratory specimens. *Chest* 1992; 102 (Suppl 1):571S–9S.

139. BELENCHIA JM, WUNDERINK RG, MEDURI GU *et al.* Alternative causes of fever in ARDS patients suspected of having pneumonia. *Am Rev Resp Dis* 1991; Abstract 683.

140. MEDURI GU, STOVER DE, GREENO R *et al.* Bilateral bronchoalveolar lavage in the diagnosis of opportunistic pulmonary infections. *Chest* 1991; 100:1272–6.

141. WIMBERLEY N, FALING LJ, BARTLETT JG. A fiberoptic bronchoscopy technique to obtain uncontaminated lower airway secretions for bacterial culture. *Am Rev Resp Dis* 1979; 117:337–43.

142. CHASTRE J, FAGON JY, SOLER P *et al.* Diagnosis of nosocomial bacterial pneumonia in intubated patients undergoing ventilation: comparison of the usefulness of bronchoalveolar lavage and the protected specimen brush. *Am J Med* 1988; 85:499–506.

143. HIGUCHI JH, COALSON JJ, JOHANSON WG JR. Bacterial diagnosis of nosocomial pneumonia in primates: usefulness of the protected specimen brush. *Am Rev Resp Dis* 1982; 125:53–7.

144. COOK DJ, FITZGERALD JM, GUYATT GH, WALTER S. Evaluation of the protected brush catheter and bronchoalveolar lavage in the diagnosis of nosocomial pneumonia. *J Intens Care Med* 1991; 6:196–205.

145. BLAVIA R, DORCA J, VERDAGUER R *et al.* Bacteriologic followup of nosocomial pneumonia by successive protected specimen brush. *Eur Resp J* 1991; 4 (Suppl):407S.

146. POTGIETER PD, HAMMOND JMJ. Aetiology and diagnosis of pneumonia requiring ICU admission. *Chest* 1992; 101:199–203.

147. TORRES A, EL-EBIARY M, PADRO L *et al.* Validation of different techniques for the diagnosis of ventilator associated pneumonia. *Am J Resp Crit Care Med* 1994; 149:324–31.

148. TIMSIT JF, MISSET B, FRANCOUL S, GOLDSTEIN FW, VAURY P, CARLET J. Is protected specimen brush a reproducible method to diagnose ICU acquired pneumonia? *Chest* 1993; 104:104–8.

149. FAGON JY, CHASTRE J, HANCE AJ *et al.* Detection of nosocomial lung infection in ventilated patients. Use of a protected specimen brush and quantitative culture technique in 147 patients. *Am Rev Resp Dis* 1988; 138:110–16.

150. DREYFUSS D, MIER L, LE BOURDELLES G *et al.* Clinical significance of borderline quantitative protected brush specimen cultures results. *Am Rev Resp Dis* 1993; 147:946–51.

151. THORPE JE, BAUGHMAN RP, FRAME PT, WESSLER TA, STANEK JL. Bronchoalveolar lavage for diagnosing acute bacterial pneumonias. *J Infect Dis* 1987; 155:855–61.

152. KAHN FW, JONES JM. Diagnosing bacterial respiratory infection by bronchoalveolar lavage. *J Infect Dis* 1987; 155: 862–9.

153. KIRPATRICK MB, BASS JB JR. Quantitative bacterial cultures of bronchoalveolar lavage fluids and protected brush catheter specimens from normal subjects. *Am Rev Resp Dis* 1989; 139:546–8.

154. TORRES A, MARTOS A, PUIG DELA BELLACASSA J *et al.* Specificity of endotracheal aspiration, protected specimen brush and broncheolar lavage in mechanically ventilated patients. *Am Rev Resp Dis* 1993; 147:952–7.

155. MEDURI GV. Ventilator associated pneumonia in patients with respiratory failure: a diagnostic approach. *Chest* 1990; 97:1208–19.

156. DOTSON RG, PINGLETON SK. Bronchoalveolar lavage and protected specimen brush cultures in ventilator-associated pneumonia. *Chest* 1991; 100:365.

157. SOLE-VIOLAN J, RODRIGUEZ DE CASTRO F, REY A, MARTIN-GONZALEZ JC, CABRERA-NAVARRO P. Usefulness of microscopic examination of intracellular organisms in lavage fluid in ventilator-associated pneumonia. *Chest* 1994; 106:889–94.

158. DOTSON RG, PINGLETON SK. The effect of antibiotic therapy on recovery of intracellular bacteria from bronchoalveolar lavage in suspected ventilator-associated nosocomial pneumonia. *Chest* 1993; 103:541–6.

159. WILSON WR, COCKERILL FR, ROSENOW II EC. Pulmonary disease in the immunocompromised host. *Mayo Clin Proc* 1985; 60:610–31.

160. ZAVALA DC, SCHOELL JE. Ultrathin needle aspiration of the lung in infectious and malignant disease. *Am Rev Resp Dis* 1981; 123:125–31.

161. DE BLIC J, MCKELVIC P, LE BOURGEOIS M, BLANCHE S, BENOIST MR, SCHEINMANN P. Value of bronchoalveolar lavage in the management of severe acute pneumonia and interstitial pneumonitis in the immunocompromised child. *Thorax* 1987; 42:759–65.

162. TORRES A, JIMENEZ P, DE LA BELLACASSA JP, CELIS R, GONZALEZ J, GEA J. Diagnostic value of non-fluoroscopic percutaneous lung needle aspiration in patients with pneumonia. *Chest* 1990; 98:840–4.

163. DIJKMAN JH, VAN DER MEER JWM, BAKKER W, WEVER AMJ, VAN DER BROEK PJ. Transpleural lung biopsy by thorascopic route in patients with diffuse interstitial pulmonary disease. *Chest* 1982; 82:76–83.

164. LEWIS RJ, CACCAVALE RJ, SISSLER GE. Imaged thorascopic lung biopsy. *Chest* 1992; 102:60–2.

165. SHURE D, MOSER KM, KONOPKA R. Transbronchial needle aspiration in the diagnosis of pneumonia in a canine model. *Am Rev Resp Dis* 1985; 131:290–1.

166. LORCH DG, JOHN JF, TOMLINSON JR *et al.* Protected transbronchial needle aspiration and protected specimen brush in the diagnosis of pneumonia. *Am Rev Resp Dis* 1987; 136:565–9.

167. PAPIN T, GRUM C, WEG J. Transbronchial biopsy during mechanical ventilation. *Chest* 1986; 89:168–70.

168. CAZZADORI A, DI PERRI G, TODESCHINI G *et al.* Transbronchial biopsy in the diagnosis of pulmonary infiltrates in immunocompromised patients. *Chest* 1995; 107:101–6.

169. WARNER DO, WARNER MA, DIVERTIE MB. Open lung biopsy in patients with diffuse pulmonary infiltrates and acute respiratory failure. *Am Rev Resp Dis* 1988; 137:90–4.

170. NELEMS JM, COOPER JD, HENDERSON MB, PENG T, PHILLIPS MJ. Emergency lung biopsy. *Ann Thorac Surg* 1976; 22:260–4.

171. COCKERILL FR, WILSON WR, CARPENTER HA, SMITH TF, ROSENOW III EC. Open lung biopsies in immunocompromised patients. *Arch Intern Med* 1985; 145:1398–404.

172. MCKENNA RJ JR, CAMPBELL A, MCMURTREY MJ, MOUNTAIN CF. Diagnosis for interstitial lung disease in patients with acquired immunodeficiency syndrome (AIDS): a prospective comparison of bronchial

washing, alveolar lavage, transbronchial lung biopsy, and open lung biopsy. *Ann Thorac Surg* 1986; 41:318–21.

173. MEDURI GU, BELENCHIA JM, ESTES RJ, LEEPER KV, WUNDERINK RG. Fibroproliferative phase of ARDS. Clinical findings and effect of corticosteroids. *Chest* 1991; 100:943–52.

174. SPRINGMEYER SC, SILVESTRI RC, SALE GE *et al.* The role of transbronchial biopsy for the diagnosis of diffuse pneumonias in immunocompromised bone marrow transplant recipients. *Am Rev Resp Dis* 1982; 126:763–5.

175. ELLIS ME, SPENCE D, BOUCHAMA A *et al.* Open lung biopsy provides a higher and more specific diagnostic yield compared to broncho-alveolar lavage in immunocompromised patients. *Scand J Infect Dis* 1995; 27:157–162.

176. WILSON WR, COCKERILL FR, ROSENOW III EC. Pulmonary disease in the immunocompromised host. *Mayo Clin Proc* 1985; 60:610–31.

177. SNYDER CL, RAMSAY NK, MCGLAVE PB, FERRELL KL, LEONARD AS. Diagnostic open lung biopsy after bone marrow transplantation. *J Ped Surg* 1990; 25:871–7.

178. TOLEDO-PEREYRA LH, DE MEESTER TR, KINCALEY I, MACMAHON H, CHURG A, COLOMB H. The benefits of open lung biopsy in patients with previous non-diagnostic transbronchial lung biopsy. A guide to appropriate therapy. *Chest* 1980; 77:647–50.

179. GURURANGAN S, LAWSON RAM, MORRIS-JONES PH, STEVENS RF, CAMPBELL RHA. Evaluation of the usefulness of open lung biopsies. *Ped Hematol Oncol* 1992; 9:107–13.

180. PROBER CG, WHYTE H, SMITH CR. Open lung biopsy in immunocompromised children with pulmonary infiltrates. *Am J Dis Child* 1984; 138:60–3.

181. GAENSLER EA, CARRINGTON CB. Open biopsy for chronic diffuse infiltrative lung disease: clinical, roentgenographic and physiological correlations in 502 patients. *Ann Thorac Surg* 1980; 30:411–26.

182. ROSSITER SJ, MILLER C, CHURG AM, CARRINGTON CB, MARCK JBD. Open lung biopsy in the immuno-compromised patient. Is it really beneficial? *J Thorac Cardiovasc Surg* 1979; 77:338–45.

183. PUKSA S, HUTCHEON MA, HYLAND RH. Usefulness of transbronchial biopsy in immunosuppressed patients with pulmonary infiltrates. *Thorax* 1983; 38:146–50.

184. FAGON JY, CHASTRE J, HANCE AJ, DOMART Y, TROUILLER JL, GIBERT C. Evaluation of clinical judgement in the identification and treatment of nosocomial pneumonia in ventilated patients. *Chest* 1993; 103:547–53.

185. MEDURI GU, MAULDIN G, WUNDERINK RG *et al.* Causes of fever and pulmonary densities in patients with clinical manifestations of ventilator associated pneumonia. *Chest* 1994; 106:221–35.

186. WINER-MURAM HT, RUBIN SA, MINIATI M, ELLIS JV. Guidelines for reading and interpreting *Chest* radiographs in patients receiving mechanical ventilation. *Chest* 1992; 102:565S–70S.

187. BRYANT LR, MOBIN-UDDIN K, DILLON ML *et al.* Misdiagnosis of pneumonia in patients needing mechanical ventilation. *Arch Surg* 1973; 286–8.

188. GATTINONI L, PRESENTI A, TORRESIN A *et al.* Adult respiratory distress syndrome profiles by computed tomography. *J Thorac Image* 1986; 1:25–30.

189. WUNDERINK RG, WOLDENBERG LS, ZEISS J, DAY CM, CLEMINS J, LACHER D. The radiological diagnosis of autopsy-proven ventilator-associated pneumonia. *Chest* 1992; 101:458–63.

190. O'REILLY MJ, REDDICK EJ, BLACK W. Sepsis from sinusitis in nasotracheally intubated patients: a diagnostic dilemma. *Am J Surg* 1984; 147:601–4.

191. GRINDLINGER GA, NIEHOFF J, HUGHES SL, HUMPHREY MA, SIMPSON G. Acute paranasal sinusitis related to nasotracheal intubation of head injured patients. *Crit Care Med* 1987; 15:214–17.

192. SALORD F, GAUSSORGUES P, MARTI-FLICH J. Nosocomial maxillary sinusitis during mechanical ventilation: a prospective comparison of orotracheal versus the nasotracheal route for intubation. *Intens Care Med* 1990; 16:390–3.

193. DESMOND P, RAMAN R, IDIKULA J. Effect of nasogastric tubes on the nose and maxillary sinus. *Crit Care Med* 1991; 19:509–11.

194. WESTERGREN V, FORSUM U, LUNGDGREN J. Possible errors in diagnosis of bacterial sinusitis in tracheal intubated patients. *Acta Anesthesiol Scand* 1994; 38:649–703.

195. HOLZAPEL L, CHEURET S, MADINIER G. Influence of long-term oro or nasotracheal intubation on nosocomial sinusitis and pneumonia: results of a prospective randomized clinical trial. *Crit Care Med* 1993; 21:1132–8.

196. ROUBY JJ, LAURENT P, GOSNACH *et al.* Risk factors and clinical relevance of nosocomial maxillary sinusitis in the critically ill. *Am J Resp Crit Care Med* 1994; 150:776–83.

197. HEFFNER JE. Nosocomial sinusitis. Den of multiresistant thieves. *Am J Resp Crit Care Med* 1994; 150:608–9.

198. PETERSDORF RG, CURTIN JA, HOEPRICH PD, PEELER RN, BENNET IL. A study of antibiotic prophylaxis in unconscious patients. *N Engl J Med* 1957; 257:1001–9.

199. MANDELLI M, MOSCONI P, LANGER M *et al.* Prevention of pneumonia in an intensive care unit: a randomized multicenter clinical trial. *Crit Care Med* 1989; 17:501–5.

200. KLASTERSKY J, HENSGENS C, NOTERMAN J, MOUAWAD E, MEUNIER-CARPENTIER F. Endotracheal antibiotics for the prevention of tracheobronchial infections in tracheostomized unconscious patients: a comparative study of gentamicin and polymyxin B combination. *Chest* 1975; 68:302–6.

201. KLICK JM, DU MOULIN GC, HEDLEY-WHYTE J, TERES D, BUSHNELL LS, FEINGOLD DS. Prevention of Gram-negative bacillary pneumonia using polymyxin aerosols as prophylaxis. Effect in the incidence of pneumonia in seriously ill patients. *J Clin Invest* 1975; 55:514–9.

202. FEELY TW, DU MOULIN GC, HEDLEY-WHYTE J, BUSHNELL LS, GILBERT JP, FEINGOLD DS. Aerosol polymyxin and pneumonia in seriously ill patients. *N Engl J Med* 1975; 293:471–5.

203. VAN SAENE HKF, STOUTENBEEK CP, HART CA. Selective decontamination of the digestive tract in intensive care patients: a critical evaluation of the clinical, bateriological and epidemiological benefits. *J Hosp Infect* 1991; 18:261–77.

204. STOUTENBEEK CP, VAN SAENE HFK, MIRANDA DR, ZANDSTRA DF. The effect of selective decontamination of the digestive tract on colonisation and infection rate in multiple trauma patients. *Intens Care Med* 1984; 10:185–92.

205. VAN DER WAAIJ D. Colonisation resistance of the digestive tract: clinical consequences and implications. *J Antimicrob Ther* 1982; 10:263–70.

206. KOLLEF MH. The role of selective digestive tract decontamination on mortality and respiratory tract infections: a meta-analysis. *Chest* 1994; 105:1101–8.

207. SELECTIVE DECONTAMINATION OF THE DIGESTIVE TRACT TRIALISTS COLLABORATIVE GROUP. Meta-analysis of randomized controlled trials of selective decontamination of the digestive tract. *BMJ* 1993; 307:525–32.

208. HAMMOND JM, POTGIETER PD, SAUNDERS GL, FORDER AA. Double blind study of selective decontamination of the digestive tract in intensive care. *Lancet* 1992; 340:5–9.

209. GASTINNE H, WOLFE M, DELATOUR F, FAURISSON F, CHEVRET S. A controlled trial in intensive care units of selective

decontamination of the digestive tract with nonabsorbable antibiotics. The French Study Group on Selective Decontamination of the Digestive Tract. *N Engl J Med* 1992; 326:594–9.

210. FERRER M, TORRES A, GONZALEZ J *et al.* Utility of selective digestive decontamination in mechanically ventilated patients. *Ann Intern Med* 1994; 120:389–95.

211. BOW EJ, RONALD AR. Antibacterial chemoprophylaxis in neutropenic patients where do we go from here? (Editorial) *Clin Infect Dis* 1993; 17:333–7.

212. WARD TT, THOMAS RG, FYE CL *et al.* Trimethoprim-sulfamethoxasole prophylaxis in granulocytopenic patients with acute leukemia: evaluation of serum antibiotic levels in a randomized, double-blind, placebo controlled Department of Veteran Affairs Cooperative Study. *Clin Infect Dis* 1993; 17:323–32.

213. DASCHNER F. Emergence of resistance during selective decontamination of the digestive tract. *Eur J Clin Microbiol Infect Dis* 1992; 11:1–3.

214. LEDINGHAM MCA, ALCOCK SR, EEASTAWAY AT, MCDONALD JC, MCKAY IC, RAMSAY G. Triple regimens of selective decontamination of the digestive tract, systemic cefotaxime, and microbiologicalal surveillance for prevention of acquired infection in intensive care. *Lancet* 1988; 16:1087–93.

215. TAYLOR M, OPPENHEIM BA. Selective decontamination of the gastrointestinal tract as an infection control measure. *J Hosp Infect* 1991; 17:271–8.

216. DE CHAMPS CL, GUELON DP, GARNIER RM *et al.* Selective digestive deconstamination by erythromycin base in a polyvalent intensive care unit. *Intens Care Med* 1993; 19:191–6.

217. LA FORCE FM. Systemic antimicrobial therapy of nosocomial pneumonia: monotherapy vs combination therapy. *Eur J Clin Microbiol Infect Dis* 1989; 8:61–8.

218. MOORE RD, SMITH CR, LIETMANN PS. Association of aminoglycoside plasma levels with therapeutic outcome in Gram-negative pneumonia. *Am J Med* 1984; 77:657–62.

219. HODSON ME, PENDETH ARL, BATTEN JC. Aerosol carbenicillin and gentamicin treatment of *Pseudomonas aeruginosa* infection in patients with cystic fibrosis. *Lancet* 1981; 2:1137–9.

220. BROWN RB, KRUSE JA, COUNTS GW *et al.* Double-blind treatment of endotracheal tobramycin in the treatment of Gram-negative bacterial pneumonia. *Antimicrob Agents Chemother* 1990; 34:269–72.

221. KUNIN CM, JOHANSEN KS, WORNING AM, DASCHNER FD. Report of a symposium on use and abuse of antibiotics worldwide. *Rev Infect Dis* 1990; 12:12–19.

222. STOBBERINGH E, JANKNEGT R, WIJNARDS G. Antimicrobial practice, antibiotic guidelines and antibiotic utilisation in Dutch hospitals. *J Antimicrobiol Chemother* 1993; 32:153–61.

223. MAKI DG, SCHUNA AA. A study of antimicrobial misuse in a university hospital. *Am J Med Sci* 1978; 275:271–82.

224. ROBERTS AW, VISCONTI JA. The rational and irrational use of systemic antimicrobial drugs. *Am J Hosp Pharm* 1972; 29:828–34.

225. LEIGH DA. Antimcrobial usage in forty-three hospitals in England. *J Antimicrobiol Chemother* 1982; 8:75–84.

226. RODER BL, NIELSEN SL, MAGNUSSEN P, ENGQUIST A, FRIMODT-MOLLER N. Antimicrobial practice. Antibiotic usage in an intensive care unit in a Danish university hospital. *J Antimicrob Chemother* 1993; 32:633–42.

227. GRASELA TH JR, SCHENTAG JJ, BOEKENOOGEN SJ, CRIST KD, LOWES WL, LUM BL. A clinical pharmacy-oriented drug surveillance network: results of a nationwide antibiotic utilisation review of bacterial pneumonia – 1987. *Ann Pharmacother* 1989; 23:162–70.

228. SINGH KP, VOOLMAN T, LANG SD. Pneumococcal bacteremia in South Auckland: a five year review with emphasis on prescribing practices. *N Z Med* 1992; 105:394–5.

229. DENTON M, MORGAN MS, WHITE RR. Quality of prescribing of intravenous antibiotics in a district general hospital. *BMJ* 1991; 302:327–8.

230. GYSSENS IC, VAN DEN BROCK PJ, KULLBERG BJ, HEKSTER YA, VAN DER MEER JWM. Optimizing antimicrobial therapy. A method for antimicrobial drug use evaluation. *J Antimicrob Chemother* 1992; 30:724–7.

231. GOULD IM. Control of antibiotic use in the United Kingdom. *J Antimicrob Chemother* 1988; 22:395–401.

232. HIRSCHMAN SZ, MEYERS BR, BRADBURY K, MEHL B, GENDELMAN S, KIMELBLATT B. Use of antimicrobial agents in a university teaching hospital. Evolution of a comprehensive control program. *Arch Int Med* 1988; 148:2001–7.

20 Anaerobic bacterial pneumonia, lung abscess, pleural effusion/empyema

JAVED KHAN* and MICHAEL E. ELLIS†
*King Fahad National Guard Hospital, Riyadh, Saudi Arabia and †King Faisal Specialist Hospital and Research Centre, Riyadh, Saudi Arabia

Introduction

Although anaerobic lung infection has been recognised for a century[1] the precise contribution of anaerobic bacteria to community- and hospital-acquired pneumonia, lung abscess and empyema has been clarified only in the last 20 years. The development of specialised sampling techniques to reduce contamination, together with dedicated anaerobic culture techniques have shown t hat the role of anaerobic bacteria as pulmonary pathogens had previously been greatly underestimated. Changes in taxonomy have impacted on the reporting of the relative contributions of different bacteria. The observation that it is more usual to find polyanaerobic and mixed anaerobic/aerobic organisms from appropriate specimens and that some organisms are resistant to antimicrobials has had major implications for treatment.

This chapter summarises the current status of anaerobes in lung infection, including the presentation and management of the post pneumonic sequelae of abscess and empyema.

Table 20.1. *Causes of lung abscess*

1.	Aspiration from oropharynx	
2.	Pyogenic pneumonia	
3.	Bloodborne infections	
4.	Secondary to bronchial obstruction	
5.	Infection of:	Pulmonary infarction
		Hydatid cyst
		Bullae
6.	Posttraumatic	
7.	Associated with:	Diabetes mellitus
		Bronchiectasis
		Coalworker's pneumoconiosis
		Primary and metastatic malignancy
8.	Transdiaphragmatic spread	

Anaerobic pulmonary infection

Pathogenesis

Aspiration of oropharyngeal secretions which contain saturated levels of anaerobes of up to 10^{12} organism per gram, which if excessively frequent and voluminous overwhelm the lungs clearance capacity (which normally removes the smaller quantities encountered in healthy people), is the major initiating mechanism in the genesis of anaerobic lung infection. Predisposing conditions have been described previously (Table 20.1 and Chapter 28) which include breaching of mechanical defence barriers, for example, by endotracheal tubes, depressed level of consciousness, for example, cerebrovascular accidents and intestinal dysmobility, for example oesophageal disease.

Major host systemic disturbances such as humoral or cell-mediated immune defects do not feature in anaerobic lung disease. However acid-chemical pneumonitis, lung infarction, bronchiectasis, mechanical bronchial obstruction, for example, by tumour, all predispose to anaerobic pneumonia. Chronic obstructive airways disease is not a factor.

The oral cavity contains over 200 bacterial species which colonise different locations within the oral cavity. Infected gingival crevices contribute a major reservoir of anaerobic bacteria implicated in anaerobic lung infection (ALI) – as deduced from the similarity of the bacteria found in the two sites and from animal experiments in which lung abscess can be induced by intratracheal inoculation of pyorrhoeic pus.[2,3] This area between tooth and gum tissue (gingival crevice) contains a high number of bacteria and has an anaerobic environment similar to that of colon.[4,5] Normal saliva from a healthy mouth contains approximately 10^7–10^8 anaerobes per ml, but saliva from patients with gingivitis may have 10^{11} per ml.[6] In 1931, Smith noted that bacteria detected in the walls of the lung abscess at autopsy resembles organisms found in gingival crevices.[7] Furthermore, anaerobic lung disease is less frequent in edentulous persons. Less commonly implicated sources include septic phlebitis via the haematogenous route and contiguous spread from a subdiaphragmatic abscess.

Unless promptly recognised and treated, an initial anaerobic pneumonitis may progress to necrotising pneumonia, abscess formation or empyema. Postulated virulence factors include the capsular polysaccharide in some *Bacteroides* spp.,[8] an immunoregulatory T-cell lymphokine[9] and inhibition of alveolar macrophage and neutrophil killing via anaerobic bacterial produced short chain fatty acids, for example butyric acid.[10] Of some interest is the observation that polymicrobial and not monomicrobial challenge is necessary to effect tissue necrosis and abscess formation in an animal model.[2,3] However, it is not clear in the human *in vivo* situation whether each organism is pathogenic *per se*.

Bacteriology

A number of taxonomic changes in the anaerobes have occurred including (i) the reclassification of previous *Peptococcus* spp. into *Peptostreptococcus* spp., (ii) several *Peptostreptococcus* spp. now known to be aerotolerant and resistant to metronidazole have been classified within the *Streptococcus* spp., for example, *Streptococcus intermedius, Streptococcus constellates* and *Streptococcus parvulus*, (iii) *Bacteroides melaninogenicus* has now been reclassified as fastidious and penicillinase-producing *Prevotella* spp. and *Porphyromonas* spp.

Currently, the major anaerobic pathogens implicated in the genesis of ALI are *Peptostreptococcus* spp., *Prevotella (Bacteroides) melaninogenicus, Fusobacterium nucleatum, Fusobacterium necrophorum, Porphyromonas (Bacteroides) asaccharolytica, Porphyromonas endodontalis* and *Porphyromonas gingivalis*.[11] These organisms originate from upper airway sources particularly the gingival crevices. The role of *B. fragilis* (which is not part of the normal oral flora) is somewhat uncertain but the increasing incidence of penicillin, cephalosporin and clindamycin resistance is of concern. *Veillonella* spp. are often found but their role is unclear. Other unusual anaerobes include *Clostridium* spp., *Eubacterium* spp., *Actinomyces* spp., *Lactobacillus* spp., *Proprionibacterium* spp., *Bifidobacterium* spp. and *Capnocytophaga* spp.[12]

In two large series, the average number of anaerobic strains per case reviewed was between 2.4 and 3.2.[11,13] However, 12% of specimens in one series of ALI had only one anaerobe isolated, indicating that in addition to their role in mixed/synergistic infections, single anaerobes may well also be virulent alone.[12] In addition to anaerobes many patients with aspiration pneumonia have aerobes – the frequency of this phenomenon is higher in patients with hospital-acquired aspiration pneumonia. These patients become colonised with Gram-negative bacilli (Chapter 8) particularly *Pseudomonas aeruginosa, Escherichia coli* and *Klebsiella pneumoniae*. Other aerobes that may be found include *Staphylococcus aureus, Streptococcus pneumoniae, Haemophilus influenzae* and *Enterococcus faecalis*.

Antibiotic resistance among anaerobic bacteria is of substantial concern. For example, up to 20% are resistant to penicillin[14] and β-lactamase production has been found in approximately half of *Fusobacterium* spp.[15] and in 30% of anaerobic rods isolated.[12] Among the *B. fragilis* group, 85% have been found to be β-lactamase positive, whilst the remainder were penicillin resistant by other mechanisms.[12]

The incidence of anaerobic bacterial infection of the lung varies with the clinical setting, for example, in hospital-acquired pneumonia anaerobes are found in 35%, in community-acquired pneumonia between 22–33%, in empyema 19–76%, aspiration pneumonia 62–100% and in pulmonary abscess 85–93%.[16]

Most studies of ALI or lung abscess have used transtracheal aspiration for specimen collection. Empyema presents a technically much easier situation for specimen collection. The available diagnostic methods have been fully reviewed in Chapter 1. Detection of characteristic volatile fatty acids in invasively obtained pulmonary specimens and more recently in an expectorated sputum by gas liquid chromatography, has been employed by research laboratories but has limited usefulness.[17] Blood cultures are rarely positive.

Clinical presentation and management of anaerobic pneumonia

Acute ALI largely occurs in the setting of aspiration. There may be evidence of poor dental hygiene. Symptoms and signs of acute anaerobic pneumonia may be indistinguishable from streptococcal pneumonia, apart from a decreased incidence of rigors and a longer duration of symptoms.[18] Thus a peak temperature of around 102–103 °F (38.9–39.4) and leukocytosis of 14×10^9/l are common.[16] Many cases of anaerobic pneumonia may have been previously diagnosed as 'atypical' pneumonia in the absence of an identifiable pathogen. Radiographically right posterior upper lobe and superior lower lobe segments are most often involved in aspiration pneumonia in patients acquiring their infection whilst in the supine position. Not uncommonly, an accompanying pleural effusion is present.

Inappropriate management may result in progression of the acute syndrome to a subacute putrifying-necrotic process, chronic destructive pneumonia, lung abscess or empyema. Subacute pneumonia often occurs in a hospital setting – tissue necrosis (pulmonary gangrene) with multiple cavitary disease spreading contiguously and associated with a foul discharge carries a dismal prognosis.[19] In chronic destructive pneumonia there is progressive airway and parenchymal destruction associated with microabscesses, haemoptysis, foul smelling sputum, chest pain, weight loss, anaemia, malnutrition and a past medical history of TB.[20] The disease may mimic pulmonary tuberculosis or other chronic pneumonias.

Lung abscess/empyema may develop after 2–6 weeks. These suppurative complications are discussed below.

Management of acute anaerobic pneumonia pivots around antibiotics. The optimal choice has evolved in recent years. Although there is little data to suggest that penicillin alone in doses of 12–24 Mu per day in acute ALI is inferior, penicillin is no longer the universally favoured antimicrobial. This is based on *in vitro* studies which indicate resistance,[12,14,15] the polymicrobial aerobic-anaerobic mix of many infections and some clinical trials. Clindamycin appears to be superior to penicillin in terms of treatment success, relapse rate, defervescence and clinical resolution in the treatment of complicated anaerobic lung infection, i.e. abscess and necrotising pneumonia.[21,22] Clindamycin also appears to enhance phagocyte killing.[23] In the setting of combined Gram-negative aerobic/anaerobic pneumonia, such as occurs in hospital-acquired pneumonia then an aminoglycoside should be added. Metronidazole, a lynch pin anti-anaerobic antibiotic has proved disappointing in the treatment of ALI and cannot be recommended as sole therapy.[24] This may be due to its inactivity against aerobes. Alternative antimicrobials include amoxicillin–clavulanate, ticarcillin–clavulanate, ampicillin–sulbactam, or imipenem (or meropenem). Tetracycline and the combination of penicillin with metronidazole are further possibilities to consider though clinical experience is rather limited. The optimal duration of antibiotic therapy for acute ALI is not known. However, in view of the potential serious complications from inappropriate treatment then treatment should not be discontinued until active radiographical changes have cleared. It is not uncommon for initial clinical and radiological deterioration to occur (Chapter 28). For patients with complications, up to 4 months therapy may be needed. The management of abscess and empyema is described below.

The outcome for anaerobic pulmonary infection in general is good with a mortality rate of around 5%. Patients with hospital-acquired anaerobic pulmonary infection do less well (mortality rate 20%) whilst approximately 10% of patients with lung abscess die.[16]

Lung abscess

Introduction

Lung abscess can be defined as a pus containing necrotic lesion of the lung parenchyma. Some authorities regard a lesion larger than 2 cm in diameter as true abscess.[25]

The problem of lung abscess was recognised by physicians in ancient times and continues to pose a challenge for contemporary practitioners because of the long duration of illness, significant mortality and diagnostic and therapeutic problems involved. In the pre-antibiotic era, lung abscess was a relatively common infection associated with considerable morbidity and mortality. Supportive care and postural drainage were the major forms of treatment. Surgical drainage was considered in the chronic stage of the disease and the results were often dismal. The mortality in this era was more than 30%; 30% of patients had significant residual symptomatic disease.[26] When early drainage of acute putrid abscess was introduced the prognosis improved significantly and the mortality rate fell to 5–10%.[27] In the late 1940s with the advent of penicillin therapy, the relative merits of surgical versus medical therapy were debated. By the late 1950s, however, most investigators agreed that patients with lung abscess should receive a trial of antibiotic therapy. Surgery was indicated in patients with 'delayed closure' – defined as persistent cavity on chest X-ray after 4–6 weeks of antibiotic treatment. Later it was shown that the majority of such patients with 'delayed closure' could also be managed medically by an extended period of antibiotic therapy.[28] As a result, surgical intervention was less often performed and considered only after failure of medical treatment. In the following decade, when antibiotics were more frequently available, most lung infections were treated early and effectively and few pyogenic pneumonias progressed to lung abscess.

However, in underdeveloped countries, the incidence of lung abscess did not change substantially.[29] Currently, in most developed countries, lung abscess is particularly common among immunocompromised by drug or disease or as a post-obstructive complication.[30]

Classifications

Lung abscess can be classified according to duration of symptoms, underlying lung disease, organisms and site of involvement.

Depending upon duration of symptoms (< or > 6–8 weeks) prior to presentation, lung abscesses are often arbitrarily classified as *acute* or *chronic*. Sixty per cent of patients present with acute abscess and 40% as chronic.

Lung abscesses can also be divided as *primary* or *secondary*. Primary lung abscess occurs in previously healthy immunocompetent individuals with no underlying local disease. Secondary lung abscess occurs in patients with local obstruction of the airways or in whom the host defence system is compromised either by disease, such as malignancy or by drug therapy such as cancer chemotherapy or chronic steroid therapy.

Lung abscess can also be classified bacteriologically. *Putrid lung abscess* refers to foul-smelling sputum indicating anaerobic infection. *Non-specific lung abscess* is an abscess where no likely pathogen is isolated by aerobic cultures of expectorated sputum. *Specific* and *pyogenic abscess* indicates specific bacterial aetiology.[31] Lung abscesses can be described as secondary to bacterial, mycobacterial, fungal, and parasitic disease.

Aetiology

Lung abscess may result from many conditions (Table 20.2) however, aspiration of organisms from oropharynx is the most common aetiological mechanism in the development of anaerobic lung abscess (Table 20.2).[32,33]

Aspiration material generally settles as gravity dictates such as in the posterior segment of right upper lobe and superior segment of right lower lobe, as in the supine position, these are the most dependent segments in which bronchi are in most direct line of upper respiratory tract. However, in the upright position, basal segments of both lower lobes are dependent.

Lung abscesses may complicate pulmonary infarction. Septic emboli from tonsillar, peritonsillar abscess or pharyngeal infection can give rise to lung abscess.

Primary and metastatic malignancy and necrotic lesions of silicosis and coal miners pneumoconiosis are occasionally associated with lung abscess.[4]

Pyogenic pneumonias may result in lung abscess especially *Staphylococcus* spp. and *Klebsiella* spp. Occasionally, if untreated, streptococcal pneumonia may progress to cavitation. Pneumonia secondary to *Pseudomonas* spp. rarely cavitates although any bacterial and fungal pneumonia may result in lung abscess.[34]

Blood-borne infection resulting in lung abscess occurs most commonly with *S. aureus* particularly in intravenous drug users where it may be associated with tricuspid valve endocarditis.[35]

Trauma is an uncommon cause of lung abscess. Haematoma secondary to lung contusion may become infected. Transdiaphragmatic spread through lymphatics or diaphragmatic defects from subdiaphragmatic or hepatic abscess can occur.

Bronchial obstruction can result in lung abscess. Bacterial infection can occur if obstruction persists for more than a week.[36,37] Malignancy should be suspected in all middle aged, especially smokers presenting with cavitating lesion on chest radiograph.

Within the area of necrosis multiple micro-abscesses may be seen. Lung abscess may be single, multiple or localised. When this parenchymal necrotic area communicates with the bronchus and drains, the typical radiological appearance of lung abscess with air fluid level can be seen. These cavities are usually located in the subpleural region of the lung.

Clinical features

The course of untreated lung abscess has been well documented in published literature prior to antibiotics.[19]

Classically, lung abscess presents as an indolent illness in patients with predilection for aspiration or with other underlying conditions, such as bronchiectasis, lung cancer, or an infected pulmonary infarction.[25] Common symptoms include cough, foul sputum, fever, chest pain, weight loss and night sweats.[38] These features may be present

Table 20.2. *Principal causes of aspiration*

1.	Decreased level of consciousness
	Alcoholism
	Seizure disorder
	Drug overdose
	Anesthesia
	Cerebrovascular accident
2.	Impaired swallowing and gastrointestinal dysfunction
	Neurological disease with bulbar dysfunction
	Oesophageal reflux

Table 20.3. *Bacteriology of lung abscess*

1.	Bacterial	
	(a)	Anaerobes:
		Fusobacterium nucleatum
		Peptostreptococci or anaerobic streptococci
		Prevotella melaninogenicus
		Bacteroides fragilis group
	(b)	Aerobes:
		Streptococcus spp.
		S. aureus
		Klebsiella spp.
		Haemophilus spp.
		Pseudomonas spp.
		Nocardia
	(c)	Mycobacteria:
		M. tuberculosis
		M. kansasii
		M. avium
2.	Fungal	
	i.e. *Aspergillus*	
3.	Parasitic	
	(a)	Hydatid
	(b)	Amoebic

several days before the patient seeks medical advice. However, when the lung abscess is associated with pneumonia or as a result of haematogenous spread, the onset is more abrupt and the patient generally is more ill and the duration of symptoms is much shorter.

Chest pain, often pleuritic, is relatively common (80%) and is often the reason the patient seeks advice. Cough is associated with copious purulent sputum occurs in almost all cases. Abscess resulting from aspiration, is typified by foul smelling sputum and may even have a foul taste. If haemoptysis is present, this may vary from streaking of sputum to a life-threatening event.[39] Chills are often noted but true rigors are rare. Fever is present in the majority of patients (mean peak fever usually 39.1 °C)[16,11]. A history of smoking is common.[38] Lung abscess can occur at any age but in one study, it was observed more commonly in middle-aged men.[38]

A good clinical history is very useful in determining the cause of lung abscess. This should include eliciting the presence of aspiration risk factors or other underlying predisposing factors (Table 20.1 and Table 20.2). Physical examination may reveal finger clubbing. If the lung abscess is close to the pleural space, signs of consolidation such as an impaired percussion note and bronchial breath sounds may be present. Clinical signs of pleural effusion may suggest an empyema.

Bacteriology

The microbiology of lung abscess reflects the mechanism by which the lung abscess has arisen. In the pre-antibiotic era, the availability of surgical and autopsy specimens from patients with lung abscess not treated with antibiotics provided an excellent opportunity for bacteriological study. These studies established the importance of anaerobes as causative organisms in lung abscess secondary to aspiration.[40] However, because of the chaotic state of bacterial taxonomy and inadequate technique of anaerobic bacterial culture, these studies are of limited value.[11] Since the early 1970s, an extraordinary period of research and with the development of new invasive techniques to obtain the uncontaminated specimens and utilising quality culture methods, the microbiology of lung abscess has been better defined. All bacteriological studies published during this period confirmed the role of anaerobes in lung abscess.[11,41]. Bartlett *et al.* in their experience with transtracheal aspirate in 93 patients with lung abscess showed that 83–93% had anaerobic bacteria in the lower airways.[11] Other investigators have found anaerobes in 62–100% of patients with aspiration pneumonia and lung abscess.[41,42] The major anaerobes involved (Table 20.3) are broadly similar to those occurring in ALI.

Bacteroides fragilis was isolated in 15–20% of patients in earlier studies.[34,43] This has important therapeutic applications, as *B. fragilis* is usually resistant to penicillin. However, other studies have found that incidence of *B. fragilis* may actually be only 5% or less[38,44] and that a major portion of patients had 'other *Bacteroides* species' but 27% of these isolates, however, also proved to be resistant to penicillin.[22,13] Brook and Finegold in studies of children with lung abscess, had observed that the distribution and resistance pattern of anaerobes isolated was similar to that in adults.[45]

Although anaerobes play a dominant role in lung abscess due to aspiration, aerobic bacteria produce suppurative lung disease in certain clinical settings: The common aerobes include *Streptococcus* spp., *Staphylococcus* spp., *Klebsiella* spp. and *Pseudomonas* spp. The most frequent cause of staphylococcal lung abscess is septic embolic lesions in intravenous drug abusers having tricuspid valve endocarditis.[46] *Klebsiella* pulmonary infections particularly occur in alcoholic, compromised hosts or as a complication of hospital-acquired pneumonia. Other less common bacterial organisms producing lung abscesses include *Streptococcus pyogenes*,[47] *Haemophilus influenzae*, *Pseudomonas pseudomallei*,[48] *Legionella, Nocardia* and *Streptococcus pneumoniae* especially type III.[49]

In neutropenic (absolute neutrophil count less than 500/mm^3) and severely debilitated patients, *Aspergillus* is an important pathogen.[50] When cell-mediated immunity is impaired, the usual pathogens are *Nocardia* spp., *Mycobacterium tuberculosis*, *Mycobacterium kansasii*, *Mycobacterium avium* and fungi (*Aspergillus, Mucor, Cryptococcus*). *Nocardia* is also common in patients on long-term corticosteroids.[51] In the acquired immunodeficiency syndrome (AIDS), the usual organisms are *M. tuberculosis, Cryptococcus, M. kansasii, Rhodococcus equi* and *Nocardia*.[52,53] In endemic areas lung abscess may be secondary to amoebic liver abscess. In this situation, the liver is almost invariably involved.

Blood borne infections are characteristically multiple. Aspiration-related infections are usually polymicrobial and anaerobes play a dominant role. Infection with a single species is uncommon but where it occurs it is usually with aerobic organisms.[35]

Approach to diagnosis

The history is very important in evaluating the predisposing factors in the development of lung abscess. It had been observed that only 10–15% of patients with anaerobic lung abscess had no predisposition to either aspiration or periodontal disease.[54] An attempt should be made to elicit features suggestive of risk factors for aspiration. Malignancy should be suspected in smokers, especially middle-aged men, as lung malignancy may be found in 7–15% of patients with lung abscess.[29,47] Lung abscess may also be associated with chronic debilitating diseases such as diabetes mellitus, bronchiectasis, immunosuppression associated with organ transplantation, cancer chemotherapy or chronic steroid therapy.[55] Patients should be asked about the travel history to certain endemic areas where fungi such as coccidioidomycosis, histoplasmosis and blastomycosis are common. Similarly, any exposure to patients with cavitary tuberculosis should be sought.

When examining a patient, particular attention should be paid to any evidence of periodontal disease, impaired gag reflux or deranged swallowing mechanism. There are no specific features of lung abscess. However, a foul or putrid smell is pathognomonic of anaerobic pulmonary disease.[56] However, the absence of foul-smelling sputum does not exclude the possibility of anaerobic disease as lung abscess may not be communicating with tracheobronchial tree and some anaerobic organisms do not produce this type of odour. Patients may have signs consistent with consolidation and or pleural effusion.

Sputum examination

The usual microbiological studies performed in patients with cavitary lung disease include stains and cultures of expectorated sputum for detection of aerobic bacteria, mycobacteria and fungi.

The expectorated sputum is contaminated by the anaerobes of the upper airways during its passage and is not suitable for the diagnosis of anaerobic lung abscess. However, a Gram's stain may show many neutrophils mixed with Gram-positive and Gram-negative rods, cocci and bacilli (polymicrobial stain). A lung abscess caused by aerobic bacteria is usually monomicrobial. Sputum is also useful for the diagnosis of noninfectious causes of lung cavity such as bronchogenic carcinoma. When there is an associated pleural effusion, appropriate cultures should be obtained. Positive blood cultures are found only if an anaerobic lung abscess is of haematogenous origin.

Bronchoscopy

The routine use of bronchoscopy in the diagnosis and management of lung abscess is controversial. Bronchoscopy specimens are usually contaminated during the passage of the bronchoscope through the upper airways.[57] Moreover, approximately one-half of the aspirated specimen consists of topical lidocaine used which may be toxic to bacteria. Part of this problem can be solved by using a protective brush catheter procedure (BFW brush Meditech Co) which utilises the concept of a telescoping catheter with a distal occluding plug of carbon wax which dissolves to avoid contamination of the brush during the passage through the inner channel.[58] In addition, use of a limited quantity of lidocaine, preparations of lidocaine without antibacterial preservative and transport of specimen in saline rather than broth, and avoidance of delay in bacteriological processing can improve the diagnostic ability. Prior antibiotic treatment may also decrease the sensitivity of the examination. With the development of new techniques such as protective specimen brush and bronchoalveolar lavage with quantitative cultures, the utility and diagnostic value of bronchoscopy has increased.[59] However, a strong commitment by bronchoscopists and microbiologists together with a rigid adherence to scrupulous techniques is crucial.[59,60] Many authorities believe that, if the diagnosis of anaerobic lung abscess is supported by a typical clinical and radiological presentation, a bronchoscopy may not need to be done as long as the patient is responding to antibiotic therapy. Bronchoscopy can even be dangerous if it is performed on a patient with a giant anaerobic lung abscess (over 4 cm in diameter) as passage of brush or biopsy forceps through the abscess cavity can cause massive endobronchial spillage with a disastrous result.[61] Bronchoscopy is indicated for patients with atypical presentations, delayed resolution or who fail to respond clinically to antibiotics (Table 20.4). Bronchoscopy is also indicated in patients with suspected anaerobic lung abscess who are not expectorating sputum in order to exclude any endobronchial obstruction. It is useful in patients when tuberculosis is suspected but sputum smear is negative. Bronchoscopy is also indicated if the diagnosis of bronchogenic carcinoma is suspected. Sosenko and Glossroth[62] retrospectively reviewed their data for 52 patients and concluded that findings suggestive of a neoplasm include (a) lack of a predisposing factor, (b) lack of systemic symptoms, (c) a white blood count less than $11 \times 10^9/l$ and d) absence of an infiltrate surrounding the abscess.

Bronchoscopy usually involves a number of diagnostic procedures such as protective specimen brushing, bronchoalveolar lavage with quantitative cultures,[58] protective transbronchial needle aspiration,[63] and a single catheter with an agar plug.[64] In most studies, bronchoalveolar lavage, protective specimen brushing and endotracheal aspirations are comparable techniques.[65]

Other techniques

The other diagnostic procedures that are sometimes advocated include transtracheal aspiration[54] and transthoracic aspiration.[42,66,67] Transtracheal aspiration has been termed 'the gold standard' for specific aetiological diagnosis of the lower respiratory tract infections. Overall, it is the easiest and safest procedure with the best diagnostic yield.[68] The incidence of false-negative findings in a patient not previously treated with antibiotics is about 1%.[54] However, there is a higher number of false-positive results (25%) especially in those with chronic bronchitis, bronchiectasis, pulmonary neoplasms and those undergoing frequent tracheal suctions.[69] In addition, non-pathogenic organisms (usually aerobic) may be isolated, especially in chronically ventilated patients as their lower airways may be colonised with microorganisms without any evident pulmonary disease.

Table 20.4. *Indications for bronchoscopy*

1.	Atypical presentation
2.	Delayed resolution
	Persistent fever after 2 weeks
	Persistent cavity after 4 weeks
3.	Suspicion of neoplasm

Transthoracic needle aspiration obtains specimens directly from the lung parenchyma suitable for microbiological examination and provides a useful alternative to fibre-optic bronchoscopy and open lung biopsy.[70,71] It can be performed under ultrasound or CT guidance. Compared with transtracheal aspiration, there is a lower incidence of false positive results (5–20%). In one study, transthoracic lung aspiration provided microbiological diagnosis in 41 out of 50 patients, however, 14% developed pneumothorax.[70] It may be a useful diagnostic tool in patients with giant lung abscess, those with persistent toxicity or in cases where bronchoscopy has failed.

Quantitative cultures of lower airway secretions seem to have improved the diagnostic accuracy of bronchoscopy aspiration,[72] bronchoalveolar lavage,[73] tracheal aspiration,[74] and expectorated sputum.[75] Most of the published data, however, documents the benefit of quantitative cultures for aerobic bacteria with only few cases reports regarding anaerobic micro-organisms.[76]

Radiology

Lung abscess may be suspected from the history or physical examination but a firm diagnosis usually depends on radiographical demonstration of a cavity containing an air–fluid level. The principal differential diagnosis of a lung abscess is shown in Table 20.5. Pneumonic consolidation usually precedes the typical cavitary disease. If the treatment is ineffective or inadequate, the infection can produce necrosis of the lung parenchyma resulting in the formation of a cavity. When this cavity communicates with a bronchus and drains the necrotic debris, air enters the cavity and creates an air–fluid level. Abscesses are generally oval or spherical. The wall of the cavity is usually irregular. At times it can be difficult to distinguish an empyema with an air–fluid level from a lung abscess. Occasionally certain radiological features may be helpful: (a) If the lateral chest radiograph shows a 'D shaped' opacity, the posterior chest wall being the vertical part of 'D', then the lesion is more likely to be an empyema[77] (b) in empyema with air–fluid level, the posterior anterior chest film usually shows a wider air–fluid level as compared to lateral view. A retrospective review of 48 patients with suppurative disease identified certain features suggesting empyema with broncho-pleural fistula rather than lung abscess[78] These included the presence of pleural effusion on earlier chest roentgenograms, extension of the air–fluid level to the chest wall, a tapering border of air–fluid collection and extension of air–fluid collections across fissure lines. Computed tomography is useful when a conventional radiograph is unhelpful. Occasionally, a lesion appears solid on plain radiography but the CT may show cavitation. Moreover, with CT additional information in defining the extent of disease can be obtained, as well as its anatomical location and in differentiating abscess from empyema (Table 20.6).

Table 20.5. *Differential diagnosis of lung abscess*

1.	Cavitating lung cancer or metastatic disease
2.	Bland pulmonary infarction
3.	Wegener's granulomatosis
4.	Hodgkin's and Non-Hodgkin's lymphoma
5.	Sarcoidosis (rare)
6.	Cavitated rheumatoid nodule
7.	Cyst bullae containing fluids

Table 20.6. *Comparison of computed tomographic features of abscess and empyema*

	Abscess	Empyema
Shape	Spherical	Lenticular
Change in shape with change in patient position	None	Possible
Wall characteristics		
Width	Thick; non-uniform	Thin, uniform
Inner surface	Irregular	Smooth
Interface with chest wall	Acute angle	Obtuse angle
Interface with adjacent lung	Poorly defined	Well defined
Lung compression	Absent	Present
Attenuation valve	Wide range	Narrow range

Stark and colleagues assessed the usefulness of CT compared with that of conventional radiography in the evaluation of lung abscess and empyema.[79] In this retrospective study, the CT diagnosis was accurate in 100% of cases and provided additional significant diagnostic information not available on plain radiographs in 47% of cases, which included presence of mediastinal or chest wall involvement, presence of contralateral lung disease and presence of pneumothorax.

Treatment

Antibiotics

Since the availability of broad spectrum antibiotics, medical therapy has become the mainstay of treatment in the management of patients with lung abscess Ideally, specific treatment should depend on the identification of causative micro-organism(s). However, in the absence of definitive bacteriology, the majority of patients with lung abscess are initially treated empirically. A reasonable choice of antibiotics can be made on the basis of clinical presentation and a Gram's stain of the sputum. The most common pathogens in lung abscess are anaerobes.[4,25,31,34] and the majority of isolates are penicillin sensitive. There are many drugs which are effective against these organisms but penicillin, clindamycin and metronidazole are commonly advocated.[22] The initial treatment for anaerobic lung abscess consists of penicillin therapy. The dose of penicillin is variable,[80] and some authorities recommend high doses (10–12 million units per day) intravenously in average-sized adults. Others believe penicillin G in doses of 5–10 million units daily is equally effective. The initial experience with penicillin was favourable with nearly all patients responding to treatment. Oral penicillin V was believed to be as effective as parenteral penicillin and the rare patient who failed to respond to penicillin, did well with tetracycline.[81,82] However, recently *in vitro* sensitivity studies have raised some concern since 15–20% of patients have anaerobic isolates resistant to penicillin.[22,83] In spite of this observation, Bartlett has shown that penicillin continues to be relatively good for anaerobic orodental or pulmonary infections.[84]

Two therapeutic trials comparing clindamycin and penicillin had shown statistically significant benefits with clindamycin in terms of failure rates, relapses, mean duration of fever and mean duration of putrid sputum.[21,85] Many authorities therefore consider clindamycin as a preferred drug for the treatment of lung abscess.[24]

Metronidazole is active against all anaerobes and as such was considered a useful drug in the treatment of anaerobic lung abscess. However, clinical experience has been very disappointing with a very high (43%) therapeutic failure rate, presumably because of the contributing role of microaerophiles and aerobic streptococci in these polymicrobial infections.[24,86,87]. Thus, metronidazole is recommended to be used only in combination with another drug, such as penicillin.[88]

Many other drugs have excellent anaerobic activity and are reasonable alternatives to penicillin or clindamycin. These include imipenem, or meropenem, ampicillin, sulbactam, cefoxitin, piperacillin, cefotaxime, cefoperazone and cefoxitin.[89] The combination of β-lactam antibiotics with β-lactamase inhibitors is also useful. Erythromycin and other macrolides such as azithromycin and clarithromycin have good activity against anaerobes in general but have relatively poor activity against fusobacteria.

In hospital-acquired infections when aerobic Gram-negative bacilli or staphylococci are consistently recovered from respiratory secretions or are suspected, then probable initial treatment should consist of ampicillin–sulbactam or ticarcillin–clavulanate. When the culture results are available, the antibiotic regimen can be altered if necessary. The initial treatment usually consists of parenteral therapy subsequently changing to oral therapy.

The duration of treatment is rather arbitrary. Chest radiographs and temperature course are useful in assessing the response to treatment.

Radiographic deterioration during the first 7–14 days of therapy is not uncommon. Non-cavitary pneumonia often evolves into cavitary lesions during appropriate antibiotic therapy[18,90] and in 50% of patients the infiltrates worsen in first three days, and may continue to worsen for at least one week in one third. This is not an indication that initial therapy is ineffective. The treatment should be continued until the fever subsides and the chest radiographs, obtained at 2–4 week intervals, show complete resolution or small stable residual scar. This often requires 6–8 weeks of treatment. Many authorities advocate short periods of therapy consisting of 3–6 weeks. Factors which herald delayed response include (a) a large cavity over 4 cm in diameter, (b) prolonged symptoms (over 8–12 weeks), (c) necrotising pneumonia as indicated by multiple abscesses, (d) advanced age, (e) compromised host status, (f) associated bronchial obstruction, (g) serious associated diseases, and (h) abscess due to aerobic bacteria.[91]

Drainage

Patients may fail to respond to standard antimicrobial therapy and require additional measures, such as drainage and surgery. Some authorities consider drainage to be the most important component of treatment of lung abscess and would recommend earlier intervention to establish drainage if there is no spontaneous drainage via the bronchial tree, and for patients who continue to have fever after 2 weeks of adequate antibiotic therapy. Abscesses can be drained via bronchoscopy[92,93] or percutaneously.[94–96] When an abscess is large, bronchoscopy and attempted endobronchial drainage may be hazardous, resulting in spillage into the normal lung with impairment of gas exchange. When percutaneous drainage is performed, appropriate care should be taken to avoid contamination of pleural space. More recently, small bore catheters (10 F gauge) have been successfully used under CT or sonography guidance in the treatment of lung abscess, thus obviating the need for surgery.[94,96]

Surgery

Operative treatment, in the form of lobectomy or sometimes pneumonectomy, is required in 12% of patients,[11,97,98] and is specifically indicated for: (a) failed medical treatment, (b) suspicion of carcinoma, (c) significant haemoptysis, (d) presence of complications such as empyema and broncho-pleural fistula.

Progress

Most patients with lung abscess respond slowly to antibiotic therapy. Fever usually subsides within one week. Persistence of fever beyond two weeks is unusual and is an indication for bronchoscopy to facilitate drainage or to diagnose an unsuspected underlying lesion. Radiological response lags behind the clinical response. Radiographic infiltration may persist for 3 months or more. If the patient is asymptomatic and the possibility of malignancy has been investigated, no further intervention is indicated; however, if the patient is symptomatic and the size of the cavity is more than 2 cm with a thickened cavity wall and the patient has received at least 5 weeks of antibiotic treatment, surgical resection is usually recommended.

Complications

The most common complication of lung abscess is the development of empyema. This may also be the presenting symptom. Empyema should be considered in patients with a delayed response to antibiotics and chest physiotherapy.

Haemoptysis is not an uncommon complication. Persistent or recurrence of haemoptysis may be an indication for elective surgery or embolisation of the bronchial artery in patients who pose a poor surgical risk. Occasionally, *Aspergillus* may colonise the residual cavity and evolve to an aspergilloma – which may be another cause of haemoptysis. Sometimes, destruction of the cavity wall by the necrotising process can lead to saccular bronchiectasis. Metastatic abscess especially to the brain is rarely seen. Amyloidosis resulting from chronic suppurative lung disease is rare after adequate antibiotic treatment.

Pleural effusion and empyema

Pleural effusion is a common complication of bacterial pneumonia occurring in 20–60% of patients with bacterial pneumonia. The majority of patients with pleural effusions resolve with effective antibiotic treatment of the underlying pneumonia. However, morbidity and mortality is higher in patients with pneumonia and para-pneumonic effusions compared to patients with pneumonia alone, which may partly reflect inadequate management of the pleural effusion.

Para-pneumonic effusion is defined as an effusion associated with bacterial pneumonia, lung abscess or bronchiectasis. An uncomplicated para-pneumonic effusion is a free-flowing effusion that resolves spontaneously with antibiotic therapy alone. A complicated para-pneumonic effusion progresses to intrapleural loculations and requires pleural space drainage for resolution of pleural sepsis. The word empyema is derived from the Greek meaning pus in the body cavity and represents the end stage of a complicated para-pneumonic effusion.

Pathogenesis

The exact mechanism by which a pleural infection develops is not known. In animal studies the introduction of bacteria into the pleural space alone is not sufficient to cause infection of the pleural space,[98] unless there is a prior injury to the pleura or bacteria is introduced absorbed to a foreign body.[99]

The pleural space is usually infected via the lung. Bacteria reaches the lung through the alveoli then gains access to the pleural cavity. Different bacterial species have different propensity to involve pleura. For example, *S. aureus* and *E. coli* are more likely to involve the pleura than *S. pneumoniae* or *Klebsiella* spp.[100]

Pleural effusion develops either as a result of increased accumulation of fluid or decreased lymphatic clearance. Pleural mesothelium is not a major barrier to the movement of low protein oedema fluid or high protein inflammatory exudate.[101,102] Once the inflammatory exudate accumulates in the lung, this can move freely by pressure gradients into the pleural space causing pleural effusion.[102]

Leckie and Tothill have shown that in patients with tuberculosis, pleural fluid absorption from the pleural space is reduced by 50%.[103] This may result from occlusion of lymphatics by fibrin or cellular debris or by external compression from infiltration of parietal pleura. In addition, endotoxins, cytokines or other products of inflammation can also contribute to pleural fluid accumulation.

The evolution of a para-pneumonic effusion can be divided into three stages which represents continuity of the process.[104] The *exudative stage* occurs during first few days in which fluid accumulates in the pleural space either by transfer of alveolar fluid induced by the pneumonic process or from increased capillary permeability of the visceral pleura.[105] Fluid volume is usually small, exudative, sterile and free flowing with normal glucose and pH levels. The predominant cellular component is polymorphonuclear leucocytes (PMN). At this stage, pleural effusion may resolve spontaneously with appropriate antibiotics. If pneumonia remains untreated, then after several days progression to second fibropurulent stage occurs. There is further accumulation of pleural fluid which becomes turbid and contains more PMN, cellular debris and bacteria. At this stage, visceral and parietal pleura are covered by fibrin deposition which may produce loculations across the pleural surface. Progression to multiple intrapleural loculations complicates effective drainage of the pleural space.[106] Pleural pH and glucose decrease as a result of leukocyte phagocytosis and bacterial metabolism.[107] The third or organisation stage is characterised by capillary proliferation and influx of fibroblasts from both visceral and parietal pleural surfaces resulting in an elastic membrane called 'pleural peel' which encases the lung and restricts pulmonary re-expansion. Atelectasis of the adjacent lung is due to both mass effect and trapping by the relatively inelastic sheets. Pleural fluid becomes viscous and purulent and is difficult to drain through a closed thoracostomy tube. It assumes this specific characteristic because of the coagulability of pleural fluid, the abundance of cellular debris and increased fibrin collagen deposition. Decreased bacterial opsonisation from complement depletion results in bacterial persistence.[108] If the patient remains untreated the empyema fluid may rupture into the lung causing broncho-pleural fistula or may drain spontaneously through the chest wall.

Pleural effusions secondary to bacterial infections are predominantly neutrophilic. The main attractant for neutrophils is interleukin-8 (IL-8).[109,110] In recent studies it has been shown that interleukin is produced by pleural mesothelial cells, macrophages and many other cells.[111] Interleukin is an important cytokine in pleural inflammation and is relatively resistant to proteolytic degradation.[112] In tuberculous pleural effusions, neutrophils are initially recruited, followed by monocytes which are attracted by another cytokine, monocyte chemotactic peptid-1 (MCP-1) produced by mesothelial cells and macrophages.[113] Small lymphocytes eventually become the predominant cell type as a result of local recruitment and clonal expansion of a population of reactive 'T' cells.[114]

Microbiology

Before the antibiotic era, streptococcal pneumonia was responsible for most empyemas.[115] The incidence of pneumococcal empyema has diminished significantly due to earlier and effective treatment of *S. pneumoniae*. In 48% of patients staphylococcal pneumonia may cause associated para-pneumonic effusion: one half of these patients develop empyema.[116] The incidence of empyema caused by anaerobic organisms varies between 17–71% of all empyemas.[117,118] However, the pleural fluid isolate in anaerobic empyema is often polymicrobial. In one study, 41% of patients had both anaerobic and aerobic organisms, 35% had anaerobes and 24% had only aerobic organisms. Anaerobic organisms includes *B. melaninogenicus,* anaerobic streptococci and *F. nucleatum*.[118] The aerobic organisms found along with anaerobes include *S. aureus* and *S. pneumoniae.* Almost any of the bacterial organisms which produce bacterial pneumonia can be implicated in empyema. However, *H. influenzae, Klebsiella pneumoniae* and *Pseudomonas aeruginosa* are most frequently isolated. In many cases because of previous treatment with antibiotics, no organisms may be identified.[119]

Clinical manifestations

Para-pneumonic effusion is more common among the elderly and infirm. The male to female ratio is 3:1. Co-morbid conditions may be seen in 62% of patients and the overall mortality is higher in such patients. 10–32% of patients may have chronic pulmonary disease.[120]

The clinical signs and symptoms of para-pneumonic effusions are usually dominated by those of the underlying lung infection. In patients with aerobic bacterial infections, the onset is usually abrupt.

Patients present with fever, pleuritic chest pain, cough and leukocytosis.[121] In contrast, patients with anaerobic lung and pleural infection usually have subacute illness. These may present with significant weight loss, chronic productive cough, mild anaemia and leukocytosis. The majority of patients have a history of aspiration or periodontal disease. Empyema occurs most often as a complication of pneumonia accounting for 40%–60% of cases in the post antibiotic era.[122] Occasionally an empyema may develop without any associated pneumonic process or obvious parenchymal infection. However, most of these are probably secondary to a subclinical pneumonic process. About 25% of cases of empyema follow a surgical procedure or trauma.[123] Abdominal infection predisposes to empyema in about 10% of cases.[124]

Approach to diagnosis

This involves clinical evaluation of predisposing conditions, radiology and pleural fluid analysis (Table 20.7). Pleural effusion may arise from many conditions. Other than infection, congestive heart failure, nephrotic syndrome and cirrhosis of the liver are responsible for all transudative pleural effusions. Pneumonia, malignant pleural disease, tuberculosis, pulmonary embolisation and gastrointestinal disease account for 90% of exudative pleural effusions. The possibility of para-pneumonic effusions should always be considered in patients presenting with bacterial pneumonia.

Table 20.7. *Diagnosis of pleural fluids*

Consider cause from pre-existing disease, e.g.
heart failure
malignancy
pneumonia
Radiology
plain
CT
US
Pleural fluid analysis
gross appearance colour, odour, viscosity, purulence, blood
cholesterol/triglyceride
electrophoresis
protein, LDH (serum/fluid ratio), pH, glucose
Gram's stain
cellular count, cytology

Radiology

A chest radiograph is usually abnormal in patients with moderate pleural effusion. If the fluid volume is small (less than 75 ml) in the upright position, fluid accumulates between the inferior surface of the lung and diaphragm: 'sub-pulmonic effusion'. Costophrenic angles are usually clear and the outline of the diaphragm sharp. However, the most convex part of the diaphragm is seen laterally instead of the usual normal medial position. With further accumulation of fluid, the posterior costophrenic angles are obliterated. The diaphragmatic outline is lost and fluid extends upwards and presents a typical meniscus shape. Unobscured diaphragmatic margins on posteroanterior and lateral radiographs exclude clinically important para-pneumonic effusions. Patients with clear diaphragms but radiographic evidence of non-dependent loculations should have further studies with computed tomography (CT), or ultrasonography. Ultrasound can demonstrate as little as 10 ml pleural fluid.[125] Ultrasound is useful for identification of an optimal site for thoracentesis or pleural biopsy.[126] CT chest is valuable in the evaluation of patients with pleural disease. It can demonstrate parenchymal abnormalities of patients with extensive pleural disease. CT scan is very useful in differentiating lung abscess from empyema.[127] In patients with para-pneumonic effusions, CT scan can demonstrate loculations adjacent to or extending into mediastinum and can guide therapy.[128]

Pleural fluid analysis

Pleural fluid analysis is a very useful test to differentiate exudative and transudative pleural effusions. A diagnostic thoracentesis should be performed in all patients with free pleural fluid of a size greater than 10 mm on the decubitus radiograph (unless the cause is obvious, such as congestive heart failure). A comprehensive and systemic approach to analysis of pleural fluid may help to diagnose the cause of pleural effusion in 75% of patients.[129] The relative contraindications to thoracocentesis include bleeding disorders, active skin infections, small volume of pleural fluid and mechanical ventilation. Complications include bleeding, pneumothorax, pleural space sepsis and injury to the liver and spleen. The incidence of pneumothorax varies from 5–19%; however, fewer than 5% of patients require chest tube drainage.[130] When the volume of pleural fluid is small on standard chest radiographs, thoracentesis should be performed under ultrasound guidance.[131] The aspirated fluid should be inspected for colour, odour, viscosity and purulence. Straw coloured fluid is typical of transudates and minimally inflammatory exudative effusions such as early malignancy, tuberculosis, tuberculous pleurisy and yellow nail syndrome.[132] A bloody effusion in the absence of trauma suggests malignancy, pulmonary infarction, or benign asbestos pleural effusion. A milky effusion suggests chylothorax, chyliform effusion or an empyema. In chylothorax, the disease process is acute, the pleural surfaces are not thickened and there are no cholesterol crystals. The triglyceride level is usually higher than 110mg/dl, whereas in chyliform effusions, the disease process is chronic, the pleural surfaces are thickened and the triglyceride level is less than 50mg/dl and cholesterol crystals can be identified.[133] Occasionally, it is difficult to differentiate between chylothorax and chyliform effusion when cholesterol crystals are absent or the triglyceride level is between 50 mg/dl and 110 mg/dl. Electrophoresis may demonstrate chylomicrons which are diagnostic of chylothorax.[134] A putrid smell is suggestive of anaerobic bacterial infection. However, 50–60% of anaerobic empyemas are not foul smelling. Frank pus confirms the presence of empyema and is an absolute indication for urgent chest tube drainage of the pleural space.

Light and co-workers have suggested that the most practical method of differentiating transudative from exudative pleural effusion is the measurement of serum and pleural fluid protein and lactic dehydrogenase concentrations (LDH). Exudative pleural effusions meet at least one of the following criteria:

(i) Pleural fluid proteins/serum protein ratio of more than 0.5.
(ii) Pleural fluid LDH/serum LDH ratio more than 0.6.
(iii) Pleural fluid LDH more than two thirds of the upper normal limit for serum.

If none of these criteria is met, the patient has a transudative pleural effusion.[135] Cholesterol measurement may be useful when protein and LDH concentrations provide equivocal results. When pleural fluid cholesterol is below 60 mg/dl, it indicates transudative effusion. However, 10% of exudative pleural effusions may have cholesterol levels below 60 mg/dl.[136]

In para-pneumonic effusions, pleural fluid analysis remains the most useful diagnostic test for identifying the stage of a para-pneumonic effusion and guiding therapy. A Gram's positive stain in non-purulent fluid is an acceptable indication for immediate pleural fluid drainage. However, the most difficult decision in managing patients with para-pneumonic effusion is determining whether Gram-negative non-purulent fluid should be drained by a chest tube, or not.

It has been observed that chemical analysis of pleural fluid can assist in the differentiation of uncomplicated para-pneumonic effusion that responds to antibiotics alone from complicated para-pneumonic effusion that may require pleural drainage.[137] The pleural pH and glucose concentrations decrease proportionately with the severity of pleural inflammation. These changes result from several reasons: metabolism of bacteria and leukocytes and the slow equilibration of CO_2 and glucose across the thickened pleural membranes.[138]

A pH of 7.20–7.30 was suggested as pleural space drainage cut points in bacteriologically negative, non-purulent free flowing effusions.[139] The pleural fluid glucose concentration correlates directly with pleural fluid pH in para-pneumonic effusions. Additional analysis of para-pneumonic pleural fluid had suggested that a pH of less than 7.0, a glucose of less than 40 mg/dl and a LDH of more than 1000 μ/l indicates a complicated para-pneumonic effusion[140] and is an absolute indication for chest tube drainage. A pH of > 7.30 and a glucose of >60 mg/dl on admission predicts good outcome with antibiotic therapy alone.[140,141] Patients presenting with pleural fluid pH between 7.10 and 7.20 and pleural fluid glucose above 40mg/dl or pleural fluid LDH > 1000 i.u./l require close monitoring. Repeated thoracenteses within 12–24 hours may assist in management. It should be noted that the pH and glucose criteria were proposed as a guide to be used in conjunction with the clinical presentation and not as an absolute indication for drainage.[142] In a retrospective study of 91 patients with empyema a positive Gram's stain, pH less than 7.0, glucose concentration less than 40 mg/dl and an LDH greater than 1000 i.u./l were each found to have high specificity (82–96%) but low sensitivity (18–53%) for eventual surgical drainage. These criteria therefore may have limited usefulness in predicting the need for eventual chest tube drainage.[143] In a meta-analysis of pleural fluid chemistry in para-pneumonic effusions involving seven primary studies, it was concluded that pleural fluid pH had the highest diagnostic usefulness. A pleural pH of 7.29 should be considered the pleural fluid decision threshold for determining the need for chest tube drainage in patients with a low clinical suspicion of pleural infection. Conversely, the decision threshold for 'high risk' patients is 7.21. The primary studies did not support the use of pleural fluid glucose or LDH as independent predictors of complicated para-pneumonic effusions.[144] A pleural fluid white cell count of $1000/ml^3$ is partially helpful in distinguishing transudative from exudative pleural effusion. A pleural fluid white cell count of $10\,000/mm^3$ is most commonly found in para-pneumonic effusions, pulmonary embolism, pancreatitis, collagen vascular disease and malignancy and occasionally tuberculosis. The differential cell count on pleural fluid is much more useful than the white cell count. The pleural fluid contains predominantly polymorphonuclear leukocytes in an acute disease process and predominantly mono-nuclear cells in chronic pleural effusions.

The demonstration of marked lymphocytosis particularly with lymphocyte counts of 85–95% of the total white cells in an exudative pleural effusion suggests tuberculous pleurisy, lymphoma, sarcoidosis, chronic rheumatoid pleurisy or chylothorax. The major clinical significance of mesothelial cells in exudates is that the presence of more than 5% mesothelial cells makes tuberculous pleurisy unlikely.[145] However, the absence of mesothelial cells is also common in other conditions in which the pleura becomes coated with fibrin such as complicated para-pneumonic effusion, chronic malignant pleural effusion, rheumatoid pleurisy and following the use of sclerosing agents.

Pleural biopsy

Needle biopsy of the pleura is very useful in diagnosing tuberculous pleuritis, and this procedure should be considered when such a diagnosis is suspected. The initial biopsy may show granulomas in 50–80% of patients.[146] Cultures of biopsy specimens for mycobacteria may be positive in over 90% of patients[147] and combined histology of pleural biopsy and culture may be diagnostic in over 90%.[148] If the initial biopsy is negative, a repeat biopsy may provide a diagnosis of tuberculous pleuritis in 10–40% of patients.[149]

Thoracoscopy

Recently, thoracoscopy has been used for the diagnosis and treatment of pleural diseases. In one study of pleural disease the sensitivity of thoracoscopy was 92–97% and specificity was 99%.[150] In another the sensitivity was higher for malignancy compared to tuberculous effusion.[151] The overall incidence of post-operative complications is between 4%–10% and mortality between 0.07–0.5% (the common complications include persistent airleak, wound infection, bleeding and intercostal neuralgia).[152]

Management

> Those cases of empyema or dropsy which are treated by incision or cautery, if water or pus flows rapidly all at once, certainly prove fatal. When empyema is treated either by cautery or incision, if pure and white pus flow from the wound, the patient recovers, but if mixed with blood, slimy and fetid, they die.[153]

Infection of the pleural space, empyema thoracis, was recognised and treated with open drainage by Hippocrates. Despite its historical significance and the development of medical science, it remains a challenging clinical entity. Successful treatment of pleural sepsis requires prompt treatment with appropriate antibiotics to cover likely organisms including anaerobes, together with drainage of frank pus. All patients with bacterial pneumonia should be monitored for the development of para-pneumonic effusion. All patients who develop para-pneumonic effusion should undergo prompt needle thoracentesis. The pleural fluid chemistry can then guide the need for drainage. Patients with loculated para-pneumonic effusion should be considered for intrapleural fibrinolytics or early surgical intervention. Treatment of pleural empyema depends on the stage of the disease, the appearance and location of pleural fluid in the pleural space and results of microbiological investigations. The various facets of management are summarised in Table 20.8.

Antibiotics

The selection of appropriate antibiotics is based on organisms identified by Gram's stain of pleural fluid, culture of the aspirated fluid or sputum. If cultures or Gram's stain are unhelpful in the intervening period while awaiting results, a broad spectrum antibiotic effective against anaerobes and aerobes should be used. Most antibiotics penetrate the pleural space well and achieve concentrations of 75% of serum level in pleural fluid.[154] Aminoglycosides and β-lactams may be inactivated in the presence of pus, low pH and β-lactamase enzymes.[155,156] Drugs that show excellent pleural penetration include cephalosporins, aztreonam, clindamycin, ciprofloxacin, cephalothin and penicillin. The single agents that are likely to be active against the wide spectrum of potential pathogens include imipenem–cilastatin (or meropenem) and ticarcillin–clavulanic acid. Combinations of antibiotics should include an effective agent against anaerobes (clindamycin, metronidazole) plus an agent active against aerobic Gram-positive cocci and Gram-negative bacilli. The duration of therapy is variable depending on specific clinical circumstances. Treatment of uncomplicated para-pneumonic effusion is that of the underlying pneumonia. Patients with empyema should receive at least 4–6 weeks of treatment. The principles of treatment with local installation of antibiotics and antiseptics into the pleural space is supported by experimental and clinical studies but there is no general agreement on their use.[157,158]

Chest tube drainage

Any patient with para-pneumonic effusion and having the following pleural fluid characteristics should be considered for tube thoracostomy:

(a) The pleural fluid is grossly purulent.
(b) The Gram's stain of the pleural fluid is positive.
(c) The pleural fluid glucose level is below 40 mg/dl.
(d) The pleural fluid pH is less than 7.00.

With free-flowing fluid, the chest tube can be placed at the bedside. The chest tube can be removed when the patient is febrile, drainage is serous and less than 50 ml to 100 ml in 24 hours. If the patient remains febrile, symptomatic and drainage is minimal, and the chest radiograph shows incomplete evacuation of pleural fluid, CT chest or ultrasound should be obtained for assessment of multiple loculations. The factors which results in failure of chest tube drainage include: tube blockage by viscous fluid, multiple pleural loculations, improper tube position and tube kinking.[159]

Table 20.8. *Management of pleural fluid*

Antibiotics
Tube thoracostomy for gross pus positive Gram's stain pleural fluid glucose < 40 mg/l pleural fluid pH < 7.00
Image-guided percutaneous catheter drainage for loculated fluid failed tube thoracostomy +/– early formation of fluid
Intrapleural streptokinase/urokinase for loculated fluid
Thoracoscopy with adhesion lysis or debridement for loculated fluid
Thoracotomy with decortication for failure of other techniques
Open tube drainage/rib resection for failure of other techniques broncho-pleural fistula
Cavity obliteration – thoracoplastics

If the pleural fluid is not free flowing, a CT of the chest should be obtained for better definition of pleural space disease. In patients with multiple pleural fluid levels, an open procedure is the best management as loculi and adhesions need to be broken down.

Image guided percutaneous catheters

With a low success rate of tube thoracostomy for loculated para-pneumonic effusion, attention has been focused on other approaches for the drainage of pleural spaces. One of the options is radiologically guided percutaneous catheter drainage using small bore 'pigtail' catheters placed with ultrasound or CT guidance. The reported success rate (72–90%) is probably related to more precise placement of chest tubes.[160] Some authorities recommend percutaneous catheters as an initial thoracic drainage technique for patients in the exudative or early fibrinopurulent stages of empyema formation who have a relatively thin pleural fluid[161,162] and as a second line therapy in those with failed chest tube drainage.[163]

Intrapleural streptokinase

Failure of chest tube drainage is usually associated with the fibropurulent stage of empyema in which the pleural fluid becomes multiloculated through formation of fibrous stands. Theoretically, the intrapleural injection of streptokinase can destroy these fibrous strands and facilitate drainage of pleural space. The initial use of fibrinolytic agents for the treatment of haemothorax and post pneumonic empyema was described in 1949.[164,165] The initial results were encouraging but its use did not gain acceptance because of the rare occurrence of intrapleural haemorrhage and systemic fibrinolysis.[166,167] With the subsequent availability of purified streptokinase there has been a resurgence in its use as intrapleural fibrinolysis.[167] Several small clinical studies have suggested that intrapleural streptokinase is a safe and effective adjunct in the management of complicated para-pneumonic effusions and pleural empyema and may reduce the need for surgery.[168,169] The technique involves daily instillation of 250 000 units of streptokinase in 100 ml of normal saline into the pleural cavity via a small catheter or chest tube which is clamped for 4 hours. The response to treatment is assessed by clinical and radiological improvement and reduction of drainage to < 60–100 ml/day. The number of streptokinase instillations for patient may vary from 2–6. Urokinase can be used instead of streptokinase because of slow antigenicity but it is expensive. As the incidence of adverse effects to purified streptokinase is low, its use will remain occasional.[167]

Surgical drainage techniques

Patients who present in the late fibrinopurulent or organisation stages, or have evidence of intrapleural pus and multiple loculations have a low probability of improvement by closed thoracostomy tube and may require other aggressive procedures for adequate drainage of the pleural space with expansion of the lung.[170] In addition, patients who fail chest tube drainage are also candidates for more a definitive surgical procedure. Many surgical procedures are available for treatment of thoracic empyema. In patients with established empyema with thickened pleura and significant loss of volume thoracotomy with decortication is the treatment of choice.[171,172] It has gained favour because surgery can be successfully performed at any stage of an empyema with a low morbidity and mortality and it has an excellent success rate. Patients do not require decortication for the management of pleural restriction alone. These procedures should only be considered for the control of pleural infection.

Thoracoscopy has been used successfully in the lysis of adhesions and debridement of empyema cavities. It is suggested that one can begin with thoracoscopy and if the procedure is not successful a decortication can be done through a formal thoracotomy.[173]

When the pleural fluid is thick and closed drainage of pleural infection is inadequate, open tube drainage should be considered if the patient is not a candidate for decortication. Open drainage can be performed by resection of ribs overlying the dependent region of the empyema and insertion of the chest tubes under direct visualisation. This procedure allows the surgeon to ensure that all intrapleural adhesions are broken down by mechanical means and that is the option if one anticipates the need for long term drainage. Open drainage can also be performed as an open window thoracostomy that avoids chest tube placement in patients with empyema and provides control of pleural infection in patients with broncho-pleural fistula.[172] This method has the advantage of providing drainage without tubes so the patient can take care of himself at home. Over a period of time the cavity gradually obliterates. Alternatively the cavities can be obliterated by transposition of muscle or omental flaps. The purpose of thoracoplasty is to remove the rigidity of the chest wall and so establish contact between either the now flexible chest wall and residual lung, or after pneumonectomy with the mediastinum in order to obliterate the empyema space. The procedure is rarely undertaken today because of the deformity that results and the success that can be achieved with other forms of management.[173]

Conclusions

Para-pneumonic effusion represents one of the diagnostic urgencies. If the pneumonias are treated appropriately, probably no pneumonia will progress to complicated para-pneumonic effusion. It is important that thoracocentesis should be performed without delay once para-pneumonic effusion develops and this will help in decision making. Free-flowing fluids can be drained by chest tubes or catheters and intrapleural streptokinase can also be used as adjunctive therapy. In cases of non-free-flowing fluid it is recommended that CT should be obtained earlier as this type of para-pneumonic effusion is unlikely to improve by simple tube drainage and would require aggressive surgical intervention.

References

1. GUILLEMOT L, HALLE J, RIST E. Recherches bacteriologiques et experimentales surles pleuresies putrides. *Arch Med Exper Pol Anat Let Path* 1904;16:571–640.
2. SMITH DJ. Fusospirochetal diseases of the lungs. *Tubercle* 1928;16:420–33.
3. SMITH DT. Fusospirochetal disease of the lungs produced with cultures from Vincent's angina. *J Infect Dis* 1930;46:303–10.
4. SCHWEPP HI, KNOWLES JH, KANE L. Lung abscess: an analysis of the Massachusetts general hospital cases from 1943 through to 1956. *N Engl J Med,* 1961;265:1039–43.
5. SLOTS J. Microflora in the healthy gingival sulcus in man. *Scand J Dental Res* 1977;85:247–54.
6. LASSCHE WJ. *Anaerobic Bacteria: Role in Disease*. Springfield K. CC Thomas; 1974;409– 34.
7. SMITH DT. Experimental aspiratory abscess. *Arch Surg* 1927;14:231–9.
8. MAYRAND D, HOLT SC. Biology of asaccharolytic black-pigmented *Bacteroides* species. *Microbiol Rev* 1988;52:134–152.
9. CRABB JH, FINBERG R, ONDERDONK AB, KASPER DL. T-cell regulation of *Bacteroides fragilis* induced intraabdominal abscesses. *Rev Infect Dis* 1990;12(suppl 2):S178–84.
10. EFTIMIADI C, TONETTI M, CAVALLERO A, SACCO O, ROSSI GA. Short-chain fatty acids produced by anaerobic bacteria inhibit phagocytosis by human lung phagocytes. *J Infect Dis* 1990;161:138–42.
11. BARTLETT JG. Anaerobic bacterial infections of the lung. *Chest* 1987; 91:901–9.
12. MARINA M, STRONG CA, CIVEN, R, MOLITORIS E, FINEGOLD SM. Bacteriology of anaerobic pleuropulmonary infections: preliminary report. *Clin Infect Dis* 1993;16(suppl 4):S256–S262.
13. FINEGOLD SM, GEORGE WL, MULLIGAN ME. Anaerobic infections. *Disease-A-Month* 1985;31:1–77.
14. MUSIAL CE, ROSENBLATT JE. Antimicrobial susceptibilities of anaerobic bacteria isolated at the Mayo Clinic during 1982 through 1987. Comparison with results from

1977 through 1981. *Mayo Clin Proc* 1989;64:392–9.

15. APPELBAUM PC, SPANGLER SK, JACOBS MR. Beta-lactamase production and susceptibilities to amoxicillin, amoxicillin-clavulanate, ticarcillin, ticarcillin-clavulanate, cefoxitin, imipenem, and metronidazole of 320 non-*Bacteroides fragilis, Bacteroides* isolates and 129 fusobacteria from 28 US centers. *Antimicrob Agents Chemother* 1990;34:1546–50.
16. BARTLETT JG. Anaerobic bacterial pleuropulmonary infections. *Semin Resp Med* 1992;13:158–66.
17. HUNTER JV, CHADWICK M, HUTCHINSON G, HODSON ME. Use of a gas liquid chromatography in the clinical diagnosis of anaerobic pleuropulmonary infection. *Br J Dis Chest* 1985;79:1–8.
18. BARTLETT JG. Anaerobic bacterial pneumonitis. *Am Rev Resp Dis* 1979;119:19–23.
19. KLINE BS, BERGER SS. Pulmonary abscess and pulmonary gangrene. Analysis of ninety cases observed in ten years. *Arch Intern Med* 1935;56:753–72.
20. CAMERON EWJ, APPELBAUM PC, PUDIFIN D, HUTTON WS, CHATTERTON SA. Characteristics and management of chronic destructive pneumonia. *Thorax* 1980;35:340–6.
21. LEVISON ME, MANGURA CT, LORBER B *et al.* Clindamycin compared with penicillin for the treatment of anaerobic lung abscess. *Ann Intern Med* 1983;98:466–71.
22. GUDIOL F, MANRESA F, PALLARES R *et al.* Clindamycin vs penicillin for anaerobic lung infections. High rate of penicillin failures associated with penicillin-resistant *Bacteroides melaninogenicus*. *Arch Intern Med* 1990;150:2525–9.
23. ASTRY CL, NELSON S, KARAM GH, SUMMER WR. Interactions of clindamycin with antimicrobial defenses of the lung. *Am Rev Resp Dis* 1987;135:1015–19.
24. PERLINO CA. Metronidazole vs clindamycin treatment of anaerobic pulmonary infection. Failure of metronidazole therapy. *Arch Intern Med* 1981;141:1424–7.
25. BARTLETT JG, FINEGOLD SM. Anaerobic infection of the lung and pleural space. *Am Rev Resp Dis* 1994;110:56.
26. ALLEN C I, BLACKMAN JF. Treatment of lung abscess with report of 100 consecutive cases. *J Thorac Surg* 1936;6:136.
27. NEUHOJ H. Acute putrid abscess of the lung. *Gyn Obst Surg* 1945;80:307.
28. WEISS W. Delayed cavity closure in acute non specific primary lung abscess. Am J Med Sci, 1968:255:313–19.
29. HAMMOND JM, POTGIETER PD, HANSLO D, SCOTT H, RODITI D. The aetiology and antimicrobial susceptibility patterns of microorganisms in acute community-acquired lung abscess. *Chest* 1995;108:937–41.
30. POHLSON EC, MCNAMARA JJ, CHAR C *et al.* Lung abscess: a changing pattern of the disease. *Am J Surg* 1985;150:97–101.
31. FOX JR, HUGHES FA, SUTCLIFF WA. Nonspecific lung abscess: experience with fifty five consecutive cases. *J Thorac Surg* 1953;26:255.
32. PERLMAN LU, LERNER E, D'ESOPO N. Clinical classification and analysis of 97 cases of lung abscess. *Am Rev Resp Dis* 1969;99:390.
33. AMBERSON JB. Aspiration bronchopneumonia. *Int Clin* 1937;3:126–38.
34. BARTLETT J, GORBACH S, TALLY F, FINEGOLD S. Bacteriology and treatment of primary lung abscess. *Am Rev Resp Dis*, 1974;109:510–18.
35. KAYE MG, FOX MJ, BARTLETT JG *et al.* The spectrum of *Staphylococcus aureus* infection. *Chest* 1992;97:788–792.
36. KIM IG, BRUMMITT W, HUMPHREY A *et al.* Foreign body in the airway: a review of 202 cases. *Laryngoscope* 1973;83:347.
37. ABDULMAJID OA, EBEID AM, MOTAWEH MH, KLEIBO S. Aspirated foreign bodies in tracheobronchial tree: a report of 250 cases. *Thorax* 1976;31:635.
38. NEILD JE, EKYN SJ, PHILLIPS I. *J Med*, 1985;57:875–82.
39. PHILPOTT NJ, WOODHEAD MA, WILSON AG, MILLARD FJ. Lung abscess: a neglected cancer of life threatening hemoptysis. *Thorax* 1993;48:674–5.
40. SMITH DT. Fuso-spirochaetal disease of the lungs, its bacteriology, pathology and experimental reproduction. *Am Rev Tubercul* 1927;16:584–98.
41. GONZALEZ CL, CALIC F. Bacteriologic flora of aspiration induced pulmonary infections. *Arch Intern Med* 1975;135:711–14.
42. BEERENS H, TAHOU-CASTEL M. Infections humaines a bacteries anaerobies nontoxigenes. Brussels, *Presses Acad Europ* 1965:91–114.
43. CORBER B, SWENSEN RM. Bacteriology of aspiration pneumonia: a prospective study of community and hospital-acquired cases. *Am Intern Med* 1974;81:329–31.
44. PENA N, MUNOZ F, VARGAS J, ALFAGEME I, UMBRIA S, FLOREZ C. Yield of percutaneous needle lung aspiration in lung abscess. *Chest* 1990;97:69–74.
45. BROOK I AND FINEGOLD SM. Bacteriology and therapy of lung abscess in children. *J Pediatr* 1979;94:10–12.
46. FISHER AM *et al.* Staphylococcal pneumonia: a review of 21 cases in adults. *N Engl J Med* 1958;258:919.
47. POHLSSON CC, MCNAMARA JJ, CHAR C, KURATA L. Lung abscess: a changing pattern of the disease. *Am J Surg* 1985;150:97–101.
48. HOWE C, SAMPATH A, SPOTNITZ M. The pseudomallu group: a review. *J Infect Dis* 1971;124:596.
49. KEEFER CS, INGLEFINGER FJ, SPINK WW. Significance of hemolytic streptococci bacteremia: study of 246 patients. *Arch Intern Med* 1937;60:1084.
50. WILLIAMS DM, KRICK JA, REMINGTON JS. Pulmonary infections in compromised host. *Am Rev Resp Dis* 1976;114:359.
51. WILSON JP, TURNER HR, KIRCHNER KA *et al.* Nocardia infections in renal transplant recipients. *Medicine* 1989;68:38–57.
52. MURRAY JF, MILLS J. Pulmonary infection complications of human immunodeficiencies virus infection. *Am Rev Resp Dis* 1990;141:1582.
53. HARVEY RL, SUNSTROM JC. *Rhodococcus equi* infection in patients with and without human immunodeficiency virus infection. *Rev Infect Dis* 1991;13:139.
54. BARTLETT JG. Diagnostic accuracy of transtracheal aspiration bacteriology. *Am Rev Resp Dis* 1977;115:779.
55. ESTERERA AJ, PLATT MR, MILLS LJ *et al.* Primary lung abscess. *J Thorac Cardiovasc Surg* 1980;79:275–282.
56. AETEMEIER WA. The cause of putrid odour of perforated appendicitis with peritonitis. *Ann Surg* 1938;107:634–6.
57. BARTLETT JG, ALEXANDER J, MAYHEW J *et al.* Should fiberoptic bronchosocpy aspirates be cultured? *Am Rev Resp Dis*. 1976;114:73–8.
58. WIMBERLY N, FALING J, BARTLETT JG. A fiberoptic bronchoscopy technique to obtain uncontaminated lower airways secretions for bacterial culture. *Am Rev Resp Dis* 1979;110:337–43.
59. BROUGHTON WA, MIDDLETON RM, KIRKPATRICK MB, BASS JB JR. Bronchoscopy protected specimen brush and bronchoalveolar lavage in the diagnosis of bacterial pneumonia. *Infect Dis Clin* 1991;5:437–45.
60. ALLEN RM, DUNN WF, LIMPER AH. Diagnosing ventilator associated pneumonia role of bronchoscopy. *Mayo Clin Proc* 1994;69:962–8.
61. HAMMER DL, ARANDA CP, GALATI V, ADAMS FV. Massive intrabronchial aspiration of contents of pulmonary abscess after fiberoptic bronchoscopy. *Chest* 1978;74:306–7.
62. SOSENKO A, GLASSROTH J. Fiberoptic bronchoscopy in the evaluation of lung abscess. Chest 1985;87:489–94.
63. LORCH DJ JR, JOHN JF JR, TOMLINSON *et al.* Protected transbronchial needle aspiration and protected specimen brush in the diagnosis

of pneumonia. *Am Rev Resp Dis*, 1987;136:565–9.

64. MARQUETTE CH, RAMON P, COURCOL R *et al.* Bronchoscopic protected catheter brush for the diagnosis of pulmonary infections. *Chest* 1988;93:746–50.

65. TORRES A, MARTOS A, PUIG DE LA BELLACASE A *et al.* Evaluation of bronchoalveolar lavage for the diagnosis of bacterial pneumonia in ventilated patients. *Am Rev Resp Dis* 1993;147:952–7.

66. BARTLETT JG, ROSENBLATT JE, FINEGOLD SM. Percutaneous transtracheal aspiration in the diagnosis of anaerobic infections. *Ann Intern Med* 1973;79:535–40.

67. CONUS DJ, SCHWENK GR, DOERING PR *et al.* Thoracic needle biopsy: improved results utilising a team approach. *Chest* 1987;91:813–16.

68. KALINSKE RW, PARKER RH, BRANDT D, HOEPRICH PD. Diagnostic usefulness and safety of transtracheal aspiration. *N Engl J Med*, 1967;276:604–8.

69. BJERKESTRAND G, DIAGNRANIS A, SCHREINER A. Bacteriological findings in transtracheal aspirates from patients with chronic bronchitis and bronchiectasis. *Scand J Resp Dis* 1975;56:201–7.

70. CONCES DJ, SCHWENK RG, DOERING PR, GLANT MD. Thoracic needle aspiration improved results utilising team approach. *Chest* 1987;91:813–16.

71. GRINAN NP, LUCENA FM, ROMERO JV *et al.* Yield of percutaneous lung aspiration in lung abscess. *Chest* 1990;9769–74.

72. LORCH DG JR, JOHN JF JR, TOMLINSON JR. Protected transbronchial needle aspiration and protected specimen brush in the diagnosis of pneumonia. *Ann Rev Resp Dis* 1987;136:565–9.

73. THORPE JE, BAUGHMAN RP, FRAME PT *et al.* Bronchoalveolar lavage for diagnosing acute bacterial pneumonia. *J Infect Dis* 1987;155:855–61.

74. BARTLETT JG, FALLING LJ, WILLEY S. Quantitative tracheal bacteriologic and cytologic studies in patients with long term tracheostomies. *Chest* 1978;74:635–9.

75. BARTLETT JG, FINEGOLD SM. Bacteriology of expectorated sputum with quantitative culture and wash technique compared to tracheal aspirates. *Am Rev Resp Dis* 1978;117;1019–27.

76. HENRIQUEZ AH, MENDOZA J, GONZALEZ PC. Quantitative cultures of bronchoalveolar lavage from patients with anaerobic lung abscess. *J Infect Dis* 1991;164:414–17.

77. LE ROUX BT, MOHALA ML, ODELL JA, WHITTON ID. Suppurative disease of the lung and pleural space Part I. *Curr Prob Surg* 1986;21:1.

78. SCHACHTER EN, KREISMAN H, PUTMAN C. Diagnostic problems in suppurative lung disease. *Arch Intern Med* 1976;136:167–71.

79. STARK DD, FEDERLE MP, GOOD PC *et al.* Differentiating lung abscess and empyema: Radiography and tomography. *AJR* 1983;141:163–7.

80. WEISS W. Delayed cavity closure in acute nonspecific primary lung abscess. *Am J Med Sci* 1968;255:313–19.

81. WEISS W. Oral antibiotic therapy of acute primary lung abscess: Comparison of penicillin and tetracycline. *Curr Ther Res* 1970;12:154.

82. WEISS W. Cavity behaviour in acute primary nonspecific lung abscess. *Am Rev Resp Dis* 1973;109:1273–75.

83. KIRBY BD, GEORGE WL, SUTER VL, CITRON DM, FINEGOLD SM. Gram-negative anaerobic bacilli their role in infection and patterns of susceptibility to antimicrobial agents: little known bacteroides species. *Rev Infect Dis* 1980;2:941–51.

84. BARTLETT GJ. Antibiotics in lung abscess. *Semin Resp Infect* 1991;6:103–11.

85. SEN P, TECSON F, KAPILA R, LOURIA D. Clindamycin in the oral treatment of putative anaerobic pneumonias. *Arch Intern Med* 1974;134:73–7.

86. SANDERS SC, HANNA BJ, LEWIS C. Metronidazole in the treatment of anaerobic infections. *Am Rev Resp Dis* 1979;120:337–43.

87. TALLY FP, SUTTER VL, FINEGOLD SM. Treatment of anaerobic infections with metronidazole. *Antimicrob Agents Chemother* 1975;7:672–5.

88. EYKYN SJ. The therapeutic use of metronidazole in anaerobic infections: six years experience in a London Hospital. *Surgery* 1983;93:209–14.

89. FINEGOLD SM. Susceptibility testing of anaerobic bacteria. *J Clin Microbiol* 1988;26:1253–6.

90. LANDAY MJ, CHRISTENSEN CE, BYNUM LJ, GOODMAN C. Anaerobic pleural and pulmonary infections. *AJR* 1980:134:233–40.

91. HAGAN JL, HARDY JD. Lung abscess revisited: a survey of 184 cases. *Ann Surg* 1983;197:755–62.

92. CONNORS JP, ROBAR CL, FERGUSON TB. Transbronchial catheterisation of pulmonary abscess. *Ann Thorac Surgery* 1975;19:254.

93. SCHMITT GS, OHAR JM, KANTER KR, NEUNHEIM KS. Indwelling transbronchial catheter drainage of lung abscess. *Ann Rev Resp Dis* 1978;117:53.

94. VAINBRUB B, MUSHER DM, GUINN *et al.* Percutaneous drainage of lung abscess. *Am Rev Resp Dis* 1978;117:53.

95. VANSONNENBERG E, D'AGOSTINO HB, CASOLA G *et al.* Lung abscess: CT guided drainage. *Radiol* 1991;178:347–51.

96. HA HK, KANG MW, PARK JM *et al.* Lung abscess. Percutaneous catheter therapy. *Acta Radiol* (4)34:362–5.

97. BAKER RB. The treatment of lung abscess – current concepts (editorial). *Chest* 1985;39:266–70.

98. MAVROUDIS C, GANZEL BL, KATZMARK S, POLK HC JR. Effect of hemothorax on experimental empyema thoracis in the guinea pig. *J Thorac Cardiovasc Surg* 1985;89:42–9.

99. SAHN SA, TARYLE DA, GOOD JT JR. Experimental empyema: time course and pathogenesis of pleural fluid acidosis and low pleural fluid glucose. *Am Rev Resp Dis* 1979;120:355–61.

100. MAVROUDIS C, GANZEL BL, COX SK *et al.* Experimental aerobic anaerobic thoracic empyema in the guinea pig. *Ann Thorac Surg* 1987; 43:295–7.

101. WEINER-KRONISH JP, BROADDUS VC. Interrelationship of pleural and pulmonary interstitial liquid. *Ann Rev Physiol* 1993;55:209–26.

102. WIENER-KRONISH JP, SAKUMA T, KUDOH I *et al.* Alveolar epithelial injury and pleural empyema in acute *P. aeruginosa* pneumonia in anesthetised rabbits. *J Appl Physiol* 1993;75:1661–9.

103. LECKIE WJH, TOTHILL P. Albumin turnover in pleural effusions. *Clin Sci* 1965;29:339–52.

104. SCERBO J, KELTZ H, STONE DJ. A prospective study of closed pleural biopsies. *JAMA*, 1971;218:377–80.

105. HAMILTON SM, JOHNSON MG, GONG A *et al.* Relationship between increased vascular permeability and extravascular albumin clearance in rabbit-inflammatory responses induced with *Escherichia coli*. *Lab Invest* 1986;55:580–7.

106. ANDREW NC, PARKER EF, SHAW RR *et al.* Management of nontuberculous empyema. *Am Rev Resp Dis* 1962;85:935–6.

107. LEW PD, ZUBLER R, VANDAUX P, FARQUET JJ, WALDVOGLE F, LAMBAR PH. Decreased heat labile opson activity and complement level associated with evidence of C_3 breakdown products in infected pleural effusion. *J Clin Invest* 1979;63:326–34.

108. SAHN SA, RELLER LB, TARYLER DA *et al.* The contribution of leukocytes and bacteria to the low pH of empyema fluids. *Am Rev Resp Dis* 1982;128:811–15.

109. BROADDERS VC, HEBERT CA, VITANGCOL RB *et al.* Interleukin-8 is a major neutrophil chemotactic factor in pleural fluids of patients with empyema. *Am Rev Resp Dis*, 1992;146:825–30.

110. ANTONY VB, GODBEY SW, KUNKLE SI *et al.* Recruitment of inflammatory cells to the pleural space: chemotactic cytokines IL-8 and monocyte chemotactic peptide-I in human pleural fluids. *J Immunol* 1993;151:7216–23.
111. PEVERI P, WALZ A, DEWALD B, BAGGIOLINI M. A novel neutrophil activating factor produced by human mononuclear phagocytes. *J Exp Med* 1988;167:1547–59.
112. JONGIC N, PERI G, BERNASCONI S *et al.* Expression of adhesion molecule and chemotactic cytokines in cultured human mesothelial cells. *J Exp Med* 1992;176:1165–74.
113. SHIMOKATA K, KAWACHI H, KISHIMOTO H *et al.* Local cellular immunity in tuberculous pleurisy. *Am Rev Resp Dis* 1982;126:822–84.
114. BARNES PF, MISTRY SD, COOPER CI, PRIMEZ C, REA TH, MODLIN RI. Compartmentalisation of CD_4 T lymphocytes subpopulation in tuberculous pleuritis. *J Immunol* 1989;142:1114–9.
115. FINLAND M, BARNES MW. Changing ecology of acute bacterial empyema: occurrence and mortality at Boston City Hospital during 12 selected years from 1935 to 1972. *J Infect Dis* 1978;137:274–91.
116. KAYE MG, FOX MJ, BARTLETT JG *et al.* The clinical spectrum of *Staphylococcus aureus* pulmonary infection. *Chest* 1990;97:788–92.
117. SMITH JA, MULLERWORTH MH, WESTLAKE GW *et al.* Empyema thoracis: 14 years experience in teaching centre. *Ann Thorac Cardiovasc Surg* 1981;18:85–90.
118. BARTLETT J, THADEPALLI H, GORBACH S *et al.* Bacteriology of empyema. *Lancet* 1974;1:338–40.
119. FORTY J, YEATMAN M, WELLS FC. Empyema thoracis: a review of a $4\frac{1}{2}$ years experience of cases requiring surgical treatment. *Resp Med* 1990;84:147–53.
120. KELLY JW, MORRIS MJ. Empyema thoracis: medical aspects of evaluation and treatment. *South Med J* 1994;87:1103–10.
121. LIGHT RW, GIRARD WM, JENKENSON SG, GEORGE RB. Parapneumonic effusions. *Am J Med* 1980;69:507–11.
122. BARTLETT JG. Bacterial infections of pleural space. *Semin Respir Infect* 1988;3:308–21.
123. LIGHT RW. *Pleural Diseases*. Philadelphia, Lea and Febiger; 1983:101–18.
124. LEMMER JH, BOTHAM MJ, ORRINGER MB. Modern management of adult thoracic empyema. *J Thorac Cardiovas Surg* 1985;90:849–55.
125. YAM LT. Diagnostic significance of lymphocytes in pleural effusion. *Ann Intern Med* 1967;66:972–82.
126. O'MOORE PU, MULLER PR, SIMEONE JF *et al.* Sonographic guidance in diagnostic and therapeutic interventions in pleural space. *AJR* 1987;149:1–5.
127. WILLIFORD ME, GODWIN D. Computed tomography of lung abscess and empyema. *Radiol Clin N Am* 1983;21:575–83.
128. HIMELMAN RB, COLLEN PW. The prognostic value of loculations in parapneumonic effusions. *Chest* 1986;90:852–6.
129. COLLIN TR, SAHN SA. Thoracentesis: complications, patients' experience and diagnostic value. *Chest* 1987;91:817–22.
130. COLLEN TR, SAHN SR, GROGAN DR *et al.* Complication associated with thoracentesis: a prospective randomised study comparing 3 different methods. *Arch Intern Med* 1990;150:893–77.
131. KOHAN JM, POE RH, ISRAEL RH *et al.* Value of chest-ultrasonography versus decubitus roentgenography for thoracentesis . *ARRG* 1986;133:1124–26.
132. SAHN SA. The diagnostic value of pleural fluid analysis. *Semin Resp Crit Care Med* 1995;16:269–277.
133. COE JE, AIKAWA JK. Cholesterol pleural effusion. *Arch Intern Med* 1961;108:763–4.
134. STAATS BA, ELLESFSON RD, BADAHN LL, DINES DE, PARKASH UBS, OXFORD D. The lipoprotein profile of chylous and nonchylous pleural effusion. *Mayo Clin Proc* 1980;55:700–4.
135. LIGHT RW, MACGREGOR MI, LUCHSINGER PC, BALL WC. Pleural effusions: the diagnostic separation of transudates and exudates. *Ann Intern Med* 1972;77:507–13.
136. HAMM H, BROHAN U, BOHMER R, MISSMAHL HP. Cholesterol and pleural effusions. A diagnostic aid. *Chest* 1987;92:296–302.
137. LIGHT RW, MACGREGOR MI, BALL WC. Diagnostic significance of pleural fluid PH and PCO_2. *Chest* 1973;64:591–6.
138. SAHN SA, RELLER LB, TARYLER DA *et al.* The contribution of leukocytes and bacteria to the low pH of empyema fluid. *ARRD* 1983;128:811–15.
139. LIGHT RW, GIRARD WM, JENKINSON SG, GEORGE PB. Parapneumonic effusions. *Am J Med* 1980;69:507–12.
140. POTTS DE, LEVIN DC, SAHN SA. Pleural pH in parapneumonic effusions. *Chest* 1976;70:328–31.
141. LIGHT S, STRANGE C, SAHN SA. Pleural fluid PH in parapneumonic effusions. *Chest* 1970;64:591.
142. SAHN SA. Management of complicated parapneumonic effusion. *ARRD* 1993;148:813–17.
143. POE RH, MARIN MG, ISRAEL RH *et al.* Utility of pleural fluid analysis in predicting tube thoracostomy decortication in parapneumonic effusion. *Chest* 1991;100:963–7.
144. HEFFNER JE, BROWN LK, BARBIERI C, DELCO JM. Pleural fluid chemical analysis in para-pneumonic effusions: a meta-analysis. *Am J Resp Crit Care Med* 1995;151:1700–8.
145. YAM LT. Diagnostic significance of lymphocytes in pleural effusion. *Ann Intern Med* 1967;66:972–82.
146. SCERBO J, KELTZ H, STONE DJ. A prospective study of closed pleural biopsy. *JAMA* 1971;218:377–80.
147. MESTITZ P, PURVES MJ, POLLARD AC. Pleural biopsy in the diagnosis of pleural effusion. *Lancet* 1958;2:1349–53.
148. LEVINE H, METZGER W, LAURA D, KAY L. Diagnosis of tuberculous pleurisy by culture of pleural biopsy specimen. *Arch Intern Med* 1970;126:269–71.
149. VON HOFF DD, LIVOLSI V. Diagnostic reliability of needle biopsy of parietal pleura. *Am J Clin Path* 1975;64:200–3.
150. BOUTIN C, LODDENKEMPER R, ASTOUL P. Diagnostic and therapeutic thoracoscopy: techniques and indications in pulmonary medicine. *Tuber Lun Dis* 1993;74:225–39.
151. JANCOVICI R, LANG-LAZDUNSKI L, PONS F *et al. Ann Thorac Surg* 1996;61:533–7.
152. YIM AP, LIU HP. Complications and failures of video-assisted thoracic surgery: experience from two centres in Asia. *Ann Thorac Surg* 1996;61:538–41.
153. HIPPOCRATES. In Major RH, ed: *Classic Description of Disease* Springfield, Illinois: Charles C. Thomas, 1965:568–9.
154. TARYLE DA, GOOD JT, MORGAN JT *et al.* Antibiotic concentration in human parapneumonic effusion. *J Antimicrob Chemother* 1981;7:171–7.
155. THYS JP, VANDERHOEFL P, HERCHRELZ A *et al.* Penetration of aminoglycosides in uninfected pleural exudate and in pleural empyema. *Chest* 1988;93:530–2.
156. RUBENIS M, KOZIJ VM, JACKSON GG. Laboratory studies in gentamicin. *Antimicrob Agents Chemother* 1963:153–6.
157. ROSENFELL FL, MCGIBREY D, BRAINBRIDGE MV, WATSON DA. Comparison between irrigation and conventional treatment for empyema and pneumonectomy space infection. *Thorax* 1981;36:272–7.
158. HUHER JA, HARARI D, BRAINBRIDGE MV. The management of empyema by thoracoscopy and irrigation. *Ann Thorac Surg* 1985;39:517–20.
159. STARK DP, FEDERLE MP, GOODMAN

PC. CT and radiographic assessment of tube thoracostomy. *AJR* 1983;141:253–8.

160. ULMER JL, CHOPLIN RH, REED JC. Image guided catheter drainage of infected pleural space. *J Thorac Imaging* 1991;6:65–73.

161. HANNAN GR, FLOWER CD. Radiographically guided percutaneous drainage of empyemas. Clin *Radiol* 1988;39:121–6.

162. SILVERMAN SG, MUELLER PR, SAINI S *et al.* Thoracic empyema: management with image guided catheter drainage. *Radiology* 1988;169:5–9.

163. VAN SONNENBERG E, NAKAMOTO SK, MUELLER PR *et al.* CT ultrasound guided catheter drainage of empyemas after chest tube failure. *Radiology* 1984;151:349–53.

164. TILLET WS, SHERRY S, READ CT. Use of streptokinase -streptodornase in treatment of postpneumonic empyema. *J Thorac Surg* 1951;21:275–95.

165. GODLEY PC, BELL RC. Major hemorrhage following the administration of intrapleural streptokinase. *Chest* 1984;84:486–7.

166. AYE RW, FROESE DP, HILL LD. Use of purified streptokinase in empyema and hemothorax. *Am J Surg* 1991;161:560–2.

167. MOULTAN JS, MOOR PT, MENCINI RA. Treatment of loculated pleural effusion with transcatheter intracavitary urokinase. *AJR* 1989;153:941–5.

168. TAYLOR RFH, RUBENS MB, PEARSON MC, BARNES NC. Intrapleural streptokinase in the management of empyema. *Thorax* 1994;49:856–9.

169. BRAUM MA, ARONSON BA, NEMCEK AA *et al.* Intracavitary fibrinolysis: effective treatment for empyema and hemothorax. *Radiology* 1993;189:156.

170. LEMMER JH, BOTHAM MJ, ORRINGER MB. Modern management of adult thoracic empyema. *J Thorac Cardiovasc Surg* 1985;90:849–55.

171. MUSKETT A, BURTON NA, KARWANDE SV *et al.* Management of refractory empyema with early decortication. *Am J Surg* 1988;156:529–32.

172. FISHMAN NH, ELLERTSON DG. Early pleural decortication for thoracic empyema in immunosuppressed patients. *J Thorac Cardiovasc Surg* 1981;74:537–41.

173. RIDLEY PD, BRAIMBRIDGE MV. Thoracoscopic debridement and pleural irrigation in the management of empyema thoracis. *Ann Thorac Surg* 1991;51:461–4.

21 Pneumonia in the immunocompromised host

MICHAEL E. ELLIS

King Faisal Specialist Hospital and Research Centre, Riyadh, Saudi Arabia

The challenge

The compromised host is an individual who has become highly predisposed to (severe) infections. As a contribution to the total medical care-seeking population, this component has escalated over the last 2–3 decades. The revolution of high technological medical care (causing breaches in mechanical host defence), changes in certain socio-behavioural phenomena (leading to immune suppressive HIV disease, for example), the increasing numbers of patients with previously classified terminal disease who now are amenable to definitive therapy and who survive longer – as a result of improved techniques and therapies (for example, organ and blood/bone transplantation), the generally increased longevity of the population which provides the backdrop of increased age-related general immune disintegration and persons with more specific immune disturbing diseases such as diabetes mellitus have all contributed to produce a population much more vulnerable to infections. The impact on pulmonary disease was recently exemplified in a study of community-acquired pneumonia.[1] In that study 57% of patients had concurrent immunosuppression – such a high figure had not been reported in previous studies. In addition to these factors, widespread appropriate and inappropriate use of antibiotics and antifungals have been associated with, and in some circumstances have selected out, difficult to treat resistant organisms, or others which would not normally have been pathogenic.

The lung is frequently involved as a target organ either primarily or secondarily to haematogenous or contiguous spread of infection in these patients. For example, 52 episodes of pneumonia among 68 patients with acute leukaemia were documented over a 19-month period in renal transplant patients[2]. In cardiac transplant, bone marrow transplant and liver transplant patients pneumonia occurs in between 15% and 50% of cases.[3–6]

The occurrence of pneumonia in this heterogenous group of patients poses a formidable health care challenge, the response best coordinated by the primary physician with a team input from infectious disease physicians and pulmonologists. As explained below the myriad of complexities involved in presentation, diagnosis and management demand an inordinate amount of physician effort and time. Pneumonia in the immunocompromised has a number of unique features (Table 21.1).

The deprived immune status of these patients will blunt the normal inflammatory response to infection. This not only removes to some extent the classical diagnostic markers of infection such as white cell response and radiographical features, but paralyses the host's ability to respond. For example, in an HIV-positive patient often the only initial feature of *Pneumocystis carinii* pneumonia is cough or dyspnoea. The radiograph may be normal at presentation in one-quarter of patients with BAL substantiated *P. carinii*. Bacterial pneumonia in a severely neutropenic patient may not be accompanied by adequate sputum production needed for analysis. A similar situation exists in profoundly granulocytopenic patients who already have established fungal infection where cough, fever and a normal chest radiograph are the only findings in subsequently proven *Aspergillus* pneumonia. These relatively common presentation scenarios often lead to delay in diagnosis and institution of appropriate and specific therapy – possible factors implicated in a worst prognosis.

Table 21.1. *Immunocompromised host with pneumonia: special features*

Blunted inflammatory response
Frequent bacteraemia
Medical emergency often
Increased spectrum microbes
Polymicrobial
Non-infectious interface/overlap
Generally more aggressive diagnostics
Empirical antimicrobial therapy
Prophylactic antimicrobials
Pre-emptive therapy
Often acute/fulminant

A sub-optimal host response limits the ability to contain infecting organisms and their consequences. For example, positive blood cultures and sepsis syndrome tend to occur more frequently in patients with neutropenia compared to those without neutropenia given the same underlying disease status.[7]

The spectrum of micro-organisms responsible for pneumonia in the compromised host is, in general, wide and complements that seen in the immunocompetent individual. In Mundy's paper of community-acquired pneumonia the incidence of *S. pneumoniae* was the same irrespective of the immune status of the host. Other Gram-negative bacillary pneumonia was more commonly seen compared to *Haemophilus influenzae* pneumonia in non-HIV immunocompromised patients, whereas *H. influenzae* was more common in immunocompetent patients. In HIV-positive individuals compared to non-HIV-positive individuals *P. carinii* pneumonia was significantly more common, and unknown agents were diagnosed significantly less frequently, and aspiration pneumonia occurred significantly less often.

Among renal transplant and oncology patients the *Pneumococcus* occurs as frequently as in the normal host.[8] However, most of the patients in whom this is observed are less intensely immunosuppressed. The greater the immunosuppression the more likely opportunistic lung pathogens such as Gram-negative bacteria, *Nocardia*, fungi, protozoa, CMV and other Herpes viruses will emerge. Multiplicity of organisms may be observed either concurrently or consecutively in immunocompromised patients as a result of the changing immune status over time, or as a result of the emergence of CMV, which is immunosuppressive *per se*.

However, non-infectious causes of pulmonary injury are common and enter into the differential diagnosis in the immunocompromised patient with febrile pneumonitis (Chapter 28). These include pulmonary oedema, ARDS, drug toxicity, thrombo-embolism, non-specific interstitial pneumonitis, underlying malignant disease infiltration, radiation injury, pulmonary haemorrhage, leucostasis, hyperleukocytosis, alveolar proteinosis, graft-versus-host disease and bronchiolitis obliterans. Some of these occur as a direct result of sepsis – for example, ARDS in bacteraemic patients, or may themselves, present a background of diffuse lung damage on which superinfection may subsequently occur.

The diagnostic approach therefore, to the immunocompromised patient with pulmonary disease is generally more aggressive compared to the immunocompetent patient. Repeated cultures of blood, sputum and antibody, antigen determination (and PCR) are commonly performed. Semi-invasive techniques such as BAL or bronchial washing are routine in many centres. Invasive procedures such as transtracheal aspiration, percutaneous needle aspiration, transbronchial biopsy and open lung biopsy are done but with a varying degree of enthusiasm. Open lung biopsy still remains the gold standard 'catch-all' method, providing the best means of diagnostically evaluating the patient, although even this technique is not totally reliable. However, it may provide some basis for rationalising antimicrobial treatment or directing treatment for non-infective conditions, for example, for pulmonary embolism.[9] Currently, it is not clear whether the outcome of such patients is improved as a result of such intensive aggressive diagnostic procedures when compared to those managed on the basis of less invasive methodology or even empirical therapy alone. If a skilful medical team is involved in such procedures, morbidity appears to be low.[9] Nevertheless, concern remains over submitting a critically ill patient with advanced respiratory disease and an uncorrectable coagulopathic status to a relatively major procedure. Clearly, this area requires clarification.

Immunocompromised patients with febrile pneumonitis are often given empirical broad spectrum antimicrobials to cover for the most likely pathogens. Initial selection of antimicrobials depends upon the immune status, timing from date of immunosuppression, clinical and radiological presentation. This approach to management is based on probability that a particular infection or a non-infectious process is present – which may be subsequently modified in the light of culture and histology results. Other approaches widely adopted include prophylaxis and pre-emptive therapy.

Prophylaxis

Over the period of immune suppression selection of a prophylactic is based upon the likelihood that particular pathogens may emerge. In the case of invasive candidiasis in patients undergoing allogeneic bone marrow transplantation, oral fluconazole has been shown to be effective in reducing fungal disease. Quinolones are widely used to prevent emergence of Gram-negative infections in haematology patients.

Pre-emptive therapy

This depends upon on detecting, pre-clinically, features that are likely to predict emergence of disease. In the situation of CMV disease, detection of blood CMV antigen before the emergence of signs and symptoms followed by treatment with intravenous ganciclovir has lead to a reduction in subsequent established CMV disease in liver transplant recipients. A similar situation exists in patients with antibiotic-resistant neutropenic fever who have haematological malignancy where administration of intravenous amphotericin B has lead to diminution in fungal disease.

This chapter will overview the pulmonary infections in such patients, apart from those with HIV which have been detailed in Chapter 22. Predisposing factors, presentation, diagnostic approaches and definitive/preventative managements will be discussed. Features of the infections special to the particular host setting will be highlighted but the individual micro-organisms, their presentation, diagnosis and management have been described in greater detail elsewhere in the book and the reader should refer to these chapters as appropriate.

Defects in host defences

These can be viewed as mechanical, biochemical or cellular which are present either locally (i.e. respiratory and pulmonary), distant from the respiratory tract (i.e. extra-pulmonary) or systematically.

Local

Mechanical abnormalities in or derangement of the naso-oropharynx and larger airways (including the mucociliary escalator) will predispose to aspiration-induced pneumonia (Chapters 20 and 28), from organisms normally only colonising the upper respiratory tract which normally would be restrained from entering the more distal airways. Immunoglobulin A and to an extent IgG and IgE production and lactoferrin/transferrin secreted by airway conducting cells may have important roles in airway defences. Defective production may result in increased bacterial adherence to respiratory epithelium, failure of antitoxins opsonising and complement fixing roles, hence predisposing to bacterial and viral infections. The precise role of respiratory-secreted immunoglobulin does, however, remain unclear.

In the lower respiratory tract the resident alveolar macrophage together with complement, surfactant and extra-cellular products (such as defensins) are of fundamental importance in the process of ingestion and intracellular killing of a variety of Gram-positive and Gram-negative bacteria, *Mycobacteria*, viruses and fungi. Defects induced, for example, in bone marrow transplant patients, will render the host highly susceptible to infection. However, it is the dendritic antigen-presenting cells in respiratory columnar epithelium, interstitial and alveolar tissue which are vital in triggering the initial pulmonary immunological response to infection. Thereafter, regional T-cell (mainly CD4+ interacting with TH-1 and TH-2) activation occurs producing a variety of cytokines which modulate infection response. Also involved are CD8 suppressor/cytotoxic cells, other cytokine producers and probably macrophages. Again, although immunoglobulins are produced in the lower respiratory tract, their precise role is unclear. Details of the pulmonary defence system have been discussed in Chapter 3.

Distant

Alteration in host defences at extra-pulmonary sites may provide a portal of entry for contiguous tissue, lymphatic or haematogenous spread to the lungs. Thus implanted vascular catheters for example are a risk for localised *S. aureus/S. epidermidis* infections, from which haematogenous dissemination may occur. Intestinal mucosal damage secondary to chemotherapy, for example, permits Gram-negative and fungal microbaemia which is a risk for haematogenous pneumonia. Obstruction of the gut, biliary system or renal tracts can also produce local infection – the focus acting as a source for onward spread to the lungs. Finally disturbance of the balance of microbes in oropharyngeal and gut flora through the use of antibiotics and antifungals will create a reservoir of pathogens.

Systemic

By far the most common and important factors that predispose to pulmonary infection are systemic defects including qualitative and quantitative dysfunction of granulocytes and alterations in cellular and humoral immunity. Examples of diseases and other situations which produce immune defects together with the major-associated infective organisms are shown in Table 21.2 and 21.3. It is important to realise that these traditional associations are never 100% true. For example, in lymphoma, although cell-mediated immunity (CMI) is typically reduced, there are additional abnormalities in polymorphonuclear functions. Disease status and other factors should not be considered separately from each other. Often, multiple interactive situations arise, for example, a patient with acute leukaemia will also have intravenous lines, chemotherapy and ultimately bone marrow transplantation all of which impair and modify the infection susceptibility.

There are additional unique features for each of the major transplantation categories. These are now discussed and summarised in Tables 21.4–21.8.

Bone marrow transplantation

In 1993, 15 000 allogeneic and autologous bone marrow transplants were performed worldwide for a variety of conditions, including non-malignant congenital immune deficiencies, aplastic anaemia, thalassaemia, and malignant conditions such as acute leukaemia, chronic myeloid leukaemia, myeloma, solid tumours and lymphomas. Survival rates in excess of 50% × 5 years are now commonplace. Intensive myelo-ablative chemoradiotherapy conditioning, degree of matching of donor marrow at HLA level to minimise differences in transplant antigen loci and subsequent graft rejection and graft-versus-host disease, use of immunosuppressives, eradication of malignant cells prior to transplant, stem cell harvesting and use of growth factors all impact on the vulnerable transplant recipient and modulate the risk of pulmonary sepsis and other pulmonary complications which occur in up to 60% of all patients.[10] In fact, bone marrow transplantation sets itself apart from solid organ transplantation as the immune system in its entirety is replaced rather than merely suppressed. This results in the most prolonged and profound immunosuppression state induced in patients with malignant disease. Consequently there is a high risk for a variety of life-threatening opportunistic sepsis. Following immune-ablation, profound neutropenia exists for up to 2–3 weeks and, although qualitative neutrophil recovery will be seen, functional impairment continues for several months thereafter. Both CMI and humoral immune defects persist for up to 1 year, longer if graft-versus-host disease (amplified further by the associated exogenous immunosuppressive drug regimens) occurs. It is useful to consider each of the three temporal phases of bone marrow transplantation as each phase tends to display a propensity for the emergence of particular micro-organisms.

First 30 days post-transplant (phase one)

Neutropenia, lymphopenia and severely damaged mucosal surfaces are the predominant host defects in this phase.

Bacterial pneumonia

This occurs relatively uncommonly nowadays, probably reflecting widespread use of prophylactic antibiotics (notably quinolones), and the administration of early broad spectrum antibiotics given for neutropenic fever in the absence of a clinical focus. However, the exact incidence varies between 12% and 50%.[10–12] Approximately 10% of the cases of pneumonia among hospitalised BMT patients are found to be bacterial.[13] The notable decline in Gram-negative bacteraemias (e.g. *Pseudomonas* spp., *E. coli*, *Klebsiella* spp. and *Enterobacter* spp.), their niche replaced with an upsurge in Gram-positive (including coagulase negative *Staphylcoccus* spp., haemolytic *Streptococcus* spp., *S. aureus*, *Cornynebacterium* spp.) has been ascribed to the widespread use of Gram-negative prophylaxis. Among these, *S. pneumoniae* is the commonest cause of acute pneumonia. Non-pneumophila *Legionella* spp., mycobacterial and other organisms are less commonly seen. HSV1, *Candida* and *Aspergillus* infections emerge with the passage of neutropenia. The presence of a necrotising process should raise the possibility in the first 30 days of *S. aureus*, *Klebsiella* spp., *Pseudomonas* spp or *Legionella* spp. pneumonia.

It is of some interest that respiratory encapsulated bacterial infections tend to occur several months after transplant. Infections with *H. influenzae* and *S. pneumoniae* emerge as a result of deficient polysaccharide antibodies. There is an association with chronic GVHD.[14, 15] Penicillin or trimethoprim-sulphamethoxazole is an effective prophylaxis for these late bacterial infections. Although IVIG also appears to be an effective prophylactic measure, active vaccination is unreliable.

Fungal pneumonia

This tends to emerge towards the end of the first phase. *Aspergillus* spp. appears to be the most common and life-threatening cause – accounting for approximately one-third of all BMT associated pneumonias[13] – though newly emerging moulds are increasingly being reported particularly *Fusarium* spp., *Alternaria* spp., *Rhizopus* spp.[16]

Table 21.2

Immune defect or disease	Immunoglobulin	Granulocyte nos/function	CMI	Mechanical	Complement	Clearance
Myeloma	+	+	+		+	
CLL	+					
ALL		+				
AML/CML		+				
Aplastic anaemia		+				
Splenectomy	+				+	+
Hodgkin's or non-Hodgkin's lymphoma	+		+			
Hyopgammaglobulinaemia	+					
Carcinoma/sarcoma			+			
Congenital immunodeficiencies, e.g. *SCID*	+		+			
Purine pathway defect	+		+			
Chronic granulomatous disease		+				
Down's syndrome		+				
Intravascular devices			+			
Skin/mucous membrane barrier disease				+		
Corticosteroids	+	+	+			
Alkylators	+		+			
Antimetabolites	+		+			
Organ transplantation	← Varies with disease and immunosuppressive given →					

Table 21.3

Immune defect or micro-organisms	Immunoglobulin	Granulocyte nos/function	CMI	Mechanical	Complement	Clearance
α *Streptococci*		+				
S. pneumoniae	+				+	+
S. aureus		+		+		+
S. epidermidis		+		+		
Gram-negative bacilli		+				+
H. influenzae	+				+	+
N. meningitidis					+	+
Listeria monocytogenes			+			
Salmonella spp			+			
Legionella spp			+			
Mycobacteria spp			+			
Nocardia spp			+			
Aspergillus spp and other filamentous fungi		+				
Candida spp and other yeasts		+				
Cryptococcus spp			+			
CMV/EBV			+			
Herpes zoster			+			
Herpes simplex			+			
P. carinii			+			
Toxoplasma/Cyptosporidium			+			
Strongyloides		+		+		
Enteroviral		+		+		
Cryptococcus			+			
Histoplasma			+			
Coccidioides			+			

Table 21.4. *Bone marrow trasnplantation: unique or commoner features*

Highly intensive immunosuppression
Prophylactic antibiotics select
e.g. *S. aureus*
S. viridans
GVHD and CMV, late bacterial pneumonia
Fungal pneumonia particularly *Aspergillus, Fusarium* and emerging species
Neutropenia: major factor
CMVIP pathogenesis and treatment (Chapter 10)
Non-infectious causes
GVHD
non-specific interstitial pneumonitis
diffuse alveolar haemorrhage
vasculopathy

Table 21.5. *Orthotopic liver transplantation: unique or commoner features*

More sepsis intra-abdominal
Selective Gram-positive microbes secondary to bowel decontamination
Complex, prolonged operations
CMVIP relatively good response
Increase in mycobacterial species and INAH prophylaxis (toxicity)
EBV lymphoproliferative disease
Non-infectious causes
pulmonary calcification
pulmonary hypertension
auto-immune phenomena
post-op atelectasis and pleural effusions

Table 21.6. *Heart transplantation: unique or commoner features*

Sternal/mediastinal sepsis
CMVIP frequent and severe
EBV lymphoproliferative disease
Non-infectious causes
post-op atelectasis (phrenic nerve)
acute pulmonary injury
acute rejection (differential of CMV, toxoplasmosis)

Table 21.7. *Heart–lung and lung transplantation: unique or commoner features*

Secondary allograft sepsis from remaining lung
Bacterial pneumonia
CMVIP very common
EBV lymphoproliferative disease
Non-infectious causes
obliterative bronchiolitis

Table 21.8. *Renal transplantation: unique or commoner features*

Most sepsis renal/abdomen
CMVIP – good response to ganciclovir
CMV and glomerulopathy
Mycobacterial disease
EBV related lymphoproliferative disease
Non-infectious causes
pulmonary malignancies – KS, renal Ca, lymphoma renal – pulmonary overlap, e.g. Wegener's

The incidence of candidaemia is increasing and candidal pneumonia may occur in a proportion of these. In endemic areas, as a result of appropriate exposure, histoplasmosis, coccidioidomycosis and cryptococccosis should be considered. Currently, early diagnosis for fungal pneumonia is imprecise. Surveillance cultures such as detection of *Candida* spp. growth on different mucosal surfaces or the detection of *Aspergillus* spp. in sputum or BAL are considered predictive for invasive fungal disease. Candidal enolase and *Aspergillus* galactomannin detection methods are being evaluated in the human clinical setting. The course of fungal pneumonia in bone marrow transplant patients is more aggressive compared to other patient groups. Mortality for pulmonary candidiasis is 60–70% and for *Aspergillus* spp. 80–90% in these patients. Use of high dose lipid formulation antifungals, for example, liposomal amphotericin B, and combination antifungal therapy, for example, amphotericin B with 5-flucytosine or rifampicin are being elaborated for optimal dosage and efficacy. Resolution of neutropenia appears to be a major factor governing outcome and has led to the use of growth factors to shorten its duration. Surgical resection has proved feasible for well-demarcated pulmonary aspergillosis. Prophylaxis of invasive fungal infections is an ideal goal. HEPA-filtered positive pressure (with/without laminar air flow) rooms and with microbe-low diets and meticulous hand-washing are among the measures routinely implemented against *Aspergillus* spp. and *Candidal* spp. infections. Although oral fluconazole (200 mg to 400 mg daily) is a safe and effective prophylaxis against invasive *Candida albicans* infections, certain non-*albicans* species could emerge although the evidence for this is not consistent. Prophylactic intravenous amphotericin B is often used to prevent *Aspergillus* infection but prophylactic studies have shown conflicting results. It appears to be useful as secondary prophylaxis, or for the management of antibiotic-resistant neutropenia (cases of cryptic fungal infection).

Days 31–90 post-transplant (second phase)

Viral pneumonias

The second phase is a risk period for these pneumonias. CMV pneumonia in bone marrow transplant patients carries a much more dismal prognosis compared to CMV pneumonia in solid organ transplant recipients. CMV infection occurs in 60% of all bone marrow transplants, more frequently in allografts compared to autografts and more often symptomatically in allografts (CMV interstitial pneumonitis is quite unusual in autografts). CMV pneumonia occurs in approximately one-third of those who become infected with CMV. However, the widespread use of prophylactic and pre-emptive antiviral treatment, and screened blood products have substantially reduced the occurrence and impact of CMV in marrow transplant patients in recent years. The incidence and severity of CMV infection, including the development of pneumonia, increases if the patient's pre-transplant serology is positive rather than negative.[17] Risk factors for CMV interstitial pneumonitis (CMVIP) include increased age, GVHD (particularly if severe) and its associated immunosuppressive treatment, pre-transplant sero-positivity, total body irradiation, and transfusion of sero-positive blood and blood products into sero-negative recipients (primary CMV infection). Often early features of CMV disease may be non-specific, e.g. fever, constitutional symptoms and leuko-thrombocytopenia. The definitive diagnosis of CMV pneumonia requires open lung biopsy. However, the association of pulmonary symptoms with viraemia shown by culture, PCR or CMV antigen is considered diagnostic. Routine surveillance for asymptomatic CMV excretion is commonly practised. The presence of CMV in blood, throat, urine or BAL is fairly strongly predictive (around 70%) for CMV interstitial pneumonia. If these patients are given intravenous ganciclovir, the risk of developing CMVIP is reduced.[18,19] Furthermore acyclovir[20] or ganciclovir[21] prophylaxis administered to all CMV sero-positive recipients of allogeneic BMTs reduces subsequent CMVIP. Toxicity, particularly severe and persistent neutropenia, associated with ganciclovir use can be really problematical. Passive immunoprophylaxis with various preparations of globulins appears to have had some effect in preventing CMV infection and CMVIP if used in sero-negative recipients who are given sero-positive products.[22] However, variations in trial methodology in heterogeneous patient groups have dominated the different studies and there is currently no consistent prophylactic approach. Most centres nevertheless do use some form of prophylaxis (see Chapter 10). Treatment of established CMVIP is problematical – mortality is over 80%. The use of the combination of ganciclovir and CMV-specific immunoglobulin appears to be the most appropriate approach, offering a survival rate of around 60% which is superior to that if GCV or immunoglobulin is used separately.[23–25] Relapse is common, however, and maintenance ganciclovir treatment has to be given following the initial response. Foscarnet is used for ganciclovir-resistant strains.

Herpes simplex pneumonia, has likewise declined in BMT patients as a result of the widespread use of acyclovir. Even prior to this *H. simplex* pneumonia was a relatively uncommon occurrence among non-bacterial pneumonia cases,[26] despite the frequent occurrence of oropharyngeal *H. simplex*. Acyclovir is the drug of choice for established pneumonia. Resistance has been described.

Varicella zoster pneumonia is rare.

HHV6 has been detected in BMT patients with pneumonitis, but is of uncertain significance.[27]

Adenovirus is an unusual cause of pneumonia in these patients. Ribavirin may have some effect, although its use is experimental.

RSV has been incriminated in outbreaks. Aerosolised ribavirin has produced mixed results.

Para-influenza and influenza rarely produce viral pneumonia in BMT patients.

Other agents

Pneumocystis carinii pneumonia is now a rarity among BMT patients following the widespread use of co-trimoxazole prophylaxis throughout the risk period, that is from transplantation to 4 months (extended for patients with GVHD). For patients intolerant to co-trimoxazole inhaled pentamidine is an alternative.

Toxoplasma pneumonia is exceedingly rare and usually occurs in the setting of multi-system disease.

Days 91–360 post-transplant (phase three)

Varicella zoster, bacterial and respiratory viral pathogens predominate.

Non-infectious complications

Graft versus-host disease (GVHD)

This is an unique complication among BMT recipients and is due to the action of donor lymphocytes on host tissues – particularly skin (exfoliative dermatitis), liver (hepatitis), gastrointestinal tract (diarrhoea) and the respiratory tract. Pre-treatment of marrow with T-cell antibodies to deplete T-lymphocytes may reduce its occurrence. GVHD can be treated or prevented with anti-lymphocyte preparations, cyclosporin, methotrexate, high dose steroids or azathioprine. GVHD and its associated immunosuppressive therapy carries with it a substantial risk for infection particularly with CMV. Patients who die with GVHD do so as a result of overwhelming sepsis. Acute GVHD normally occurs in the late first or second phase but chronic GVHD may become established later. Although most clinical features involve the skin and gastrointestinal tract, bronchopulmonary manifestations are found. These include airway obstruction, obliterative bronchiolitis and lymphocytic bronchitis. They are related directly or indirectly to chronic GVHD.[28–30]

Interstitial pneumonitis

This is defined as the presence of interstitial infiltrates in association with hypoxaemia, dyspnoea and absence of fungal/bacterial organisms. It occurs in 40% of allografts and less than 20% of autografts.[17,26] It occurs during the second phase. CMV is associated in about 50% of cases; the remainder are idiopathic. The precise aetiology is unknown. However, age, TBI, use of methotrexate rather than cyclosporin, severe GVHD and CMV infections are risk factors. Possibly cumulative pulmonary toxicity secondary to combined radiochemotherapy and CMV immunologically mediated pulmonary damage is responsible. Clinically, the presentation is indistinguishable from CMVIP or PCP. Mediastinal emphysema may complicate the picture particularly in patients who have received larger doses of TBI, who are malnourished or receiving high dose steroids.[31] Mortality is between 60% and 90%, being higher in patients who also have CMVIP. Corticosteroids have no benefit. The use of IVIG in patients who have a CMV aetiology appears to confer some benefit.[25]

Other pulmonary complications

Chemotherapy-induced cardiac/renal dysfunction can lead to pulmonary oedema which is accentuated by large volume fluid infusions. Early treatment with diuretics is beneficial and clearing of pulmonary infiltrates and weight reduction following such treatment helps to differentiate the condition from sepsis.

Diffuse alveolar haemorrhage occurs in at least 10% of bone marrow transplants.[32] This non-specific lung injury currently is thought to result from chemotherapy in some cases, worsened by coagulopathy and infection such as *Aspergillus*. Some cases are relatively asymptomatic. Others masquerade as infection with fever, diffuse alveolar infiltrates, cough and hypoxaemic respiratory distress. Frank haemoptysis is unusual. Diagnosis is based upon clinical, radiographical and alveolar macrophage haemosiderin laden content. The latter however may be less sensitive than histological examination. The mortality is up to 80%,[32] slightly better in patients without infection.

Sub-clinical pulmonary pan-vasculopathy (endothelial swelling and thrombosis) is common but of unknown significance.[33]

Pulmonary embolisation of transplanted bone marrow fragments, marrow fat and thrombi occasionally occurs.

Pulmonary veno-occlusive disease related to high dose chemotherapy and repeated bone marrow transplantation is also described. There is some response to steroids.[34]

A variety of restrictive and obstructive ventilatory defects are found post transplant, possibly related to chemoradiotherapy and to graft-versus-host disease. These include mild restrictive changes, progressive fatal obstruction and severe obliterative bronchiolitis.

Orthotopic liver transplantation (OLT)

Currently, almost 3000 OLTs are performed annually in the USA for a variety of terminal liver diseases including alcoholic or viral cirrhosis. Since Starzl in the 1960s, there have been tremendous technical and medical improvements (particularly with the introduction of cyclosporin) and these have resulted in at least 75% of patients surviving 1 year of whom most will survive at least several more years. However, prolonged operation duration (in excess of 7 hours)[35] increases the infection risk from less than one episode per patient for an operation of between 5 and 10 hours to three episodes per patient for a total operation time in excess of 25 hours. Other risk factors include large blood volume replacement, repeated hypotensive episodes, enterostomal procedures and post-operative intra-abdominal surgical complications necessitating re-operation. A pre-transplant poor liver function status and post-operative allograft and renal dysfunctions are further risk factors for infection.[35–38] Differences in study design, however, plague definite uniform conclusions. The use of cyclosporin, FK 506, prednisone and azathioprine for immunosuppression, and high dose steroids or anti-lymphocytic preparations for rejection episodes further impede the immune system's capability of defence against infection.[35]

Infectious complications occur in 70% of patients and are mainly intra-abdominal, relating to liver graft technicalities such as bile duct obstruction producing ascending cholangitis, CMV hepatitis, liver abscess or fungal peritonitis. The respiratory tract is the second most common target site for infection. Most infections occur within the first 2 months following transplant. As for bone marrow transplantation, it is convenient to examine their occurrence in a temporal fashion.

First 30 days post-transplant (phase one)

Bacterial pneumonia

Bacterial sepsis accounts for around 50–60% of all major infections.[39] The incidence of bacterial pneumonia varies considerably from less than 5% to around 25% of all patients.[6] Although most episodes occur in the first month, they can appear at any time after transplant, though by 6 months post-transplant the incidence per year has fallen from 4–5 to less than 0.5.[35] In Kusne's series there were 15 episodes among a total of 136 major infections occurring among 101 patients (15% incidence per patient).[35] In Paya's series the incidence of bacterial pneumonia was 8%.[39] Pulmonary infections account for between 7 and 19% of all bacterial infections in OLT patients.[35,36,39,54] Although most series report Gram-negative bacillary pneumonias (commonly due to *Pseudomonas* spp.), others have underscored the predominance of Gram-positive cocci, particularly *S. aureus* and *S. viridans*,[39] which may arise from the use of prophylactic selective antimicrobial or bowel decontamination.[40] Most bacterial pneumonias are nosocomial and directly related to IPPV-mechanical and post-operative atelectasis.

Fungal pneumonia

This usually occurs in this first phase although up to 50% of all cases may not present until the second month. The most common pneumonia is due to *Candida* spp. Candidal infections occur in approximately 20% of OLTs[35,37,41,43] though some series report a much lower incidence about 4%.[39] Previously, over 40% of OLT recipients developed invasive fungal disease before surgical techniques improved, operative time diminished and bowel decontamination was employed.[45] Candidal infections mainly present as intra-abdominal sepsis, candidaemia/disseminated candidiasis occurring more frequently than pneumonia. Prolonged operation or re-operation, steroid use, prolonged broad spectrum antibiotics and multiple mucosal site colonisation are risks for candidal infection.[35,41,42] *Candida* spp. commonly originate from the gastro-intestinal tract. The mortality rate from candidaemia is 25% rising as high as 75% if tissue invasion occurs.[44] Infection due to *Aspergillus* spp. is seen less often. As *Aspergillus* is transmitted via the airborne route, primary pneumonia is therefore much more likely than other system involvement. However, dissemination for example to the brain, can occur from the primary lung focus. Mortality is high – approaching 100%.[44] However, localised pulmonary involvement carries a better prognosis compared to diffuse pulmonary involvement. Other fungal diseases occasionally seen include cryptococcosis, or the disease indigenous endemic fungi limited to certain geographical regions, e.g. histoplasmosis.

Days 31–90 post-transplant (phase two)

Viral pneumonias

Cytomegalovirus is the most frequent pathogen seen in OLT patients. Asymptomatic infection occurs twice as frequently as symptomatic disease (60% versus 30%, respectively).[46] Acquisition from the donor graft or blood is the usual route of transmission. Reactivation of latent virus is also seen. The heightened immunosuppression necessary for treatment of allograft rejection, particularly with OKT3, is thought to be a major factor in primary CMV disease, less so for reactivation. Although symptomatic CMV infection can be diagnosed within the first month post-transplant, symptomatic CMV disease is commonly seen during the second phase. Low grade fever, myalgia, arthralgia and pancytopenia are common. Hepatitis and gastrointestinal involvement are seen frequently, occurring in 4% of liver transplant recipients, and which often resolve. The vanishing bile duct syndrome is also described.[47] Pulmonary involvement is less common but is important as it carries a substantial mortality. Co-infection with *P. carinii* and other pathogens is not uncommon. Unlike the situation with bone marrow transplant patients, OLT patients with CMV pneumonitis appear to respond more favourably to intravenous ganciclovir. The combination with IVIG has not been examined as it has in BMT patients. The use of pre-emptive short course ganciclovir treatment in patients with asymptomatic CMV shedding appears to substantially reduce symptomatic CMV disease in OLT patients.[48]

EBV infection mainly manifests as an asymptomatic sero-conversion phenomenon (approximately one-third of patients) but individuals with primary infection or who have received anti-lymphocytic globulin may develop a lymphoproliferative disorder. This occurs in approximately 2% of OLT cases.[52] This entity may present as a glandular fever-like syndrome. Alternatively tumours may develop in many organs, including the lung.

Other viral infections include adenovirus pneumonia. This is rare in adults[39] but as many as 10% of paediatric OLT patients develop infection[53] in whom one-fifth develop fatal lung disease.

Herpes simplex virus and Varicella zoster virus infections are uncommon if acyclovir prophylaxis has been used.

Day 91–360 post-transplant (phase three)

Less common bacterial infections including *Legionella* spp. particularly *L. pneumophila* and *L. micdadei* may occur at this time.[49] These may be sporadic or nosocomial if improperly chlorinated hospital hot water supplies are contaminated. *Nocardia* spp. have rarely been described.[50] When infections do occur, they may be part of a disseminated picture involving, for example, the skin and the central nervous system.

M. tuberculosis and non-tuberculosis mycobacteria are unusual, both in their frequency of occurrence and mode of presentation.[51] OLT patients who reside in or travel to highly endemic areas for TB who have a positive PPD skin test, or who have a past history of inadequately treated TB should be offered isoniazid prophylaxis. This, however, carries a risk of INAH hepatotoxicity which may be confused with other causes of hepatitis. It is therefore not usually given until 4 weeks post-transplant.

Nocardia spp., *Mycoplasma* spp. and community-acquired pathogens such as *S. pneumonia* and *H. influenzae* tend to occur after 30–60 days post-transplant.

P. carinii pneumonia is seen between 3 and 5 months after OLT in up to 10% of patients but the incidence varies between centres and with the use of prophylaxis.[35,39,54] Focal rather than the usual diffuse infiltrates may be found.[35]

Non-infective complications

These include post-operative atelectasis, pleural effusions, ARDS and pulmonary calcification. Atelectasis arises as a result of the extensive regional right upper quadrant surgery, previous ascites and poor muscle mass status. This is managed with physiotherapy. Pleural effusions, usually right thoracic, occur secondary to pre-existing ascites, right upper quadrant surgery or secondary to lower respiratory tract infections. Most resolve spontaneously. A few are large, persistent and re-accumulate requiring tube thoracostomies. ARDS occurs in up to 20% of patients and is multifactorial – usually secondary to sepsis, prolonged surgery, re-transplantation or after hypotension. Most cases occur in the first 2 weeks. Mortality is usually well in excess of 5%.[55]

A later complication is the development of pulmonary calcification, secondary to viral pneumonia or ARDS. Interstitial deposits of calcium microcrystals mediated by parathormone may be extensive enough to cause restrictive lung disease, fibrosis or progressive respiratory failure.[56]

Prior to their transplantation, patients with chronic liver disease may have arterial hypoxaemia[57] secondary to ascites, pleural effusion, diaphragmatic dysfunction, pulmonary vasoconstriction, intrapulmonary vascular dilatation or arterio-venous anomalies, which if severe enough may be accompanied by cyanosis, clubbing and dyspnoea. Some degree of reversal of shunt fraction may occur following OLT.

Pulmonary hypertension following liver disease associated portal hypertension and possibly due to the failure of the diseased hepatic vascular system to inactivate humoral mediators, is also well developed.[58]

Other pre-existing chronic liver disease associated pulmonary conditions include auto-immune phenomena such as lymphocytic bronchitis associated with primary biliary cirrhosis/Sjörgen's syndrome, interstitial lung disease associated with primary biliary cirrhosis and bronchiectasis with sclerosing cholangitis.[57] Atelectasis and pleural effusions may occur secondary to larger ascites, e.g. via peritoneal-pleural transport. These may pre-dispose to the retention of secretions and hence secondary pneumonia. Pre-existing restrictive and ventilatory defects are commonly found in patients with chronic lung disease but may be more related to smoking habits.[59]

Heart transplantation

This procedure now offers reasonable survival to over two-thirds of patients with otherwise terminal cardiac function secondary to coronary artery disease, cardiomyopathies, etc. The lung and thoracic cavity are the most frequently targeted sites for infections and non-infectious complications.

Pre-operatively a number of pulmonary manifestations of heart disease necessitates a balanced differential diagnostic approach. The existence of congestive heart failure may be associated with restrictive lung disease which can pre-dispose to pneumonia. Furthermore congestive heart failure *per se* may mimic pneumonia, at least radiographically. Patients are at risk for developing arrhythmias, DVT and pulmonary emboli from congestive cardiac failure. Their complications also pre-dispose the patients to secondary infection. Haemoptysis secondary to pulmonary embolism or to CCF will raise the possibility of differential diagnoses which encompass non-infectious/infectious aetiologies. Finally drugs given in the management of dysrhythmias have been associated with pulmonary toxicity (Chapter 28).

Similarly in the post-transplant phase a plethora of pulmonary complications both infective and non-infective (and sometimes both) demand a thorough, well-balanced diagnostic approach. Again, non-infective cardiopulmonary complications can themselves pre-dispose to secondary infections. In the immediate post-operative period, atelectasis mainly of the left lower lobe due to per-operative phrenic nerve injury or lung trauma from surgical manipulation leads to retained secretions which may become secondarily infected. An acute pulmonary injury syndrome complex develops within one to two days in 1–2% of patients. This is multifactorial involving post-operative ventricular dysfunction, renal dysfunction, pump-related, complement-mediated, pulmonary capillary endothelial injury and prior use of amiodarone. The resulting ARDS and pulmonary oedema not only pre-dispose to secondary bacterial sepsis but themselves carry a substantial mortality.[60–62]

Chest drains, sternotomies and tracheostomies cause defects in the local mechanical defence barriers. Intravenous catheters, intra-aortic balloon pumps and left ventricular support devices are other potential extra-pulmonary sources of infection, from which subsequent haematogenous dissemination to the lungs may occur.

All patients receive a basic immunosuppressive regimen including steroids, cyclosporin, azathioprine, ATG and additional pulse immune suppressive bolus therapy for rejection which includes high dose steroids, ATG and OKT3.

First 30 days post-transplant (phase one)

Bacterial pneumonia

This is particularly common, and the predominant hospital pathogens, namely Gram-negative rods are frequently incriminated. Occasionally, community acquired pathogens are found. Less usual is *L. pneumophila* which may be sporadic or as part of a common source outbreak. Radiographically, *L. pneumophila* is characterised by nodular, necrotising or cavitary pneumonia which may be further complicated by the development of empyema. However, non-specific alveolar infiltrates are also seen.[63] Relapses tend to occur even after initial successful treatment with erythromycin ± rifampicin. Initial administration of antimicrobials should be intravenous followed immediately by secondary prophylaxis with oral erythromycin for between 6 and 12 months.[63]

Haematogenous staphylococcal pneumonias (both methicillin sensitive *S. aureus* and methicillin resistant *S. aureus*) can occur secondary to infected intravascular devices (Fig. 21. 1(a), (b)). The rounded multiple sited lung lesions typical of haematogenous pneumonia should alert the physician to the high possibility of an intravenous device source – valvular endocarditis, however, is distinctly unusual in these patients.

A unique thoracic infection associated with heart transplantation is sternal wound associated mediastinitis occurring in up to approximately 10% of patients (Fig. 21.2).[64] Risk factors include insertion of mechanical devices such as tubes, certain artificial hearts and emergency thoracotomy. Although Gram-positive organisms such as *S. aureus* and *S. epidermidis* predominate, *Pseudomonas* spp., *Mycoplasma* spp., *Legionella* spp. and fungal organisms may also be responsible. Prior sternal wound sepsis may well evolve to mediastinitis. Often the presenting signs are subtle such as an isolated elevated white cell count. Chest wall erythema, tenderness and discharge along the sternal operative site are the more classical signs which may be present at some stage. However, their absence or modification in such highly immunocompromised patients may lead to

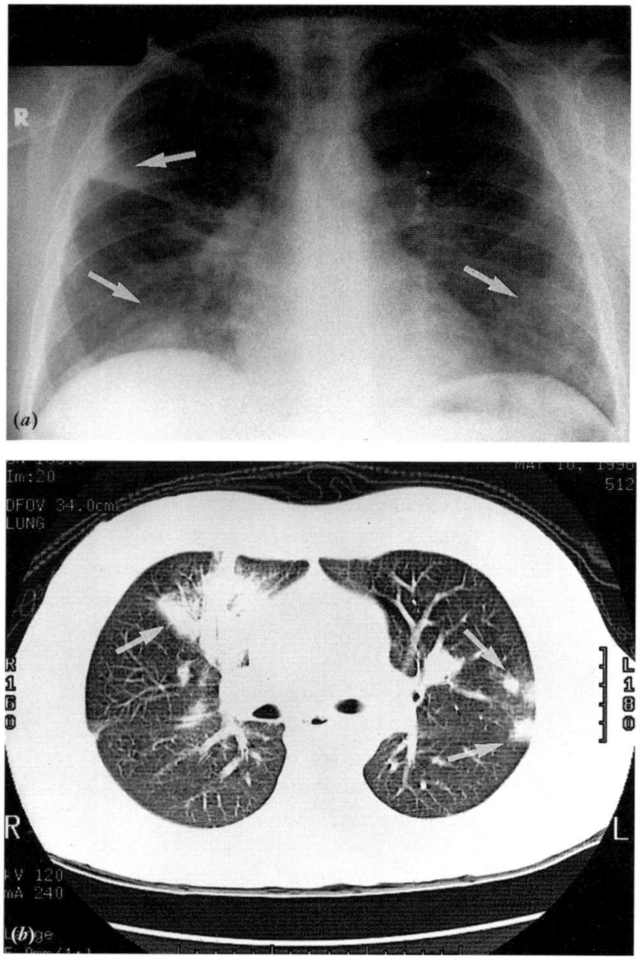

FIGURE 21.1 (*a*) Plain chest radiograph, blood culture positive MRSA (source-infected Hickman line) and multiple areas of consolidation (arrowed). (*b*) CT scan of same patient.

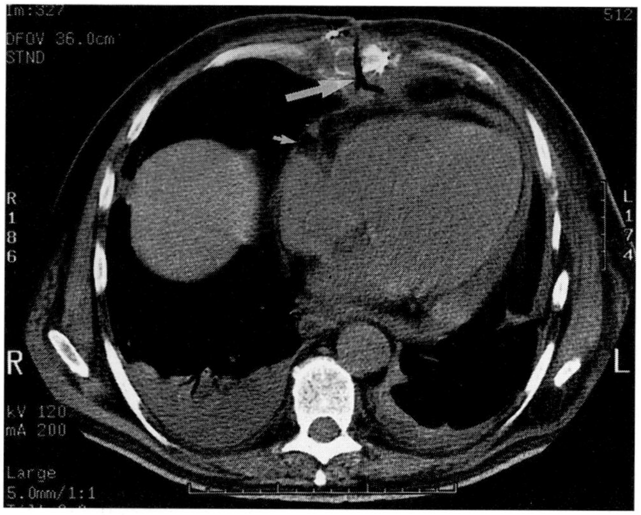

FIGURE 21.2 CT chest: pericardial effusion (small arrow) with sinus tract (large arrow) through sternum: MRSA mediastinitis.

days – weeks delay in diagnosis. The presence of pericardial effusion with tracking through the sternum is often found (Fig. 21.2). Treatment of established mediastinitis should be aggressive with antimicrobials, surgical drainage, debridement of sternum and tissues and irrigation with povidone-iodine.

Day 31–90 post-transplant (phase two)

All of the infective complications occurring in the first month can also present though less frequently throughout this second phase.

Up to 13% of patients develop pulmonary nocardiosis at any time up to 2 years or so after transplant.[65] A lone pulmonary nodule in the absence of fever may be the sole presentation in almost half of all patients with this infection. Otherwise, cough, fever and dyspnoea occur in association with a variety of radiographical features, including interstitial infiltrates and multiple rounded lesions. Occasionally the disease is overwhelming. Extrapulmonary manifestations can also be seen. Treatment is usually with long term co-trimoxazole.

Although infection with *M. tuberculosis* is unusual, infections with non-tuberculous mycobacteria have been seen in 3% of some series,[66] of which half are part of a disseminated presentation. The use of cyclophosphamide rather than azathioprine/steroids for immunosuppression seems to be associated with a lower incidence of such infections.

Viral pneumonias

CMV pneumonia occurs particularly frequently and more severely in heart and more so in heart-lung transplantations than in other types of transplantations. The incidence and severity is somewhat variable and related in part to prior immune status, type of immunosuppression, use of hyperimmunoglobulin preparations, rejection episodes and CMV status of the donor heart and blood products. A broad figure is that between 50% and 80% develop CMV infection of which one-third develop CMV symptomatic disease.[67,68] Primary CMV infection (see Chapter 10) tends to be more severe than secondary superinfection or reactivation infection. Patients receiving ATG, azathioprine and steroids are more likely to become infected when compared to those receiving cyclosporin. The route of secondary infection is as previously detailed (Chapter 10), but in addition the donor heart may be a source.[69] Symptomatic CMV disease presents between 1 and 4 months after transplantation, commonly as an atypical mononucleosis syndrome or occasionally as part of disseminated disease or pneumonia alone. CMV pneumonia is particularly common and features are non-specific. The illness carries a mortality of around 15% despite treatment with ganciclovir.[70] Respiratory failure and other critical organ involvement is common. Prior to ganciclovir usage the mortality rate was fourfold higher. CMV pneumonitis in heart transplant recipients carries a better prognosis compared to CMV interstitial pneumonitis occurring in bone marrow transplant patients. CMV infection is itself intensely immunosuppressive leading to superinfection with a variety of other organisms. CMV infection leads to graft rejection and accelerates coronary arthrosclerosis in the graft.[71] Tissue is required for firm diagnosis. Treatment is with ganciclovir alone and has been described in detail in Chapter 10. Prophylactic issues have not been studied as extensively as in BMT patients but ganciclovir may be useful.[72]

Pulmonary involvement with Herpes simplex (usually reactivation rather than primary infections) and with VZV is unusual. However, extrapulmonary infections should be treated with acyclovir to reduce the risk of pulmonary involvement and the attendant high mortality rate.

EBV infection is very common but often sub-clinical. EBV-related B-cell lymphoproliferative disease such as lymphoma is less common (approximately 7%)[73] and appears to be related to the particular immunosuppressive regimen. Management involves reduction in immunosuppressive therapy, since antivirals, cytotoxics and surgery are in general ineffective.

Fungal pneumonia

Pneumonia due to fungi occurs with considerable variation in frequency between centres. For example, invasive fungal disease was reported in 30% of patients from Stanford compared to 10% in Zurich.[74,75] Candidiasis is the commonest fungal infection and is particularly associated with intravenous lines, broad spectrum antibiotic pressure and diabetes mellitus, though pneumonia is an unusual manifestation. *A. fumigatus* and *A. flavus* pneumonia are less common and may be sporadic or linked to outbreaks associated with renovation/construction building works. The mortality rate from aspergillosis is in general higher than from candidiasis. Cryptococcosis is usually meningitic in presentation with pneumonia being uncommon. Pneumonia due to geographically limited fungi such as histoplasmosis and coccidioidomycosis are by definition seen only in patients who have been resident in those areas.

Day 91–360 post-transplant (phase three)

P. carinii is now found infrequently in the setting of co-trimoxazole prophylaxis and cyclosporin usage. Current reported incidences are of the order of 4%.[75] Response to co-trimoxazole treatment is in general good.

Primary *Toxoplasma* infection arising from blood products or the donor heart is generally more severe than secondary or reactivation toxoplasmosis. The risk for symptomatic infection following transplantation of a heart from a positive donor to a negative recipient is of the order of 50%. Infection can be life-threatening.[76] In general, extrapulmonary involvement is more common than pulmonary. Myocarditis is one such manifestation which may be mistaken for rejection. Serological changes presage clinical symptoms by several weeks. Precise diagnosis is made by histological demonstration of tachyzoites or by culture. Co-trimoxazole prophylaxis given primarily against PCP will also protect against toxoplasmosis and should be given to high risk patients. Established treatment is within 2 months of sulphadiazine and pyrimethamine, together with folinic acid host rescue.

Heart/lung and lung transplants (HL/L transplants)

Combined HL, double L and single L transplants are now performed for a variety of terminal cardiopulmonary and pulmonary conditions including primary pulmonary hypertension, congenital cardiac defects, chronic obstructive pulmonary disease and cystic fibrosis.

Survival rates of around 70% at 2 years are currently reported[77]. These particular transplant procedures are associated with the greatest vulnerability to thoracic and pulmonary infection among all transplants. Reasons which are over and above the continual background of regular and pulse drug immunosuppressive therapy are multifactorial. Particular mechanical factors include stasis of pulmonary secretions secondary to diaphragmatic paralysis (phrenic nerve injury), pulmonary oedema consequent on impaired lymphatic drainage, absence of cough reflex distal to the tracheal anastomosis, and reduction of mucociliary clearance. In addition, TLC, FEV1, FVC are reduced due to post-operative alterations in the thoracic cage. Recipient alveolar macrophages migrate to the donor lung and problems of incompatibility arise.[78] In the setting of single LT for chronic pulmonary sepsis, infection often arises secondary to immune suppression and spreads from the recipient's remaining lung.

The prevalence of CMV infection and disease is particularly high in this group of patients. Pulmonary CMV disease not only closely mimics acute lung rejection but itself leads to superinfection with other pulmonary pathogens.

Finally, obliterative bronchiolitis, possibly due to chronic rejection has been associated with recurrent pulmonary infections. Several infections are similar to, and share the same pathogenesis as, heart transplant patients, for example, sternal wound infections.

First 30 days post-transplant (phase one)

Bacterial pneumonia

This is particularly common in these patients and a substantial contributor to early mortality. Previously at least 50% of HLT/LT patients developed bacterial pneumonia.[79,80] The routine use of antimicrobial prophylaxis (usually ceftazidime with clindamycin) immediately post-operatively, with subsequent antibiotic tailoring to the microbiological results of per-transplant donor/recipient airway samples, has lead to the dramatic fall in this complication with its attendant mortality.[79] Antimicrobial cover is intensified if L transplant is performed in a frankly septic field. Immunosuppressive therapy is reduced as much as possible. Established bacterial pneumonia most often is due to *P. aeruginosa*, *Serratia marcescens* and *S. aureus*. In patients with cystic fibrosis, multi-resistant *Burkholderia cepacia* may be a problem. Semi-invasive/invasive diagnostic approaches are similar (e.g. quantitative BAL) for other patients with hospital acquired pneumonia (Chapter 19) but have not been formally verified in these patients.

Day 31–90 post-transplant (phase two)

Viral pneumonia

Among all solid organ transplant patients both CMV infection and CMV disease occur most frequently among HLT/LT patients. As with other transplant patients the incidence and severity varies with pre-transplant donor/recipient CMV serologic status and CMV mismatch, CMV status of blood/products, antiviral prophylaxis and immunosuppressive therapy. CMV infection/disease and mortality are highest (60% and 16%, respectively) if the donor is CMV positive and recipient CMV negative (D+R–) (primary infection) and CMV disease is lowest for D–R– status (19%).[81] The widespread practice of using sero-negative blood products in sero-negative recipients reduces but does not eliminate the risk of primary infection. However, if CMV disease does occur it is usually more severe than that occurring in CMV-positive recipients. A recent prophylactic approach has focused on the use of ganciclovir/acyclovir. CMV hyperimmunoglobin has also been used. Limited studies are available but inhomogenous population groups and problems with study design are common confounds, curtailing precise interpretation. However, results suggest that ganciclovir prophylaxis when compared to no prophylaxis in LT patients is effective in reducing CMV illness and is more effective than acyclovir. Thus ganciclovir given in R–D+ or R+D– situations from day 7 to day 28 followed by acyclovir from day 29 to day 90 reduces CMV infection and disease from around 84% to 52%.[81] CMV prophylaxis not only reduces the frequency of CMV disease but delays its onset from the first 2–3 months to greater than 3–4 months post-transplant. This is well beyond the period of acute lung rejection and reduces any confusion that arises from its earlier occurrence. However, further studies concerning optimal dosages require to be delineated. Diagnosis of CMV pneumonia requires BAL samples and a rapid detection test (See Chapter 10). Transbronchial biopsy is necessary to differentiate CMV disease from acute lung rejection. Treatment is with high dose ganciclovir or foscarnet, possibly adding immunoglobulin for severe or refractory cases.

The use of acyclovir prophylaxis has substantially reduced the incidence of Herpes simplex pneumonitis.[82]

Fungal pneumonia

Fungal respiratory tract infection prior to the widespread use of antifungal prophylaxis occurred in approximately 15% of patients particularly in the graft lung, although dissemination was also present in about three-quarters of those patients who did develop pneumonia. Many cases are only diagnosed post-mortem. Candidal pneumonia is uncommon among fungal pneumonias and among patients with invasive candidiasis. Aspergillosis and cryptococcosis occur less commonly than candidal infections but tend to involve the lower respiratory tract more often than *Candida* spp. If airway secretions are found to contain fungi, either colonising or even contaminating, aggressive appropriate antifungal therapy (i.e. fluconazole for most *Candida* spp. and amphotericin B for *Aspergillus* spp.) is instituted by some centres, and continued until after follow-up cultures are negative (a month for *Candida* spp. and 6 months for *Aspergillus* spp.). A low incidence (around 5%) of invasive fungal infections has been achieved with this approach.[81] However, correctly designed prospective studies of antifungal prophylaxis involving sentinel surveillance cultures have not been performed.

Other agents

Mycobacterial disease due both to *M. tuberculosis* and the non-tuberculous mycobacteria are rare problems in HLT/LT. *M. tuberculosis* is treated with standard anti-tuberculous therapy. However, rifampicin and cyclosporin or FK 506 interactions occur and alternative drugs used for a longer period may be necessary. Non-tuberculous mycobacteria may be found in the absence of clinical signs and symptoms.

Some centres do not routinely treat such patients in this setting and follow up does not indicate clinical disease.[81] However, clinical disease does require treatment (see Chapter 11).

The major effect of Epstein–Barr virus infection is the development of lymphoproliferative disease. An overall incidence of 5% of recipients is found of which two-thirds occur in the allograft. Treatment involves reduction of immunosuppressive therapy, α-interferon or re-transplantation. Despite these measures, obliterative bronchiolitis, recurrent lymphoproliferative disease, rejection or death occurs in about two-thirds of patients.

Day 91–360 post-transplant (phase three)

The widespread use of co-trimoxazole prophylaxis has lead to a substantial reduction in *P. carinii* pneumonia. A 1–3% incidence is now common. *P. carinii* may be an incidental finding on occasions.

Renal transplantation

Renal transplantation has one of the best survival profiles with over 90% of recipients being alive at 1 year. Major infections relate to the graft and abdomen but pulmonary infections are also an important source of mortality and morbidity. There is a considerable overlap between renal and pulmonary disease in these patients, producing dilemmas for differential diagnosis. Non-infectious pulmonary disease may pre-dispose to or coincide with pulmonary infection. Thus ventilatory and diffusion abnormalities exist in patients with chronic renal failure and some of these persist even after transplantation. The cause of these is not always clear but inter-related contenders include pulmonary oedema secondary to ventricular dysfunction, capillary membrane permeability abnormalities, pulmonary haemorrhage, pulmonary calcification and chronic pulmonary hypertension. Various causes of chronic renal disease may in addition have a pulmonary component of the syndrome such as occurs in Goodpasture's syndrome (pulmonary infiltrates) and Wegener's granulomatosis (cavitary lung disease) (see Chapter 28). This further challenges the differential diagnostic exercise. In the period after transplantation these non-infective pulmonary complications may persist or others may arise *de novo* and include pulmonary oedema, thrombo-embolism and malignancies such as lymphoma, Kaposi's sarcoma and metastatic renal cancer. An added complication in the renal transplant patient profile is the concern over antimicrobial–renal function interactions in terms of renal toxicity and appropriate serum level attainment.

First 30 days post-transplant (phase one)

Community-acquired bacterial pneumonia is predominantly due to *S. pneumoniae* and to *H. influenzae*. The onset is often acute and the course fulminating. Hospital-acquired pneumonia is usually caused by Gram-negative rods or staphylococcal infection. Steroid pulse therapy given for acute rejection seems to be a particular risk factor.[8] Super-infection with fungi and other organisms may occur and worsen the prognosis. *Legionella* spp. as with other transplant patients can also occur at this time.

Day 31–90 post-transplant (phase two)

The widespread use of co-trimoxazole prophylaxis used primarily for urinary tract infection prophylaxis has reduced the incidence of PCP in this patient population. The incidence is positively influenced by cyclosporin use.[3,83] The use of co-trimoxazole both for prophylaxis and for treatment may produce trimethoprim associated hypercreatinaemia and confuse the issue of allograft rejection. Appropriate dosing may thus be compromised. In this situation nebulised pentamidine is indicated. It is presumed to be efficacious by extrapolation from the experience in other patient populations.

Viral pneumonia

Cytomegalovirus infection and disease share characteristics seen in other transplant populations; namely CMV may be acquired in the previously non-immune patient, reactivated or occur as a super-infection with a different strain. CMV infection occurs in around 70% of allograft recipients of which one-third develop disease. Immune suppression with OKT3, ALG and ATG will promote reactivation. Cyclosporin by inhibiting host response will lead to loss of containment of CMV. Often non-specific features presage pneumonia such as fever of uncertain origin, neutropenia, thrombocytopenia and flu-like symptoms. Bilateral diffuse interstitial infiltrates characterise the chest radiographic presentations. CMV immunosuppressive driven secondary infection with *P. carinii*, fungi and Gram-negative organs may then occur. CMV has been associated with glomerulopathy and rejection.[84] The response of CMV pneumonitis to ganciclovir in renal transplant patients is encouraging with around two-thirds of treated patients surviving. The outcome is not so good in patients who require IPPV. The role of immunoglobulin is unclear but could be useful.[85] Prophylactic issues using high dose acyclovir have been discussed (see Chapter 10). A pre-emptive approach using ganciclovir for high risk CMV sero-positive patients at risk for CMV disease because of potent immunosuppressive therapy with ALG recently has been shown to reduce the incidence of CMV disease.[86]

Fungal pneumonia

This may occur as a primary infection or secondary to another lung infection. The frequency of occurrence in renal transplantation is low relative to other organ transplant settings but mortality particularly due to *Aspergillus* spp. is over 80%[87] and is specially dismal in the context of secondary infection.

Day 91–360 post-transplant (phase three)

Mycobacterial disease is more common in patients with chronic renal failure and in those who proceed to renal transplant, when compared to the general population. The incidence varies with geographical location and endemicity of mycobacterial disease.[88] *M. tuberculosis* is the causative agent in two-thirds, non-tuberculous mycobacteria in one-third. Pulmonary symptomatology may be mild. Extra-pulmonary mycobacterial disease is quite common. The mortality rate may be high in patients with disseminated disease. Dosages of ethambutol, pyrazinamide and ethionamide have to be reduced in patients with reduced glomerular filtration rate, to avoid toxicity. Streptomycin is nephrotoxic. Rifampicin can reduce cyclosporin levels with the attendent risk of graft rejection through induction of liver enzymes. Controversy exists over isoniazid dosing in patients with diminished renal function. However the consensus of opinion is that dose reduction or determination of acetylator phenotype is unnecessary in patients with impaired renal function.[89] The role of isoniazid prophylaxis is also conjectural. Isoniazid prophylaxis is sometimes offered to patients with a positive tuberculin test or a past history of untreated TB undergoing renal transplant. However, reactivation of TB in patients with a positive tuberculin test has not always been experienced. In addition, isoniazid toxicity can occur in renal patients – a group of individuals who are prone to a high incidence of chronic liver disease following transplantation.

EBV-related lymphomas including pulmonary lymphoma is unusual. Common manifestations of EBV infection are atypical mononucleosis, fever and hepatitis. Focal nodular pulmonary infiltrates should however lead to a suspicion of this complication. The mechanisms include OKT3 promotion of EBV growth, and cyclosporin reduction of T-cell dependent responses to EBV transformed B-cells.[90,91] The management pivots around reduction of immunosuppressive therapy and the use of high dose intravenous acyclovir, ganciclovir or interferon. However, the outcome is poor.

Pulmonary infections in patients with leukaemia and lymphoma

Pneumonia is one of the most common causes of morbidity and mortality in this patient group.[92] The spectrum of infection seen in these patients arises consequent to the similar risk factors described in patients undergoing bone marrow transplantation, but modified as the result of variation in the type and degree of immunosuppresive therapy given and for the particular predominant host defect. The presence of profound and protracted granulocytopenia is a fundamental governing factor particularly in the emergence of bacterial and fungal opportunistic infections[93] Cell-mediated immune derangements in the presence of normal granulocyte counts also tend to favour bacterial sepsis but emergence of protozoal, parasitic and viral diseases tend to be more common whilst fungal infections are less often encountered. Therefore, the likelihood of a particular pathogen emerging will to an extent be governed by the predominant immune defect given all the other risk factors present, e.g. mechanical defects. However, it has to be emphasised that it is somewhat facile to categorise in an over-rigid fashion the risk for a particular pathogen, since overlap is common and risk factors are usually heterogeneous and include cytotoxic treatment, steroids, continuing antimicrobial prophylaxis, etc.

Patients with a predominant granulocytopenic effect

Bacterial pneumonia

This arises either primarily or secondarily to haematogenous spread from an extrapulmonary source. Formerly, Gram-negative infections especially *P. aeruginosa, E. coli* and *Klebsiella* spp. predominated. Data from serial EORTC international antimicrobial therapy trials and others have shown a progressive fall in the incidence of Gram-negative bacteraemia, accompanied by a rise in Gram-positive bacteraemia in granulocytopenic patients over the last 20 years.[94] Nowadays Gram-positive sepsis particularly *S. epidermidis* and *S. viridans* are more frequently seen and may outnumber those due to Gram-negatives.[95] This may be due to the more widespread use of antimicrobial prophylactics particularly the quinolones, and the increased prevalence of mucositis associated with modern chemotherapeutic regimes. The more widespread use of broad spectrum antibiotics, in general has also been responsible for the emergence of multiply resistant organisms. These may transfer between patient populations. This epidemiological shift has implications for empirical therapy of neutropenic fever and early non-specific pneumonia. Many workers now include Gram-positive antibiotic cover to supplement the initial Gram-negative antibiotic regimens.

Fungal pneumonia

The second most common opportunistic pathogenic process in these patients is fungal pneumonia. Candidal pneumonia is not nearly as common as that due to *Aspergillus* spp. However, the emergence of fluconazole resistant *C. albicans* strains and non-*albicans* species provides challenges for initial therapy. Although *Aspergillus* spp. remains the most likely pathogenic mould in the appropriate radiological clinical setting, other species are emerging. These include *Fusarium* spp. and *Scopulariopsis* spp.[96] Their presentation is usually indistinguishable from disease due to *Aspergillus* spp. but antifungal susceptibility may be different. Early invasive diagnostic techniques are crucial in these patients, but are limited by technical problems, accuracy and specificity. The outcome for invasive pulmonary aspergillosis in such patients is dismal with a mortality rate approaching 100%. Certainly correction of neutropenia appears paramount for cure. Exogenous growth factors, high doses of amphotericin B and surgery are sometimes combined in an attempt to maximise therapeutic efficacy but scientific data is lacking. In patients originally responding with apparent cure relapse may be seen if the patient experiences subsequent neutropenic episodes.

Viral pneumonia

Herpes simplex is the most common viral infection observed in these patients. Most often the presentation is mucocutaneous and Herpes simplex pneumonia is rare. Chickenpox pneumonia occasionally occurs and can be life-threatening in leukaemic/lymphoma patients. CMV pneumonia is also seen but is less common than in transplant patients.

Patients with a predominant CMI defect

Bacterial pneumonia

In these patients with encapsulated species such as *H. influenzae* and *S. pneumoniae*, pneumonia can occur. *Listeria* spp., *Legionella* spp., *Mycobacteria* spp., *Salmonella* spp. and *Nocardia* spp., also occur in this patient group. Often systemic features predominate or frank extrapulmonary manifestations occur, for example, subcutaneous abscess with *Nocardia* spp.

Protozoa and parasitic infections
These are features of patients with CMI defects albeit pneumonia is a relatively rare manifestation, for example, in the case of *Toxoplasma, Strongyloides*.

Others
Fungal pneumonia is unusual apart from cryptococcosis. However, *P. carinii* is seen, the presentation sometimes atypical.

Viral pneumonia due to Varicella zoster and cytomegalovirus is also encountered.

Other immunocompromised patients

Patients with solid tumours (apart from lymphoma)

The pre-disposition to pulmonary infection in patients with these malignancies is in general less than occurs in the other immunocompromised patients described previously. This reflects their relatively well-preserved immune status when compared, for example, to bone marrow transplant patients. However, many of these individuals are malnourished. Malnutrition produces selective IgA deficiency, defective complement function, natural killer cell and thymus-mediated T-cell abnormalities. Associated trace element, mineral and vitamin deficiencies also impact on immune function. These include iron deficiency (granulocyte and T-lymphocyte dysfunction), zinc deficiency (phagocytic and T-lymphocyte dysfunction) and phosphate deficiency (granulocyte dysfunction). Patients with cancer may also be elderly and these individuals experience a general decline in both neutrophil and CMI function. The net effect on immune function in patients with miscellaneous solid non-lymphoma cancers is one of a predominantly diminished cell mediated immune function. Vulnerability to a range of organisms as detailed in Table 21.3 occurs, particularly with *Legionella* spp., *Nocardia* spp., *Mycobacteria* spp., *Listeria* spp., CMV and other Herpes viruses, *Toxoplasma* and *Cryptococcus*.

Pulmonary metastatic carcinoma may not only masquerade on occasions as pulmonary infection (see Chapter 28) but may cause bronchial obstruction and lead to post-obstructive pneumonia. Carcinomatous oesophagus involvement may also favour aspiration pneumonitis. The same process will occur in patients with centrally driven impaired gag reflex abnormalities such as in patients with cerebral metastases.

The additional immunosuppressive insult provided by chemoradiotherapy, steroids, etc. given to these patients will, of course, amplify and expand the spectrum of infecting pathogens.

Miscellaneous disease states

Several other acquired diseases and infections have adverse effects which are often subtle on host defences and pre-dispose patients to infections. Diabetes mellitus impairs chemotaxis, complement C3, phagocytosis and myeloperoxidase functions. Iron metabolism is also effected. Vulnerability to tuberculosis, *S. aureus* and pneumococcal pulmonary infections exist particularly. Candidal and other infections such as mucormycosis are also seen.

Alcoholism and alcoholic liver disease impairs gag reflex, nutritional status, macrophage, chemotaxis, natural killer and T-cell functions. Tuberculosis and a wide range of bacterial sepsis are seen.

Auto-immune diseases include SLE and rheumatoid arthritis in which complement chemotaxis, phagocytosis, lymphocyte and cell-mediated immune functions are impaired. These result in varicella zoster virus, CMV and fungal diseases.

In patients with chronic renal failure there is a diminished marrow granulocyte reserve. This with partial inhibition of phagocytosis and iron overload (in haemodialysis) pre-disposes to bacterial sepsis. Mucormycosis has been associated with desferrioxamine treatment.

Patients undergoing splenectomy, either surgical/traumatic or induced, such as autosplenectomy in sickle cell disease experience pneumococcal infections.

Finally, certain microbes per se diminish host resistance. HIV has been discussed fully in Chapter 22. CMV, EBV, HCV and *Capnocytophaga* are further examples of organisms which can lead to secondary infection with other micro-organisms.

Key issues in the management of the immunocompromised host with febrile pneumonitis

The following summary points need to be borne in mind when these patients present (see Table 21.9)

- The immunocompromised patient with clinical/radiological signs of lower respiratory tract infection is a medical emergency and should receive urgent, comprehensive diagnostic approach attention.
- Making a diagnosis entails assimilating such factors as the host defect profile. This, in turn, requires information regarding status of underlying disease, immunosuppressive therapy, transplant status and the interval from transplant and pre-existing/baseline microbial immune status. This will provide a template on which a diagnostic differential can be constructed. Thus the particularly aggressive chemo-radiotherapy regimens used in bone marrow transplantation lead to the most profound neutropenia seen in any patient, accompanied by a propensity for infections such as filamentous fungi which are unique in these patients in the early post-transplant period.
- In an era of high technological medicine the crucial importance of a complete history can be underestimated. Details of travel, occupation, exposure to ill persons/animals and pre-transplantation vaccination status may provide important diagnostic clues. Such epidemiological factors are importance since they will partly determine the pool of potential pathogens. Thus, if the patient has developed respiratory signs and symptoms whilst in the community, *S. pneumoniae*, *H. influenzae*, or *Legionella* spp. are probable. If the patient has hospital-acquired pneumonia, coagulase-negative *S. aureus*, MRSA and *Pseudomonas* spp. are more likely. Recent travel to areas endemic for specific mycoses

Table 21.9. *Key issues of management*

Epidemiological history
travel
exposure
vaccination
Immune status and profile
History and physical
Broad multi-factorial approach
Appropriate invasive diagnostics
Laboratory expertise
Empirical antimicrobials/revision
Adjunctive therapies

such as coccidioidomycoses should lead to the inclusion of geographically linked pathogens in the differential diagnosis. Similarly, a thorough physical examination is mandatory in a patient with neutropenic febrile pneumonitis. Multiple nodular necrotic skin rashes should entertain the differential of disseminated fungal disease. The many non-infective causes of lung injury as defined and described in Chapter 28 should also be borne in mind. Therefore, an itchy palmar rash in conjunction with dyspnoea and crepitations in the bone marrow transplantation patient should suggest graft-versus-host disease.

- It is vital to remember that the presentation of infective pulmonary complications often does not follow the pattern or course elaborated by the same pathogen in immune competent patients.
- The supportive technologic diagnostic approach in immunocompromised patients with fever and pulmonary infiltrates should be swift, comprehensive and appropriately aggressive, since early features are often non-specific and delay in achieving a correct diagnosis is undesirable. Plain chest radiography is, in general, inferior to CT scanning in arriving at a correct diagnosis in bone marrow transplant patients.[97] A blunderbuss approach involving polypharmacy is also unsatisfactory for reasons of cost, imprecision, toxicity issues, emergence of resistant organisms and the possibility that the correct diagnosis will still be missed.
- The types and quality of specimens are of paramount importance if laboratory studies are to be optimally helpful. Limitations of sputum sampling and guidelines for collection and processing have been extensively discussed (Chapter 1). These are sometimes helpful in diagnosing some bacterial pneumonias but much less so for other bacteria, for example, *Legionella* spp. and in protozoal, viral and fungal pneumonias.
- Recourse to more invasive techniques has become the norm in the diagnostic work up of such patients in whom the pneumonic process cannot be precisely specified. Flexible bronchoscopy combined with BAL and protective specimen brushing with quantitative counts is a complex, conjectural subject (Chapters 1 and 19). Transbronchial biopsy has found a place in the diagnostic management of patients suspected to have *P. carinii* pneumonia, tuberculosis, diffuse interstitial pneumonitis and tumour, whereas open lung biopsy still remains the sampling method able to provide most diagnostic information. Of course, all these procedures are limited by hypoxia and coagulopathies which preclude many patients. Recently, precise sub-regional thoracoscopic guided lung biopsy has extended the invasive armamentarium with promising results in terms of safety and efficacy.
- Once adequate material has been sampled, processing should be accomplished by a comprehensive laboratory, confident and conversant in the current diagnostic art of all the major opportunistic pathogens, such as DFA testing for *Legionella* spp., early antigen detection for CMV and the use of DNA analysis and other molecular probes.
- However, in many patients for a variety of reasons, for example, contra-indications to invasive procedures or negative findings therefrom, or lack of expertise, a specific cause for the patient's fever and pulmonary infiltrates cannot be readily identified. Empirical therapy has to be given in these situations. The approach is not uniform from centre to centre, although published guidelines do exist.[98,99] Choice of antimicrobials take into account all of the aforementioned variables as well as foreknowledge of that particular institution's risk for particular pathogens with their antimicrobial susceptibility pattern. In patients developing neutropenic fever without pulmonary symptoms and signs, initial antibiotic treatment will be broad spectrum, for example, ceftazidime, to which an aminoglycoside is added for sepsis syndrome, or vancomycin if a risk for *S. viridans* bacteraemia exists. The comprehensive management of fever in immunocompromised patients without an obvious pulmonary focus is outside the aims of this text – the approach is described elsewhere.[98] If pulmonary features develop, the initial regime may be modified. For example, occurrence of focal circumscribed lung lesions in the profoundly neutropenic patient would suggest *Aspergillus* spp. and amphotericin B should be started. Appearance of diffuse infiltrates would raise the spectre of PCP, CMV etc. depending on timing and other risk factors. This should prompt a rapid search for a precise diagnosis, whilst concurrently modifying antimicrobial cover with co-trimoxazole, ganciclovir, etc.
- The vast majority of units managing immunocompromised patients offer a programme of antimicrobial prophylaxis. This may reduce, but not eliminate, some pathogens but at the expense of risking the emergence of resistant organisms, inducing drug toxicity and not always with clear survival or overall morbidity improvements. In certain areas, however, the use of prophylactic antimicrobials has been shown to significantly reduce the emergence of certain pathogens, for example, acyclovir for Herpes zoster, Herpes simplex and CMV disease.
- Finally, adjunctive therapeutic manipulation with, for example, haematopoietic growth factors, passive immunoglobulins, interferons, and active immunisations have variably improved host defences, though translation into clinical benefit is not always seen.

References

1. MUNDY LM, AUWAERTER, PG, OLDACH D, WARNER ML, BURTON A, VANCE E, GAYDOS CA, JOSEPH JM, GOPALAN R, MOORE RD, QUINN TC, CHARACHE P, BARTLETT JG. Community-acquired pneumonia: Impact of immune status. *Am J Resp Crit Care Med* 1995;152:1309–15.
2. SICKLES EA, YOUNG VM, GREENE WH, WIERNIK PH. Pneumonia in acute leukaemia. *Ann Intern Med* 1973;79:528–34.
3. RAMSEY PG, RUBIN RH, TOLKOFF-RUBIN NE, COSIMI AB, RUSSELL PS, GREENE R. The renal transplant patient with fever and pulmonary infiltrates: aetiology, clinical manifestations, and management. *Medicine* 1980;59:206–22.
4. NEIMAN PE, THOMAS ED, REEVES WC *et al.* Opportunistic infection and interstiatial pneumonia following marrow transplantation for aplastic anaemia and haematologic malignancy. *Transpl Proc* 1976;8:66.
5. REMINGTON JS, GAINES JD, GRIEPP RB *et al.* Further experience with infection after cardiac transplantation. *Transpl Proc* 1972;4:699.
6. KROWKA MJ, CORTESE DA. Pulmonary aspects of liver disease and liver transplantation. *Clin Chest Med* 1989;10:593–616.
7. BODEY GP, BUCKLEY M, SATHE YS *et al.* Quantitative relationships between circulating leukocytes and infection in patients with acute leukaemia. *Am J Roentgenol*, 1966;64:328–40.
8. RAMSEY PG, RUBIN RH, TOLKOFF-RUBIN NE *et al.* The renal transplant patient with fever and pulmonary infiltrates: aetiology, clinical manifestations, and management. *Med (Baltimore)* 1980;59:206–22.
9. ELLIS ME, SPENCE D, BOUCHAMA A, ANTONIUS J, BAZARBASH M, KHOUGEER F, DE VOL E, FUNGAL STUDY GROUP. Open lung biopsy provides a higher and more specific diagnostic yield compared to broncho-alveolar lavage in immunocompromised patients. *Scand J Infect Dis* 1995;27:157–62.
10. KROWKA MJ, ROSENOW EC, HOAGLAND HC. Pulmonary complications of bone marrow transplantation. *Chest* 1985;87:237–46.
11. WINSTON DJ, GALE RP, MEYERS DV, YOUNG LS. Infectious complications of human bone marrow transplantation. *Medicine* 1979;58:1–31.
12. CORDONNIER C, BERNAUDIN JF, BIERLING P, HUET Y, VERNANT JP. Pulmonary complications occurring after allogeneic bone marrow transplantation. *Cancer* 1986;58:1047–54.
13. PANNUTI CS, GINGRICH RD, PFALLER MA *et al.* Nosocomial pneumonia in adult patients undergoing bone marrow transplantation: a 9 year study. *J Clin Oncol* 1991;9:77–84.
14. WINSTON DJ, SCHIFFMAN G, WANG DC *et al.* Pneumococcal infections after human bone marrow transplantation. *Ann Intern Med* 1979;91:835–41.
15. LUM LG. Immune recovery after bone marrow transplantation. *Haematol Oncol Clin N Am*, 1990;4:659–75.
16. MORRISON VA, HAAKE RJ, WEISDORF DJ. Non-*candida* fungal infections after bone marrow transplantation: risk factors and outcome. *Am J Med* 1994;96:497–503.
17. WINSTON DJ, HO WG, CHAMPLIN RE. Cytomegalovirus infections after allogeneic bone marrow transplantation. *Rev Infect Dis* 1990;12 (suppl 7): S776–92.
18. SCHMIDT GM, HORAK DA, NILAND JC *et al.* A randomised, controlled trial of prophylactic ganciclovir for cytomegalovirus pulmonary infection in recipients of allogeneic bone marrow transplantation. *N Engl J Med* 1991;324:1005–11.
19. GOODRICH JM, MORI M, GLEAVES CA *et al.* Early treatment with ganciclovir to prevent cytomegalovirus disease after allogeneic bone marrow transplantation. *N Engl J Med* 1991;325:1601–7.
20. GRANT PRENTICE H, GLUCKMAN E, POWLES RL *et al.* Impact of long-term acyclovir on cytomegalovirus infection and survival after allogeneic bone marrow transplantation. *Lancet* 1994;343:749–53.
21. GOODRICH JM, BOWDEN RA, FISHER L *et al.* Ganciclovir prophylaxis to prevent cytomegalovirus disease allogeneic marrow transplant. *Ann Intern Med* 1993;118:173–8.
22. WINSTON DJ, HO WG, LIN C *et al.* Intravenous immune globulin for prevention of cytomegalovirus infection and interstitial pneumonia after bone marrow transplantation. *Ann Intern Med* 1987;106;12–18.
23. REED EC, BOWDEN RA, DANDLIKER PS *et al.* Treatment of cytomegalovirus pneumonia with ganciclovir and intravenous cytomegalovirus immunoglobulin in patients with bone marrow transplants. *Ann Intern Med* 1988;109:783–8.
24. SCHMIDT GM, KOVACS A, ZAIA JA *et al.* Gangiclovir/immunoglobulin combination therapy for treatment of human cytomegalovirus associated interstitial pneumonia in bone marrow allograft recipients. *Transplantation* 1988;46:905–7.
25. EMANUEL D, CUNNINGHAM I, JULES-ELYSEE K *et al.* Cytomegalovirus pneumonia after bone marrow transplantation successfully treated with the combination of gangiclovir and high-dose intravenous immunoglobulin. *Ann Intern Med* 1988;109:777–82.
26. MEYERS JD, FLOURNOY N, THOMAS ED. Non bacterial pneumonia after allogenic transplantation: a review of ten year's experience. *Rev Infect Dis* 1982;4:1119–32.
27. CONE RW, HACKMAN RC, HUANG M-LW *et al.* Human herpes using virus-6 in lung tissue from patients with pneumonitis after bone marrow transplantation. *N Engl J Med* 1993;329:155–61.
28. PRINCE DS, WINGARD JR, SARAL R, SANTOS GW, WISE RA. Longitudinal changes in pulmonary function following bone marrow transplantation. *Chest* 1989;96:301–6.
29. CLARK JG, CRAWFORD SW, MADTES DK, SULLIVAN KM. Obstructive lung disease after allogeneic marrow transplantation: Clinical presentation and course. *Ann Intern Med* 1989;111:368–76.
30. BESCHORNER WF, SARAL R, HUTCHINS GX, TUTSEHKA PJ, SANTOS GW. Lymphocytic bronchial associated with graft-versus-host disease in recipients of bone marrow transplants. *N Engl J Med* 1978;299:1030–6.
31. HILL G, HELENGLASS G, POWLES R, PERREN T, SELBY P. Mediastinal emphysema in marrow transplant recipients. *Bone Marrow Transpl* 1987;2:315–20.
32. ROBBINS RA, LINDER J, STAHL MG, THOMPSON AB *et al.* Diffuse alveolar haemorrhage in autologous bone marrow transplant recipients. *Am J Med* 1989;87:511–18.
33. SLOANE JP, DEPLEDGE MH, POWLES RL, MORGENSTERN GR, TRICKEY BS, DABY PJ. Histopathology of the lung after bone marrow transplantation. *J Clin Pathol* 1983;36:546–54.
34. HACKMAN RC, MADTES DK, PETERSON FB, CLARK JG. Pulmonary veno-occlusive diesease following bone marrow transplantation. *Transplantation* 1989;47:989–92.
35. KUSNE S, DUMMER JS, HO M *et al.* Infections after liver transplantation: an analysis of 101 consecutive cases. *Medicine* 1988;67:132–43.
36. GEORGE DL, ARNOW PM, FOX AS *et al.* Bacterial infection as a complication of liver transplantation: Epidemiology and risk factors. *Rev Infect Dis* 1991;13:387–96.

37. BRIEGEL J, FORST H, SPILL B, HAAS A, GRABEIN B, HALLER M, KILGER E, JAUCH KW, MAAG K, RUCKDESCHEL G, PETER K. Risk factors for systemic fungal infections in liver transplant recipients. *Eur J Clin Microbiol Infect Dis* 1995;14:375–82.
38. CUERVAS-MONS V, MILLAN I, GAVALER JS, STARZL TE, VAN THIEL DH. Prognostic value of pre-operatively obtained clinical and laboratory data in predicting survival following orthotopic liver transplantation. *Hepatology* 1986;6:922–7.
39. PAYA CV, HERMANS PE, WASHINGTON (II) JA, SMITH TF, ANHALT JP, WIESNER RH, KROM RAF. Incidence, distribution and outcome of episodes of infection in 100 orthotopic liver transplantations. *Mayo Clin Prod* 1989;64:555–64.
40. WIESNER RH, HERMANS PE, RAKELA J *et al.* Selective bowel decontamination to decrease Gram-negative aerobic bacterial and candida colonisation and prevent infection after orthotopic liver transplantation. *Transplantation* 1988;45:570–4.
41. WAJSZCZUK CP, DUMMER JS, HO *et al.* Fungal infections in liver transplant recipients. *Transplantation* 1985;347–53.
42. TOLLEMAR J, ERICZON BG, HOLMBERG K, ANDERSSON J. The incidence and diagnosis of invasive fungal infections in liver transplant recipients. *Transpl Proc* 1990;22:242–4.
43. COLLINS LA, SAMORE MH, ROBERTS MS, LUZZATI R, JENKINS RL, LEWIS WD, KARCHMER AW. Risk factors for invasive fungal infections complicating orthotopic liver transplantation. *J Infect Dis* 1994;170:644–52.
44. PAYA CV. Fungal infections in solid-organ transplantation. *Clin Infect Dis* 1993;16:677–88.
45. DUMMER JS, HARDY A, HO M. Early infections in kidney, heart and liver transplant recipients on cyclosporine. *Transplantation* 1983;36:259–67.
46. SINGH N, DUMMER JS, KUSNE *et al.* Infections with cytomegalovirus and other herpes viruses in 121 liver transplant recipients: Transmission by donated organ and the effects of OKT3 antibodies. *J Infect Dis* 1988;158:124–31.
47. O'GRADY JG, ALEXANDER GJM, SUTHERLAND S, DONALDSON PT, HARVEY F, PORTMANN B, CALNE RY, WILLIAMS R. Cytomegalovirus infection and donor/recipient HLA antigens: interdependent co-factors in pathogenesis of vanishing bile duct syndrome after liver transplantation. *Lancet* 1988;2:302–5.
48. SINGH N, YU VL, MIELES L, WAGENER MM, MINER RC, GAYOWSKI T. High dose acyclovir compared with short course pre-emptive ganciclovir therapy to prevent cytomegalovirus disease in liver transplant recipients: a randomised trial. *Ann Intern Med* 1994;120:375–81.
49. TOKUNGA Y, CONCEPCION, W, BERQUIST WE *et al.* Graft involvement by legionella in a liver transplant recipient. *Arch Surg* 1992;127:475–7.
50. FORBES GM, HARVEY FAH, PHILPOTT-HOWARD JN *et al.* Nocardiosis in liver transplantation: Variation in presentation, diagnosis and therapy. *J Infect* 1990;20:11–19.
51. HIGGINS RSD, KUSNE S, YOUSEM RJ *et al.* Mycobacterium tuberculosis after liver transplantation: Management and guidelines for prevention. *Clin Transpl* 1992;6:81–90.
52. NALESNIK MA. Lymphoproliferative disease in organ transplant recipients. *Springer Semin Immunopathol*, 1991;13:199–216.
53. MICHAELS MG, GREEN M, WALD ER *et al.* Adenovirus infection in paediatric liver transplant recipients. *J Infect Dis* 1992;165:170–4.
54. ASCHER NL, STOCK PG, BUMGARDNER GL, PAYNE WD, NAJARIAN JS. Infection and rejection of primary hepatic transplant in 93 consecutive patients treated with triple immunosuppressive therapy. *Surg Gyn. Obst*, 1988;167:474–84.
55. TAKAOKA F, BROWN MR, PAULSEN W, RAMSAY MAE, LINTMALM GB. Adult respiratory distress syndrome following orthotopic liver transplantation. *Clin Transp* 1989;3:294–9.
56. MUNOZ SJ, NAGELBERG SB, GREEN PL *et al.* Ectopic soft tissue calcium deposition following liver transplantation. *Hepatology* 1988;8:476–83.
57. KROWKA MJ, CORTESE DA. Hepatopulmonary syndrome: an evolving perspective in the era of liver transplantations (Editorial). *Hepatology*, 1990;11:138–141.
58. LOCKHART A. Pulmonary arterial hypetertension in portal hypertension. *Clin Gastroenterol* 1985;14:123–38.
59. HOURANI J, BELLAMY P, BATRA P, BUSUTTIL R, SIMMONS M, TASKIN D. Lung function and chest radiographic abnormalities in patients with severe liver failure. *Chest* 1988;94 (Suppl): 54.
60. BYRICK RJ, NOBLE WH. Postperfusion lung syndrome. *Thoraic Cardiovasc Surg* 1978;76:685–93.
61. CHENOWETH DE, COOPER SW, HUGLI TE, STEWART RW, BLACKSTONE EH, KIRKLIN JW. Complement activation during cardiopulmonary bypass. Evidence of generation of C3a and C5a anaphylatoxins. *N Engl J Med* 1981;304:497–503.
62. NALOS PC, KASS RM, GANG ES, FISHBEIN MC, MANDEL WJ, PETER T. Life-threatening post-operative pulmonary complications in patients with previous amiodarone pulmonary toxicity undergoing cardiothoracic operations. *J Thorac Cardivoasc Surg*, 1987;93:904–12.
63. FULLER J, LEVINSON MM, KLINE JR *et al.* Leginnaires' disease after heart transplantation. *Ann Thorac Surg* 1985;39:308–13.
64. TRENTO A, DUMMER GS, HARDESTY RL, BAHNSOA HT, GRIFFITH BP. Mediastinitis following heart transplantation: Incidence, treatment and results. *Heart Transpl* 1984;3:336–40.
65. SIMPSON GL, STINSON EB, EGGER MJ *et al.* Nocardial infections in the immunocompromised host: a detailed study in a defined population. *Rev Infect Dis* 1981;3:492–9.
66. NOVICK RJ, MORENO-CABRAL CE, STINSON EB *et al.* Non-tuberculous mycobacterial infections in heart transplant recipients: a 17 year experience. *J Heart Transp* 1990;9:357–65.
67. DUMMER JS, WHITE LT, HO M, GRIFFITHS BP, HARDESTY RL, BAHNSON HT. Morbidity of cytomegalovirus infection in recipients of heart or heart–lung transplants who received cyclosporine. *J Infect Dis* 1985;152:1182–91.
68. HOFFLIN JM, PATASMAN I, BALDWIN JC *et al.* Infectious complications in heart transplant recipients receiving cyclosporine and corticosteroids. *Ann Inter Med* 1987;106:209–12.
69. WILSON EJ, MEDARIS DN, BARRETT LV, BAHNA, RUBIN RH. The effects of donor pre-treatment on the transmission of murine cytomegalovirus with cardiac transplants and explants. *Transplantation* 1986;41:781–2.
70. WATSON FS, O'CONNELL JB, AMBER IJ *et al.* Treatment of cytomegalovirus pneumonia in heart transplant recipients with 9 (1.3-dihydroxy-2-propoxymethyl)-guanine (DHPG). *J Heart Transpl* 1988;7:102–5.
71. GRATTAN MT, MORENO-CABRAL CE, STARNES VA *et al.* Cytomegalovirus infection is associated with cardiac allograft rejection and atherosclerosis. *JAMA* 1989;261:3661–3668.
72. LASKE A, GALLINO A, MOHACSI P *et al.* Prophylactic treatment with ganciclovir for cytomegalovirus infection in heart transplantation. *Transpl Proc* 1991;23: 1170–3.
73. PENNOCK JL, OYER PE, REITZ BA, JAMIESON SW, BIEBER CP, WALLWORK J, STINSON EB, SHUMWAY NE. Cardiac transplantation in perspective for the future:

survival, complications, rehabilitation, and cost. *J Thorac Cardiovasc Surg* 1982;83:168–77.

74. JAMIESON SW, OYER PE, REITZ BA *et al.* Cardiac trasnplantation at Stanford. *Heart Transp* 1981;1:86–92.

75. WASER N, MAGGIORINI M, LUTHY A, LASKE A, VON SEGESSER L, MOHACSI P, OPRAVIL M, TURINA M, FOLLATH F, GALLINO A. Infectious complications in 100 consecutive heart transplant recipients. *Eur J Clin Microbiol* 1994;13:12–18.

76. SPEIRS GE, HAKIM M, CALNE RY *et al.* Relative risk of donor-transmitted *Toxoplasma gondii* infection in heart, liver, and kidney transplant recipients. *Clin Transpl* 1988;2:257–60.

77. HUTTER JA, DESPINS P, HIGENBOTTAM T, STEWART S, WALLWORK J. Heart–lung transplantation: better use of resources. *Am J Med* 1988;85:4–11.

78. PARADIS IL, MARRARI M, ZEEVI A *et al.* HLA phenotype of lung lavage cells following heart-lung transplantation. *Heart Transpl* 1985;422–5.

79. ZENATI M, DOWLING RD, DUMMER JS *et al.* Influence of donor lung on the develoment of early infections in heart–lung transplant recipients. *J Heart Trasnpl* 1990:5:502–9.

80. DAUBER JH, PARADIS IL, DUMMER JS. Infectious complications in pulmonary allograft recipients. *Clin Chest Med* 1990;11:291–308.

81. PARADIS IL, WILLIAMS P. Infection after lung transplantation. *Semin Resp Infect* 1993;8:207–15.

82. SMYTH RL, HIGENBOTTAM TW, SCOTT JP *et al.* Herpes simplex virus infection in heart–lung transplantation recipients. *Transplantation* 1990;49:735–9.

83. HARDY AM, WAJSZCZUK CP, SUFFREDINI AF, HAKALA TR, HO M. *Pneumocystis carinii* pneumonia in renal-transplant recipients treated with cyclosporine and steroids. *J Infect Dis* 1984;149:143–7.

84. RICHARDSON WP, COLVIN RB, CHEESEMAN SH *et al.* Glomerulopathy associated with cytomegalovirus viremia in renal allografts. *N Engl J Med* 1981;305:57–63.

85. LAUTENSCHLAGER I, AHONEN J, EKLUND B *et al.* Hyperimmune globulin therapy of clinical cytomegalovirus infection in renal allograft recipients. *Scand J Infect Dis,* 1989;21:139–43.

86. HIBBERD PL, TOLKOFF-RUBIN NE, CONTI D, STUART F, THISTLETHWAITE JR, NEYLAN JF, SYNDMAN DR, FREEMAN R, LORBER MI, RUBIN RH. Pre-emptive ganciclovir therapy to prevent cytomegalovirus disease in cytomgalovirus antibody-positive renal transplant recipients. A randomised controlled trial. *Ann Int Med* 1995;123:18–26.

87. WEILAND D, FERGUSON RM, PETERSON PK, SNOVER DC, SIMMONS RL, NAJARIAN JS. Aspergillosis in 25 renal transplant patients. *Ann Surg* 1983;198:622–9.

88. MALHOTRA KK, DASH SC, DHAWAN IK, BHUYAN UN, GUPTA A. Tuberculosis and renal transplantation-observations from an endemic area of tuberculosis. *Postgrad Med J* 1986;62:359–62.

89. ELLARD GA. The potential clinical significance of the isoniazid acetylator phenotype in the treatment of pulmonary tuberculosis. *Tubercle*, 1984;65:211–27.

90. WALZ G, ZANKER B, MELTON LB *et al.* Possible association of the immunosupressive and B-cell lymphoma-promoting properties of cyclosporine. *Transplantation* 1990;49:191–4.

91. GOLDMAN M, GERARD M, ABRAMOWICZ D *et al.* Induction of interleukin-6 and interleukin-10 by the OKT3 monoclonal antibody: possible relevance to post-transplant lymphoproliferative disorders. *Clin Transpl* 1992;6:265–8.

92. EASTEY EH, KEATING MJ, MCCREDIE KB *et al.* Causes of remission and failure in acute myelogenous leukaemia. *Blood* 1982;60:309–15.

93. BODEY GP, BUCKLEY M, SATHE YS *et al.* Quantitative relationships between circulating leukocytes and infection in patients with acute leukaemia. *Ann Intern Med*, 1966;64:328–40.

94. EORTIC International Antimicrobial Therapy Co-operative Group. Single daily dosing of amikacin and ceftriaxone is as efficacious and no more toxic than multiple daily dosing of amikacin and ceftazidime. Ann Int Med, 1993;115:584–93.

95. EORTIC International Antimicrobial Therapy Co-operative Group. Gram-positive bacteraemia in granulocytopenic cancer patients: results of a prospective randomised therapeutic trial. *Eur J Cancer Clin Oncol* 1990;26:569–74.

96. NEGLIA JP, HURD DD, FERRIERI P *et al.* Invasive scopulariopsis in the immunocompromised host. *Am J Med* 1987;83:1163–6.

97. JANZEN DL, PADLEY SPG, ADLER BD *et al.* Acute pulmonary complications in immunocompromised non-AIDS patients: comparison of diagnostic accuracy of CT and chest radiography. *Clin Radiol* 1993;18:385–9.

98. HUGHES WT, ARMSTRONG D, BODEY GP, FELD R, MANDELL GL, MEYERS JD, PIZZO PH, SCHIMPFF SC, SHENEP JL, WADE JC, YOUNG LS, YOW MD. Guidelines for the use of antimicrobial agents in neutropenic patients with unexplained fever. *J Infect Dis* 1990;161:381–96.

99. PIZZO PA. Management of fever in patients with cancer and treatment neutropenia. *N Engl J Med* 1993;328:1323–32.

22 HIV-associated respiratory infections

EDMUND L.C. ONG

Infectious Diseases Unit, University of Newcastle Medical School, UK

Opportunistic pulmonary infections are the most common cause of acute illness and death in patients with HIV infection[1]. The first recognised cases of the acquired immune deficiency syndrome (AIDS) occurred in the summer of 1981 in America. Cases of *Pneumocystis carinii* pneumonia (PCP) and Kaposi's sarcoma (KS) were documented in young men who it was subsequently realised were both homosexual and immunocompromised[2]. Since then there has been increasing knowledge of the natural history of HIV infection[3] and the microbial spectrum of disease that involved the lungs[4]. However, it is important to recognise that the causes of pulmonary infections in the HIV-infected population are changing as demographics, widespread practice of prophylaxis and life expectancy change.

Infection with HIV causes a progressive and ultimately profound reduction in the host immune response. This is best measured by the progressive loss of T helper lymphocyte (CD4) as shown in Fig. 22.1. The development of secondary infections in patients with HIV infection results from interactions between specific organisms and host defences. The infections that are AIDS defining such as PCP tend to occur later in the course of HIV infection when there has been substantial depletion of CD4 cells[5]. The late emergence of PCP relates to its relatively low pathogenicity as compared to other organisms like *Mycobacterium tuberculosis* (MTB) which appear to cause disease earlier in the course of HIV infection as shown by the higher CD4 count

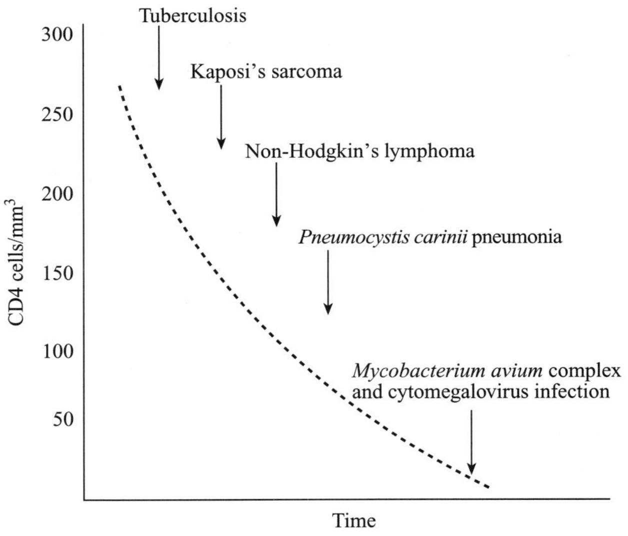

FIGURE 22.1 Occurrence of AIDS-defining conditions in the natural history of HIV infection according to CD4 cell count.

in these patients. Encapsulated bacteria such as *Streptococcus pneumoniae* and *Haemophilus influenzae* are also much more virulent than *P. carinii* and may cause disease at any point in the course of HIV infection.

Despite the pulmonary infections which are characteristic of the advanced phases of HIV infection, the lungs can be infected by the virus itself even in the asymptomatic period. This concept is substantiated by the observation that HIV-1 sequences can be demonstrated in pulmonary cell populations recovered from the respiratory tract of HIV-1 sero-positive subjects at all stages of infection at different levels and influenced by several factors[6,7].

About 25% of subjects with early infection and 50% of individuals with advanced disease show a high intensity alveolitis that is initiated and sustained by HIV-1 specific cytotoxic T lymphocytes[8], natural killer cells[9] and alveolar macrophages and mediated by a number of cytokines[10].

Clinical approach

The multiple infective causes of pulmonary disease in patients with HIV are listed in Table 22.1. The clinical manifestations of these pneumonias overlap considerably but to some extent the nature of the disease progression, the presence of fever, the radiographic pattern and the white cell count may assist to narrow the differential diagnosis. However, it must be borne in mind that each infectious process particularly in the context of severe immunosuppression and prophylactic antibiotics has the potential to present atypically. Moreover, some processes are occasionally caused by a mixed infection or reflect infection superimposed on another process such as neoplastic disorder like Kaposi's sarcoma. Thus it is mandatory in the management of such patients to establish the specific aetiology by a relevant microbiological test when an infective process is suspected. Geography is an important issue in predisposing patients from endemic areas to specific infectious agents as in Indianapolis, for example, pulmonary histoplasmosis is almost as common as PCP and may present identically[11].

As with any other patient population, HIV-infected patients with respiratory symptoms should have a chest radiograph and sputum specimen stain and culture. If breathlessness is a prominent feature, blood gas measurement allows determination of the degree of respiratory failure, the need for oxygen therapy and calculation of the alveolar oxygen gradient. Oximetry may be an alternative and it avoids the inconvenience of arterial puncture but gives less precise information than arterial blood gases. Simple pulmonary function

Table 22.1. *Pulmonary infections associated with HIV infection*

Fungi	Mycobacteria
Pneumocystis carinii	*Mycobacterium* tuberculosis
Cryptococcus neoformans	*Mycobacterium avium* complex
Histoplasma capsulatum	*Mycobacterium genavense*
Coccidioides immitis	Other non-tuberculous mycobacteria
Bacteria	Viruses
Streptococcus pneumonia	Cytomegalovirus
Haemophilus influenzae	Herpes simplex virus
Staphylococcus aureus	Epstein–Barr virus
Branhamella catarrhalis	Respiratory syncytial virus
Rhodococcus equi	Influenza A and B virus
Mycoplasma pneumoniae	
Legionella species	
Bordella pertussis	

tests such as forced vital capacity and transfer factor are quick to perform and are a readily available way to screen HIV patients for pulmonary disease.

If no adequate sputum specimen is obtained, most patients should be able to undergo induction of sputum using hypertonic 3% saline via an ultrasonic nebuliser. The diagnostic sensitivity and specificity for *P. carinii* should be over 75% using published methods[12]. Other opportunistic pathogens such as *Mycobacteria* spp., *Histoplasma* spp., *Cryptococcus* spp. or *Coccidiomycosis* spp. can be recognised morphologically. If induced sputum analysis is negative, flexible fiberoptic bronchoscopy with bronchoalveolar lavage should be performed to obtain good quality specimen and the sensitivity for *P. carinii* is 87–89%[13] and when combined with transbronchial biopsies, the diagnostic sensitivity increases to 94–100%[14]. This technique should rarely fail to diagnose PCP even if the patient has received several days of empirical therapy.

Reassessment of the patient should occur if the bronchoalveolar lavage and transbronchial biopsies are unrevealing for a specific pulmonary process. If further deterioration occurs clinically or radiographically, a repeat bronchoscopy or open lung biopsy should be performed. This is often necessary to establish a diagnosis of lymphoma, Kaposi's sarcoma, cytomegalovirus or fungus infection (see Fig. 22.2).

DIAGNOSIS, THERAPY AND PREVENTION OF SPECIFIC INFECTIONS

Pneumocystis carinii pneumonia

The emergence of *P. carinii* (see also Chapter 30) as a major pathogen of individuals with AIDS has revolutionised the approach to diagnosis and management of patients with PCP. Molecular studies of the organisms have suggested that pneumocystis may be more closely related to the fungi than to the protozoan parasites[15–18]. The appearance of the organism *in vivo* is most similar to that of the protozoa, including the thick walled cyst form with multiple internal sporozoites and the small, thin-walled trophozoites (Fig. 22.3). By contrast, the cyst wall contains b-1,3-glucans and stains with both methenamine silver and the periodic acid-Schiff (PAS) stains typically used for fungi.

PCP is the most common life-threatening infection in patients with AIDS in the United States and Europe and in the initial years of the epidemic was responsible for up to 85% of all respiratory episodes[19]. The incidence of PCP as the first AIDS-defining condition still remains substantial although, because of widespread prophylaxis, it is progressively declining[20]. The disease ranges in severity from a mild infection with a normal chest radiograph and an indolent course to respiratory failure requiring assisted ventilation where the mortality may exceed 90%[21]. PCP usually presents as a diffuse pulmonary infiltrate associated with fever, chest tightness, cough and breathlessness (Fig. 22.4). Some patients may complain of wheeze[22]. It is important therefore not to discount symptoms in patients even with a normal chest radiograph as 5–14% of patients

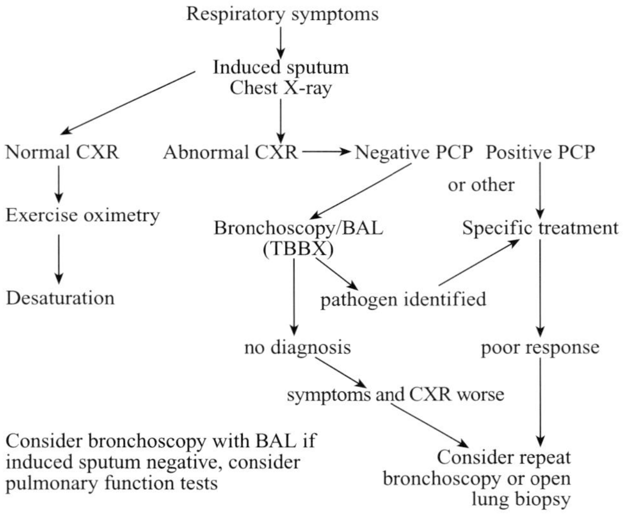

FIGURE 22.2 Algorithm for respiratory symptoms in HIV. RX, treatment; CXR, chest radiograph; PCP, *P. carinii* pneumonia; BAL, bronchoalveolar lavage; TBBX, transbronchial biopsy.

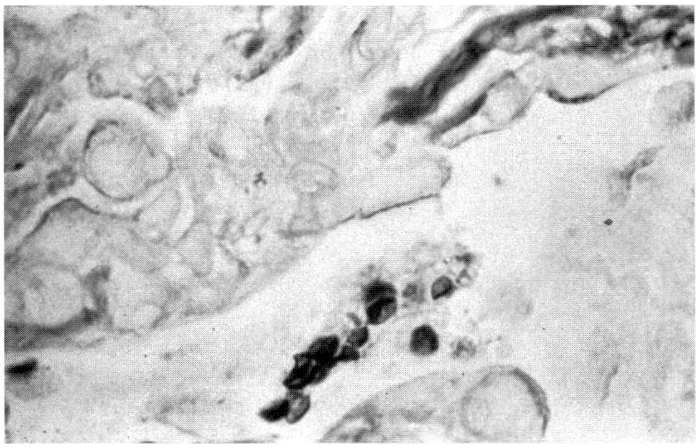

FIGURE 22.3 Methenamine silver stain of *P. carinii*.

subsequently found to have respiratory disease had a normal chest radiograph at presentation[23].

Such a normal appearance may result not only in PCP but also in mycobacterial and cytomegalovirus infection[24]. Severe cases of PCP frequently show extensive consolidation with air bronchograms and 5–10% of cases show atypical features (Fig. 22.5), including cystic changes[25], localised upper zone changes and miliary pattern mimicking tuberculosis[26,27], hilar and mediastinal lymphadenopathy[28] and pleural effusion[29].

The role of nosocomial transmission of *P. carinii* remains controversial. A surveillance study from Switzerland suggested a higher risk of PCP in HIV-negative immunocompromised patients in contact with AIDS patients with PCP[30]. Interestingly, although *P. carinii* has long been thought to be distributed worldwide, a seroprevalence study has shown variation from 63.8% to 82.8% in adults from the United States, Haiti, Mexico, Africa and Korea[31].

Measurement of arterial oxygenation is important in the detection and treatment of the rapidly progressive and potentially fatal hypoxaemia which indicates severe PCP. Exercise induced arterial desaturation detected by oximetry may be a sensitive index for PCP[32]. Pulmonary function tests such as single breath carbon monoxide transfer factor (TLCO), transfer coefficient (KCO), total lung capacity (TLC), vital capacity (VC), and forced vital capacity (FVC) have been reported to be reduced in patients with PCP whereas other simple measures of airway function (peak expiratory flow, forced expiratory volume in one second, maximum expiratory flow rate at 50% of vital capacity) are often normal[33]. A reduction in TLCO is the most sensitive of these indices for PCP[34] and may correspond with the degree of histological abnormality in the lung[35]. It, however, lacks specificity as such low values may be detected in many AIDS-related lung disorders including Kaposi's sarcoma and *M. tuberculosis* infection.

Gallium-67 citrate lung scans have been shown to have a high sensitivity of more than 90% but low specificity of 51%[36]. In contrast to gallium-67 which is selectively taken up by inflammatory cells, the clearance of aerosolised 99mTC DTPA from the lung is a measure of pulmonary epithelial permeability[37]. DTPA clearance from the lung is greatly increased in patients with PCP[38]. Both techniques are time consuming and costly and require the assistance of a nuclear medicine department.

PCP is most readily diagnosed by induced sputum examination. The yield ranges from 70–95%, although the sensitivity is reduced by 20% if patients are on prophylaxis particularly aerosolised pentamidine[39]. Almost all cases of PCP can be diagnosed by BAL; transbronchial and open lung biopsy are rarely necessary. Giemsa, toluidine blue-0, methenamine silver, Gram's stain and immunofluorescent monoclonal antibody techniques are all sensitive and specific at varying degrees[12]. Several groups have used polymerase chain reaction (PCR) to diagnose PCP[40,41]. However, both the specificity of identifying active infection by detection of DNA sequences and the pathogenesis of active PCP (reinfection versus reactivation of latent infection) are uncertain.

Treatment of PCP

Co-trimoxazole (trimethoprim-sulphamethoxazole – TMP/SMX) is the treatment of choice for patients who can tolerate it. This combination was first shown to be effective in man in 1975[42]. The recommended dose of trimethoprim is 20 mg/kg/day and sulphamethoxazole 100 mg/kg/day

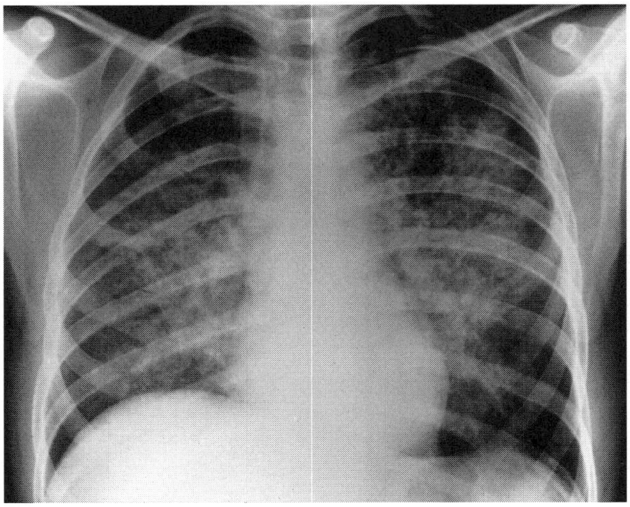

FIGURE 22.4 Chest radiograph showing typical diffuse pulmonary infiltrate of PCP.

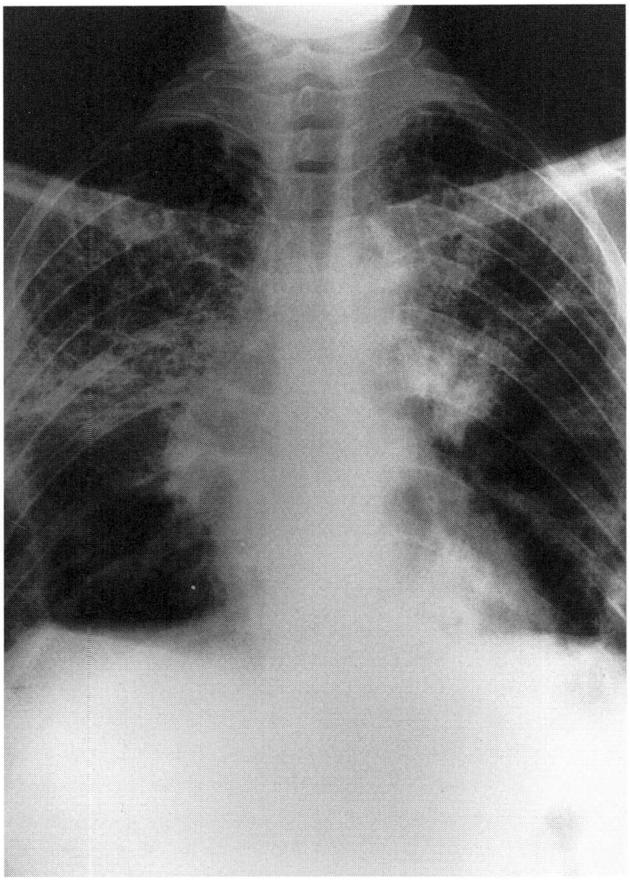

FIGURE 22.5 Chest radiograph showing atypical cystic changes of PCP.

administered intravenously in divided doses or as a continuous infusion. Although TMP/SMX is the most effective combination, side effects are common and occur in 50–80% of patients with AIDS[43]. The reason for this high incidence is not understood, but generally a high incidence of adverse drug reactions particularly hypersensitivity reactions is observed in individuals with HIV infection. Bone marrow suppression is frequently seen with neutropenia, thrombocytopenia and megaloblastic anaemia[44]. Folinic acid supplementation may minimise the myelotoxicity. Other side-effects are hepatotoxicity, tremor, nephrotoxicity and rarely Stevens–Johnson syndrome. The duration of treatment required for PCP is 3 weeks and, as TMP/SMX is well absorbed, oral treatment can usually be started after a few days of treatment when defervescence has occurred; mild cases may be treated with oral TMP/TMX from the outset.

Pentamidine was shown to be effective in the treatment of the epidemic childhood form of PCP in 1958[45]. It should be given either intravenously (4 mg/kg) or by inhalation for mild infection. Adverse reactions are common occurring in about half of patients and may be severe; they include nausea and vomiting, rash, flushing, tachycardia, hypertension, hypoglycaemia and hyperglycaemia, pancreatitis, nephrotoxicity and hepatotoxicity[46].

Against this background of severe adverse events with parenteral administration, aerosolised pentamidine was developed as an alternative treatment for mild infections. The drug is delivered directly to the lungs and few systemic adverse effects had been observed[47]. The dosage used in a number of studies[48] was 600 mg daily up to 21 days. It is important to note that the delivery nebulising system has to generate particle size suitable for alveolar deposition[49,50].

The combination of dapsone and trimethoprim is also effective in the treatment of PCP though no comparative prospective studies with TMP/SMX have been done[51]. This combination is particularly useful when severe side-effects occur with pentamidine or TMP/SMX. It should not, however, be used in patients with glucose 6-phosphate dehydrogenase deficiency. The recommended dose is dapsone 100 mg a day and trimethoprim 20 mg/kg a day. Side-effects include nausea, vomiting, marrow suppression, haemolytic anaemia and methaemoglobinaemia.

Clindamycin and primaquine have been shown to be effective for PCP[52]. In this particular study clindamycin was given intravenously (600 mg four times daily) and primaquine (15 mg base daily). Of episodes of PCP occurring in 25 patients unresponsive or intolerant to first line treatment 28 were treated with this combination. There were two episodes with no improvement. Rash was observed with nausea and leucopenia. Oral therapy may be just as effective[53]. Tolerability of clindamycin may be a problem[54].

Trimetrexate (lipid soluble analogue of methotrexate) has been shown to be effective in patients (response rate 69%) who had failed to improve with first line treatment with TMP/SMX or pentamidine[55]. The drug has to be administered intravenously at a dose of 30–60 mg/m^2. A dose escalation study[56] using oral piritrexim at 150 and 250 mg/m^2 showed that four of 23 patients failed to improve, four suffered dose limiting toxicity and seven patients had a recurrent episode within 2 months of completing the therapy.

Difluoromethylornithine (DFMO), a polyamine synthesis inhibitor, in one study[57] among patients who had failed to respond to first line treatment, was shown to be of some benefit with an overall survival of 36%. This included patients receiving intermittent positive pressure ventilation. Adverse events such as thrombocytopenia, leucopenia, anaemia and diarrhoea were common.

Atovaquone, a hydroxynaphthoquinone which is a selective and potent inhibitor of the eukaryotic mitochondrial electron chain in parasitic protozoa had been shown to be less effective than TMP/SMX in randomised trials[58] for mild and moderately severe PCP cases. Treatment-limiting adverse effects were less frequent in the atovaquone arm and it seems reasonable to attribute part of the lower efficacy of atovaquone to poor bioavailability. The presence of food particularly high fat food increases bioavailability to two to four fold[59].

On current evidence trimetrexate, piritrexim, difluoromethylornithine and atovaquone should only be used in patients who cannot tolerate standard therapy (TMX/SMX and parenteral pentamidine) or regimens with substantial evidence of activity such as trimethoprim dapsone and clindamycin and primaquine.

Adjunctive therapy with corticosteroids has been shown to be of benefit if administered in the early stages of PCP. The California Collaborative Treatment Group conducted an open study[60] of adjunctive prednisone therapy in which 251 patients with PCP were randomly allocated to treatment with prednisone (40mg twice a day for 5 days, continued at tapering doses over the 21-day course of therapy) or no therapy. Patients were eligible if adjunctive therapy was begun within 36 hours of antimicrobial therapy and if the ratio of arterial oxygen pressure to the fraction of oxygen in inspired air (P_aO_2:F_i0_2) was >75. The three primary end points were respiratory failure (P_aO_2:F_i0_2 <75), ventilatory failure and death and these were reduced by 50% in those allocated to the steroid arm. The results were most striking in subjects whose gas exchange ability was most severely impaired at entry. There were no increases in life threatening infections, Kaposi's sarcoma or other serious complications of steroid therapy in the steroid group. Another randomly allocated double blind placebo-controlled trial[61] demonstrated that a 21-day course of prednisone (60 mg by mouth daily) begun within 48 hours of initiating antimicrobial therapy reduced the early deterioration on oxygenation (defined as decrease of 10% in oxygen saturation). A National Institute of Health (NIH, USA) consensus panel has since recommended that patients with PCP with an arterial $p0_2$ of <70–75 mmHg on room air should be treated with corticosteroids at the same time as antimicrobial therapy is begun[62].

In all individuals with HIV for whom critical care is being considered, the goals of such care must be defined clearly at the outset and be continuously reviewed during the course of the individual's treatment. They should be counselled as to what they might expect and presented their options in realistic terms. This should be done if at all possible before they are severely ill. Appropriate intensive care should be provided if the individual so desires after being presented the facts and, if in the judgement of the responsible physician such intervention would not be futile, at least in the short term. On the other hand, individuals who decline critical care should understand that all necessary measures will be taken for their continuing medical care and that they will not be abandoned. Care should be equally intense but in keeping with the individual's wishes and prognosis[50].

Prophylaxis of PCP

In patients with HIV infection, lifelong primary prophylaxis is warranted for all patients with CD4 cell counts below 200 cells/mm^3; for patients with unexplained persistent fever (>37.8 °C) for 2 weeks or oropharyngeal candidiasis (unrelated to antibiotic or corticosteroid therapy) regardless of CD4 cell count[63]. Following successful treatment, PCP recurs in more than 65% of patients with AIDS who receive zidovudine therapy alone. Therefore secondary prophylaxis is advocated. Whereas in adults the development of PCP becomes increasingly likely with decreasing CD4 lymphocyte count, in children the value of the CD4 count is limited especially during the first year of life[64].

TMP/SMX (960 mg daily) is the drug of choice which was shown in a large trial conducted by the ACTG (AIDS Clinical Trial Group) 021 comparing it with aerosolised pentamidine 300 mg monthly as prophylaxis for secondary PCP[65]. TMP/SMX has a higher efficacy with the risk of recurrent PCP being less than 3.25 times less than aerosolised pentamidine. However, the rate of toxicity (27%) was higher in the TMP/SMX arm than in the aerosolised pentamidine arm. Because the high incidence of TMP/SMX related side effects appears to be at least dose related, lower dose regimens have been investigated. Although no randomised comparative large trials have been reported, several studies have suggested that an intermittent dosage such as 960 mg three times weekly could be as effective and better tolerated than the higher dose[66,67]. Although TMP/SMX is highly effective, the high frequency of adverse reactions in patients with HIV infection has led to extensive efforts to find alternatives. Dapsone with or without pyrimethamine at varying doses[68–70] pyrimethamine with sulfadoxine[71] and nebulised pentamidine[72] have shown some efficacy. It should be noted that there is increasing evidence that a higher dosage of the currently recommended 300 mg monthly inhaled pentamidine may be needed to provide better efficacy for primary and secondary prophylaxis[73]. The administration of aerosol pentamidine should be delivered in an environment with negative pressure ventilation to avoid chemical irritation of the skin and the risk of nosocomial pathogen transmission.

There is concern about the increasing number of reports of extrapulmonary pneumocystis infections, atypical pulmonary recurrences, a lower diagnostic yield from bronchoalveolar lavage, pneumothoraces and cystic changes, pancreatitis and disturbances in glucose metabolism in patients taking aerosolised pentamidine[74–76].

Tuberculosis

Tuberculosis (see Chapter 15) can be one of the earliest infections to occur in the course of HIV infection[77] and therefore may be diagnosed before the patient is known to be HIV positive. HIV testing should be considered in all cases of tuberculosis and undertaken after appropriate counselling in those with risk factors for HIV infection. Most cases of tuberculosis are likely to be due to reactivation of previous infection[78] although HIV infection may predispose individuals to new infections. HIV-associated tuberculosis is dependent on three factors: (i) prevalence of tuberculous infection in general population; (ii) prevalence of infection with HIV; (iii) the extent to which these two segments of the population overlap.

Early in the course of HIV infection, before marked immunodeficiency develops, tuberculosis usually presents with upper zone changes on chest radiographs (with or without cavitation), the tuberculin test is usually positive and acid fast bacilli may be seen on direct sputum smear microscopy. As HIV-induced immunodeficiency increases, the presentation of tuberculosis may become increasingly non-specific and atypical, chest radiographs may be unusual with lower zone changes and diffuse or miliary shadowing and, less often, cavitation. Extrapulmonary manifestations involving the gastrointestinal and central nervous systems are more common, particularly lymph node disease[77]. Tuberculin test is often negative. It is important to note that chest radiographs may be normal[79].

Several reports have documented the nosocomial transmission of multiple drug resistant (MDR) strains of *M. tuberculosis* and the rapid progression to life threatening disease among patients with HIV particularly in the United States[80]. Nearly all the patients in these outbreaks have had organisms resistant to both isoniazid and rifampicin, the two most effective antituberculosis drugs[81]. Such infection with MDR strains is associated with widely disseminated disease and rapid progression, poor treatment response with an inability to eradicate the organism and substantial mortality (72–89%).

Induction of sputum and bronchoscopy with bronchoalveolar lavage may show acid-fast bacilli on smear and culture in patients unable to produce sputum[79]. Other sites such as bone marrow, blood culture, liver biopsy specimens may also provide bacteriological confirmation[82].

The development of cutaneous anergy to tuberculo-protein with the progression of the immunodeficiency associated with HIV infection greatly reduces the value of the tuberculin skin test as measure of previous tuberculous infection. However, even with such a limitation, tuberculin testing should still be undertaken at time of diagnosis of HIV infection, a careful history of BCG vaccination taken and the presence or absence of a BCG scar recorded. Skin tuberculin testing is best performed by the Heaf method with the disposable head. Management should be as indicated in the flow diagram (Fig. 22.6). If an HIV-positive person with or without a history of BCG vaccination is negative to other recall antigens as well as tuberculin and has a CD4 count of <200/mm^3, he or she should receive chemoprophylaxis if there is a history of contact with tuberculosis or a history of, or radiographic evidence of, previous tuberculosis[83].

Treatment

Generally the treatment regimen recommended for immunocompetent hosts also appears to be effective in achieving sputum conversion in HIV-infected tuberculosis patients[77,83]. However, cases of failure have been reported in the literature with fully susceptible strain[84]. The Centers for Disease Control recommends that patients with HIV infection should be treated with isoniazid, rifampicin, and pyrazinamide during the first 2 months and that ethambutol should be added if drug resistance is suspected[85]. The continuation phase with rifampicin and isoniazid should be continued for a minimum of 9 months and for at least 6 months beyond documented culture conversion as evidenced by three negative cultures. The issue regarding lifelong chemoprophylaxis with isoniazid following initial treatment is controversial and on the basis of current evidence should be judged on each patient's clinical status and stage of their HIV disease. As tuberculosis can be one of the earliest infections to occur in the course of HIV infection, such patients should not be universally subjected to chemoprophylaxis with isoniazid following treatment[86]. There is a high incidence of cutaneous adverse effects associated with therapy in HIV positive patients[87,88]. Haematological and hepatic reactions to rifampicin, isoniazid and pyrazinamide are commoner[89] and occasional anaphylactoid reactions to rifampicin can occur. Drug interactions such as rifampicin and isoniazid with ketoconazole and fluconazole are well documented. Thiacetazone is widely implicated in severe life-threatening reactions like exfoliative dermatitis and Steven–Johnson syndrome and in one series the mortality rate due to this drug was 3%[87]. Such a finding has major implications for the National Tuberculosis Control Programmes that utilise thiacetazone, particularly in the developing countries.

Chemoprophylaxis with isoniazid has been demonstrated to reduce the risk of developing tuberculosis in HIV-positive injecting drug users without clinical tuberculosis[78]. Chemoprophylaxis may need to be given for longer than the six months recommended for HIV negative patients. The flow diagram indicates which patients should be given chemoprophylaxis. If chemoprophylaxis is not given 3-monthly clinical and chest radiograph monitoring for tuberculosis should be undertaken. There is currently no epidemiological evidence that previous BCG vaccination will protect individuals who subsequently acquire HIV infection from developing tuberculosis[79]. BCG vaccination should not be given to individuals known to be HIV positive.

Patients with tuberculosis and those suspected of having the disease should be cared for in rooms that are adequately ventilated and kept at negative pressure relative to surrounding areas. Ideally, air

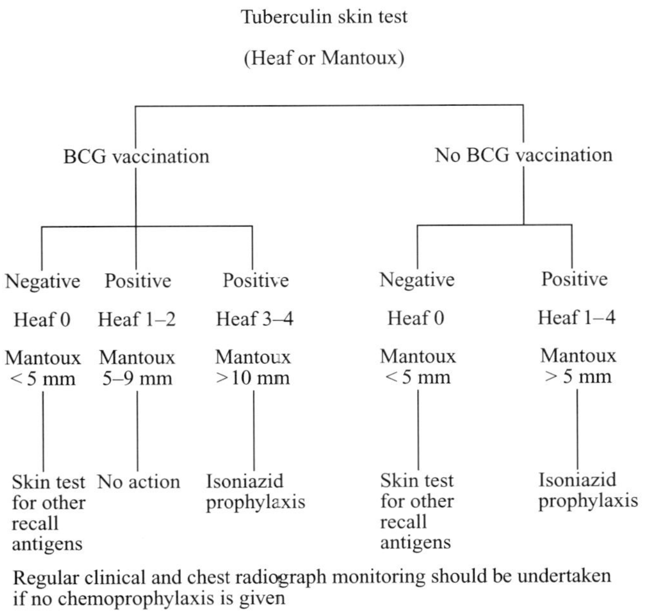

FIGURE 22.6 Management of asymptomatic HIV-positive patients. (Adapted from (83)).

from such rooms should be vented to the outside of the building not recirculated. All cough-producing procedures such as bronchoscopy, the induction of sputum and the administration of aerosolised pentamidine should be performed in well ventilated areas or in booths occupied only by the patient to contain infection at the source.

Mycobacterium avium complex infection

Mycobacterium–avium complex (MAC) infection is among the most common opportunistic diseases observed in patients with AIDS (see also Chapter 11). *M. avium*, specifically serovars 1, 4 or 8 predominates as the causative agent. MAC is ubiquitous; the organism is frequently found in water, soil and foodstuffs. Data from United States has shown that the incidence of disseminated MAC (DMAC) has increased from approximately 6% between 1985 and 1988 to approximately 23% between 1989 and 1990. The risk of developing DMAC increases as the CD4 count declines. The incidence of DMAC bacteremia increases as the CD_4 count declines, particularly to less than 100 cells/mm^3 when it exceeds 40% at 2 years[90]. The incidence of DMAC infection is unrelated to age, sex, race or risk group for HIV infection[91].

MAC can be occasionally isolated from respiratory and stool culture specimens obtained from patients with severe HIV disease and such isolation should prompt investigation for evidence of focal or disseminated disease[92,93]. Distinction between primary infection without disease (colonisation), primary infection with disease, and secondary infection as a manifestation of dissemination is at times difficult. Patients may have transient respiratory colonisation with a single positive culture or episodic excretion of MAC without disease. Therapy in such circumstances may not be of any benefit.

Signs and symptoms of MAC pulmonary disease, including cough, breathlessness, and fever are non-specific but the presentation is generally milder than that of tuberculosis[94,95]. Recommended diagnostic criteria for patients with noncavitary pulmonary disease caused by non-tuberculous mycobacteria include: (i) the presence of two or more sputum specimens that are AFB smear positive or that produce heavy growth on culture, and (ii) failure to clear cultures with good pulmonary toilet or 2 weeks of antimycobacterial therapy[75]. These guidelines may not apply to severely immunocompromised patients as therapy should be strongly considered in such a population group where the risk of dissemination is high.

The symptoms and signs of DMAC are also non-specific, but patients typically present with recurrent daily episodes of fever, frequently with very high temperature, chills, profuse night sweats, weakness, malaise, anorexia and marked weight loss[96].

Diarrhoea occurs in almost one-half of the patients[97,98]. Severe anaemia may be a predictor of DMAC and patients may require transfusion. Physical examination may show hepatomegaly. Other sites of infection include skin, bone and joints, eyes and large airways and brain.

Chest radiographs are abnormal in only 4–9% of patients with MAC showing evidence of pneumonitis with patchy or nodular infiltrates[99]. Mediastinal and hilar lymphadenopathy is unusual and cavitary disease and pleural effusions are rare in patients with MAC.

Blood cultures are frequently positive in DMAC using both systems such as radiometric BACTEC TB or Septi Chek AFB[100].

Treatment

Although studies have not identified an optimal regime or confirmed that any therapeutic regime produces sustained clinical benefit for individuals with DMAC, available evidence suggests that there is a need for treatment[98,101]. To date the agents most commonly used in clinical trials include azithromycin, clarithromycin, ciprofloxacin, clofazimine, ethambutol, rifabutin, rifampicin and parenterally administered amikacin.

Because of the genetic diversity of strains isolated from patients[102], the large organism burden and rapid emergency of resistance to antimicrobial agents like clarithromycin, therapy with two or more drugs is recommended[103]. Every regimen should contain either azithromycin or clarithromycin. Isoniazid and pyrazinamide are not effective for the therapy of MAC. Clinical manifestations of DMAC should be monitored several times during the initial weeks of therapy and microbiological response as assessed by blood culture every 4 weeks during initial therapy can be useful in interpreting the efficacy of a therapeutic regimen. Most patients show substantial clinical improvement in the first 4–6 weeks of therapy although elimination of the organisms from blood cultures may take longer.

MAC prophylaxis

Patients with HIV infection and less than 100 CD4 T-lymphocytes/mm^3 should be considered for prophylaxis against MAC. Prophylaxis should be continued life-long unless multiple drug therapy for MAC becomes necessary because of the development of DMAC. While the use of clofazimine alone appeared ineffective[104] two identical studies[90] demonstrated that rifabutin prophylaxis showed a 50% reduction in the rate of MAC bacteraemia. These two studies were designed to determine whether MAC bacteraemia could be prevented or delayed but not to evaluate the impact of prophylaxis on symptoms of survival. But, when additional analyses were done there was no clear survival advantage. However, it should be noted that the duration of prophylaxis in these studies was limited – a mean of 185 and 231 days, respectively and therefore there are no long-term data on the durability of the preventative effect or on the emergence of resistance. Widespread use may not only influence resistance development in MAC which would affect the treatment of DMAC but may result in rifampicin resistance in MTB. Rifabutin, like rifampicin, induces hepatic metabolism of other drugs. A one third reduction in zidovudine time-concentration levels and similarly rifabutin has been shown to lower clarithromycin area under the curve by >50%[105]. Fluconazole a cytochrome p450 inhibitor may increase rifabutin levels by up to 80% potentially increasing the risk of rifabutin associated uveitis[107]. Clinicians therefore, must weigh the potential benefits of MAC prophylaxis against the potential for toxicities and drug interactions, the cost and the potential to produce resistance in a community with a high rate of *M. tuberculosis* infection.

Other mycobacterial infections

Infections with *Mycobacterium kansasii*, *Mycobacterium gordonae*, *Mycobacterium xenopi*, *Mycobacterium chelonae*, *Mycobacterium fortuitum*, *Mycobacterium haemophilum*, and *Mycobacterium genavense* have been reported in the literature in association with HIV infection. Disseminated infection with *M. genavense* was first described in 1990. Cases reported from Europe presented with a chronic illness with fever, diarrhoea and marked weight loss[108]. In a series of 53 cases, the mean CD4 count was 24/mm^3 and the 1 year mortality rate was 75%[109], similar to patients with DMAC. *M. genavense* was widely disseminated as demonstrated by identification in the gastrointestinal tract, bone marrow, lymph nodes, and blood. Because DNA sequences had identified a unique pattern, *M. genavense* can be considered a new member of the genus Mycobacterium. The organism appears to be ubiquitous with reported cases from three continents[110].

Bacterial pneumonias

Bacterial pulmonary infections appear to be more common among patients with HIV infection than among the general population accounting for 2.5% to 10% of cases. The yearly incidence of pneumococcal pneumonia among HIV patients who have a low CD4 count is about 17.6/1000 as compared to the general population of 2.6/1000. The annual incidence of pneumococcal pneumonia among intravenous HIV drug users is 10% compared to 2% among non-HIV intravenous drug users[111].

Community-acquired pneumonias in patients with HIV are caused by *Streptococcus pneumoniae*, *Haemophilus influenzae*, *Staphylococcus aureus*, *Moraxella catarrhalis*, *Legionella* spp. and *Mycoplasma pneumoniae*. The rate of recurrence after an episode is high[112]. Hospital-acquired pneumonias in this population are usually caused by Gram-negative rods or staphylococci[113].

The presentation of bacterial pneumonia in HIV infected patients is fairly similar to that of immunocompetent individuals.

Features of fever, productive cough, frequent occurrence of pleuritic chest pain and consolidation are well described. The duration of symptoms is usually less than 1 week. Laboratory testing generally reveals relative leukocytosis with a left shift. Among HIV-positive patients, bacteraemia develops more frequently in pneumococcal pneumonia than in HIV-seronegative patients. Chest radiography shows a segmental or lobar infiltrate in most cases, although diffuse infiltrates may be seen in up to 40%. The diagnosis of bacterial pneumonia is made on clinical grounds with a diagnostic gram stain or culture of sputum in 50% of cases. The antimicrobial therapy is similar to that administered to HIV-negative patients with bacterial pneumonia[111].

Nocardial infection is a rarely reported opportunistic infection in HIV-infected individuals and typically occurs in advanced immunodeficiency. It is usually disseminated at the time of diagnosis and is characterised by an indolent course that may be difficult to differentiate from other systemic infections. Invasive procedures to obtain tissue or fluid for culture are frequently necessary to make the diagnosis, although a Gram's or modified acid-fast stain of sputum or other infected material may suggest the aetiological agent. Trimethoprim-sulfamethoxazole is the treatment of choice and consideration should be given to life-long maintenance therapy[114–116].

Rhodococcus equi has been reported to cause pneumonia in patients with AIDS[117,118]. This coccobacillus is Gram's stain positive and partially alcohol acid fast. In contrast to other community-acquired pneumonias, the onset of symptoms is rather gradual. The chest radiograph usually shows a localised infiltrate (frequently in the upper lobes) that can cavitate. It may disseminate and cause extrapulmonary disease. Macrolides (erythromycin, azithromycin, clarithromycin) rifampicin, vancomycin and imipenem are among the antibiotics that have the most activity against *R. equi*[119,120].

Fungal infections

Pulmonary fungal infections affecting patients with HIV infection include those caused by *Cryptococcus neoformans*, *Histoplasma capsulatum*, *Coccidioides immitis*, *Penicillium marneffei*, *Blastomyces dermatitidis*, *Nocardia asteroides*, *Aspergillus* spp. and *Candida* spp. (See also Chapters 16 and 18.)

C. neoformans is widely distributed throughout the world and is isolated most frequently from the excreta of pigeons and chickens. It is the most common life-threatening fungal infection in patients with AIDS occurring in about 6–10% of such individuals in North America and up to 30% in Africa. Meningitis is the initial manifestation of crytococcosis in 70–85% of patients with AIDS[121,122] and is associated with simultaneous pulmonary involvement in 30% of these patients. Primary pulmonary involvement has been reported in only 5% of patients. Clinical manifestations are non-specific and only 60–70% of patients have fever lasting for days to months[123]. Pleuritic chest pain is relatively common and is occasionally associated with pleural effusion[124,125]. Other chest radiograph findings include either a localised or diffuse interstitial infiltration. Laboratory evaluation may show lymphopenia in most cases. Assays for serum cryptococcal antigen are positive in 75% to 90% of cases. Bronchoscopy with BAL has diagnostic sensitivity of 67% that increases to 100% when transbronchial biopsies are included[13]. When *C. neoformans* is recovered from pulmonary secretions, CSF obtained by lumbar puncture should be performed.

The treatment of choice is amphotericin B (0.5–1.0 mg/kg per day) with the addition of flucytosine (75–150 mg/kg per day as four divided doses) as initial therapy in the moderately to severely ill patient. The serum flucytosine concentration should be within the range of 25–50 mg/l. In milder cases either fluconazole or itraconazole may be used as initial treatment. Patients with high CSF antigen level and continuing clinical signs of infection and who cannot tolerate conventional amphotericin should be treated with liposomal amphotericin. A randomised trial compared amphotericin B with the oral azole fluconazole for treatment in cryptococcal meningitis; the overall rate of survival was similar with the two agents although the mortality was higher among recipients of fluconazole during the first 2 weeks[126]. A smaller randomised study compared amphotericin B plus flucytosine with fluconazole and found that the combination therapy was significantly more effective by both mycological and clinical criteria[127]. After mycological and clinical responses have been achieved, fluconazole (200–400 mg daily) or itraconazole (200–400 mg daily) can be used for chronic suppressive therapy to prevent relapse as about 50% of AIDS patients will relapse within 6 months of successful completion of their initial therapy[128].

Histoplasmosis in patients with HIV infection is nearly always a disseminated disease. Between 4% and 5% of patient with AIDS in endemic areas have disseminated histoplasmosis and in more than 50% of this group histoplasmosis is the first manifestation of the syndrome[11,129]. The clinical presentation includes high fever (75%) weight loss (49%) lymphadenopathy (30%) and hepatosplenomegaly (30%). Cough or breathlessness is noted in about 64%[130]. Chest radiographs show diffuse interstitial infiltrates in the majority of patients. Pleural effusion is seen in fewer than 4% of patients. In patients with progressive disseminated histoplasmosis, bone marrow biopsy, buffy coat smear and blood culture by means of a lysis centrifugation system are helpful diagnostic measures. Leukopenia and thrombocytopenia are well-recognised features and the CD4 count is generally very low (33–75 cells/mm^3) at the time of diagnosis.

At present amphotericin B is used for the treatment of histoplasmosis and chronic suppression is needed since there is high rate of relapse. A protocol suggested an initial course of 1000 mg followed by 50–80 mg once weekly to a total dose of 2000 mg. Bi-weekly doses of 50–80 mg were then given indefinitely[131]. The risk of long-term toxicity must be borne in mind. Oral itraconazole (200 mg daily) appears promising as an alternative.

AIDS patients who have coccidioidomycosis present with fever and dyspnoea. Generally they have a CD4 count of <150 cells/mm^3. In 40% of cases chest radiographs show diffuse reticulonodular pulmonary infiltrates[132]. Meningitis and extrapulmonary involvement are common. Positive blood cultures are associated with a high mortality and in one series was shown to be positive in 12% of cases. Coccidioidal serological assays (both tube-precipitin and complement fixation) give positive results in about 90% of cases[133].

Despite therapy with amphotericin B (1.0–1.5 mg/kg per day), mortality is 70% with a median survival time of only 1 month. This initial therapy should be continued until a total dose of 1 gram has been given. Thereafter, itraconazole (400 mg/day) or fluconazole (400 mg/day) may be substituted if the patient has shown a clinical response[134]. Overall, coccidioidomycosis is an uncommon disease but nevertheless the diagnosis must be considered when patients have clinical findings and either reside or travel in endemic areas.

Aspergillus spp. is only rarely encountered as a primary pulmonary pathogen in patients with HIV and is a late cause of pulmonary disease usually in patients receiving corticosteroids or broad spectrum antibiotics and who are neutropenic[135,136].

Blastomycosis spp. is rarely described in patients with HIV infection but in a series of 15 cases, 13 had pulmonary involvement. The majority had CD4 count <200 cells/mm^3 and had AIDS when the diagnosis was made[137].

Penicillium marneffei, a diamorphic fungus indigenous to South East Asia causes disseminated infection with protean features in natives or travellers to the area[138].

Viral infection

The viruses that cause significant pulmonary disease in HIV infection include cytomegalovirus, herpes simplex type I and type II, Epstein–Barr virus, respiratory syncytial virus and influenza virus.

Cytomegalovirus (see also Chapter 10) is the major opportunistic pathogen in patients with AIDS causing choroido-retinitis, colitis, hepatitis, adrenitis, radiculitis, and oesophagitis. It is also frequently isolated in broncho alveolar lavage specimens in patients with AIDS and pneumonitis being commonly found with *Pneumocystis carinii* pneumonia. It is now well established that cytomegalovirus causes a frequently fatal pneumonitis in recipients of allogenic renal[139], liver[140], heart[141] and bone marrow transplants[142]. However, whether cytomegalovirus causes significant pneumonitis in patients with AIDS remains controversial. In a study in 1983 nearly 100% of asymptomatic homosexual men have serological evidence of CMV infection[143]. CMV is usually latent in the body and is re-activated by the suppression of cell mediated immunity and it produces a spectrum of manifestation ranging from chronic viral shedding detectable in the urine or saliva to overt disease. More than 30% of homosexual men who were seropositive for CMV shed CMV in urine or semen and up to 90% of AIDS patients have evidence of active CMV infection at autopsy[144]. CMV pulmonary infection is defined as the isolation of CMV from respiratory secretions and CMV pulmonary disease, on the other hand, is defined as evidence of cytopathic effects of CMV on pulmonary tissue with alveolar macrophages or epithelial cells containing intranuclear or intracytoplasmic inclusions[145]. CMV has been isolated from 30% of patients with PCP and its isolation in this setting is associated with a poor outcome. Mortality among patients with PCP alone is 14% but the rate increases to 92% when CMV is also present[146].

Viral cultures of BAL fluid are frequently positive for CMV with a high degree of sensitivity but a low specificity. Demonstration of cells with intranuclear or intracytoplasmic inclusion bodies in cytological or histological specimens is the most widely accepted means of documenting CMV pneumonia in patients with AIDS. Other criteria that have been suggested include the following:

(i) Isolation of CMV from cultured pulmonary tissue or BAL fluid.
(ii) Demonstration in tissue of cells of intranuclear inclusion bodies or with CMV antigen or nucleic acid.
(iii) Failure to find other pathogenic organism.

Treatment with ganciclovir decreases the quantity of virus isolated but does not appear to affect the outcome of CMV pneumonia[147].

Infection with herpes simplex type I or type II manifests as one of three syndromes: chronic mucocutaneous, localised visceral, or disseminated disease. The syndromes depend upon the site of inoculation and immune status of the patient[148]. Pneumonitis can be either focal or diffuse. Mucocutaneous reactivation into the tracheobronchial tree usually produces a focal necrotising process while haematogenous spread gives rise to diffuse interstitial pneumonia. The diagnosis is suggested by the finding of typical multinucleated giant cells with typical inclusion body of the BAL fluid or biopsied pulmonary tissue. The diagnosis is further supported by specific immunofluorescence staining for HSV and its subsequent growth from biopsied lung. The agent of choice currently is intravenous acyclovir (dosage 10 mg/kg every 8 hours) for 10 days. There have been a number of reports of infections due to acyclovir resistant strains of HSV 1 and HSV 2 in AIDS patients and in those circumstances foscarnet is a useful alternative[149].

Primary targets for Epstein–Barr virus are the B cells which have specific surface receptors for the virus. In HIV-infected patients, EBV infection may manifest as Burkitt-like non-Hodgkin's lymphoma or hairy leukoplakia (with asymptomatic replication in the oral epithelium) or lymphocytic interstitial pneumonitis where EBV DNA is found in 80% of biopsied pulmonary samples[150]. No effective therapy is currently available.

Respiratory syncytial virus infection occurs more often in children than in adults and can present alone or along with infection due to other pathogens. Chest radiograph shows diffuse interstitial infiltrates and the virus can be isolated from BAL fluid by growth in cell culture. Repeat identification can be done using direct staining of the BAL cell pellet with fluorescein-conjugated monoclonal antibody to RSV[150]. Severe diffuse disease can develop in immunocompromised or cardiopulmonary-compromised children and aerosolised ribavirin is a potentially effective agent for treatment.

Human herpes 6 (HHV-6), the first T-lymphotropic human herpes was isolated in 1986 from hosts with lymphoproliferative disorders and AIDS[151]. The pathogenic role of this virus is poorly understood, as the disease that has been conclusively linked to HHV-6 is exanthem subitum[152], a benign febrile illness associated with primary infection in early childhood. At least 90% of individuals are infected by HHV-6 by the age of 2 years[153]. It can therefore activate in immunocompromised hosts[154] and cause pneumonitis[155] and marrow suppression in bone marrow transplant hosts. HIV-infected hosts represent a rapidly growing immunocompromised population at risk for developing serious HHV-6 infections[156] and this virus has been proposed as a cofactor in the pathogenesis of AIDS[157,158]. Ganciclovir and foscarnet are effective therapy.

HIV infected patients with influenza virus infection have a typical clinical presentation in a rate of secondary complications similar to those of normal subjects. However, it can cause considerable morbidity and mortality and consideration should be given to influenza immunisation and chemoprophylaxis in this enlarging population of patients[159,160].

NON-INFECTIVE PULMONARY DISEASES

Neoplastic diseases

Pulmonary Kaposi's sarcoma (KS) is seen almost exclusively in homosexual men and can be encountered at any stage of HIV infection. Symptomatic pulmonary disease has a poor prognosis as the median duration of survival is approximately 3 months[161]. The symptoms of pulmonary KS usually consist of dyspnoea, cough, chest tightness and sometimes fever. Bronchoconstriction is also a feature. About a third of patients with cutaneous KS or other organ involvement will develop pulmonary involvement; only rarely will the lungs be affected exclusively. The chest X-ray findings in pulmonary KS tend to show a more nodular pattern with less even infiltration than is typical of PCP[162]. Pleural effusions are also more suggestive of pulmonary KS. These effusions are frequently bloody. Bronchoscopy provides the strongest evidence of pulmonary KS. Endobronchial lesions can be easily visualised although the pulmonary parenchyma is the principal site of disease. Biopsy is relatively contra-indicated because of possible haemorrhage but transbronchial biopsy has been used to diagnose KS in some difficult cases[163].

Non-Hodgkin's lymphoma is the second most common HIV-related malignant neoplasm and affects all groups of patients. It is usually an aggressive, high grade B-cell variety and commonly involves the central nervous system, gastrointestinal tract and liver and rarely the lung[164].

Non-neoplastic diseases

Interstitial pneumonitis in association with HIV infection is predominantly of two types: non-specific interstitial pneumonitis (NIP) and lymphoid interstitial pneumonitis (LIP). NIP can occur for up to 32% of episodes of pneumonitis in adults and can be present in nearly half of asymptomatic patients[165].

LIP is primarily a disease in children with HIV infection. Symptoms are usually more severe and extrathoracic involvement including adenopathy and lymphocytic infiltrations of the kidney, liver, bone marrow and gastrointestinal tract is common. Corticosteroid therapy may benefit some patients[166].

Both NIP and LIP can mimic other conditions. Their diagnosis requires a tissue specimen that is pathologically consistent with these conditions and the absence of other pathogens.

References

1. MURRAY JF, MILLS J. Pulmonary infectious complications of human immunodeficiency virus infection. *Am Rev Resp Dis* 1990;141:1356–1372, 1582–98.
2. JAFFE HW, BREGMAN DJ, SELIK RM. Acquired immune deficiency syndrome in the United States; first 1000 cases. *J Infect Dis* 1983;148:339–45.
3. MUNOZ A, SCHRAGER LK, BACELLAR H *et al.* Trends in the incidence of outcomes defining acquired immunodeficiency syndrome (AIDS) in the Multicenter AIDS Cohort Study: 1985–1991. *Am J Epidemiol* 1993;137:423–38.
4. MEDURI GU, STEIN DS. Pulmonary manifestations of acquired immunodeficiency syndrome. *Clin Infect Dis* 1992;14:98–113.
5. MASUR H, OGNIBENE FP, YARCHOAN R *et al.* CD4 counts as predictors of opportunistic pneumonias in human immunodeficiency virus infection. *Ann of Int Med* 1989;lll:223–31.
6. AGOSTINI C, TRENTIN L, ZAMBELLO R, SEMENZATO G. State of the art. HIV-1 and lung. Infectivity, pathogen mechanisms and cellular immune response taking place in the lower respiratory tract. *Am Rev Resp Dis* 1993; 147:1038–41.
7. CLARKE JR, TAYLOR IK, FLEMING J, NUKUNA A, WILLIAMSON JD, MITCHELL DM. The epidemiology of HIV-1 infection of the lung in AIDS patients. *AIDS* 1993;7:555–60.
8. AUTRAN B, MAYAUD C, RAPHAEL M, PLATA F, DENIS M, BOURGUIN A *et al.* Evidence for a cytotoxic T lymphocyte alveolitis in human immunodeficiency virus-infected patients *AIDS* 1988;2:179–83.
9. AGOSTINI C, ZAMBELLO R, TRENTIN L, FERUGLIO C, MASCIARELLI M, SIVIERO F *et al.* Cytotoxic events taking place in the lung of patients with HIV-1 infection. Evidence for an intrinsic defect of the MHC- unrestricted killing partially restored by the incubation with rIL-2. *Am Rev Resp Dis* 1990; 142; 516–22.
10. MAYAUD CM, CADRANEL J. HIV in the lung: guilty or not guilty. *Thorax* 1993;48:1191–5.
11. JOHNSON PC, KHARDORI N, NAJJOR AF, BUTT F, MANSELL PW, SAROSI GA. Progressive disseminated histoplasmosis in patients with acquired immunodeficiency syndrome. *Am J Med* 1988;85:152–8.
12. KOVACS JA, NG V, MASUR H *et al.* Diagnosis of *Pneumocystis* carinii pneumonia; improved detection in sputum using monoclonal antibodies. *N Engl J Med* 1988;318:589–93.
13. BROADDUS C, DAKE MD, STULBARG MS *et al.* Bronchoalveolar lavage and transbronchial biopsy for the diagnosis of pulmonary infections in the acquired immunodeficiency syndrome. *Ann of Int Med* 1985;102: 747–52.
14. OGNIBENE FP, SHELHAMER J, GILL V. The diagnosis of *Pneumocystis carinii* pneumonia in patients with the acquired immunodeficiency syndrome using subsegmental bronchoalveolar lavage. *Am Rev Resp Dis* 1982;129: 929–32.
15. LUNDGREN B, COTTON R, LUNDGREN JD *et al.* Identification of *Pneumocystis carinii* chromosomes and mapping of five genes. *Infect Immun* 58 1990;1705–10.
16. EDMAN JC, KOVACS JA, MASUR H *et al.* Ribosomal RNA sequence shows *Pneumocystis carinii* to be a member of the fungi. *Nature (London)* 1988;134:519–22.
17. SOGIN ML, EDMAN JC. A self-splicing intron in the small subunit rRNA gene of *Pneumocystis carinii. Nucl Acids Res* 1989;17: 5349–59.
18. STRINGER SL, STRINGER JR, BLASE MA *et al. Pneumocystis carinii*: sequence from ribosomal RNA implies a close relationship with fungi. *Exp Parasitol* 1989;68: 450–61.
19. MURRAY JF, FELTON CP, GARAY SM *et al.* Pulmonary complications of the acquired immunodeficiency syndrome: report of a National Heart, Lung and Blood Institute Workshop. *N Engl J Med* 1984;310:1682–8.
20. MURRAY JF, GARAY SM, HOPEWELL PC *et al.* NHLBI workshop summary. Pulmonary complications of the acquired immunodeficiency syndrome: an update. *Am Rev Resp Dis* 1987;135: 504–9.
21. WACHTER RM, LUCE JM, TURNER J *et al.* Intensive care of patients with the acquired immunodeficiency syndrome. Outcome and changing patterns of utilisation. *Am Rev Resp Dis* 1986;134: 891–6.
22. ONG ELC, HANLEY SP, MANDAL BK. Bronchial responsiveness in AIDS patients with *Pneumocystis carinii* pneumonia. *AIDS* 1992;6: 1331–3.
23. RANKIN JA, COLLMAN R, DANIELE RP. Acquired immune deficiency syndrome and the lung. *Chest* 1988;94: 155–64.
24. GOODMAN PC, BROADDUS VC, HOPEWELL PC. Chest radiographic patterns in the acquired immune deficiency syndrome. *Am Rev Resp Dis* 1984;130:689–94.
25. DE LORENZO LJ, HUANG CT, MAGUIRE GP, STONE DJ. Roentgenographic patterns of Pneumocystis carinii pneumonia in 104 patients with AIDS. *Chest* 1987;91:323–7.
26. MILLIGAN SA, STULBARG MS, GAMSU G, GOLDEN JA. Pneumocystis carinii pneumonia radiographically simulating tuberculosis. *Am Rev Resp Dis* 1985;132: 1124–6.

27. ONG ELC, MURRAY H, ELLIS ME. Miliary *Pneumocystis carinii* pneumonia in AIDS. *Int J STD, AIDS* 1992;3: 54–5.

28. STERN RG, GAMSU G, GOLDEN HA, HIRJI M, WEBB WR. *Am J Roentgenol* 1984;142: 689–92.

29. NAIDICH DP, GARAY SM, LUTMAN BS, MCCAULEY DI. Radiographic manifestations of pulmonary disease in the acquired immunodeficiency syndrome (AIDS). *Semin Roentgenol* 1987;22: 14–30.

30. ITEN A, CHAVE JP, WAUTERS JP *et al.* *Pneumocystis carinii* pneumonia in HIV negative patients: nosocomial transmission? *IX International Conference on AIDS/IV STD World Congress*, Berlin. June 1993 (abstract PO-B10–1461).

31. SMULIAN AG, SULLIVAN DW, LINKE MJ *et al.* Geographic variation in the humoral response to *Pneumocystis carinii*. *J Infect Dis* 1993: 167; 1243–7.

32. SMITH DE, MCLUCKIE H, WYATT J, GAZZARD B. Severe exercise hypoxaemia with normal or near normal X-rays: a feature of *Pneumocystis carinii* infection. *Lancet* 1988;ii: 1049–51.

33. COLEMAN DL, DODEK PM, GOLDEN JA. Correlation between serial pulmonary function tests and fibreoptic bronchoscopy in patients with *Pneumocystis carinii* pneumonia and the acquired immune deficiency syndrome. *Am Rev Resp Dis* 1984;129:491–3.

34. SHAW RJ, ROUSSAK C, FORSTER SM, HARRIS JW, PINCHING AJ, MITCHELL DM. Lung function abnormalities in patients infected with the human immunodeficiency virus with and without overt pneumonitis. *Thorax* 1988;43: 436–40.

35. SANKARY RM, TURNER J, LIPAVSKY A, HOWES EL, MURRAY JF. Alveolar capillary block in patients with AIDS and *Pneumocystis carinii* pneumonia. *Am Rev Resp Dis* 1988;137:443–9.

36. KRAMER EL, SANGER JJ, GARAY SM. Gallium-67 scans of the chest in patients with acquired immune deficiency syndrome. *J Nucl Med* 1987;28:1107–14.

37. O'DOHERTY MJ, PAGE CJ, CROFT DM, BATEMAN NT. Regional lung epithelial leakiness in smokers and non-smokers. *Nucl Med Commun* 1985;6:353–7.

38. MASON GR, DUANE GB, EFFROS RM, MENA I. Rapid clearance of inhaled aerosols of technetium-99m DTPA in patients with *Pneumocystis carinii* pneumonia. *J Clin Med* 1985;26:59.

39. LEVINE SJ, MASUR H, GILL VJ *et al.* Effect of aerosolised pentamidine prophylaxis on the diagnosis of *Pneumocystis carinii* pneumonia by induced sputum examination in patients infected with the human immunodeficiency virus. *Am Rev Resp Dis* 1991;144:760–76.

40. LIPSHIK GY, GILL VJ, LUNDGREN JD *et al.* Improved diagnosis of *Pneumocystis carinii* infection by polymerase chain reaction on induced sputum and blood. *Lancet* 1992;340:203–6.

41. OLSSON M, ELVIN K, LOFDAHL S, LINDER E. Detection of *Pneumocystis carinii* DNA in sputum and bronchoalveolar lavage samples by poylmerase chain reaction. *J Clin Microbiol* 1993;31:221–6.

42. HUGHES WT, FELDMAN S, SANYAL SK. Treatment of *Pneumocystis carinii* pneumonitis with trimethoprim-sulphamethoxazole. *Can Med Assoc J* 1975;112S:47–50.

43. SATTLER FR, COWAN R, NIELSEN DM *et al.* Trimethoprim-sulphamethoxazole compared with pentamidine for treatment of *Pneumocystis carinii* pneumonia in the acquired immunodeficiency syndrome. *Ann Intern Med* 1988;109:280–1.

44. GORDIN FM, SIMON GL, WOFSY CB *et al.* Adverse reactions to trimethoprim-sulphamethoxazole in patients with the acquired immunodeficiency syndrome. *Ann Intern Med* 1984;100:495–9.

45. IVADY G, PALDY L. A new form of treatment of interstitial plasma cell pneumonia in premature infants with pentavalent antimony and aromatic diamidines. *Mschr Kinderheilk* 1958;106:10–14.

46. WHARTON JM, COLEMAN DL, WOFSY CB *et al.* Trimethoprim-sulphamethoxazole or pentamidine for *Pneumocystis carinii* pneumonia in the acquired immunodeficiency syndrome. A prospective randomised trial. *Ann Intern Med* 1986;105:37–44.

47. MONTGOMERY AM, LUCE JM, TURNER J *et al.* Aerosolised pentamidine as sole therapy for *Pneumocystis carinii* pneumonia in patients with acquired immunodeficiency syndrome. *Lancet* 1987;ii:480–3.

48. CONTE JE, HOLLANDER H, GOLDEN JA. Inhaled or reduced dose intravenous pentamidine for *Pneumocystis carinii* pneumonia. A pilot study. *Ann Intern Med* 1987;07:495–8.

49. ARMSTRONG D, BERNARD E. Aerosol pentamidine. *Ann Intern Med* 1988;109:852–4.

50. ONG E. Infection with the human immunodeficiency virus. An overview. *Care Crit ill* 1993;9:7–10.

51. LEOUNG GS, MILLS J, HOPEWELL PC *et al.* Dapsone-trimethoprim for *Pneumocystis carinii* pneumonia in the acquired immunodeficiency syndrome. *Ann Intern Med* 1986;105:45–8.

52. TOMA E, FOURNIER S, POISSON M *et al.* Clindamycin with primaquine for *Pneumocystis carinii* pneumonia. *Lancet* 1989;i: 1046–8.

53. BLACK JR, FEINBERG J, MURPHY RL *et al.* Clindamycin and Primaquine therapy for mild to moderate episodes of *Pneumocystis carinii* pneumonia in patients with AIDS: AIDS Clinical Trials Group 044. *Clin Infect Dis* 1994;18: 905–13.

54. DORRELL L, FIFE A, SNOW MH, ONG ELC. Toxicity of clindamycin in HIV infected patients. *Scand J Infect Dis* 1992;24:689.

55. ALLEGRA CJ, CHABNER BA, TUAZON CU *et al.* Trimetrexate for the treatment of *Pneumocystis carinii* pneumonia in patients with acquired immunodeficiency syndrome. *N Engl J Med* 1987;317:978–85.

56. FALLON J, KOVACS J, ALLEGRA C *et al.* A pilot study of piritrexim with leucovorin for the treatment of *Pneumocystis* pneumonia (Abstract ThB. 399). *VI International Conference on AIDS*, San Francisco, USA. 1990.

57. GOLDEN JA, SJOERDSMA A, SANTI DV. *Pneumocystis carinii* pneumonia treated with alpha-difluoromethylornithine. *West J Med* 1984;141:613–23.

58. HUGHES W, LEOUNG G, KRAMER F *et al.* Comparison of atovaquone (566C80) with trimethoprim-sulphamethoxazole to treat *Pneumocystis carinii* pneumonia in patients with AIDS (1993). *N Engl J Med* 1993;21:1521–7.

59. HUGHES W, KENNEDY W, SHENEP JL *et al.* Safety and pharmacokinetics of 566C80, a hydroxynaphthoquinone with anti-*Pneumocystis carinii* activity. A phase I study in HIV-infected men. *J Infect Dis* 1991;163:843–8.

60. BOZZETTE SA, SATTLER F, CHIN J *et al.* A controlled trial of early adjunctive treatment with corticosteroids for *Pneumocystis carinii* pneumonia in the acquired immunodeficiency syndrome. *N Engl J Med* 1990;323:1451–1457.

61. MONTANER JS, LAWSON LM, LEVITT M *et al.* Oral corticosteroids prevent early deterioration in patients with moderately severe AIDS-related *Pneumocystis carinii* pneumonia. *Ann Intern Med* 1990;113:14–20.

62. The National Institutes of Health-University of California Expert Panel for corticosteroids as adjunctive therapy for *Pneumocystis* pneumonia consensus statement on the use of glucocorticoids as adjunctive therapy for *Pneumocystis* pneumonia in the acquired immunodeficiency syndrome. *N Engl J Med* 1990;323:1500–4.

63. CENTERS FOR DISEASE CONTROL. Recommendations for prophylaxis against *Pneumocystis carinii* pneumonia for adults and adolescents infected with human immunodeficiency virus. *MMWR* 1992;41 (RR-4):1–11.

64. EUROPEAN COLLABORATIVE STUDY. CD4 T cell count as a predictor of pneumonia

in children of mothers infected with HIV. *Br Med J* 1994;308:437–40.

65. HARDY D, FEINBERG J, FINKELSTEIN DM *et al.* A controlled trial of trimethoprim-sulphamethoxazole or aerosolized pentamidine for secondary prophylaxis of *Pneumocystis carinii* pneumonia in patients with the acquired immunodeficiency syndrome. *N Engl J Med* 1992;327: 1842–8.

66. RUSKIN J, LARIVIERE M. Low dose co-trimoxazole for prevention of *Pneumocystis carinii* pneumonia in human immunodeficiency virus disease. *Lancet* 1991;337: 468–71.

67. CARR A, TINDALL B, PENNY R, COOPER DA. Trimethoprim – sulphamethoxazole appears more effective than aerosolized pentamidine as secondary prophylaxis against *Pneumocystis carinii* pneumonia in patients with AIDS. *AIDS* 1992;6:165–71.

68. SLAVIN MA, HOY JF, STEWART K, PETTINGER MB, LUCAS CR, KENT SJ. Oral dapsone versus nebulised pentamidine for *Pneumocystis carinii* pneumonia prophylaxis: an open randomized prospective trial to assess efficacy and haematological toxicity. *AIDS* 1992;6: 1169–74.

69. GIRARD P-M, LANDMAN R, GAUDEBOUT C *et al.* Dapsone-pyrimethamine compared with aerosolized pentamidine as primary prophylaxis against *Pneumocystis carinii* pneumonia and toxoplasmosis in HIV infection. *N Engl J Med* 1993;328:1514–20.

70. DORRELL L, SNOW MH, ONG ELC. Dapsone-pyrimethamine vs aerosolised pentamidine as prophylaxis against *Pneumocystis carinii* pneumonia in HIV infection (Abstract B10-1420). *International Conference on AIDS*, Berlin. 1993.

71. SAINT-MARC T, LIVROZET JM, MOREAU J, GARNIER JL, SELLEM C, TOURAINE JL. Safety and efficacy of pyrimethamine - sulfadoxine in primary and secondary prophylaxis of pneumocystosis. Abstract WB 2242 *VII International Conference on AIDS*, Florence, Italy. 1991.

72. LEOUNG GS, FEIGAL DW JR, MONTGOMERY AB *et al.* Aerosolized pentamidine for prophylaxis against *Pneumocystis carinii* pneumonia. The San Francisco Community Prophylaxis Trial. *N Engl J Med* 1990;323:769–75.

73. ONG ELC, DUNBAR EM, MANDAL BK. Efficacy and effects on pulmonary function tests of weekly 600 mg aerosol pentamidine as prophylaxis against *Pneumocystis carinii* pneumonia. *Infection* 1992;20:136–9.

74. JULES-ELYSEE KM, STOVER DE, ZAMAN MB *et al.* Aerosolized pentamidine: effect on diagnosis and presentation of *Pneumocystis carinii* pneumonia. *Ann Intern Med* 1990;112:750–7.

75. TEIZAK EE, COTE RJ, GOLD JWM, CAMPBELL SW, ARMSTRONG D. Extrapulmonary *Pneumocystis carinii* infections. *Rev Infect Dis* 1990;12: 380–6.

76. NORTHFELT D, SAFRIN S. Extrapulmonary pneumocystis clinical features in human immunodeficiency virus infection. *Medicine* 1990;69:392–8.

77. BARNES PF, BLOCH AB, DAVIDSON PT, SNIDER DE. Tuberculosis in patients with human immunodeficiency virus. *N Engl J Med* 1991;324:1644–50.

78. SELWYNN PA, HARTEL D, LEWIS VA *et al.* A retrospective study of the risk of tuberculosis among intravenous drug users with human immunodeficiency virus infection. *N Engl J Med* 1989;320:545–50.

79. ONG ELC, MANDAL BK. Tuberculosis in patients infected with the human immunodeficiency virus. *Quart J Med* 1991;2291: 613–17.

80. DOOLEY SW, VILLARINO ME, LAWRENCE M *et al.* Nosocomial transmission of tuberculosis in a hospital unit for HIV infected patients. *J Am Med Assoc* 1992;276:2632–4.

81. DALEY CL, SMALL PM, SCHECTER GF *et al.* An outbreak of tuberculosis with accelerated progression among persons infected with the human immunodeficiency virus. *N Engl J Med* 1992;326:231–5.

82. HOPEWELL PC. Impact of human immunodeficiency virus infection on the epidemiology, clinical features, management and control of tuberculosis. *Clin Infect Dis* 1992;15:540–7.

83. SUBCOMMITTEE OF THE JOINT TUBERCULOSIS COMMITTEE OF THE BRITISH THORACIC SOCIETY. Guidelines on the management of tuberculosis and HIV infection in the United Kingdom. *Br Med J* 1992;304:1231–3.

84. SUNDERAM G, MANGURA BT, LOMBARDO JM, REICHMAN LB. Failure of optimal four drug short-course tuberculosis, chemotherapy in a compliant patient with human immunodeficiency virus. *Am Rev Resp Dis* 1987;36:1475–8.

85. CENTERS FOR DISEASE CONTROL. Tuberculosis and human immunodeficiency virus infection; recommendations of the Advisory Committee for the Elimination of Tuberculosis (ACET). *MMWR* 1989;38:236–50.

86. ONG ELC. Managing tuberculosis and HIV infection. *Br Med J* 1992;304:1567.

87. NUNN P, FIBUGA D, GATHUA S *et al.* Cutaneous hypersensitivity reactions due to thiacetazone in HIV-1 seropositive patients treated for tuberculosis. *Lancet* 1991;337:627–30.

88. ONG ELC, MANDAL BK. Multiple drug reactions in a patient with AIDS. *Lancet* 1989;ii:976–7.

89. SMALL PM, SCHECTER GF, GOODMAN PC *et al.* Treatment of tuberculosis in patients with advanced human immunodeficiency virus infection. *N Engl J Med* 1991;324:289–94.

90. NIGHTINGALE SD, CAMERON DW, GORDIN FM *et al.* Two controlled trials of rifabutin prophylaxis against *Mycobacterium avium* complex infection in AIDS. *N Engl J Med* 1993;329:828–33.

91. HORSBURGH CR, SELIK RM. The epidemiology of disseminated nontuberculous mycobacterial infection in the acquired immunodeficiency syndrome. *Am Rev Resp Dis* 1989;139:4–7.

92. HAWKINS CC, GOLD JWM, WHIMBY E *et al. Mycobacterium avium* complex infections in patients with the acquired immunodeficiency syndrome. *Ann Intern Med* 1986;105:184–8.

93. YOUNG LS. *Mycobacterium avium* infection. *J Infect Dis* 1988;157:863–7.

94. MODILEVSKY T, SATTLER FR, BARNES PF. Mycobacterial disease in patients with human immunodeficiency virus infection. *Arch Intern Med* 1989;149:2201–5.

95. WALLACE RJ, OBRIEN R, GLASSROTH J, RALEIGH J, DUTT A. Diagnosis and treatment of disease caused by non-tuberculous mycobacteria. *Am Rev Resp Dis* 1990;142:940–53.

96. WALLACE JM, HANNAH JB. *Mycobacterium avium* complex infection in patients with the acquired immunodeficiency syndrome: a clinico-pathologic study. *Chest* 1988;93: 926–32.

97. CHAISSON RE, KERULY J, RICHMAN DD, CREAGH-KIRK T, MOORE RD. Incidence and natural history of *Mycobacterium avium* complex infection in advanced HIV disease treated with zidovudine. *Am Rev Resp Dis* 1991;143:A278.

98. HORSBURGH CR. *Mycobacterium avium* complex infection in the acquired immunodeficiency syndrome. *N Engl J Med* 1991;324:1332–8.

99. RUF B, SCHUERMANN D, BREHMER W, POHLE HD. Pulmonary manifestations due to *Mycobacterium avium-Mycobacterium intracellulare* (MAI) in AIDS patient. *Am Rev Resp Dis* 1991;141: A611.

100. KIEHN TE, CAMMARATA RC. Laboratory diagnosis of mycobacterial infections in patients with acquired immunodeficiency syndrome. *J Clin Microbiol* 1986;24;708–11.

101. HOY J, MIJCH A, SANDLAND M, GRAYSON L, LUCAS R, DWYER B Quadruple drug therapy for *Mycobacterium*

avium bacteraemia in AIDS patients. *J Infect Dis* 1990;161:801–5.

102. ARBEIT RD, SLUTSKY A, BARBER TW *et al.* Genetic diversity among strains of *Mycobacterium avium* causing monoclonal and polyclonal bacteraemia in patients with AIDS. *J Infect Dis* 1993;167:1384–90.

103. MASUR H and the Public Health Service Task Force on prophylaxis and therapy for *Mycobacterium avium* complex. Recommendations on prophylaxis and therapy for disseminated *Mycobacterium avium* complex in patients infected with the human immunodeficiency virus. *N Engl J Med* 1993;329:898–904.

104. ABRAMS DI, MITCHELL TF, CHILD CC *et al.* Clofazimine as prophylaxis for disseminated *Mycobacterium avium* complex infection in AIDS. *J Infect Dis* 1993;167:1459–63.

105. NARANG P, NIGHTINGALE S, MANZONE C *et al.* Does rifabutin affect zidovudine disposition in HIV+ patients? Abstract POB 3888. VIII International Conference on AIDS/111. STD World Congress, Amsterdam. 1992.

106. DATRI 001 STUDY GROUP. Clarithromycin plus rifabutin for MAC prophylaxis; evidence for a drug interaction, Abstract 291. *The First National Conference on Human Retroviruses and Related Infections*, Washington. 1993.

107. SIEGAL FD, EILBOTT D, BURGER H *et al.* Dose limiting toxicity of rifabutin in AIDS-related complex: syndrome of arthralgia/arthritis. *AIDS* 1990;4: 433–41.

108. BOTTGER E, TESKE A, KIRSCHNER P *et al.* Disseminated *Mycobacterium genavense* infection in patients with AIDS. *Lancet* 1992;340:76–80.

109. PECHERE M, EMLER S, WALD A *et al.* Infection with *Mycobacterium genavense*: clinical features in 44 cases. Abstract WS-B10-2 *IX International Conference on AIDS/IV STD World Congress*, Berlin. 1993.

110. COYLE MB, CARLSON LDC, WILLIS CK *et al.* Laboratory aspects of *Mycobacterium genavense*, a proposed species isolated from AIDS patients. *J Clin Microbiol* 1992;30:2934–7.

111. CHAISSON RE. Bacterial pneumonia in patients with human immunodeficiency virus infection. *Semin Respir Infect* 1989;4:133–8.

112. POLSKY B, GOLD JWM, WHIMBEY E *et al.* Bacterial pneumonia in patients with the acquired immunodeficiency syndrome. *Ann Intern Med* 1986;104: 38–41.

113. LEVINE SJ, WHITE DA, ELLIS AO. The incidence and significance of *Staphylococcus aureus* in respiratory cultures from patients infected with the human immunodeficiency virus. *Am Rev Resp Dis* 1990;141:89–93.

114. JAVALY K, HOROWITZ HW, WORMSER GP. Nocardiosis in patients with human immunodeficiency virus infection. Report of 2 cases and review of the literature. *Medicine (Baltimore)* 1992 May 71[3]:128–38.

115. MIRALLES GD. Disseminated *Nocardia farcinica* infection in an AIDS patient. *Eur J Clin Microbiol Infect Dis* 1994;13:497–500.

116. CASTY FE WENCEL M Endobronchial nocardiosis. *Eur Respir J* 1994;10:1903–5.

117. PRESCOTT JF. *Rhodococcus equi*: an animal and human pathogen. *Clin Microbiol Rev* 1991;4:2–34.

118. WEINGARTEN JS, HUANG DY, JACKMAN JD. *Rhodococcus equi* pneumonia; an unusual early manifestation of the acquired immunodeficiency syndrome (AIDS). *Chest* 1988;94:195–6.

119. MAGNANI G, ELIA G, MCNEIL M *et al.* *Rhodococcus equi* cavity pneumonia in HIV infected patients: an unsuspected opportunistic pathogen. *J Acq Immunodef Syn* 1992;5:1059–64.

120. GINER C, DE RAFAEL, RUIZ LM *et al.* *Rhodococcus equi*: antimicrobial susceptibility pattern. Abstract 1338 XXX11 *Interscience Conference on Antimicrobial Agents and Chemotherapy*, Anaheim. 1992.

121. KOVACS JA, KOVACS AA, POLIS M *et al.* Cryptococcosis in the acquired immunodeficiency syndrome. *Ann Intern Med* 1985;103:533–8.

122. ZUGER A, LOUIE E, HOLZMAN RS, SIMBERKOFF MS, RAHAL JJ. Cryptococcal disease in patients with the acquired immunodeficiency syndrome. Diagnostic features and outcome. *Ann Intern Med* 1986;104:234–40.

123. CLARK RA, GREER D, ATKINSON W, VALAINIS GT, HYSLOP N. Spectrum of *Cryptococcus neoformans* infection in 68 patients infected with human immunodeficiency virus. *Rev Infect Dis* 1990;12:768–77.

124. NEWMAN TG, SONI A, ACARON S, HUANG CT. Pleural cryptococcosis in the acquired immune deficiency syndrome. *Chest* 1987;91:459–603.

125. WASSER L, TALAVERA W. Pulmonary cryptococcosis in AIDS. *Chest* 1987;92: 692–5.

126. SAAG MS, POWDERLY WG, CLOUD GA *et al.* Comparison of amphotericin ß with fluconazole in the treatment of acute AIDS-associated cryptococcal meningitis. *N Engl J Med* 1992;326:83–89.

127. LARSEN RA, LEAL MAE, CHAN LS. Fluconazole compared with amphotericin B plus flucytosine for cryptococcal meningitis in AIDS. A randomized trial. *Ann Intern Med* 1990;113:183–7.

128. POWDERLY WG, SAAG MS, CLOUD GA *et al.* A controlled trial of fluconazole or amphotericin ß to prevent relapse of cryptococcal meningitis in patients with the acquired immunodeficiency syndrome. *N Engl J Med* 1992;326:793–8.

129. NIGHTINGALE SD, PARKS JM, POUNDERS SM, BURNS DK, REYNOLDS J, HERNANDEZ JA. Disseminated histoplasmosis in patients with AIDS. *South Med J* 1990;83:624–30.

130. JOHNSON PC, HAMIL RJ, SAROSI GA. Clinical review: progressive disseminated histoplasmosis in the AIDS patient *Semin Resp Infect*, 1989;4:139–46.

131. MCKINSEY DS, GUPTA MR, RIDDLER SA, DRIKS MR, SMITH DL, KURTIN PJ. Long term amphotericin ß therapy of disseminated histoplasmosis in patients with the acquired immunodeficiency syndrome (AIDS). *Ann Intern Med* 1989;111:655–9.

132. GALGIANI JN, AMPEL NM. Coccidioidomycosis in human immunodeficiency virus infected patients. *J Infect Dis* 1990;162:1165–9.

133. FISH DG, AMPEL NM, GALGIANI JN *et al.* Coccidioidomycosis during human immunodeficiency virus infection: A review of 77 patients. *Medicine* (*Baltimore*) 1990;69:334–91.

134. TUCKER RM, DENNING DW, DUPONT B, STEVENS DA. Itraconazole therapy for chronic coccidiodal meningitis. *Ann Intern Med* 1990;112:108–12.

135. DENNING DW, FOLLANSBEE SE, SCOLARO M, EDELSTEIN H, STEVENS DA. Pulmonary aspergillosis in the acquired immunodeficiency syndrome. *N Engl J Med* 1991;324:654–62.

136. KLAPHOLZ A, SALOMON N, PERLAMN DC, TALAVERA W. Aspergillosis in the acquired immunodeficiency syndrome. *Chest* 1991;100:1614–18.

137. PAPPAS PG, POTTAGE JC, POWDERLY WG *et al.* Blastomycosis in patients with the acquired immunodeficiency syndrome. *Ann Intern Med* 1992;16: 847–53.

138. TSANG DN, LI PC, TSUI MS, LAU YT, MA KF, YEOH EK. Penicillium marneffei: another pathogen to consider in patients infected with the human immunodeficiency virus. *Rev Infect Dis* 1991;13:766–7.

139. RUBIN RH, TOKOFF-RUSTIN NE, OLIVER D *et al.* Multicentre seroepidemiologic study of the impact of CMV infection on renal transplantation. *Transplantation* 1985;40:243–9.

140. SINGH N, DRUMMAR JS, KUME S *et al.* Infections with cytomegalovirus and other herpes viruses in 121 liver transplant recipients:

transmission by donated organ and the effect of OKT3 antibodies. *J Infect Dis* 1988;158:124–31.

141. GOVENSEK MJ, STEWART RW, KEYS TF *et al.* A multivariate analysis of the risk of cytomegalovirus infection in heart transplant recipients. *J Infect Dis* 1988;157:515–22.

142. WINGARD JR, MEILLITIS ED, SOSTRIM MB *et al.* Interstitial pnuemonitis after bone marrow transplantation; nine year experience at a single institution. *Medicine* (*Baltimore*) 1988;67:175–86.

143. MINTZ L, DREW WL, MINER RC, BRAFF EH. Cytomegalovirus infections in homosexual men: an epidemiologic study. *Ann Intern Med* 1983;99:326–9.

144. REICHERT CM, O'LEARY TJ, LEVENS DL, SIMRELL CR, MACHER AM. Autopsy pathology in the acquired immune deficiency syndrome. *Am J Path* 1983;12:357–8.

145. DREW WL. Cytomegalovirus infection in patients with AIDS. *J Infect Dis* 1988;158:449–56.

146. STORER DE, WHITE DA, ROMANO PA, GELLENE RA, ROBESON WA. Spectrum of pulmonary diseases associated with the acquired immune deficiency syndrome. *Am J Med* 1985;78:429–37.

147. COLLABORATIVE DHPG TREATMENT STUDY GROUP. Treatment of serious cytomegalovirus infections with 9-C(1, 3 - dihydroxy-2-propoxymethyl) guanine in patients with AIDS and other immunodeficiences. *N Engl J Med* 1986;314:801–5.

148. COREY L, SPEAR PG. Infections with herpes simplex viruses. *N Engl J Med* 1986;314:749–57.

149. ENGLUND JA, ZIMMERMAN ME, SWIERKOSZ EM, GOODMAN JL, SCHOLL DR, BALFOUR HH. Herpes simplex virus resistant to acyclovir. A study in a tertiary care center. *Ann Intern Med* 1990;112:416–22.

150. WALLACE JM. Pulmonary infections in human immunodeficiency disease: viral pulmonary infections. *Semin Resp Infect* 1989;4: 147–54.

151. SALAHUDDIN SZ, ABIASHI DV, MARKHAM PD *et al.* Isolation of a new virus, HBLV, in patients with lympho-proliferative disorders. *Science* 1986; 234:596–601.

152. YAMANISHI K, OKUNA T, SHIRAKI K *et al.* Identification of human herpesvirus 6 as a causal agent for exathem subitum *Lancet* 1988;1:1065.

153. PELLET PE, BLACK JB, YAMAMOTO M. Human herpesvirus 6: the virus and the search for its role as a human pathogen. *Adv Virus Res* 1992; 41:1–51.

154. DROBYSKI WRR, DUNNE WM, BURD EM *et al.* Human herpesvirus 6 (HHV-6) infection in allogenic bone marrow transplant recipients 1: evidence for a marrow suppression role for HHV-6 *in vivo*. *J Infect Dis* 1993:167:735–9.

155. CARRIGAN DR, DROBYSKI WR, RUSSLER SK, TAPPER MA, KNOX KK, ASH RC. Interstitial pneumonitis associated with human herpesvirus-6 infection in marrow transplantation. *Lancet* 1991:338:147–9.

156. ONG E. Viral infections in the immunocompromised host. *Hosp Update* 1995; April Suppl: 18–24.

157. LUSSO P, ENSOLI B, MARKHAM PD *et al.* Productive dual infection of human CD4+ T lymphocytes by HIV-1 and HHV-6. *Nature* 1989;337:370–3.

158. CORBELLINO M, LUSSO P, GALLO RC, PARRAVICINI C, GALLI M, MORONI M. Disseminated human herpesvirus 6 infection in AIDS. *Lancet* 1993;342:1242.

159. SAFRIN S, RUSH J, MILLS J. Influenza in patients with human immunodeficiency virus. *Infect Chest* 1990; 98:33–7.

160. CENTERS FOR DISEASE CONTROL (Immunisation Practices Advisory Committee). Prevention and control of influenza. *MMWR* 1987;36:373–12.

161. OGNIBENE FP, STEIS RG, MACHER AM *et al.* Kaposi's sarcoma causing pulmonary infiltrates and respiratory failure in the acquired immunodeficiency syndrome. *Ann Intern Med* 1985;102:471–5.

162. KAPLAN LD, HOPEWELL PC, JAFFE HW *et al.* Kaposi's sarcoma involving the lung in patients with the acquired immunodeficiency syndrome. *J AIDS* 1988;1:23–30.

163. NASH G, FLIGIEL S. Kaposi's sarcoma presenting as pulmonary disease in the acquired immunodeficiency syndrome: diagnosis by lung biopsy. *Hum Pathol* 1984;15:999–1001.

164. WHITE DA, MATTHAY RA. Non infectious pulmonary complications of infection with human deficiency virus. *Am Rev Resp Dis* 1989;140:1763–87.

165. SUFFREDINI AF, OGNIBENE FP, LACK EE *et al.* Non-specific interstitial pneumonitis: a common cause of pulmonary disease in the acquired immunodeficiency syndrome. *Ann Intern Med* 1987;107:7–13.

166. TRAVIS WD, FOX CH, DEVANEY KO *et al.* Lymphoid pneumonitis in 50 adult patients infected with the human immunodeficiency virus: lymphocytic interstitial pneumonitis versus non-specific interstitial pneumonitis. *Hum Pathol* 1992;23: 529–41.

23 Infection in children

JONATHAN COURIEL
Booth Hall Children's Hospital, University of Manchester School of Medicine, UK

Introduction

Acute infections of the respiratory tract are the commonest illnesses of childhood. In Britain, respiratory infections are the most common reason for a child to be taken to a doctor, accounting for a third of all consultations between general practitioners and children[1]. They are also the most frequent cause of acute hospital admission in childhood and account for 8–18% of acute paediatric admissions[1–3].

Most respiratory infections affect only the nose, ears and throat (the upper respiratory tract), causing a minor, self-limiting illness. But in 5–20% of infections, the lower respiratory tract is involved, often leading to more serious illness. Although the mortality from respiratory infections in children from developed countries continues to fall steadily, deaths do still occur, particularly in infants. For example, there were 204 deaths from acute respiratory infection in children in England and Wales in 1992: 63% of these were in infants less than 1 year old[4]. By contrast, in developing countries, acute respiratory infections remain one of the commonest causes of death in children: it is estimated that, worldwide, four million children die of acute respiratory infections every year[5].

Children are not miniature adults. The patterns of respiratory infections in children, and the pathogens causing these infections, differ markedly from those in adults. For example, the commonest serious respiratory infection in infancy is acute viral bronchiolitis caused by the respiratory syncytial virus (RSV), a disease not seen in immunocompetent adults: the bacteria that cause life-threatening pneumonia in newborn infants are harmless bowel commensals in adults, such as group B beta-haemolytic streptococci and *Escherichia coli*: viral infection of the larynx and trachea is a minor illness in adults but can lead to fatal upper airway obstruction in children.

Why are children different?

These striking differences between respiratory infections in children and adults, and the specific and characteristic age ranges of many childhood infections, reflect the immature structure and function of the respiratory and immune systems of the developing child.

The *smaller airways* of children are easily obstructed by mucosal swelling or secretions. As airways resistance is inversely proportional to the fourth power of the radius of the airway, halving airway calibre increases resistance 16-fold. Thus 1 mm of mucosal oedema in an infant trachea 5 mm in diameter increases the resistance to airflow eightfold, whereas the same degree of oedema in an older child's trachea of 10 mm diameter will double resistance.

The *thoracic cage* of young children is much more compliant than that of adults. If there is airways obstruction and increased fluctuations in the intrathoracic pressures during the respiratory cycle, this increased compliance results in severe chest wall recession, reduced efficiency and increased work of breathing, and increased oxygen consumption.

The *respiratory muscles* of young children are also relatively inefficient. In infancy, the diaphragm is the main respiratory muscle: the intercostal and accessory muscles make relatively little contribution. Muscle fatigue can develop rapidly in the tachypnoeic child and result in respiratory failure and apnoea[6,7].

The *ventilatory control mechanisms* of young infants, and particularly those born prematurely, are immature. This immaturity is manifested clinically as recurrent central apnoea with certain infections, notably RSV bronchiolitis and pertussis[8].

Children, and particularly young infants, are *immunologically vulnerable*. Their immune function is very different from that of an adult who has been exposed to, and has developed immunity against, many organisms. For example, the newborn infant has negligible amounts of IgM and IgA class antibodies, as these are not produced by the foetus and do not cross the placenta from the mother. Serum IgG levels are 60–80% of adult levels at term as maternal IgG does cross the placenta in late pregnancy. These maternal IgG antibodies confer some degree of passive immunity but are catabolised by 3–6 months. Although the infants start to synthesise their own IgG about this age, the serum IgG level is only 30–40% of the adult level at 6 months, rising to 70% by 2 years of age[9]. Several aspects of cellular immunity are also immature in early infancy.

All of these normal developmental phenomena mean that children, and particularly infants, are especially vulnerable to infections and that they respond to these infections very differently from adults.

Host and environmental risk factors

As well as these factors which affect all children, there are other influences which place certain children at increased risk of respiratory infection (Table 23.1).

The *age of the child* has a major influence on the type, frequency and severity of respiratory infection to which the child is susceptible. The overall incidence of acute respiratory infections peaks in early childhood and steadily declines with age, reflecting the pattern of exposure to infection and the development of the child's immunity[2,10]. Certain infections are seen only in children within a narrow age band. For example, viral bronchiolitis occurs almost exclusively in infants aged between 4 weeks and 8 months; epiglottitis is uncommon in the first year of life and has its peak incidence in the third year of life. Two-thirds of deaths due to respiratory infections occur in infancy[4]. The incidence of most lower repiratory infections is

Table 23.1. *Risk factors for lower respiratory infections in children*

Age
Male sex
Prematurity
Parental smoking
Large family size
Congenital abnormalities
Immunodeficiency

significantly higher in boys than in girls in early life, for reasons that are not understood[2].

We have known for over 25 years that *parental smoking* increases the risk of all respiratory illnesses, and particularly lower respiratory tract infection, in children[11]. The effect is greater in infants than in older children, is related more to maternal than paternal smoking habits, and is dose-related (the greater the number of cigarettes the mother smokes, the higher the risk of the infant having lower respiratory tract infection). Both maternal smoking during pregnancy and post-natal passive exposure of the infant predispose the children of smokers to respiratory disease.

The degree of a child's *exposure* to other children or adults with infections influences the number of infections they develop. For example, infants with older siblings, and those living in over-crowded homes, have more frequent respiratory infections. When children first attend school or nursery, the number of infections they contract rises[2].

Breast feeding, which protects against gastrointestinal infection in the first year of life, also significantly reduces the incidence of respiratory illness in infancy, when compared to the incidence in children who are bottle-fed with artificial cows' milk formulae[12,13]. This protective effect, which is presumed to be immune mediated, is most important in developing countries but is also evident in industrialised societies.

Children with congenital defects of the respiratory tract, such as tracheo-oesophageal fistula or lobar sequestration, and children with congenital heart disease, are at increased risk of lower respiratory tract infection. Neurologically handicapped children, and those with impaired immunity or ciliary dyskinesia, are also particularly vulnerable. Recurrent or persistent chest infections are a common presenting feature of cystic fibrosis, the commonest cause of chronic respiratory infection in children. Infections in all of these groups of children are not only more common, but also tend to be more severe than in normal infants, with a greater risk of respiratory failure and of death.

Infants who are *born prematurely*, and particularly those who have developed bronchopulmonary dysplasia (chronic lung disease of prematurity) after neonatal ventilation, frequently require hospital admission for respiratory infections in early childhood. The mortality from respiratory infection in these infants is higher than in term infants.

Aetiology of respiratory infections in childhood

The spectrum of pathogens that cause respiratory infections in children is wider and different from that in adults. Furthermore, children's susceptibility to particular organisms and to certain infections changes as they grow older.

Viruses

Over 90% of respiratory infections are caused by viruses[2]. In developed countries with temperate climates, most upper respiratory tract infections (URTIs) are caused by rhinoviruses (30–50%), coronaviruses (5–20%), influenza, parainfluenza and adenoviruses, RSV and enteroviruses[2,14]. The commonest causes of lower respiratory infections are RSV and parainfluenza viruses: influenza and adenoviral infections are less common but important[2,10,14,15].

It is important to appreciate that a single viral pathogen can cause several different clinical illnesses, and that several different pathogens can produce a clinically identical illness. For example, RSV infection can cause bronchiolitis, croup, pneumonia, otitis media or simple pharyngitis in different children. On the other hand, RSV, parainfluenza and influenza viruses can all cause acute bronchiolitis. Dual infections (two viruses or one virus and one bacterium) are being increasingly recognised[15].

Respiratory syncytial virus (RSV)

This is the most important respiratory pathogen of early childhood. Virtually all children have at least one RSV infection by the age of 2. Re-infection is common: 75% of children infected in the first year have a second milder infection in the second year[2]. This may reflect antigenic variation of the virus[16]. By the age of 5 years, RSV infections are much less common and rarely severe.

RSV causes 70–80% of cases of bronchiolitis, 10–15% of croup, 15% of bronchitis and a third of episodes of pneumonia in early childhood[2,14]. It is a common cause of URTIs, including acute otitis media. In young infants, and especially those born preterm, it can cause life-threatening central apnoea[17,18]: RSV infection has been associated with the sudden infant death syndrome (cot-death). There are two strains of the virus, A and B. Their clinical features are indistinguishable.

There are annual epidemics of RSV infection in late autumn and winter which last for 3-5 months[2,10]. These epidemics have a major impact on local health services: for example in the author's children's hospital, in one 8-week period during a typical winter epidemic there were 179 admissions of infants with RSV bronchiolitis, with a mean length of stay of 4.5 days[19].

Parainfluenza viruses

Although the five serotypes of parainfluenza virus (1, 2, 3, 4a and 4b) have different seasonal patterns, all can produce a wide range of respiratory infections from mild pharyngitis to severe croup[2,10]. It is not possible to identify the particular serotype on clinical grounds. Infections caused by types 1 and 3 are more common than those due to the other strains. Some strains cause autumn epidemics every second year, whereas others are endemic with added annual spring epidemics. By the age of 2 years, 90% of children will have had one type 3 infection, and 30% will have had two or more. Para-influenza viruses are the commonest cause of infective croup (laryngotracheobronchitis), and important pathogens in pneumonia and bronchiolitis.

Influenza viruses

Influenza types A and B are less common and important pathogens in childhood than RSV and parainfluenza. They commonly cause an URTI with high fever and myalgia, but can also cause serious lower respiratory tract infection, including pneumonia.

Adenoviruses

Of these viruses 42 different serotypes have been identified[20]. Some affect primarily the gastrointestinal tract but others are respiratory pathogens. Types 1–3 can be isolated from children with febrile URTIs. Types 3, 4, 7, and 21 can cause severe bronchiolitis and pneumonia[2,20,21]. There is a significant risk of death with such infections and as many as 70% of survivors are left with permanent damage to the airways (bronchiolitis obliterans)[22].

Bacteria

Bacterial infections account for a much lower proportion of lower respiratory tract infections in children than in adults. Because of the difficulties of obtaining suitable bacteriological specimens from the lower tract and of interpreting the results obtained of nasal, throat, or sputum cultures, where contamination by commensals can occur, the role of bacteria in lower respiratory infection remains controversial.

In the newborn infant, Gram-negative organisms and group B β-haemolytic streptococci are the commonest bacterial pathogens. In infants, pneumococcus and to lesser extent *Haemophilus influenzae* and *Staphylococcus aureus*, are important. In some regions, *Chlamydia trachomatis* is a frequent cause of pneumonia in the first two months of life. In older children, HiB, pneumococcus, *Mycoplasma pneumoniae* and *Bordetella pertussis* are the commonest bacterial causes of lower respiratory infection.

Classification of respiratory infections

Respiratory infections in children are classified anatomically, depending on which part of the respiratory tract is most severely affected. Although this classification is artificial, as several levels of the tract may be involved in a single infection, it is more useful than a classification based on aetiology.

The five major clinical categories of infection are:

(i) Upper respiratory tract infection
  e.g. common cold, pharyngitis, tonsillitis, otitis media
(ii) Laryngeal and tracheal infection
  e.g. croup, epiglottitis, bacterial tracheitis
(iii) Acute bronchitis
  e.g. viral bronchitis, pertussis
(iv) Acute bronchiolitis
(v) Pneumonia
  e.g. viral, bacterial, chlamydial pneumonia

In the remainder of this chapter, infections of the lower respiratory tract will be described in detail. Upper respiratory tract infections are discussed in Chapter 25.

Infections of the larynx and trachea

Infections of the upper airway (larynx and trachea) are common in childhood. They are important because the small diameter and cross-sectional area of the upper airway renders young children vulnerable to life-threatening obstruction by the mucosal oedema and inflammatory secretions of these infections. Although infection is the commonest cause of acute upper airways obstruction in children, non-infectious causes such as an inhaled foreign body or angioneurotic oedema must always be considered in the differential diagnosis (Table 23.2).

Clinical features

Stridor is the cardinal feature of upper airway obstruction[23]. This is heard predominantly on inspiration, but may also be audible on expiration. Like wheeze in asthma, the intensity of stridor does not indicate the severity of narrowing[24]. As well as stridor, there may be hoarseness due to inflammation of the vocal cords, and a barking or seal-like tracheal cough.

The severity of obstruction is assessed by the degree of sternal and subcostal recession, and the respiratory and heart rate. Increasing agitation or drowsiness, or central cyanosis, indicate severe hypoxaemia and the need for urgent intervention. The degree of systemic disturbance varies with the infection that is present.

Croup

Croup is the commonest cause of acute upper airways obstruction in children. Croup is defined as an acute clinical syndrome with inspiratory stridor, barking cough, hoarseness, and variable degrees of respiratory distress, due to laryngeal or tracheal obstruction. This definition embraces several distinct disorders with different pathophysiology and clinical courses, which require quite specific and different management[23–25].

Viral croup (viral laryngotracheitis, viral laryngotracheobronchitis) is the commonest form of croup, accounting for over 95% of acute laryngotracheal infections. Para-influenza viruses types I, II, and III are the commonest pathogens but the respiratory syncytial virus, influenza A and B viruses, adeno- and rhino-viruses can produce a similar illness[2,10,26,27]. Spread is by droplet and the hand-to-nose routes.

Viral invasion of the nasopharynx is followed by spread to the laryngeal and tracheal mucosa. Destruction of the ciliated tracheal epithelium, inflammatory oedema and a fibrinous exudate lead to tracheal narrowing, particularly in the sub-glottis where the annular cricoid cartilage limits expansion[27]. There is associated inflammation of the vocal cords.

In an 11-year study of children attending a paediatric practice in North Carolina, croup accounted for 15% of lower respiratory tract infections[10,25]. The peak incidence of viral croup is in the second year of life. Approximately 2–3% of all young children are admitted to hospital with croup on at least one occasion[2]: most admissions are in children aged between 6 months and five years[2,27,28]. Although viral croup occurs throughout the year, it is more common in the autumn and winter. As with other respiratory infections, viral croup is commoner in boys than in girls (ratio 1.5:1)[28].

Table 23.2. *Differential diagnosis of acute upper airways obstruction in children*

Croup	viral laryngotracheitis	(very common)
	recurrent or spasmodic croup	(common)
	bacterial tracheitis	(rare)
Epiglottitis		(uncommon)
Diphtheria		(rare)
Retropharyngeal abscess		(rare)
Infectious mononucleosis		(rare)
Laryngeal foreign body		(rare)
Angioneurotic oedema		(rare)
Inhalation of hot gases		(rare)
Trauma		(rare)

The typical features of a barking cough, harsh stridor and hoarseness are usually preceded by fever and coryza for 1–3 days. The symptoms often begin, and are worse, at night. Many children have stridor and a mild fever (<38.5 °C), with little or no respiratory difficulty. If tracheal narrowing is minor, stridor is present only when the child hyperventilates or is upset. With more severe narrowing, the stridor becomes both inspiratory and expiratory and is present even when the child is at rest. Some children, and particularly those below the age of 3, develop the features of increasing upper airway obstruction and hypoxaemia, with marked sternal and subcostal recession, tachycardia, tachypnoea and agitation. If the infection extends distally to the bronchi, wheeze may also be audible.

Investigations are of little value. A differential white cell count and microbiological tests are not diagnostic and need not be performed as a routine. Lateral or postero-anterior radiographs of the neck may show widening of the hypopharynx and narrowing of the sub-glottic trachea (the 'steeple sign'), but these features are seen in only 40–50% of cases of croup and do not correlate with clinical severity[29,30].

Other forms of croup

Some children have repeated episodes of croup without fever or coryza. Symptoms appear suddenly at night, and may persist for only a few hours. This recurrent or spasmodic croup is often associated with atopic diseases such as asthma, eczema or hay-fever: it may represent hyperreactivity of the upper airway[31,32]. The episodes can occasionally be severe, but are usually self-limiting. It can be difficult to distinguish clinically between viral and recurrent croup: there is debate about whether they are two distinct entities or merely different presentations of a single condition[30,33].

Bacterial tracheitis (pseudomembranous croup), an uncommon but life-threatening form of croup, is described below.

Management of acute viral croup

Accurate diagnosis, gentle handling and careful observation are the mainstays of good management[23]. Children with croup are often frightened, miserable and uncomfortable: they may be happier on their parent's lap than lying flat in a cot. Disturbing the child should be kept to a minimum as crying increases their oxygen demand, increases laryngeal swelling, and accelerates respiratory muscle fatigue. Most cases of viral croup resolve spontaneously within 2–4 days, but in others, increasing dyspnoea necessitates hospital admission.

Oxygen

Many children admitted to hospital with croup have hypoxaemia as a result of alveolar hypoventilation secondary to airways obstruction, and ventilation-perfusion imbalance. The degree of hypoxaemia correlates poorly with clinical signs: the respiratory rate and the degree of sternal recession are the most reliable indicators[24]. Ideally, oxygen saturation should be monitored with a pulse oximeter on admission and continuously thereafter if there is evidence of severe obstruction. Humidified oxygen can be given through a face-mask. Inhalation of warm moist air (mist) is widely used but of unproven benefit[34]. Croup tents are uncomfortable, frightening, impair observation, and are also of dubious value[33].

Nebulised adrenaline

Although nebulised adrenaline (epinephrine) has been used in the treatment of severe croup for 30 years, its role remains controversial. Adrenaline's alpha-adrenergic activity causes mucosal vasoconstriction and reduces subglottic oedema. Adair *et al.*[35] suggested that inhalation of an aerosol of racemic adrenaline through an intermittent positive pressure breathing device reduced the need for intubation or tracheostomy (racemic adrenaline is a mixture of the L- and R-isomers of the drug). Subsequent prospective studies have failed to replicate these findings[33]. Aerosols from simple nebulisers are as effective and better tolerated[36,37]. The more widely available and cheaper l-adrenaline is as effective as the racemic preparation[38].

Nebulised l-adrenaline (5 ml of 1:1000) given with oxygen through a face-mask reduces the clinical severity of obstruction and respiratory resistance[39], but does not improve arterial blood gases, reduce the duration of hospitalisation, or the need for intubation[30,36,37]. The improvement from a single dose lasts for only 30–60 minutes. The dose can be repeated after 2–3 hours. Tachycardia is increased but other side effects are uncommon. This treatment should be given only to children with severe obstruction in a setting where they can be observed closely with continuous ECG and oxygen saturation monitoring, as they may need endotracheal intubation.

Corticosteroids

There has been even more debate about the value of corticosteroids in the treatment of croup[23,30,40]. This controversy reflects serious deficiencies in many published studies and a failure to define clearly the condition being studied and clinically important outcome measures[25,40,41]. Over the last five years, better designed studies[42,43] and meta-analysis[44] have clarified the role of steroids in children admitted to hospital with croup. For example, Super *et al.*, showed that children given dexamethasone in a single parenteral dose of 0.6 mg/kg on admission had a more rapid resolution of symptoms in the first 24 hours than children in the placebo group[42]. However, there were no differences between oxygen saturation levels or the duration of hospitalisation between the two groups. Tibbals showed that, in children who needed endotracheal intubation for croup, the duration of intubation was much less in those given naso-gastric prednisiolone (1 mg/kg every 12 hours) than in the placebo group[43].

The need for reintubation was markedly less in the prednisolone group.

Steroids are assumed to act by reducing inflammation and capillary endothelial permeability, with a reduction in mucosal oedema. Dexamethasone, which has a half-life of 36–54 hours, has been the steroid most widely studied. Adverse effects appear to be uncommon, but it needs to be given either intravenously or intramuscularly. Two recent studies of nebulised budesonide have shown a reduction in clinical scores in children with croup over the first 2–4 hours after administration[33,45,46]. However, in one study, children with severe croup, the patients in whom such therapy might be most valuable, were excluded, and 60% of the children also subsequently received dexamethasone[46]. In the other study, which did include children with severe croup, there were no data presented to indicate any benefit beyond the 2-hour assessment period[45].

Endotracheal intubation

About 2–5% of children admitted with croup require endotracheal intubation to maintain an adequate airway[28]. The decision to intubate is based on increasing tachycardia, tachypnoea and chest recession, or the appearance of cyanosis, exhaustion or confusion. Intubation should be performed under general anaesthetic by an experienced paediatric anaesthetist unless there has been a respiratory arrest. Most pass an orotracheal tube initially and then replace this with a naso-tracheal tube once adequate oxygenation and tracheal suction have been performed. It is important to avoid using an excessively large tube as there is a risk of pressure necrosis and subsequent sub-glottic scarring[47]. If there is doubt about the diagnosis, or difficulty in intubation is anticipated, an ENT surgeon who can perform a tracheostomy should be present.

Intubated children need meticulous care if complications such as tube-blockage or displacement are to be avoided[48]. There is a small but real risk of hypoxic brain damage associated with upper airway obstruction in this group of children. Pulmonary oedema, pneumothorax and pneumomediastinum are other uncommon complications. The median duration of intubation is 4–7 days: the younger the child, the longer intubation is required[28,43]. If there are difficulties in extubation, then bronchoscopy under a general anaesthetic is appropriate: if this reveals severe obstruction or inflammatory necrosis, tracheostomy may be necessary[2]. Secondary bacterial infection with *S. aureus*, *Haemophilus* or *Streptococcus*, is seen in over 50% of children who are intubated for viral croup. Tracheal secretions should be sent for bacterial studies and an appropriate antibiotic, such as cefotaxime, given[2,28].

Bacterial tracheitis

Bacterial tracheitis (membranous or pseudomembranous croup) is an uncommon but life-threatening cause of upper airways obstruction in children[49,50]. Infection of the tracheal mucosa results in copious thick purulent secretions, the formation of an adherent inflammatory membrane in the sub-glottic region, and mucosal necrosis[51,52]. *S. aureus* is the most frequently identified pathogen, but *H. influenzae* B, alpha-haemolytic streptococci, *Moraxella catarrhalis*, *Pseudomonas aeruginosa* and *Klebsiella spp* have all been isolated from tracheal secretions[51–53]. In some affected children, parainfluenza or influenza virus have been isolated as well as the bacterial pathogen, suggesting bacterial infection may be secondary to viral tracheitis[53].

Diagnosis

Early diagnosis and treatment are essential if fatal obstruction is to be avoided[54]. The diagnosis can usually be made on the basis of the clinical features. However, children with bacterial tracheitis exhibit features common to both viral croup and epiglottitis (Table 23.3). Children with bacterial croup appear more toxic than children with viral croup, with a high fever and the signs of progressive upper airways obstruction. The presence of a prominent croupy cough and the absence of drooling help distinguish bacterial croup from epiglottitis. Most affected children are aged between 1–5 years, but children up to the age of 12 have been reported.

Radiographs of the major airways may show irregularities of the tracheal wall due to oedema and mucosal sloughing, and sub-glottic narrowing[50,52] but these signs are not always present[51]. Bronchoscopy under general anaesthetic is used in some centres to confirm the diagnosis and to perform tracheal toilet, but this approach is far from universal[52,53,55]. A chest X-ray should be performed as there is radiological evidence of pneumonia in over 50% of children[50].

Management

Once the diagnosis is made, the child should be urgently transferred to a paediatric intensive care unit. Four-fifths of affected children require tracheal intubation to maintain an adequate airway. At intubation, the epiglottis and aryepiglottic folds appear normal, but copious purulent secretions containing fragments of necrotic tracheal mucosa are aspirated from the trachea. These should be sent for bacterial culture: blood cultures should also be sent, but these are usually sterile. Intravenous cefotaxime and flucloxacillin should be given for 7–14 days, unless bacteriological studies indicate another antibiotic is more appropriate. Nebulised adrenaline or steroids are not effective.

Meticulous care of the endotracheal tube and continuous monitoring of ECG, respiration and oxygen saturation are essential. Even with frequent endotracheal suction and careful humidification, blockage of the endotracheal tube by the tenacious secretions is common[52]. In one series of 17 children with bacterial tracheitis, seven had life-threatening episodes of obstruction, four had cardiorespiratory arrests and two died[53]. Replacement of the endotracheal tube, or occasionally, tracheostomy may be needed to maintain the airway. An artificial airway is normally required for 5–14 days, depending on the severity of the infection and the age of the child. Providing severe hypoxic episodes, with their attendant risk of hypoxic-ischaemic encephalopathy are avoided, the child can be expected to make a full recovery.

Acute epiglottitis

Epiglottitis (supraglottitis) is the most acute and dangerous infection of the respiratory tract in children. Infection with *H. influenza* B (HiB) causes acute inflammation, hyperaemia and submucosal oedema of the epiglottis and aryepiglottic folds, with progressive narrowing of the supra-glottic airway. If untreated, this swelling leads within hours to total obstruction, respiratory arrest, and death.

Table 23.3. *Comparison of clinical features of viral and bacterial croup and epiglottitis*

	Viral croup	Epiglottitis	Bacterial tracheitis
Onset	over days	over hours	hours to days
Preceding coryza	yes	no	yes
Cough	severe, barking	absent or slight	marked
Drooling saliva	no	yes	no
Appearance	unwell	toxic, v ill	toxic
Fever	mild	marked	marked
Stridor	harsh, rasping	soft, whispering	marked
Voice, cry	hoarse	muffled	normal

As well as the features of upper airway obstruction, there is marked systemic disturbance due to the associated bacteraemia.

Incidence

Epiglottitis is predominantly a disease of the preschool child. Although it occurs in infants and in adults[2,56,57], four-fifths of cases occur in children aged between 1 and 5 years. The mean age in a national Swedish study of 485 children with epiglottitis was 3.7 years: over 90% of affected children were more than 18 months of age (56). The overall annual age-specific incidence in children was 10/100 000 children, but in the most commonly affected 0–4 years age-group, the incidence was 25/100 000. Most studies report a male preponderance[2].

Unlike other respiratory infections, there is no clear seasonal pattern of incidence: some studies have reported that it is more common in the summer whilst others have reported a winter preponderance. In countries where routine immunisation of infants with the conjugate vaccine against HiB has been introduced, there has been a dramatic reduction in the incidence of epiglottitis[58,59].

Aetiology

H. influenzae type B (HiB) is the causative pathogen in virtually all cases of acute epiglottitis. In the Swedish study, *H. influenzae* was isolated from 92% of the blood cultures sent[56]. All serotyped isolates were type B. In this and several other large studies, no other bacterial pathogens were isolated in the children, although there are occasional case reports of epiglottitis being caused by Group A beta-haemolytic streptococci and other streptococci.

Clinical features

Although epiglottitis shares many of the clinical features of viral and bacterial croup, it must be recognised as a separate entity[2,60–62]. It is far less common than croup, but prompt diagnosis and management are essential if death is to be avoided.

The onset of the illness is acute, with high fever, lethargy, noisy breathing (inspiratory stridor) and rapidly increasing respiratory difficulty developing over 3–6 hours. There may have been a preceding coryzal illness but this is less common than with croup. In contrast to croup, cough is minimal or absent (Table 23.3). Because the throat is so painful, the child is reluctant to speak and unable to swallow drinks or saliva.

Typically the child sits immobile with the neck extended, the chin slightly raised and the mouth open, drooling saliva[62]. There is usually a soft whispering inspiratory stridor and sometimes a quiet snoring expiratory stridor. The voice is muffled rather than hoarse. There is marked sternal, subcostal and supraclavicular recession. The child appears toxic and pale and may have poor peripheral circulation, with cool peripheries and delayed capillary refill, due to the associated bacteraemia. There is usually a high fever (>39 °C) and marked tachycardia. Disturbance of the child, such as attempting to lie him/her down to examine the throat with a spatula, or inserting an intravenous cannula, can precipitate total obstruction and should be avoided.

Management

The diagnosis is based on the characteristic history and clinical signs. Lateral X-rays of the neck, which may show thickening of the epiglottis ('thumb sign') and distention of the hypopharynx, are unreliable and should be avoided. Between 25 and 50% of chest X-rays show evidence of consolidation, atelectasis, or less often, pulmonary oedema. Radiographs should not be performed before there is a secure airway.

Once the diagnosis is made, urgent admission to a paediatric intensive care unit should be arranged. Any disturbance or upset of the child should be avoided. Between 70 and 100% of children with epiglottitis require intubation[63]. They should be given humidified oxygen sitting on their parent's knee while arrangements are made for intubation. The child should be intubated under halothane and oxygen anaesthesia to stabilise the airway. Endotracheal intubation may be difficult because of the intense swelling and inflammation of the epiglottis ('cherry red epiglottis'). Once intubated, most children require only sedation: paralysis and mechanical ventilation are needed in only a minority[63]. Very rarely, intubation is not possible and an emergency tracheostomy is required. There is no evidence that nebulised adrenaline or steroids are beneficial.

Once the airway is secured, blood and throat swabs should be sent for culture and intravenous antibiotic therapy started. In the past, chloramphenicol was used and was very effective, but nowadays a third generation cephalosporin such as cefotaxime, ceftriaxone or cefuroxime is preferred[60,63,64]. Ampicillin is not adequate because of the increasing incidence of β-lactamase strains of HiB. As there is a small risk of HiB infection in those in close contact with children with epiglottitis, rifampicin prophylaxis is given to these contacts.

With appropriate treatment, fever and tachycardia normally resolve within 12–18 hours[63]. Most children can be extubated within 24–36 hours and have recovered fully within 3–5 days. Complications such as hypoxic cerebral damage, pulmonary oedema and other serious haemophilus infections such as pneumonia, are uncommon. Nevertheless there is still a significant mortality associated with this infection: six of the 485 children in the Swedish study died of acute obstruction[56].

Other causes of upper airways obstruction

Although croup and epiglottitis account for over 98% of cases of acute upper airways obstruction, other less common conditions need to be considered in the differential diagnosis (Table 23.2).

Diphtheria is nowadays extremely rare and is seen only in children who have not been immunised against the disease. Nevertheless, it is important to ask about immunisations in any child with fever and the signs of upper airways obstruction, particularly if they have been abroad recently. Marked tonsillar swelling in *infectious mononucleosis* or *acute tonsillitis* can rarely compromise the upper airway. *Retropharyngeal abscess* is very uncommon nowadays, but can present with fever and the features of upper airways obstruction[65]. Surgical drainage and intravenous antibiotics are needed. Laryngeal oedema can develop over minutes as part of an *anaphylactic reaction*, often with angioneurotic oedema of the face and mouth. Food allergies, drug reactions and insect stings are the common causes. The inquisitive toddler is at risk of inhaling a *foreign body*. Small toys, batteries, coins and foodstuffs (nuts, sweets, meat) are the commonest offending items[2].

Acute bronchitis

Although acute viral bronchitis is common in children, there has been little research into the condition. This reflects the lack of a clear definition of the disease and the fact that it is normally a minor self-limiting infection which rarely merits hospital admission.

Aetiology and epidemiology

Viruses and *M. pneumoniae* are the commonest pathogens. Adenoviruses, influenza A and B viruses, para-influenza viruses, RSV and rhinoviruses can all produce a similar illness. Acute bronchitis due to *Mycoplasma* spp. or *C. pneumoniae* infection is more common in older children and adolescents[66]. Primary bacterial bronchitis is uncommon in otherwise healthy children[2].

Acute bronchitis accounts for between 10–40% of acute lower respiratory infections in children[10,66]. The peak incidence is in the second year of life and when the child first attends school or nursery. Up to the age of six, RSV and parainfluenza are the commonest pathogens: after this age, influenza viruses and *Mycoplasma* spp. are more common: (acute bronchitis is also a common feature of measles). Acute bronchitis is more frequent in the autumn and winter.

Clinical features

The characteristic features of acute bronchitis are fever and cough following an upper respiratory tract infection. In the prodromal phase, there is fever with pharyngitis or rhinitis for 1–2 days. A cough appears which is initially dry, but then becomes productive of mucoid or purulent sputum. There may be vomiting if the cough is particularly vigorous, and older children may suffer chest pain due to the coughing. The cough gradually disappears over 1–2 weeks.

Examination is often normal. There may be evidence of rhinitis or pharyngitis. Auscultation reveals scanty scattered wheezes or a few crackles. Investigations are unhelpful and unnecessary: a chest X-ray, if performed, shows no abnormality.

Differential diagnosis

It can be difficult to distinguish between an episode of acute asthma triggered by a viral URTI and acute bronchitis. If there is breathlessness, widespread wheeze or evidence of hyperinflation, and particularly if there have been previous similar episodes, the diagnosis is likely to be asthma and appropriate treatment should be given. In infancy, bronchiolitis is another possibility. If coughing and wheeze occur without a preceding fever or URTI, aspiration of feeds or an inhaled foreign body should be considered.

Management

In most cases, no treatment is necessary. Paracetamol or ibuprofen reduce fever and chest pain. Decongestants, expectorants and cough suppressants are widely used but are of unproven benefit. Antibiotics are often prescribed but are rarely indicated or beneficial: secondary bacterial infection in viral bronchitis is uncommon[2]. However, it is reasonable to give a 7–10 day course of an antibiotic if the fever returns, if a purulent cough persists for more than 7–10 days or if there is persistent systemic upset. As HiB or pneumococcus are the likeliest causes of secondary infection, co-amoxyclav, a cephalosporin, or erythromcin are appropriate.

Pertussis (whooping cough)

Pertussis is a particular form of acute bronchitis that merits attention: it remains an important cause of respiratory morbidity in children despite its reduced incidence since the introduction of immunisation.

Aetiology and pathophysiology.

B. pertussis is almost always the causative pathogen. Adenoviruses, *Bordetella parapertussis* and *M. pneumoniae* occasionally cause an illness which mimics pertussis[2]. The bacterium invades the tracheal and bronchial epithelium, causing inflammation and damage to the respiratory microcilia. Tenacious mucus is produced, which can lead to bronchial obstruction and atelectasis. Occasionally, pneumonia develops, either due to infection with *B. pertussis* or due to secondary pathogens such as *S. aureus* or pneumococcus.

Epidemiology

The infection is endemic with occasional epidemics. It is highly infectious: 60–70% of non-immunised children develop the disease[67]. The commonest sources are family members and school contacts[68]. In one community-based survey, the peak incidence was at the age of three[69]. Unlike other respiratory infections, girls are more commonly affected than boys[2].

The incidence of pertussis is inversely related to the level of immunisation in the community. Although there is controversy about the efficacy of the vaccine and the duration of the protection it gives, non-immunised children are 3–4 times more likely to develop the disease than immunised children. However, by the age of 12, over 90% of children immunised in infancy are susceptible to infection[2].

Recently there have been reports of sudden increases in the number of cases of pertussis. In one report from Cincinnati, there was an increase of 260% in the number of confirmed cases diagnosed in a single regional centre between 1992 and 1993[70]. Although 80% of affected children were less than 5 years old, more older children were infected than in previous series. Four-fifths of the children had been immunised with the whole-cell vaccine, indicating the limitations of this vaccine in this population.

Clinical features

There is a broad spectrum of severity of this illness: many cases are mild and probably pass undiagnosed[69,71], but in others hospital admission and mechanical ventilation are necessary.

The incubation period of pertussis is 7–14 days. Initially there is a coryzal or catarrhal stage lasting 3–14 days, where there is a dry cough and sometimes a nasal discharge[69]. At this stage there are no characteristic features to suggest the diagnosis, but the child is highly infectious.

There then follows the *paroxysmal* or *spasmodic phase*. There are increasingly frequent and severe paroxysms of coughing, in which the child becomes red in the face or cyanosed, with tears streaming and mucus coming from the mouth. These paroxysms are more common at night, on exertion, or if the child is upset. They may end with a characteristic sharp inspiratory breath (whoop), but this is often not present, particularly in infants. Vomiting is seen in over half of cases, but there is little constitutional upset between paroxysms[69]. In infants less than 6 months old, the group at highest risk, recurrent apnoeas may be present in as many as 25% of cases, either at the end of paroxysms, or as an early feature of the illness[72].

In a study of 500 consecutive cases of pertussis seen in a single general practice, this distressing phase lasted for between 2 days and 24 weeks, with a mean of 52 days[69]. The paroxysms gradually become less frequent and less severe. If the child develops a viral infection during this recovery period, an unwelcome but less severe encore of the symptoms can appear.

Diagnosis

Most cases can be diagnosed from the history of a prolonged paroxysmal cough, particularly if a whoop has been heard[68,69]. Other diagnoses that should be considered include asthma, mycoplasmal infection, an inhaled foreign body, or less commonly, a chronic respiratory disease such as cystic fibrosis.

In most cases, investigations are unnecessary. A chest X-ray is usually normal, but in a sixth of cases in one series, segmental or lobar collapse was noted[2]. This resolved spontaneously. *B. pertussis* can be identified by culture of a pernasal or nasopharyngeal swab early in the course of the illness unless antibiotics have been given[68,73]. Alternatively, an immunofluorescent antibody test can be used to detect the antigen but this test has a lower sensitivity and specificity than the clinical history[73]. An absolute lymphocytosis of more than 10 000/mm^3 (occasionally extremely high), is suggestive of pertussis.

Management

Mild cases in older children can be safely treated at home. Admission is indicated in children aged less than six months, and in those with apnoeic attacks or severe paroxysms with cyanosis. It is important to maintain an adequate fluid intake: suction and supplementary oxygen may be required.

Although *Bordetella* is sensitive to several antibiotics, there is no convincing evidence that giving an antibiotic once the paroxysmal stage has been reached improves outcome. Erthromycin does reduce the period of infectivity of affected children and it can prevent the disease developing in susceptible contacts if given during the incubation period. Corticosteroids, salbutamol, inhaled cromoglycate and phenobarbitone have all been used to treat paroxysms, but their value remains unproven.

The most effective management is prevention by immunisation. The current whole-cell vaccine offers 80–90% protection. In immunised children who develop pertussis, the infection is less severe and prolonged[71]. Immunisation rates have varied dramatically during the last 20 years as a result of concern about possible rare, but irreversible, neurological damage caused by the vaccine. The current consensus is that there is no convincing evidence of a causal relationship between the vaccine and permanent neuro-developmental sequelae[2,68]. (It is noteworthy that not all developed countries have universal vaccination for pertussis, for example, Sweden[67].)

Outcome/complications

Although the illness runs a protracted course, most children make a full recovery[74]. The major risks are recurrent apnoeas, seen almost exclusively in infants less than 6 months of age, encephalopathy which is probably secondary to cerebral hypoxia during paroxysms, and secondary pneumonia. In several series of hospitalised patients with pertussis, up to 5% have needed intensive care and mechanical ventilation for these complications[75]. In the past, pertussis was an important cause of bronchiectasis, but this is now rare[2].

Acute viral bronchiolitis

Acute bronchiolitis is the commonest lower respiratory tract infection of young children. Around 10% of infants develop bronchiolitis: a fifth of these are admitted to hospital[2]. Winter epidemics of bronchiolitis occur each year. Over 80% of affected children are aged between one and eight months.

Aetiology and pathophysiology

Acute bronchiolitis is due to viral colonisation of the bronchiolar mucosa. Respiratory syncytial virus (RSV) is the pathogen in 70–85% of cases, the remainder being caused by parainfluenza, influenza and adenoviruses[2,76]. Dual infection with other viruses, or organisms such as *Chlamydia trachomatis* or *M. pneumoniae*, may be more common than previously thought, occurring in at least 5–10% of cases of RSV infections[15,77].

The virus replicates rapidly in the bronchiolar epithelium, causing necrosis of the ciliated cells and proliferation of non-ciliated cells. The ciliary damage impairs clearance of secretions. This combined with increased mucus secretion and desquamation of cells, leads to bronchiolar obstruction, atelectasis and hyperinflation. The peribronchial tissues show inflammatory infiltration, submucosal oedema and congestion. An associated interstitial pneumonia may occur. Structural recovery usually occurs in 2–3 weeks[76]. Occasionally, and particularly if adenovirus serotype 7 or 21 is the pathogen, there is permanent bronchiolar damage with persistent segmental or lobar atelectasis and hyperinflation (bronchiolitis obliterans).

The acute functional consequences of these changes are small airways obstruction, gas trapping and impaired gas exchange. Thoracic gas volume and respiratory resistance rise, and expiratory flow rates and dynamic compliance fall[2,76,78]. The work of breathing and oxygen consumption are increased[79]. Impaired ventilation, combined with ventilation-perfusion imbalance, and in some infants, hypoventilation due to apnoea or fatigue, lead to hypoxaemia and hypercarbia[80,81].

Diagnosis

Accurate diagnosis is based on the clinical features (Table 23.4). Fever and a nasal discharge precede a dry cough and increasingly rapid, distressed breathing. Wheezing is often, but not always, audible. Feeding difficulties due to dyspnoea are often the reason for admission. Central apnoea with cyanosis is seen in 10–20% of babies admitted with bronchiolitis[17,18]. Apnoeas usually occur early in the illness and may be the presenting feature, preceding the features of airways obstruction.

On examination there is tachycardia and tachypnoea, with subcostal, intercostal and supraclavicular recession (Table 23.4). Unlike the breathing pattern seen in croup or pneumonia, there is little sternal recession, as gas-trapping prevents this. The sternum is prominent, the chest appears barrel-shaped, and the liver is displaced downwards, indicating hyperinflation. The child has a short, dry, wheezy cough. There are fine inspiratory crackles and/or high pitched expiratory wheezes in all lung fields. In severe cases there may be irregular breathing, cyanosis or pallor. Fever is present in most infants; conjunctivitis, pharyngitis or otitis media occur in a minority.

Identifying the high risk infant

Certain infants are at increased risk of severe illness, respiratory failure requiring ventilatory support, and of death from bronchiolitis (Table 23.5). Children with chronic lung disease, congenital heart disease or immunodeficiency, are at particularly high risk[82–85]. Infants aged less than 6 weeks and those born prematurely are also at risk: apnoea is common in these babies[86].

In a case-control study of 33 infants ventilated for RSV-bronchiolitis and 99 RSV-positive infants who were not ventilated, 39% of the ventilated infants had apnoea before admission and 63% had apnoea before ventilation was started[86]. Apnoea was significantly more frequent in infants born prematurely. The median age, after correction for prematurity, was 19 days in the ventilated group and 122 days in the controls. Others have shown that low birthweight, preterm delivery, neonatal respiratory disease and young age are risk factors for respiratory failure[87]. Infants with any of these factors need close observation.

Differential diagnosis

Other serious conditions can mimic bronchiolitis and may be overlooked (Table 23.6): for example, previously unsuspected cystic fibrosis, aspiration pneumonitis, congenital cardiac and lung defects, or immunodeficiency. It can be impossible to distinguish between the first episode of asthma and acute bronchiolitis. Careful attention to the preceding history, examination, and chest radiograph usually allows other causes to be identified.

Even if the diagnosis of bronchiolitis is certain, an associated underlying congenital abnormality or dual infection should be considered if the illness is severe, prolonged, or atypical. For example, babies with congenital heart defects or immunodeficiency may be asymptomatic until they develop bronchiolitis, when they deteriorate rapidly.

Table 23.4. *Clinical features of bronchiolitis*

Tachypnoea: 50–100 breaths/minute
Subcostal and intercostal recession
Sharp, dry cough
Hyperinflation: sternum prominent, liver depressed
Tachycardia (120–170 beats/minute)
Fine end-inspiratory crackles
High-pitched wheezes: expiratory > inspiratory
Cyanosis or pallor
Irregular breathing/apnoea

Table 23.5. *Risk factors for severe bronchiolitis*

Age less than 6 weeks at presentation
Apnoea
Preterm birth
Underlying disorders
lung disease, e.g. bronchopulmonary dysplasia, CF
congenital heart disease
immunodeficiency (congenital or acquired)
multiple congenital abnormalities
severe neurological disease

Table 23.6. *Differential diagnosis of acute bronchiolitis*

Pulmonary
Asthma
Pneumonia
infective e.g. RSV, *Chlamydia trachomatis*
aspiration, e.g. with gastro-oesophageal reflux
opportunistic, secondary to immunodeficiency
e.g. *Pneumocystis carinii*, cytomegalovirus
Congenital lung disease
e.g. congenital lobar emphysema, lung cysts
Cystic fibrosis
Inhaled foreign body
Non-pulmonary
Congenital heart disease
e.g. obstructed pulmonary venous drainage, VSD[a]
Septicaemia
Severe metabolic acidosis

[a] VSD, ventricular septal defect.

Investigations

Investigations often add relatively little to management. A chest X-ray typically shows hyperinflation, with depressed and flattened diaphragms. A third of infants have collapse or consolidation, particularly in the upper lobes. There is no correlation between these findings and the severity of the illness[88]. Chest X-rays are not required routinely in bronchiolitis and should be reserved for infants with severe disease, sudden deterioration, or an underlying cardiac or respiratory disorder[88]. Full blood counts and serum electrolytes are normal in over 80% of children admitted with bronchiolitis[89]. Electrolyte disturbances, most notably hyponatraemia, are uncommon except in severe disease[90,91]. Arterial blood gases should be performed only in severe cases. Arterial CO_2 levels are commonly above 10 kPa in hospitalised infants[2,80].

RSV and the other respiratory viruses can be identified by fluorescent antibody techniques or by culture of nasopharyngeal secretions. Although rapid viral identification has been used to isolate RSV-positive children[92], the lack of a positive result does not preclude a diagnosis of bronchiolitis or affect outcome. Viral identification can be regarded as desirable rather than essential.

Assessing and monitoring progress

Hypoxia is the most important physiological consequence of bronchiolitis. However, this can be difficult to detect clinically in infants[93]. Mulholland compared blood gases with oxygen saturation measured by pulse oximetry (S_aO_2) and clinical signs in infants with bronchiolitis[81]. Crackles and cyanosis correlated with arterial oxygen levels, but respiratory rate, heart rate and recession did not predict hypoxaemia. Others have found that clinical signs correlate poorly with hypoxaemia[80,93–95]. Pulse oximetry is the most reliable way to assess severity and oxygen needs in bronchiolitis.

Pulse oximeters are not universally available, and serial clinical assessments are still essential to monitor progress. Pulse oximetry has important limitations[96–98]. Errors in S_aO_2 can occur with poor application of the sensor[96], with the movement artefact that can occur during crying or procedures[97], or with anaemia, hypotension or hypothermia. Monitors are inaccurate if the S_aO_2 falls below 80%. Nevertheless, the advantages of oximeters in providing continuous, instantaneous, and non-invasive measures of arterial oxygen levels outweigh their limitations.

S_aO_2 should be measured at presentation in all infants with bronchiolitis and monitored continuously in infants with moderate to severe disease, particularly those receiving oxygen or with risk factors (Table 23.4). In high risk infants and especially those born prematurely, respiration ('apnoea') monitors should be used to detect central apnoea which can present suddenly and fatally.

Preventing cross-infection

Many children admitted to hospital without RSV infection acquire the disease from other infants. Cross-infection is an important cause of morbidity and death, particularly in children with pre-existing cardiorespiratory disease. Cross-infection rates of 15–30% have been recorded[99]. The virus is shed in large quantities in respiratory secretions and is easily passed from patient to patient by health professionals or family members.

One study showed that a combination of rapid virus identification, cohort nursing, and the use of gowns and gloves, reduced the cross-infection rate from 26% to 9%[92]: Isolation of RSV-positive babies and hand-washing were ineffective by themselves. Others have found isolation and handwashing can reduce hospital-acquired RSV infections and have stated that viral identification, gloves and gowns are unnecessary[100,101].

Treatment

There is currently no treatment which has convincingly been shown to reduce the severity or duration of viral bronchiolitis[2]. Many different treatments are used but most are of unproven benefit[86]. Adequate hydration and oxygenation, minimal handling, and the early recognition and treatment of complications remain the foundations of good care.

Fluids

Despite poor feeding, dehydration is uncommon in bronchiolitis. Hyponatraemia due to increased secretion of anti-diuretic hormone (ADH) and water retention occurs in severe RSV infections, particularly in infants with hypercapnoea and those needing ventilation[90,91]. Seizures and severe apnoeas can be associated with hyponatraemia[90]. Fluid intake should be restricted to two-thirds of the normal allowance and electrolyte levels monitored in infants with severe bronchiolitis[91].

In theory, obstructing a nostril with a naso-gastric tube will increase respiratory resistance and the work of breathing and should be avoided in respiratory distress. Gastric dilatation may further embarrass ventilation. In practice, most infants with mild-moderate disease tolerate a nasogastric tube well. In infants requiring oxygen, and those with marked tachpnoea or recurrent apnoeas, intravenous fluids are indicated.

Oxygen

Oxygen is the only agent that consistently reduces hypoxaemia in bronchiolitis[2]. As clinical assessment is not reliable, the infant's oxygen needs should be assessed by S_aO_2 levels. The S_aO_2 should be maintained above 92–95% by adjusting the inspired oxygen concentration. Oxygen should be warmed, humidified, and given into a head-box. Most babies tolerate masks or nasal prongs poorly. Nasopharyngeal oxygen is effective in children with respiratory distress[102], but has not been assessed specifically in acute bronchiolitis.

Bronchodilators

The value of bronchodilators in bronchiolitis remains controversial. In North America, nebulised beta-agonists or adrenaline are widely used[103], but in Britain they are regarded as ineffectual[104,105]. These views reflect differences in the definitions of the disease: many American studies of bronchiolitis include children who would be diagnosed as having asthma in the UK[2,105].

Several studies have shown improved lung mechanics after bronchodilators. Soto-Quiros found a significantly improved specific conductance in 30% of infants with RSV-bronchiolitis given nebulised salbutamol[106]. Tepper showed improved expiratory flow rates with orciprenaline in some infants[107]. Nebulised ipratropium reduced the work of breathing but produced no clinical improvement[79,108]. The clinical response to bronchodilators has also been studied. Two studies showed a transient improvement in respiratory signs after nebulised salbutamol[109,110]. However, these studies included children up to the age of 21 months, only half the subjects had proven RSV infection, and the observation lasted only 2–4 hours. Wang showed no improvement in S_aO_2 or clinical score with nebulised salbutamol and/or ipratropium in infants with mild bronchiolitis[111]. Ho found a fall in S_aO_2 with nebulised salbutamol in RSV-positive infants[112]. Sanchez compared salbutamol to nebulised racemic adrenaline in patients with acute bronchiolitis. Salbutamol had no effect on clinical score, S_aO_2 or respiratory resistance. Adrenaline improved respiratory rate and airway resistance[113]. Oral or intravenous methylxanthines are not beneficial[114].

On balance, there is no convincing evidence that bronchodilators produce a significant clinical improvement in bronchiolitis[103,104] and no justification for their routine use. A trial of nebulised salbutamol or ipratropium is reasonable in older infants where distinction from asthma may be difficult. As bronchodilators may paradoxically worsen hypoxaemia in wheezy infants, they should be given in oxygen with careful clinical and S_aO_2 monitoring.

Ribavirin

Ribavirin is a synthetic nucleoside with virostatic activity against many viruses including RSV. An aerosol from a small particle generator is delivered to a head box, face mask, or oxygen tent for 12–20 hours a day for 3–5 days. It can be given through a ventilator circuit if special precautions are taken to prevent deposition within the ventilator[115,116]. Side-effects are rare but because of a theoretical risk of teratogenicity, pregnant women should avoid exposure[85].

Early studies of ribavirin in bronchiolitis showed improved signs and oxygenation, but these studies were flawed[117,118]. In previously-well children with RSV bronchiolitis, there is no convincing evidence ribavirin hastens recovery or reduces complications.

The American Academy of Paediatrics recommends the use of ribavirin in certain infants with RSV infection[85]. These include infants with congenital heart or chronic lung disease, impaired immunity, multiple abnormalities, preterm infants and those aged less than six weeks, and infants ventilated for RSV infection. There is little evidence to support several of these recommendations. For example, whilst prematurity and young age are undoubtedly risk factors, it is not known that giving ribavirin to infants with these factors is beneficial.

Several studies have suggested that ribavirin benefits infants with bronchiolitis and underlying cardiopulmonary disease[117]. In babies with bronchopulmonary dysplasia or heart disease, clinical scores improved more rapidly with ribavirin, but there was no reduction in hospital stay or need for oxygen[119]. Groothuis studied early ribavirin treatment in children with RSV infection and bronchopulmonary dysplasia or heart disease[120]. After 3 days, the improvements in S_aO_2 and oxygen needs were greater with ribavirin than placebo, but clinical scores and length of admission were not improved.

In another study, ventilated infants with RSV bronchiolitis received either ribavirin or water aerosols[116]. The duration of ventilation, supplementary oxygen, and hospital stay were less in the ribavirin group[120]. The mean length of ventilation in the placebo group was 10 days, but other studies have reported a mean length of ventilation of 4 days in infants not given ribavirin[84]. Because it was thought possible that the nebulised water, a known bronchial irritant, had prolonged ventilation in the placebo group, another group studied ventilated infants who received either ribavirin or saline aerosol. The ribavirin and placebo patients did not differ in duration of ventilation, oxygen therapy, or hospital stay[115]. Both studies excluded infants presenting with apnoea: there are no studies to show ribavirin reduces apnoea.

There is clearly a need for a multicentre controlled trial of nebulised ribavirin in infants with cardio-pulmonary disease and babies under 6 weeks old with RSV infection[118], given the uncertain efficacy and the high cost of ribavirin. Until then, it is reasonable to use ribavirin only in patients with proven RSV infection and underlying chronic lung disease, immunodeficiency, or congenital heart disease.

Corticosteroids

Corticosteroids are of no value in viral bronchiolitis. In one controlled study, betamethasone had no effect on respiratory signs or length of admission[121]. In another study, where infants with bronchiolitis received intravenous hydrocortisone, oral prednisolone, or placebo, steroids had no effect on length of admission, lung function or clinical recovery[122].

Antibiotics

Acute bronchiolitis is always viral in origin. The risk of secondary bacterial infection in 565 children hospitalised with RSV infection, who had no underlying pulmonary or immune disorder, was less than 2%[123]. Thirteen infants had concurrent bacterial infection (e.g. meningitis, urinary tract infection) at presentation. Although secondary bacterial infection is uncommon, dual infection should be considered if there are atypical clinical or radiological features[15,77]. It is prudent to give intravenous antibiotics to infants with recurrent apnoea, particularly if there is circulatory impairment, as the possibility of septicaemia cannot be excluded. Antibiotics should be considered in infants with an acute deterioration, a high white cell count, a high C-reactive protein, or progressive infiltrative changes on chest X-ray[124]. Cefotaxime, or erythromycin if there is suspicion of chlamydial infection, are appropriate.

Assisted ventilation

The decision to ventilate in bronchiolitis is based on clinical grounds. Recurrent apnoea with severe hypoxaemia and progressive and persistent acidosis (pH < 7.20) are absolute indications. Most paediatricians ventilate infants with a disturbed conscious level, deteriorating chest movement, or persistently low oxygen saturation levels ($S_aO_2 < 85\%$) despite high inspired oxygen concentrations ($> 60\%$). Increasing tachypnoea and tachycardia indicate deterioration but are not in themselves indications for ventilation. There is no absolute value of arterial pCO_2 which indicates the need for ventilation: infants with pCO_2 levels greater than 12 kPa can be managed without ventilation[2].

Both pressure-limited ventilation and volume-controlled ventilators are used. Ventilator settings are tailored to the patient's response. Expiration is dependent on airway resistance and pulmonary compliance. As infants with bronchiolitis have poor compliance and increased resistance, adequate expiratory times are needed to avoid hyperinflation. Slow rates (10–25 breaths per minute) with long expiratory (2–3 seconds) and inspiratory times (1–1.5 seconds) are used. Peak inspiratory pressures are kept as low as possible but pressures over 40 cm H_2O may be needed[125]. The value of positive end expiratory pressure (PEEP) is unproven and it may be harmful[126].

The objective is to maintain arterial pH greater than 7.28 and arterial pO_2 greater than 10 kPa. Provided a high pCO_2 does not reflect tube blockage, pneumothorax or ventilator failure, and as long as the arterial pH is acceptable, high pCO_2 levels can be safely tolerated (permissive hypercapnoea). Active weaning from ventilation is vital[86].

In infants whose condition deteriorates despite maximal ventilation, extra-corporeal membrane oxygenation (ECMO) should be considered. A preliminary report of ECMO in 12 infants with bronchiolitis and refractory hypoxia despite maximal ventilation is encouraging[127]. Current trials should clarify the role of ECMO in bronchiolitis.

Vaccination

Attempts to produce an effective safe vaccine over the last 25 years have failed. Early formalin-inactivated or live vaccines failed to protect against RSV infection and enhanced rather than reduced the severity of subsequent natural infection[128]. These failures reflect the complex immune processes involved in RSV infection and the antigenic variation of the virus. Despite our increased understanding of the immuno-pathological process which molecular biology has brought, and advances in vaccine design, active immunisation against RSV remains a distant, perhaps unattainable, goal. Passive immunisation with intravenous high titre RSV immunoglobulin[129,130] may reduce the severity of infection in certain high-risk groups, but is not practicable for the general population.

Outcome of bronchiolitis

Although the acute phase of RSV bronchiolitis normally lasts 10–20 days, many children suffer from recurrent episodes of cough, wheeze and breathlessness for many months, and in some cases, for years after the acute illness[105]. These recurrent episodes of airways obstruction can be indistinguishable from exacerbations of infantile asthma and indeed the children often respond to bronchodilator and anti-inflammatory inhaled treatment. The complex relationship between asthma and post-bronchiolitic wheeze continues to be a source of intense debate[2,105,131].

Pneumonia

Studies of community-acquired pneumonia in adults have shown that almost 90% of episodes are caused by just three organisms: *Streptococcus pneumoniae* (60–75%), *M. pneumoniae* (5–18%), and *H. influenzae* B (4–5%)[132,133]. Apart from pneumonia caused by the influenza virus during epidemics (6–8%), other viruses account for only 2–8% of all adult episodes. Bases on these studies, clear guidelines on the management of pneumonia in adults have been established[134,135].

Unfortunately, there are few similar studies of childhood pneumonia[10,15,136]. Many questions about the incidence, aetiology and optimal management of pneumonia in children remain unanswered. This ignorance reflects the lack of a practical clinical definition of pneumonia, the wide spectrum of viruses, bacteria and other micro-organisms that cause pneumonia in different age groups of children, and the difficulties in identifying causative pathogens in children.

Incidence

Pneumonia is defined pathologically as acute inflammatory consolidation of the alveoli or infiltration of the interstitium of the lung with inflammatory cells, or a combination of both of these. Frequently there is associated inflammatory exudate in the small bronchi and bronchioles[2]. This definition is of limited clinical value. In children, and especially in infants, the clinical signs of pneumonia are quite non-specific and diagnosis depends on radiological evidence of inflammation and consolidation. Many cases of pneumonia pass undiagnosed in the community as the children are not seriously ill and chest radiographs are not performed.

In an 11-year study in an American paediatric group practice, Murphy *et al.* showed that the peak incidence of pneumonia (40 episodes/1000 children/year, was between 6 months and 5 years of age, falling to a rate of 11 episodes/1000 children/year over the age of nine[136]. Pneumonia accounted for 23% of 6000 episodes of lower respiratory infection[10]. The incidence is influenced by many factors which makes comparison of data from different populations difficult. Poor socioeconomic status, the number of siblings within the home[137], parental smoking[11] and preterm delivery[138] are all associated with an increased incidence of pneumonia in early childhood. Children from urban communities are twice as likely to be admitted to hospital with pneumonia as those from rural populations[137]. In general, pneumonia is more common in the winter months, but the seasonal incidence varies with the responsible pathogen[2,10]: RSV causes annual winter epidemics of pneumonia, whereas *M. pneumoniae* is endemic, with epidemics every 4 years[139].

Although the mortality from pneumonia has steadily fallen in developed countries, deaths do still occur. In 1992, there were 125 deaths from pneumonia in children in England and Wales: 78% were in children less than a year old, and the male to female ratio was 1.66 :1. Pneumonia accounted for more childhood deaths than all other respiratory illnesses put together[4].

Age and aetiology

The spectrum of organisms which cause pneumonia in children is different and wider than that in adults: in childhood, viruses and *Mycoplasma* are much more common causes of pneumonia than bacteria. Age has a marked influence on the susceptibility to a particular pathogen (Table 23.6): an understanding of the different organisms that cause pneumonia at different ages is essential to manage the episode appropriately.

Neonatal pneumonia

In the newborn period, pneumonia is usually caused by organisms acquired from the mother's genital tract during or immediately before delivery[140,141]. Group B streptococcus (*Streptococcus galactiae*), a vaginal commensal in 10–20% of pregnant women, and Gram-negative bacteria such as *E. coli* or *Klebsiella pneumoniae*, are the most frequent pathogens. *Listeria monocytogenes*, pneumococcus, *H. influenzae*, and *S. aureus* and *Staphylococcus epidermidis* are less common causes of pneumonia in the newborn period[140]. Pneumonia due to viruses such as cytomegalovirus or herpes simplex infection in the mother during pregnancy is uncommon and usually part of a multisystem intrauterine infection of the foetus. Infection due to the usual childhood respiratory viruses are notably uncommon in this age group.

In some populations in the United States, *C. trachomatis* is the commonest cause of pneumonia in the first two months of life[142–144]. As this organism is acquired from the maternal genital tract during birth, the low incidence of chlamydial pneumonia in Britain, which was two cases per thousand live-births in one prospective study[145], reflects the low incidence of genital carriage of *Chlamydia* in British mothers.

Pneumonia in the first 3 years

Between 1 month and 3 years of age, most pneumonias are viral in origin[2,10,15,136]. RSV is the most common pathogen, but parainfluenza types 1 and 3, influenza A and B and adenoviruses types 1, 3, 7 and 21 are also important. Pneumococcus is the most common bacterial pathogen. *H. influenzae* B (HiB) is an important cause of pneumonia in the United States, but was rarely recognised in Britain or Australia[2,136], even before HiB vaccination programmes were introduced. Although infection with *M. pneumoniae* occurs frequently in this age group, mild infection without pneumonia is the usual manifestation[139,142]. The severe cavitating pneumonia caused by *S. aureus* is now rare[2].

Pneumonia in older children

Above 4 years of age, *M. pneumoniae* and the pneumococcus are the most frequently identified organisms and viruses become progressively less important. The role of *Chlamydia pneumoniae* in lower respiratory infections in older children and adolescents is as yet unclear[144,146,147].

Clinical features

Diagnosing pneumonia in a child is often more difficult than in an adult. The classical features of bronchial breathing, impaired percussion, and pleuritic pain, are uncommon in children. Often the only signs in a child are fever, tachypnoea, chest wall recession and scattered crackles. The younger the child, the less specific the clinical signs[148]. For example, in the newborn infant with pneumonia, recurrent apnoea, hypotension, tachypnoea and lethargy are the common presenting features[140].

In a few patients, distinctive clinical features suggest a specific pathogen. For example, the insidious onset of fever, headache and abdominal pain, followed by cough and crepitations in a previously well 8-year old suggest mycoplasmal infection. However, mycoplasmal pneumonia can also be clinically and radiologically indistinguishable from pneumococcal or staphylococcal infection[149,150]. *C. trachomatis* classically causes an afebrile pneumonia with a dry, staccato cough in the first 2 months of life[143], but viruses can produce an identical clinical picture.

The limitations of clinical diagnosis were illustrated in one study of 98 children with pneumonia[151]. Symptoms such as cough, dyspnoea, rhinorrhoea and abdominal pain, and signs such as fever, crepitations and otitis media, were present in similar proportions of children with viral and bacterial pneumonia. Wheeze was more frequent in viral infection but it is also common with mycoplasma.

A chest X-ray is usually essential to confirm pneumonia. Different patterns of inflammation, varying from lobar or segmental consolidation, to poorly defined alveolar shadowing (bronchopneumonia), or the 'ground-glass' appearance with air bronchograms seen in some neonatal pneumonias, may be present. It is not possible to distinguish reliably between viral and bacterial pneumonia[152,153]. This distinction is further hampered by the phenomenon of dual or multiple infection, where two or more organisms are present[15,77]. Pleural effusions and abscess formation are highly suggestive of bacterial infection.

Features of some specific pneumonias

Viral pneumonia

There is a wide spectrum of severity: many mild cases are treated as 'chest infections' at home. It is rarely possible to distinguish between the different viruses on clinical grounds. Systemic upset and high fever, sometimes with febrile convulsions, are more common with influenza and adenoviral pneumonias[2,154,155]. Severe adenoviral infections start with pharyngitis, conjunctivitis, a measles-like rash, and a high fever. Tachypnoea, wheezing and crackles on auscultation then appear. There may be evidence of widely disseminated infection with encephalitis, coagulation defects and myocardial involvement. The chest X-ray initially shows hyperinflation with patchy consolidation: atelectasis secondary to the associated severe bronchiolitis is common as the disease progresses. Dual infection is present in over a quarter of cases[154,155]. There is a high mortality, particularly in young or malnourished children[154].

Mycoplasmal pneumonia

This is the commonest pneumonia in children[2,10,139]. There is an insidious onset of dry cough, after a prodrome with coryza, marked constitutional upset and fever, and in some cases bullous myringitis, arthralgia and transient urticarial or maculopapular rashes. The cough becomes productive of mucoid sputum and is protracted: wheeze and crackles are present on examination. The chest X-ray typically shows perihilar infiltrates and widespread patchy shadowing, but pleural effusions and lobar consolidation can also occur[2,150].

C. trachomatis pneumonia

In developed countries, pneumonia due to this organism is seen only in young infants whose mothers are genital carriers of the organism[143]. The mothers are often asymptomatic, but may suffer from vaginal discharge or premature labour. The onset is usually when the child is 4–12 weeks of age[142,143], but a fulminating illness in the first two weeks of life has also been described[156]. The earliest respiratory signs in the affected infant are snuffles due to the associated naso-pharyngitis, conjunctivitis and a dry staccato cough. There is tachypnoea but the child is usually afebrile. A chest X-ray shows hyperinflation and interstitial infiltrates.

Bacterial pneumonias

Pneumococcus is the commonest bacterial cause of pneumonia, particularly in children aged between one month and three years[2,157]. It classically causes lobar consolidation, but it can also lead to bronchopneumonia. There is a rapid onset of high fever and dry cough: older children may complain of pain in the chest, abdomen or neck. *H. influenzae* causes a similar illness but the onset is often more insidious, and the defervescence with antibiotics less dramatic.

In the past *S. aureus* was a common cause of an acute and severe pneumonia, particularly in young children. It presented with rapidly progressive tachypnoea and respiratory distress, often accompanied by peripheral circulatory failure and acidosis. Radiologically there was evidence of bilateral consolidation. Abscess formation, empyema and pyopneumothoraces were common complications, and the mortality from the condition was higher than other forms of pneumonia. Nowadays, this infection is very uncommon unless there is a predisposing cause such as an underlying congenital abnormality of the lung, prematurity or recent measles[2].

Identifying the causative organism

There are serious limitations to the techniques used to identify pathogens in childhood pneumonia. Bacterial culture of nasal or pharyngeal swabs is unreliable as asymptomatic carriage of possible pathogens is common: for example, pneumococci can be isolated from the nasopharynx of a third of healthy children[157]. Few young children can expectorate sputum: if it is produced, it is easily contaminated with pharyngeal commensals. In newborn infants with pneumonia, culture of gastric and tracheal aspirates or of maternal cervical swabs should be performed, but is often unhelpful. Blood cultures are positive in 40% of cases of neonatal pneumonia[140] but in only 10–20% of older children with bacterial pneumonia[158,159]. Needle aspiration of the lung is positive in four-fifths of such children[158], but because of concerns about airleaks, this technique is rarely used. Culture of aspirated pleural fluid may be diagnostic if this is present.

The detection of pneumococcal or HiB antigen in serum or urine by counter immuno-electrophoresis, latex agglutination or co-agglutination is more sensitive than blood culture in childhood pneumonia[157,159]. Unfortunately, the high rates of both false-positive and false-negative results with these techniques limit their value.

Mycoplasmal infection is diagnosed by a fourfold rise in the complement fixation titre or a single titre of 1/128 or more: specific IgM antibody can be detected with enzyme-linked immunosorbent assay, and enzyme-linked immunoassays (EIA) and PCR techniques are also being used[139]. Serum cold agglutinins are detectable in 33–76% of patients, but are not specific for mycoplasmal infection[149]. Chlamydial infection is diagnosed by immunofluorescence, culture or serology. Viruses can be identified by immunofluorescence or culture of naso-pharyngeal aspirates, or by an increase in specific antibody titre. The total and differential white cell count and the C-reactive protein are of limited value in distinguishing between bacterial and viral infection[151].

Which investigations are of value in clinical management? Children who are well enough to be treated at home need no investigations provided there is a prompt response to therapy[160]. All children admitted to hospital with pneumonia should have blood cultures and a chest radiograph as an absolute minimum. Only if the child is severely ill on admission, or if there is an unsatisfactory response to treatment, are further investigations indicated. Bacterial antigen tests can give results within hours, but the results must be regarded with caution. The aspiration of pleural fluid and needle lung biopsy should be reserved for the severely ill child. The results of viral investigations rarely alter management and, apart from immuno-fluorescent studies, are often not available until after the acute phase of pneumonia. A single high titre of mycoplasma antibody can confirm recent infection. Even after extensive investigation, no pathogen is identified in 40–50% of cases of childhood pneumonia (in 14–53% of patients more than one pathogen is found)[151,159].

Management

Antibiotics

Because it is impossible to exclude the presence of bacterial infection, all children diagnosed as having pneumonia should be given antibiotics. As the identity of the causative pathogen is rarely known at the time the child presents, the initial choice of antibiotic is based mainly on the child's age and a knowledge of the likely pathogens in that age group.

In the newborn period, initial treatment should be with an aminoglycoside, such as gentamicin or netilmicin, and penicillin or ampicillin, to cover infection with group B streptococcus and Gram-negative organisms[140]. Cefotaxime is an alternative: if there is concern about staphylococcal infection, flucloxacillin should be added. Erythromycin is the antibiotic of choice for *C. trachomatis* infection.

In infants who are not severely ill, oral penicillin or amoxycillin with or without clavulanic acid, are effective. In severely ill children, an intravenous cephalosporin such as cefotaxime, or a penicillin, and an anti-staphylococcal agent, such as flucloxacillin, should be given. Over the age of 1 year, penicillin is the drug of choice: however, if there is no significant improvement within the first 48 hours of treatment, the possibility of HiB infection should be covered by using ampicillin or amoxycillin with or without clavulanic acid[160]. Over the age of 5 years, erythromycin should be considered if there are features suggesting mycoplasmal pneumonia, otherwise oral penicillin is appropriate. Antibiotic therapy may need to be changed when the results of bacteriological studies become available. Depending on the severity of the illness and the response to treatment, antibiotics should be given for 7–10 days: it is recommended that erythromycin is taken for 10–14 days. In staphylococcal pneumonia, intravenous and then oral antibiotics are required for 4–6 weeks[2].

General supportive care

As with bronchiolitis, children admitted to hospital with pneumonia require close observation. Oxygen should be given by face-mask, nasal cannulae or into a headbox if the child is distressed. Oxygen saturation should be measured on admission and continuously in children with severe respiratory distress.

Intravenous or nasogastric fluids may be required: as in bronchiolitis, excessive ADH secretion can lead to hyponatraemia in severe pneumonia, and some degree of fluid restriction may be necessary[90,91]. Anti-pyretics such as paracetamol or ibuprofen are effective. Mist therapy was used in the past but is of no proven benefit[2]. Physiotherapy is not valuable in the early phases of pneumonia, and indeed the disturbance involved can lead to worsening of respiratory distress and hypoxaemia. In the recovery phase of the illness, postural drainage and percussion is helpful in clearing secretions.

Complications and outcome

The prognosis for most children with pneumonia is of full recovery unless there is some underlying disorder such as immunodeficiency, cystic fibrosis or a congenital lung anomaly.

It often takes longer for the radiological abnormalities to recover than the child. For example, after staphylococcal pneumonia, there may be areas of consolidation or pneumatocoeles that persist for many months although the child is well. However, even in this illness, one of the most destructive and extensive pneumonias of childhood, full functional and radiological recovery is normal.

Permanent lung damage can occur after severe mycoplasmal infection or adenoviral pneumonia. Persistent collapse, bronchiolitis obliterans, bronchiectasis, and Swyer–James or MacLoed's syndrome, where there is a small hyperlucent lobe with impaired perfusion and ventilation, have been described after these infections in early childhood. Up to 40–70% of children with adenovirus type 7 pneumonia and bronchiolitis are left with some functional abnormality[22].

Acute respiratory infections in the developing world

The patterns of acute respiratory infection described so far in this chapter are those seen in children living in developed countries, where the mortality rates for these infections are significant but relatively low. It is important to appreciate that only 1–2% of all childhood deaths from respiratory infection occur in the developed world: the remaining 98–99% of deaths occur in developing countries[14]. Globally, it is estimated that 3.5–4 million of the 13 million children aged less than 5 years who die each year die from an acute respiratory infection (ARI)[161].

Over 80% of these respiratory deaths are due to pneumonia. Deaths from bronchiolitis and measles laryngotracheitis are also important, but deaths from epiglottitis and simple viral croup are relatively uncommon in the developing world. It is estimated that approximately half a million of the respiratory deaths in this age group are a complication of measles and that a further 200 000 are the result of pertussis[161]. As in the developed world, 75–80% of these childhood deaths occur in children who are less than a year old. Malnutrition increases both the frequency and severity of respiratory infections, whilst breast-feeding confers some protection[12,13]. Overcrowding, poverty, poor parental education and pollution are all important adverse influences[14].

Aetiology and treatment

Over the last 15 years, research into acute respiratory infections in the developing world has led to important recommendations about appropriate management[162]. In contrast to the developed world, bacterial pneumonia is the most common serious respiratory infection. *S. pneumoniae*, and both typable and non-typable strains of *H. influenzae*, are the most frequent pathogens, accounting for over half of all cases[14,163]. *S. aureus*, *K. pneumoniae* and *H. para-influenzae* are also important (Table 23.7). Dual infections with two bacterial pathogens or, more commonly, with a bacterial and a viral pathogen are common. Infection with viruses, particularly with RSV, is common, but secondary bacterial infection occurs much more commonly than in the developed world[14,161]. Infections with *Pneumocystis carinii* and *Mycobacterium tuberculosis* are of ever-increasing importance in areas where HIV infection is prevalent, such as parts of East Africa.

Table 23.7. *Aetiology of pneumonia in children*

Age	Common pathogens	Uncommon pathogens
Neonate (<4 weeks)	Group B streptococci *E. coli* *S. aureus*	*H. influenzae* *S. pneumoniae* *Listeria monocytogenes* *C. trachomatis* *P. aeruginosa*
1 m – 2 years	RSV Parainfluenza viruses Influenza viruses *S. pneumoniae*	Respiratory viruses Adenoviruses *H. influenzae* B *S. aureus* *C. trachomatis*
2 – 12 years	*S. pneumoniae* *M. pneumoniae*	Respiratory viruses *H. influenzae* B

The overall incidence of acute infections is surprisingly similar to that in the developed world, indicating that the markedly higher specific mortality rates in the developing countries reflect severity rather than frequency[14]. One reason for these high mortality rates is the limited availability of both diagnostic and therapeutic resources for the management of affected children[164]. This lack of resources has stimulated the development of management protocols that can be easily implemented by local health workers.

Several simple clinical assessments have been developed to diagnose and assess the severity of pneumonia accurately[162]. These depend on the recognition of rapid breathing, such as greater than 50–60 breaths a minute in infants or more than 40 breaths a minute in children aged between 12 and 25 months, and recession of the lower chest wall[165]. Expiratory grunting is a less reliable screening sign. Cyanosis can be difficult to detect in dark-skinned children or in those with anaemia, and is a late sign of severe disease[166]. In older children and in the newborn the diagnosis of pneumonia is more difficult: distinction from other illnesses such as malaria or heart failure can present problems.

The introduction of internationally accepted guidelines for diagnosis and treatment has led to reductions in mortality rates of 25–67% in different studies[161]. Oral antibiotics such as chloramphenicol with or without penicillin V, cotrimoxazole or amoxycillin have all been used successfully. It is recognised that children with significant hypoxaemia at presentation are at higher risk of death and the use supplemental oxygen has been assessed. It is difficult to assess the degree of hypoxaemia clinically but objective measures such as pulse oximetry are often unavailable[166]. Oxygen given through a nasopharyngeal feeding catheter is more efficient than delivery through a face-mask or head-box[102]. Oxygen concentrators are much more cost-effective than oxygen cylinders but require capital and electricity to function[166].

As well as management guidelines for acute episodes, preventative approaches are being pursued. More effective immunisation programmes against *S. pneumoniae*, HiB, pertussis and measles are difficult to implement in poor countries but could significantly reduce the toll of acute respiratory infections. Better nutrition, with the promotion of breast feeding and vitamin supplementation, and improved education of health workers and the general population also merit investment.

The child with recurrent lower respiratory tract infections

Although all children suffer from respiratory infections, they vary greatly in the number they develop. This variation often reflects the environmental and host factors described earlier in this chapter, but in some children repeated infections indicate an abnormal predisposition to respiratory illness. Parental concern about repeated chest infections or a recurrent or persistent cough is a common reason for referral to a paediatrician.

Causes of recurrent cough

There are many different causes of a recurrent cough in a child (Table 23.8). One of the commonest is asthma. Community surveys have consistently shown that many children with asthma have been labelled as suffering from recurrent chest infections or bronchitis. As viral URTIs are the commonest trigger of acute asthmatic episodes in children, it is not surprising that infection of the lower respiratory tract is overdiagnosed. The presence of recurrent wheeze and breathlessness as well as cough, or a personal or family history of atopic conditions such as allergic rhinitis or eczema, and the classical trigger factors for childhood asthma, all support a diagnosis of asthma.

Many children for whom there is concern about recurrent infections are simply experiencing the number that occur at different ages in normal healthy children[10,167]. In others, a persistent cough is the result of an acute infection with pertussis, mycoplasma, or in the younger child, with RSV. With these infections, a cough, sometimes associated with wheeze or the production of clear mucus, can persist for several months. An inhaled foreign body or recurrent aspiration of feeds may also present as recurrent or persistent infection. Some children develop a debilitating habit or psychogenic cough after a minor acute infection. Cough is more common in children whose mothers smoke and in those who actively smoke themselves[11].

Chronic suppurative lung disease

An important minority of children with a recurrent or persistent cough produce purulent sputum or have repeated episodes of pneumonia. (The term bronchiectasis is sometimes used to describe some of these children but this is strictly a radiological or histological diagnosis.) These children merit detailed assessment to establish the cause of their infections, to decide on appropriate treatment and to prevent the progression of lung damage (Table 23.9).

Table 23.8. *Causes of recurrent or persistent cough*

Asthma
Recurrent 'normal' infections
Prolonged infection (e.g. pertussis, *Mycoplasma*)
Aspiration (Gastro-oesophageal reflux, inco-ordinate swallowing)
Habit/psychogenic cough
Cigarette smoking (active/passive)
Intrabronchial foreign body
Suppurative lung disease

Table 23.9. *Causes of suppurative lung disease*

Cystic fibrosis
Post-infective (e.g. adenovirus, pertussis)
Tuberculosis
Ciliary abnormalities
Congenital abnormalities
Foreign body
Immunodeficiency

Cystic fibrosis

Cystic fibrosis is the commonest cause of chronic suppurative lung disease in children, affecting one in 2500 births in Caucasians (see Chapter 24). Most affected children present with recurrent chest infections in early childhood and over 90% also have malabsorption and failure to thrive due to exocrine pancreatic insufficiency. About 10–20% present with intestinal obstruction due to meconium ileus in the first days of life: others are diagnosed because of a family history of this autosomal recessive condition. Viscid mucus in the small airways predisposes to chronic infection, initially with *S. aureus* or *Haemophilus* spp., but later with *P. aeruginosa*. The infection, and the inflammatory response to it, lead to progressive damage of the bronchial wall and bronchiectasis.

Bronchial obstruction

In the past, many cases of childhood bronchiectasis followed acute infections, classically pertussis or measles[168]. This is now rare, but permanent airway damage, with persistent atelectasis, bronchiolitis obliterans and chronic infection is seen after severe adenoviral pneumonia[155]. In other children, persistent lobar or segmental collapse after an acute infection becomes a focus for chronic inflammation and suppuration. The possibility of an inhaled foreign body should always be considered in a young child who develops a persistent productive cough, particularly if there has been an acute onset of respiratory symptoms after an episode of choking.

Ciliary abnormalities

An increasing number of defects of the structure or function of the cilia of the respiratory epithelium have been recognised in recent years[169]. Children with immotile or dyskinetic cilia have abnormal mucociliary clearance and present with a persistent productive cough and later with the features of bronchiectasis. As the epithelium of the upper respiratory tract is also affected, chronic purulent rhinitis, sinusitis, and middle ear disease are often also present. Half the children with classical Kartagener's syndrome have situs inversus with dextrocardia in addition to these features[169]. Affected males are infertile because of immotile spermatozoa.

Congenital abnormalities of the lung

Recurrent or persistent chest infections are common in children with congenital abnormalities of the airways or lung parenchyma. For example, repeated episodes of pneumonia affecting one lobe are often the presenting feature of lobar sequestration, lung cysts, bronchial stenosis and cystadenomatoid malformations of the lung. Children born with oesophageal atresia and tracheo-oesophageal fistula often have repeated episodes of pneumonia and bronchitis in early life as a result of persisting abnormalities of airway and oesophageal function[170].

Tuberculosis

Tuberculosis should be considered in any child with a persistent productive cough, particularly if there are associated systemic features such as nocturnal fever, weight loss or general malaise. However, many infected children are asymptomatic and their infection may only be detected on contact or school screening.

The pulmonary manifestations of TB in children are similar to those described in adults (see Chapter 15). Since most tuberculous infections are transmitted by inhalation, primary lesions occur in the lungs in over 95% of infected children[171]. As with adults there are several different possible clinical and radiological patterns of lung disease that can develop from the primary complex[171,172]. These include the development of effusions, cavitation, bronchial obstruction due to mediastinal lymphadenopathy with atelectasis or distal emphysema, tuberculous pneumonia, endobronchial tuberculosis, or miliary disease. Extrapulmonary manifestations, of which tuberculous meningitis is the most serious, are more common in children than in immunocompetent adults. As in adults diagnosis depends on a high index of suspicion, skin testing, radiology, and the bacteriological assessment of appropriate specimens.

Immunodeficiency disorders

The respiratory tract is the organ system most commonly involved in a wide variety of immunodeficiency disorders. A defect of immune function should be considered in all children who have respiratory infections that are unusually severe, recurrent, unresponsive to conventional treatment, or atypical[173]. Common associated features in immunodeficiency disorders include failure to thrive, which is often associated with gastrointestinal disease, severe atopy, and auto-immune disease. Many primary immunodeficiencies are inherited disorders and a family history of severe infections or early death should be sought.

A detailed description of the complex aetiology of immunodeficiencies and their management in children has been provided by Haeney and Kattan[173,174]. Conventionally, these disorders are separated into primary (congenital) or secondary (acquired) immunodeficiencies.

Primary immunodeficiencies can be classified[173] into

(i) Defects of antibody production
  e.g. a-gamma-globulinaemia
  IgG subclass deficiency

(ii) Defects of cellular immunity
  e.g. DiGeorge syndrome

(iii) Abnormalities of phagocytic function
  e.g. chronic granulomatous disease
  cyclical neutropenia

(iv) Complement disorders.

In the past, secondary immunodeficiencies were most commonly the consequence of serious diseases such as malignancy, or sickle cell anaemia, immunosuppressive treatment, measles, malnutrition or prematurity, but in many countries, infection with human immunodeficiency virus (HIV) is now by far the commonest cause of an acquired immunodeficiency (see below).

The nature of the immune defect determines the susceptibility to particular microorganisms (Table 23.10) and the nature and the severity of the clinical features. Identifying the pathogen is therefore not only important in deciding on what appropriate treatment should be, but it may also indicate which component of the immune system is defective. For example, identification of *P. carinii* and CMV in bronchial lavage fluid from a child with interstitial pneumonia would suggest a defect of T-cell mediated function, whilst recurrent cavitating staphylococcal pneumonia which was refractory to appropriate antibiotic treatment might suggest a neutrophil defect, such as chronic granulomatous disease. Further clues as to the nature of the immune defect may be provided by the coexistence of associated defects, such as thymic aplasia and congenital heart disease in DiGeorge syndrome, or severe eczema and thrombocytopenia in children with the Wiskott–Aldrich syndrome.

Assessment of the child with chronic suppurative lung disease

The history often gives valuable clues to the cause of a chronic purulent cough. The examination may reveal important signs such as wheeze, crackles, hyperinflation, digital clubbing, hepatosplenomegaly or nasal disease.

The plain chest X-ray is valuable in assessing the severity and distribution of lung involvement. Widespread changes such as bronchial wall thickening or inflammation involving several lobes would suggest cystic fibrosis, immotile cilia or an immunodeficiency disorder. Focal changes are more common if there is a congenital abnormality, an inhaled foreign body or bronchial obstruction for some other reason. Computerised tomography is helpful for assessing congenital anatomical abnormalities, such as a sequestration. High resolution CT is also more sensitive than plain radiographs at revealing bronchiectatic changes and has largely replaced bronchography. Isotope scans can provide useful regional evidence about ventilation and perfusion.

All children with persistent cough should have their sweat electrolytes measured. The sweat test remains the standard diagnostic test for CF, although DNA analysis is being used increasingly. Other investigations include bacteriological and viral studies on sputum if this can be produced; viral and mycoplasmal antibody levels; and in selected cases, immune function tests. The latter should ideally be planned with a clinical immunologist. Which immune tests are performed will depend on the nature and severity of the respiratory symptoms (Table 23.11). For example, in the child who has repeated

Table 23.10. *Immunodeficiencies: predominant infective organisms*

Antibody deficiency (B-cell)	HiB, pneumococcus other pyogenic bacteria *Giardia lamblia* ECHO virus
Defective cellular immunity (T-cell)	Viruses (CMV, Herpes, RSV, measles, entero) *Pneumocystis carinii* *Candida, Aspergillus* *Mycobacteria*
Phagocyte disorders	*Staphylococcus, Klebsiella* *Candida, Aspergillus*
Complement deficiencies	Pneumococcus Meningococcus

Table 23.11. *Immunodeficiencies: investigations*

Antibody deficiency	Immunoglobulins (G, A, M, E) IgG subclasses Specific antibodies B-cell populations
Defective cellular immunity	White cell differential Chest X-ray (thymic shadow) Lymphocyte populations Mitogen responses
Phagocyte defects	White cell differential Chemotaxis, phagocytosis, Nitroblue tetrazolium test
Complement deficiency	C3, C4, CH 50 levels

episodes of cough with purulent sputum containing *pneumococcus*, but who is otherwise well with no clinical or radiological evidence of lung damage, measurement of immunoglobulin and immunoglobulin sub-class levels, and specific antibody levels against pneumococcus and HiB would be appropriate, as a specific antibody deficiency is the most likely diagnosis. By contrast, a child with severe opportunistic pneumonia demands a detailed assessment of cellular and humoral immune function.

Flexible fibreoptic bronchoscopy is playing an increasingly important role in the assessment of children with chronic lung sepsis or suspected immunodeficiency. Microbiological and cellular specimens can be obtained by suction, by the use of a protected brush, or by bronchoalveolar lavage. Bronchoscopy also allows a detailed evaluation of airway anatomy and dynamics.

Pulmonary infection in the child with HIV infection

Soon after AIDS was first described in adults and the human immunodeficiency virus (HIV) was identified as its cause, it became evident that children could also be affected and that their clinical course and manifestations were different from those seen in adults. HIV infection has been dealt in Chapter 22: in this section the different characteristics of HIV infection in children are addressed.

Table 23.12. *Pulmonary complications of HIV infection*

Infections		
	Protozoa	*Pneumocystis carinii*
	Viruses	Cytomegalovirus
		RSV
		Adenovirus
		Influenza and parainfluenza
		Herpes simplex, Varicella zoster
	Bacteria	Encapsulated (e.g. HiB, *Pneumococcus*)
		Gram-negative (e.g. *E. coli, Klebsiella*)
		Mycobacteria
	Fungi	*Candida*
		Aspergillus
Malignancies		
Interstitial pneumonitis		
		e.g. Lymphoid interstitial pneumonitis
		Pulmonary lymphoid hyperplasia

Epidemiology

Although they account for only 2% of cases of AIDS in the developed world, in the developing world up to 25% of infected individuals are children[174,175]. As vertical transmission from mother to infant is by far the commonest mode of infection, the prevalence of HIV infection in child-bearing women is important. This varies from 0.15% in the United States, to 3% in parts of New York, to between 5 and 30% in parts of Africa[175]. The transmission rates from infected mother to infant are also much higher in Africa (45%) than in Europe (13%). The other important method of infection has been through infected blood products, but with screening this is now less common.

Pathogenesis

The virus infects the CD4 helper-inducer subset of T-lymphocytes: B-lymphocytes and macrophages are also involved[175]. The impaired cellular immunity predisposes the child, who already has a relatively immature immune system, to opportunistic infections with a wide range of organisms (Table 23.12). In adults, serious infection is likely once the CD4 count is less than 200/mm^3, but in children, who normally have much higher absolute numbers of CD4 cells, infections such as *P. carinii* pneumonia (PCP) can occur with CD4 counts of over 1000/mm^3. B-cell dysfunction is also much more prominent than in adults, and overwhelming bacterial infections, such as pneumococcal sepsis, are common.

Clinical features

Children have a much shorter incubation period for clinical disease than adults: half the children with perinatally acquired HIV infection become symptomatic within the first year of life[174,175].

Respiratory illnesses are the leading presenting feature of AIDS in children (Table 23.12), but lymphadenopathy, hepatosplenomegaly, failure to thrive and bacterial sepsis are also important.

PCP is the commonest pulmonary infection. The median age at presentation is 4–5 months. In some children the classical features of tachypnoea, cough, fever and cyanosis, with a chest X-ray that shows a ground-glass appearance, are present, but in others the features are non-specific. Diagnosis depends on identification of the organism on broncho-alveolar lavage fluid. Treatment is with high-dose co-trimoxazole for 3 weeks. The mortality in children is approximately 50%.

Other important opportunistic infections include CMV and herpes simplex pneumonitis and fungal infections. The respiratory viruses normally encountered in childhood, such as RSV and parainfluenza, represent major risks for these children. Mycobacterial infection, with *M. tuberculosis*, or less commonly *Mycobacterium avium–intracellulare*, are also important in populations where infection with these organisms is prevalent, such as parts of Africa.

Other non-infective lung diseases are common in children with AIDS. Several forms of interstitial pneumonitis are now recognised. In one of these, lymphoid interstitial pneumonitis (LIP), Epstein–Barr viral infection of lung tissue has been demonstrated: the significance of this is unclear.

Management

As PCP is the commonest lung infection in this group of children, prophylaxis is of vital importance. Co-trimoxazole remains the agent of choice, but pentamidine and dapsone have both been used in children. The role of zidovudine in lung disease remains unclear. The incidence of infection in children with low CD4 counts can be reduced by giving regular intravenous immunoglobulin infusions. In children who develop an acute lung infection, prompt identification of the causative organism is essential, if necessary by BAL or even open lung biopsy. A number of anti-viral agents have been successfully used including ribavirin (for RSV), gancyclovir and foscarnet (for CMV), and acyclovir (for HSV). In children exposed to varicella zoster or measles, hyperimmune globulin if given before infection is well established can be effective. Bacterial infections are treated in the normal fashion.

References

1. LUNG AND ASTHMA INFORMATION AGENCY. The burden of respiratory disease. *Factsheet 95/3* Lung and Asthma Information Agency, Dept of Public Health Sciences, St George's Hospital, London;1995.
2. ACUTE RESPIRATORY INFECTIONS. In Phelan PD, Olinsky A, Robertson CF. *Respiratory Illness in Children*. Oxford: Blackwell, 1994, pp 27–93.
3. HILL AM. Trends in paediatric medical admissions. *Br Med J* 1989;298:1479–83.
4. OFFICE OF POPULATION CENSUSES AND SURVEYS. *Mortality Statistics 1992: Childhood, DH6 no. 6* HMSO London;1994.
5. GARENNE M, RONSMANS C, CAMPBELL H. The magnitude of mortality from acute respiratory infections in children under five years of age in developing countries. *World Health Stat Q* 1992;45:180–91.
6. NICHOLS DG. Respiratory muscle performance in infants and children. *J Pediatr* 1991;118:493–502.
7. DAVIES GM, COATES AL. Maturation of airway mechanics. In Loughlin GM, Eigin H, eds. *Respiratory Disease in Children*. Baltimore: Williams and Wilkins; 1994: Chapter 1.
8. GAULTIER C. Maturation of respiratory control. In Loughlin GM, Eigin H, eds. *Respiratory Disease in Children*. Baltimore: Williams and Wilkins;1994: Chapter 2.
9. IMMUNOLOGICAL SYSTEM. In Behrman RE, Vaughan VC, eds *Nelson Textbook of Pediatrics*, Philadelphia: WB Saunders; 1987: Chapter 10:456.
10. DENNY FW, CLYDE WA. Acute lower respiratory tract infections in non-hospitalised children. *J Pediatr* 1986;108:635–46.
11. COURIEL JM. Passive smoking and the health of children. *Thorax* 1994;49:731–4.
12. HOWIE PW, FORSYTH JS, OGSTON SA, CLARK A, FLOREY C. Protective effect of breast feeding against infection. *BMJ* 1990;300:11–6.
13. BEAUDRY M, DUFOUR R, MARCOUX S. Relation between infant feeding and infections during the first six months of life. *J Pediatr* 1995;126:191–7.
14. GRAHAM NMH. Respiratory infections. In Pless IB, ed. *The Epidemiology of Childhood Disorders*. Oxford: Oxford University Press; 1994: Chapter 7:173–210.
15. RAY CG, HOLBERG CJ, MINNICH LL *et al.* Acute respiratory illnesses during the first three years of life; potential roles for various etiologic agents. *Pediatr Infect Dis J* 1993;12:10–14.
16. TOMS GL. Respiratory syncytial virus – how soon will we have a vaccine? *Arch Dis Child* 1995;72:1–5.
17. ANAS N, BOETTRICH C, HALL CB, BROOKS JG. The association of apnea and respiratory syncytial virus infection in infants. *J Pediatr* 1982;101:65–8.
18. CHURCH NR, ANAS NG, HALL CB, BROOKS J. Respiratory syncytial virus-related apnea in infants. *Am J Dis Child* 1984;138:247–50.
19. RAKSHI K, COURIEL JM. The management of bronchiolitis. *Arch Dis Child* 1994;71:463–9.
20. RUUSKANEN O, VAAHTORANTA-LEHTONEN, MEURMAN O. Adenovirus infection of the respiratory tract. In David TJ, ed. *Recent Advances in Paediatrics* Edinburgh: Churchill Livingstone;1994: Vol. 11:19–31.
21. MURTAGH P, CERQUIEO C, HALAC A, AVILA M, KAJON A. Adenovirus type 7h respiratory infections: a report of 29 cases of acute lower respiratory disease. *Acta Paediat* 1993;82:557–61.
22. SLY PD, SOTO-QUIROS ME, LANDAU LI, HUDSON I, NEWTON-JOHN H. Factors predisposing to abnormal pulmonary function after adenovirus type 7 pneumonia. *Arch Dis Child* 1984:59:935–9.
23. COURIEL JM. Management of croup. *Arch Dis Child* 1988;63:1305–8.
24. NEWTH CJL, LEVISON H, BRYAN AC. The respiratory status of children with croup. *J Pediatr* 1972;81:1068–73.
25. CHERRY JD. The treatment of croup: continued controversy due to failure of recognition of historic, ecologic, etiologic and clinical perspectives. *J Pediatr* 1979;94:352–4.
26. CHERRY JD. Croup (laryngitis, laryngotracheitis, spasmodic croup, and laryngotracheobronchitis). In Feigin RD, Cherry JD, eds. *Pediatric Infectious Diseases*, Philadelphia: WB Saunders, 1992: vol. 1:209–20.
27. DENNY FW, MURPHY TF, CLYDE WA. Croup: an 11-year study in a pediatric practice. *Pediatrics* 1983;71:871–6.
28. WAGENER J, LANDAU LI, OLINSKY A, PHELAN PD. Management of children hospitalised for laryngo-tracheobronchitis. *Pediat Pulmonol* 1986;2:159–62.
29. MILLS JL, SPACKMAN TJ, BORNS P

MANDELL GA, SCHWARTZ MW. The usefulness of lateral neck roentgenograms in laryngotracheo-bronchitis. *Am J Dis Child* 1979;133:1140–2.

30. SKOLNIK NS. Treatment of croup: a critical review. *Am J Dis Child* 1989;143:1045–9.

31. ZACH M, ERBEN A, OLINSKY A. Croup, recurrent croup, allergy, and airways hyperreactivity. *Arch Dis Child* 1981;56:331–41.

32. ZACH M, SCHNALL RP, LANDAU LI. Upper and lower airway hyperactivity in recurrent croup. *Am Rev Respir Dis* 1980;121:979–83.

33. LANDAU LI, GEELHOED GC. Aerosolised steroids for croup. *NEJM* 1994;331:322–3.

34. BOURCHIER D, DAWSON KP, FERGUSSON DM. Humidification in viral croup: a controlled trail. *Aust Paediatr J* 1984:20:289–91.

35. ADAIR JC, RING WH, JORDAN WS, ELWYN RA. Ten-year experience with intermitent positive pressure breathing in treatment of acute laryngotracheobronchitis. *Anesth Analg* 1971;50:649–55.

36. TAUSSIG LM, CASTRO O, BEAUDRY PH, FOX WW, BUREAU M. Treatment of laryngotracheobronchitis (croup). *Am J Dis Child* 1975;129:790–3.

37. FOGEL JM, BERG J, GERBER MA, SHERTER CB. Racemic epinephrine in the treatment of croup: nebulization alone versus nebulization with intermittent positive pressure breathing. *J Pediatr* 1982;101:1028–31.

38. WAISMAN Y, KLEIN BL, BOENNING DA, YOUNG GM, CHAMBERLAIN JM, O'DONNELL R, OCHSENSCHLAGER DW. Prospective randomised double-blind study comparing L-epinephrine and racemic epinephrine aerosols in the treatment of laryngotracheitis (croup). *Pediatrics* 1992;89:302–6.

39. LENNEY W, MILNER AD. Treatment of acute viral croup. *Arch Dis Child* 1978;53:704–6.

40. ANON. Steroids and croup (Editorial). *Lancet* 1989;2:1134–6.

41. TUNNESSEN WW, FEINSTEIN AR. The steroid-croup controversy: an analytic review of methodologic problems. *J Pediatr* 1980;96:751–6.

42. SUPER DM, CARTELLI NA, BROOKS LJ, LEMBO RM, KUMAR ML. A prospective randomised double-blind study to evaluate the effect of dexamethasone in acute laryngotracheitis. *J Pediatr* 1989;115:323–9.

43. TIBBALLS J, SHANN FA, LANDAU LI. Placebo-controlled trial of prednisolone in children intubated for croup. *Lancet* 1992;340:745–8.

44. KAIRYS SW, OLMSTEAD EN, O'CONNOR GT. Steroid treatment of laryngotracheitis: a meta-analysis of the evidence from randomised trials. *Pediatrics* 1989;83:683–3.

45. HUSBY S, AGERTOFT L, MORTENSEN S, PEDERSEN S. Treatment of croup with nebulised steroid (budesonide): a double blind, placebo controlled trial. *Arch Dis Child* 1992;68:352–5.

46. KLASSEN TP, FELDMAN ME, WATTERS LK, SUTCLIFFE T, ROWE PC. Nebulised budesonide for children with mild-to-moderate croup. *NEJM* 1994;331:285–9.

47. MCENIERY J, GILLIS J, KILHAM H, BENJAMIN B. Review of intubation in severe laryngotracheobronchitis. *Pediatrics* 1991;87:847–53.

48. LEAR GH, MCKENZIE SA, BORALESSA H. Management of acute upper airway obstruction in an intensive care unit in a district general hospital. *Arch Dis Child* 1990;65:241–6.

49. CRESSMAN ER, MYER CM. Diagnosis and management of croup and epiglottitis. *Pediatr Clin N Am* 1994;41:265–76.

50. FRIEDMAN EM, JORGENSEN K, HEALY GB, MCGILL TJI. Bacterial tracheitis. *Laryngoscope* 1985:95:9–11.

51. HAN BK, DUNBAR JS, STRIKER TW. Membranous laryngotracheo-bronchitis (membranous croup). *Am J Roentgenol* 1979;133:53–8.

52. HENRY RL, MELLIS C, BENJAMIN B. Pseudomembranous croup. *Arch Dis Child* 1983;58:180–3.

53. LISTON SL, GEHRZ RC, SIEGEL LG, TILELLI J. Bacterial tracheitis. *Am J Dis Child* 1983;137:764–7.

54. GALLAGHER PG, MYER CM. Membranous laryngotracheo-bronchitis in infants and children. *Pediatrics Emerg Care* 1991;7:337–42.

55. ECKEL HE, WIDEMANN B, DAMM M, ROTH B. Airway endoscopy in the diagnosis and treatment of bacterial tracheitis in children. *Int J Pediatr Otorhinolaryngol* 1993;27:147–57.

56. TROLLFORS B, NYLEN O, STRANGERT K. Acute epiglottitis in children and adults in Sweden 1981–3. *Arch Dis Child* 1990;65:491–4.

57. MAYO-SMITH MF, HIRSCH PJ, WODZINSKI SF, SCHIFFMAN FJ. Acute epiglottitis in adults: an eight-year experience in the state of Rhode Island. *NEJM* 1986;314:1133–9.

58. TAKALA AK, PELTOLA H, ESKILA J. Disappearance of epiglottitis during large scale vaccination with *Haemophilus influenzae* type B conjugate vaccine among children in Finland. *Laryngoscopy* 1994;104:731–5.

59. GORELICK MH, BAHER MD. Epiglottitis in children, 1979–1992. Effects of *Haemophilus influenzae*e type B immunisation. *Arch Pediatrics Adolesc Med* 1994;148:47–50.

60. COURIEL JM. Respiratory emergencies. In Advanced Life Support Group, eds. *Advanced Paediatric Life Support*. London: *BMJ Publications* 1993:61–72.

61. MAURO RD, POOLE SR, LOCKHART CH. Differentiation of epiglottitis from laryngotracheitis in the child with stridor. *Am J Dis Child* 1988:142:679–82.

62. LOSECK JD, DEWITZ-ZINK BA, MELZER-LANGE M *et al.* Epiglottitis: comparison of signs and symptoms in children less than two years old and older. *Ann Emerg Med* 1990;19:99–102.

63. BUTT W, SHANN F, WALKER C *et al.* Acute epiglottitis: a different approach to management. *Crit Care Med* 1988;16:43–7.

64. SAWYER SM, JOHNSON PD, HOGG G, ROBERTSON CF, OPPEDISANO F, MCINNES SJ, GILBERT GL. Successful treatment of epiglottitis with two doses of ceftriaxone. *Arch Dis Child* 1994;70:129–132.

65. COULTARD M, ISAACS D. Retropharyngeal abscess. *Arch Dis Child* 1991;66:1227–30.

66. CHERRY JD. Acute bronchitis. In Feigin RD, Cherry JD, eds *Pediatric Infectious Diseases*, 3rd ed, Philadelphia: WB Saunders;1992: vol. 1:197–209.

67. ISACSON J, TROLLFORS B, TARANGER J, ZACKRISSON G, LAGERGARD T. How common is whooping cough in a non-vaccinating country? *Pediatr Infect Dis J* 1993;12:284–8.

68. ANON. Pertussis, infants, and herds (Editorial). *Lancet* 1992:339:526–7.

69. JENKINSON D. Natural course of 500 consecutive cases of whooping cough: a general practice population study. *BMJ* 1995:310:299–302.

70. CHRISTIE CD, MARX ML, MARCHANT CD, REISING SF. The 1993 epidemic of pertussis in Cincinnati. Resurgence of the disease in a highly immunised population of children. *NEJM* 1994;331:16–21.

71. GROB PR, CROWDER MJ, ROBBINS JF. Effect of vaccination on severity and dissemination of whooping cough. *BMJ* 1981;282:1925–8.

72. GAN VN, MURPHY TV. Pertussis in hospitalised children. *Am J Dis Child* 1990;144:1130–4.

73. STREBEL PM, COCHI SL, FARIZO KM, PAYNE BJ, HANAUER SD, BAUGHMAN AL. Pertussis in Missouri: evaluation of nasopharyngeal culture, direct fluorescent antibody testing and clinical case definitions in the diagnosis of pertussis. *Clin Infect Dis* 1993;16:276–85.

74. KRANTZ I, BJURE J, CLAESSON I, ERIKSSON, SIXT R. TROLLFORS B. Respiratory sequelae and lung function after pertussis in infancy. *Arch Dis Child* 1990;65:569–73.

75. GORDON M, DAVIES HD, GOLD R.

Clinical and microbiologic features of children presenting with pertussis to a Canadian pediatric hospital during an eleven year period. *Pediatr Infect Dis J* 1994;13:617–22.
76. WOHL MEB, CHERNICK V. Bronchiolitis. *Am Rev Resp Dis* 1978;118:759–81.
77. TRISTRAM DA, MILLER RW, MCMILLAN JA, WEINER LB. Simultaneous infection with respiratory syncytial virus and other respiratory pathogens. *Am J Dis Child* 1988;142:834–6.
78. SEIDENBERG J, MASTERS IB, HUDSON I, OLINSKY A, PHELAN PD. Disturbance in respiratory mechanics in infants with bronchiolitis. *Thorax* 1989;44:660–7.
79. STOKES GM, MILNER AD, HODGES IGC, HENRY RL, ELPHICK MC. Nebulised therapy in acute severe bronchiolitis in infancy. *Arch Dis Child* 1983;58:279–83.
80. SIMPSON H, MATTHEW D, INGLIS JM, GEORGE EL. Virological findings and blood gas tensions in acute lower respiratory tract infections in children. *Br Med J* 1974; ii:629–32.
81. MULHOLLAND EK, OLINSKY A, SHANN FA. Clinical findings and severity of acute bronchiolitis. *Lancet* 1990;335:1259–61.
82. HALL CB, POWELL KR, MACDONALD NE, GALA CL, MENEGUS ME, SUFFIN SC, COHEN HJ. Respiratory syncytial virus infection in children with compromised immune function. *N Engl J Med* 1986;315:77–81.
83. MACDONALD NE, HALL CB, SUFFIN SC, ALEXSON C, HARRIS PJ, MANNING JA. Respiratory syncytial virus infection in infants with congenital heart disease. *N Engl J Med* 1982;307:397–400.
84. STRETTON M, AJIZIAN SJ, MITCHELL I, NEWTH CJ. Intensive care course and outcome of patients infected with respiratory syncytial virus. *Pediatr Pulmonol* 1992;13:143–50.
85. AMERICAN ACADEMY OF PEDIATRICS. Use of ribavirin in the treatment of respiratory syncytial virus infection. *Pediatrics* 1993;92:501–4.
86. RAKSHI K, COURIEL JM. The management of bronchiolitis. *Arch Dis Child* 1994;71:463–69.
87. LEBEL MH, GAUTHIER M, LACROIX J, ROUSSEAU E, BUITHIEU M. Respiratory failure and mechanical ventilation in severe bronchiolitis. *Arch Dis Child* 1989;64:1431–7.
88. DAWSON KP, LONF A, KENNEDY J, MOGRIDGE N. The chest radiograph in acute bronchiolitis. *J Paediatr Child Health* 1990;26:209–11.
89. WELLIVER RC, CHERRY JD. Bronchiolitis and infectious asthma. In Feigin RD, Cherry JD, eds, *Textbook of Pediatric Infectious Diseases*, 3rd Ed, 1992: Philadelphia: WB Saunders;1992:245–54.
90. RIVERS RPA, FORSLING ML, OLVER RP. Inappropriate secretion of antidiuretic hormone in infants with respiratory infections. *Arch Dis Child* 1981;56:358–63.
91. STEENSELL-MOLL HA, HAZELZET JA, VAN DER VOORT E, NEIJENS HJ, HACKENG WHL. Excessive secretion of antidiuretic hormone in infections with respiratory syncytial virus. *Arch Dis Child* 1990;65:1237–9.
92. MADGE P, PATON JY, MCCOLL JH, MACKIE PLK. Prospective controlled study of four infection-control procedures to prevent nosocomial infection with respiratory syncytial virus. *Lancet* 1992;340:1079–83.
93. BERMAN S, SIMOES EAF, LANATA C. Respiratory rate and pneumonia in infancy. *Arch Dis Child* 1991;66:81–4.
94. WANG EEL, MILNER RA, NAVAS L, MAJ H. Observer agreement for respiratory signs and oximetry in infants hospitalised with lower respiratory infections. *Am Rev Resp Dis* 1992;145:106–9.
95. SHAW KN, BELL LM, SHERMAN NH. Outpatient assessment of infants with bronchiolitis. *Am J Dis Child* 1991;145:151–5.
96. STEBBENS VA, POETS CF, ALEXANDER JR, ARROWSMITH WA, SOUTHALL DP. Oxygen saturation and breathing patterns in infancy. 1: Full term infants in the second month of life. *Arch Dis Child* 1991;66:569–73.
97. SOUTHALL DP, SAMUELS M. Inappropriate sensor application in pulse oximetry. *Lancet* 1992;340:481–2.
98. POETS CP, SAMUELS M, NOYES JP, JONES KA, SOUTHALL DP. Home monitoring of transcutaneous oxygen tension in the early detection of hypoxaemia in infants and young children. *Arch Dis Child* 1991;66:676–82.
99. ANON. Nosocomial infection with respiratory syncytial virus. *Lancet* 1992;340:1071–2.
100. ISAACS D, DICKSON H, O'CALLAGHAN C, SHEAVES R, WINTER A, MOXON ER. Handwashing and cohorting in the prevention of hospital acquired infection with respiratory syncytial virus. *Arch Dis Child* 1991;66:227–31.
101. O'CALLAGHAN C. Prevention of respiratory syncytial virus infection. *Lancet* 1993;341:182.
102. SHANN F, GATCHALIAN S, HUTCHINSON R. Naso-pharyngeal oxygen in children. *Lancet* 1988; ii:1238–40.
103. NEWCOMBE R W. Use of adrenergic bronchodilators by pediatric allergists and pulmonologists. *Am J Dis Child* 1989;143:481–5.
104. GOODMAN BT, CHAMBERS TL. Bronchodilators for bronchiolitis? *Lancet* 1993;341:1380.
105. MILNER AD, MURRAY M. Acute bronchiolitis in infancy: treatment and prognosis. *Thorax* 1989;44:1–5.
106. SOTO-QUIROS ME, SLY PD, UREN E, TAUSSIG LM, LANDAU LI. Bronchodilator response during acute viral bronchiolitis in infancy. *Pediatrics Pulmonol* 1985;l:85–90.
107. TEPPER RS, ROSENBERG D, EIGEN H, REISTER T. Bronchodilator responsiveness in infants with bronchiolitis. *Pediatr Pulmonol* 1994;17:81–5.
108. HENRY RL, MILNER AD, STOKES GM. Ineffectiveness of ipratropium bromide in acute brochiolitis. *Arch Dis Child* 1983;58:925–6.
109. KLASSEN TP, ROWE PC, SUTHCLIFFE T *et al*. Randomized trial of salbutamol in acute bronchiolitis. *J Pediatrics* 1991;118:807–11.
110. SCHUH S, CANNY G, REISMAN JJ *et al*. Nebulized albuterol in acute bronchiolitis. *J Pediatr* 1990:117:633–7.
111. WANG EEL, MILNER R, ALLEN U, MAJ A. Bronchodilators for treatment of mild bronchiolitis: a factorial randomised trial. *Arch Dis Child* 1992;67:298–93.
112. HO L, COLLIS G, LANDAU LI, LE-SOUEF PM. Effect of salbutamol on oxygen saturation in bronchiolitis. *Arch Dis Child* 1991;66:1061–4.
113. SANCHEZ I, DEKOSTER J, POWELL RE, WOLSTEIN R, CHERNICK V. Effect of racemic epinephrine and salbutamol on clinical score and pulmonary mechanics in infants with bronchiolitis. *J Pediatr* 1993;122:145–51.
114. SCHENA JA, CRONE RK, THOMPSON JE. The use of aminophylline in severe bronchiolitis. *Crit Care Med* 1984;12:225.
115. MEERT KL, SARNAIK AP, GELMINI MJ, LIEH-LAI MW. Aerosolised ribavirin in mechanically ventilated children with respiratory syncytial virus lower respiratory tract disease: a prospective double blind, randomised trial. *Crit Care Med* 1994;22:566–71.
116. SMITH DW, FRANKEL LR, MATHERS LH, TANG ATS, ARIAGNO RL, PROBER CG. A controlled trial of aerosol ribavirin in infants receiving mechanical ventilation for severe respiratory syncytial virus infection. *N Engl J Med* 1991;325:24–9.
117. WALD ER, DACHEFSKY B, GREEN M. In re ribavirin: a case of premature adjudication. *J Pediatr* 1988;112:154–8.
118. ISAACS D, MOXON ER, HARVEY D *et al*. Ribavirin in respiratory syncytial virus infection. A double blind placebo controlled trial is needed. *Arch Dis Child* 1988;63:986–90.
119. HALL CB, MCBRIDE JT, GALA CL *et al*. Ribavirin treatment in infants with underlying cardio-pulmonary disease. *JAMA* 1985;254:3047–51.
120. MOLER FW, BRANDY KP, CUSTER JR. Ribavirin for severe RSV infection. *N Engl J Med* 1991;325:1884.

121. LEER JA, BLOOMFIELD NJ, GREEN JL *et al.* Corticosteroid treatment in bronchiolitis: A controlled collaborative study in 297 infants and children. *Am J Dis Child* 1969:117:495–503.
122. SPRINGER C, BAR-YISHAY E, UWAYYED K *et al.* Corticosteroids do not affect the clinical or physiological status of infants with bronchiolitis. *Pediatr Pulmonol* 1990;9:181–5.
123. HALL CB, POWELL KR, SCHNABEL KC, GALA CL, PINCUS PH. Risk of secondary bacterial infection in infants hospitalised with respiratory syncytial virus infection. *J Pediatr* 1988;113:266–71.
124. RUUSKANEN O, PUTTO A, SARKKINEN H, MEURMAN O, IRJALA K. C-reactive protein in respiratory virus infection. *J Pediatr* 1985;107:97–100.
125. FRANKEL LR, LEWISTON NJ, SMITH DW, STEVENSON DK. Clinical observations on mechanical ventilation for respiratory failure in bronchiolitis. *Pediatr Pulmonol* 1986;2:307–11.
126. SMITH PJ, EL KHATIB MF, CARLO WA. PEEP does not improve pulmonary mechanics in infants with bronchiolitis. *Am Rev Resp Dis* 1993;147:1295–8.
127. STEINHORN RH, GREEN TP. Use of extra corporeal membrane oxygenation in the treatment of respiratory syncytial virus bronchiolitis: the national experience, 1983–1988. *J Pediatrics* 1990;116:337–42.
128. TOMS GL. Respiratory syncytial virus – how soon will we have a vaccine? *Arch Dis Child* 1995;72:1–5.
129. GROOTHUIS JR, SIMOES EAF, LEVIN MJ *et al.* Prophylactic administration of respiratory syncytial virus immunoglobulin to high risk infants and young children. *N Engl J Med* 1993;329:1524–30.
130. LEVIN MJ. Treatment and prevention options for respiratory syncytial virus infections. *J Pediatr* 1994;l24:S22–S27.
131. LANDAU LI. Bronchiolitis and asthma: are they related? *Thorax* 1994;49:293–96.
132. BRITISH THORACIC SOCIETY. Community-acquired pneumonia in adults in British Hospitals 1982–1983: a survey of aetiology, mortality, prognostic factors and outcome. *Quart J Med* 1987;62:195–220.
133. WOODHEAD MA, MACFARLANE JT, MCCRACKEN JS, ROSE DH, FINCH RG. Prospective study of the aetiology and outcome of pneumonia in the community. *Lancet* 1987; i: 671–4.
134. HARRISON BDW, FARR BM, CONNOLLY CK, MACFARLANE JT, SELKON JB, BARTLETT CLR. The hospital management of community-acquired pneumonia. *J Roy Coll Phys* 1987;21:267–9.
135. BRITISH THORACIC SOCIETY. Guidelines for the management of community-acquired pneumonia in adults admitted to hospital. *Br J Hosp Med* 1993;49:346–50.
136. MURPHY TH, HENDERSON FW, CLYDE WA, COLLIER AM, DENNY FW. Pneumonia: an eleven-year study in a pediatric practice. *Am J Epidemiol* 1981;113:12–21.
137. CLARKE SKR, GARDNER PS, POOLE PM, SIMPSON H, TOBIN JO. Respiratory syncytial virus infection: admissions to hospital in industrial, urban and rural areas. *Br Med J* 1978; ii:796–8.
138. MCCORMICK M, SHAPIRO S, STARFIELD BH. Rehospitalisation in the first year of life for high risk survivors. *Pediatrics* 1980;66:991–6.
139. ANON. Mycoplasma pneumoniae (Editorial). *Lancet* 1991;337:651–2.
140. ISAACS D. Pneumonia. In Isaacs D, Moxon ER, eds. *Neonatal Infections*, Oxford: Butterworth Heinemann; 1991: 70–83.
141. WEBBER S, WILKINSON AR, LIDESLL D, HOPE PJ, DOBSON SRM, ISAACS D. Neonatal pneumonia. *Arch Dis Child* 1990;65:207–11.
142. RETTIG PJ. Infections due to *Chlamydia trachomatis* from infancy to adolescence. *Pediatrics Infect Dis* 1986;5:449–57.
143. SUTHERLAND S. *Chlamydia trachomatis.* In Greenough A, Osborne J, Sutherland S. eds. *Congenital, Perinatal and Neonatal Infections.* Edinburgh: Churchill Livingstone, 1992;35–48.
144. BOURKE SJ. Chlamydial respiratory infections. *Br Med J* 1993;306:1219–20.
145. PREECE PM, ANDERSON JM, THOMPSON RG. *Chlamydia trachomatis* infection in infants: a prospective study. *Arch Dis Child* 1989;64:525–9.
146. MARRIE TJ. *Chlamydia pneumoniae. Thorax* 1993;48:1–4.
147. TORRES A, EL-EBIARY M. Relevance of *Chlamydia pneumoniae* in community-acquired respiratory infections. *Eur Resp J* 1993;6:7–8.
148. SINGHI S, DHAWAN A, KARAIA S, WALIA BNS. Clinical signs of pneumonia in infants under 2 months. *Arch Dis Child* 1994;70:413–7.
149. BROUGHTON RA. Infections due to *Mycoplasma pneumoniae* in childhood. *Pediatr Inf Dis* 1986;5:71–85.
150. HUTCHISON AA, LANDAU LI, PHELAN PD. Severe *Mycoplasma* pneumonia in previously healthy children. *Med J Aust* 1981;1:126–9.
151. TURNER RB, LANDE AE, CHASE P, HILTON N, WEINBERG D. Pneumonia in pediatric outpatients: cause and clinical manifestations. *J Pediatr* 1987;111:194–200.
152. FRIIS B, EIKEN M, HORNSLETH A, JENSEN A. Chest X-ray appearances in pneumonia and bronchiolitis. *Acta Paediatr* 1990;79:219–25.
153. KORPPI M, KIEKARA O, HEISKANEN-KOSMA T, SOIMAKALLIO S. Comparison of radiological findings and microbial aetiology of childhood pneumonia. *Acta Paediatr* 1993;82:360–63.
154. MURTAGH P, CERQUIEO C, HALAC A, AVILA M, KAJON A. Adenovirus type 7h respiratory infections: a report of 29 cases of acute lower respiratory disease. *Acta Paediatr* 1993;82:557–61.
155. RUUSKANEN O, VAAHTORANTA-LEHTONEN, MEURMAN O. Adenovirus infection of the respiratory tract. In *Recent Advances in Paediatrics*, Edinburgh: Churchill Livingstone; 1994: vol. 11:19–31.
156. ATTENBURROW AA, BARKER CM. Chlamydia pneumonia in the low birth-weight neonate. *Arch Dis Child* 1985;60:1169–72.
157. VENKATESAN P, MACFARLANE JT. Role of pneumococcal antigen in the diagnosis of pneumococcal pneumonia. *Thorax* 1992;47:329–31.
158. SILVERMAN M, STRATTON D, DIALLO A, EGLER LJ. Diagnosis of acute bacterial pneumonia in Nigerian children. *Arch Dis Child* 1977;52:925–31.
159. RAMSEY BW, MERCUSE EK, FOY HM *et al.* Use of bacterial antigen detection in the diagnosis of pediatric lower respiratory tract infections. *Pediatrics* 1986;78:1–9.
160. ANON. Pneumonia in childhood (Editorial). *Lancet* 1988; i:741–3.
161. CAMPBELL H. Acute respiratory infection: a global challenge. *Arch Dis Child* 1995;73:281–6.
162. WORLD HEALTH ORGANISATION. Technical bases for the WHO recommendations on the management of pneumonia in children at first level health facilities. *WHO/ARI/91.20* Geneva : WHO; 1991.
163. SHANN F, GRATTEN M, GERMER S, LINNEMANN V, HAZLETT D, PAYNE R. Aetiology of pneumonia in children in Goroka hospital, Papua New Guinea. *Lancet* 1984:ii:537–41.
164. CHERIAN T, JOHN TJ, SIMOES E, STEINHOFF MC, JOHN M. Evaluation of simple clinical signs for the diagnosis of acute lower respiratory tract infection. *Lancet* 1988; ii:125–8.
165. DYKE T, BROWN N. Hypoxia in childhood pneumonia: better detection and more oxygen is needed in developing countries. *BMJ* 1994;308:119–20.
166. WORLD HEALTH ORGANISATION. Oxygen therapy in the management of children with acute respiratory infections in developing countries. *WHO/ARI/93.28* Geneva: WHO, 1993.

167. RUBIN BK. Evaluation of the child with recurrent chest infections. *Pediatr Infect Dis* 1985;4:88–98.
168. SUPPURATIVE LUNG DISEASE. In Phelan PD, Olinsky A, Robertson CF, eds. *Respiratory Illness in Children*. Oxford: Blackwell; 1994:Chap. 9:196–206.
169. STILLWELL PC. Cilia Dyskinesia Syndrome. In Loughlin GM, Eigin H, eds. *Respiratory Disease in Children*. Baltimore: Williams and Wilkins, 1994: Chap. 33: 411–15.
170. COURIEL JM, HIBBERT M, OLINSKY A, PHELAN PD. Long term pulmonary consequences of oesophageal atresia. *Acta Paediat Scand* 1982:71:973–8.
171. TUBERCULOSIS. In Phelan PD, Olinsky A, Robertson CF, eds, *Respiratory Illness in Children*. Oxford: Blackwell; 1994: Chap. 12:269–84.
172. INSELMAN LS. TUBERCULOSIS. IN LOUGHLIN GM, EIGIN H, eds. *Respiratory Disease in Children*. Baltimore: Williams and Wilkins; 1994: Chap. 30:373–82.
173. HAENEY M. The detection and management of primary immunodeficiency. In David TJ, ed. *Recent Advances in Paediatrics*, Edinburgh: Churchill Livingstone: 1991:Vol 9:Chap. 2:21–40.
174. KATTAN M. AIDS and other immune deficiency states. In Loughlin GM, Eigin H, eds. *Respiratory Disease in Children*. Baltimore: Williams and Wilkins; 1994: Chap. 49:657–69.
175. MELLINS RB, BERDON WE. The lung in human immunodeficiency virus infection. In Phelan PD, Olinsky A, Robertson CF, eds. *Respiratory Illness in Children*. Oxford: Blackwell; 1994: Chap. 14:309–18.

24 Pulmonary infection in cystic fibrosis

ANTHONY KEVIN WEBB, JAMES MOORECROFT and MARY DODD

Bradbury Cystic Fibrosis Unit, Wythenshawe Hosptial, Manchester, UK

Introduction

Cystic fibrosis (CF) is a multisystem disease. The basic genetic defect affects epithelial cells lining ductal systems. Consequently, significant pathology occurs in the bronchial and biliary trees, the gastrointestinal tract, the pancreatic ducts and the vas deferens. However, chronic pulmonary infection is responsible for almost the total mortality of patients with cystic fibrosis[1]. Currently, medical management is palliative rather than curative. Patient care may be shared but should primarily be located in centres of expertise[2,3]. Treatment of pulmonary infection is directed at delaying and diminishing the chronic pulmonary sepsis which leads to lung destruction and terminal respiratory failure[4]. Death can be predicted to occur within two years for half of those patients whose lung function has fallen to a third of predicted values[5].

Improved management of CF lung disease has produced survival into adulthood (16 years old) for 90% of paediatric patients[6,7]; a profound change from three decades ago when the majority of patients died in early childhood[8]. It has been predicted that better care will increase median survival into the fourth decade of life by the year 2000[9]. However, current medical treatment is not curative. Our current knowledge of the pathogenesis of CF pulmonary infection coupled with aggressive treatment is insufficient to halt the relentless advance of lung sepsis. Recent medical advances and scientific breakthroughs need to be translated into therapy to produce survival to a pensionable age.

Cystic fibrosis: the disease

The basic defect

Cystic fibrosis is the most common lethal autosomal recessive genetic disorder among Caucasians.

In the UK, 1 in 20–40 people carry the gene for cystic fibrosis, there is an annual incidence 1 in 2500 live births of babies with cystic fibrosis, 290 babies are born with cystic fibrosis each year and there are 140 deaths[7]. In 1991 the average age of CF patients was 13 years with a mean age of survival into the third decade of life. By the year 2000 there will be 7000 CF patients in the United Kingdom[7] with equal numbers of adult and paediatric patients.

The race to discover and identify the CF gene reached a conclusion in September 1989 with the cloning and sequencing of the gene. The gene is located on the long arm of chromosome 7[10–12]. It is a 1480 amino acid protein. A single amino acid deletion, phenylalanine at position 508 (delta F508) is the most frequent mutation but over 300 further mutations have been identified[13]. In Europe and America the incidence of delta F508 has been comprehensively studied and the overall incidence is approximately 70%[13].

European genetic gradients for delta 508 are recognised with the lowest incidence in Turkey and the highest incidence in Denmark. Less common mutations may be higher for some ethnic groups with the mutation G551D being more common in Celts. Although cystic fibrosis is usually described in Caucasians, it has been reported to a small but significant degree in Asians where the diagnosis may be overlooked or delayed.

The occurrence of so many mutations makes it an unlikely prospect that the disease can be eliminated by screening programmes over the next three decades. The occurrence of unidentified mutations can cause diagnostic difficulty when a patient has the characteristic phenotype of cystic fibrosis and an uninformative genetic test.

The protein encoded by the mutant gene in cystic fibrosis has been elaborately named the cystic fibrosis transmembrane conductance regulator (CFTR)[11]. The CFTR protein is located in the apical membrane of epithelial cells and is a member of the ABC (ATP-binding cassette) family of transporter proteins. The main biochemical difference between normal and CF cells is a decreased permeability of chloride ion transport across the epithelium[14,15]. In normal cells, chloride transport is activated by cyclic AMP. In CF cells this process is impaired[16]. This cyclic AMP related chloride transport defect is characterised by an increased negative potential difference across epithelial cells and can be measured[17]. It is now accepted that CFTR functions as a chloride channel[18,19]. Incorporation of CFTR into non-epithelial invertebrate cells produces a chloride channel where none existed previously[20]. Normal CFTR incorporated into cultured CF cells has corrected the ion channel defect, restoring chloride permeability[21,22]. The construction of a normal chloride channel in CF epithelial tissue by genetic reconstitution has crystallised the direction and potential of future molecular biological research for correcting and treating respiratory and gastrointestinal disease; those tissues where the organ pathology is the most severe and yet the most accessible.

Pulmonary pathophysiology

The aphorism drawn from folklore that ‘the child will die soon, whose forehead tastes salty when kissed’ recognised the lethal consequences of having cystic fibrosis[23]. In 1953,the collapse of several CF children during a New York heat wave was correctly attributed to excessive loss of salt in their sweat[24]. Occasionally CF patients will crystallise salt on to their skin during the course of exercise. These clinical observations led to the development of the sweat test as a diagnostic tool[25]. It is reliable and reproducible when performed by experienced technicians.

Epithelial cells lining ductal systems usually have a secretory and reabsorptive function. The correct composition of electrolyte,protein and water in epithelial secretions is essential to fulfil the cellular function of protection, lubrication and digestion. In the CF respiratory epithelium it is suggested that chloride impermeability leads to an increased uptake of sodium ions into the cell. An excessive passage of water osmotically follows sodium into the cells. This leads to a decrease in water content of mucus on the luminal surface of the bronchi.

Alteration in the volume and quality of the bronchial water disturbs mucociliary clearance[26]. Although the lungs of CF neonates dying at birth are structurally and functionally normal[27], plugging is found in the small ducts of the serous and submucosal glands[28] (Figs. 24.1 (*a*), (*b*). Mucous gland hypertrophy, hypersecretion and mucus stasis produce a favourable environment for early bacterial colonisation and infection. Although the cilia are structurally normal, escalatory function is grossly diminished by the increased viscosity of mucus which contains large numbers of bacteria and cellular debris. Inspissated secretions in small airways become chronically infected, inciting a self damaging exhuberant local cellular and humoral host inflammatory response. A chronic neutrophilic bronchiolitis ensues leading to bronchiectasis. Pus is found in the airways and the bronchial epithelium becomes ulcerated and infiltrated by inflammatory cells (Figs 24.1 (*c*)–(*f*)). Smooth muscle also becomes hypertrophied with associated infiltration by inflammatory cells (Fig. 24.1 (*g*), (*h*)). In the airways the cartilage is damaged (Fig. 24.1 (*i*)) and there is loss of elastic tissue and the airways become floppy and unstable. Initially,these changes predominate in the upper lobes but then extend to the lingula and middle lobes. Local areas of emphysema or bullae occur in sites of lung destruction often underlying thickened pleura (Fig. 24.1 (*j*)).

A rich plexus of vessels proliferate around the bronchi forming communications between bronchial and pulmonary arterial circulations. Bronchial arteries become hypertrophied and tortuous. Progressive airway narrowing, lung destruction and an abnormal pulmonary circulation lead to gross ventilation perfusion mismatch with increasing hypoxia and consequent pulmonary hypertension

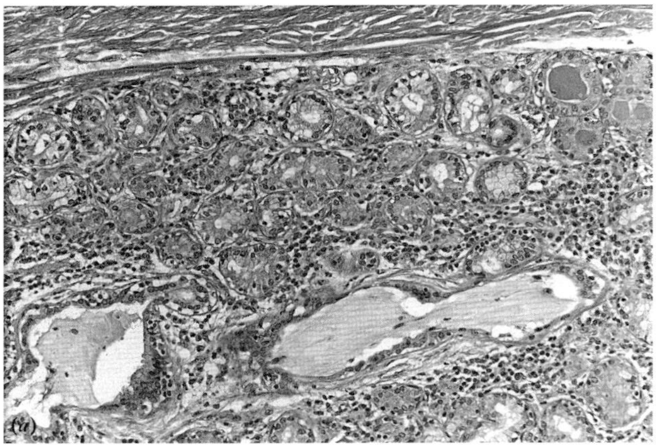

FIGURE 24.1 (*a*) Serous and mucous gland hyperplasia with dilated glands containing viscid mucus. (H & E).

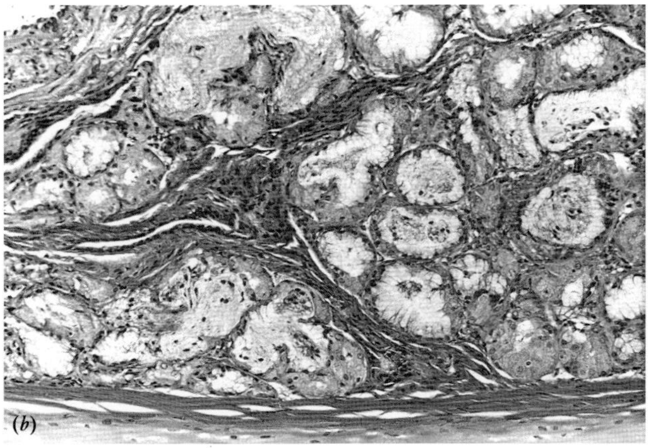

FIGURE 24.1 (*b*) Dilated bronchial mucous glands (H & E).

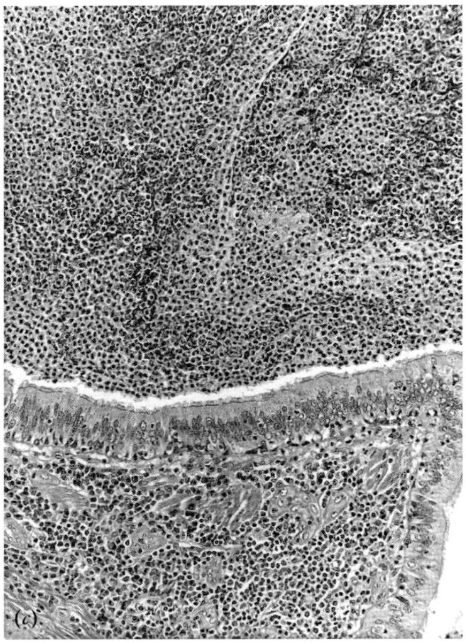

FIGURE 24.1 (*c*) Intact bronchial epithelium with pus in the the lumen and chronic inflammation in the wall. (H & E).

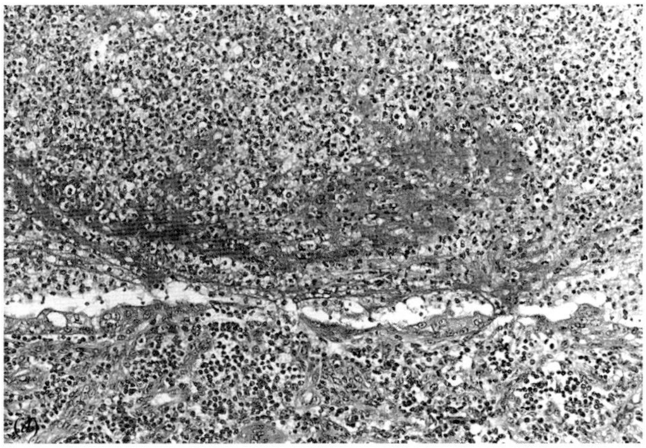

FIGURE 24.1 (*d*) Ulceration and loss of bronchial epithelium with pus in the airways. (H & E).

(Fig. 24.1 (*k*)). Inability to ventilate leads to carbon dioxide retention. Respiratory failure (Type 1 or 2) ensues and leads to death.

Why impermeability to the chloride ion in the apical membrane of respiratory epithelial cells should lead to chronic pulmonary infection with specific organisms such as *Staphylococcus aureus* and *Pseudomonas aeruginosa* is unclear but the combination of abnormal CF mucins[29], a higher osmolality in CF lungs[30], an abnormal electrolyte transport mechanism and bacterial virulence factors may act synergistically to produce bacterial adherence. Furthermore, a recent paper has suggested the correlation of high risk and low risk genotypes for the acquisition of *P.aeruginosa*[31]. Predisposition to chronic colonisation being correlated with CFTR mutation genotype.

Microbiology of lung infection

Principal pathogens

Cystic fibrosis lungs provide a favourable environment for bacterial colonisation and subsequent chronic infection. Some of the reasons for this process are discussed below. The percentage of different organisms isolated on sputum culture, over a period of six months, in a 150 adult CF patients are shown in Fig. 24.2. The principal infecting pathogens usually follow a chronological sequence of colonisation but several different organisms may be found in a single sputum culture at one time. Initial colonisation usually takes place with *S. aureus*. Another early childhood pathogen is *Haemophilus influenzae*. Both *S.aureus* and *H.influenzae* are also found in adults. By early adolescence,the majority of CF patients are infected with *P.aeruginosa* the

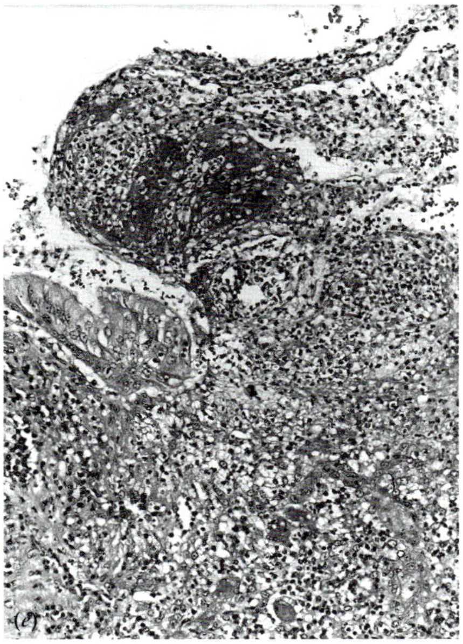

FIGURE 24.1 (*e*) Ulceration in bronchial wall with fibrosis and polymorphs. (H & E).

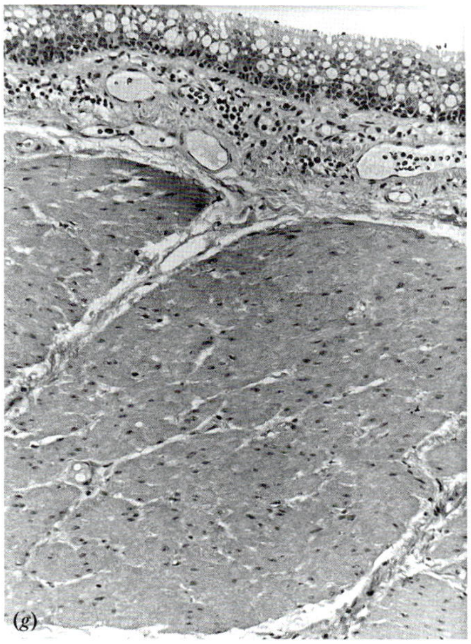

FIGURE 24.1 (*g*) Bronchial wall with less smooth muscle but an acute or chronic inflammatory reaction in the wall. (H & E).

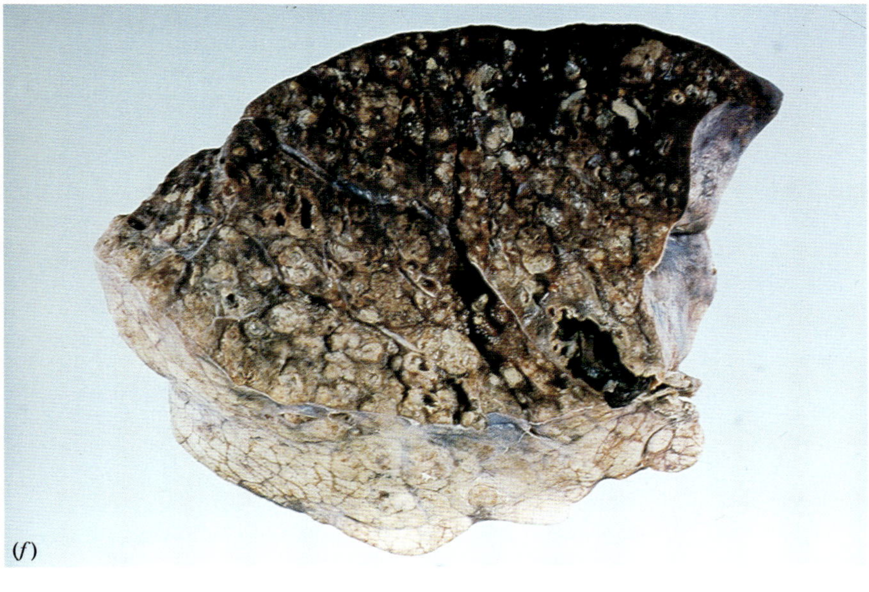

FIGURE 24.1 (*f*) Gross bronchiectasis in sectioned lung.

principal pathogen of the disease. Survival is longer in patients not infected with *P.aeruginosa*[32].

Over the last decade, a small but significant number of adults have become infected with *Burkholderia cepacia*. The increased incidence and prevalence of infection with *B.cepacia* occurs when CF patients are in close personal contact. The organism may be associated with a greater morbidity and mortality in some but not all CF patients.

Viral infections have an important role by introducing and orchestrating bacterial colonisation and infection. They cause seasonal infective pulmonary exacerbations and consequently may accelerate lung disease.

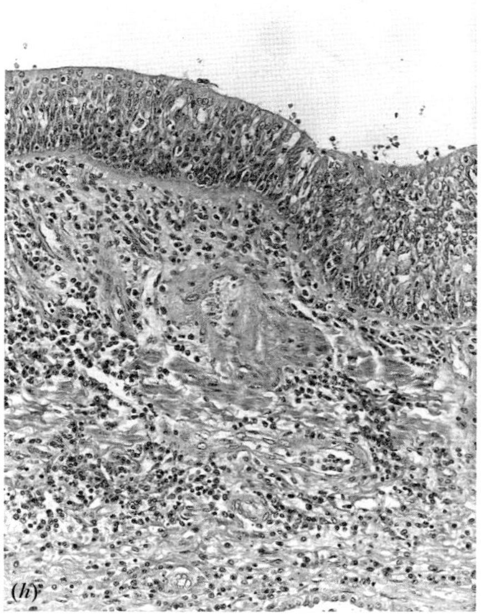

FIGURE 24.1 (*h*) Bronchial wall with marked increase in smooth muscle (H & E).

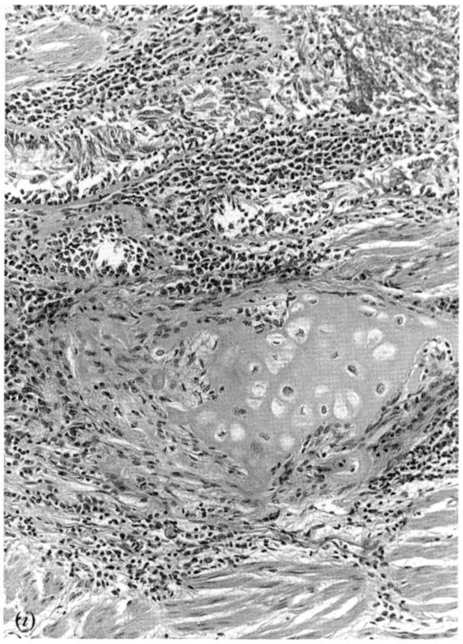

FIGURE 24.1 (*i*) Destruction of cartilage in bronchial wall infiltrated by inflammatory cells. (H & E).

Additional infecting pathogens include other *Pseudomonas* species, *Aspergillus fumigatus,* mycobacteria, community-acquired and atypical pneumonias.

Staphylococcus aureus

S.aureus was the classic initiating pathogen during the early pre antibiotic era of the disease and the principal cause of mortality in infancy and childhood[33,34].

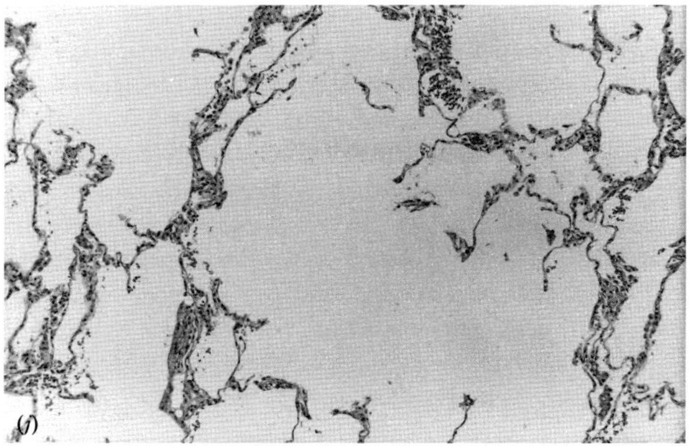

FIGURE 24.1 (*j*) Alvelolar lymphocytes with dilated air spaces (H & E).

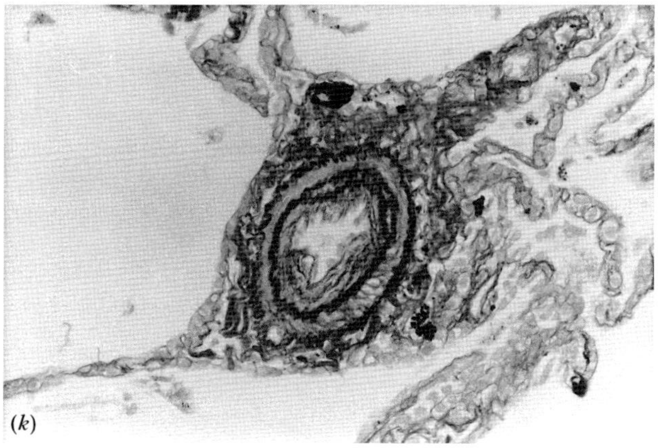

FIGURE 24.1 (*k*) Muscular pulmonary artery with intimal longditudinal and medial muscle wall hypertrophy. (H & E).

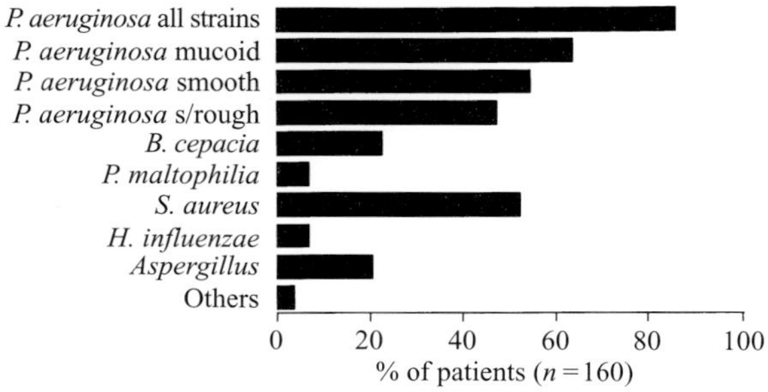

FIGURE 24.2 Organisms found in the sputum of 160 adults with cystic fibrosis over a period of 6 months. Sputum cultures often contained more than one organism.

No specific phage type has been associated with CF[35] but capsular typing has suggested a predominance of type 8. Some of the virulence factors produced by *S.aureus* include exopolysaccaride,enterotoxins, haemolysins, coagulases and teichoic acid. Some of these factors may initiate epithelial damage thereby promoting adhesion and persistence of bacteria in the airways[36].

The introduction in childhood of high dose prophylactic anti-staphylococcal therapy resulted in a considerable increase in survival. Controversy continues as to the length of time that long-term prophylactic anti-staphylococcal antibiotics should be prescribed and whether maintenance is responsible for delaying or accelerating subsequent colonisation with *P.aeruginosa*[37]. Prevalence of the organism decreases with age but its presence as the only infecting organism in the older patient should not be ignored. Serum precipitins to *S.aureus* persist in adult life[38]. Persistent colonisation of CF sputum by staphylococcus should be treated. In one centre,the policy is to treat infective exacerbations associated with high sputum carriage of *S.aureus* (>10 cfu/ml)[39]. This restricted usage of anti-staphylococcal antibiotics was felt to be responsible for only a 30% incidence of colonisation with *P.aeruginosa*[40]. It is a common observation that older patients colonised only by *S.aureus* usually have better pulmonary function.

Haemophilus Influenzae

H.influenzae is the third most commonly cultured organism in CF sputum (after *S.aureus* and *P.aeruginosa*). The organism is non-encapsulated and sometimes non-typable although biotype 1 predominates[41]. The organism has fastidious growth characteristics and may be difficult to isolate in the presence of *P.aeruginosa*. However, improved culture techniques have resulted in an increased isolation, emphasising its role as an important contributor to lung damage[42]. The organism often persists in sputum after cessation of antibiotics. This may be due to the favourable environment of CF airways but there is considerable variation in the protein and liposaccharide composition of the outer membrane proteins resulting in considerable antigenic heterogeneity which may allow non-typable *H.influenzae* to avoid host immune defences.

One study has reported the presence of *H.influenzae* in sputum to be a negative prognostic indicator for 5-year survival[43]. A further study has reported increased isolation during infective exacerbations in children[44]. A marked increase in the inflammatory marker C-reactive protein has been reported in association with infective exacerbations[45]. Serum precipitins to *H.influenzae* are found in 30–40% of older patients[38].

H.influenzae found in CF sputum should be treated aggressively. The organism, even when penicillin sensitive, may be difficult to eliminate from CF lungs due to poor sputum penetration of antibiotics[46].

Pseudomonas aeruginosa

Epidemiology and acquisition

Mucoid *P.aeruginosa* is the most important bacterial pathogen affecting CF patients. Chronic infection of the lungs with *P.aeruginosa* is the major cause of morbidity and mortality for CF patients[47]. In the early descriptions of the disease, isolation of the organism was unusual[34] but, in the late 1950s isolation was described with increasing frequency. The classical mucoid phenotype of *P.aeruginosa* was described in 1966 and is found in 60–70% of CF patients (Fig 24.3)[48].

Currently, in large CF adult centres, the prevalence of *P.aeruginosa* may reach 80–90%. In the majority of patients intermittent colonisation precedes chronic colonisation[49]. This is a crucial period where early prophylactic treatment provides a therapeutic opportunity to delay chronic colonisation.

The sources from which CF patients initially acquire and become colonised with *P.aeruginosa* have not been clearly identified. Acquisition from an environment contaminated by other CF patients has been discussed[50,51] but it is considered an uncommon source. The possibility of direct cross-infection between patients has caused concern[52]. Cross infection occurs between siblings and they usually carry the same strain of *P. aeruginosa*[53]. The risk of cross-infection between patients at holiday camps is low[54]. The evidence of cross-infection with *P.aeruginosa* between patients in the Danish CF centre[55] resulted in a policy of segregating patients colonised with *P.aeruginosa* from other patients. Following the inception of this policy there was a reduction in the incidenc of patients acquiring *P.aeruginosa*[56]. Improved methods of 'tracking' *P.aeruginosa* have followed the use of pyocin typing and analysis using DNA probes and genomic finger printing[57–59]. Collectively, these methods of epidemiological surveillance would suggest that the majority of CF patients harbour and keep their own strains of *P.aeruginosa* although there may be considerable phenotypic variation.

The observation that initial (66%) and chronic colonisation (68%) of 300 Danish patients with *P.aeruginosa* occurred during the winter months suggested that infection with respiratory viruses may predispose to, or aggravate, bacterial infection[49].

It has been suggested there may be synergism between respiratory syncytial viral infections and *P.aeruginosa*[60].

The nasal epithelium shares the same basic defect as the bronchial epithelium. The upper airways are similarly diseased. The majority of CF patients have chronic sinusitis and nasal polyps. It has been suggested that colonisation of the upper respiratory tract may precede infection of the lower airways[61]. Although the upper airways can act as reservoirs for bacterial infection, it has not been possible to

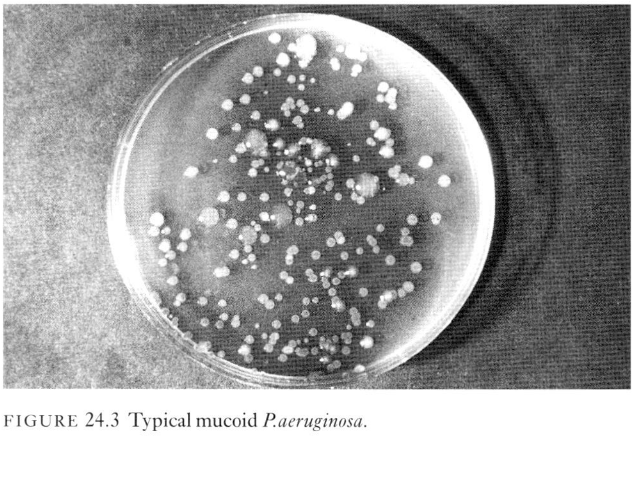

FIGURE 24.3 Typical mucoid *P.aeruginosa*.

demonstrate colonisation in these sites prior to pulmonary infection. An exception to this observation occurs following transplantation when the donor lungs may become colonised with *P.aeruginosa*, the source being the reservoir sites in the CF recipient's upper airways.

Adherence,colonisation and chronic infection

Multiple factors influence the persistence of *P.aeruginosa* in a favourable bronchial environment.

As discussed, preceding bacterial and viral infections will have already chronically damaged respiratory epithelium. In addition, purulent blood stained secretions, impermeable to antibiotics are a rich culture medium for *P.aeruginosa*. Above all, *P.aeruginosa* demonstrates a remarkable ability to adapt and persist in a potentially hostile environment. The organism produces its own bacterial adhesins (alginate, pili, lectins and exoenzyme S)[62–64] and virulence factors (elastases, pyocyanin pigments, proteases and rhamnolipids)[65,66]. The continuing damage created by these virulence factors may expose surface receptors which further encourage adhesion[67]. The damage created by numerous bacterial products is matched by an exuberant host inflammatory response which maintains and amplifies local tissue damage further encouraging the chronicity of *P.aeruginosa* infection.

Chronicity of *Pseudomonas* infection

Colonisation with *P.aeruginosa*, despite aggressive treatment with antibiotics, always becomes chronic. Some of the adaptive characteristics of *P.aeruginosa*, as discussed above, contribute to this chronicity. However, the principal reason for the persistence of *P.aeruginosa*, is its ability to form alginate,an exopolysaccaride consisting of mannuronic and guluronic acids. The alginate produced by mucoid *P.aeruginosa* protects the bacteria within an ionised biofilm from antibiotic penetration[39]. Bacterial microcolonies enmeshed in alginate are protected against neutrophil damage which 'in frustration' damages host tissue (Fig. 24.4). The ability of *P.aeruginosa* to alter its phenotype by the biosynthesis of alginate,loss of surface O-specific lipopolysaccharide and polyagglutination with O-specific sera reflects the adaptability of the organism to ensure its survival in the CF lung. Early work demonstrated that alginate biosynthesis in *P.aeruginosa* has a controlling chromosomal locus[68]. A rapid expansion in genetic and molecular studies of alginate biosynthesis in the 1980s has shown that alginate biosynthesis is controlled by a complex sensory regulating system which responds to local pulmonary stimuli including the dehydration and raised osmolarity associated with the CF lung[69]. The pathways by which mucoid *P.aeruginosa* regulates alginate biosynthesis have been characterised[70].

Alginate biosynthesis is physiologically demanding but provides *P.aeruginosa* with both offensive and defensive properties, enabling it to adapt to its micro-environment. It stimulates an ineffectual antibody response[71] and a neutrophilic oxidative response[72]. It inhibits chemotaxis[73] and frustrates phagocytosis[74]. It is not surprising that alginate interferes with the efficacy of antibiotics[75]. Alginate may specifically bind cationic aminoglycosides[76]. The inhibitory concentration of antibiotics for mucoid strains of *P.aeruginosa* may be considerably higher than for non-mucoid strains.

Burkholderia cepacia

In the 1980s several North American clinics reported an increased isolation of the organism *B.cepacia* from the sputum of CF patients[77,78]. In the last 5 years there has been an increased incidence and prevalence of the organism in some large CF centres in the UK[79].

Several factors cause *B.cepacia* to be of equal concern to doctors and CF patients; the most important include accelerated lung disease in some patients, cross-infection between patients in close contact and increased antibiotic resistance. The rapid emergence of this organism has drastically altered the social fabric of CF society and medical management.

Microbiology

B.cepacia was first isolated in the 1950s and is recognised as a plant pathogen typically causing bulb rot in onions (Fig. 24.5). It can contaminate antiseptics, disinfectants and even utilises penicillin G as a carbon source. Culture of *B.cepacia* may present difficulties and it is a fundamental tenet that a bacteriology laboratory supporting a CF unit should now routinely use selective media and conditions appropriate for culture of the organism. A suitable multitest system for identifying *B.cepacia* would be API 2ONE[39]. When adopting the correct culture media for the first time, some laboratories have found *B.cepacia* present in their patient population when it was not considered to be a problem. A quality control exercise found that only 36 of 115 laboratories using non-selective media could correctly isolate *B.cepacia* from infected sputum whereas 14 of 15 laboratories using *B.cepacia* selective media were able to isolate the organism correctly[80].

B.cepacia also displays a higher level of antibiotic resistance than *P.aeruginosa*. There appears to be a low level of porin-mediated antibiotic uptake and an absence of self-promoted antibiotic uptake. Some strains of *B.cepacia* become totally antibiotic resistance making a correct choice of drug extremely difficult. Non-oxidative killing of *B.cepacia* by neutrophils is diminished although oxidative killing for *B.cepacia* and *P.aeruginosa* appears to be similar.

B.cepacia colonisation usually follows infection with *P.aeruginosa*. As a preterminal event, it may be the only pathogen found in CF sputum but may also be found as the only infecting organism in well

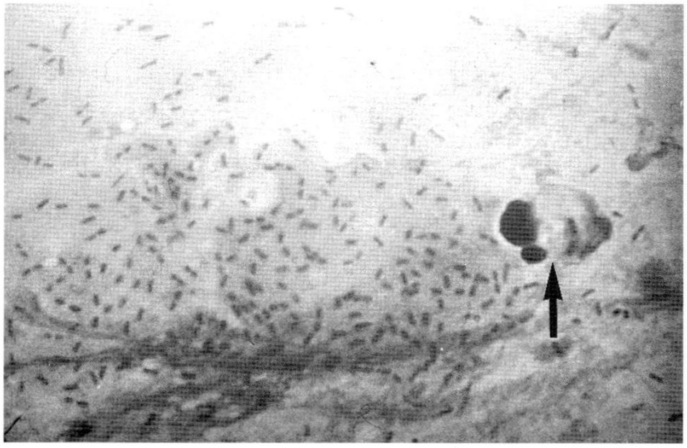

FIGURE 24.4 Frustrated neutrophil failing to penetrate alginate enmeshing a microcolony of *P. aeruginosa*. Slide courtesy of Dr J. Govan.

patients. The adhesion of piliated strains of *B.cepacia* to mucins and epithelial cells appears to increase with disease severity and may be enhanced by the presence of *P.aeruginosa*[81].

Epidemiology and cross-infection

B.cepacia differs from that of *P.aeruginosa* in one crucial aspect; cross-infection with this organism takes place between CF patients when they are in close contact, either in hospital or socially. Previous studies have suggested possible risk factors associated with colonisation[82] but a further study suggests that close patient contact is the principal cause of transmission of *B.cepacia*[79]. However, a recent study emphasised that person-to-person transmission was unusual and that patients retained their own strain of *B.cepacia* even after transplantation[83].

It has been found that *B.cepacia* can contaminate environmental surfaces providing the potential for an indirect source of transmission[84]. It may also be found on the hands of carers. However there is no scientific proof that medical personnel are an intermediary source for transmitting *B.cepacia* infection between patients.

The route by which transmission of *B.cepacia* takes place is not clear. However, improved methods of typing different strains of *B.cepacia* which include selective culture media, bacteriocin typing, ribotype analysis and genomic finger printing have proved invaluable epidemiological surveillance tools. An early study, which utilised some of these methods suggested cross-infection had occurred between two adults by person-to-person transmission when they attended a summer educational camp[85]. Cross-infection did not relate to length of close contact and some *P.aeruginosa* patients with prolonged contact did not acquire the organism. In a more detailed study, which a included a large number of patients from two regional adult CF centres (Edinburgh and Manchester) the spread of a highly transmissible epidemic strain of *B.cepacia* was described within and between the two units[79]. The strain had the same phenotypic and genotypic typing patterns, morphological appearance on culture and possessed multiple antibiotic resistance. The link between the two geographically separated clinics was attendance by patients from both units at a CF selection camp in the UK before going to Canada. Intial cross-infection to the Manchester clinic was provided by a source case from the Edinburgh clinic. This epidemic strain subsequently spread within both units. (Fig. 24.6 (*a*), (*b*)). Within the Edinburgh group, a significant number of *P.aeruginosa* patients became colonised with *B.cepacia* by a single *B.cepacia* individual attending a communal evening training exercise programme. At the Manchester clinic, a female (*B.cepacia*) infected six males (*P.aeruginosa*) when she kissed them under the mistletoe at Christmas. The details of this study provide some clues as to the mode of cross-infection. Close patient contact allows the interchange of salivary or respiratory secretions. There is no information as to whether *B.cepacia* has an incubation period before being cultured in sputum, although some patients have shown a fourfold increase in *B.cepacia* antibodies several weeks before the first culture of the organism (Nelson, personal communication). Appreciation of the cross-infectivity of *B.cepacia* has led to patient segregation policies.

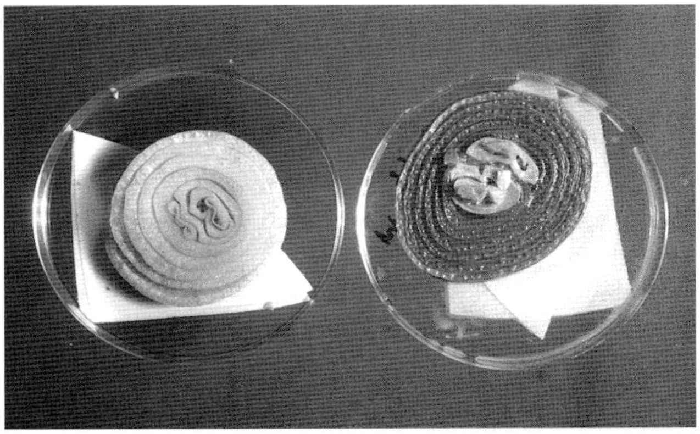

FIGURE 24.5 *Burkholderia cepacia* is pathogenic to onions. A blackened onion infected with *B.cepacia*. Slide courtesy of Dr J.Govan.

Virulence and immune responses

There appear to be different clinical responses to pulmonary colonisation with *B.cepacia*. Some patients may have asymptomatic or transient carriage of the organism. Others have an accelerated

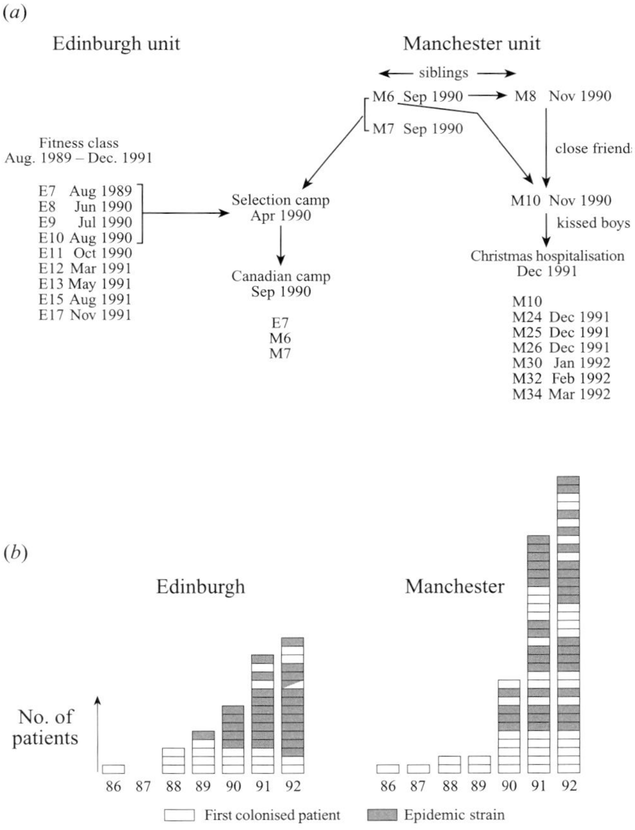

FIGURE 24.6 (*a*) Demonstrates the index *B.cepacia* case (E7) in the Edinburgh clinic in 1989. E7 passes B.cepacia to M6 and M7 at the Canadian selection camp. M6 returns to Manchester. She infects her sister (M8). Their close friend M10 is infected who infects other patients who she kisses under the mistletoe. (*b*) Demonstrates the increasing annual incidence in the Manchester and Edinburgh clinics of an epidemic strain of *B.cepacia*. Published with permission of the *Lancet*.

progression of lung disease when compared to those patients colonised by *P. aeruginosa*. In those patients with mild to moderate disease severity, progress is over years but in severely diseased patients acquisition may lead to death in months. Finally, infection may be associated with rapid death over weeks irrespective of initial disease severity. A profound host response in CF patients is characterised by a necrotising pneumonia, septicaemia, a swinging pyrexia, rapid wasting and no clinical response to medical therapy[86] (Fig. 24.7 (*a*), (*b*)). This rapid clinical decline is not described with *P.aeruginosa*.

The virulence characteristics of *B.cepacia* are poorly characterised. Unlike *P.aeruginosa*, *B.cepacia* does not produce alginate or elastases.

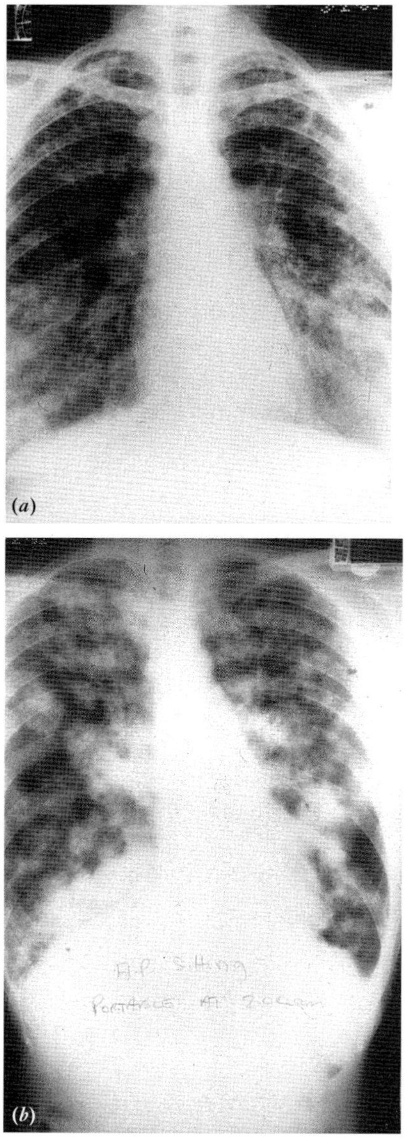

FIGURE 24.7 (*a*) Chest radiograph taken on day one of an infective exacerbation in a clinically stable CF male infected with *B.cepacia* for two years. (*b*) Chest radiograph on day fourteen when he died. Radiograph is typical of necrotising pneumonia associated with *B.cepacia*.

Virulence factors produced inlude proteases, lipases, haemolysins and lecithinases but none of these factors has specifically been identified as the cause of bacterial virulence. Even less is published about the cellular and humeral host responses to *B.cepacia*. Increased levels of specific *B.cepacia* antibodies have been associated with clinical deterioration and are presumably non-protective[87]. A recent short-term study showed no difference in improvement following a course of antibiotics for inflammatory markers and lung function between patients with *B.cepacia* and *P.aeruginosa*[88].

The degree of antibiotic resistance to *B.cepacia* has stimulated research to look for alternative therapies such as immunotherapy to treat this difficult organism. Some of these research results are promising but are unlikely to be clinically useful for some time[89].

Other *Pseudomonas* species

Other *Pseudomonas* species may be found on culture from the sputum of cystic fibrosis patients; These include *P.maltophilia* (now known as *Xanthomonas maltophilia*), *P.gladioli*, *P.fluorescens*, *P.putida*, and *P.stutzeri*. Their clinical significance is unknown. The prevalence of *P.maltophilia* has increased in some units to 8%. and selective media is required to maximise its isolation[90,91].The incidence is greater in large CF centres. Cross-infection may occur but increased knowledge of the organism has not equalled that of *B.cepacia*. *P.maltophilia* does not seem to have the same pathogenicity as *B.cepacia*.

Viruses and atypical organisms

Respiratory viral infections increase the morbidity in patients with pulmonary disease. The respiratory viruses which have commonly been isolated from the lower respiratory tract of CF patients include influenza A and B, parainfluenza, respiratory syncytial virus, rhinovirus, adenovirus, Coxsackie virus, herpes simplex and varicella. It has been postulated that viral infections are the initiator of damage to CF lungs which then predisposes to subsequent bacterial infection. An increased incidence of chronic colonisation with *P.aeruginosa* has been reported during the winter months concurrent with an increase in viral infections[49].

Acute deterioration in pulmonary disease has been described with influenza A virus infections[92]. A prospective study found that although viral infections were not more common in CF patients there was a strong correlation between decline in pulmonary function, clinical status and the frequency of viral infections[93].

There are several reasons why virus infections promote pulmonary damage; viruses can impair host defences by increasing epithelial cell damage, reducing bacteriocidal activity and retard mucociliary clearance[93]. A synergistic interaction between viruses and bacteria increases pulmonary damage. Viral infections have been associated with increased isolation of *P.aeruginosa* antibodies in CF patients[60].

Early treatment of viral infections is important. Specific available antiviral agents include acyclovir,amantidine,ribavarin and gancyclovir. The early introduction of acyclovir to varicella infection in five CF adults prevented pulmonary deterioration[94], whereas three untreated CF children deteriorated[95].

Prospective studies of viral infections in the community have been confounded by the inability to make an early diagnosis. Measurement of serological conversion is useful for epidemiological studies but not for institution of early treatment. Enthusiasm to establish an earlier diagnosis has increased with the advent of specific antiviral drugs. Recent improved diagnostic techniques include enzyme-linked and radioimmune assays which will detect viral antigens[96] nucleic acid hybridisation,Western blotting and specicfic viral monoclonal antibodies[97]. However not all these techniques are readily available in current clinical practice.

CF adults[98] and children[99] can readily mount a satisfactory antibody response to vaccination against influenza A and B. Although significant antibody memory is retained a year later,viral drift occurs requiring annual reconstitution of vaccines. Influenza viral infection is potentially lethal for CF patients and there should be an active annual vaccination programme. The vaccine is well tolerated.

Atypical microorganisms may also cause respiratory infections in equal proportion to the normal population. The principal organisms include *Mycoplasma pneumoniae*, *Legionella pneumophila* and *Chlamydia*. Serodiagnosis may be difficult with concurrent *Pseudomonas* infection due to antigenic cross-reactivity[100,101].

Mycobacterial infections

Mycobacterial infections are a rare but serious pulmonary complication in cystic fibrosis[102]. Increased isolation of atypical mycobacteria may be associated with established severe lung damage[103]. Diagnosis may be delayed as many of the symptoms of cystic fibrosis are common to those with tuberculosis; chronic sputum production, fatigue,weight loss and occasional fever. However, night sweats are uncommon in cystic fibrosis and more typical of tuberculosis. It is important to send frequent sputum cultures for acid fast bacilli when patients are deteriorating and unresponsive to routine anti-pseudomonal antibiotic therapy. Repeated isolation of acid fast bacilli will also distinguish occasional harmless colonisation from significant pathological infection. Isolation of mycobacteria from purulent sputum of may be impaired by overgrowth of the culture with *P.aeruginosa* which is present in 90% of CF patients[104]. Recovery of mycobacteria can be improved by bacterial decontamination of CF sputum with NACl–Naoh–oxalic acid which results in an impressive reduction in bacterial overgrowth[105].

In one unit,following the introduction of routine smears and culture for mycobacteria, 7 out of 233 patients were found to have positive sputum samples[102]. In the Manchester unit we have identified only two atypical mycobacterial infections (2/200 patient population) over the period of a decade. However a recent study by Kilby *et al.* has reported a 20% increased isolation of non-tuberculous mycobacteria (NTM) from CF patients[104]. The usual organism being *Mycobacterium avium–intracellulare* complex. There are no published studies of the optimum chemotherapy for CF patients infected with NTM but in addition to routine antituberculous drugs the new macrolides (clarithromycin and azithromycin) offer useful addtional therapy for these difficult organisms.

Aspergillus and other fungi

In a recent study, stainable fungi were found in the lungs at autopsy in 13 of 63 CF patients[106]. Hyphae consistent with *Aspergillus* species were detected in 5 out of 63 patients and yeast like cells consistent with Candida in 8 out of 63 patients. Aggressive medical therapy was more likely to be associated with fungal infection.

Bronchopulmonary aspergillosis was first described in CF patients in 1965[107]. However, making the clinical diagnosis of allergic bronchopulmonary *Aspergillosis* (ABPA) in CF patients is difficult for several reasons; (a) the chest radiograph which is already abnormal,may display transient shadowing due to an infective exacerbation, (b) in CF patients with chronic lung damage there is a high incidence of positive aspergillus precipitins, (c) *Aspergillus fumigatus* may be recovered from the sputum cultures of up to 20–30% of patients (Table 24.1), (d) CF patients may have some of the diagnostic criteria of ABPA such as positive precipitins and immediate skin tests without displaying any clinical features of the disease[108]. It is not surprising that estimates of ABPA in CF are wide ranging (0.5%–11%) depending upon the criteria used[109–111]. It has been proposed that a scoring system is used combining clinical and laboratory criteria to reach a working diagnosis[112]. (Table 24.1.) Perhaps the best immunological evidence for ABPA are elevated IgE levels of greater than 500 in association with a positive RAST test. It is important to treat ABPA with oral steroids (Fig. 24.8(*a*)–(*b*)) in cystic fibrosis. Repeated measurements of IgE levels can be used to assess the response to steroids.There are anecdotal case histories of good responses to treatment with the antifungal agent itraconazole[113]. Documented good clinical responses to both steroids and antifungal agents highlights the therapeutic dilemma as to what is the best option for treating *A. fumigatus* in cystic fibrosis.

There has been some concern that CF patients awaiting transplantation, who are colonised with *Aspergillus* in their sputum, will develop disseminated aspergillosis following transplantation. However, despite the association of *A. fumigatus* and CF, invasive aspergillosis following transplantation for CF patients is not increased when compared with non-CF patients receiving transplants[114]. If *Aspergillus* is found in sputum prior to transplantation, prophylactic antifungal drugs may eradicate colonisation.

Inflammatory lung disease in cystic fibrosis

Systemic immunity in cystic fibrosis is normal.However chronic bacterial infection (usually *P.aeruginosa*) leads to an exuberant but localised host response in the CF lung. The immune response is inadequate and fails to eradicate lung infection. As a consequence the inflammatory response is amplified and 'frustrated'. This persistent stimulus provokes interacting cellular and humeral responses which lead to immune mediated lung damage and a perpetuation of chronic infection.

Humoral responses

Elevated antibody levels in CF patients are associated with poor lung function, declining clinical status and ultimately a worse prognosis[115]. In this study IgG and IgA antilipolysaccharide antibodies started to rise at the onset of chronic infection and increased during the later stages of infection. The antibody reponse is primarily to antigenic components of *P.aeruginosa*. Extracellular components

Table 24.1. *Indicators of bronchopulmonary aspergillosis in cystic fibrosis*

(a)	Elevated IgE levels with a positive RAST (radioallergosorbent test) to *A. fumigatus*.
(b)	Pulmonary shadows which resolve with steroids and not with antibiotics
(c)	Blood eosinophilia
(d)	Persistent *Aspergillus* species cultured from sputum
(e)	Positive *Aspergillus* precipitins
(f)	Immediate skin test reaction to *A.fumigatus*

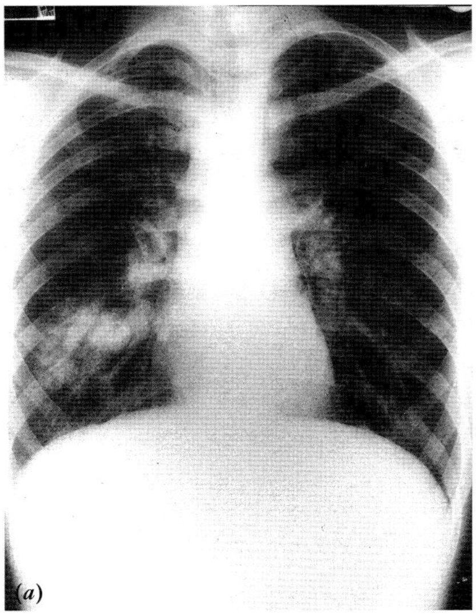

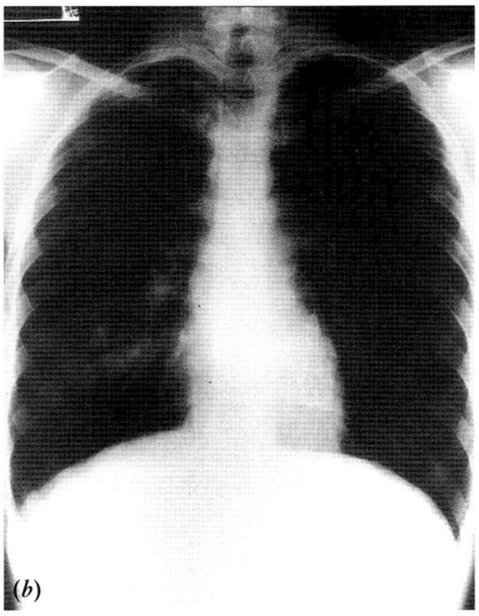

FIGURE 24.8 (*a*) Radiograph demonstrating infiltrating shadows in right middle lobe which failed to resolve with antibiotics. Patient had elevated IgE levels, a positive RAST test to *Aspergillus* and positive *Aspergillus* precipitins. (*b*) Radiograph demonstrating radiological resolution of shadowing following treatment with oral steroids, supporting a diagnosis of bronchopulmonary aspergillosis.

include alkaline protease,elastase,exotoxin A,phospholipase C and exoenzyme S[116–119]. Antibodies to cellular components included alginate, outer membrane proteins, pili and flagella[120–122]. Anti-*P.aeruginosa* flagellar antibodies have been demonstrated in the saliva and sputum of CF patients[123]. Alginate produced by *P.aeruginosa* is also immunogenic and IgA antibodies,usually the first to be detected following colonisation, have been associated with a poor prognosis[124]. The detection of *P.aeruginosa* antibodies in serum before being cultured in sputum has been described[125]. This finding may be a useful indicator for initiating treatment during the early period of colonisation and then monitoring antibody level responses to the routine treatment of subsequent chronic infection.

A failure of opsonisation is an observed feature of immunological inefficiency in CF. High levels of the sublcass immunoglobulin IgG2 has been reported with severe disease[126]. This immunoglobulin subclass is non-opsonising and may have a direct antiphagocytic effect and form immune complexes. Phagocytosis of bacteria by macrophages is promoted by high affinity receptors on IgG1 and IgG3 globulins and a shift to the production of IgG2 and IgG4 may contribute to this inhibition of opsonisation[127]. Pier *et al.*[74] found that a group of patients who resisted *P.aeruginosa* infection formed antibodies against mucoexopolysaccharide which promoted opsonophagocytic killing of *P.aeruginosa* by neutrophils.

It is not surprising that immune complex overload spills into systemic circulation and accounts for the arthritis, cutaneous and occasional cerebral vasculitis.

Cellular responses

The cellular response in CF is primarily mediated by neutrophils producing proteolytic enzymes and macrophages producing cytokines. The neutrophils produce an array of potent enzymes that break down lung connective tissue. Histology of the small airways reveals a neutrophilic bronchiolitis. Free radicals are produced in excessive amounts compared to controls[128]. Leukocytes are the main source of DNA found in CF sputum[129]. Neutrophil products are normally protective but when frustrated they damage lung tissue as an innocent bystander. There is a failure of neutrophil apoptosis. Other neutrophil products include collaginases,gelatinases and metalloproteinases. The lung is normally protected against neutrophil proteolytic activity by alpha-1-protease inhibitor and secretory leukocyte protease inhibitor. Although the levels of these enzymes are normal in CF they are overwhelmed by damaging neutrophil products. The degree of lung damage can be measured by the level of neutrophil elastase found in CF sputum during infective exacerbations[130] and elastic degradation products in urine[131].

In addition to the neutrophil,pulmonary macrophages (alveolar, interstitial and intravascular) play a major role in orchestrating the CF host response to infection. They release the cytokines which are mediators of inflammation but also produce proteinases,lipid products and oxidants which will degrade lung tissue in the same way as neutrophil products. They will also signal and attract other inflammatory cells[132].

Cytokines are intercellular messengers; The most clearly defined cytokines in CF are tumour necrosis factor alpha (TNF-a), the interferons and the interleukins. TNF-a is found in considerable quantities in CF serum[133] and is reported to augment the inflammatory process and to be the cause of anorexia and weight loss in severe disease[134].

A more recently descibed cytokine IL-8 is the main neutrophil chemoattractant produced by stimulated macrophages. It is found in high quantities in blood, bronchial washings and sputum and increased levels correlate with disease severity[135].

The role of cytokines in cystic fibrosis lung disease is complex and still evolving[136].

Clinical management of pulmonary infection

Symptoms and signs

The progress of CF lung disease is slow and insidious occurring over many years. In early childhood, diagnosis is suggested either by failure to thrive or recurrent respiratory tract infections. Once the steatorrhea has been corrected with pancreatic replacement nutritional status is considerably improved. Childhood infective respiratory problems cause suspicion when they are slow to resolve and reoccur. Diagnosis of CF is rapidly established when there is a previously affected sibling in the family. In later years respiratory symptoms and signs predominate.

Morning cough productive of white sputum may be the initial respiratory complaint. The sputum becomes purulent with chronic infection. The volume of sputum increases and purulence fails to resolve with antibiotic therapy. Cough may become persistent, troubling sleep.

Small haemoptyses are common and require reassurance. Infrequently haemoptysis may be massive and life threatening (500 ml of blood over 24 hours) requiring active intervention[137,138].

Variable wheezing occurs with infective exacerbations,associated asthma and progressive airways narrowing. Bronchial hyperreactivity can be correlated with increasing disease severity[139]. Pleuritic pain is extremely common in moderate to severe disease. Breathlessnes occurring during moderate exercise is common but persisting at rest despite treatment is an ominous symptom. Morning headaches suggest overnight carbon dioxide retention. Sinusitis and polyps cause facial discomfort and nasal stuffiness[140]. Sinus disease is always present radiologically with nasal polyps being the most common problem in younger patients. In older patients constant nasal blockage with a purulent post nasal drip is more frequent.

The pulmonary clinical signs of cystic fibrosis are often deceptively few and do not reflect disease severity. Clubbing occurs in nearly all older patients[141]. Hypertrophic pulmonary osteoarthropathy is uncommon (2%) but may be painful[1]. Patients can become grossly barrel chested and kyphotic with hyperinflated lungs. Ausculation may be singularly unhelpful despite radiological changes of severe disease. Coarse inspiratory and expiratory crackles can be heard over the upper lobes which may resolve with treatment but sometimes persist. During an infective exacerbation, transient pleural rubs are commonly auscultated and often may be palpable. Wheezing may be heard during infective exacerbations. Sudden acute breathlessness usually suggests the development of a pneumothorax.

As the disease progresses in severity patients can lose weight rapidly unless corrected actively with aggressive nutritional support.

The signs (facial and peripheral oedema) of right heart failure associated with carbon dioxide retention indicate preterminal disease.

Location of care

Although patient care may be shared, treatment of CF patients should primarily be located in recognised centres of expertise from the time of diagnosis. Patient survival is longer in centres[6,142]. In a centre the benefits of innovative treatments can be assessed in a larger number of patients. An experienced CF team can quickly distinguish between CF and non CF complications of the disease. In this setting,patients receive from a team better education and improved knowledge of their disease. As a consequence, patient self-care should be maximised. Finally audit of treatment practice and research outcomes can be qualitatively scrutinised in a well organised centre.

Monitoring treatment

The treatment of pulmonary infection requires a team of experts who will collectively review and contribute to all aspects of CF care. This care will include severity of infection, bacteriology, diabetes, nutrition, physiotherapy, exercise, patient compliance and social problems. Decisions will be made as to whether treatment changes are required and when to refer patients for transplantation when medical treatment is failing. Established protocols should assist in the management of various complications which may arise such as haemoptysis, pneumothorax, intestinal obstruction, respiratory failure and pregnancy.

It is essential to record and repeatedly measure the immediate and long term responses to treatment of individual patients. During inpatient stay, objective measurements should be made to assess the response to intravenous antibiotics (Table 24.2); bacteriological measurements should include sputum culture and 24-hour sputum weight (Fig. 24.9) at the beginning and end of a course of intravenous antibiotics. Other clinical measurements should include spirometry (Fig. 24.10), body weight, blood gas analysis, exercise capacity and host responses. All patients should have their airways reversibility assessed to inhaled bronchodilators, also their bronchoconstricter responses to nebulised antibiotics. Bronchodilator responses to inhaled and oral steroids should be measured. Physiotherapy technique should be assessed and tailored to lifestyle. Compliance with self care and correct taking of medication should be reviewed. Optimising nutrition and controlling established diabetes is essential for the maturing patient. Equally all patients should be screened for the onset of diabetes. Failure to establish a timely diagnosis may result in unnecessary clinical deterioration.

There are many aspects of patient care but the above mentioned are specific to monitoring and assessing the progress and severity of pulmonary infection and ensuing lung damage. Use of these parameters will determine whether treatment needs to be altered as an outpatient or inpatient. Sicker patients in borderline or established respiratory failure should have overnight oximetry, transcutaneous carbon dioxide levels and an assessment of response to titrated oxygen. Radical treatments may need to be instituted in these rapidly declining patient awaiting transplantation, such as overnight non-invasive ventilation or the siting of a permanent feeding gastrostomy.

Table 24.2. *Indicators to measure reponse to a course of intravenous antibiotics in hospital*

Indicator	Timing
Chest radiograph Spirometry Body weight 24 hour sputum weight Arterial blood gases Sputum culture and sensitivities Inflammatory markers	Beginning and end of treatment
Exercise test Transcutaneous overnight oxygen and carbon dioxide saturation on air if $p_aO_2 < 60$ mm Hg during the day	End of treatment

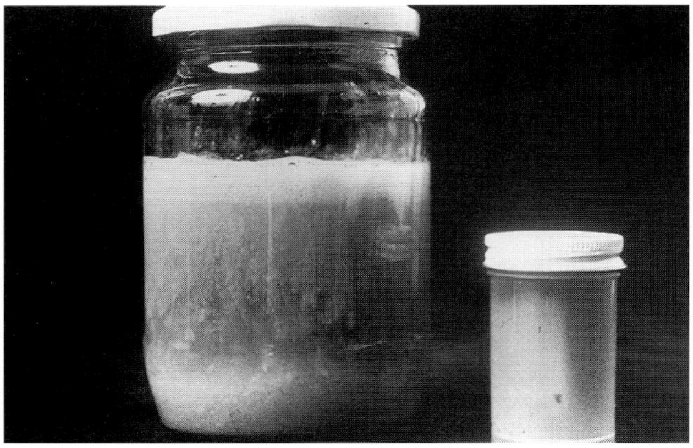

FIGURE 24.9 Large jar used to collect 24-hour sputum from CF patient. Small jar represents chronic sputum pot.

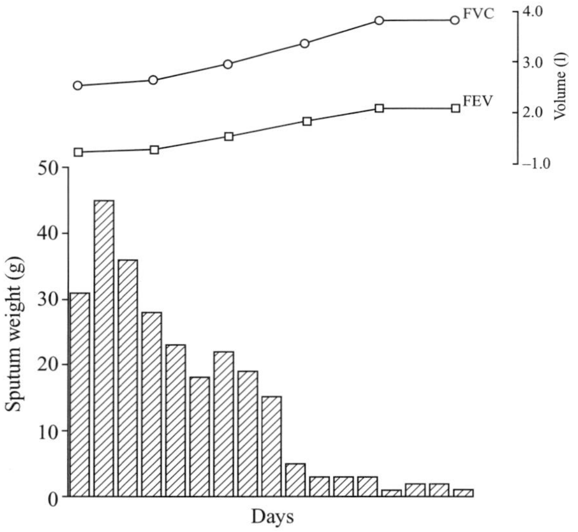

FIGURE 24.10 Reduction in daily 24-hour sputum weight and increase in spirometry with a course of intravenous antibiotics.

Antibiotic therapy

Prevention of *Pseudomonas aeruginosa* colonisation

The goal of CF therapy is to delay chronic colonisation with *P.aeruginosa*. Survival is longer in CF patients not infected with *P.aeruginosa* compared to patients who harbour the organism[32].

The quality and intensity of treatment provided by paediatricians may determine the degree of well being of the CF child referred to the adult physician. During childhood, therapy can be most opportunely directed at preventing or delaying infection with *P.aeruginosa*. Naturally many other factors may influence disease severity such as the acquisition of *B.cepacia* and adverse social circumstances.

During childhood,the principal pathogen is *S.aureus*. The administration of prophylactic antistaphylococcal antibiotics was undoubtedly the factor responsible for improved survival in the early years of the disease.It has been suggested that the long term use of antistaphylococcal antibiotics may have been a factor in the early colonisation of patients with *P.aeruginosa*[37]. Uncertainty still remains as to how long prophylactic antistaphylococcal antibiotics should be maintained when *P.aeruginosa* becomes the dominant infecting pathogen.

Several strategies have been developed to prevent or delay *P.aeruginosa* infection. The observation that *P.aeruginosa* infection is higher in large CF units has led one CF unit to segregate patients infected with *P.aeruginosa* from non-colonised patients with a reduction in *P.aeruginosa* colonisation[56]. A further approach was to vaccinate patients against acquiring *P.aeruginosa*. An initial study was unsuccessful and indeed suggested a more rapid pulmonary deterioration in vaccinated patients[143]. More recently, a polysaccharide-exotoxin A conjugate vaccine, which produces opsonic anti LPS and toxin A neutralising antibodies[144] has been evaluated with greater success. Self evidently this vaccine will only be efficacious against non colonised *P.aeruginosa* patients and will not be beneficial to 90% of adult CF patients. Woods and Bryan[145] immunised rodents with a *P.aeruginosa* alginate vaccine with an appropriate alginate antibody response and enhanced bacterial clearance.

Almost a decade ago, a brief report suggested that early colonisation with *P.aeruginosa* could be delayed with nebulised colistin[146]. The study was not controlled and patient numbers were small. A recent study has administered a combination of nebulised colistin and oral ciprofloxacin to patients at time of initial isolation of *P.aeruginosa* resulting in significantly less patients becoming chronically colonised with *P.aeruginosa* over a period of two years[147]. This clinical practice is likely to be most effective in paediatric clinics where less patients are infected by *P.aeruginosa*.

Efforts have been made to detect the transition from early benign colonisation to invasive infection with *P.aeruginosa* by a rise in antpseudomonal antibodies before detecting the organism in sputum culture[125]. It would seem reasonable that rising antipseudomonal antibodies are a good indicator for commencing oral or intravenous antibiotic therapy,whether or not the organism is present in sputum.

Patients would then receive intravenous antibiotics on the basis of a rising *P.aeruginosa* antibody titre. However patients may be unwilling to submit to the rigours of hospitalisation and intravenous antibiotics on the basis of a blood test and when they feel well.

Treatment of chronic *Pseudomonas aeruginosa* colonisation

Once the CF lung has become chronically infected with *P.aeruginosa*, the organism is impossible to eradicate permanently with intravenous antibiotics. Following treatment there may be a reduction in bacterial colony count or transient elimination of *P.aeruginosa* but reinfection within months is inevitable.

Treatment frequency and intensity

Although the treatment of CF patients embraces a multidisciplinary team approach, the cornerstone of patient care is the administration of oral, intravenous and nebulised antibiotics (Table 24.3). How frequently CF patients infected with *P.aeruginosa* should receive intravenous antibiotics is much debated. It has been suggested that inpatients can derive equal and sufficient benefit from the other modalities of care (physiotherapy, nutrition, exercise) and the addition of intravenous antibiotics is not crucial[148,149]. The majority of double-blind studies have not supported this thesis, demonstrating an improved clinical outcome following a course of intravenous antibiotics[150,151]. An infective exacerbation with clinical deterioration can usually be clearly defined by a decline in spirometry and body weight with an increase in sputum weight and purulence. Serial measurements of acute phase reactants such as C-reactive protein may be useful[45]. Charting these reproducible and easily measured indicators, complemented by close knowledge of the patient's usual clinical status nearly always accurately predict the need for intravenous antibiotics.

The majority of CF centres treat patients chronically colonised by *P.aeruginosa* with intravenous antibiotics approximately every 3 months. This policy was initiated by the Danish group on a prophylactic basis when the patients were often clinically stable. Improved survival was reported although the data were confounded by the absence of a control group[152]. However, several studies measuring *Pseudomonas* antibodies,free radical activity and breakdown products of lung proteolysis have shown that the exuberant host inflammatory response persists during the asymptomatic phase of patients chronically infected with *P.aeruginosa*[128,153]. Although some of these markers declined following a course of antibiotic treatment, they quickly rose following a treatment phase when the patient was clinically stable and asymptomatic, suggesting that lung damage is still silently progressing. Current evidence suggests that CF patients chronically infected with *P.aeruginosa* should receive regular intravenous antibiotics, although a minority of patients clearly remain clinically well for many years without this intervention. Frequent intravenous antibiotic therapy can create the problems of bacterial drug resistance, antibiotic allergy, damaged veins resulting in poor venous access and interference with quality of life.

Antibiotic choice

Intravenous antibiotics for CF patients are conventionally administered in large doses 3–4 times a day for a two week period. The choice of antibiotics is determined by the sensitivity of cultured *P.aeruginosa*.This choice may be confounded by the growth of multiple Pseudomonads with phenotypic differences (rough, smooth and mucoid) and different resistance patterns for each organism. *B.cepacia* with a multiple antibiotic resistance pattern may accompany the growth of *P.aeruginosa*.

Table 24.3. *Antibiotics for* Pseudomonas aeruginosa *colonisation in adults*

Drug	Route	Dosage	
Ciprofloxacin	Oral	750 mg	bd.
Colistin	nebulised	2 million units	bd
Gentamicin	nebulised	80 mg–160 mg	bd
Tobramycin	nebulised	80 mg–160 mg	bd
Aminoglycoside	Intravenous	80–120 mg	tds[a]
combined with			
either			
Ceftazidime	Intravenous	3 g	qds
or			
a monobactam			
Aztreonam	Intravenous	2–3 g	qds
or			
a carbapenem			
Imipenem	Intravenous	500 m	tds
Meropenem	Intravenous	2 g	tds
or			
a penicillin			
Azlocillin	Intravenous	5 g	qds
Timentim	Intravenous	3.2 g	qds

[a]Determine dose against peak levels of 10–12 μg/ml and trough levels of < 2 μg/ml.

A course of intravenous antibiotics usually combines an aminoglycoside with either an antipseudomonal penicillin or a third-generation cephalosporin. Peak levels for tobramycin or gentamicin should be measured after initiation of therapy; Satisfactory peak levels of aminoglycosides should be 10–12 micrograms/ml with a trough (preadministration) level of less than 2 micrograms/ml to minimise ototoxicity. Dosage of aminoglycosides in adults is related to serum levels rather than the usual indices of body weight and surface area due to the ability of CF patients to rapidly eliminate drugs from the circulation. Nephrotoxicity is singularly unusual. For these reasons, intravenous antibiotics are given frequently in divided doses rather than a single daily dose. Tobramycin is preferred to other aminoglycosides because of greater sputum penetration and less antibiotic resistance[154] but it is more expensive than gentamicin. Ceftazidime is the most commonly employed cephalosporin and has good MIC activity against the majority of *P.aeruginosa* isolates[155].

The monobactams (aztreonam) have been demonstrated to have equal efficacy against *P.aeruginosa*[156] but they have a narrower spectrum of activity being limited to gram negative organisms. The carbapenems (imipenem and meropenem) are a useful addition to the anti-pseudomonal antibiotics especially if there is resistance or allergy to cephalosporins or penicillins. The commonly used antibiotics and dosage are indicated in Table 24.3. Large doses of antibiotics are extremely well tolerated by CF patients probably due to the rapid metabolism. The development of allergic reactions to penicillins and cephalosporins can occur with repeated antibiotic courses. It is then appropriate to substitute a monobactam or a carbapenem.

Although antibiotic monotherapy can be as effective as a two drug combination of a β-lactam and an aminoglycoside[157], concern has been expressed that monotherapy will encourage antibiotic resistance and a two drug combination may have a synergistic effect against bacteria.

Metabolism of most drugs in CF patients is increased and there is a rapid clearance from the circulation. The result is a shorter half-life where there is a low serum peak concentration of drugs and a potential for serum drug free intervals. As a consequence, large dosages are prescribed and where possible drug levels measured and adjusted for the individual patients.

Despite the rapid elimination of drugs in CF patients, continuing clinical improvement has been observed following a course of intravenous antibiotics. The suppression of bacterial growth following a course of antimicrobial therapy has been recognised since the 1940s and has been called the post-antibiotic effect (PAE). Interest in this concept has recently reawakened[158]. The PAE has been described for the quinolones and the aminiglycosides[159]. Which factors influence the PAE are still being evaluated but include drug dose and dosing interval. The PAE may differ for individual antibiotics and different bacteria[160]. Further work is required in this sphere, which may influence prescribing practices of oral and intravenous antibiotics for CF patients.

Antibiotic delivery

The mode of antibiotic delivery should optimise maximum bacteriocidal effect but also has to fit in with the patient's lifestyle.

Bolus dose administration has the disadvantages of patient discomfort, vein damage, low serum levels,inaccurate dosage intervals and drug wastage. Antibiotics are made up in mini-infusion bags by the pharmacy and they are infused over 15–20 minutes. Equally adult patients or parents can be taught to make up antibiotics for home or hospital treatment. Some pharmaceutical companies have devised a home delivery service of preprepared antibiotic infusion bags which patients have found efficient and suitable to their lifestyle.

Venous access, using peripheral veins for multiple intravenous antibiotic courses becomes increasingly difficult, due to local thrombophlebitis. Improved venous access has been achieved with the development of totally implantable venous access systems (TIVAS)[161]. They are located under the skin with local anaesthetic by an experienced surgeon either on the chest wall (Port-a-Cath) or a P.A.S port on the upper arm. The device located on the arm is smaller and preferred by females for cosmetic reasons. Following insertion, they only need removal if complications ensue. They are safer than other central venous line systems[162]. The provision of secure and safe venous access has improved and enabled more home intravenous antibiotic therapy. When the access systems are in use for a course of intravenous antibiotic therapy the insertion,flushing and removal of the needles requires a full aseptic technique. Infection (usually fungal) is uncommon, but is the most commonly reported complication[163]. If this occurs it is essential to remove the device and treat the infecting organism on the basis of catheter and blood culture results.

Other complications of TIVAS include, catheter displacement, blockage or large vessel thrombosis[164].

Antibiotic treatment: home or hospital?

The dilemma between trying to lead a normal quality life and accommodate intensive intravenous antibiotic therapy several time a year has been partly resolved by teaching patients to administer their drugs at home. This has been facilitated by the increasing use of long lines or permanently sited 'porta-caths'. Patients prefer home therapy which is less costly when compared with hospital treatment. Several studies comparing home therapy to inpatient therapy have reported no difference in outcome for pulmonary function and reinfection if physiotherapy is maintained[165–167]. However, patients must be carefully selected for their known compliance rates and sicker patients may need hospital admission for a much more comprehensive assessment and repeated changes of treatment during a 2-week course of antibiotics. This is not readily achieved on a domiciliary basis. However,it is possible, when treatment has been programmed in hospital for the sickest patient awaiting transplantation to successfully receive continuing care at home. This care will include continuous intravenous antibiotics, nocturnal ventilation and a feeding gastrostomy.

Lifelong administration of intravenous antibiotics can result in resistance, allergic reactions and considerable expense; they prolong life but not for a normal life-span. It is evident from previous discussion that antibiotics have considerable limitations in controlling lifelong pulmonary infection with *P.aeruginosa* (Table 24.4). However, survival continues to improve in CF adults and although there are other factors which have improved prognosis such as better nutrition and improved compliance undoubtedly more expert use of an expanding armamentorium of antibiotics has played a significant role.

Oral antibiotics for *Pseudomonas aeruginosa*

No effective oral antibiotics to treat *P.aeruginosa* were available until the advent of the quinolones. Ciprofloxacin concentrates well in bronchial secretions and has been used satisfactorily as an alternative to intravenous antibiotic therapy[168]. However resistance and a declining clinical response follows repeated usage[169]. Some recovery of drug sensitivity has been reported[170]. Occasionally patients will respond to broad spectrum oral antibiotics other than the quinolones when only *P.aeruginosa* is cultured. This may be due to the concealed presence of *S.aureus*,routine 'bronchitic type' pathogens or non-typeable *Haemophilus influenzae*[42]. A more subtle antimicrobial effect may occur with the inhibition of pseudomonas virulence factors and interference of alginate biosynthesis by levels of antibiotics below a bacteriocidal MIC level[39].

It is apparent that *in vitro P.aeruginosa* resistance and sensitivity does not always predict clinical response. Sublethal nebulised concentrations of antibiotics and synergy between two resistant drugs are sometimes surprisingly effective against *P.aeruginosa*.

Nebulised antibiotics

Currently, the two main clinical indications for the prescription of nebulised antibiotics for CF patients are (i) To delay or prevent chronic colonisation with *P.aeruginosa*. CF patients who receive a combination of nebulised colistin and oral ciprofloxacin at the time of initial colonisation with *P.aeruginosa* will have a mean delay of two years to chronic infection[147]. (ii) To delay and prevent clinical deterioration in CF patients already chronically infected with *P.aeruginosa*. A previous study has shown that nebulised antibiotics can reduce

Table 24.4. *How antibiotics fail*

Fail to prevent bacterial adherence,colonisation and chronic infection
Fail to prevent exuberant host responses
Fail to prevent alginate formation
Fail to eradicate bacteria
May promote other bacteria

Table 24.5. *Requirements for an efficient compressor\nebuliser system*

Sufficient flow rate through the system to ensure rapid delivery
Maximum drug delivery to small airways
Particle size less than 5 μm
Minimal patient respiratory effort by using a system with a low resistance
Small residual volume in nebuliser to maximise drug release
Ease of cleaning by patient
Easy access to a nebuliser\compressor service for repair and exchange

admissions to hospital and reduce a decline in lung function[171]. Some scientific support as to why nebulised antibiotics (of which only 10–15% of the dose is delivered to purulent secretions in small airways) should be efficacious is answered by the observation that sublethal concentrations of antibiotics will decrease bacterial virulence factors and binding to epithelial surfaces[172].

In our unit we prescribe nebulised colistin for CF adults chronically colonised with *P.aeruginosa* when it is difficult to maintain pulmonary function between regular courses of intravenous antibiotics. No controlled trials are published to support this strategy and patient clinical response is unpredictable.

In order to optimise drug deposition and compliance it is important to use an efficient and effective compressor-nebuliser delivery system which should fulfil specific requirements (Table 24.5). Preferably antibiotics are nebulised using a low flow compressor with an active Venturi nebuliser. Guide-lines have been produced advising on good clinical practice for the use of nebulised antibiotics in cystic fibrosis.

Severely diseased patients with reduced spirometry who are eligible and most appropriate for prescription of colistin may develop breathlessness and chest tightness on commencing the drug. It is important to formally measure bronchoconstrictor responses and breathlessness prior to initiating colistin[173]. If patients are intolerant of nebulised colistin it may be possible to continue therapy by reducing the dose of the drug and concentration of the solution by dilution with water.

Treatment of *Burkholderia cepacia*

The emergence of *B.cepacia*, which may have multiple antibiotic resistance and is readily transmissible has created dilemmas as to the best management approach.

The degree of antibiotic resistance of *B.cepacia* has made it extremely difficult to adopt a rational intravenous antibiotic policy to this organism. Uncontrolled studies have suggested that a combination of several antibiotics may be synergistically effective against *B.cepacia* when there is *in vitro* drug resistance[174,175]. Sometimes, *B.cepacia* may have similar sensitivity patterns as *P.aeruginosa* and will respond to intravenous antibiotics satisfactorily. It has been suggested that *P.aeruginosa* promotes the adherence of *B.cepacia* to epithelial cells[176]. It is unclear whether treating a patient colonised with both *P.aeruginosa* and *B.cepacia* will alter this bacterial synergy.

The best medical treatment of *B.cepacia* is to provide a similar approach to that taken with *P.aeruginosa*, which is to maximise all facets of care provided by an experienced team. Patients infected with *B.cepacia* require a greater medical input and more medical admissions than patients with *P.aeruginosa*. The clinical responses to intravenous antibiotic therapy may be similar for both *B.cepacia* and *P.aeruginosa* despite *in vitro* antibiotic resistance to *B.cepacia*[88].

Colonisation with *B.cepacia* is currently as high as 40% in some units[177]. Perception of the ready transmissability of *B.cepacia* has led to the institution of segregation policies. In clinical practice, patients with *B.cepacia* have been segregated both as inpatients and outpatients from *P.aeruginosa* patients. Patients are informed which organisms they grow in their sputum. It is recommended that good clinical practice should include the following hygienic measures; meticulous hand washing by staff,that the two groups should use separate lung function, humidification, nebuliser and exercise equipment. Currently, there is no evidence that medical and paramedical staff are a third party source for transmitting *B. cepacia* between patients. However respiratory equipment has been implicated as a source for transmitting *B.cepacia* between CF patients[178] and immune compromised patients[179].

Ideally, there should be separate wards for each patient group. If this is not practical there should be separate eating areas and no sharing of kitchen facilities.

Out of hospital it has also been recommended that *B.cepacia* patients do not socialise with other CF patients. This includes close relationships,holiday camps, national and international meetings. The responsibility for fulfilling these measures has been made the responsibility of the patients. Despite a rigourous hospital isolation approach and support for social separation by most CF centres, patients continue to socialise resulting in the continuing transmission of *B.cepacia*[180]. The majority of units have reported a decline in the incidence of infection with *B.cepacia* following the establishment of a policy of strict patient segregation[181,79].

Segregating CF patients from each other has caused considerable anger and fear. The ethos of cystic fibrosis, directed at providing mutual moral support and advancing collective knowledge has disintegrated.

A further concern has been expressed that following organ transplantation, *B.cepacia* patients do worse than *P.aeruginosa* patients[182,183]. This has created ethical issues where some transplant centres are not listing patients for transplantation if colonised with multiple antibiotic resistant *B.cepacia*. However, it is these severely ill patients who are most in need of early transplantation.

A current survey of three transplant centres in the UK has not supported this opinion. No significant difference in outcome following transplantation was found for patients colonised with *B.cepacia* or *P.aeruginosa*[184].

Complications of pulmonary infection

The common clinical problems and complications which may exacerbate chronic pulmonary infection include pneumothoraces, recurrent large haemoptyses, abdominal surgery, pregnancy and diabetes. Each complication requires a different clinical management but intervention must be prompt to prevent pulmonary deterioration.

The incidence of pneumothorax in the older patient reflects disease severity and is associated with a poor prognosis[185]. A large pneumothorax (Fig. 24.11) requires prompt insertion of a drainage tube. A small pneumothorax not requiring drainage presents a difficult management problem. Physiotherapy is difficult and thickening secretions may prevent re-expansion of the lung. It is important to institute intravenous antibiotics at an early stage. If medical treatment is unsuccessful after approximately 10 days the patient should undergo videothoracoscopy to seal the leak[186].

Large haemoptyses make physiotherapy difficult. Patient positioning is limited and coughing discouraged. Oral or intravenous antibiotic should be instituted at an early stage. Temporary relief can be provided with vasopressor agents[137] and if the haemoptyses are continuing then bronchial artery embolisation is the treatment of choice[138,187]. Rebleeding does occur and rembolisation may be necessary for a small number of patients.

Pregnancy and abdominal surgery present similar problems with elevation of the diaphragm limiting lung expansion.

Pregnancy limits the use of some drugs due to potential teratrogenicity but continuous intravenous antibiotics and hospitalisation may be required during the last trimester for those patients with severe disease. Post-partum, patients may produce large quantities of sputum and some lung function may lost. Mothers with moderate to severe pre-pregnant lung disease disease (FEV1 < 60% predicted) do worse,producing preterm infants and increased loss of lung function and mortality compared with mildly affected mothers[188].

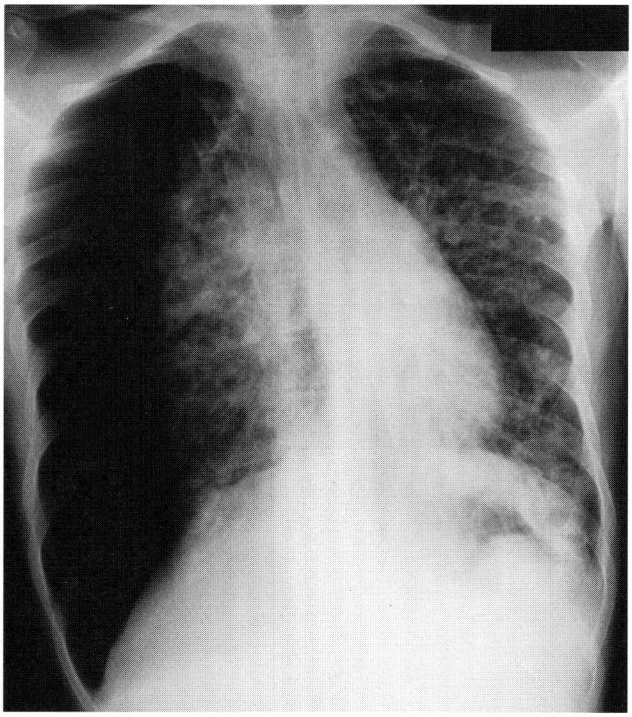

FIGURE 24.11 Large tension pneumothorax in a young 24-year-old male.

Following delivery, CF mothers may neglect their self-care in order to look after their child. The median survival for CF females adults is the late twenties and by adolescence the child is likely to be motherless.

As patients grow older endocrine pancreatic function declines. Impaired glucose tolerance in CF adults may be as high as 40%[189]. Glucose intolerance may increase during infective exacerbations, with the introduction of steroids and supplemental nutrition. At the Manchester unit 25% (40/160) of patients are clinically diabetic and require insulin or oral hypoglycaemic tablets. Insulin is the treatment of choice. Diabetes may increase morbidity but an adverse effect upon survival is disputed[190,191]. Poorly controlled CF diabetes is associated with a decline in pulmonary function[192].

Poor control of CF diabetes results in polyuria, polydipsia and weight loss. Morning secretions are thickened and difficult to expectorate.

Supportive therapy

In addition to antibiotics and anti-inflammatory therapy, the routine essential components of care include physiotherapy, bronchodilator therapy, patient education, monitoring compliance with self-care, maximised nutrition and adequate control of diabetes (see above). Self-care may be very demanding of patients trying to lead a busy normal life (Table 24.6). Inevitably, the focus of care becomes sharper and more traumatic for patient and carers during the preterminal stages of the disease when tremendous efforts are made to keep the patient alive especially if they are listed for transplantation.

Physiotherapy: the role of the physiotherapist

Physiotherapy is fundamental for long-term management of the chest in CF. It should commence at time of diagnosis and be performed daily. The most actively researched and validated physiotherapy technique is the active cycle of breathing exercises which includes the forced expiration technique (FET)[193]. The demonstrated virtues of this technique are the efficient mobilisation of secretions from small to large airways, it can be performed independent of assistance for both children and adults,does not exaggerate airways obstruction and is less tiring than coughing. There has been considerable debate about the comparative benefits of different physiotherapy techniques[194]

The prescription and monitoring of exercise should also be considered the remit of the physiotherapist. It has been reported that prognosis is improved for fitter CF patients[195]. The corollary that regular exercise programmes alter prognosis is unproven. However, exercise studies have demonstrated that patients feel less breathless and can improve cardiorespiratory fitness[196–198]. CF patients enjoy exercise and prefer it to other treatment modalities; it is recreational and sociable, body image is improved and the sense of benefit is immediate. Unfortunately it has sometimes been suggested that exercise can effectively replace the daily discipline of physiotherapy. Anecdotal support is provided by patients who remark they cough

Table 24.6. *Daily timetable of self-care*

	am	pm
Physiotherapy	20 min	20 min
Exercise	10 min	10 min
Nebulisation (antibiotics broncdodilators)	15 min	15 min
Total 1.5 hours		

In addition, oral medication and sometimes insulin.The sicker patients may need to self-care nocturnal ventilation, oxygen supplementation and gastrostomy feeding.

and produce sufficient sputum during exercise. This belief is disproved by two studies which have shown that, although exercise does increase sputum expectoration, a greater amount is produced with physiotherapy[199,200] and (Fig. 24.12). Sufficient sputum may be produced by combining exercise and physiotherapy modalities; an option preferred by the majority of patients. Physiotherapy and exercise should be considered to have complementary rather than exclusive roles.

The physiotherapist also has further important roles in contributing to patient care (Table 24.7). The physiotherapist also will assess reversibility to nebulised bronchodilators and the response to the institution of oral and inhaled steroids and bronchodilators on the home or hospital peak flow charts.

The physiotherapist is also ideally placed to monitor some aspects of compliance. Physiotherapy has a reported adherence rate of only 40–50%[201–203].

Nutrition

CF is a wasting disease. The causes are multifactorial and include a high energy demand probably related to the basic defect[204,205], the catabolic effect of gross pulmonary sepsis and poorly controlled pancreatic steatorrhoea. The patients require a high calorific intake which is difficult to achieve in the face of anorexia and progressive disease although it has been shown that a non-restricted diet is associated with a better

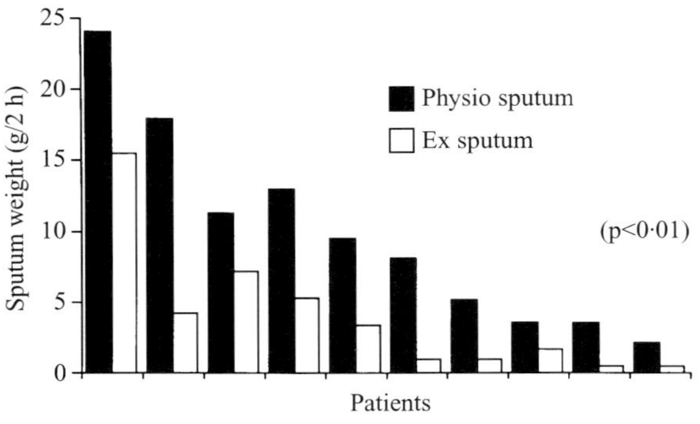

FIGURE 24.12 Physiotherapy and exercise increase sputum expectoration but physiotherapy produces more sputum than exercise. Exercise should not replace physiotherapy. Reproduced with permission of *Thorax*.

Table 24.7. *Role of the physiotherapist*

Educate, tailor, monitor and reinforce physiotherapy techniques for the individual patient
Assess reversibility to nebulised bronchodilators
Assess bronchoconstritor responses to nebulised antibiotics at time of prescription
Assess and monitor peak expiratory flow charts
Assess exercise capacity,prescribe safe enjoyable exercise programmes; monitor progress
Assess long-term compliance with above aspects of care

prognosis[142]. An increasingly aggressive approach is being adopted to maintain body weight for those patients listed for heart–lung transplantation. Wasted patients need to be nourished for the rigours of transplantation and the aftercare which is dominated by infection and rejection. The majority of underweight patients may need a feeding gastrostomy at time of acceptance for a transplantation.

Treatment of preterminal disease

Preterminal disease can be defined as failure of CF patients to respond to treatment following repeated admissions to a recognised CF centre. When FEV1 % predicted has fallen below 30%, a significant number of these patients will die within 2 years[5]. Consequently the majority of these patients will be considered and listed for organ transplantation. At time of transplantation, CF patients receive either a double lung or heart and lung transplant according to the practice of the transplant centre. Double lung transplantation is becoming more popular than heart–lung transplantation and there are probably more donors for this procedure. The donor lung retains the physiological characteristics of the donor following transplantation. Following a successful transplant CF patients can recover considerable body weight and will no longer require a feeding gastrostomy.

Patient selection and exclusion,operative techniques and complications require lengthy discussion and are outside the scope of this chapter. The actuarial survival for 69 CF patients undergoing heart–lung transplantation at a centre was 69% at 1 year and 52% at 2 years[206]. The commonest causes of death following transplantation are infection and chronic rejection. Following transplantation, the common infecting organisms are listed in Table 24.8. The transplanted lung is more susceptible to infection than other transplanted organs; it is in contact with the environment,postoperative pain and inefficient mucociliary clearance which inhibit chest drainage. The allograft lung of CF patients is especially vulnerable to infection as the sinuses and upper airways remain persistently colonised by resistant organisms which may subsequently reinfect the new lungs. Of particular concern to some transplant centres has been the occurrence of early post operative death due to sepsis with *B.cepacia*[182,183]. However, CF patients are the largest patient group requiring and receiving organ transplantation with results as good as those patients transplanted for other end stage lung diseases[206]. For those patients who receive a successful organ transplant, quality of life is enormously improved[207].

Table 24.8. *Common infecting pathogens following lung transplantation*

Bacterial	*Pseudomonas aeruginosa* and *B.cepacia*
	Streptoccus pneumoniae
Viral	Cytomegalovirus
Protozoa	*Pneumocystis carinii* and *Toxoplasma gondii*

Gross malnutrition can be combated by aggressive interventional feeding. All patients in our unit have a feeding gastrostomy site following acceptance for transplantation.

Non-invasive ventilation may control nocturnal hypoventilation and associated carbon dioxide retention. At the same time nocturnal oxygen can be administered safely[208]. It may be a successful bridge to transplantation[209,210]. Some patients do not adapt easily to learning the technique of nasal intermittent positive pressure ventilation (NIPPV), sometimes it is difficult to match patient breathing pattern and ventilator. NIPPV ventilation is usually instituted for patients developing carbon dioxide retention. A recent paper has suggested that nocturnal nasal continuous positive airway pressure (nCPAP) may forestall nocturnal oxygen desaturation[211]. This is not current clinical practice in transplant centres and the two methods have not been compared.

CF patients when obviously dying despite optimal management should not be placed on continuous positive pressure ventilation in the anticipation of organ donation. However, CF patients should receive intensive medical care,even with ventilation on an intensive care unit if there is a reversible situation.

Excessive zeal should be avoided in attempting to keep alive patients when a dignified and peaceful death is the appropriate management. Unfortunately, organ donor shortage and modern technology sometimes combine to produce different ways of dying.

Treating the inflammatory disease

A complicated exuberant host inflammatory response to chronic infection has a major role in causing progressive lung damage[131]. Therapeutic strategies used to diminish the inflammatory response currently include steroids, non-steroidal anti-inflammatory agents (NSAIDS), inhalation of aerosols of DNase to breakdown sputum and anti-elastases to combat lung proteolysis.

Oral steroids and non-steroidals as anti-inflammatory drugs

An initial study, treated paediatric patients with alternate day (2 mg/kg body weight) oral prednisone for four years and reported improved pulmonary function with few side-effects[212]. Unfortunately, a further study observed unacceptable high side-effects (cataracts, glucose intolerance and diminished growth) with the high dose arm (2 mg/kgm body weight) leading to termination of this part of the study. Subsequently the low dose arm (1 mg/kg) was concluded due to lack of demonstrable efficacy[213].

Steroids can be used for short courses as an addition to intravenous antibiotic therapy. In this role the patient may feel better and there may be both an anti-inflammatory and bronchodilator effect.

Non-steroidal anti-inflammatory drugs which do not exhibit the side effects of steroids are currently being evaluated with marginal benefits[214,215]. In animals it has been found that ibuprofen inhibits the generation of leukotriene 4 a neutrophil chemotaxin[216].

DNase

Purulent CF sputum contains excessive amounts of deoxyribonucleic acid (DNA) reflecting neutrophil breakdown. Purulent sputum is more viscous,protects bacteria from antibiotic penetration and may act as a vehicle for proteolytic enzymes. Human DNase, the enzyme responsible for the breakdown of DNA has successfully been cloned using recombinant technology. It has been shown that the enzyme can reduce CF sputum viscosity and increases pourability[217] resulting in a liquefying effect. Two recent short-term studies in CF patients with mild to moderate disease have shown that nebulised DNase is safe, increases sputum volume (33%) and improves spirometry (15%)[218,219]. The questions that future trials must address are long-term safety, benefit during infective exacerbations for patients with severe and moderate disease, reduction in bacterial load,infectivity and consequent amelioration of the progression of pulmonary disease. The drug is expensive and its cost-effectiveness needs evaluating.

Elastase inhibitors

The inability of the host CF lung to eliminate chronic bacterial infection results in continuous neutrophil infiltration. Excessive protease activity and in particular neutrophil elastase exceeds the activity of the protease inhibitors; alpha-1-antitrypsin and secretory leukoproteinase inhibitor (SLPI). Therapeutic strategies have led to the development of locally applied antiproteases to combat the inflammatory response. A short-term study demonstrated that the delivery of aerosolised alpha-1-antitrypsin to the bronchi elevated the levels in epithelial lining fluid (ELF) three to sixfold, inhibited neutrophil elastase activity and restored to normal neutrophil killing of *P.aeruginosa*[220]. Parenteral administration was ineffective.

The future management of pulmonary infection

Future research into improving the treatment of established pulmonary infection should be directed at greater understanding of the pathogenesis of *B.cepacia* and *P.aeruginosa*. Genetic and molecular technology should provide some of these insights. There is a need for more effective antibiotics with different mechanisms of bacterial destruction.

Inevitably the future treatment of cystic fibrosis depends upon (a) the application of screening techniques to eliminate the disease, (b) the success of gene therapy and (c) the development of novel drugs which will correct impermeability of the chloride channel.

There has been considerable debate about the merits of population screening of heterozygotes since the cloning of the gene in 1989. The main problem has been the considerable degree of genetic heterogeneity with only 70% of CF chromosomes being accounted for by the same allele. Currently, screening can be offered very usefully to relatives of affected individuals. In a similar manner,genetic screening can be offered to normal males in close partnership with a CF female when pregnancy is being planned.

Concern has also been expressed that population screening may cause psychosocial problems and do more harm than good[221], but a recent population study has suggested that the majority of people (90%) are in favour of screening[222].

Pharmacological correction with novel drugs which alter chloride impermeability has been tried but delivery and maintenance of delivery present logistic problems. Correction of the basic genetic defect is still the ultimate goal. Potential fields currently being explored are viral vectors,liposomal transfer of CFTR and artificial chromosomes. The cystic fibrosis mouse has been cloned and liposomal transfer of CFTR to a mouse has successful[223]. We live in exciting times but caution dictates that the successful transfer of scientific success to medical cure may be a decade away and these advances will help the paediatric rather than the adult patients.

Acknowledgements

I am indebted to Dr J. Govan and Dr M. Super for helpful criticism of the manuscript. I am extremely grateful to Dr P. Hasleton for the pathology illustrations.

References

1. PENKETH ARL, WISE A, MEARNS MB, HODSON ME, BATTEN JC. Cystic fibrosis in adolescence and adults. *Thorax* 1987; 42:526–32.
2. ROYAL COLLEGE OF PHYSICIANS OF LONDON. *Cystic Fibrosis in Adults. Recommendations for the Care of Patients in the UK.* London Royal College of Physicians; 1990.
3. NIELSEN H, SCHIOTZ PO. Cystic fibrosis in Denmark in the period 1945–1981. Evaluation of centralised treatment. *Acta Paediatr Scand* 1982; (Suppl 301):107–19.
4. RYLAND D, REID L. The pulmonary circulation in cystic fibrosis. *Thorax* 1975; 30:285–92.
5. KEREM E, REISMAN J, COREY M, CANNY GJ, LEVISON H. Prediction of mortality in patients with cystic fibrosis. *N Engl J Med* 1992; 326:1187–91.
6. DODGE JA. Cystic fibrosis in the United Kingdom. 1977–1985: an improving picture. *Br Med J* 1988; 297:1599–602.
7. DODGE JA, MORISON S, LEWIS PA *et al.* Cystic fibrosis in the United Kingdom, 1968–1988: incidence, population and survival. *Paediatr Perinatal Epidemiol* 1993; 7:157–66.
8. MAY DM, LOWE CU. The treatment of fibrosis of the pancreas in infants and children. *Paediatrics* 1948; 59:377–9.
9. ELBORN JS, SHALE DJ, BRITTON JR Cystic fibrosis: Current survival and population estimates to the year 2000. *Thorax* 1991; 46:881–5.
10. ROMMENS JM, IANNUZZI MC, KEREM B *et al.* Identification of the cystic fibrosis gene: chromosome walking and jumping. *Science* 1989; 245:1059–65.
11. RIORDAN JR, ROMMENS J, KEREM B *et al.* Identification of the cystic fibrosis gene: cloning and characterisation of complementary DNA. *Science* 1989; 245:1066–73.
12. KEREM B, ROMMENS JM, BUCHANAN JA *et al.* Identification of the cystic fibrosis gene: genetic analysis. *Science* 1989; 245:1073–80.
13. CYSTIC FIBROSIS GENETIC ANALYSIS CONSORTIUM Worldwide Survey of the Delta F508 mutation; report from the cystic fibrosis genetic analysis consortium. *Am J Hum Genet* 1990; 47:354–359.
14. MITCHELL-HEGGS P, MEARNS N, BATTEN JC. Cystic fibrosis in adolesence and adults. *Quart J Med* 1976; 179:479–504.
15. QUINTON PM. Cystic fibrosis: a disease in electrolyte transport. *FASEB J* 1990; 4:2709–17.
16. WELSH MJ. Abnormal regulation of ion channels in cystic fibrosis epithelia. *FASEB J* 1990; 4:2718–25.
17. KNOWLES M, GATZY J, BUCHER R. Increased bioelectric potential difference across respiratory epithelia in cystic fibrosis. *N Engl J Med* 1981; 305:1489–95.
18. BEAR CE, LI CH, KARTNER N *et al.* Purification and functional reconstruction of the cystic fibrosis transmembrane conductance regulator (CFTR). *Cell* 1992; 68:809–18.
19. ANDERSON MP, RICH GP, GREGORY RJ, SMITH AE, WELSH MJ. Generation of cAMP-activated chloride currents by expression of CFTR. *Science* 1991; 251:679–82.
20. KARTNER N, HANRAHAN JW, JENSEN TJ *et al.* Expression of the cystic fibrosis gene in non-epithelial invertebrate cells produces a regulated anion conductance. *Cell* 1991; 64:681–92.
21. DRUMM ML, POPE HA, CLIFF WH *et al.* Correction of the cystic fibrosis defect *in vitro* by retrovirus-mediated gene transfer. *Cell* 1990; 62:1227–33.
22. RICH DP, ANDERSON MP, GREGORY RJ *et al.* Expression of cystic fibrosis transmembrane conductance regulator corrects defective chloride channel regulations in cystic fibrosis airway epithelial cells. *Nature* 1990; 347:358–63.
23. BUSCH R. The history of cystic fibrosis. *Acta Univ Carol (Med)* 1990; 36:13–15.
24. DI'SANT'AGNESE PA, DARLING RC, PERERA GA, SHEA E. Abnormal electrolyte composition of sweat in cystic fibrosis of the pancreas, its clinical significance and relationship to the disease. *Paediatrics* 1953; 12:549–63.
25. GIBSON LE, COOKE RE. A test for concentration of electrolytes in sweat in cystic fibrosis of the pancreas utilising pilocarpine by ionophoresis. *Paediatrics* 1959; 23:545–9.
26. WELSH MJ. Electrolyte transport by airway epithelia. *Physiol Rev* 1987; 67:1143–84.
27. CLAIREAUX AE. Fibrocystic disease of the pancreas in the newborn. *Arch Dis Child* 1956; 31:22–7.
28. STURGESS JM. Morphological characteristics of the bronchial mucosa in cystic fibrosis. In Quinton PM, Martines JR, Hopfer U., eds. *Fluid and Electrolyte Abnormalities in Exocrine Glands in Cystic Fibrosis*. San Francisco Press; 1982: 254–70.
29. RAMPHAL R, VISWANATH S. Why is *Pseudomonas* the coloniser and why does it persist. Infect 1987; 14(4):281–7.
30. CACALANO G, KAYS M, SAIMAN L, PRINCE A. Production of the *Pseudomonas aeruginosa* neuraminidase is increased under hyperosmolar conditions and is regulated by genes involved in alginate expression. *J Clin Invest* 1992; 89:1866–74.
31. KUBESCH P, DORK T, WULBRAND U *et al.* Genetic determinants of airways colonisation with *Pseudomonas aeruginosa* in cystic fibrosis. Lancet 1990; 341:189–93.
32. WILMOTT RW, TYSON SL, MATTHEW DJ Cystic fibrosis survival rate: the influence of allergy and *Pseudomonas aeruginosa*. *Am J Dis Child* 1985; 139:669–71.
33. ANDERSEN DH. Cystic fibrosis of the pancreas and its relation to coeliac disease: A clinical and pathological study. *Am J Dis Child* 1938; 56:344–99.
34. DI'SANT'AGNESE PA, ANDERSON DL. Coeliac syndrome: chemotherapy of infection of the respiratory tract associated with cystic fibrosis of the pancreas: observations with penicillin and drugs of the sulphonamide

groups, with special reference to penicillin aerosol. *Am J Dis Child* 1946; 72:17–61.

35. HOFF GE, HOIBY N. *Staphylococcus aureus* in cystic fibrosis: antibiotic sensitivity and phage types during the last decade. *Acta Pathol Microbiol* 1975; (B)83:219–25.

36. ALY R, LEVIT S. Adherence of *Staphylococcus aureus* to squamous eipthelium: role of fibronectin and teichoic acid. *Rev Infect Dis* 1987; 94(suppl 4):341–50.

37. KULCZYCKI LL, WIENTZEN RL, HELLER T, BELLANTI JA. Factors influencing *Pseudomonas* colonisation in cystic fibrosis. *Ann Allergy* 1988; 60:423–8.

38. MEARNS MB, HUNT GH, RUSHWORTH R. Bacterial flora of the respiratory tract in patients with cystic fibrosis 1950–1971. *Arch Dis Child* 1972; 47:902–7.

39. GOVAN JR, NELSON JW. Microbiology of lung infection in cystic fibrosis. *Br Med Bull* 1992; 48:912–30.

40. GOVAN JRW, DOHERTY C, GLASS S. Rational parameters for antibiotic therapy in patients with cystic fibrosis. *Infection* 1987; 15:300–7.

41. HOIBY N, KILIAN M. *Haemophilus* from the lower respiratory tract of patients with cystic fibrosis. *Scand J Resp Dis* 1976; 57:103–7.

42. BILTON D, PYE A, JOHNSON MM, MITCHELL JL, DODD ME, WEBB AK, STOCKLEY RA, HILL S. The isolation and characterisation of non-typeable *Haemophilus influenzae* from the sputum of adult cystic fibrosis patients. *Eur J Resp Med* 1995; 8:948–53.

43. KNOKE JD, STERN RC, DOERCHUK CF, BOAT TF, MATTHEWS LW. Cystic fibrosis: the prognosis for five-year survival. *Pediatr Res* 1978; 12:676–9.

44. RAYNER RJ, HILLER EJ, ISPAHANI P, BAKER M. *Haemophilus* infection in cystic fibrosis. *Arch Dis Child* 1990; 65:255–8.

45. GLASS S, HAYWARD C, GOVAN JRW. Serum C-reactive protein in assessment of pulmonary exacerbation and antimicrobial therapy in cystic fibrosis. *J Pediatr* 1988; 113(1):76–9.

46. PRESSLER T, SZAFF M, HOIBY NM. Antibiotic treatment of *Haemophilus influenzae* and *Haemophilus parainfluenzae* infection in patients with cystic fibrosis. *Acta Paediatr Scand* 1984; 73:541–7.

47. HOIBY N. Microbiology of lung infections in cystic fibrosis patients. *Acta Paediatr Scand* 1982; (Suppl 301):33–54.

48. DOGGETT RG, HARRISON GM, STILLWELL RN, WALLIS ES. An atypical *Pseudomonas aeruginosa* associated with cystic fibrosis of the pancreas. *J Pediatr* 1966; 68:215–21.

49. JOHANSEN HK, HOIBY N. Seasonal onset of initial colonisation and chronic *Pseudomonas aeruginosa* infection in Danish cystic fibrosis patients. *Thorax* 1992; 47:109-11.

50. ZIMAKOFF J, HOIBY N, ROSDENAL K, GUILBERT JP. Epidemiology of *Pseudomonas aeruginosa* infection and the role of contamination of the environment in a cystic fibrosis clinic. *J Hosp Infect* 1983; 4:31–40.

51. DORING G, ULRICH M, MULLER T. Generation of *Pseuodomonas aeruginosa* aerosols during hand washing from contaminated sink drains, transmission to hands of hospital personnel, and its prevention by use of a new heating device. *Zbl Hyg* 1991; 191:494–505.

52. KELLY NM, FITZGERALD MX, TEMPANY E, O'BOYLE C, FALKINER FR, KEANE CT. Does *Pseudomonas* cross-infection occur between cystic fibrosis patients? *Lancet* 1982; ii: 688–90.

53. THOMASSEN MJ, DEMKO CA, DOERCHUK CF, ROOT JM. *Pseudomonas aeruginosa* isolates: comparisons of isolates from campus and from sibling pairs with cystic fibrosis. *Paediatr Pulmonol* 1985; 1:40–5.

54. SPEERT DP, LAWTON D, DAMM S. Communicability of *Pseudomonas aeruginosa* in a cystic fibrosis summer camp. J *Paediatr* 1982; 101:227–9.

55. PEDERSON SS, KOCH C, HOIBY N, ROSENDAL K. An epidemic spread of multi-resistant *Pseudomonas aeruginosa* in a cystic fibrosis centre. *J Antimicrob Chemother* 1986; 17:505–16.

56. HOIBY N, PEDERSEN SS. Estimated risk of cross-infection with *Pseudomonas aeruginosa* in Danish cystic fibrosis patients. *Acta Paediatr Scand* 1982; 78:395–404.

57. FYFE JAM, HARRIS H, GOVAN JRW. Revised pyocin typing method for *Pseudomon as aeruginosa*. *J Clin Med Microbiol* 1984; 20:47–50.

58. OGLE JW, JANDA JM, WOODS DE, VASIL ML. Characterisation and use of a DNA probe as an epidemiological marker for *Pseudomonas aeruginosa*. *J Infect Dis* 1987; 155:119–26.

59. OJENIYI B, HOIBY N, ROSDAL VT. Genome fingerprinting as a typing method used on polyagglutinable *Pseudomonas aeruginosa* isolates from cystic fibrosis patients. *APMIS* 1991; 99:492–8.

60. PETERSEN NT, HOIBY N, MORDHORST CH, LIND K, FLENSBORG EW, BRUN B. Respiratory infections in cystic fibrosis patients caused by a virus, *Chlamydia* and *Mycoplasma* – possible synergism with *Pseudomonas aeruginosa*. *Acta Paediatr Scand* 1981; 70:623–8.

61. KOMIYAMA K, TYANAN JJ, HABBICK BF, DUNCAN DE, LIEPERT DJ. *Pseudomonas aeruginosa* in the oral cavity and sputum of patients with cystic fibrosis. *Oral Surg* 1985; 59:590–4.

62. BAKER NR, SVANBORG-EDEN C. Role of alginate in the adherence of *Pseudomonas aeruginosa*. *Antibiot Chemother* 1989; 42:72–9.

63. BAKER NR. Adherence and the role of alginate. In Gacesa P, Russell NJ, *Pseudomonas Infection and Alginates. Biochem Genet Pathol* 1990. London: Chapman and Hall; 1990:95–108.

64. BAKER NR, MINOR V, DEAL C, SHAHRABDI MS, SIMPSON DA, WOODS DE. *Pseudomonas aeruginosa* exoenzyme S is an adhesin. *Infect Immun* 1991; 59:2859–63.

65. WILSON R, ROBERTS D, COLE P. Effect of bacterial products on human ciliary function *in vitro*. *Thorax* 1985; 40:125–31.

66. HINDLEY ST, HASTIE AT, KUEPPERS F, HIGGINS M, WEINBAUN G. Ciliostatic factors from *Pseudomonas aeruginosa*. *Chest* 1989; 95:(Suppl)214S–15S.

67. PLOTKOWSKI MC, BECK G, TOURNIER JM. Adherence of *Pseudomonas aeruginosa* to respiratory epithelium and the effect of leucocyte elastase. *J Med Microbiol* 1989; 30:285–93.

68. FYFE JAM, GOVAN JRW. Alginate synthesis in mucoid *Pseudomonas aeruginosa*: a chromosomal locus involved in control. *J Gen Microbiol* 1980; 119:443–50.

69. GOVAN JRW, MARTIN DW, DERETIC VP. Mucoid *Pseudomonas aeruginosa* and cystic fibrosis: the role of mutations in the muc loci. FEMS Microbiol 1992; letters 100:323–30.

70. RUSSEL NJ, TATNELL PJ, GACESA P. The regulation of alginate biosynthesis by mucoid *Pseudomonas aeruginosa*. In Hoiby N, Pedersen SS, eds. *Cystic Fibrosis, Basic and Clinical Research*. Excerpta Medica Elsevier Science Publ: 1992: 81–92.

71. PEDERSEN SS, HOIBY N, ESPERSEN F, KHARAZMI A. Alginate in infection. *Antibiot Chemother* 1991; 44:68–79.

72. JENSEN EP, KHARAZMI A, LAMB K, COSTERTON JW, HOIBY N. Human polymorphonuclear leucocyte response to *Pseudomonas aeruginosa* grown in biofilm. *Infect Immun* 1990; 58:2383–5.

73. PEDERSEN SS, KHARAZAMI A, ESPERSEN F, HOIBY J. *Pseudomonas aeruginosa* alginate in cystic fibrosis sputum and the inflammatory response. *Infect Immun* 1990; 58:3363–8.

74. PIER G *et al.* Opsonophagocytic killing antibody to *Pseudomonas aeruginosa* mucoid exopolysaccharide in older non-colonised patients with cystic fibrosis. *N Engl J Med* 1989; 317:793–8.

75. GOVAN JR. Alginate and antibiotics. *Antibiot Chemother* 1989; 42:88–96.

76. NICHOLS WW, DORRINGTON SM,

SLACK MEP, WALMSLEY HL. Inhibition of tobramycin diffusion by binding to alginate. *Antimicrob Agents Chemother* 1988; 32:518–23.

77. THOMASSEN MJ, DEMKO CA, KLINGER JD, STERN RC. *Pseudomonas cepacia* colonisation among patients with cystic fibrosis: a new opportunist. *Am Rev Resp Dis* 1985; 131:791–6.

78. ISLES A, MACLUSKY I, COREY M *et al.* *Pseudomonas cepacia* infection in cystic fibrosis:an emerging problem. *J Pediatr* 1984; 104:206–10.

79. GOVAN JR, BROWN PH, MADDISON J *et al.* *Pseudomonas cepacia* – evidence for transmission by social contact in patients with cystic fibrosis. *Lancet* 1993; 342:15–19.

80. TABLAN OC, CARSON LA, CUSICK LB, BLAND LA, MARTONE WJ, JARVIS WR. Laboratory proficiency tests results on the use of selective media for isolating *Pseudomonas cepacia* from simulated sputum specimens of patients with cystic fibrosis. *J Clin Microbiol* 1987; 25:485–7.

81. SIMAN AL, CACALANO G, PRINCE A. *Pseudomonas cepacia* adherence to respiratory epithelial cells is enhanced by *Pseudomonas aeruginosa*. *Infect Immun* 1990; 58:2578–84.

82. SIMMONDS EJ, CONWAY SP, GHONEIM ATM, ROSS H, LITTLEWOOD JM. *Pseudomonas cepacia*: a new pathogen in patients with cystic fibrosis referred to a large centre in the United Kingdom. *Arch Dis Child* 1990; 65:874–7.

83. STEINBECK S, SUN L, JIANG RZ *et al.* Transmissibility of *Pseudomonas cepacia* infections in clinic patients and lung transplant recipients with cystic fibrosis. *N Engl J Med* 1994; 331:981–7.

84. NELSON JW, DOHERTY CJ, BROWN PH, GREENING AP, KAUFMANN ME, GOVAN JRW. *Pseudomonas cepacia* in inpatients with cystic fibrosis. *Lancet* 1991; 338:1525.

85. LIPUMA JJ, DASEN SE, NEILSON DW, STERN RC, STULL TL. Person-to-person transmission of *Pseudomonas cepacia* between patients with cystic fibrosis. *Lancet* 1990; 336:1094–6.

86. GLASS S, GOVAN JRW. *Pseudomonas cepacia*: fatal pulmonary infection in a patient with cystic fibrosis. *J Infect* 1986; 13:157–8.

87. BROWN P, BUTLER S, NELSON J *et al.* *Pseudomonas cepacia* in adult cystic fibrosis: accelerated decline in lung function and increasing mortality. *Thorax* 1993; 48:425.

88. PECKHAM DG *et al.* Effect of antibiotic treatment on inflammatory markers and lung function in cystic fibrosis patients with *Pseudomonas cepacia Thorax* 1994; 49:803–7.

89. BURNIE J P, AL-WARDI E J, WILLIAMSON P, MATHEWS R C, WEBB K, DAVID T. Defining potential targets for immunotherapy in *Burkholderia cepacia* infection. *FEMS* 1994; 1–8.

90. GLADMAN G, CONNOR PJ, WILLIAMS RF, DAVID TJ. Controlled study of *Pseudomonas cepacia* and *Pseudomonas maltophilia* in cystic fibrosis. *Arch Dis Child* 1992; 67:192–5.

91. HOLMES B, LAPAGE SP, EASTERLING BG. Distribution in clinical material and identification of *Pseudomonas maltophilia*. *J Clin Pathol* 1979; 32:66–72.

92. CONWAY SP, SIMMONDS EJ, LITTLEWOOD JM. Acute severe deterioration in cystic fibrosis associated with influenza A virus infection. *Thorax* 1992; 47:112–14.

93. WANG EEL, PROBER CJ, MANSON B, COREY M, LEVISON H. Association of respiratory viral infections with pulmonary deterioration in patients with cystic fibrosis. *N Engl J Med* 1984; 311:1653–1658.

94. ONG ELC, MULVENNA P, WEBB AK. Varicella-zoster infection in adults with cystic fibrosis: role of azyclovir. *Scand J Infect Dis* 1991; 23:283–5.

95. MACDONALD NE, MORRIS RF, BEAUDREY PH. Varicella in children with cystic fibrosis. *Pediatr Infect Dis J* 1987; 6:414–16.

96. SARKINEN HK, HALONEN PE, ARSTILA PP, SALMI AA. Detection of respiratory syncytial, para-influenza type 2, and adenovirus antigens by radio immuno-assay and enzyme immuno-assay on nasopharyngeal specimens from children with acute respiratory disease. *J Clin Microbiol* 1989; 13:258–65.

97. VOLPI A, WHITLEY RJ, CEBALLOS R, STAGNO S, PEREIRA L. Rapid diagnosis of pneumonia due to cytomegalovirus with specific monclonal antibodies. *J Infect Dis* 1983; 147:119–1120.

98. ONG ELC, BILTON D, ABBOTT JV, WEBB AK, MCCARTNEY RA, CAUL EO. Influenza vaccination in adults with cystic fibrosis. *Br Med J* 1991; 303:557.

99. ADLARD P, BRYETT K. Influenza immunization in children with cystic fibrosis. *J Int Med Res* 1987; 15:344–51.

100. ONG ELC, ELLIS ME, WEBB AK *et al.* Infective respiratory exacerbations in young adults with cystic fibrosis: role of viruses and atypical micro-organisms. *Thorax* 1989; 44:739–42.

101. EFTHIMIOU J, HODSON ME, TAYLOR AJ, BATTEN JC. Importance of viruses and *Legionella pneumophilia* in respiratory exacerbations in young adults with cystic fibrosis. *Thorax* 1984; 39:150–4.

102. EFTHIMIOU J, SMITH MJ, HODSON ME, BATTEN JC. Fatal pulmonary infection with *Mycobacterium fortuitum* in cystic fibrosis. *Br J Dis Chest* 1984; 78:299–302.

103. HJELTE L, PETRINI B, KALLENIUS G, STRANDVIK B. Prospective study of mycobacterial infections in patients with cystic fibrosis. *Thorax* 1990; 45:397–400.

103. SMITH MJ, EFFTHMIOU J, HODSON ME, BATTEN JC. Mycobacterial isolations in young adults with cystic fibrosis. *Thorax* 1984; 39:369–75.

105. WHITTIER S, HOPFER RL, KNOWLES MR, GILLIGAN PH. Improved recovery of *Mycobacteria* from respiratory secretions of patients with cystic fibrosis. *J Clin Microbiol* 1993; 31:861–4.

106. BHARGAVA V, TOMASHEFSKI JF, STERN C, ABRAMOWSKY CR. The pathology of fungal infection and colonisation in patients with cystic fibrosis. *Hum Pathol* 1989; 20:977–86.

107. MEARNS MB, YOUNG W, BATTEN JC. Transient pulmonary infiltrations in cystic fibrosis due to allergic aspergillosis. *Thorax* 1965; 20:385–92.

108. MEARNS MB, LONGBOTTOM J, BATTEN JC. Persisting antibodies to *Aspergillus fumigatus* in cystic fibrosis. *Lancet* 1967; i:538–9.

109. BRUETON MJ, ORMEROD LP, SHAH KJ, ANDERSON CM. Allergic bronchopulmonary aspergillosis complicating cystic fibrosis in childhood. *Arch Dis Child* 1980; 55:348–53.

110. MAGUIRE S, MORIARTY B, TEMPANY E, FITZGERALD M. Unusual clustering of allergic bronchopulmonary aspergillosis in children with cystic fibrosis. *Paediatrics* 1988; 82:835–9.

111. ZEASKE R, BRUNS WT, FINK JN *et al.* Immune responses to *Aspergillus* in cystic fibrosis. *J Allergy Clin Immun* 1988; 82:73–7.

112. HILLER JC. Pathogenesis and management of aspergillosis in cystic fibrosis. *Arch Dis Child* 1990; 65:397–8.

113. DENNING DW, VAN WYE JEV, LEWISTON NJ, STEVENS DA. Adjunctive therapy of allergic pulmonary aspergillosis with itraconazole. *Chest* 1991; 100:813–19.

114. MADDEN BP, CHAN CM, KAMALVAND K *et al.* *Aspergillus* infection in patients with cystic fibrosis following lung transplantation. In Escobar H, Baquero S, Suarez, L, eds. *Clinical Ecology of Cystic Fibrosis. Excerpta Medica* Elsevier Sciences; 1993.

115. PEDERSEN SS, ESPERSEN F, HOIBY N. Diagnosis of chronic *Pseudomonas aeruginosa* infection in patients with cystic fibrosis. *J Clin Microbiol* 1987; 25:1830–6.

116. DORING G, HOIBY N. Longditudinal study of immune responses to *Pseudomonas aeruginosa* antigens in cystic fibrosis. *Infect Immun* 1983; 42:197–201.

117. DORING G, GOLDSTEIN W, ROELL A, SCHIOTZ PO, HOIBY N, BOTZENHART K. Role of *Pseudomonas aeruginosa* exoenzymes in lung infections of patients with cystic fibrosis. *Infect Immun* 1985; 49:557–62.

118. HOLLSING A, GRANSTOM M, VASIL ML, WRETLIND B, STRANDVIL B. Prospective longditudinal study of serum antibodies to *Pseudomonas aeruginosa* exoproteins in cystic fibrosis. *J Clin Microbiol* 1987; 25:1868–74.

119. WOODS D, TO M, SOKOL PA. *Pseudomonas aeruginosa* exoenzyme S as a pathogenetic determinant in respiratory infection. In Hoiby N, Pedersen SS, Shand G H, Doring G, Holder IA, eds. *Pseudomonas aeruginosa* infection. *Antibiot Chemother* 1989; Vol 42, Basel-Karger.

120. PIER GB. Immunological properties for *Pseudomonas aeruginosa* mucoid exopolysaccharide (alginate). *Antibiot Chemother* 1989; 80–7.

121. HANCOCK REW, MOAT ECA, SPEERT DP. Quantitation and identification of antibodies to outer-membrane proteins of *Pseudomonas aeruginosa* in sera of patients with cystic fibrosis. *J Infect Dis* 1984; 49:220–6.

122. ANDERSON TR, MONTIE TC, MURPHY MD, MCCARTHY VP. *Pseudomonas* flagellar antibodies in patients with cystic fibrosis. *J Clin Microbiol* 1989; 27:2789–93.

123. NELSON JW, GOVAN JRW, BARCLAY GR. *Pseudomonas* flagellar antibodies in serum, saliva and sputum from patients with cystic fibrosis. Serodiagnosis and immunotherapy. *Infect Dis* 1990; 4:351–61.

124. PEDERSEN SS, HOIBY N, ESPERSEN F, KOCH C. Role of alginate in infection with mucoid *Pseudomonas aeruginosa* in cystic fibrosis. *Thorax* 1992; 47:6–13.

125. BRETT MM, GHONHEIM AT, LITTLEWOOD JM. Prediction and diagnosis of early *Pseudomonas aeruginosa* infection in patients with cystic fibrosis: a follow up study. *J Clin Microbiol* 1988; 26:1565–70.

126. PRESSLER T, PEDDERSEN SS, ESPERSEN F, HOIBY N, COCH C. IgG subclass antibodies to *Pseudomonas aeruginosa* in serum from patients with chronic *Ps. aeruginosa* infection investigated by ELISA. *Clin Exper Immun* 1990; 81:428–34.

127. BERGER M, NORVELL T, TOSI M, KONSTAN M, SCHRIEBER J. Lack of complement receptor expression by alveolar macrophages (AM) correlates with poor enhancement of phagocytosis of *P. aeruginosa* by complement (C). *Pediatr Res* 1990; 27:154A.

128. SALH W, WEBB AK, GUYAN PM *et al.* Aberrant free radical activity in cystic fibrosis. *Clin Chim Acta* 1989; 181:65–74.

129. BARTON AD, RYDER K, LOURENCO RV, DRALLE W, WEISS SG. Inflammatory reaction and airways damage in cystic fibrosis. *J Lab Clin Med* 1976; 88:423–6.

130. SUTER S, SCHAAD UB, TEGNER H, OHLSSON K, DESGRANDCHAMPS D, WALD-VOGEL FA. Levels of free granulocyte elastase in bronchial secretions from patients with cystic fibrosis: effect of antimicrobial treatement against *Pseudomonas aeruginosa*. *J Infect Dis* 1986; 153(5):902–9.

131. BRUCE MC, PONCZ L, KLINGER JD, STERN RC, TOMASHEFSKI JF, DEARBORN DG. Biochemical and pathologic evidence for proteolytic destruction of lung connective tissue in cystic fibrosis. *Am Rev Resp Dis* 1985; 132:529–35.

132. OZAKI T *et al.* Role of alveolar macrophages in the neutrophil-dependendent defence system against *Pseudomonas aeruginosa* infection in the lower respiratory tract. *Am Rev Resp Dis* 1989; 140:1595–601.

133. NORMAN D, ELBORN JS, CORDON SM *et al.* Plasma tumour necrosis factor alpha in cystic fibrosis. *Thorax* 1991; 46:91–5.

134. SUTER S, SCHAAD, UB, ROUX-LOMBARD P, GIRARDIN E, GRAU G, DAYER JM. Relation between tumour necrosis factor alpha and granulocyte elastase-alpha 1–proteinase inhibitor complexes in the plasma of patients with cystic fibrosis. *Am Rev Resp Dis* 1989; 140:1640–4.

135. ASSADULLAHI TP, CHURCH MK, DAI Y, WARNER J. Interleukin 8 concentrations are elevated in children with cystic fibrosis. *Am Rev Resp Dis* 1992; 145:(4), A118.

136. SHALE D. Cytokines in cystic fibrosis. In Dodge JA, Brock DJH, Widdicombe JH, eds. *Cystic Fibrosis Current Topics*. Chichester: Wiley, Sons; 1994.

137. BILTON D, WEBB AK, FOSTER H, MULVENNA P, DODD ME. Life threatening haemoptysis in cystic fibrosis; an alternative therapeutic approach. *Thorax* 1990; 45:975–6.

138. COHEN AM, DOERCSHUK CF, STERN RC. Bronchial artery embolisation to control haemoptysis in cystic fibrosis. *Radiology* 1990; 175:401–3.

139. EGGLESTON PA, ROSENSTEIN BJ, STACKHOUSE CM, ALEXANDER MF. Airway hyperreactivity in cystic fibrosis. Clinical correlates and possible effects on the course of the disease. *Chest* 1998; 94:360–5.

140. STERN RC, BOAT TF, WOOD RE, MATHEWS LW, DOERSHUK CF. Treatment and prognosis of nasal polyps in cystic fibrosis. *Am J Dis Child* 1982; 136:1067–70.

142. COREY J, MCLOUGHLIN FJ, WILLIAMS M, LEVISON H. A comparison of survival, growth and pulmonary function in patients with cystic fibrosis in Boston and Toronto. *J Clin Epidemiol Metab* 1988; 41:583–91.

143. LANGFORD DT, HILLER J. Prospective, controlled study of a polyvalent pseudomonas vaccine in cystic fibrosis – three year results. *Arch Dis Child* 1984; 59:1131–4.

144. SCHAAD UB, LANG AB, WEDGEWOOD J *et al.* Safety and immunogenicity of *Pseudomonas aeruginosa* conjugate A vaccine in cystic fibrosis. *Lancet* 1991; 338:1236–7.

145. WOODS DE, BRYAN LE. Studies of the ability of alginate to act as a protective immunogen against infection with *Pseudomonas aeruginosa* in animals. *J Infect Dis* 1985; 581–8.

146. LITTLEWOOD JM, MILLER MG, GHONHEIM AT, RAMSDEN CH. Nebulised colomycin for early *Pseudomonas* colonisation in cystic fibrosis. *Lancet* 1985; I:865.

147. BRETT MM, GHONHEIM AT, LITTLEWOOD JM. Serum IgA antibodies against *Pseudomonas aeruginosa* in cystic fibrosis. *Arch Dis Child* 1990; 65:259–63.

148. BEAUDRY PH, MARKS MI, MCDOUGALL D, DESMOND K, RANGEL R. Is anti-*Pseudomonas* therapy warranted in acute respiratory exacerbations in children with cystic fibrosis? *J Pediatr* 1980; 97:144–77.

149. GOLD R, CARPENTER S, HEURTER H, COREY M, LEVISON H. Randomised trial of ceftazidime versus placebo in the management of acute respiratory exacerbations in patients with cystic fibrosis. *J Pediatr* 1987; 111:907–13.

150. WIENTZEN R, PRESTIDGE CB, KRAMER RI, MCCRACKEN GH, NELSON JD. Acute pulmonary exacerbations in cystic fibrosis. *Arch J Dis Child* 1980; 134:1134–8.

151. HYATT AC, CHIPPS BE, KUMOR KM, MELLITIS ED, LIETMAN PS, ROSENSTEIN BJ. A double- blind controlled trial of anti-*Pseudomonas* chemotherapy of acute respiratory exacerbations in patients with cystic fibrosis. *J Pediatr* 1981; 99:307–11.

152. SZAFF M, HOIBY N, FLENSBORG EW. Frequent antibiotic therapy improves survival of cystic fibrosis patients with chronic *Pseudomonas aeruginosa* infection. *Acta Pediatr Scand* 1983; 72:651–7.

153. RAYNER RJ, WEISEMAN MS, CORDON SM, NORMAN D, HILLER EJ, SHALE DJ. Inflammatory markers in cystic fibrosis. *Resp Med* 1991; 85:139–45.

154. PAPORISZ U, POSSELT HG, WOENNE R *et al.* Evaluation of long term tobramycin therapy in patients with cystic fibrosis and advanced pulmonary disease. *Eur J Pediatr* 1979; 130:259–69.

155. PADOAN R, BRIENZA A, CROSSIGNANI RM *et al.* Ceftazidime in the treatment of pulmonary exacerbations in patients with cystic fibrosis. *J Pediatr* 1983; 103:320–6.

156. SALH W, BILTON D, DODD M, ABBOT J, WEBB AK. A comparison of aztreonam and ceftazidime in the treatment of respiratory infections in adults with cystic fibrosis. *Scand J Infect Dis* 1992; 24:215–18.

157. GOLD R, OVERMEYER A, KNIE B, FLEMING PC, LEVISON H. Controlled trial of ceftazidime vs ticarcillin and tobramycin in the treatment of acute respiratory exacerbations in patients with cystic fibrosis. *Pediatr Infect Dis* 1985; 4:172–7.

158. VOGELMAN BS, CRAIG WA. Post antibiotic effects. *J Antimicrob Chemother* 1985; 15:37–46.

159. PASTOR A, PEMAN J, CANTON E. *In-vitro* postantibiotic effect of sparfloxacin and ciprofloxacin against *Pseudomonas aeruginosa* and *Enterococcus faecalis J Antimicrob Chemother* 1994; 34:679–85.

160. KUMAR A, MARSHALL BH, MAIER GA, DYKE JW. Post-antibiotic effect of eftazidime, ciprofloxacin, imipenem, piperacillin and tobramycin for *Pseudomonas cepacia*. *J Antimicrob Chemother* 1992; 30:597–602.

161. STEAD RJ, DAVIDSON TI, DUNCAN FR *et al.* Use of totally implantable system for venous access in cystic fibrosis. *Thorax* 1987; 42:149–50.

162. SHAW JF, DOUGLAS R, WILSON T. Clinical performance of Hickman and Portacath atrial catheters. *N Z J Surg* 1988; 58:657–9.

163. HORN CK, CONWAY SP. Candidaemia: risk factors in patients with cystic fibrosis who have totally implantable venous access systems. *J Infect* 1993; 26:127–32.

164. PECKHAM DG, HILL J, MANHIRE AR, KNOX AJ. Resolution of superior vena cava obstruction following thrombolytic therapy in a patient with cystic fibrosis and a long-term indwelling catheter. *Resp Med* 1994; 88:627–9.

165. DONATI MA, GUENETTE G, AUERBACH H. Prospective controlled study of home and hospital therapy of cystic fibrosis pulmonary disease. *J Pediatr* 1987; 111:28–33.

166. DAVID TJ. Intravenous antibiotics at home in children with cystic fibrosis. *J Roy Soc Med* 1989; 82:130–1.

167. KUZEMKO JA. Home treatment of pulmonary infections in cystic fibrosis. *Chest* 1988; 94:1625–55.

168. HODSON M, ROBERTS CM, BUTLAND RJA, SMITH MJ, BATTEN JC. Oral ciprofloxacin compared with conventional intravenous treatment of *Pseudomonas aeruginosa* infection in adults with cystic fibrosis. *Lancet* 1987; i:235–7.

169. CAMBELL IA, JENKINS J, PRESCOTT RJ. Intermittent ciprofloxacin in adults with cystic fibrosis and chronic *Pseudomonas* pulmonary infection. *Med Sci Res* 1989; 17:797–8.

170. GOLDFARB J, STERN RC, READ MD, YAMASHITA TS, MYERS CM, BLUMER JL. Ciprofloxacin monotherapy for acute pulmonary exacerbations of cystic fibrosis. *Am J Med* 1987; 82 (Suppl 4A):174–8.

171. HODSON ME, PENKETH ARL, BATTEN JC. Aerosol carbenicillin and gentamicin treatment of *Pseudomonas aeruginosa* infections in patients with cystic fibrosis. *Lancet* 1981; ii:1137–9.

172. GEERS TJ, BAKER NR. The effect of sub-lethal levels of antibiotics on the pathogenicity of *Pseudomonas aeruginosa* from tracheal tissue. *J Antimicrob Chemother* 1987; 19:569–78.

173. MADDISON J, DODD M, WEBB AK. Nebulised colistin causes chest tightness in adults with cystic fibrosis. *Resp Med* 1994; 88:145–7.

174. KUMAR A, WOFFORD J, MCQUEEN R, GORDON RC. Ciprofloxacin, imipenem and rifampicin: *in-vitro* synergy of two and three drug combinations against *Pseudomonas cepacia*. *J Antimicrob Chemother* 1989; 23:831–5.

175. COHN RC, JACOBS ML, ARONOFF SC. *In vitro* activity of amiloride combined with tobramycin against *Pseudomonas* isolates from patients with cystic fibrosis. *Antimicrob Agents Chemother* 1988; 32:395–6.

176. SAIMAN L, CACILANO GC, PRINCE A. *Pseudomonas cepacia* adherence to respiratory epithelial cells is enhanced by *Pseudomonas aeruginosa*. *Infect Immun* 1990; 58:2578–84.

177. SAJJAN US, COREY M, KARMALI KA, FORSTNER SF. Binding of *Pseudomonas cepacia* to normal intestinal mucin and respiratory mucin from patients with cystic fibrosis. *J Clin Invest* 1992; 89:646–56.

178. BURDGE DR, NAKIENA EM, NOBLE MA. Case-control and vector studies of nosocomial acquisition of *Pseudomonas cepacia* in adult patients with cystic fibrosis. *Infect Control Hospital Epidemiol* 1993; 14,127–30.

179. YAMAGISHI Y, FUJITA J, TAKIGAWA K, NEGEYAMA K, NAKAZAWA T, TAKAHARA J. Clinical features of *Pseudomonas cepacia* pneumonia in an epidemic among immune compromised patients. Chest 1993; 103:1706–9.

180. SMITH DL, SMITH EG, GUMERY LB, STABLEFORTH DS *Pseudomonas cepacia* infection in cystic fibrosis. *Lancet* 1992; 339:252.

181. THOMASSEN MJ, DEMPKO CA, DOERSHUQ CF, STERN RC, KLINGER JD. *Pseudomonas cepacia*: Decrease in colonisation in patients with cystic fibrosis. *Am Rev Resp Dis* 1986; 134:669–71.

182. RAMIREZ JC, PATTERSON GA, WINTON TL, HOYOS AL, MILLER, JD MAURER JR. Bilateral lung transplantation for cystic fibrosis. *J Cardiothor Surg* 1992; 103:287–94.

183. SNELL GI, HOYOS A, KRAJDEN M, WINTON T, MAURER JR. *Pseudomonas cepacia* in lung transplant recipients with cystic fibrosis. *Chest* 1993; 103:466–71.

184. EGAN J, MCNEIL K, BOOKLESS K *et al.* Transplantation for *Pseudomonas cepacia*. *Lancet* 1994; (letter):344–5.

185. SPECTOR ML, STERN RC. Pneumothorax in cystic fibrosis: a 26 year experience. *Ann Thor Surg* 1989; 47:204–7.

186. DONNELLY RJ, PAGE RD, COWEN ME. Endoscopy assisted microthoracotomy: initial experience. *Thorax* 1992; 47:490–3.

187. COHEN AM. Haemoptysis–role of angiography and embolisation. *Pediatr Pulmonol* 1992; (Supp 8):85–6.

188. EDENBOROUGH FP, STABLEFORTH DE, WEBB AK, MACKENZIE WE, SMITH DL. The outcome of pregnanacy in woman with cystic fibrosis. *Thorax* 1995; 50:170–4.

189. HANDVERGER S, ROTH J, GORDON P. Glucose intolerance in cystic fibrosis. *N Engl J Med* 1969; 281:451–61.

190. REISMAN J, COREY M, CANNY G, LEVISON H. Diabetes mellitus in patients with cystic fibrosis: Effects on survival. *Paediatrics* 1990; 86:374–7.

191. FINKELSTEIN SM, WIELINSKI CL, ELLIOT GJ. Diabetes mellitus associated with cystic fibrosis. *J Pediatr* 1988; 112:373–7.

192. LANG S, THORSTEINSSON B, ERICHSEN G, NERUP J, KOCH C. Glucose tolerance in cystic fibrosis. *Arch Dis Child* 1991; 66:612–16.

193. PRYOR JA, WEBBER BA, HODSON ME, BATTEN JC. Evaluation of the forced expiration technique as an adjunct to postural drainage in the treatment of cystic fibrosis. *Br Med J* 1979; 2:417–18.

194. PRYOR JA, WEBBER BA. Physiotherapy in cystic fibrosis – which technique? *Physiotherapy* 1992; 78:105–8.

195. NIXON PA, ORENSTEIN DM, KELSEY SF, DOERSHUK CF. The prognostic value of exercise testing in patients with cystic fibrosis. *N Engl J Med* 1992; 237:1785–8.

196. O'NEILL PA, DODD ME, PHILLIPS B, POOLE J, WEBB AK. Regular exercise and reduction of breathlessness in patients with cystic fibrosis. *Br J Dis Chest* 1987; 81:62–9.

197. ORENSTEIN DM, FRANKLYN BA, DOERSHUK CF. Exercise conditioning and cardiopulmonary fitness in cystic fibrosis. *Chest* 1981; 80:392–8.

198. CROPP GJ, PULLANO TP, CERNY CJ, NATHANSON T. Exercise tolerance and cardiorespiratory adjustment at peak work capacity in cystic fibrosis. *Am R Resp Dis* 1982; 126:211–16.

199. SALH W, BILTON D, DODD ME, WEBB

AK. Effect of exercise and physiotherapy in aiding sputum expectoration in adults with cystic fibrosis. *Thorax* 1989; 44:1006–8.

200. BILTON D, DODD ME, ABBOTT JV, WEBB AK. The benefits of exercise combined with physiotherapy in the treatment of adults with cystic fibrosis. *Resp Med* 1992; 86:507–11.

201. PASSERO MA, REMOR B, SALOMON J. Patient reported compliance with cystic fibrosis therapy. *Clin Pediatr* 1981; 20:264–8.

202. SHEPHERD SL, HOVEL MF, HARWOOD IR *et al.* A comparative study of the psychosocial assets of adults with cystic fibrosis and their healthy peers. *Chest* 1990; 97:1310–16.

203. ABBOTT J, DODD M, BILTON D, WEBB AK. Treatment compliance in adults with cystic fibrosis. *Thorax* 1994; 49:115–20.

204. O'RAWE A, DODGE JA, REDMAN AOB, MACINTOSH I, BROCK DJH. Increased energy expenditure in cystic fibrosis is associated with specific mutations. *Clin Sci* 1991; 82:71–6.

205. SHAPIRO BL. Mitochondrial dysfunction, energy expenditure in cystic fibrosis. *Lancet* 1988; ii:289.

206. MADDEN BP, HODSON ME, TSANG V, RADLEY-SMITH R, KHAGHANI A, YACOUB MY. Intermediate-term results of heart–lung transplantation for cystic fibrosis. *Lancet* 1992; 339:1583–7.

207. CAINE N, SHARPLES LD, SMYTH R, WALLWORK J. Survival and quality of life of cystic fibrosis patients before and after heart–lung transplantation. *Transpl Proc* 1991; 23:1203–4.

208. TORZILLO PJ, SULLIVA CE, BYE BT. Nocturnal nasal IPPV stabilises patients with cystic fibrosis and hypercapnic respiratory failure. *Chest* 1992; 102:846–50.

209. PIPER AJ, PARKER S, TORZILLO PJ, SULLIVAN CE, BYE PT. Nocturnal nasal IPPV stabilises patients with cystic fibrosis and hypercapnic respiratory failure. *Chest* 1992; 102:846–50.

210. HODSON ME, MADDEN BP, STEVEN MH, TSANG VT, YACOUB MH. Non-invasive mechanical ventilation for cystic fibrosis patients – a potential bridge to transplantation. *Eur Resp J* 1991; 4:524–7.

211. REGNIS JA, PIPER AJ, KENKE KG, PARKER S, BYE PT, SULLIVAN CE. Benefits of nocturnal nasal CPAP in patients with cystic fibrosis. *Chest* 1994; 106:1717–24.

212. AUERBACH HS, KIRKPATRICK JA, WILLIAMS M, COLTEN HR. Alternate day Prednisone reduces morbidity and improves pulmonary function in cystic fibrosis. *Lancet* 1985; ii:686–8.

213. ROSENSTEIN BJ, EIGEN H. Risks of alternate-day Prednisone in patients with cystic fibrosis. *Paediatrics* 1991; 87:245–6.

214. SORDELLI DO, MACRI CM, MAILLIE AJ. A study of the effect of Piroxican (PIR) treatment to prevent lung damage in cystic fibrosis patients with *Pseudomonas aeruginosa* (Pa) pneumonia. *Paediatr Pulmonol* 1990; (Suppl 5):247–8.

215. KONSTAN MW, HOPPEL CL, CHAI DL, DAVIES PB. Ibuprofen in children with cystic fibrosis: pharmacokinetics and adverse affects. *J Pediatr* 1991; 118:956–64.

216. KONSTAN M W, VARGO KM, DAVIS PB. Ibuprofen attenuates the inflammatory response to *Pseudomonas aeruginosa* in a rat model of chronic pulmonary infection. Am *Rev Resp Dis* 1990; 141:186–92

217. SHAK S, CAPON DJ, HELLIMSS R, MASTERS SA, BAKER CL. Recombinant human DNase 1 reduces the viscosity of cystic fibrosis sputum. *Proc Nat Acad Sci, USA* 1990; 87:9188–92.

218. HUBBARD RC, MCELVANEY NG, BIRRER P *et al.* A preliminary study of aerosolised recombinant human deoxyribonuclease 1 in the treatment of cystic fibrosis. *N Engl J Med* 1992; 326:812–15.

219. AITKEN M L, BURKE W, MACDONALD G. SHAK S, MONTGOMERY AB, SMITH A. Recombinant human DNase. Inhalation in normal subjects and patients with cystic fibrosis. A Phase One Study. *Am J Med* 1992; 267:1947–51.

220. MCELVANEY NG, HUBBARD RC, BIRRER P *et al.* Aerosol alpha-1-antitrypsin treatment for cystic fibrosis. *Lancet* 1991; 337:392–4.

221. MARTEAU TM. Psychological aspects of screening. *Br Med J* 1989; 299:527.

222. WILLIAMSON R. Universal community carrier screening for cystic fibrosis. *Nature Genet* 1993; 3:195–201.

223. HYDE SC, GILL DR, HIGGINS CF *et al.* Correction of the ion transport defect in cystic fibrosis transgenic mice by gene therapy. *Nature* 1993; 362:250–5.

25 Upper respiratory tract infections

MICHAEL E. ELLIS and PETER McARTHUR
King Faisal Specialist Hospital and Research Centre, Riyadh, Saudi Arabia

Introduction

This chapter describes infections which affect the upper respiratory tract from its origin in the nasal passages as far as the trachea. It covers the common cold, nasopharyngotonsillitis syndrome, epiglottitis, laryngitis, tracheitis, sinusitis, and otitis media. Particular emphasis is given to adults. Chapter 23 details respiratory tract infections in the paediatric group.

The common cold

The common cold (actually a collection of symptoms) is probably the most frequently encountered acute disabling illness (Table 25.1). Although self-limiting, tens of millions of school or working days in developed countries are sacrificed annually, self-medication with costly over-the-counter drugs is widespread despite lack of marked efficacy in many, physician visit time is enormous and abuse of antibiotic prescriptions common. It is estimated that most individuals have between two and ten colds per year[1,2], the frequency being twofold higher in children compared to adults, in women and in crowded environments.

Table 25.1. *The common cold*

Causative agents	Rhinoviruses (40%) coronaviruses (15%)	
	adenovirus, parainfluenza, RSV, influenza	(45%)
	enterovirus, rubeola, rubella, varicella	
Risk factors	Overcrowding	
	Smoking	
	Stress	
Complications	Sinusitis	
	Otitis media	
	Secondary bacterial infection	
	Mild CNS disorders	
	Obstructive airways disorder	
Management	Antihistamines ±	
	Sympathomimetics ±	
	Topical decongestants +	
	Intranasal anticholinergics ±	
	Naproxen/NSAIDS ±	
	Vitamin C ±	
	Steam inhalations ±	
	Interferons ±	
	Other antivirals ±	

± = Questionable efficacy.
+ = Effective.

Aetiology/pathology

The common cold is caused by a number of agents. The aetiological agents are, in 40% of cases rhinoviruses (>100 serotypes), coronaviruses (>three types) 15%, adenovirus (>30 serotypes), parainfluenza (four types), RSV (two types), influenza A, B and C and enterovirus/rubeola/rubella/varicella in up to 5% each. Presumptive but unknown viruses may be responsible for approximately one-quarter of cases of the common cold, whilst some bacteria, notably group A β-haemolytic *Streptococcus* may present with common cold symptomatology.

Coronavirus appears only to produce the 'common cold' in the respiratory tract, the other common cold aetiological agents can also produce either respiratory tract target disease such as bronchitis (particularly rhinovirus) pharyngitis (particularly adenovirus), laryngitis/croup (parainfluenzae), bronchiolitis (RSV) or pneumonia (RSV, parainfluenzae).

The transmission of the viruses occurs through large droplets, small aerosols, by direct hand-to-hand/mouth/nose contact or via infected fomites. Although all the viruses may be transmitted by any route, rhinovirus and RSV transmission appear to be particularly facilitated by hand-to-hand or hand to respiratory/mucosal contact rather than by air. However, evidence exists in support of an aerosol route for rhinovirus, at least in adults[3]. Rhinoviral disease can be interrupted by the use of virucidal finger tissues[4]. On the other hand, Coxsackie and probably influenza/adenovirus appear to utilize the aerosol route mainly. Other factors contributing to viral transmission include over-crowding and lack of ventilation and ambient relative humidity (depending on whether the virus is enveloped). A cold and/or a chilly environment does not appear to facilitate the transmission of common cold viruses[5].

The usual incubation period is between 1 and 3 days. Viral shedding lasts for between a few days (coronavirus) and three weeks (rhinovirus) – the maximum amount of shedding paralleling the clinical symptoms. However, asymptomatic shedding has been documented over a longer period.

Some studies have indicated that smoking increases the risk for the common cold[6], whilst others have not confirmed that, although symptoms are accentuated[7]. High levels of environmental cigarette smoke may also increase the susceptibility to respiratory tract infections[8]. Moderate alcohol consumption appears to diminish the risk for non-smokers[6]. Psychological stress enhances susceptibility[9]. Outbreaks are seasonal with rises in cases for the common cold in August and September, peaking between October and February and declining thereafter.

Attachment of virus to a cell surface glycoprotein receptor is the first crucial step in infection. These receptors for rhinovirus are situated on the nasopharyngeal epithelial cells. Recently, the complex of the human rhinovirus type 16 with a portion of its receptor, the intercellular adhesion molecule or ICAM-1 has been studied by cryoelectronmicroscopy, which reveals canyons – a strategic point of contact with the virus[10]. Such analysis might provide a basis for rational antirhinoviral drug therapy. There is little evidence of cell necrosis or mucosal damage in rhinoviral infections[11]. However, it is the marked host inflammatory response which produces submucosal oedema and polymorph infiltration which leads to the classical features of rhinorrhoea and nasal stuffiness. In addition, mucociliary function is compromised as a result of acquired ciliary defects. Among the inflammatory mediators kinins[12] such as bradykinin, histamine, interleukin-1 and prostaglandins have been implicated and have been the basis of some drug therapies. Parasympathetic and α-adrenergic neuronal mechanisms also contribute.

It has generally been assumed that the common cold involves only the nasal passages and that spread outside these anatomical areas is unusual. However, a recent CT study has demonstrated ethmoid, frontal, sphenoid and maxillary sinusitis in many patients with the common cold[13]. The isolation of rhinovirus, and subsequent resolution of these features without antibiotic use provides good evidence for widespread involvement of the upper airways in the common cold. Further support for this has been provided by measurement of middle ear pressures which were found to be abnormal in 72% of patients–which resolved in all patients within two weeks[14]. However, *clinically* apparent middle ear disease occurred in less than 5%. The isolation of rhinovirus from middle ear fluid in some cases of otitis media provides further evidence for the role of the virus in some patients with otitis media[15]. Extra-respiratory manifestations of the common cold include mild central nervous system disorders, particularly slowness of choice reaction times[16].

Secondary bacterial colonisation and infection can occur as a result of viral-induced Eustachian tube inflammatory obstruction and mucociliary dysfunction, but in general appears to be unusual.

Abnormalities in pulmonary function have been documented following viral upper respiratory tract infections and clinically these have manifest as asthma exacerbations[17]. The precise role of the common cold viruses in the pathogenesis of asthma, however, remains – a subject of intense debate[18]

Clinical features

The clinical features include rhinorrhea which is often purulent and profuse, sore throat, sneezing, itchy nose and cough. There may be hoarseness. High grade fever and systemic disturbance do not usually feature prominently in adults, being more commonly observed in children. Symptoms may be worse in smokers. Anorexia, and ear or facial discomfort may also be found. Conjunctival involvement or marked pharyngeal erythema suggests an adenoviral or enteroviral aetiology rather than rhinoviral. However, the clinical features are not sufficiently unique to identify specific viral pathogens. Only the duration of the incubation period may differ between viruses but the majority of common colds still have an incubation period of between 1 and 3 days[19].

Management

Modalities of treatment include symptomatic relief, antivirals and prophylactic measures. Poorly controlled studies, small population samples, reliance on subjective rather than objective response parameters, and the use of the experimental common cold rather than natural cold models have limited the interpretation of the outcome of different treatments.

Symptomatic measures

Since histamine levels do not change appreciably in the common cold[20], it is not surprising that, in general, various antihistamines have not been proven effective. Those that do show some efficacy may be due to associated anticholinergic rather than their antihistaminic properties. However, this viewpoint is challenged. At least one study with terfenadine which has no anticholinergic activities has shown significant improvement in symptoms and rhinoscopical appearances[21].

Oral sympathomimetic drugs such as phenylpropanolamine and pseudoephedrine have been shown to have brief antisecretory activity as estimated by rhinomanometry, occurrences of sneezing and congestion parameters[22]. However, there are fears over the rebound vascular dilatation phenomena when these agents are used in excess of four days. Concern over hypertensive or tachycardic side-effects with high doses has also been voiced.

Topical decongestants such as oxymetazoline have been shown objectively and subjectively to have dose response effects[23].

Cholinergic mechanisms are at least partially responsible for nasal mucus production in rhinoviral colds. Intranasally administered anticholinergic agents such as ipatropium have shown some activity in reducing nasal hypersecretion but *not* nasal symptoms in experimental colds[24], and reducing rhinorrhea symptoms and nasal discharge weights in natural colds[25].

Recently the non-steroidal inflammatory agent naproxen – a prostaglandin inhibitor – was shown to be beneficial in reducing headache, myalgia and cough in the experimental rhinoviral cold, but without altering the viral shedding or serum neutralising antiviral responses[26]. Aspirin has modest benefit, but in one study was associated with an increase in viral shedding, although the relevance of this to transmission was not clear[27].

Combined anticholinergics and sympathomimetics have shown modest benefits[28].

The therapeutic role of vitamin C is a controversial issue. There is evidence of disordered vitamin C metabolism in the common cold[29], and of oxidants mediating the symptoms of the common cold[30]. Although there is little consistent evidence that the antioxidant vitamin C reduces the incidence of the common cold, 21 studies involving over 6000 subjects who had received in excess of 1 g/day of vitamin C have shown an average reduction in the duration of common cold episodes and a reduction in their severity by 23%[31]. Nevertheless, the large variations of the benefits observed still clouds the clinical significance of the use of supplemental vitamin C.

Other traditional modalities of treatment such as steam inhalations seem ineffective[32]. However, immediate symptom relief may be produced[33].

Antivirals

Interferons, their inducers, capsid binding agents, zinc salts and miscellaneous agents possessing antiviral properties such as benzimidazole and quinolones have been studied extensively. When used therapeutically, intranasal recombinant interferon α2a and α2b spray preparations appear to have negligible efficacy but prominent side-effects including blood tinged nasal mucus, nasal ulceration and discomfort[34,35]. However, when they are used prophylactically at 5 mega units/day for one week following exposure for natural colds they appear to reduce the incidence by 40%[36]. Use of recombinant interferon β-serine nasal drops, however, has not been shown to be an effective prophylactic[37], possibly due to the different method of drug delivery or to peculiar properties of that type of interferon. Combination intranasal interferon α2b with ipratropium and naproxen significantly reduces viral shedding, the development of colds, rhinorrhea and malaise when compared to placebo in an experimental rhinoviral study[38].

Orally administered capsid binding agents appear ineffective, possibly due to their poor excretion into nasal secretions. However, intranasal pirodavir was shown recently to reduce the chance of infection sevenfold in an experimental rhinoviral common cold model[39]. Similarly zinc, although inhibiting *in vitro* viral polypeptide cleavage has generally not been clinically effective in most studies[40], though a few studies have shown a reduction in the duration of common cold symptoms[41]. Other antiviral agents with uncertain, unproven or no effects include the benzimidazoles such as enviroxime and intranasally administered monoclonal rhinoviral antibodies.

Prophylaxis

The large number of serotypes and mutation of surface residues of the human rhinovirus limits the development of an effective vaccine. Prophylactic administration of nasal recombinant interferon, together with non-steroidal anti-inflammatories and other drugs appears moderately effective when used short term, and this is associated with a reduction in side-effects.

Interruption of the transmission routes also appears modestly effective in reducing the incidence for example, by the rigorous use of malic acid/citric acid/sodium lauryl sulphate impregnated viricidal tissues[42], or by training to reduce hand-to-nose or hand-to-eye contact[43].

Naso-pharyngo-tonsillitis syndrome

Inflammation of the mucosal surfaces of the soft palate, uvula, tonsils and adenoids is called pharyngotonsillitis (Table 25.2). Co-involvement of the nasal passages or dominance of particular sites determines the specific description, for example, nasopharyngitis or tonsillitis. Although a wide spectrum of microbial organisms is implicated, viruses predominate in nasal areas whilst bacteria tend to occur more frequently at the tonsillar gate area.

Table 25.2. *Nasopharyngotonsillitis*

Associated agents[a]	Rhinovirus > GABHS > group C + other streptococci, >[b] coronavirus > influenza > parainfluenza > herpes simplex > EBV > others (see text)
Antimicrobials for streptococcal infection	Penicillin V for 10 days Cure rate may increase with β-lactamase-stable or non-β-lactam antibiotics used due to 'protecting' flora, penicillin tolerance Newer cephalosporins, macrolides > more effective Anti-anaerobic cover better for chronic/recurrent tonsillitis
Complications	Peritonsillar abscess Otitis media, mastoiditis, osteomyelitis Pustulosis palmaris et plantaris IgA nephropathy Sleep apnoea Rheumatic fever Crohns? Sarcoid? Tonsillar haemorrhage

[a]Varies with sampling technique, site, age of patient and acute/chronic presentation.

[b]In children, *H. influenzae* or *S. aureus* may be more commonly found.

Immunopathological highlights

The pharyngeal mucosal surface is endowed with several anti-microbial defence mechanisms. These include mechanical means such as swallowing, sneezing, coughing and the mucosal epithelial integrity. Saliva and tears contain certain substances capable of directly or indirectly inhibiting micro-organisms, for example, lysozyme which lyses bacterial cell wall peptidoglycan and fungal wall chitin, peroxidase, betalysin and lactoferrin (free iron binder). The so-called colonisation resistance factor of the pharynx provided by normal commensal resident flora is purported to prevent overgrowth of potentially more pathogenic microorganisms via their competition for microbial nutrients, ecological manipulation and production of competitor organism inhibitors (bacteriocins) and even antibiotics produced from these bacteria. These organisms are acquired progressively after birth. They include *Staphylococcus*, coagulase negative *Staphylococcus*, diphtheroids, *Streptococcus viridans* and non-capsulated *Neisseria*, *Hemophilus*, *Pneumococcus*, *Meningococcus*, β-haemolytic *Streptococcus*, *Branhamella*, α haemolytic *Streptococcus* and Gram-negative *Diplococcus*. It has been shown that therapeutic recolonisation with α streptococci significantly reduces the recurrence of β-haemolytic *Streptococcus* Group A throat infections[44]. Note, however, that given the correct conditions, even these organisms may become pathogenic, for example, in the context of severe depressed host immunity. Antimicrobial use facilitates the emergence of pathogens such as β-lactamase producing *Staphylococcus* spp, *Haemophilus* spp, *Moraxella*, *Fusobacterium* spp and also fungi including *Candida albicans*.

The mucosal surface itself with the tonsils and adenoids in particular are active in immune defence. Sub-epithelial lymphocytes, macrophages and other cells interact with antigens. The adenoids and tonsils are sentinels to the respiratory and gastrointestinal tracts and are home to T- and B-lymphocytes, which circulate to and from the lower respiratory tract interacting with lymphocytes from other extra-respiratory sources. It is thought that tonsil dependent lymphocytes preferentially seed the upper body mucosal sites[45]. Micropore (M) cells transport antigen from tonsillar crypt epithelium into the tonsillar B cell follicles and extrafollicular T cell areas[46]. Secretory Ig production, stimulated following follicular dendritic cell presentation of antigens to the B cells, demonstrates some notable differences from serum immunoglobulins. For example, IgA is in a dimeric form and that derived from adenoids is protected from enzymic digestion by a 'secretory piece'[47]. Secretory IgA and IgM inhibit uptake of soluble antigens and block epithelial colonisation of microorganisms. Most of the IgA is IgA1 which can be cleaved by certain bacteria. Recurrent tonsillitis leads to over-production of IgA and possible nephropathy. IgA can also neutralise viruses and toxins and inhibit bacterial adherence. IgD acts as a bacterial receptor for protein D producing bacteria such as the colonising *Haemophilus influenzae* and *Moraxella* spp and these bacteria may act by increasing the number of tonsillar B cells. IgE production reflects the participation of the tonsils in upper airway allergic diatheses. Other immunological defences include natural killer cells and cytokines. There is an age-associated marked decline in tonsillar Ig positive and Ki 67 positive monoclonal antibody-activated cells, and in patients with recurrent tonsillitis an increase in IgD positive cells is found[48]. With age, the number of M cells also decrease resulting in reduced antigen presentation and a resultant reduced expansion of B cell clones[49].

Continual low grade subclinical pharyngeal or tonsillar inflammation occurs secondary to the constant presence of microbial antigens. If pathogenic microbes become entrapped in tonsillar tissue, up-regulation of this background physiological process occurs. The degree and extent of inflammation depends on a number of microbe/host factors. Initial bacterial contact and entry is dependent on the presence of adhesins and fibronectin (may enhance Gram-positive adhesion and reduce Gram-negative adhesion), suitable host cell receptors, bridging between the adhesins and the receptor, local factors (including competitive resident flora population – for example, prior infection by viruses enhances the presence of Gram-negative and staphylococcal adherence), diet, for example, lectin content, and chemical/oxygen requirements of the pharyngeal milieu. Strain-associated virulence of the organism, ability to produce β-lactamase within the tonsil environment, production of proteases to destroy fibronectin and cleave secretory IgA1, stimulation of the release of mast cell histamine which contributes to the magnitude of the inflammatory response and alteration in lymphocyte suppressor : helper ratio are other factors. Other extracellular enzymes and other mediators of the inflammatory response are also important. These latter include hyaluronidase, fibrin, antiphagocytic M protein production, streptolysin, haemolysin, streptokinase, deoxyribonuclease, proteases and rhinoviral production of bradykinin/lysyl-bradykinin (for pain receptor stimulation).

Microbiology

Recognised microorganisms incriminated in acute pharyngitis are, in order of relative frequency, rhinovirus, group A β-haemolytic streptococci (GABHS) Group C β-haemolytic streptococci and other non-Group A streptococci, coronavirus, influenza, parainfluenza and herpes simplex. The presence of Group A *Streptococcus* may not always indicate disease but rather colonisation or healthy carriage. It has been demonstrated in patients with acute tonsillitis (AT) due to GABHS disease, but not in asymptomatic patients who have GABHS, that massive attachment of streptococcal chains, positive for FITC labelled antibodies, to tonsillar epithelial cell membrane occurs via cell projections[50]. Furthermore, fine needle aspiration or culture of tonsil core removed at tonsillectomy for recurrent tonsillitis has not always shown good bacteriological correlation with specimens obtained by superficial swabbing[51,52]. There is also some difference in the bacteriological spectrum between adults and children. For example, *Haemophilus influenzae* tends to be found more frequently in the 2–7 years age-group, *Staphylococcus aureus* at 8–14 years and anaerobes in older age groups[53]. Less frequently (each contributing to not more than 1% of all cases) are EBV/CMV, anaerobes, *Corynebacterium diphtheriae/Corynebacterium ulcerans/Corynebacterium haemolyticum*, *Neisseria gonorrhoea*, *Treponema palladium*, *Mycoplasma pneumoniae*, Coxsackie and primary HIV infection. The precise contribution of two recently implicated pathogens namely, *Chlamydia pneumoniae* and *Mycoplasma hominis* is unknown[54,55].

Most cases of pharyngitis due to bacteria, adenovirus and coronavirus occur in the winter, influenza in the winter/spring and adenovirus associated pharyngoconjunctival fever in the summer. Tonsillitis appears to be more common in children whose parents smoke suggesting that tobacco smoke may alter oropharyngeal flora, mucociliary function or be associated with an increased cross-infection rate[56].

Clinical features

The presence and severity of the presenting features of acute pharyngitis depend upon the organism and the host immune integrity. Most patients have an acute onset of fever and sore or scratchy throat accompanied by a variable degree of systemic features including anorexia, headache, fever, chills, myalgia or malaise. Accompanying local physical findings include a degree of tonsillar hypertrophy, exudation, erythema, oedema, and regional lymphadenopathy. In many cases it is possible to predict the aetiology by a global assessment of these features, but overlap and variability does occur. Mild pharyngeal discomfort suggests rhinoviral, or coronaviral aetiology. This may be supported by accompanying rhinorrhea or nasal stuffiness, little systemic disturbance, local inflammation or lymphadenopathy. Mild non-exudative pharyngitis is typical for most cases of HIV infection, diphtheria, cytomegalovirus and mycoplasma. Gonococcal pharyngitis is usually asymptomatic. Pharyngeal erythema without exudation but with systemic features and nasal symptoms suggest influenza. Prominent soreness, systemic symptoms, erythema and a streptococcal-like exudate with conjunctivitis should raise the possibility of adenovirus. Severe soreness is found in cases due to herpes, *Streptococcus*, peritonsillar abscess complication, or Epstein–Barr virus-associated infectious mononucleosis. In adults, the presence of extra-pharyngeal symptoms, fiery red erythema, extensive confluent exudate with oedema and enlarged regional lymph nodes, suggests *Streptococcus pyogenes*. However, children often do not have such a characteristic exudate. Streptococci groups B, C, F and G, not thought to be implicated previously do, in fact, cause painful exudative tonsillitis, although still somewhat uncommonly[57]. Ulcers or vesicles, particularly if they are also present elsewhere in the oral cavity, suggest herpes simplex, Coxsackie or HIV. A thick exudative tonsillitis with associated marked tonsillar hypertrophy, generalised lymphadenopathy, splenomegaly and malaise is found in Epstein–Barr virus infection. Nasal phonation, marked difficulty in swallowing or stridor may suggest a peritonsillar abscess or extensive tonsillar enlargement as in EBV. A greyish firmly adherent pseudomembrane is found in diphtheria. An associated erythematous skin rash may be present in streptococcal, HIV, EBV or arcanobacterial infections. Severe systemic toxicity suggests streptococcal, EBV, *Fusobacterium* spp., diphtheria (occasionally) or *Yersinia* spp. aetiologies. Palatal petechiae suggests β-haemolytic *Streptococcus* Group A, EBV/CMV, measles or Rubella.

In most patients, the illness lasts from between 4 (viral) and 10 (bacteria) days. A longer course occurs in infections due to EBV, gonorrhoea, influenza or syphilis or may be suggestive of unusual aetiologies such as *Actinomyces, Candida* or non-infective causes, which include chronic irritation, Kawasaki's disease, SLE, Behçet's or aphthous ulceration.

The basic laboratory investigation is aerobic and anaerobic bacterial culture of a superficial pharyngeal swab. However, there is some discrepancy between the bacteriological findings provided by such a specimen and that from a fine needle aspiration or core culture[51,52]. In recurrent adenotonsillitis, deep tissue specimens produce a higher yield of β-lactamase organisms in general, and certain other species may be found such as *Streptococcus* groups C, G and *H. influenzae*[58]. Other appropriate investigations include viral cultures, specific culture media stains or techniques for other suspected pathogens (for example, Thayer-Martin for *Neisseria*, crystal violet for *Fusobacterium*, Löffler's for diphtheria), serology such as monospot for EBV, and acute and convalescence sera for viruses and *Mycoplasma*. Rapid diagnostic high specificity antigen tests for *Streptococcus* may prove useful in the initial antibiotic decision-making, but the low sensitivity may yield several false-negatives. Hence negative antigen testing results should be backed up with a formal culture result.

Management

General measures include pain relief with aspirin gargles, xylocaine elixir or systemic analgesics such as acetaminophen or ibuprofen. A combination of 800 mg of aspirin with 64 mg of caffeine as an analgesic adjuvant has been found to be highly effective[59]. Maintenance of fluid balance is important, particularly in children. If the initial presentation suggests streptococcal infection, then antimicrobials are indicated on the grounds that (a) suppurative complications can be reduced; (b) rheumatic fever risk is reduced; (c) symptoms are more rapidly resolved; and (d) intrafamilial spread is curtailed. Despite reports that occasional therapeutic failures occur, penicillin V at a dose of 250 mg three to four times a day for an adult for 10 days is still the recommended approach. For patients with penicillin allergy, erythromycin is an alternative. Clinical cure, subsequent relapse and reinfection rates are similar to those for penicillin[60]. Should the signs and symptoms not be typical of streptococcal infection, then either penicillin can be started and discontinued if bacteriology proves negative, or symptomatic management can be given alone pending the bacteriology results. Recurrence or risk of rheumatic fever is not increased through a day or two delay of instituting antibiotic therapy. In the presence of mild pharyngitis, debate has been generated over whether *all* cases of streptococcal pharyngitis require antibiotic treatment. For other aetiologies appropriate definitive therapy may be offered, for example, amantadine or rimantadine for influenzal pharyngitis (Chapter 9), acyclovir or foscarnet for herpes simplex, cotrimoxazole for *Yersinia*, etc.

Antimicrobial management of streptococcal infections

Oral penicillin is still the most popular antibiotic for use in suspected bacterial pharyngitis. Following treatment defervescence occurs at a mean of 2–3 days and bacterial or clinical response is seen in 80–90% of patients. However, concern has been generated over the increasing frequency of documented microbiological and clinical failures occurring with penicillin V. For example, it is currently believed that up to 30% of patients with β-haemolytic *Streptococcus* Group A tonsillitis may not achieve microbiological eradication[61,62], a figure much higher than seen in previous years. Reduced patient compliance could be responsible – it was found that 16% of patients receiving penicillin V for tonsillitis were poorly compliant, although clinical and bacteriological response was still in excess of 90% in one series[63]. Reduction in dosage frequency to twice or three times from four times daily still achieves a very high rate of success[64]. The old adage that the duration of penicillin V should be 10 days still appears to hold true and that clinical cure and bacteriological failure is up to threefold higher in patients receiving less than 10 days' therapy[65–67]. An increase in the numbers of β-lactamase producing normal resident flora may offer protection from antibiotics to otherwise susceptible pathogens. Some support from this comes from observations of an increased bacteriological eradication when β-lactamase stable or other antibiotics are used instead of penicillin V, for example, augmentin, penicillin with rifampicin or cefadroxil[68]. During treatment with cefprozil, a significantly lower return of β-lactam *S. aureus* strains were encountered, compared to patients treated with penicillin V[69]. Using a subcutaneous mouse abscess model, it was shown that β-lactamase producing *S. aureus* protected GABHS from penicillin[70] and that cefprozil obviated this protection. Whether this always translates into clinical relevance remains conjectural[61,68,69], although patients treated with clindamycin for recurrent acute tonsillitis were found to have a strikingly significant reduction in episodes of AT and subsequent tonsillectomy[71]. Another mechanism for the failure of penicillin may be related to increased reports of penicillin tolerance. There does not appear to be any convincing evidence to suggest that delayed institution of antibiotics is associated with higher failure rates. In fact, it has been suggested that a 2-day delay might actually be beneficial by permitting development of host immunity. Recent information that deep tissue specimens provide a different bacteriological spectrum compared to superficial sampling may have some bearing on the lack of response to penicillin V[51,52,72]. Tonsillitis caused by pathogens resistant to penicillin V is another reason for antimicrobial failure[51–53,58]. Unusual infectious diseases may occasionally be encountered and prove resistant to therapy, for example, *Actinomycoses*[73], botryomycosis[74], EBV, *Corynebacterium*, herpes simplex[75], chlamydial organisms or *Mycoplasma*[54,55,76], *Prevotella intermedia*[77] or *Toxoplasma gondii*[78]. Complications such as peritonsillar abscess, a defective host immune system or non-infectious causes such as SLE should also be considered in apparent treatment failures.

Although penicillin V still remains the antibiotic of choice for most cases of acute tonsillitis, there is a move towards using alternative antimicrobials with excellent tonsillar drug concentration availability, β-lactamase resistance and broader spectrum. There is increasing support for their greater clinical efficacy. Azithromycin, one of the 'new' macrolides has a prolonged half-life and achieves high tonsillar drug concentrations. This may enable once daily, 5-day courses[79]. A recent comparative study of azithromycin versus clarithromycin showed similar clinical and bacteriological eradication success rates and post treatment reinfection rates of 96%, 95% and 3–8%, respectively, for each treatment, and that a 3-day course of azithromycin was highly effective[80]. This was confirmed in a comparative prospective trial of penicillin V given for 10 days versus azithromycin given for 3 days: clinical/bacteriological cure was equivalent but bacteriological recurrence was twice as common in azithromycin treated patients[81]. In one multicentre study of 377 patients with GABHS tonsillitis, the cephalosporin cefpodoxime given twice daily for 5 days or daily for 10 days was significantly superior to penicillin V given for 10 days in achieving bacteriological eradication and a better (though not significant) clinical response[61]. This better response was not confirmed by others[63]. Cefprozil is another cephalosporin which has received recent attention. It can remove interfering β-lactamase *S. aureus* strains[69,70] and also achieves a more satisfactory clinical response compared to penicillin V[69], though again this has not been repeatedly confirmed[68]. In two recent comparative studies of once daily cefixime (an extended spectrum cephalosporin) or cephalexin versus penicillin V in streptococcal A pharyngitis, penicillin V returned significantly inferior bacteriological clinical cure and relapse rates[82,83]. Clindamycin appears to be another useful and effective alternative antimicrobial agent to use in recurrent acute tonsillitis[71].

Epstein–Barr virus tonsillitis

The anginose variety of EBV viral associated infectious mononucleosis often presents with profound prostration, toxaemia and massive exudative tonsillitis. There may be extra-respiratory features supportive of the diagnosis, such as generalised lymphadenopathy, hepatitis, splenomegaly, haemolytic anaemia, thrombocytopenia and rash (particularly if the patient had recent antibiotics). Laboratory confirmatory evidence includes a high atypical mononucleosis count, presence of positive heterophil red cell antibodies (monospot test) and other appropriate serological investigations. An immense increased bacterial colonisation and attachment of the tonsillar surfaces with, for example, β-haemolytic streptococci occurs[84]. In addition, a high percentage of anaerobes including *Fusobacterium* spp. and *Prevotella* may be found[85] though their contribution to the overall disease process is not precisely known. Response to intravenous corticosteroids is often (but not always) dramatic, with a rapid reduction in tonsillar signs occurring within 1–2 days. Acute complete airways obstruction requires emergency crico-thyroidotomy. Concomitant antibiotics may be given if a secondary infection is judged present, but this carries a high risk of drug rash which is rarely fatal. Patients with airways obstruction who fail to respond to corticosteroids should undergo acute tonsillectomy which is highly effective[86].

Complications of tonsillitis and their management

Peritonsillar abscess or quinsy (PTA) is suggested by the presence of severe pain and dysphagia. Examination reveals marked swelling and displacement of the tonsil. A 'hot potato' voice change due to velopharyngeal insufficiency from palatal muscle dysfunction[87] is characteristic of PTA or peritonsillar cellulitis (PTC). Bilateral involvement can produce pharyngeal obstruction. Occasionally, further extension with evolution to life-threatening necrotising mediastinitis occurs. It is important to distinguish PTA from PTC since antimicrobials are more likely to be successful in PTC. Differentiating clinical features are in general unhelpful. However, complete pharyngeal occlusion, increased age, dysphagia, drooling, absent trismus and unilaterality have been suggested by some to suggest PTA rather than PTC[88] but the findings have not been confirmed by others[89]. CT scanning[90] appears to be highly sensitive in identifying abscess formation. Mandibular angle ultrasound[91] has been shown to differentiate PTC from PTA with 90% certainty[92]. Successful management of PTC with parenterally administered antibiotics is the norm. Established PTA may fail medical treatment and surgery is often indicated – either aspiration with incision/drainage or tonsillectomy. Single occasion three-point puncture aspiration of pus has been found to be as successful as formal incision or drainage[93]. The presence of *S. pyogenes* rather than other aerobic or anaerobic mixed flora in the setting of recurrent tonsillitis would favour tonsillectomy rather than aspiration. Recurrent PTA may be unacceptably high in simple aspiration procedures compared to incision and drainage[94]. Additionally, although it has been done successfully in children[95], non-co-operation may be a problem. In general, abscess tonsillectomy appears preferable on the grounds of reduced hospitalisation, reduction in recurrence, avoidance of interval tonsillectomy and is more acceptable to the patient[96]. Tonsillectomy should be bilateral to remove the risk of recurrence (in the contralateral tonsil), particularly in patients less than 30 years[97]. Complicated extensive abscess formation, e.g. with mediastinitis requires an aggressive surgical approach together with broad spectrum antibiotics directed towards aerobes and anaerobes[98].

Other suppurative complications

These include otitis media, mastoiditis, bacteraemia, osteomyelitis, venous thrombosis and pneumonia. Other less common suppurative conditions include Lemierre's disease associated with *Fusobacterium* species, bacteremia and pulmonary involvement and other soft tissue abscesses[99,100], non-immunologically mediated perimyocarditis[101], regional necrotising fasciitis[102] and pseudoaneurysm of the internal carotid artery[103].

Non-suppurative complications

Pustulosis palmaris et plantaris (PPP)

PPP is a refractory recurrent pustular dermatosis. Considerable interest in this related complication comes mainly from the East. One theory of pathogenesis evokes focal tonsillar infection with tonsillar derived autoantibody Arthus type/cytotoxic tonsillar lymphocytic tissue injury. Tonsillectomy has been effective in approximately three-quarters of these cases[104]. A raised medullasin protease level may predict patients' response[105].

IgA nephropathy

Chronic tonsillitis may be associated with IgA nephropathy and tonsillectomy has been shown to reduce proteinuria in about 65% of patients[106].

Sleep apnoea and alveolar hypoventilation

Although this is not a complication of tonsillitis *per se*, adenotonsillar hypertrophy can occur in association with chronic tonsillitis, and this is the commonest cause of obstructive sleep apnoea syndrome and alveolar hypoventilation in children[107]. Sleep and behavioural disturbances, excessive daytime somnolence, snoring, respiratory pauses or apnoea during sleep, chest wall retractions, skeletal (chest and facial) deformity and cardiopulmonary sequelae are features. The diagnosis is substantiated by polysomnographical recordings or observations of snoring, air flow disturbance, respiratory movement abnormalities, diminished oxygen saturation and alterations in meso-pharyngeal pressures. Treatment is with tonsillo-adenoidectomy[108]. Additional surgical correction may be required for associated maxillo-facial deformations.

Miscellaneous associated complications

The course of sarcoidosis has been suggested to be adversely affected by chronic tonsillitis and may be improved by tonsillectomy[109]. Focal tonsillar infection has also been suggested to be causative of some cases of sternocostoclavicular hyperostosis and rheumatoid arthritis, and partly responsive to tonsillectomy[110]. Crohn's disease and its earlier onset has been associated with an increased frequency of childhood pharyngitis[111]. Spontaneous tonsillar haemorrhage, a rare but potentially dangerous complication of adenotonsillar hypertrophy, has recently been described[112].

Rheumatic fever

Streptococcus Group A exudative tonsillitis present for 21 days carries an appreciable risk for rheumatic fever – approximately 2.5% as described in 1961[113], but the incidence is very low nowadays. However, this is tempered by the age of the patient, environmental factors, genetic and the organism strain. It is mediated by a hypersensitive autoimmune process based on cross-reactivity between streptococcal constituents such as the cell wall or M protein, and myocardial sarcolemmal membranes. Eradication of β-haemolytic *Streptococcus* Group A prevents primary and recurrent attacks of rheumatic fever.

Recurrent and chronic tonsillitis

Culture isolates from tonsil core tissue in patients with recurrent tonsillitis (RT) or tonsillar hypertrophy (TH) indicate that over 70% of patients harbour *H. influenzae* which is often not present on surface cultures[114]. An aetiological role or *H. influenzae* in the genesis of TH has been suggested[115]. Other organisms which may be found in such tonsils include *S. pyogenes* in 20%, *S. aureus*, *M. catarrhalis*, *B. fragilis*, streptococci Groups C and G, and *S. pneumoniae*. Many of these organisms are β-lactamase producing and resistant to ampicillin, penicillin, erythromycin and other antibiotics.

Anaerobes are being increasingly implicated in chronic tonsillitis. In fact, a shift from a predominance of viruses, Group A β-haemolytic *Streptococcus* and *H. influenzae* towards *Bacteroides* spp., *Fusobacterium* spp., *Prevotella* spp. and anaerobic cocci occurs as a result of changes in the chronically infected tonsil. Many of these organisms are capsulated and possess virulence factors such as lipopolysaccharides, neutrophil cytotoxins and DNAase. Agreement as to the frequency of occurrence of these organisms is difficult due to differences in methods of sample collection (contamination and surface sterilisation, scissor chopping of tonsils, whether core or surface samples are collected, unilateral or bilateral tonsillar sampling, prior antibiotic use, and variably sensitive microbiological techniques). Nevertheless, between 33% and 88% of organisms are found to be anaerobes in recurrent tonsillitis[116]. Increased levels of antibodies to specific anaerobes in patients with chronic tonsillitis supports their causative role[117]. One of the mechanisms by which anaerobes may play an important clinical role in chronic or recurrent tonsillitis is that of β-lactamase production which mediates protection of pathogenic/streptococci from antibiotics. This has been suggested by a number of *in vitro* studies[118]. Clinical studies showing increased cure rates of recurrent Group A β-hemolytic streptococcal tonsillitis using amoxyl with a β-lactamase inhibitor clavulanic acid, compared to penicillin alone supports this theory[116,119]. Nevertheless, treatment failures still occur and other mechanisms of resistance must therefore exist.

Histological changes suggest that antibiotic penetration into the core tissue of such tonsils will be suboptimal. Indeed, the incidence of recurrent episodes does not, in general, appear to be influenced by standard antimicrobial treatment, although there are some documented successes, for example, with clindamycin[71].

There is considerable debate on the optimal antimicrobial approach in the patient with chronic tonsillitis. On the basis of the role of anaerobes some authors are strongly advocating broad spectrum antibiotic therapy directed at both aerobes and anaerobes, for example, amoxycillin with clavulanic acid or clindamycin, cefoxitin or imipenem. A few studies do support this[116,120].

To some extent, however, antibiotics may be deleterious by removing the normal protective flora such as α *Streptococcus* which interferes with GABHS. Therapeutic recolonisation with an aerosol spray of selected α haemolytic streptococcal strains following antibiotic treatment of acute tonsillitis appears to reduce the recurrence rate[44].

In addition, overgrowth by fungi, enterococci, *Clostridium difficile* and other organisms may occur. Clearly, further controlled randomised clinically scientific studies are required.

The germinal cell sclerosis which accompanies RT will undoubtedly produce local immunocompromisation. Immunomodulatory treatment is a possibility and pidotiniod (a biological response modifier which increases blastogenesis, activates neutrophils and increases the T4:T8 ratio) has apparently had some clinical success in terms of reducing the number and severity of recurrences[121].

Tonsillectomy has its opponents and proponents but, in general, most ENT surgeons have agreed on the following indications: (i) recurrent symptomatic disabling tonsillitis (e.g. local problems – pain, regional problems – hearing difficulties), (ii) quinsy, (iii) refractory PPP, IgA nephropathy, etc., (iv) upper airways obstruction including infectious mononucleosis refractory to steroids, (v) obstructive sleep-apnoea syndrome. The benefits of tonsillectomy have to be balanced against the procedural risks (bleeding, anaesthesia related morbidity and mortality including infection, and unknown long-term immune disturbances), and the likelihood of self-limitation of tonsillitis. However, during a mean waiting list period of 7 months, resolution of tonsillitis was not observed[122]. In adults in contrast to children, continuing symptoms over several years is relatively common, and can be effectively terminated by tonsillectomy. More than 90% of the tonsils removed are pathological. In adults, the procedure has a very low morbidity and is cost-effective[123]. For children with well-documented recurrent pharyngitis, tonsillectomy significantly reduces subsequent throat infections for at least 2 years[124].

Table 25.3. *Comparison of paediatric and adult epiglottitis*

	Paediatric	Adults
Aetiology	Hib > 90%	Hib << 50% Other organisms and culture -ve ≥ 50%
Epiglottic abscess	±	++
Incidence/100 000	Approx 1 and falling	10–39 stable
Clinical features		
drooling	+++	+
stridor	+++	+
sore throat	+	+++
Need for airway rescue	Most	<< 50%
Safety of direct laryngoscopy	–	+
Classical cherry red epiglottitis	+	±

Acute epiglottitis or supraglottitis in adults

This section highlights the current status of AE in adults – there are important clinical, microbiological and management differences from AE in children (Table 25.3). Furthermore, the influence of widespread Hib vaccination of the paediatric population, whilst having a dramatic impact on paediatric *Haemophilus* infections is as yet unclear for adults.

The cartilaginous epiglottis serves to prevent aspiration of food and secretions into the lower airway. Inflammation of this structure, epiglottitis, usually does not occur in anatomical isolation – the adjoining arytenoids, aryepiglottic folds, uvula, tongue base and false vocal cords may also be involved and the infection is more appropriately described as supraglottitis. Anatomical evolution occurs from a curved structure covering a narrow subglottic opening found in infants to a more laterally developed and flatter cover for a larger opening in adults. Microbial infection of the epiglottis results in an intense inflammatory infiltrate composed of polymorphs, mucosal ulceration, hyperaemia and oedema which places the patient at risk from the most feared complication namely, airways obstruction from glottic closure. However, more inflammatory oedema appears to be necessary to produce airways disease in adults compared to children.

Regional suppurative complications can occur including epiglottic and prevertebral abscess and mediastinitis[125,126]. Epiglottic abscess appears to be much more common in adults[126]. Although bacteraemia occurs in many cases, distal suppurative complications are rare[125] but include meningitis, pneumonia, and thoracic empyema[127]. An interesting observation is that, in some patients with AE, the hypoxaemia is apparently unrelated to the degree of glottic obstruction, implying a V/Q imbalance at alveolar level. Some of these cases may be related to the development of adult respiratory distress syndrome[128] itself secondary to systemic infection, obstructive hypoxia, high negative alveolar pressures or to associated pneumonia. However, in some patients there is no clinically or radiological apparent pneumonic infiltrate and the mechanism of hypoxaemia is unknown.

Epidemiology

AE was previously believed to be rare in adults, this concept reflected by the sparse publication of isolated case reports[129]. The current reported incidence in adults reflects that a substantial increase in the number of reported cases has occurred in recent years. The incidence of AE has increased from three cases/year prior to 1985 to nine thereafter with almost half being greater than 30 years of age in one study[130]. In a 25-year period in Copenhagen county, 168 of 279 patients treated for AE were adults, the adult preponderance reflected throughout Denmark[131]. Others have noted trends in the increase of the number of adult cases with adult AE[132], often accompanied by a decrease in the number of paediatric cases[133]. The annual incidence of adult AE is variably estimated at 10–39/1 000 000 adults[134–138]. Some more recent figures show a decline of paediatric AE from 3.5 to 0.6/100 000 over 10 years ending 1990, whilst that in adults remaining stable at 1.8[125]. The reasons for the changing epidemiology are unknown. Increase recognition of previously unidentified cases is a possibility since the disease may have a variable and different presentation and course compared to children[125,131]. Other possibilities include the influence of Hib vaccination in children[139], the growing number of immunocompromised adults who may be at risk from AE[125] or a real increase in cases. In addition the risk of epiglottitis may not be uniform in all populations despite a similar exposure risk for *H. influenzae*[138]. Some studies have indicated a summer or autumnal season predominance[125,130,132,138] but this has not been reported in all studies. Although the usual age incidence among adults is 20–40 years, the age range can be from 20–90 years[140].

Microbiology

In contrast to the paediatric population where *H. influenzae* type B (Hib) is isolated from swabs or blood cultures in almost all cases[141–143], this organism is less frequently implicated in adult AE. Documentation of Hib bacteraemia in adults has usually varied between 0% and 23%[134,144], although some studies have shown a higher incidence, e.g.

53% of adults compared to 92% of children with *H. influenzae* bacteraemia[137]. The most recent study found Hib bacteraemia in 15% and a positive Hib upper respiratory culture in 20% only[125], although cultures were not performed in all patients. Some cases of Hib adult epiglottitis have been described in patients having close contact with children colonised with Hib and this underscores the need to consider rifampicin prophylaxis even for adult household contacts of such cases[145]. A variety of other pathogens are found in adult AE, including *S. aureus*, β-haemolytic *Streptococcus* Group A and non Group A, *S. pneumoniae*, *Candida albicans*, *Neisseria* spp., *E. coli*, *Enterobacter cloacae*, *Mycobacterium tuberculosis*, *Pasteurella* spp., *Moraxella* spp., *Klebsiella* spp., *Bacteroides melanogenogenicus*, other anaerobes and *H. parainfluenzae*[125,130,132,146,147]. A particularly severe necrotising epiglottitis in the pregnant female due to Epstein–Barr virus infection has been described[148]. *S. pneumoniae* AE is highly indicative of an immunocompromised status. However, *H. influenzae* type B remains the most commonly *identified* aetiological agent. In addition the presence of Hib bacteremia is associated with more severe disease in adults[134,149]. More than 50% of all cases of adult AE have negative bacterial cultures though this may be an overestimate since routine culturing is not always performed. Other possibilities which may limit the usefulness of cultures[150] incorrect swab cultures, for example, from the throat rather than from the epiglottis, infection being submucosal rather than superficial or the use of prior antibiotics. Furthermore, some cases of bacteriologically negative adult AE may actually be viral in aetiology – Coxsackie B has been implicated for example[141], and some patients have a 'viral' blood picture[150].

Clinical features

The clinical picture of AE in adults is variable and deceptive[151,152]. The classical common paediatric presentation (Chapter 23) with a 'tripod posture', drooling mouth or stridor is a presentation infrequently found in adults. Many adults appear less ill or toxic and for that reason are probably underdiagnosed or the diagnosis is delayed. Nevertheless, the death of George Washington reminds us that AE can be a serious and life-threatening illness. Males usually outnumber females. In an analysis of 129 cases[125] sore throat (95%) and odynophagia (94%) predominated, whereas drooling or a sitting erect posture were found in only 30% and 16%, respectively. Sometimes the degree of soreness is extraordinarily severe. Although muffled phonation was present in 54%, stridor occurred in only 12%. A broadly similar presentation profile has been described by others[130]. Other symptoms include fever or chills, dyspnoea, cervical adenopathy in approximately 30–40% and less commonly cough or haemoptysis in less than 5%[125,130,151]. Hoarseness is uncommon but aphasia could indicate imminent airway obstruction. Examination of the oral cavity may be unremarkable in as many as half of all patients, with pharyngitis or lingual tonsillar inflammation the most common abnormalities found on physical examination[125,130]. The degree of pharyngitis may also be disproportionately mild compared to the pharyngeal pain. The presence of pharyngitis has often led to mistaken diagnosis in several cases of tonsillar pharyngitis, the patients later presenting with airways obstruction[132,142,152]. Occasionally, uvulitis may be the only physical abnormality[153]. Adults as children can sometimes present with acute respiratory embarrassment, stridor with rapid (within a few hours) progression to upper airways obstruction, but this occurs less frequently compared to children[125,130,132,151,152]. The unfavourable anatomical structure of the paediatric larynx or epiglottis may in part account for the overall less severe presentation in adults. Of some interest is that a paediatric type epiglottis may be found in some cases of adult AE who progress to glottic obstruction[141]. Laboratory features include leukocytosis of between 10–25 $\times 10^9$/l and occasionally higher in 70–80% of patients[130] or a mean of approximately 15×10^9/l[125,132]. Rarely patients with epiglottitis can present with accompanying features of ARDS typified by bilateral diffuse pulmonary infiltrates associated with respiratory distress relatively refractory to oxygen and with no evidence for cardiogenic pulmonary oedema or chronic obstructive pulmonary disease[128]. Both transient and life-threatening non-cardiogenic pulmonary oedema may also occur following relief of the upper airways obstruction from AE[154,155] despite the maintenance of an adequate airway.

The overall mortality rate in adult AE as gleaned from most series is of the order of 1%[136]. A more recent study indicated a mortality rate of 2/356 adults and 6/485 children[137]. The presence of respiratory distress may substantially increase this risk as may the presence of an epiglottic abscess. Underlying immunocompromisation or co-morbid medical conditions appear to occur more frequently in adults. These include diabetes mellitus, HIV positivity, neutropenia, myeloma, alcoholism, asthma, leukaemia and other malignancies[125,146]. Nevertheless, epiglottitis is rare in these severely immunocompromised patients. The finding of unusual organisms such as *Kingella kingae* or *Candida* spp. or the presence of pneumococaemia should suggest an underlying immunodeficiency including HIV[156,157,158]. Although severe immunocompromisation does not always presage an acute fulminating course requiring airways rescue, it nevertheless occurred in all five patients with AIDS reported by Rothstein[158] so aggressive airway intervention should be considered in these patients.

The importance of not misdiagnosing AE as tonsillo-pharyngitis, foreign body impaction, tumours, retropharyngeal abscess, drug reactions, angioneurotic oedema, inhalation of toxic gases or superheated steam, and the need to differentiate from other infectious aetiologies including infectious mononucleosis, diphtheria, pertussis, and anaerobic infections has led to better efforts to establish an early definitive diagnosis.

Characteristic radiographical findings include the thumbprint sign of epiglottic enlargement with an extremely narrow airway and vellecular obliteration – seen on lateral neck radiography[159]. Other radiographical features include swelling of aryepiglottic folds, arytenoid, uvula and supraglottic tissue, oedema of the prevertebral/retropharyngeal soft tissues and hypopharyngeal ballooning. CT might be useful if local complications such as abscess are suspected[160]. However, lateral neck radiography is of variably limited diagnostic usefulness. Whereas some workers report a high correlation between radiology and laryngoscopy findings[159], the false-negative rate can be between 10% and 21%[134,161,162]. However, if careful fold thickness measurements are taken at the midpoint or basal areas and near the false vocal cords, the sensitivity and specificity can be of the order of 95%. A negative radiological examination therefore cannot reliably exclude the diagnosis. There is a growing tendency to avoid this examination both because of underdiagnosis and by promoting delay in instituting appropriate airways management.

Quite unlike the situation in children, indirect and direct laryngoscopy in adults with AE can be safely performed in most adults without precipitating total airways obstruction, and thus allow a definitive diagnosis to be made[134,151,164]. The fibreoptic nasolaryngoscope offers technical advantages in diagnosis[131,165]. This should therefore, be undertaken in adults in whom there is strong suspicion for AE particularly as evidenced by the patient who has odynophagia, disproportionately severe to the degree of visible oropharyngeal inflammation. However, indirect laryngoscopy may still be dangerous in adults who have severe respiratory distress such as stridor[166]. The cherry red, swollen and oedematous epiglottis is diagnostic though such a classical appearance may be less dramatic in adults, the epiglottis often appearing as pale and oedematous.

Management

The two main management objectives in adult AE are the monitoring and establishment of an airway, and antimicrobials. In paediatric AE, an artificial airway is required in nearly all patients (Chapter 23). In adults, the risk of total respiratory obstruction is significantly less with most patients recovering without the need to establish an airway. Of 543 adults with AE 13% required an airway compared to 71% of 357 children[125–131,132,136,137]. Nevertheless, some adults do present with advanced airways obstruction and others deteriorate and require emergency airway intervention. In addition, the mortality rate is substantially increased in patients presenting with respiratory distress[167]. There is controversy as to whether to establish an artificial airway in *all* adult patients or to be more selective thereby avoiding unnecessary tracheostomies with their attendant morbidity and mortality risk by attempting to predict which patients are at risk for subsequent airways closure. Of course, it is mandatory to observe closely *all* adult patients with AE in a unit with close proximity facilities for expert guided emergency intubation/cricothyroidomy if needed. Some patients deteriorate rapidly and without warning[134] even after a period of steady improvement[147]. Patients with a short history (less than 8 hours)[168] or those who are toxic or drooling with stridor/sitting erect posture/dyspnoea/higher mean leukocyte count are more likely to require airways intervention[125,161,168], with stridor/sitting erect posture on multivariate logistic regression analysis significantly predicting for airway intervention[125]. The presence of *H. influenzae* bacteraemia has been shown in some studies to predict a hazardous course with risk for obstruction[134]. If patients are going to deteriorate, they usually move gradually and sequentially to increasing stages of respiratory difficulty (Freedman stages I–IV), and sudden respiratory arrest is said not to occur in patients who have no previous airway compromise[169]. However, occasional reports indicate that sudden airways obstruction *does* occur even in the absence of prior signs of airways embarrassment[152] and this has lead to some clinicians proposing artificial airways in *all* adult patients with AE[141,170]. Clearly, without clinical expertise, close monitoring and immediate equipment, monitoring of patients having no respiratory embarrassment without securing an airway can be hazardous. One reasonable approach to airway management in adults with AE has been summarised[171] as follows. In cases with no respiratory complaint the patient should be carefully monitored in an ICU setting with facilities for immediate intubation/tracheostomy available. Repeated flexible nasoendoscopy might be useful to monitor the airway in such patients[165]. Patients with *any* degree of initial or subsequent respiratory embarrassment (however mild) should have their airway secured by a planned but urgent intubation/tracheostomy. The wisdom of this approach is reflected by occasional reports of sudden unexpected and fatal deterioration even in stable and improving patients closely monitored even in an ICU setting[149]. Finally, in patients with impending respiratory embarrassment or severe respiratory distress immediate intubation, cricothyroidotomy or tracheostomy in the ER should be performed. Inhalational induction is recommended[171]. The choice of airway is also controversial – the trend is definitely away from tracheostomy to oral/nasal tracheal intubation under direct visual control, since the course of AE is often only a few days.

AE has also been described in pregnancy. In such a situation where the foetus may also be at risk from hypoxia, more aggressive airways management with planned artificial airway at presentation might be wise[172].

Patients often receive corticosteroid adjunctive therapy despite the absence of clinical trials showing benefit. Adrenalin is sometimes given but the suggestion that improvement in stridor or respiratory distress or avoidance of tracheostomy occurs[151,173] requires testing in a controlled setting.

Antimicrobials should be chosen to cover β-lactamase producing *H. influenzae*, *S. aureus*, Group A, β-hemolytic *Streptococcus* and *S. pneumoniae.* Chloramphenicol has been the gold standard antimicrobial for AE in the past but fears over its toxicity and concern over reports of resistant organisms have emerged. Ampicillin is no longer suitable due to the high incidence of β-lactamase strains. Currently a second- or third-generation cephalosporin such as cefuroxime is recommended although its antistaphylococcal activity is limited[125]. Occasional reports of multiply resistant pneumococcal isolates indicate that even β-lactams, extended spectrum cephalosporins and cotrimoxazole may not be effective on occasions[174]. Amoxicillin with clavulanic acid is an effective alternative and active against *S. aureus*.

Final remarks

It will be of some considerable interest and importance to monitor the impact of widespread Hib vaccination on the incidence of adult AE. Evidence has emerged that this has already had a significant impact in reducing paediatric AE due to Hib[139,175]. However, cases of paediatric AE still occur but often in older children and caused by organisms other than Hib, particularly group A β-haemolytic *Streptococcus*[139]. Given the fact that documented Hib-associated AE in adults is relatively uncommon it would be surprising if Hib vaccination substantially reduced the number of adult cases. Major immediate challenges in the management of adult AE include elucidation of microbial aetiology, improvement in early diagnoses, and rationalising/unifying the approach to management.

Laryngitis

The larynx is a complex structure composing cartilages and muscles containing the vocal cords and joints whose functions are maintenance and protection of the airway, involvement in deglutition and

Table 25.4. *Laryngitis: causes*

Influenza virus, rhinovirus > bacterial (*M. catarrhalis, H. influenzae*)	
Rarely staphylococcal	
Tuberculosis	
Fungal:	*Candida*, *Cryptococcus*, blastomycosis, coccidiomycosis, histoplasmosis
Actinomycosis	
H. simplex, H. zoster	
Non-infective : SLE, GI reflux	

phonation[176]. Infectious inflammation of the larynx can result in local pain, dysphonia/aphonia, haemoptysis and airways obstruction. In addition, it is quite possible that if the vocal cords themselves are uninvolved, the signs and symptoms may be vague and go undetected. Of all symptoms, hoarseness due to involvement of at least the anterior two-thirds of the vocal cords is the commonest respiratory symptom of laryngeal infection. The majority of patients experience laryngitis as part of a more generalised upper respiratory tract illness but occasionally primary infectious laryngitis does occur.

Most of the viral respiratory pathogens can involve the larynx (Table 25.4). Hoarseness is the predominant symptom occurring in between 2% and 40% of patients, typically as part of the earlier ($\leq$ 1 week) constellation of symptoms. Influenza and rhinovirus are the most frequently incriminated pathogens.

Bacterial aetiologies are generally less commonly implicated. For example, only a few patients with streptococcal tonsillo-pharyngitis have laryngeal involvement. However, recently, *M. catarrhalis* and *H. influenzae* have been found in approximately 50% and 10% of cases of adult acute laryngitis, respectively, whereas they are rarely isolated in age-matched healthy patients[177]. These findings together with the more rapid elimination of *Moraxella* with erythromycin compared to placebo and associated subjective improvement of voice disturbance and cough, suggest a pathogenic role for *Moraxella*. However, objective improvement as measured by laryngoscopy and voice scores did not parallel these findings. As most cases of laryngitis resolve spontaneously, erythromycin is not routinely indicated in most cases of adult laryngitis but might have a role to play in patients whose voice is professionally precious[177]. Penicillin V on the other hand has no impact on symptoms or microbiological eradication in such patients[178].

Rarely staphylococcal laryngotracheitis occurs. If so patients may develop the toxic shock syndrome, with a widespread confluent macular erythematous rash, hypotension and presence of TSS toxin I[179]. This is a life threatening event requiring aggressive supportive treatment and antibiotics which include clindamycin or cloxacillin. Other rare bacterial etiologies include diphtheria and tuberculosis. In the prechemotherapeutic era tuberculous laryngitis was almost always associated with advanced pulmonary cavitary disease among patients in their 30s, and hoarseness in such a setting was usually promptly recognised as tuberculous. Nowadays, tuberculous laryngitis, without pulmonary involvement is a more common presentation[180,181]. As a cause of extrapulmonary tuberculosis, however, it is rare[182]. Associated with this changing presentation is the changing anatomical site from the posterior laryngeal commissure (thought to reflect the physical impaction of highly positive sputum in a recumbent patient) to involvement of the true or false cords[181]. Endoscopically the appearance can mimic chronic non-specific laryngitis or tumour with ulcerations, oedema and granulation tissue. Biopsy for histological examination, AFB stain and culture is necessary for definitive diagnosis. Unrecognised or untreated, fibrosis, stenosis or laryngeal incompetence may occur.

Fungal laryngitis is of relatively greater importance nowadays in the light of the increasing immunocompromised host population. In absolute terms, however, mycotic laryngitis is uncommon. Of all the diagnosed mycoses in a major hospital in New Orleans, 14% had laryngeal involvement[183]. Nevertheless, many of these fungi can masquerade as carcinoma in their appearance and patients have undergone total laryngectomy on such suspicion. It is therefore important to consider a fungal aetiology in the differential diagnosis of hoarseness. *Laryngeal candidiasis* most often occurs in association with pharyngeal or oesophageal candidiasis. However, sole laryngeal involvement with no oral or pharyngeal disease has been described[184]. The patients are usually predisposed due to antibiotics, corticosteroids, endotracheal intubation, leukaemia, alcohol abuse, cytotoxic disease and debilitation[184,185]. Chronic mucocutaneous candidiasis characterised by skin and mucous membrane involvement is due to a narrow T-cell defect and may produce candidal laryngitis whose symptoms may be minimal[186]. In a review of 399 patients with AIDS, 51 had oropharyngeal or oesophageal or laryngeal candidiasis and included three patients who had isolated laryngeal candidiasis[187]. In fact, *Candida albicans* appears to be the most common cause of laryngeal infection in AIDS. Nevertheless, patients with laryngeal candidiasis may occasionally be otherwise quite healthy[188]. Candidal laryngitis also may be part of, and perhaps even the source of, a much wider involvement namely, disseminated candidiasis. Prosthetic candidal infections have also been documented, for example, on silicone voice prosthesis[189]. Hoarseness and painful dysphagia are the two most common presenting features although these may be poorly correlated with the degree of laryngeal involvement. Airways obstruction is an uncommon complication – it may also be the presenting symptom[190]. Laryngoscopy reveals thick white laryngeal exudates sometimes accompanied by gross ulceration and oedema. It may be mistaken for carcinoma[188]. Untreated, chronic laryngeal candidiasis can lead to scar tissue. The management of laryngeal candidiasis is with oral nystatin (gargles), fluconazole, itraconazole or intravenous amphotericin B.

Although disease due to *Cryptococcus neoformans* most often presents with neurological involvement, widely disseminated disease is also described. A primary pulmonary focus usually precedes these presentations. Approximately one-third of patients with cryptococcosis do not have a detectable underlying predisposition. The majority are associated with HIV infection or with other immunosuppressive conditions[191]. No cases of laryngeal involvement were reported in a recent large series of cryptococcosis[191]. Thus, cryptococcosis of the larynx is a rare entity. The first reported case was in a middle-aged immune competent man who developed chronic hoarseness and respiratory distress which required tracheostomy[192]. Another occurred in an immunocompromised young lady[193]. The first AIDS-related case was published in 1992 masquerading as Kaposi's sarcoma[194]. Laryngoscopy may reveal laryngeal oedema which may be so extensive as to produce glottic obstruction and warty white lesions on the cords which may prove to be pseudoepitheliomatous on biopsy. Bronchoscopy may show cryptococcal ulcerative lesions in the endobronchial tree. Diagnosis is made by biopsy and treatment is with amphotericin B.

Blastomycosis can also present with chronic hoarseness, cough and occasionally haemoptysis. Approximately 5% of all cases of blastomycosis have laryngeal involvement[195]. The laryngoscopy appearance of erythematous granulomas which have irregular borders initially suggests carcinoma, but biopsy (which may need to be performed multiply) is mandatory to show and culture the typical double contoured organisms, and hence to avoid radical surgery or radiotherapy. There may be a positive past travel history, or a chest radiograph indicating a previous pulmonary infection which could provide a valuable diagnostic clue. Untreated, fibrosis, laryngeal stenosis or laryngocutaneous fistula occurs[196,197]. Treatment is with amphotericin B.

Coccidiomycosis of the larynx usually occurs as part of a disseminated picture[198] in which there is a prominent pulmonary clinical component, in which laryngitis most often occurs either through erosion of paratracheal nodes or via a haematogenous route. Rarely, primary laryngeal coccidiomycosis has been described[199]. In addition to the systemic features of cough, chest pain, fever and skin lesions, hoarseness, throat pain and features of airways obstruction can ensue. Biopsy for histology and culture, skin testing and serology are necessary for the diagnosis. Treatment is with itraconazole or amphotericin B.

Similarly, *histoplasmosis* of the larynx usually presents as part of a chronic disseminated picture particularly in patients with underlying immunosuppression such as HIV, leukaemia, etc.[200]. Oropharyngeal or laryngeal involvement occurs in approximately a third of such patients. Usually there are anterior laryngeal ulcers and biopsy is a highly sensitive diagnostic manoeuvre[201]. Amphotericin B is the treatment of choice.

Other *unusual infections* include actinomycosis[202], herpes simplex and zoster[203]. Syphilis should also be considered. Even the so-called endemic treponemal infection can produce severe disease including gummatous laryngitis[204].

Chronic laryngitis may also have a non-infective cause, for example, tumours, voice abuse and autoimmune diseases such as SLE[176,205]. Gastrointestinal reflux is a well recognised but often overlooked cause of chronic laryngitis. These patients have chronic cough especially at night, throat clearing and burning. A spectrum of posterior laryngoscopic findings are found ranging from interarytenoid erythema to contact ulceration and granuloma formation over the vocal processes of the arytenoid cartilages[206]. The condition should be recognised since response to omeprazole or surgical correction, e.g. Nissen fundoplication is often helpful[206,207].

Whilst most cases of microbial laryngitis are benign and due to self-limiting infections, occasionally more severe or therapeutically challenging problems occur. These should be entertained in patients with underlying immunodeficiency or comorbid illness, a history of appropriate foreign travel and in all patients with chronic symptoms. In these situations all patients should undergo laryngoscopy with biopsy not only for histological examination but to exclude pseudocarcinomatous mimics such as tuberculosis and fungal diseases.

Tracheitis

It is curious that bacterial tracheitis described in the 1940s in children did not feature again in the literature until the 1970s. The condition is characterised by extensive inflammation of the infra-glottic region but remarkable sparing of the epiglottis, supraglottis and the glottic larynx. Mucosal ulceration, purulent debris and oedema make up the gross pathological findings. Although there are some clinical features resembling viral laryngotracheobronchitis or epiglottitis, it is a separate entity – previous cases may have therefore been overlooked[208]. Unlike viral laryngotracheobronchitis it does not respond to racemic epinephrine. Detailed paediatric aspects are covered in Chapter 23.

Bacterial tracheitis was first described as such in adults by Johnson[209]. The key presenting features are stridor, dyspnoea, sometimes accompanied by wheeze. Absence of drooling and severe dysphagia are pointers against epiglottitis[210], whilst a high white count and high fever are against viral croup. Sudden respiratory distress due to subglottic airways obstruction is a major life threatening complication and is due to the intense tracheal oedema and inflammatory exudate. Complications include pneumonia, pneumothorax, toxic shock syndrome and cardiopulmonary arrest[208]. Radiology may show irregular subglottic narrowing due in part to pseudomembranous formation. The lung parenchyma is usually clear. Endoscopy often reveals large amounts of mucopurulent material which cultures *S. aureus*, *S. pyogenes*, *S. pneumoniae* or *H. influenzae*.

There may be a preceding history of a viral respiratory tract infection, particularly with influenza or parainfluenza. Theories of pathogenesis have involved viral-induced impairment of mucociliary clearance, decreased formation of fibronectin and disorganised neutrophil function[208]. These mechanisms may be more important in individuals already predisposed to bacterial infection, e.g. dysgammaglobulinaemia, oesophageal-tracheal fistulas[208] and in patients infected with HIV[211].

The management involves prevention of airways obstruction by removal of inspissated inflammatory debris and airway oedema, maintenance of an effective airway and systemic antibiotics[212]. Carinal resection may be needed in severe airway stenosis[213].

In recent years, fungal tracheitis has been increasingly described. *Aspergillus*, *Candida*, mucoralis and others have been implicated (in descending order of frequency). *Aspergillus* affects the respiratory tract in a number of ways but in several studies, localised *Aspergillus* infection of the trachea and/or bronchi occurred in about 5% of patients[214] (see also Chapter 16). As with invasive pulmonary aspergillosis there is almost always underlying immunocompromisation but the degree of this is relatively mild. There is therefore less pronounced neutropenia, less exposure to steroids and it is these factors which may have resulted in a more localised form of aspergillosis. However, heart–lung transplant, solid tumour, bone marrow transplantation, haematological malignancy, HIV infection and

Table 25.5. *Tracheitis: causes*

Bacterial	*S. aureus*
	S. pyogenes
	S. pneumoniae
	H. influenzae
	Rare, e.g. *Corynebacterium pseudodiphtheriticum*, TB
Viral	Influenza
	Parainfluenza
	Rare, e.g. H. simplex, measles
Fungal	*Aspergillus*
	Candida
Non-infectious	Ventilator associated

lymphoma have all been described as risk factors[214]. In the setting of lung transplantation, disease is initially limited to the anastomosis site, or in the case of single lung transplants to the transplanted site – suggesting the role of abnormal local defence mechanisms[215]. Other risk factors include local disturbance of the airways structure or function, for example, luminal bronchial carcinoma, disorders of mucociliary function and endotracheal intubation. Fungal tracheitis can manifest pathologically either as a superficial intraluminal process resulting in pseudomembrane formation, a fungal airways plug or as localised plaques with a degree of ulcerative tissue invasion limited at first to the mucosa but later bridging the bronchial wall to involve lung parenchyma or even dissemination[214].

Clinically the patients may complain of cough, fever, dyspnoea and chest pain. Acute airways obstruction may occur and this can present as a unilateral wheeze and may in fact be the first localising sign of *Aspergillus* tracheo-bronchitis[216]. Patients may also be asymptomatic and the process recognised as an incidental finding at post-mortem. The chest radiograph is normal in a third of patients. Complications include fistula formation, for example, tracheoesophageal fistula[214], tracheo-pulmonary fistula with fatal haemorrhage[217] and airways obstruction[217].

Fungal tracheitis is now also recognised in AIDS patients[218], the clinical and histological features being similar to those patients without AIDS. Airway disease in AIDS related aspergillosis appears to be more common (occurring in about a quarter of all cases) than in non-HIV patients[219], and possibly reflects abnormalities of mucus production or ciliary dysfunction in AIDS patients.

The outcome of fungal tracheobronchitis is guarded with a mortality rate of up to 40% reported[218]. Treatment involves systemic amphotericin B or itraconazole, removal of the fungal burden endoscopically[220] and reduction of immunosuppression. The ideal approach has yet to be defined.

Some other unusual processes and organisms have been incriminated in adult tracheitis. These include mechanical ventilator associated necrotising tracheobronchitis[221] in which parainfluenzae 3 may have contributed. However, bacterial tracheitis has also been recognised as a complication of endotracheal intubation[222]. Airway mucosal ischaemia may play an important role in ventilator associated necrotising tracheobronchitis. Angiotensin converting enzyme inhibitors may prevent lesions in animal models[223]. Ulcerative tracheobronchitis has also been described in association with inflammatory disease often years after colectomy[224]. Necrotising tracheitis has been seen secondary to *Corynebacterium pseudodiphtheriticum* in a patient with COAD treated with prednisone but not otherwise immunocompromised[225]. Necrotising tracheobronchitis has also occurred secondary to *Herpes simplex* in both compromised and normal patients[226], in tuberculous tracheitis[227], and following measles[228].

Adult croup syndrome

There had been no reports of acute laryngotracheobronchitis or croup in adults until a few years ago[229]. This entity is of course well recognised in children (see Chapter 23). Seven patients aged 25–73 years were described. They had acute inflammatory swelling of the subglottic space and presenting symptoms of an antecedent common cold followed by barking cough and upper airways obstruction (stridor, retractions, narrowed subglottic space on radiography). All patients received airways humidification, nebulised racemic epinephrine and steroids whilst three required airways intervention. There were no deaths. The aetiology is presumed viral but this has not been proven. It has to be differentiated from other non-infectious causes of subglottic airways narrowing including prolonged intubation, sarcoid and Wegener's granulomatosis.

Rhinoscleroma

This disease was first described by Hebra in 1874; however, little advancement in the understanding of the immunopathogenesis, mechanisms of transmission and optimal therapy of the condition has since emerged.

The microbial agent is *Klebsiella rhinoscleromatis* recognised by Von Frisch in 1882. The organism is a facultative anaerobic Gram-negative encapsulated diplobacillus not normally present in the respiratory tract. An intense host response results in an inflammatory spectrum and the subsequent clinical picture ranges from rhinitis to upper or lower respiratory tract deformity and obstruction.

Most patients are young adults (more female than male) of low socioeconomic status characterised by overcrowding, poor hygiene and malnutrition. Patients originate from rural areas of the tropics particularly Egypt, Africa, India as well as from Central and Southern America, Eastern Europe and the Middle East[230–234]. Immigration has led to a resurgence of the disease in parts of the world where it had previously been uncommon or had disappeared from[235] and this may lead to delays in diagnosis. It seems likely that close and prolonged contact with the person having active disease is necessary for transmission.

Following infection with *K. rhinoscleromatis*, there is an initial intense mixed inflammatory cell response which commences usually at epithelial interfaces, e.g. at the stratified squamous epithelium/respiratory epithelium in the larynx[236]. This consists of neutrophils, eosinophils, lymphocytes and plasma cells. Later epithelial hypertrophy with numerous monocytes, lymphocytes and histiocytes occurs. Sheets of highly vacuolated histiocytes called Mikulicz's cells together with eosinophilic Russell bodies may also be present[237]. The intracellular–intravacuolar organism may be identified by Giemsa or other silver stains or by an immunoperoxidase technique. Ultimately the inflammatory response switches to a predominantly non-specific picture with extensive fibrosis and diminution in lymphocyte and plasma cell infiltrates. Humoral immunity appears to be normal but a cell-mediated immune defect is present. Thus, the CD8 cell count is increased and the T-cell mitogen response diminished[238]. Although macrophages appear able to phagocytose the bacteria, they cannot inhibit their proliferation or kill them[234] and produce histiocytic rather than epidermoid cell granuloma.

Over 90% of cases involve the upper respiratory tract and usually the nose[239]. Patients usually give a long history of rhinitis which later becomes purulent and fetid (catarrhal stage). There may be atrophy and crusting of the nasal mucosa. A granulomatous stage ensues in which nodular swellings may be found at rhinoscopy. Epistaxis may occur. Local tissue invasion of the nasal septum, turbinates and lip produces deformity such as broadening of the nose (Hebra's nose)[240] as well as other abnormalities (Fig.25.1(*a*)). Stenosis characterises the third or sclerotic stage.

Extension from the original affected areas may occur through lymphatics or contiguous routes, possibly aided by surgical or bronchoscopic procedures[240]. This can result in a progressive destructive and obliterative involvement of the sinuses, orbit, pharynx, larynx, and trachea as well as spread to the regional lymph nodes[237]. Thus, in late stage disease, the patient may present with chronic sinusitis, hoarseness, dysphagia or the orbital apex syndrome[241]. Respiratory obstruction is a dreaded complication. Routine pan-upper and lower respiratory tract endoscopy in rhinoscleroma which on presentation is apparently confined to the nose indicates secondary site involvement, e.g. trachea and sinus are extraordinarily frequent[241]. The late presentations may mimic malignancy[242]. Rarely, primary involvement of sites apart from the nose are found, e.g. antroscleroma. Skin lesions are also well described which may either be primary or occur as direct extensions from intranasal lesions[243]. Complications include malignant change and airways stenosis.

Diagnosis is based upon the endoscopical findings and biopsy and demonstration of the organism in tissue is pathognomonic. The characteristic Mikulicz cells on imprint smears or by formal histology may be demonstrable[244]. CT of the nose and nasopharynx[236] may show homogenous soft tissue masses which are non-enhancing and have distinct edges. In the more distal airways, crypt-like irregularities or concentric irregular narrowing which produce stenosis may be present. Marked thickening of the attachment of the soft to the hard palate – the so-called 'palatal sign' – may be a useful diagnostic feature[245]. Other causes of granulomatous inflammation have to be considered in the differential diagnosis including non-infectious granulomatous disease such as sarcoid, Wegener's granulomatosis, tumours, syphilis, leprosy, *Leishmania* and fungal disease.

The management is difficult and involves a protracted course (months to years) of antimicrobials and surgery. Antibiotics frequently used are streptomycin, tetracycline, gentamicin, cotrimoxazole, second or third generation cephalosporins, clofazimine, topical acriflavine, rifampicin (topical or systemic) and ciprofloxacin[231,237,246]. Sometimes the response to antibiotics is dramatic (Fig.25.1(*a*), (*b*)). Corticosteroids, silver nitrate and radiotherapy have also been used. However, relapse or progression is not uncommon and surgical debridement which may be followed by plastic reconstruction is a major treatment modality particularly in cases of respiratory embarrassment. Endoscopic laser therapy has also proved useful since this is associated with less postoperative oedema and may reduce the risk of dissemination[237,247]. The precise cause of the immunological defect is unknown and the role of immunomodulatory therapy has not been investigated.

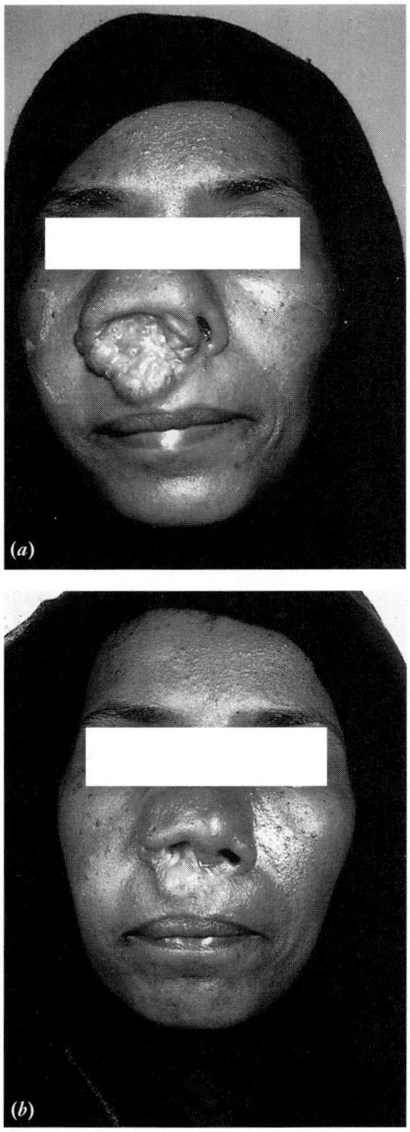

FIGURE 25.1 Rhinoscleroma before (a) and after (b) antibiotic treatment.

Sinusitis

Sinusitis is one of the most common health care complaints seen by primary care physicians and accounts for an enormous expenditure in clinical expertise, technical support, and pharmaceuticals, affecting more than 31 million people in the United States[248]. Advances in computed tomography have contributed valuable information of the normal and pathological states of the paranasal sinuses, encouraging a more scientific approach to the understanding and management of sinus infections.

Anatomical considerations

All the paranasal sinuses are present at birth in a rudimentary form, but only the maxillary, anterior and posterior ethmoid sinuses are pneumatised sufficiently in childhood to play a role in infection. The frontal and sphenoid sinuses undergo later pneumatisation and are significant after the age of 6 and 5 years, respectively. The ethmoids are adult size by approximately age 14, while the maxillary sinus reaches full maturation following the descent of the secondary teeth sometime in adolescence[249]. In both children and adults, the critical anatomical area is termed the osteomeatal unit (Fig.25.2) described by Naumann in 1965[250]. Blockage in this middle meatus-anterior ethmoid complex can lead to obstruction-induced inflammation in the maxillary and frontal sinuses, with reduced ventilation and disruption of normal vehicle ciliary clearance[251].

The sinuses are lined with ciliated pseudo-stratified columnar epithelium continuous with the nasal mucosa. This is covered by a mucous blanket that is continuously propelled by ciliary action through the sinus ostea. Besides acting as a humidification and lubrication agent, this blanket is a macro-molecular sieve, entrapping micro-organisms and particulates and transporting them for expulsion into the pharynx. In addition, it has a host defence function as an extra-cellular source of IgA/IgG, multiple enzyme actions and antimicrobial functions. Of proteins in nasal secretions, 15–30% are lysozymes which prevent infection for most air-borne bacteria, and 4% are lactoferrin which binds iron and kills bacteria[252].

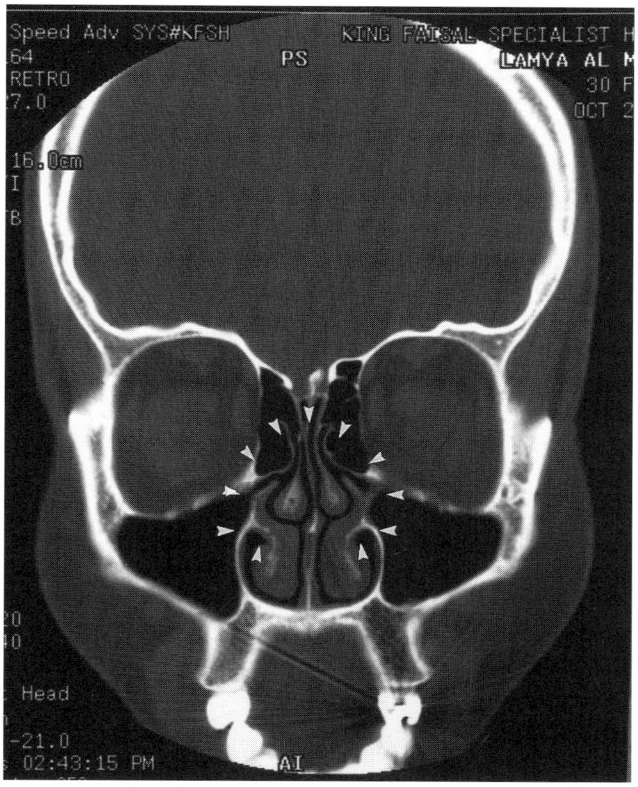

FIGURE 25.2 CT coronal section head showing osteomeatal unit (arrowed).

The middle meatus is bathed in the major portion of inspiration airflow and is the site where the flow changes from vertical to horizontal convection, and as such, has particulate matter deposited there. The ostea leading into the maxillary frontal sinuses are not direct openings but tubular and are prone to functional obstruction in a variety of clinical scenarios[253].

Pathophysiology

Occlusion of the sinus ostea initiates the sinusitis cycle. Upper respiratory viral infection usually precedes bacterial sinusitis. The resultant mucosal congestion blocks airflow and drainage initiating stagnation of secretions, changes in pH and mucosal gas metabolism and results in damage to the cilia and epithelium. This creates an environment for bacterial growth in a closed cavity, further inflammation, mucosal thickening and continuing obstruction. The hypoxic environment can lead to a change from predominately aerobic flora to anaerobes. Ciliary function becomes impaired as well as the bactericidal granulocyte function[254].

Clinical profile

Acute sinusitis is usually defined as an infliction lasting up to 3 weeks, while persistence of symptoms of sinus disease for longer than this period, constitutes chronic disease[255].

Acute sinusitis in adults classically presents with nasal congestion, rhinorrhoea, fever, and various degrees of headache or facial pain dependent upon the sinus site affected.

Ethmoid involvement is characterised by periorbital headache, exacerbated by straining or coughing and bending forward. The headache is worse in the morning and improves during the day. Other sinuses are usually involved to some degree. The presence of sore throat and allergy symptoms are often noted.

Maxillary sinusitis may present as a 'toothache', periorbital pain or pain and tenderness over the involved maxilla made worse in the upright position. Discomfort usually lasts throughout the day.

Acute frontal sinus infection presents with a severe frontal headache, worse in the supine position, with tenderness over the involved sinus. Due to its proximity to the brain and orbit, pus under pressure in this sinus can be a medical emergency.

A deep-seated headache may herald a sphenoid sinus infection. Difficult to diagnose and also close to vital structures, it too may necessitate early medical and surgical intervention[256]. Children with acute sinusitis usually have less specific complaints. They frequently have little pain as there is less pressure because of the relatively larger ostium size to sinus volume. Wald has described two clinical entities. Most commonly patients present with a clear mucoid or purulent nasal discharge and cough lasting over ten days. This is accompanied by a low-grade fever, very little pain, fetid breath and a periorbital swelling in the morning. The second entity, much rarer, is profiled by 'a bad cold', fever, periorbital swelling, facial pain and copious purulent nasal discharge[257].

Due to the development and anatomy of the sinuses with progressing age, children under the age of six rarely suffer from sphenoid or frontal sinus infections. Chronicity is less common in children as sinus disease tends to be of short duration and is reversible with conservative treatment.

Predisposing factors are important in both acute and chronic sinusitis. Local factors which play an important role include nasal obstruction, septal deviation, polyps, foreign bodies, tumours, trauma and baro-trauma, and teeth infections. Adults suffer from three to four upper respiratory viral infections per year, while children have an average of six to eight per year and more if frequenters of daycare centres, increasing the likelihood of chronic sinusitis. A number of systemic diseases are associated with an increase in the incidence of chronic sinusitis. Although most patients with sinus disease are not immunodeficient, immunodeficiency diseases are often characterised by sinusitis as part of their clinical presentation. Of immunodeficiency disease patients, 30% develop sinusitis sometime in their clinical course[255]. Allergy is more common in acute and chronic sinusitis than in controls, particularly IgE-initiated allergy[258].

Nasal polyps and sinusitis are not uncommon in cystic fibrosis. The thick, tenacious secretions tend to block the ostea leading to secondary bacterial infection[259].

Patients with the immotile cilia syndrome are predisposed to acute sinusitis due to ultrastructural defects in the cilia of the mucosa[260].

There is a frequent association of paranasal sinus disease and bronchial asthma. Of asthmatic patients, 40–60% have radiographic evidence of sinusitis[261,262]. Studies show that difficult to control asthma will improve when coexistent sinusitis is treated[263]. This is particularly true in corticosteroid dependent children[264].

Adjunctive tests in sinusitis

Plain sinus-radiography

Plain standard views of the sinus is a sensitive diagnostic technique for detecting acute sinus inflammation of the maxillary antrum. Patients with air-fluid levels, total opacity, and thickened mucosa more than 6 mm in adults or 4 mm in children have a high probability of having an infection[265]. These views, however, are inadequate for evaluation of the anterior ethmoid air cells, the upper two-thirds of the nasal cavity and the infundibular middle meatus and frontal recess air passages[266].

Computed tomography

CT scans better demonstrate disease in the ethmoid sinuses, and are used for evaluation when response to medical treatment has not been satisfactory. Optimal demonstration of the anterio-ethmoid sinuses and osteomeatal structures is performed in the coronal plane. CT scanning is essential in cases complicated by extension into the orbit or brain[267].

Magnetic resonance imaging

Despite offering the best soft-tissue contrast, MRI is expensive, needs long imaging times, and does not demonstrate boney landmarks, and therefore should be reserved as a secondary or tertiary examination for the small number of patients with complex infectious disorders, particularly when known intracranial extension of disease exists[268].

Ultrasonography

Advantages of this technique include an absence of ionising radiation, rapid test time, and patient convenience. Reports of the accuracy of diagnosis utilising A-Mode ultrasonography have been mixed, however, and in practice it has been reserved for evaluation for fluid in the maxillary sinuses in pregnant women[269,270].

Nasal endoscopy

Nasal endoscopy utilising the use of rigid telescopes, popularized by Kennedy[271] and Stammberger[272] has helped immeasurably in the diagnosis and the management planning of sinusitis. Of patients with sinus symptoms and negative CT scan findings, 9% were diagnosed with infection by Vinning *et al.*[273]. In patients with positive CT scans, telescopic examination was important in identifying anatomical abnormalities predisposing to infection and subsequently correctable by surgery, demonstrating the compatibility between CT and nasal endoscopy. The use of the flexible endoscopes is useful in the investigation of symptoms related to post-nasal discharge[274].

Transillumination

Transillumination as part of the routine examination may be useful in adolescents and adults if light transmission is either normal or absent, but is of little value in children under the age of ten due to the relative thickness of the mucosa and boney vault[275]. Absence of light in either the frontal or maxillary sinuses indicates that further imaging techniques may be needed and suggests that antral puncture will probably yield positive culture results[276]. Normal light transmission following empirical treatment, with symptom improvement, may herald a successful treatment regime, without the need of follow-up X-rays.

Nasal cytology

A predominance of polymorphonuclear cells is found in patients with sinus infections, even in the presence of allergy[277]. Wilson *et al.* demonstrated that if the smear was positive for greater than six neutrophils per high power field, the radiograph was positive 90% of that time[278]. Other authors have concluded that nasal cytology should not be considered an adequate alternative to sinus radiography, due to the technique's non-specificity[279].

Microbiology

Brook studied the bacterial flow in normal non-inflamed sinuses and demonstrated the presence of aerobic and anaerobic organisms (Table 25.6). The anaerobic isolates included *Bacteroides* spp., anaerobic Gram-positive cocci and *Fusobacterium*. Aerobes isolated were predominately beta and alpha haemolytic streptococci, *S. pneumoniae, H. influenzae*, and *S. aureus*[280]. Other studies have confirmed these findings[281,282], demonstrating the non-sterility of the sinus cavity. Proliferation of these bacteria present in low titre, under conditions predisposing the sinus to infection, may be the cause of sinusitis. Supporting this assumption is the fact that, in acute sinusitis, these are

Table 25.6. *Sinusitis*

Causes	Bacterial	*S. pneumoniae*, *H. influenzae*, *S. aureus*
		M. catarrhalis (children)
		Bacteroides spp. *Fusobacterium* spp.
		(especially in chronic)
	Viral	Rhinoviruses, Parainfluenzae,
		Adenovirus, Influenza
	Fungal	*Aspergillus*
		fungal ball
		allergic
		chronic indolent
		fulminant
		Mucormycosis
		Candida and others (see text)
Management	Antibiotics	Amoxycillin ± clavulanate
		Erythromycin – sulfisoxazole
	Co-trimoxazole	
	Steam/hot decongestants	
	α-adrenergics	
	Saline irrigation	
	Topical steroids	
	Surgery	

the same bacteria found in high titres in purulent aspirates, as noted by a number of authors[283,284]. In adults and children *S. pneumoniae* and *H. influenzae* are the most common pathogens, while in children *M. catarrhalis* is also prominent.

In chronic sinusitis anaerobes play a large role in both adults and children,[285,286] predominately *Bacteroides* spp., anaerobic Gram-positive cocci, and *Fusobacterium* spp. Aerobic pathogens are alpha-haemolytic streptococci, *Haemophilus* spp. and *S. aureus*.

Viruses can be isolated in up to 15% of aspirates from patients with signs and symptoms of sinusitis, including rhinovirus, para influenza, adenovirus and influenza. The role of viruses in causing acute sinusitis remain unclear.

Medical management

Management goals (Table 25.6) should be established and should include:

(i) Control of infection
(ii) Reduction of tissue oedema
(iii) Maintenance of patency of the sinus ostia[287]

As nasal swab cultures are unreliable, empiric antibiotic therapy directed at the most common pathogens is appropriate except in complicated or refractory cases when antral puncture and aspiration may be indicated.

Patients with acute sinusitis have a spontaneous cure rate of 40%, and therefore half of patients who harbor β-lactamase-producing organisms will recover even if they are not receiving an optimal antimicrobial agent[288]. As such, amoxycillin, 500 mg q 8hrly (or 40 mg/ kg/day in three divided doses in children), is the antimicrobial of choice, being effective in most patients, relatively inexpensive and generally free of side-effects. In communities where there is a proven high incidence of β-lactamase producing organisms, or as a second course following failure of amoxycillin, amoxycillin potassium clavulanate (augmentin) is indicated.

If an allergy to penicillin exists, erythromycin-sulfisoxazole (50/150/mg/kg/day in four divided doses) is appropriate in children and adults. A broad spectrum of antimicrobial activity is also provided by sulfamethoxazole-trimethoprim (40 mg/8 mg/kg/day in two divided doses), but it is not effective against resistant *S. pneumoniae* or group A streptococci, important coinfecting organisms in 20% of patients with acute sinusitis[289]. First generation cephalosporins are not active against *H. influenzae* and are therefore not indicated empirically. Cefaclor, a second generation cephalosporin, is susceptible to β-lactamases produced by *H. influenzae* and *M. catarrhalis*, limiting its usefulness under these conditions[290].

The initial course of antibiotics should be continued for 10 to 14 days, or at least 7 days beyond the time at which they improve substantially or become symptom free. If, in the first 72 hours no clinical improvement is noted, an alternative antibiotic regimen should be considered[291].

In refractory cases and in chronic sinusitis, aspiration and cultures should be done to facilitate antibiotic choice, but often surgical management may be necessary to provide adequate drainage and ostia patency.

Adjunctive measures in medical management

Steam inhalation liquefies and softens crusts and moisturises inflamed mucosa often providing effective relief of symptoms. The addition of astringents and aromatics to this treatment has not been scientifically proven to be beneficial, but most patients subjectively state that it is helpful. Several controlled studies using hyperthermia in sinusitis have been sited[292], to support the observation that supraphysiologic temperatures block rhino-viral replication *in vitro*, but the conclusions are divergent. Nevertheless, steam inhalation remains the most popular adjunctive treatment modality.

Respiratory epithelial ciliary beat frequency increases in response to increasing temperatures may be responsible for the objective decongestant effect noticed by patients after ingesting hot tea with lemon, hot water or hot chicken soup[293,294].

As maxillary ostia diameter is reduced by 20% in the recumbent position, elevation of the head of the bed when supine will relieve some of the functional obstruction[295].

The use of alpha-adrenergic decongestants, both topical and oral, reduce nasal mucosa oedema and improve microciliary clearance, but should be used in the acute phase of disease only, to minimise the risks of rebound rhinitis medicomentosa and atrophic rhinitis[296].

Warm saline irrigations are useful in removing crusts, pus and thick secretions[297].

There is no rational reason for the use of antihistamines or anticholinergics in the treatment of acute or chronic sinusitis, as histamine does not appear implicated in these disorders[298]. In chronic sinusitis, complicated by a local nasal environment of seasonal and perennial allergic rhinitis, perennial nonallergic eosinophilic rhinitis, or nasal polyps, topical corticosteroids may be effective as an adjunctive measure in the medical management.

Surgery for sinusitis

Surgery for acute sinusitis is limited to diagnostic and therapeutic drainage procedures, trephination of the frontal sinus and sphenoid sinuses to relieve pus under pressure and wash out procedures of the maxillary sinuses where empiric treatment has failed, to obtain cultures and mobilize obstructing mucus plugs in the middle meatae.

Modern approaches to surgery for chronic sinusitis focus on the debridement of the osteomeatal complex, opening up the mucociliary tracts from the frontal sinus recess and anterior ethmoid. Classically, this is termed an ethmoidectomy, and can be accomplished by the intranasal or external approach. Mosher, in 1912, described the anterior ethmoidectomy as 'the bloodiest and most dangerous (operation) in all of surgery,[299] but more recent advances in computed axial tomography and endoscopic instrumentation have converted this technique into a relatively safe and effective approach in experienced hands. Nevertheless, numerous complications have been described, including CSF leaks, injury to the lacrimal apparatus, meningitis, severe haemorrhage, orbital haematoma, and blindness[300–302]. Probably the most common complication is scarring between the middle turbinate and the lateral nasal wall, a problem that can be controlled by meticulous dissection and post-operative scab debridement.

External ethmoidectomy is relatively safer affording better visualisation of the base of the skull and orbit, but leaving a scar and making anterior sinusotomy as an extension to the procedures, more difficult.

In summary, the role of surgery in chronic sinusitis is to provide decompression and aeration of the affected sinus in order to allow the reconstitution and restoration of normal mucociliary function of the nasal and paranasal complex. This requires a thorough understanding of the functional anatomy of the osteomeatal complex of the anterior ethmoid and its relationships with the other ethmoid, sphenoid and frontal sinuses[303,304].

Fungal disease of the sinuses

Fungal infection of the paranasal sinuses is rare. Infections with *Aspergillus* spp., *Candida* spp., *Penicillium* spp., *Fusarium* spp., *Paecilomyces* spp., *Schizophyllum* spp., *Bipolaris* spp., *Exserohilum* spp., *Curvularia* spp., *Cladosporium* spp., *Rhizopus* spp., *Cunninghamella* spp., *Conidiobolus* spp., *Basidiobolus* spp. *and Absidia* spp. have been reported[305]. The immune status of the host, the environmental load of fungi present, and local structural conditions of the sinuses causing tissue hypoxia predispose toward the development of a particular fungal disease[306].

Diagnosis depends on histopathology, as fungal culture may or may not be positive. Fungal hyphae may be seen on haematoxylin-eosin staining or more clearly on special stains such as Gomori–methenamine or Fontana–Masson[307].

Aspergillosis is the most common fungal infection of the paranasal sinus in both compromised and non-compromised hosts[308]. The fact that this organism cannot actively penetrate undamaged and intact mucous membrane and skin, for lack of keratolytic enzymes, separates the four forms of clinical aspergillosis involvement into two groups: extramucosal (saprophytic growth in retained secretions in a sinus cavity) and mucosal or penetrating fungal sinusitis. The aspergilloma and allergic aspergillosis sinusitis form the first group, and chronic indolent and fulminant fungal sinusitis form the second group.

The aspergilloma or cavitary 'fungus ball' is confined to a single sinus (usually the maxillary), is non-invasive, and usually occurs in a healthy host. The treatment is surgical removal of the fungal mass itself and establishment of adequate sinus drainage. No local or systemic anti-fungal chemotherapy is required[309].

Allergic aspergillosis sinusitis presents as an 'allergic' inspissated mucin ball or plug, is non-invasive, and usually occurs in an atopic healthy host with asthma and nasal polyps. Histological examination reveals eosinophils and eosinophil degradation products known as Charcot-Leydin crystals[310]. Surgical removal of the allergic mucin, sinus aeration, polypectomy and amelioration of osteomental obstruction are indicated. Systemic antifungal medications are not indicated, but local amphotericin and saline suspensions, internasal steroids or cromolyn may be of benefit[311].

Chronic indolent fungal sinusitis is always potentially invasive, affects the maxillary and ethmoid sinuses, and may be found in the compromised or non-compromised host. It should be suspected in a previously healthy patient presenting with chronic sinusitis resistant to conventional therapy. CT scanning typically shows hyperdense foci due to calcification in necrotic areas. This appearance can also be seen in thick pus, thrombus or malignancy. MRI may be more definitive as the fungal material has a greater iron and manganese composition than bacterial, producing a signal activity that is sharply decreased in T2 images while T1 images remain isodense[312]. These patients are not atopic and usually respond to surgical debridement. If, however, there is clinical, radiological or pathological evidence of invasion (Fig. 25.3), most, if not all patients should be treated by surgical extirpation of diseased tissue and a total dose of amphotericin B not exceeding 2 g for adults. Because of reported relapses after this intensive intravenous antifungal treatment, a 1-year follow-up course with an oral anti-fungal such as ketoconazole has been advocated[313]. (See Chapter 16.)

Fulminant fungal sinusitis is rare[314] and is found mainly in immune compromised hosts, especially in immunodeficiencies with severe neutropenic and T-cell defects. The highest incidence is in patients with acute leukemia,[315] but it is also seen in patients with lymphoma and other malignancies, patients with AIDS and congenital immunodeficiencies, patients who have received bone marrow or solid organ transplants, and those who have undergone chemotherapy. Once established, fulminant fungus sinusitis progresses rapidly, sometimes leading to death within hours, as a result of local and systemic spread of the disease. An aggressive approach needs to be taken with antifungal and antibacterial agents given at the onset of symptoms, coupled with early surgical debridement and drainage[316].

Mucormycosis (see also Chapter 16)

Mucormycosis is a rare fungal disease resulting from infection with fungi of class Phycomycetes, order Mucorales. It is an airborne infection starting in the lower and upper airways, associated with the clinical development of sinusitis, rhino-cerebral mucormycosis, or pulmonary infection. An opportunistic infection, it is associated with patients with diabetic ketoacidosis[317,318], corticosteroid treatment, burns[319], organ transplantation[320], neutropenia[321], and iron overload, with or without the concomitant use of desferrioxamine in patients undergoing haemodialysis[322]. It has also been reported rarely in an apparently normal host[323], complicating septic abortion[324] and in intravenous drug use[325].

This disease characteristically begins in the nose, paranasal sinuses or palate, spreading into the orbit and eventually the intracranial structures. The fungi invade the arterial vessels, and later lymphatics and veins, causing tissue necrosis secondary to arterial occlusion[326]. Necrotic ulceration of nasal mucous and hard palate, with black turbinates and unilateral proptosis occurs. The ethmoid sinuses are most likely to be involved. Biopsies of the affected turbinates should be carried out as soon as possible to confirm the diagnosis. Microscopic findings are coagulative and haemorhagic necrosis with non septate hyphae, moderate suppurative inflammation and vascular thrombosis[327]. Cultures are non-diagnostic as these organisms frequently present as saprophytes of the upper respiratory tract[328].

Recommended imaging techniques are computed tomography[329] and magnetic resonance imaging[330], the latter especially important if intra-cranial extension is suspected, or for the diabetic patient for whom intravenous contrast agents may be contraindicated.

Amphotericin B is usually ineffective in eradicating the primary lesion but can control early micrometastases. It should be given initially at doses from 1 mg/kg/day to 1.5 mg/kg/day until the patient is stabilised, when lower doses in the range of 0.8–1.0 mg/kg/day should be maintained[331].

The underlying predisposing condition should be reversed if possible.

Extensive surgical debridement of all non-vitalised tissues should be carried out as soon as the diagnosis is established, the type of surgical procedure individualised according to the underlying disease and extension of the infective process.

The synergistic effects of *in vitro* antifungal activity when amphotericin B is combined with 5-fluorocytosine or rifampin and the use of azole antifungal agents (e.g. itraconazole or fluconazole) is still under evaluation[332].

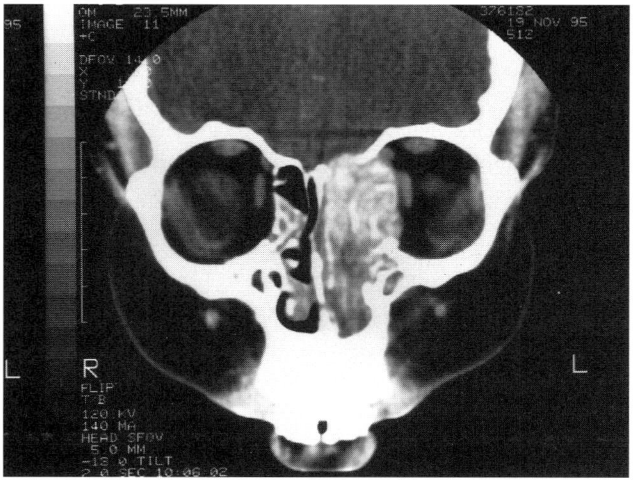

FIGURE 25.3. Ethmoid Aspergillus sinusitis with extension into anterior cranial fossa and orbit. Note hyperdense foci due to calcification.

Controversy continues to exist on the role of hyperbaric oxygen therapy but results appear to be encouraging[333–335]

Aggressive and timely medical and surgical treatment, based on a high index of suspicion, should increase the survival rate for these patients to 70% or 80%[336].

Nosocomial sinusitis

Nosocomial sinusitis differs from community-based sinusitis, in that it is a reflection of conditions related to the immunocompromised host. Predisposing factors include nasogastric and nasoendotracheal tubes, nasal packing, severe facial and cranial injuries, corticosteroid therapy, prior antibiotic therapy and mechanical ventilation[337]. In these instances, the normal flora of the sinus becomes pathogenic. In patients with sepsis of undetermined origin, sinusitis should be suspected.

Arens[338] reported a 2% incidence in patients intubated for less than 48 hours, while Stauffer[339] and Knodel[340] noted a higher rate in patients with longer intubation time, suggesting that the frequency of sinusitis is dependent on the length of nasal intubation. Furthermore, patients intubated quickly under less than ideal conditions tended to grow *Staphylococcus epidermidis*, while patients electively intubated demonstrated a clear-cut predominance of polymicrobial Gram-negative organisms[341].

If the diagnosis is suspected (fever, presence of a predisposing factor, and purulent nasal discharge), a radiological examination may confirm the diagnosis. Plain films have adequately demonstrated maxillary sinusitis[342], while sphenoid and ethmoid involvement is better shown on CT[343,344].

Removal of the nasogastric or nasotracheal tube[345] with or without surgical drainage is usually curative[346].

Orbital complications of sinusitis

The sinuses surround the thin porous walls of the orbit. Congenital or traumatic dehiscences in these walls provide a path of least resistance to infection[347]. A rich plexus of veins represent valveless communications between the facial, sinus, orbital and intracranial pathways as they drain directly to the cavernous sinus, providing a haematogenous route for the spread of infection[348,349].

Orbital infection in patients over the age of four is most commonly secondary to paranasal infection, usually because of ethmoid infection, less often due to maxillary sinus infection, and rarely as a result of frontal or sphenoid infection[350].

Acute ethmoid sinusitis may lead to subperiosteal abscess of the orbit, especially in childhood[351,352].

Extension of sphenoethmoiditis into the orbital apex can result in visual loss and ophthalmoplegia, termed 'the orbital apex syndrome', a clinical picture with minimal signs of orbital pathology such as proptosis, chemosis or lid oedema[353].

Chronic maxillary sinusitis with resultant sinus hypoplasia may lead to enophthalmus and hypoglobus, the 'silent sinus syndrome'[354].

Optic neuritis is usually thought to be a rare complication of paranasal sinusitis, but a causal relationship should be entertained, the neuritis postulated to be caused by direct extension of infection from the sinus to the optic nerve, a compressive optic neuropathy secondary to pressure from a pyocoele or mucocoele, or a sinusitis antigenically stimulating the immune system to cause a demyelinating optic neuritis[355].

Trauma or surgery to the sinuses is a common antecedent to orbital cellulitis. Visual loss following chronic sinusitis secondary to naso-orbital trauma has been reported[356]. The cellulitis may present itself years after the original insult[357].

Functional sinus endoscopic surgery has generated numerous reports of complications related to the orbit, including extraocular muscle injury[358], lacrimal drainage system injury,[359] and retro-orbital haematoma with resultant blindness[360]. Rarely, retro-orbital haematoma can be secondary to acute sinusitis[361] or chronic sinusitis[362] without preceding trauma.

Computed tomography (CT) has proved to be the radiological workhorse in the diagnosis and treatment planning for orbital infections secondary to sinusitis, although X-ray and operative findings do not always correlate[363]. The CT demonstrates the status of the bony partition shared by the orbit and sinuses and the source of the orbital sepsis, influencing the therapeutic approach. Magnetic resonance imaging (MRI) effectively demonstrates inflammatory changes in the paranasal sinuses and orbit, and extension of disease into the cavernous sinus[364].

Orbital complications of sinusitis are medical emergencies. Treatment modalities range from appropriate drainage procedures and antibiotics, to radical removal of the involved diseased tissues, depending on the clinical situation. Clinical awareness, and a team approach to the problem with active participation and communication between otolaryngologists, ophthalmologists and radiologists will enhance a successful outcome dependent upon early diagnosis and expedient medical and surgical treatment[365,366].

Osteomyelitis

Infection in the sinus can cause osteomyelitis by direct extension or by thrombophlebitis of the diploëtic veins, with resultant infection of the marrow[367]. As the maxilla lacks diploë, osteomyelitis is rare, except following dental infection[368]. The frontal sinus is more commonly involved, as first recognised as Potts puffy tumour, with erosion of the anterior sinus wall and subperiosteal abscess formation[369]. *S. aureus*, non-enterococcal *Streptococcus* and oral *anaerobes* are the usual pathologic organisms involved[370]. Long-term antibiotics, adequate drainage, and occasionally debridement of diseased tissue are necessary[371].

Intracranial complications

Acute or sub-acute exacerbations of chronic sinusitis may lead to intracranial complications including meningitis, epidural abscess, subdural abscess, brain abscess and venous sinus thrombosis[372,373]. Since the advent of the computerised axial tomography, early recognition and treatment has lowered the mortality rate to between 5% and 10%[374]. Antibiotic therapy without surgical drainage is seldom adequate in the treatment of loculated intracranial infections[375].

Sinusitis and AIDS

Sinusitis is an important and under-recognized cause of morbidity in patients with HIV disease[376]. Retrospective analysis has placed its incidence at 20% to 30% of HIV patients[377], and this incidence appears to be on the increase[378], perhaps due to the fact that patients affected with HIV are living longer with increased use of antiretroviral therapy and prophylaxis against *Pneumocytis carinii.*

There appears to be significant association between sinusitis severity and stage of HIV infection. HIV causes an allergic diathesis with increased IgE levels and sinusitis severity. IgE levels in AIDS patients increase with progression of disease[379].

Pathogens are similar to those of patients without HIV – *S. pneumoniae, H. influenzae* and less commonly, *S. aureus and Pseudomonas aeruginosa*[380]. Unusual microbiology has also been reported with opportunistic organisms including the microsporidian *Encephalitozoon E. cuniculi*[381], *Myobacterium kansasii*[382], mushroom *Schizophyllum commune*[383], *Legionella pneumophila*[384], *Candida albicans*[385], cytomegalovirus[386] and others.

Opportunistic fungal infections occur due to multiple abnormalities in local host defences, immunological functions and phagocytic activity[387].

Fungal sinusitis in patients with HIV or AIDS generally occurs late in the primary disease with low CD4 lymphocyte counts (less than 50/mm^3) unlike bacterial sinusitis which can occur at any time[388].

Differentiation between invasive and non invasive aspergillosis is not important in contrast to fungal infections in the noncompromised host – an early combined approach is indicated.

In all patients with AIDS, a high level of suspicion should be held for the presence of sinusitis. Aggressive early medical treatment is necessary, with surgery reserved for medical failures, recurrent sinusitis and sepsis and other complications related to the infection.

Otitis media

Otitis media is defined as an inflammation of the middle ear. It may present simply as a myringitis, or inflammation of the tympanic membrane, or with a middle ear effusion of varying consistency, denoted as otitis media with effusion (OME). Suppurative or purulent acute otitis media presents with one or more local or systemic signs including otalgia, otorrhea, fever, and in infants and children, a recent onset of irritability, anorexia, vomiting or diarrhoea. A middle ear effusion that persists longer than three months is termed chronic otitis media with effusion[389,390].

The estimated direct and indirect costs of care to the family has been stated to be approximately $3.5 billion a year in the United States[391]. Of children under the age of 10 years, 15% have frequent or recurrent ear infection[392], the peak incidence occurring from seven to nine months of age[393], and 65% experience otitis media by 24 months of age[394]. The incidence declines in adults, but is still substantial, with histories of otitis and/or otorrhoea of long duration reported as high as 20% to 30%[395]. The incidence of effusion persisting after an attack of otitis media is high, but varies with age, with 50% of children 2 years of age or younger, and 20% of children over two years of age, demonstrating effusion lasting more than 4 weeks[396]. Of these effusions, 90% will resolve spontaneously by 3 months[397].

Pathogenesis

The central hypothesis of the pathogenesis of acute otitis media centres around abnormal function of the Eustachian tube. The

Eustachian tube protects the middle ear from reflux from the nasopharynx, drains the contents of the middle ear into the nasopharynx, and as a ventilatory effect, equibrilates the pressure between the middle ear and nasopharynx[398]. Obstruction of the Eustachian tube by allergy or infection in the upper respiratory tract leads to stasis of secretions with resultant bacterial proliferation in the middle ear. The length of the Eustachian tube is significantly shorter in children and those at risk for otitis media, providing less effective protection and contributing to the increased incidence in these populations[399]. Studies have concluded that the ventilation defect caused by tube obstruction is the most important factor in the production of effusion, and not an initial abnormality of clearance function[400].

Children with anatomically abnormal Eustachian tubes, such as children with cleft palates, bifid uvulas, and cranial facial abnormalities, have an increased incidence of otitis media. Males have more tympanotostomy insertions and tympanoplasties, suggesting that gender may play a role in severity of disease[401]. Although the incidence of otitis media in native races of North America and Aborigines in Australia (as well as other selected indigenous areas) is extremely high[402,403], the reason for this extraordinary incidence may be more related to poor social and economic conditions than to intraracial factors[404].

Attendance at day care centres where there is a greater potential for sharing viral infections predisposes to acute otitis media[405].

Children who have recurrent otitis media are more likely to have siblings with similar disease[406].

Breast-fed children have a lower incidence of otitis media, as demonstrated in several studies, although the roles of immunoglobulins in breast milk and the different positioning techniques remain unclear[407,408].

Seasonal variations have been documented and correspond to increased incidences of viral upper respiratory infection in winter and spring[409].

Second-hand smoke has been implicated as an important factor in environmental factors causing ear infections[410].

Microbiology

Researchers have demonstrated respiratory viruses in the middle ear effusion at the time of the initial diagnosis of otitis media in 42% of patients[411], rhinoviruses and respiratory syncytial virus being the most common pathogens isolated[412] (Table 25.7). Adenoviruses have been associated with persistence of symptoms despite antimicrobial therapy[413]. Viral isolates from the middle ear, however, are relatively rare[414].

Over the last 20 years, studies of cultures obtained by tympanocentesis have shown that the most common bacterial pathogens in acute otitis media are *S. pneumoniae*, *H. influenzae* and *M. catarrhalis*, in an approximate ratio of 3:2:1[415]. *Streptococcus* A and *S. aureus* isolates are less common and anaerobic organisms are rare. *H. influenzae* and *M. catarrhalis* can produce β-lactamase, and increasing resistance of these bacteria to penicillin has been reported. In recurrent and chronic otitis media with effusion, non-typeable *H. influenzae* is more prominent[416].

Cultures of the nasopharynx in patients with otitis media have shown that they are generally identical to middle ear pathogens, supporting the hypothesis that the disease may involve spread to the middle ear space following initial nasopharyngeal colonisation[417].

Table 25.7. *Otitis media – organisms*

Viruses:	Rhinovirus, RSV, Adenovirus
Bacteria:	*S. pneumoniae*, *H. influenzae*, *M. catarrhalis*
	Streptococcus A, *S. aureus*, *M. pneumoniae*
	Gram-negative bacilli (children)
	Chlamydia trachomatis (infants)
	M. tuberculosis (rare)
Other	*P. carinii* (in HIV), fungal (in HIV)

Gram-negative bacilli are responsible for about 20% of otitis media in young infants, but are rarely found in older children or adults[418]. These bacteria are more typically found in chronic suppurative otitis media with tympanic membrane perforations or draining tympanostomy tubes, and may be secondary contaminants from the external ear canal.

Mycoplasma pneumoniae is a rare cause of otitis media and is not necessarily associated with bullous myringitis[419].

Infants with *Chlamydia trachomatis* pneumonitis often have an accompanying otitis media culturing the same pathogen[420].

Myobacterium tuberculosis infection is uncommon except in underdeveloped regions and in immunocompromised patients. Few patients exhibit the classical features of painless otorrhea, multiple perforations, facial paralysis and bony necrosis[421]. When facial palsy in the absence of cholesteatoma occurs, however, the diagnosis of tuberculous otitis media should be entertained[422]. Chronic otorrhoea is the most consistent finding[423] and a history of previous or active TB is found in about 50% of the patients[424]. As mixed infections are often present, histological examination of the granulation tissue from the middle ear and mastoid is the best diagnostic procedure[425]. Treatment should be directed toward a medical regimen, utilising a 6-month anti-tuberculous therapy, with surgery reserved for diagnostic, drainage and eventual reconstructive procedures[426].

Diagnosis

Pneumatoscopy is the minimum diagnostic procedure, and is easily (and inexpensively) performed by using a hermetically sealed otoscope to visualize the tympanic membrane with magnification while the pressure in the external auditory canal is varied. It offers a diagnostic accuracy of 85% sensitivity and 75% specificity[427]. Combinations of the different tympanic membrane findings of colour, position and mobility are the most reliable indicators of the presence or absence of OME[428].

Tympanometry, utilising the electroaccoustic emittance audiometer, provides an objective assessment of the mobility of the tympanic membrane, as well as the dynamics of ossicular chains, the intra-aural muscles and the middle ear cushion. As other conditions produce similar findings to middle ear effusion, this instrument should be used in conjunction with pneumotoscopy, raising the sensitivity and specificity to 90%[429].

Pure tone audiometry measures the functional consequences of the OME and contributes to decision-making in surgical versus non-surgical management. As a stand-alone tool, however, it has a sensitivity of only 50%[430].

Acoustic reflexes may be absent in normal infants and children, and should not be used as a sole indicator of disease[431].

Tympanocentesis is useful where other diagnostic tools are equivocal, when there is excessive scarring of the membrane, or to diagnose specific pathogens, when initial empirical treatment has failed.

Antimicrobial treatment for acute otitis media

A meta-analysis of 33 randomised trials determined that the rate of acute otitis media resolution without antibiotics or tympancentesis was 81%, while antibiotic treatment increased the rate of resolution to 95%[432]. Despite the high rate of natural resolution, there is a concomitantly high rate of intra-temporal and extra-temporal complications in those patients who do not resolve and are not treated with antibiotics, justifying their use.

Changing patterns of antimicrobial susceptibilities to middle ear pathogens such as *S. pneumoniae* and *H. influenzae* have encouraged the use of more expensive, broad spectrum antibiotics, but without a concurrent increase in effectiveness. Amoxicillin and trimethoprim–sulphamethoxazole remain effective first-line empiric treatment regimes for acute otitis media (for dosages see p. 469).

In areas with proven high β-lactamase producing organisms, in high risk patients, and in treatment failures, the use of β-lactamase-resistant antimicrobials such as amoxicillin-clavulanate, TMP-SMX, cefixime, cefuroxime axetil, cefaclor, and erythromycin-sulphisoxazole may be utilised, although TMP-SMX is the least expensive and is twice daily dosing[433].

Early recurrence of acute otitis media is caused more often by a new organism and not by a relapse of the original strain[434]. Tympanocentesis, if practical, is helpful in therapeutic decisions for the neonatal age-group and other high risk patients.

Management of chronic otitis media with effusion

A 2-week course of TMP-SMX or amoxicillin–clavulanate may be a desirable medial intervention before placing tympanostomy tubes[435]. If given concurrently with a β-lactamase-stable antibiotic, oral prednisone or prednisone can be used as a therapeutic trial in cases that are resistant to other medical management[436].

Tympanostomy tubes

Insertion of a short-acting tympanostomy tube, *in situ* from 6 to 18 months, permits mucosal recovery, disappearance of mucous glands, and opening of the mastoid air system, in children requiring immediate reversal of hearing loss secondary to chronic effusion[437].

Adenoidectomy

Adenoidectomy does modify the natural history of chronic secondary otitis media in severely affected children 4 years of age and older[438], and in children who had failed tympanostomy tubes for recurrent acute otitis media[439]. The adenoids of children with recurrent acute otitis media contain pathogenic bacteria in clinically significant amounts[440], and removal of this reservoir of pathogenic bacteria theoretically prevents ascending infection from the nasopharynx into the Eustachian tube. Adenoid size, however, does not appear to be a factor in recommending surgery and tonsillectomy does not offer any effect on middle ear effusion beyond that of adenoidectomy alone[441].

Chemoprophylaxis

Antibiotic prophylaxis has proven to be more effective than long-term tympanostomy tube placement in the prevention of repeated attacks of otitis media[442]. Prophylactic use of once-a-day, half therapeutic dose of sulphisoxazole and amoxicillin for up to a period of 6 months in children who have three attacks of otitis media in 6 months, or four attacks documented in 1 year, has reduced the incidence of attacks of otitis media up to 90%[443,444].

Decongestants and antihistamines probably have no place in the treatment of chronic secretory otitis media[445].

In children where respiratory allergy appears to play a role, control of these allergies by environmental manipulation or immunotherapy, enhances the management of chronic otitis media[446].

Disease prevention in the future may be centered around the development and use of specific vaccines targeted against otitis media-causing bacteria and viruses.

Complications of otitis media

Antibiotics have reduced the complications of acute otitis media (AOM) although bacterial resistance to some antimicrobial agents have renewed concern that some patients remain only partially treated and become increasingly vulnerable to both intratemporal and intracranial sequelae. Although 10% to 35% of children will experience recurrent otitis media or chronic otitis media with effusion, the incidence of complication sequelae is much lower, in the range of 5% to 15%[447]. The most common complication is spread of disease into the mastoid atrium and air cells, one study showing that 96% of 222 temporal bones had associated fluid and/or pathologic tissue in the mastoid[448]. Persistence of infection can lead to acute mastoiditis, with or without periostitis, coalescent mastoiditis, subperiostal abscesses and petrositis.

Perforations of the tympanic membrane secondary to increased pressure from purulent material in the middle ear can occur, and are deemed chronic if they persist for longer than two months, often requiring surgical closure. Other pathologic changes include ossicular bony changes, cholesterol granuloma, cholesteatoma and tympanosclerosis[449]. Data suggests that chronic otitis media (COM) may be associated with degeneration of the facial nerve, with or without clinical impairment of function[450]. Fatty cell infiltration and degenerative changes in the tensor tympani muscle fibres, secondary to inflammatory cell infiltration and fibroblastic reactions, can also occur[451].

Although a number of animal experiments have demonstrated a relationship between otitis media and sensory neural hearing loss (SNHL)[452,453], clinical studies have concluded that neither acute otitis media or its treatment appear to cause a permanent SNHL[454] unless there was a spread of inflammation through the round window membrane[455], a perilymphatic fistula through the oval window[456], or as a suppurative complication of labyrinthitis[457]. Contradictory reports linking SNHL with the use of antibiotic topical drops exists, some showing that local treatment with a mixture of neomycin and polymyxin B contributes to a worsening of SNHL in patients with chronic otitis media[458], and others reporting no evidence of ototoxic inner ear damage[459].

Conductive hearing loss, secondary to middle ear effusion, is usually reversed with the resolution of the effusion unless irreversible changes secondary to chronic inflammation occur, causing adhesive otitis media, ossicular discontinuity, or chronic tympanic perforation.

Discharge from the middle ear via a perforation of the tympanic membrane or an indwelling tympanostomy tube may lead to an infection of the skin of the external ear canal. The pathogens are usually a mixture of the contents of the middle ear space and external ear canal, *Pseudomonas* and *Proteus* frequently being present. Fungus, typically *Aspergillus niger* may also be found. Medical or surgical means should be employed to control the middle ear or mastoid infections, while combination anti-inflammatory, anti-infective topical drugs are utilised to treat the external dermatitis after careful suctioning and debridement.

The incidence of intracranial complications of otitis media have decreased since the pre-antibiotic era when 2.3% of patients with acute or chronic suppurative otitis media developed intracranial sequalae[460]. Today, the incidence is relatively rare. Meningitis is the most common intracranial complication, usually concurrent with an otitis media and other upper respiratory focus, and caused by bacteraemia from the latter. Commonly the infection may spread from the middle ear to the meninges via congenital pre-formed pathways or by thrombophlebitis. The most common pathogens are *S. pneumoniae* and *H. influenzae* type b[461]. Appropriate medical management of both the meningitis and supporative focus is necessary, despite which, a considerable mortality is still reported[462].

Other intracranial complications that do occur include lateral sinus thrombosis, otitic hydrocephalus, extradural and subdural empyema, focal otitis encephalitis and brain abscess.

AIDS and otitis media

Inflammatory ear disease has been reported to occur in up to 80% of patients with the Acquired Immunodeficiency Syndrome[463]. In addition, there appears to be a strong association between seropositivity, adenoid hypertrophy and secretory otitis media in adults[464]. Children with AIDS have a higher age-specific incidence of acute otitis media compared to uninfected children or children who have seroreverted[465].

Besides the usual pathogens found in acute and chronic otitis media, other opportunistic pathogens have been isolated. Progressive involvement of the temporal bone with osteomyelitis and aspergillosis has lead to facial paralysis, sixth nerve palsy and sensorineural hearing loss. *P. carinii* has been reported in the middle ear and mastoid, and is thought to have spread via a haematogenous route from the lungs[466] or directly in a retrograde fashion from the nasopharynx[467]. Morris and Prasad[468] list otosyphilis as a clinical entity in HIV, and Smith and Canalis[469] have proposed that HIV may alter the course of latent syphilis and hasten the development of otosyphilis.

Light and electron microscopic findings have included severe petrositis with narrow replacement, mastoiditis otitis media, ossicular destruction, precipitations in the perilymphatic and endolymphatic spaces in the vestible and of the semicircular canals, and subepithelial elevation of the neurosensory epithelium of the saccule and utricle[470].

Early surgical intervention is recommended if standard antibiotic therapy fails[471].

References

1. GWALTNEY JM JR, HENDLEY JO, SIMON G, JORDAN WS JR. Rhinovirus infections in an industrial population. The occurrence of illness. *N Engl J Med* 1966;275:1261–8.
2. VAN CAUWENBERGE PB. Epidemiology of common cold. *Rhinology* 1985;23:273–82.
3. DICK EC, JENNINGS LC, MINK KA, WARTGOW CD, INHORN SL. Aerosol transmission of rhinovirus colds. *J Infect Dis* 1987;156:442–8.
4. HENDLEY JO, GWALTNEY JM JR. Mechanisms of transmission of rhinovirus infections. *Epidemiol Rev* 1988;10:242.
5. WARSHAUER DM, DICK EC *et al.* Rhinovirus infections in an isolated Antarctica station. *Am J Epidemiol* 1989;129:319–40.
6. COHEN S, TYRRELL DA, RUSSELL MA, JARVIS MJ, SMITH AP. Smoking, alcohol consumption, and susceptibility to the common cold. *Am J Public Health* 1993;83:1277–83.
7. GWALTNEY JM JR, HENDLEY JO, SIMON G *et al.* Rhinovirus infections in an industrial population. Characteristics of illness and antibody response. *JAMA* 1967;202:494.
8. WU-WILLIAMS AH, SAMET JM. Environmental tobacco smoke: exposure response relationships in epidemiologic studies. *Risk Anal* 1990;10:39–45.
9. COHEN S, TYRRELL DAJ SMITH AP. Psychological stress and susceptibility to the common cold. *N Engl J Med* 1991;325:606–12.
10. HARRISON SC. Common cold virus and its receptor. *Proc Natl Acad Sci USA* 1993;90:783.
11. WINTHER B. Effects on the nasal mucosa of upper respiratory viruses (common cold). *Dan Med Bull* 1994;41:193–204.
12. PROUD D, NACLERIO RM, GWALTNEY JM, HENDLEY JO. Kinins are generated in nasal secretions during natural rhinovirus colds. *J Infect Dis* 1990;161:120–3.
13. GWALTNEY JM JR, DOUGLAS PHILLIPS C, DAVID MILLER R, RIKER DK. Computed tomographic study of the common cold. *New Engl J Med* 1994;330:25–30.
14. ELKHATIEB A, HIPSKIND G, WOERNER D, HAYDEN FG. Middle ear abnormalities during natural rhinovirus colds in adults. *J Infect Dis* 1993;168:618–21.
15. CHONMAITREE T, HOWIE V, TRUANT A. Presence of respiratory viruses in middle ear fluids and nasal wash specimens from children with acute otitis media. *Pediatrics* 1985;77:698–702.
16. SMITH AP, TYRRELL DA, AL-NAKIB W *et al.* Effects and after-effects of the common cold and influenza on human performance. *Neuropsychobiology* 1989;21:90–3.
17. HALPERIN SA, EGGLESTON PA, BEASLEY P *et al.* Exacerbations of asthma in adults during experimental rhinovirus infection. *Am Rev Resp Dis* 1985;132:976–80.
18. OPENSHAW PJM, O'DONNELL DR. Asthma and the common cold: can viruses imitate worms? *Thorax* 1994;49:101–3.
19. TYRRELL DA, COHEN S, SCHLARB JE. Signs and symptoms in common colds. *Epidemiol Infect* 1993;111:143–56.
20. NACLERIO RM, PROUD D, KAGEY-SOBOTKA A *et al.* Is histamine responsible for the symptoms of rhinovirus colds? A look at the inflammatory mediators following infection. *Pediatr Infect Dis J* 1988:7:218–22.

21. HENAUER SA, GLUCK U. Efficacy of terfenadine in the treatment of common cold. A double-blind comparison with placebo. *Eur J Clin Pharm* 1988;34:35–40.

22. BYE CE, COOPER J, EMPEY DW *et al.* Effects of pseudo-ephedrine and tripolidine, alone and in combination, on symptoms of the common cold. *Br Med J* 1980;281:189–90.

23. AKERLUND A, KLINT T, OLEN L, RUNDCRANTZ H. Nasal decongestant effect of oxymetazoline in the common cold: an objective dose-response study in 106 patients. *J Laryngol Otol* 1989;103:743–6.

24. GAFFEY MJ, HAYDEN FG, BOUD JC, GWALTNEY JM JR. Ipratropium bromide treatment of experimental rhinovirus infection. *Antimicrob Agents Chemother* 1988;32:1644–7.

25. DOCKHORN R, GROSSMAN J, POSNER M, ZINNY M, TINKLEMAN D. A double-blind, placebo-controlled study of the safety and efficacy of ipratropium bromide nasal spray versus placebo in patients with the common cold. *J Allergy Clin Immunol* 1992;90:1076–82.

26. SPERBER SJ, HENDLEY JO, HAYDERN FG, RIKER DK, SORRENTINO JV, GWALTNEY JM JR. Effects of naproxen on experimental rhinovirus colds. A randomized, double-blind, controlled trial. *Ann Intern Med* 1992;117:37–41.

27. STANLEY ED, JACKSON GG, PANUSARN C, RUBENIS M, DIRDA V. Increased virus shedding with aspirin treatment of rhinovirus infection. *J Am Med Assoc* 1975;231:1248–51.

28. DOYLE WJ, RIKER DK, MCBRIDE TP *et al.* Therapeutic effects of an anticholinergic–sympathomimetic combination in induced rhinovirus colds. *Ann Otol Rhinol Laryngol* 1993;102:521–7.

29. HEMILA H. Vitamin C and the common cold. *Br J Nutr* 1992;67:3–16.

30. MAEDA H, AKAIKE T. Oxygen free radicals as pathogenic molecules in viral diseases. *Proc Soc Exp Biol Med* 1991;198:721–7.

31. HEMILA HARRI. Does Vitamin C alleviate the symptoms of the common cold? – a review of current evidence. *Scand J Infect Dis* 1994;26:1–6.

32. FORSTALL GJ, MACKNIN ML, YEN-LIEBERMAN BR, MEDENDROP SV. Effect of inhaling heated vapor on symptoms of the common cold. *JAMA* 1994;271:1109–11.

33. TYRRELL D, BARROW I, ARTHUR J. Local hyperthermia benefits natural and experimental common colds. BMJ 1989;298:1280–3.

34. WERNER GH. Chemoprophylaxis and chemotherapy of common colds caused by rhinoviruses: overview and outlook. *Bull Acad Nat Med* 1992;176:669–81.

35. FARR BM, GWALTNEY JM JR, ADAMS KF, HAYDEN FG. Intranasal interferon-α2 for prevention of natural rhinovirus colds. *Antimicrob Agents Chemother* 1984;26:31–4.

36. HAYDEN FG, ALBRECHT JK, KAISER DL, GWALTNEY JM. Prevention of natural colds by contact prophylaxis with intranasal alpha$_2$-interferon. *N Engl J Med* 1986;314:71–5.

37. SPERBER SJ, LEVINE PA, SORRENTINO JV, RIKER DK, HAYDEN FG. Ineffectiveness of recombinant interferon-β_{serine} nasal drops for prophylaxis of natural colds. *J Infect Dis* 1989;160:700–5.

38. GWALTNEY JM JR. Combined antiviral and antimediator treatment of rhinovirus colds. *J Infect Dis* 1992;166:776–82.

39. HAYDEN FG, ANDRIES KM JANSSEN PA. Safety and efficacy of intranasal piodacir (R77975) in experimental rhinovirus infection. *Antimicrob Agents Chemother* 1992;36:727–32.

40. FARR BM, CONNER EM, BETTS RF, OLESKE J, MINNEFOR A, GWALNEY JM JR. Two randomized controlled trials of zinc gluconate lozenge therapy of experimentally induced rhinovirus colds. *Antimicrob Agents Chemother* 1987;31:1183–7.

41. GODFREY JC, CONANT SLOANE B, SMITH DS, TURCO JH, MERCER N, GODFREY NJ. Zinc gluconate and the common cold: a controlled clinical study. *J Int Med Res* 1992;20:234–46.

42. FARR BM, HENDLEY JO, KAISER DL, GWALTNEY JM. Two randomized controlled trials of virucidal nasal tissues in the prevention of natural upper respiratory infections. *Am J Epidemiol* 1988;128:1162–72.

43. CORLEY DL, GEVIRTZ R, NIDEFFER R, CUMMINS L. Prevention of post infectious asthma in children by reducing self-inoculatory behavior. *J Pediatr Psychol* 1987;12:242–58.

44. ROOS K, GRAHN E, HOLM SE, JOHANSSON H, LIND L. Interfering alpha-streptococci as a protection against recurrent streptococcal tonsillitis in children. *Int J Pediat Otorhinolaryngol* 1993;25:141–8.

45. NADAL D, ALBINI B, CHEN C, SCHLAPFER E, BERNSTEIN JM, OGRA PL. Distribution and engraftment patterns of human tonsillar mononuclear cells and immunoglobulin secreting cells in mice with severe combined immunodeficiency. Role of the Epstein–Barr virus. *Int Arch Allergy Appl Immunol* 1991;95:341–51.

46. OLAH I, SURJAN L JR, TORO I. Electronmicroscopic observations on the antigen reception in the tonsillar tissue. *Acta Acad Sci Biol Hung* 1972;23:61–73.

47. SCADDING GK. Immunology of the tonsil: a review. *J Roy Soc Med* 1990;83:104–7.

48. RUAN M, AKKOYUNLU M, GRUBB A, FORSGREN A: protein D of *Haemophilus influenzae*. A novel bacterial surface protein with affinity for human IgD. *J Immunol* 1990;145:3379–84.

49. YAMANAKA N, MATSUYAMA H, HARABUCHI Y, KATAURA A. Distribution of lymphoid cells in tonsillar compartments in relation to infection and age. A quantitative study using image analysis. *Acta Otol Laryngol* 1992;112:128–37.

50. STENFORS LE, RAISANEN S. *In vivo* attachment of beta-haemolytic streptococci to tonsillar epithelial cells in health and disease. *Acta Oto-Laryngol* 1991;111:562–8.

51. TIMON CI, CAFFERKEY MT, WALSH M. Fine-needle aspiration in recurrent tonsillitis. *Arch Otolaryngol* 1991;117:653–6.

52. BRODSKY L, NAGY M, VOLK M, STANIEVICH J, MOORE L. The relationship of tonsil bacterial concentration to surface and core cultures in chronic tonsillar disease in children. *Int J Pediatr Otorhinolaryngol* 1991;21:33–9.

53. GAFFNEY RJ, FREEMAN DJ, WALSH MA, CAFFERKEY MT. Differences in tonsil core bacteriology in adults and children: a prospective study of 262 patients. *Resp Med* 1991; 85:383–8.

54. HUMINER D, PITLIK S, LEVY R, SAMRA Z. *Mycoplasma* and *Chlamydia* in adenoids and tonsils of children undergoing adenoidectomy or tonsillectomy. *Ann Otol Rhinol Laryngol* 1994;103:135–8.

55. HONE SW, MOORE J, FENTON J, GORMLEY PK, HONE R. The role of *Chlamydia pneumoniae* in severe acute tonsillitis. *J Laryngol Otol* 1994;108:135–7.

56. HINTON AE, HERDMAN RC, MARTIN-HIRSCH D, SEED SR. Parental cigarette smoking and tonsillectomy in children. *Clin Otolaryngol* 1993;18:178–80.

57. DUDLEY JP, SERCARZ J. Pharyngeal and tonsil infections caused by non-group A Streptococcus. *Am J Otolaryngol* 1991;12:292–6.

58. MEVIO E, GIACOBONE E, GALIOTO P, PERANO D, BULZOMI AG. Evaluation of the bacterial flora in recurrent adenotonsillitis. *Adv Otorhinlaryngol Basel Karger* 1992;47:134–41.

59. SCHACHTEL BP, FILLINGIM JM, LANE AC, THODEN WR, BAYBUTT RI. Caffeine as an analgesic adjuvant. A double-blind study comparing aspirin with caffeine to aspirin and placebo in patients with sore throat. *Arch Int Med* 1991;151:733–7.

60. SODERSTROM M, BLOMBERG J, CHRISTENSEN P, HOVELIUS B. Erythromycin and phenoxymethylpenicillin (penicillin V) in the treatment of respiratory tract infections as related to microbiological findings and serum C-reactive protein. *Scand J Infect Dis* 1991;23:347–54.

61. PICHICHERO ME, GOOCH WM, RODRIGUEZ Q *et al.* Effective short-course treatment of acute group A betahemolytic streptococcal tonsillopharyngitis. Ten days of penicillin V vs 5 days or 10 days of cefpodoxime therapy in children. *Arch Ped Adolesc Med* 1994;148:1053–60.

62. SCHONHEYDER HC. Streptococcal tonsillitis: failure of penicillin therapy. *Ugeskrift for Laeger* 1994;156:1931–4.

63. SAFRAN C. Five versus ten days treatment of streptococcal pharyngotonsillitis: a randomized controlled trial comparing cefpodoxime proxetil and phenoxymethyl penicillin. *Scand J Infect Dis* 1994;26:59–66.

64. FYLLINGEN G, ARNESEN AR, RONNEVIG J. Phenoxymethylpenicillin two or three times daily in bacterial upper respiratory tract infections: a blinded, randomized and controlled clinical study. *Scand J Infect Dis* 1991;23:755–61.

65. SCHWARTZ RH, WIENTZEN RL JR. PEDREIRA F. Penicillin V for group A streptococcal pharyngitis: a randomised trial of seven vs. ten days' therapy. *JAMA* 1981;246:1790–975.

66. GERER MA, RANDOLPH MF, CHANATRY J, WRIGHT LL, DEMEO K, KAPLAN EL. Five vs. ten days of penicillin V therapy for streptococcal pharyngitis. *AJDC* 1987;141:224–7.

67. KIELMOVITCH IH, KELETI G, BLUESTONE CD, WALD ER, GONZALEZ C. Microbiology of obstructive tonsillar hypertrophy and recurrent tonsillitis. *Arch Otolaryngol Head Neck Surg* 1989;115:721–4.

68. DEETER RG, KALMAN DL, ROGAN MP, CHOW SC. Therapy for pharyngitis and tonsillitis caused by group A beta-hemolytic streptococci: a meta-analysis comparing the efficacy and safety of cefadroxil monohydrate versus oral penicillin V. *Clin Therap* 1992;14:740–54.

69. MCCARTY JM, RENTERIA A. Treatment of pharyngitis and tonsillitis with cefprozil: review of three multicenter trials (Review). *Clin Infect Dis* 1992;14 Suppl 2:S224–30; discussion S231–2.

70. BROOK I, GILMORE JD. Evaluation of bacterial interference and beta-lactamase production in management of experimental infection with group A betahemolytic streptococci. *Antimicrob Agents Chemother* 1993;37:1452–5.

71. JENSEN JH, LARSEN SB. Treatment of recurrent acute tonsillitis with clindamycin. An alternative to tonsillectomy? *Clin Otolaryngol* 1991;16:498–500.

72. MEVIO E, GIACOBONE E, GALIOTO P, PERANO D, BULZOMI AG. Evolution of the bacterial flora in recurrent adenotonsillitis. *Adv Otorhinolaryngol* 1992;47:134–41.

73. PRANSKY SM, FELDMAN JI, KEARNS DB, SEUD AB, BILLMAN GF. Actinomycosis in obstructive tonsillary hypertrophy and recurrent tonsillitis. *Arch Otolaryngol Head Neck Surg* 1991;117:883–5.

74. MARTINS RH, HESHIKI Z, LUCHESI NR, MARQUES ME. Actinomycosis and botryomycosis of the tonsil. *Auris, Nasus, Larynx* 1991;18:377–81.

75. WAT PJ, STRICKLER JG, MYERS JL, NORDSTROM MR. Herpes simplex infection causing acute necrotizing tonsillitis. *Mayo Clin Proc* 1994;69:269–71.

76. NORDAHL SH, HOEL T, SCHEEL O, OLOFSSON J. Tularemia: a differential diagnosis in oto-rhino-laryngology. *J Laryngol Otol* 1993;107:127–9.

77. BROOK I, FOOTE PA JR, SLOTS J, JACKSON W. Immune response to Prevotella intermedia in patients with recurrent nonstreptococcal tonsillitis. *Ann Otol, Rhinol, Laryngol* 1993;102:113–16.

78. EL-FAKAHANY AF, ABDALLA KF, YOUNIS MS, HASSAN OA, EL-SHANTOURY M. Tonsillar toxoplasmosis. *J Egypt Soc Parasitol* 1992; 22:375–80.

79. FOULDS G, CHAN KH, JOHNSON JT, SHEPARD RM, JOHNSON RB. Concentration of azithromycin in human tonsillar tissue. *Eur J Clin Microb Infect Dis* 1991;10:853–6.

80. MULLER O. Comparison of azithromycin versus clarithromycin in the treatment of patients with upper respiratory tract infections. *J Antimicrob Chemother* 1993;31 Suppl E:137–46.

81. HAMIL J. Mulicentre evaluation of azithromycin and penicillin V in the treatment of acute streptococcal pharyngitis and tonsillitis. *J Antimicrob Chemother* 1993;31: Suppl E:89–94.

82. BLOCK SL, HEDRICK JA, TYLER RD. Comparative study of the effectiveness of cefixime and penicillin V for the treatment of streptococcal pharyngitis in children and adolescents. *Pediatr Infect Dis J* 1992;11:919–25.

83. DISNEY FA, DILLON H, BLUMER JL *et al.* Cephalexin and penicillin in the treatment of group A β-hemolytic streptococcal throat infections. *Am J Dis Child* 1992;146:1324–7.

84. STENFORS LE, RAISANEN S. The membranous tonsillitis during infectious mononucleosis is nevertheless of bacterial origin. *Int J Ped Otorhinolaryngol* 1993;26:149–55.

85. BROOK I, DE LEYVA F. Microbiology of tonsillar surfaces in infectious mononucleosis. *Arch Ped Adolesc Med* 1994;148:171–3.

86. STEVENSON DS, WEBSTER G, STEWARD IA. Acute tonsillectomy in the management of infectious mononucleosis. *J Laryngol Otol* 1992;106:989–91.

87. FINKELSTEIN Y, BAR-ZIV J, NACHMANI A, BERGER G, OPHIR D. Peritonsillar abscess as a cause of transient velopharyngeal insufficiency. *Cleft Palate-Craniofacial J* 1993;30:421–8.

88. SHOEMAKER M, LAMPE RM, WEIR WR. Peritonsillitis: abscess or cellulitis. *Paediatr Infect Dis* 1986;5:435–9.

89. SNOW DG, CAMPBELL JB, MORGAN DW. The management of peritonsillar sepsis by needle aspiration. *Clin Otol* 1991;16:245–7.

90. PATEL KS, AHMAD S., O'LEARY G, MICHEL M. The role of computed tomography in the management of peritonsillar abscess. *Otolaryngol-Head Neck Surg* 1992;107:727–32.

91. BOESEN T, JENSEN F. Preoperative ultrasonographic verification of peritonsillar abscesses in patients with severe tonsillitis. *Eur Arch Oto-Rhino-Laryngol* 1992;249:1313–3.

92. AHMED G, JONES AS, SHAH K, SMETHURST A. The role of ultrasound in the management of peritonsillar abscess. *J Laryngol Otol* 1994;108:610–2.

93. SAVOLAINEN S, JOUSIMIES-SOMER HR, MAKITIE AA, YLIKOSKI JS. Peritonsillar abscess. Clinical and microbiologic aspects and treatment regimens. *Arch Otolaryngol-Head Neck Surg* 1993;119:521–4.

94. WOLF M, EVEN-CHEN I, KRONENBERG J. Peritonsillar abscess: repeated needle aspiration versus incision and drainage. *Ann Otol Rhinol Laryngol* 1994;103:554–7.

95. WEINBERG E, BROOSKY L, STANIEVICH J, VOLK M. Needle aspiration of peritonsillar abscess in children. *Arch Otolaryngol Head Neck Surg* 1993;119:169–72.

96. CHOWDHURY CR, BRICKNELL MC. The management of quinsy – a prospective study. *J Laryngol Otol* 1992;106:986–8.

97. SORENSEN JA, GODBALLE C, ANDERSEN NH, JORGENSEN K. Peritonsillar abscess: risk of disease in the remaining tonsil after unilateral tonsillectomy a chaud. *J Laryngol Otol* 1991;105:442–4.

98. BAKER AR. Life-threatening peripharyngeal sepsis with mediastinitis. *BJCP* 1990;44:640–1.

99. WOLF RF, KONINGS JG, PRINS TR, WEITS J. *Fusobacterium* pyomyositis of the shoulder after tonsillitis. Report of a case of Lemierre's syndrome. *Acta Orthopaediat Scand* 1991;62:595–6.

100. MORENO S, ALTOZANO JG, PINILLA B *et al.* Lemierre's disease: postanginal bacteremia and pulmonary involvement caused by *Fusobacterium necrophorum Rev Infect Dis* 1989;11:319–24.

101. PUTTERMAN C, CARACO Y, SHALIT M. Acute nonrheumatic perimyocarditis complicating streptococcal tonsillitis. *Cardiology* 1991;78:156–60.

102. SCOTT PM, DHILLON RS, MCDONALD PJ. Cervical necrotizing fascitis and tonsillitis. *J Laryngol Otol* 1994;108:435–7.

103. WATSON MG, ROBERTSON AS, COLQUHOUN IR. Pseudoaneurysm of the internal carotid artery: a forgotten complication of tonsillitis? *J Laryngol Otol* 1991;105:588–90.

104. TSUBOTA H, KATAURA A, KUKUMINATO Y *et al.* (Efficacy of tonsillectomy for improving skin lesions of *Pustulosis palmaris et plantaris* – evaluation of 289 cases at the Department of Otolaryngology of Sapporo Medical University) (Japanese). *Nippon Jibiinkoka Gakkai Kaiho (J Oto Rhino Laryngol Soc Jap)* 1994;97:1621–30.

105. NAKAMURA T, ONO T, AOKI Y. Medullasin levels in neutrophils of patients with *Pustulosis palmaris et plantaris*. *J Derm* 1993;20:201–7.

106. SUGIYAMA N, SHIMIZU J, NAKAMURA M, KIRIU T, MATSUOKA K, MASUDA Y. Clinicopathological study of the effectiveness of tonsillectomy in IgA nephropathy accompanied by chronic tonsillitis. *Acta Oto-Laryngol* (Suppl) 1993;508:43–8.

107. BROUILETTE RT, FEMBACH SK, HUNT CE. Obstructive sleep apnoea in infants and children. *J Pediatr* 1982;100:31–40.

108. POTSIC WP, PASQUARIELLO PS, BARANAK CC. Relief of upper airway obstruction by adenotonsillectomy. *Otolaryngol Head Neck Surg* 1986;4:476–80.

109. IKEDA T, DAIMARU N, INUTSUKA S *et al.* Adverse effect of chronic tonsillitis on clinical course of sarcoidosis. *Sarcoidosis* 1991;8:120–4.

110. OHGURO S, KATAURA A, KUKUMINATO Y *et al.* (Tonsillectomy and osteoarthritic disease) (Japanese). Nippon Jibiinkoka Gakkai Kaiho (*J Oto Rhino Laryngol Soc Jap*) 1994;97:1601–7.

111. WURZELMANN JI, LYLES CM, SANDLER RS. Childhood infections and risk of inflammatory bowel disease. *Digest Dis Sci* 1994;39:555–60.

112. JAWAD J, BLAYNEY AW. Spontaneous tonsillar haemorrhage in acute tonsillitis. *J Laryngol Oto* 1994;108:791–4.

113. SIEGAL AC, JOHNSON EE, STOLLERMAN GH. Controlled studies of streptococcal pharyngitis in a pediatric population. Factors related to the attack rate of rheumatic fever. *NEJM* 1961;265:559–64.

114. FRANCOIS M, BINGEN E, SOUSSI TH, NARCY PH. Bacteriology of tonsils in children: comparison between recurrent acute tonsillitis and tonsillar hypertrophy. *Adv Otorhinolaryngol* 1992;47:146–50.

115. BRODSKY L, MOORE L, STANIEVICH J. The role of *Haemophilus influenzae* in the pathogenesis of tonsillar hypertrophy in children. *Laryngoscope* 1988;98:1055–60.

116. NORD CE. The role of anaerobic bacteria in recurrent episodes of sinusitis and tonsillitis. *Clin Infect Dis* 1995;20:1512–24.

117. BROOK I, FOOTE PA JR, SLOTS J, JACKSON W. Immune response to P. intermedius in patients with recurrent nonstreptococcal tonsillitis. *Ann Otol Rhinol Laryngol* 1993;102:113–16.

118. BROOK I, YOCUM P. *In vitro* protection of group A β-hemolytic streptococci from penicillin and cephalothin by *Bacteroides fragilis*. *Chemotherapy* 1983;29:18–23.

119. BROOK I. Treatment of patients with acute recurrent tonsillitis due to group A-haemolytic streptococci: a prospective randomized study comparing penicillin and amoxycillin/ clavulanate potassium. *J Antimicrob Chemother* 1989;24:227–33.

120. PICHICHERO ME, MARGOLIS PA. A comparison of cephalosporins and penicillins in the treatment of group A β-hemolytic streptococcal pharyngitis: a meta-analysis supporting the concept of microbial pathogenicity. *Pediatr Infect Dis* 1991;10:275–81.

121. CAREDDU P, BIOCHINI A, ALFANO S, ZAVATTINI G. Pidotimod in the prophylaxis of recurrent acute tonsillitis in childhood. *Adv Otorhinolaryngol* 1992;47:328–31.

122. DONN AS, GILES ML. Do children waiting for tonsillectomy grow out of their tonsillitis? *N Z Med J* 1991;104:161–2.

123. LAING MR, MCKERROW WS. Adult tonsillectomy. *Clin Otolaryngol* 1991;16:21–4.

124. PARADISE JL, BLUESTONE CD, BACHMAN RZ *et al.* Efficacy of tonsillectomy for recurrent throat infection in severely affected children: results of parallel randomised and non-randomised clinical trials. *N Engl J Med* 1984;310:674–83.

125. FRANTZ TD, RASGON BM, QUESENBERRY CP JR. Acute epiglottitis in adults. *JAMA* 1994;272:1358–60.

126. SHIH L, HAWKINS DB, STANLEY RB JR. Acute epiglottitis in adults. A review of 48 cases. *Ann Otol Rhinol Laryngol* 1988;97:527–9.

127. HUSSAN WU, KEANEY NP. Bilateral thoracic empyema complicating adult epiglottitis. *J Laryngol Otol* 1991;105:858–9.

128. STERNBACK GL, GOLDSCHIMID D. Adult respiratory distress syndrome associated with adult epiglottitis. *J Emerg Med* 1993;11:23–6.

129. JOHNSON J, LAWY HS. Acute epiglottitis in adults due to infection with *Haemophilus influenzae* type b. *Lancet* 1967;2:134.

130. NAVARRETE ML, QUESADA P, GARCIA M, LORENTE J. Acute epiglottitis in the adult. *J Laryngol Otol* 1991;105:83–41.

131. ANDREASSEN UK, BAER S, NIELSEN TG, DAHM SL, ARNDAL H. Acute epiglottitis – 25 years experience with nasotracheal intubation, current management policy and future trends. *J Laryngol Otol* 1992;106:1072–5.

132. KASS EG, MCFADDEN EA, JACOBSON S, TOOHILL RJ. Acute epiglottitis in the adult: experience with a seasonal presentation. *Laryngoscope* 1993;103:841–4.

133. RYAN M, HUNT M, SNOWBERGER T. A changing pattern of epiglottitis. *Clin Ped* 1992;532–5.

134. MAYO-SMITH MF, HIRSCH PJ, WODZINSKI SF, SCHIFFMAN FJ. Acute epiglottitis in adults: an eight year experience in Rhode Island. *N Engl J Med* 1986;314:1133–9.

135. TVETERAS K, KRISTENSEN S. Acute epiglottitis in adults: bacteriology and therapeutic principles. *Clin Otolaryngol* 1987;12:337–43.

136. CARENFELT C, SOBIN A. Acute epiglottitis in children and adults: annual incidence and mortality. *Clin Otolaryngol* 1989;14:489–93.

137. TROLLFORS B, NYLEN O, STRANGERT K. Acute epiglottitis in children and adults in Sweden. *Arch Dis Child* 1990;65:491–94.

138. WURTELE P. Acute epiglottitis in children and adults: a large-scale incidence study. *Otolaryngol Head Neck Surg* 1990;103:902.

139. GORELICK MH, BAKER MD. Epiglottitis in children, 1979 through 1992. Effects of *Haemophilus influenzae* type b immunization. *Arch Ped Adolesc Med* 1994;148:47–50.

140. SINGER JI, MCCABE JB. Epiglottitis at the extremes of age. *Am J Emerg Med* 1988;6:228–31.

141. MORGENSTEIN KM, ABRAMSON AL. Acute epiglottitis in adults. *Laryngoscope* 1971;81:1066.

142. OSSOFF RH, WOLFF AP, BALLENGER JJ. Acute epiglottitis in adults: experience with 15 cases. *Laryngoscope* 1980;90:1155–61.

143. WETMORI RF, HANDLER SD. Epiglottitis. Evolution in management during the last decade. *Ann Otol Rhinol Laryngol* 1979;88:822–6.

144. SHAPIRO J, ROLAND DE, BAKER AS. Adult supraglottitis. *JAMA* 1988;4:563–8.

145. GLODE MP, HALSEY NA, MARTHA M, BALLARD TL, BARENKAMP S. Epiglottitis in adults: association with *Haemophilus influenzae* type b colonization and disease in children. *Ped Infect Dis* 1984;3:548–51.

146. VERNHAM GA, CROWTHER JA. Acute

myeloid leukaemia presenting with acute *Branhamella catarrhalis* epiglottitis. *J Infect* 1993;26:93–5.

147. LEUNG R. Pasteurella epiglottitis. *Aust NZ J Med* 1994;24:218.

148. BIEM J, ROY L, HALIK J, HOFFSTEIN V. Infectious mononucleosis complicated by necrotizing epiglottitis, dysphagia, and pneumonia. *Chest* 1989;96:204–5.

149. MAYO-SMITH M. Fatal respiratory arrest in adult epiglottitis in the intensive care unit. Implications for airway management. *Chest* 1993;104:964–5.

150. TVETERAS K, KRISTENSEN S. Acute epiglottitis in adults: bacteriology and therapeutic principles. *Clin Otolaryngol* 1987;12:337–43.

151. RIVRON RP, MURRAY JAM. Adult epiglottitis: is there a consensus on diagnosis and treatment? *Clin Otolaryngol* 1991;16:338–44.

152. STUART MJ, HODGETTS TJ. Adult epiglottitis: prompt diagnosis saves lives. *BMJ* 1994;308:329–30.

153. SHORT DG, KITAIN DS. Acute uvulitis in combination with acute epiglottitis: a case presentation. *Ear Nose Throat J* 1991;70:458–60.

154. LEUNG R, JASSAL J. Pasteurella epiglottitis. *Aust NZ J Med* 1994;24:218.

155. WIESEL S, GUTMAN JB, KLEIMAN SJ. Adult epiglottitis and postobstructive pulmonary edema in a patient with severe coronary artery disease. *J Clin Anesth* 1993;5:158–62.

156. KENNEDY CA, ROSEN H. Kingella kingae bacteremia and adult epiglottitis in a granulocytopenic host. *Am J Med* 1988;85:701–2.

157. COLMAN M. Epiglottitis in immunocompromised patients. *Head Neck Surg* 1986;8:466–8.

158. ROTHSTEIN SG, PERSKY MS, EDELMAN BA, GITTLEMAN PE, STROSCHEIN M. Epiglottitis in AIDS patients. *Laryngoscope* 1989;99:389–92.

159. SCHUMAKER HM, DORIS PE, BIRNBAUM G. Radiographic parameters in adult epiglottitis. *Ann Emerg Med* 1984;13:588–90.

160. WALDEN CA, ROGERS LF. Case Report. CT evaluation of adult epiglottitis. *J Comp Ass Tomogr* 1989;13:883–5.

161. CHAISSON RE, ROSS J, GERBERDING JL, SANDE MA. Clinical aspects of adult epiglottitis. *West J Med* 1986;144:700–3.

162. FONTANAROSA PB, SCOTT POLSKY S, GOLDMAN GE. Adult epiglottitis. *J Emerg Med* 1989;223–31.

163. HOEKELMAN RA. Epiglottitis: another dying disease? *Pediat Ann* 1994;23:229–30.

164. STAIR TO, HIRSCH BE. Adult supraglottitis. *Am J Emerg Med* 1985;3:512–18.

165. COX GJ, BATES GJ, DRAKE-LEE AB, WATSON DJ. The use of flexible nasoendoscopy in adults with acute epiglottitis. *Ann Roy Coll Surg Engl* 1988;70:361–2.

166. SARANT G. Acute epiglottitis in adults. *Ann Emerg Med* 1981;10:58–61.

167. KHILANANI U, KHATIB R. Acute epiglottitis in adults. *Am J Med* Sci 1984;287:65–70.

168. DAEB ZE, YENSON AC, DEFRIES HO. Acute epiglottitis in the adult. *Laryngoscope* 1985;95:289–91.

169. FRIEDMAN M. TORIUM DM, GRYBAUSKAS V, APPLEBAUM EL. A plea for uniformity in the staging and management of adult epiglottitis. *Ear Nose Throat J* 1988;67:873–80.

170. HINGORANI AD, DZERSK J, JONES AT, GOLDING-WOOD D, LEIGH JM Establish an airway early. *BMJ* 1994;308:719.

171. CROSBY E, REID D. Acute epiglottitis in the adult: is intubation mandatory? *Cam J Anaesth* 1991;38:914–8.

172. GLOCK JL, MORALES WJ. Acute epiglottitis during pregnancy. *South Med J* 1993;86:836–8.

173. DENHOLM S, RIVRON RP. Acute epiglottitis in adults: a potentially lethal cause of sore throat. *J Roy Coll Surg Edin* 1993;38:265.

174. DAUM RS, NACHMAN JP, LEITCH CD, TENOVER FC. Nosocomial epiglottitis associated with penicillin and cephalosporin-resistant *Streptococcus* pneumonia bacteremia. *J Clin Microbiol* 1994;32:246–8.

175. TAKALA AK, PELTOLA H, ESKOLA J. Disappearance of epiglottitis during large-scale vaccination with *Haemophilus influenzae* type B conjugate vaccine among children in Finland. *Laryngoscope* 1994;104:731–5.

176. PROCTOR DF. The upper airways. *Am Rev Resp Dis* 1977;115:315–42.

177. SCHALEN L, ELIASSON I, KAMME C, SCHALEN C. Erythromycin in acute laryngitis in adults. *Ann Otol Rhinol Laryngol* 1993;102:209–14.

178. SCHALEN L, CHRISTENSEN P, ELIASSON I, FEX S, KAMME C, SCHALEN C. Inefficacy of penicillin V in acute laryngitis in adults. Evaluation from results of double blind study. Ann Oto Rhino Laryngol 1985;94:14.

179. DANN EJ, WEINBERGER M, GILLIS S, PARSONNET J, SHAPIRO M, MOSES AE. Bacterial laryngotracheitis associated with toxic shock syndrome in an adult. *Clin Infect Dis* 1994;18:437–9

180. ELLIS ME, DUNBAR EM, HUSSAIN M. Paediatric laryngeal tuberculosis. *Tubercle* 1983;64:37–9.

181. GERTLER R, RAMAGES L. Tuberculous laryngitis – a one year harvest. *J Laryngol Otol* 1985;99:1119–25.

182. Report from the medical research council tuberculosis and *Chest* diseases unit. National survey of tuberculosis notifications in England and Wales 1978–9. *Br Med J* 1980;281:895–8.

183. LYONS GD. Mycotic disease of the larynx. *Ann Otol Rhinol Laryngol* 1966;75:162–75.

184. TASHJIAN LS, PEACOCK JE. Laryngeal candidiasis. Report of seven cases and review of the literature. *Arch Otolaryngol* 1984;110:806–9.

185. YONKERS AJ. Candidiasis of the larynx. *Ann Otol* 1973;82:812–15.

186. KOBAYASHI RH, ROSENBLATT HM, CARNEY JM *et al.* Candida esophagitis and laryngitis in chronic mucocutaneous candidiasis. *Pediatrics* 1980;66:380–4.

187. MARCUSEN DC, SOOY CD. Otolaryngologic and head and neck manifestations of acquired immunodeficiency syndrome (AIDS). *Laryngoscope* 1985;95:401–5.

188. HICKS JN, PETERS GE. Pseudocarcinomatous hyperplasia of the larynx due to *Candida albicans*. *Laryngoscope* 1982;92:644–7.

189. MAHIEN HF, VAN SAENE HKF, ROSINOH HJ *et al.* *Candida* vegetations on silicone voice prosthesis. *Arch Otolaryngol* 1986;112:321–5.

190. JACOBS RF, YASUDA K, SMITH AL, BENJAMIN DR. Laryngeal candidiasis presenting as inspiratory stridor. *Pediatrics* 1982;69:234–6.

191. ROZENBAUM R, GONCALVES AJR. Clinical epidemiological study of 171 cases of cryptococcosis. *Clin Infec Dis* 1994;18:369–80.

192. REESE MC, COLCLASURE JB. Cryptococcosis of the larynx. *Arch Otolaryngol* 1975;101:698–701.

193. SMALLMAN LA, STORES OPR, WATSON MG, PROOPS DW. Cryptococcosis of the larynx. *J Laryngol Otol* 1989;103:214–5.

194. BROWNING DG, SCHWARTZ DA, JURADO RL. Cryptococcosis of the larynx in a patient with AIDS: an unusual cause of fungal laryngitis. *South Med J* 1992;85:762–4.

195. DUMICH PS, NEEL HB. Blastomycosis of the larynx. *Laryngoscope* 1983;74:1266–70.

196. PAYNE J, KOOPMAN CF. Laryngeal carcinoma – or is it laryngeal blastomycosis? *Laryngoscope* 1984;94:608–11.

197. MIKAELIAN AJ, VARKEY B, GROSSMAN TW, BLATNIK DS. Blastomycosis of the head and neck. *Otolaryngol Head Neck Surg* 1989;101:489–95.

198. PLATT MA. Laryngeal coccidioidomycosis. *JAMA* 1977;237:1234.

199. GARDNER S, SEILHEIMER D, CATLIN F, ANDERSON DC, HERNRIED L. Subglottic

coccidioidomycosis presenting with persistent stridor. *Pediatrics* 1980;66:623–5.

200. SMITH JW, UTZ JP. Progressive disseminated histoplasmosis. A prospective study of 26 patients. *Ann Intern Med* 1972;76:557–65.

201. BICKARD RE, KOTZEN S. Histoplasmosis of the larynx. *South Med J* 1973;66:1311–12.

202. SHAHEEN SO, ELLIS FG. Actinomycosis of the larynx. *J Roy Soc Med* 1983;76:226–8.

203. KARNAUCHOW PN, KAUL WH. Chronic herpetic laryngitis with oropharyngitis. *Ann Otol Rhinol Laryngol* 1988;286–8.

204. PACE JL, CSONKA GW. Late endemic syphilis: case report of bejel with gummatous laryngitis. *Genitourin Med* 1988;64:202–4.

205. RAZ E, BURSZTYN M, ROSENTHAL T, RUBINOW A, KAREM E. Severe recurrent lupus laryngitis. *Am J Med* 1992;92:109–10.

206. KAMEL PL, HANSON D, KAHRILAS PJ. Omeprazole for the treatment of posterior laryngitis. *Am J Med* 1994;96:321–6.

207. DEVENEY CW, BENNER K, COHEN J. Gastroesophageal reflux and laryngeal disease. *Arch Surg* 1993;128:1021–7.

208. DONNELLY BW, MCMILLAN JA, WEINTER LB. Bacterial tracheitis: report of eight new cases and review. *Rev Infect Dis* 1990;12:729–35.

209. JOHNSON JT, LISTON SL. Bacterial tracheitis in adults. *Arch Otolaryngol Head Neck Surg* 1987;113:204–5.

210. RUDDY J. Bacterial tracheitis in a young adult. *J Laryngol Otol* 1988;102:656–7.

211. VALOR RR, POLNITSKY CA, TANIS DJ, SHERTER CB. Bacterial tracheitis with upper airway obstruction in a patient with the acquired immunodeficiency syndrome. *Am Rev Resp Dis* 1992;146:1598–9.

212. SEIGLER RS. Bacterial tracheitis: recognition and treatment. *J South Carolina Med Assoc* 1993:89:83–7.

213. NATKUNAM R, TSE CY, ONG BH, SRIRAGAVAN P. Carinal resection for stenotic tuberculous tracheitis. *Thorax* 1988;43:492–3.

214. CLARKE A, SKELTON J, FRASER RS. Fungal tracheobronchitis. Report of 9 cases and review of the literature. *Medicine* 1991;70:1–14.

215. KRAMER MR, DENNING DW, MARSHALL SE *et al.* Ulcerative tracheobronchitis after lung transplantation. A new form of invasive aspergillosis. *Am Rev Resp Dis* 1991;144:552–6.

216. TAIT RC, O'DRISCOLL BR, DENNING DW. Unilateral wheeze caused by pseudomembranous *Aspergillus* tracheobronchitis in the immunocompromised patient. *Thorax* 1993;48:1285–7.

217. PUTNAM JB JR, DIGNANI C, MEHRA RC, ANAISSE EJ, MORICE RC, LIBSHITZ HI. Acute airway obstruction and necrotizing tracheobronchitis from invasive mycosis. *Chest* 1994;106:1265–7.

218. KEMPER CA, HOSTETLER JS, FOLLANSBEE SE *et al.* Ulcerative and plaque-like tracheobronchitis due to infection with *Aspergillus* in patients with AIDS. *Clin Infect Dis* 1993;17:344–52.

219. DENNING DW, FOLLANSBEE SE, SCOLARO M, NORRIS S, EDELSTEIN H, STEVENS DA. Pulmonary aspergillosis in the acquired immunodeficiency syndrome. *N Engl J Med* 1991;324:654–62.

220. ANGELUCCI E, UGOLINI M, LUCARELLI G *et al.* Endobronchial aspergillosis in marrow transplant patients. *Bone Marrow Transpl* 1991;8:328–9.

221. CHECHANI V, VASUDEVAN VP, KAMHOLZ SL. Necrotizing tracheobronchitis: complication of mechanical ventilation in an adult. *South Med J* 1991;84:271–3.

222. FARBER HJ, BERG RA. Bacterial tracheitis as a complication of endotracheal intubation. *Pediatrics Pulmonol* 1991;11:87–9.

223. CORDER L, TALLMAN RD JR, QUALMAN S, GARDNER D, MCCLEAD R. Necrotizing tracheobronchitis (NTB) following high frequency ventilation: role of an angiotensin converting enzyme inhibitor. *Pediatrics Path* 1991;11:49–61.

224. VASISHTA S, WOOD JB, MCGINTY F. Ulcerative tracheobronchitis years after colectomy for ulcerative colitis. *Chest* 1994;106:1279–81.

225. CRAIG TJ, MAGUIRE FE, WALLACE MR. Tracheobronchitis due to *Corynebacterium pseudodiphtheriticum*. *South Med J* 1991;84:504–6.

226. SHERRY MK, KLAINER AS, WOLFF M, GERHARD H. Herpetic tracheobronchitis. *Ann Intern Med* 1988;109:229–33.

227. NATKUNAM R, TSE CY, ONG BH, SRIRAGAVAN P. Carinal resection for stenotic tuberculous tracheitis. *Thorax* 1988;43:492–3.

228. LABAY MV, RAMOS R, HERVAS JA, RYENES J, GOMEZ B. Membranous laryngotracheobronchitis, a complication of measles. *Intens Care Med* 1985;11:326–7.

229. DEEB ZE, EINHORN KH. Infectious adult croup. *Laryngoscope* 1990;100:455–7.

230. ALFARO-MONGE JM, FERNANDEZ-ESPINOSA J, SODA-MERPHY A. Scleroma of the lower respiratory tract: case report and review of literature. *J Laryngol Otol* 1994;108:161–3.

231. TAPIA A. Rhinoscleroma: a naso-oral dermatosis. *Tropical Dermatol* 1987;40:101–3.

232. OKOTH-OLENDE AND BJERREGAARD B. Scleroma in Africa: a review of cases from Kenya. *East Afr Med J* 1990;67:231–6.

233. SAAD EF. Antroscleroma. *J Laryngol Otol* 1988;102:362–4.

234. AKHTAR M, MCARTHUR PD, ALI MA. Rhinoscleroma: ultrastructural study of a case before and after treatment. *KFSH Med J* 1982;2:23–30.

235. BATSAKIS JG, EL-NAGGAR AK. Rhinoscleroma and rhinosporidiosis. *Ann Otol Rhinol Laryngol* 1992;101:879–82.

236. ABOU-SEIF SG, BAKY FA, EL-EBRASHY F, GAAFAR HA. Scleroma of the upper respiratory passages: a CT study. *J Laryngol Otol* 1991;105:198–202.

237. LENIS A, RUFF T, DIAZ JA, GHANDOUR EG. Rhinoscleroma. *South Med J* 1988;81:1580–2.

238. BERRON P, BERRON R, ORTIZ-ORTIZ L. Alterations in the T-lymphocyte subpopulation in patients with rhinoscleroma. *J Clin Microbiol* 1988;26:1031–3.

239. WABINGA HR, WAMUKOTA W, MUGERWA JW. Scleroma in Uganda: a review of 85 cases. *East Afr Med J* 1993;70:186–8.

240. DAWLATLY EE, ANIM JT, BARAKA ME. Local iatrogenic complications in nasopharyngeal rhinoscleroma. *J Laryngol Otol* 1988;102:1115–18.

241. GAMEA AM. Role of endoscopy in diagnosing scleroma in its uncommon sites. *J Laryngol Otol* 1990;104:619–21.

242. EDWARDS MB, ROBERTS GD, STORRS TJ. Scleroma (rhinoscleroma) in a Nigerian maxillo-facial practice. Review and case reports. *Int J Oral Surg* 1977;6:270–9.

243. GAAFAR HA, EL-ASSI MH. Skin affection in rhinoscleroma. A clinical, histological and electron microscopic study on four patients. *Acta Otolaryngol* 1988;105:494–9.

244. DHARAN M, NACTIGAL D, ROSEN G. Intraoperative demonstration of Mikulicz cells in nasal scleroma. A case report. *Acta Cytolog* 1993;37:732–4.

245. DAWLATLY EE. Radiological diagnosis of rhinoscleroma – the 'palatal sign.' *J Laryngol Otol* 1991;105:968–70.

246. TRAUTMANN M, HELD T, RUHNKE M, SCHNOY N. A case of rhinoscleroma cured with ciprofloxacin. *Infection* 1993;21:403–6.

247. MASHER AI, EL-KASHLAN HK, SOLIMAN Y, GALAL R. Rhinoscleroma: management by carbon dioxide surgical laser. *Laryngoscope* 1990;100:783–8.

248. MOSS AJ, PARSONS VL. Current estimates from the National Health Interview Survey, United States – 1985. Hyattsville, Maryland: National Center for Health Statistics, 1986:66–7.

249. REILLY JS. The sinusitis cycle. *Otolaryngol Head Neck Surg* 1990;103(5)2:856–861.

250. NAUMAN H. Pathologische Anatomie der chronichen Rhinitis und sinusitis. *Proceedings VIII International Congress of*

Oto-rhino-laryngology, Amsterdam, Excerpta Medica 1965, p 80.

251. KENNEDY DW, ZINREICH J, ROSENBAUM AE, JOHNS ME. Functional endoscopic sinus surgery, *Arch Otolarynol* 1985;III.

252. KALIVER MA. Human nasal host defense and sinusitis. *J Allergy Clin Immunol* 1992;424–9.

253. WAGENMANN M, NALERIO RM. Anatomic and physiologic considerations in sinusitis. *J Allergy Clin Immunol* 1992;419–23.

254. REILLY JS. The sinusitis cycle. *Otolaryngol Head Neck Surg* 1990;103:856–61.

255. FIREMAN P. Diagnosis of sinusitis in children: emphasis on the history and physical examination. *J Allergy Clin Immunol* 1992;90(3)2:433–36.

256. KENNEDY DW. Overview of sinusitis. *Otolarynology Head Neck Surg* 1990;103(5)2:847–54.

257. WALD ER. Sinusitis in infants and children. *Ann Otol Laryngol* 1992;101:37–41.

258. SPECTOR SL. The role of allergy in sinusitis in adults. *J Allergy Clin Immunol* 1992;90:518–20.

259. DRAKE-LEE AB, MORGAN DW. Nasal polyps and sinusitis in children with cystic fibrosis. *J Laryngol Otol* 1989;103:753–55.

260. ELIASSON M, MOSSBERG B, CAMNER P *et al.* The immotile cilia syndrome: a congenital ciliary abnormality as an etiologic factor in chronic airway infections and male sterility. *N Engl J Med* 1977;297:1–6.

261. BONMAN S. Maxillary sinusitis and bronchial asthma: correlation of roentgenograms, cultures and thermograms. *J Allergy Clin Immunol* 1974; 53:311–18.

262. KATZ R. Sinusitis in children with respiratory allergy. *J Allergy Clin Immunol* 1978;61:190–5.

263. RACHELEFSKY GS, KATZ RM, SIEGEL SC. Chronic sinus disease with associated reactive airway disease in children. *Paediatrics* 1984;73:526–29.

264. SLAVIN RG, CANNON RE, FREEDMAN WH *et al.* Sinusitis and bronchial asthma. *J Allergy Clin Immun* 1980;66:250–7.

265. EVANS FO, SYDNER JB, MOORE WED, MOORE GR. Sinusitis of the maxillary antrum. *N Engl J Med* 1995;293:735–39.

266. ZINREICH SJ. Paranasal sinus imaging. *Otolaryngol Head and Neck Surg* 1990; 103:863.

267. CARTER BL, BONBOFF MS, FISK JD. Computed tomographic detection of sinusitis responsible for intracranial and extracranial infections. *Radiology* 1983;147:739–42.

268. DIAMENT MJ. The diagnosis of sinusitis in infants and children: X ray, computed tomography and magnetic resonance imaging. *J Allergy Clin Immunol* 1992; 90:442–4.

269. REVINTA M. Ultrasound in the diagnosis of maxillary and frontal sinusitis. *Acta Otolaryngol* 1980;370(suppl):1–54.

270. BERG O, CARENFELT C. Etiological diagnosis in sinusitis: ultrasonography as clinical component. *Laryngoscope* 1985;95:851–3.

271. KENNEDY DW. Functional endoscopic sinus surgery. *Arch Otolaryngol* III, 1985:643–9.

272. STAMMBERGER H. *Functional Endoscopic Sinus Surgery*. Philadelphia: BC Decker: 1991.

273. VINING EM, YANAGISAWA K, YANAGISAWA E. The importance of preoperative nasal endoscopy in patients with sinonasal disease. *Laryngoscope* 1993;103:512–19.

274. DRUCE HM. Diagnosis of sinusitis in adults: history, physical examination, nasal cytology, echo and rhinoscope. *J Allergy Clin Immunol* 1982;90(3)2:436–41.

275. WALD ER, CHIPONIS D, LEDESMIA-MEDINA J. Corporative effectiveness of amoxicillin and amoxicillin-clavalanate potassium in acute paranasal sinus infections in children: a double-blind, placebo-controlled trial. *Paediatrics* 1986;77:795–800.

276. GWALTNEY J JR. Diagnostic and medical management of acute sinusitis. Presentation at the American Academy of Allergy and Immunology, San Antonio, Texas, 4 Feb 1989.

277. RACHELEFSKY GS, KATZ RM, SIEGEL SC. Chronic sinusitis in children with respiratory allergy: the role of antimicrobials. *J Allergy Clin Immunol* 1982;69:382–7.

278. WILSON NW, JALOWAYSKI AA, HOMBERGER RN. A comparison of nasal cytology with sinus X-rays for the diagnosis of sinusitis. *Am J Rhinol* 1988;2:55–9

279. GILL FF, WEIBERGER JB. The role of nasal cytology in the diagnosis of chronic sinusitis. *Am J Rhinol* 1989:13–15.

280. BROOK I: Aerobic and anaerobic bacterial flora of normal maxillary sinuses. *Laryngoscope* 1981;91:372.

281. EVANS FO JR, SYDNOR JB, MOORE WE *et al.* Sinusitis of the maxillary antrum. *N Engl J Med* 1974;290:135.

282. DALEY CL, SANDE M: The runny nose: infection in the paranasal sinuses. *Infect Dis Clin North Am* 1988;2:131.

283. WALD ER, Microbiology of acute and chronic sinusitis in children. *J Allergy Clin Immunol* Sept 1992:452–56.

284. MALOW JB, CRETICO'S CM. Non surgical treatment of sinusitis. *Otolaryngol Clin N Am* 22 (4): 1989; 22 (4): 809–18.

285. FREDERICK J, BRAUDE AL: Anaerobic infection of the paranasal sinuses. *N Engl J Med* 1974;290:135.

286. OTTEN FWA, GROTTE JJ. Treatment of chronic maxillary sinusitis in children. *Int J Pediatr Otorhinolarygol* 1988;15:269–78.

287. STAFFORD CT. The clinicians view of sinusitis. *Otolaryngol Head and Neck Surg* 1990;103(5):870–5.

288. WALD ER, CHIPONIS D, LEDESOMA-MEDINA J. Comparative effectiveness of amoxicillin and amoxicillin-clavulanate potassium in acute paranasal sinus infection in children: a double blind, placebo-controlled trial. *Pediatrics* 1986;77:795–800.

289. HENDERSON FW, GILLIGAN PH, WART K, GOFF D A. Nasopharyngeal carriage of antibiotic-resistant pneumocci by children in group day care. *J Infect Dis* 1988; 157:256–63.

290. GWALTNEY JM, SYDNOR A., SONDI MA. Etiology and antimicrobial treatment of acute sinusitis. *Ann Otol Rhinol Laryngol* 1981;90(Suppl 84):68–71.

291. WALD ER. Antimicrobial therapy in pediatric patients with sinusitis. *J Allergy Clin Immunol* 1992:469–73.

292. LWOFF A. Death and transfiguration of a problem. *Bacteriol Rev* 1969;33:390–403.

293. INGELS KJAO, KORTMAN MJW, NIJZIEL MR *et al.* Factors influencing ciliary beat measurements. *Rhinology* 1991;29:17–26.

294. SAKETKHOO D, JANUSZKIEWICZ A, SACHNER MA. Effects of drinking hot water, cold water, and chicken soup on nasal mucus velocity and nasal airflow resistance. *Chest* 1978;74:408.

295. COLE P, HAIGHT JSJ. Posture and nasal patency. *Am Rev Resp Dis* 1984; 129:351–54.

296. ZIEGLER RS. Prospects for ancillary treatment of sinusitis in the 1990s. *J Allergy Clin Immunol* 1992;90(3)2:478–92.

297. BOND BC, MUKHERJEE AC, BANG FB. Human nasal mucous flow rates. *Johns Hopkins Med J* 1967;121:38–48.

298. ZIEGLER RS. Prospects for ancillary treatment of sinusitis in the 1990s. *J Allergy Clin Immunol* 1992;90(3)2:478–92.

299. MOSHER H.P. The applied anatomy in the intranasal surgery of the ethmoid labyrinth. *Trans Am Laryngeal Assoc* 1912;34:25–39.

300. FREEDMANN WH, KERN EB. Complications of mitranasal ethmoidectomy: a review of 1000 consecutive operations. *Laryngoscope* 1979;89:421–34.

301. KENNEDY DW. Functional endoscopic sinus surgery: technique. *Arch Otolaryngol* 1985;111:643–9.

302. LUSK RP. Endoscopic approach to sinus disease. *J Allergy Clin Immunol* 1992;(30):496–504.

303. SCHAEFER SD, MANNING S, CLOSE LG. Endoscopic paranasal sinus surgery: indication and considerations. *Laryngoscope* 1989;99, 1–5.

304. RICHTSMEIER WJ. Medical and surgical

management of sinusitis in adults. *Ann Otol Rhinol Laryngol* 1992;101:46–50.

305. LAWSON W, BLITZER A. Fungal infection of the nose and paranasal sinuses. *Otolaryngol Clin N Am* 93;26(6):1037–68.

306. CONEY JP, ROMBERGER CF, SHAW GY. Fungal diseases of the sinuses. *Otolaryngol Head Neck Surg* 1990;103:1012–15.

307. GOLSTEIN MF. Allergic fungal sinusitis: an underdiagnosed problem. *Hosp Pract* 1992; 27:73–92.

308. STAMMBERGER H, JASKE R, BEUFORT F. Aspergillosis of the paranasal sinuses. X-ray diagnosis, histopathology and clinical aspects. *Ann Otol Rhinol Laryngol* 1984; 93:251–6.

309. STAMMBERGER H. Endoscopic surgery for mycotic and recurring sinusitis. *Ann Otol Rhinol Laryngol* 1985;94(Suppl 119):1–11.

310. HARTWICK RW, BATSAKIS JG. Sinus aspergillosis and allergic fungal sinusitis. *Ann Otol Rhinol Laryngol* 1991;100:427–30.

311. WAITZMAN AA, BIRT BD. Fungal sinusitis. *J Otolaryngol* 1994;23(4):244–9.

312. ZINREICH SJ, KENNEDY DW, MALAT J *et al.* Fungal sinusitis: diagnosis with CT and MR imaging. *Radiology* 1988;169:439–44.

313. WASHBURN RG, KENNEDY DW, BEGLEY MG, HENDERSON DK, BENNETT JE. Chronic fungal sinusitis in apparently normal hosts. *Medicine* 1988;67(4):231–47.

314. MCGILL TJ, SIMPSON G, HEALEY GB: Fulminant aspergillosis of the nose and paranasal sinuses: a new clinical entity. *Laryngoscope* 1980; 90:748–54.

315. MIRSKY HS, CUTTNER J: Fungal infection in acute leukemia. *Cancer* 1972; 30:348–52.

316. KAVANAGH KT, PARHAM DM, HUGHES WT. Fungal sinusitis in immunocompromised children with neoplasms. *Ann Otol Rhino Laryngol* 1991; 100:331–6.

317. BLITZER A, LAWSEN W, MYERS BR *et al.* Patient survival factors in paranasal sinus *Mucormycosis Laryng* 1980;90:635–48.

318. MCNULTY JS. Rhino cerebral mucormycosis: predisposing factors. *Laryngoscope* 1982;92:1140–3.

319. RABIN ER, LUNDBERG GD, MITCHELL ET. Mucormycosis in severely burned patients. *N Engl J Med* 1977;264:1286–9.

320. KAPLAN AH, POZA-JUNICAL E, SHAPIRO R, STAPLETON JT. Cure of mucormycosis in a renal transplant patient receiving cyclosporin with maintenance of immunosuppression. *AMJ Nephrol* 1988;8(2):139–42.

321. BAVER H. Sheldon WH. Leukopenia and experimental mucormycosis. *Am J. Pathol* 1957;33:617–18.

322. WINDUS DW, SOKES TJ, JULIAN BA *et al.*: Fatal-rhizopus infections in haemodialysis patients receiving deferoxamine. *Ann Int Med* 1987;107:678–80.

323. CASTELLI JB, PALLIN JL. Lethal rhinocerebral phyomycosis in a healthy adult: a case report and review of the literature. *Otolaryngology* 1978;86:696.

324. SHWENI PM, MOODLEY SC, BISHOP BB. Septic abortion complicated by rhino cerebral phycomycosis. A case report. *S Afr Med J* 1986;69(8):515–16.

325. FONG KM, SERENVIRATNE. EM, MCCORMECK JG. Mucor cerebral abcess associated with intravenous drug abuse. *Aust NZJ Med* 1990;20(1):74–7.

326. ABEDI E, SINUANIS A, CHOI K, PASTORE P. Twenty-five years experience treating cerebro-rhino-orbital mucormycosis. *Laryngoscope* 1984;94:1060–3.

327. SMITH HW, KIRCHNER JA. Cerebral mucormycosis. *Arch Otolaryngol* 1958;68:715.

328. MANIGLIA AJ, MINTZ DH, NOVAK S. Cephalic phycomycosis: a report of eight cases. *Laryngoscope* 1982;92:755–9.

329. GAMBA JL, DJANG WT, YEATES AE. Cranial facial mucormycosis: assessment with CT. *Radiology* 1986;160:207–12.

330. YOUSEM DM, GALETTA SL, GUSNARD DA, GOLDBERG HI. MRI findings in rhino cerebral mucormycosis. *J Comput Assist Tomogr* 1989;13(5):878–82.

331. SUGAR A. Mucormycosis. *Clin Infect Dis* 1992;14 (Suppl 1): S 126–9.

332. CHRISTENSEN JC, SHALIT I, WELCH DF *et al.* Synergistic action of amphotericin B and rifampin against *Rhizopus* species. *Antimicrob Agents Chemother* 1987;31:1775–8.

333. FERGUSON BJ, MITCHELL TG, MOON R *et al.* Adjunctive hyperbaric oxygen for treatment of rhinocerebral mucormycosis. *Rev Infect Dis* 1988;10:551–9.

334. PRICE JC, STEVENS DL. Hyperbaric oxygen in the treatment of rhino cerebral mucormycosis. *Laryngoscope* 1980;90:737–47.

335. ANAND VK, ALEMAR G, GRISWALD JA. Intracranial complications of mucormycosis: an experimental model and clinical review. *Laryngoscope* 1992;102:656–62.

336. PARFREY NA. Improved diagnosis and prognosis of mucormycosis: a clinicopathologic study of 33 cases. *Medicine* (*Baltimore*) 1986;65:113–23.

337. CAPLAN ES, HOYT NJ. Nocosomial sinusitis. *JAMA* 1982; 247:639–41.

338. ARENS JF, LEJEUNE FE, WEBRE DR. Maxillary sinusitis: a complication of nasotracheal intubation. *Anesthesiology* 1974;40:415–16.

339. STAUFFER JL, OLSON DE, PETTY TL. Complications and consequences of endotracheal intubation and tracheostomy. *Am J Med* 1981;70:65–76.

340. KNODEL AR, BECKMAN JF. Unexplained fever in patients with nasotracheal intubation. *JAMA* 1982; 248:868–70.

341. DEUTSCHMAN CS, WILTON P, SIMON J, DIBBELL D. Paranasal sinusitis associated with nasotracheal intubation: a frequently unrecognized and treatable source of infection. *Crit Care Med* 1985;14:111–14.

342. POPE TL, STELLING CB, LEITNER YB. Maxillary sinusitis after nasotracheal intubation. *South Med J* 1981;74:610–12.

343. ABRAMOVICH S, SMELT GJC. Acute sphenoiditis, alone and in concert. *J Laryngol Otol* 1982; 96:751–7.

344. LEW O, SOUTHWICK F, MONTGOMERY W, WEBER A, BAKER A. Sphenoid sinusitis. *N Engl J Med* 1983;309:1149–54.

345. DEUTSCHMAN CS, WILTON P, SIMON J, DIBBELL D. Paranasal sinusitis associated with nasotracheal intubation: a frequently unrecognized and treatable source of infection. *Crit Care Med* 1985;14:111–14.

346. O'REILLY MJ, REDDICK EJ, BLACK W *et al.* Sepsis from sinusitis in nasotracheally intubated patients: a diagnostic dilemma. *Am J Surg* 1984; 147:601.

347. LESSNER A, STERB GA. Preseptal and orbital cellulitis. *Infect Dis Clin N Am* 1992; 6(4):933–52.

348. BATSON OV. Relationship of the eye to the paranasal sinuses. *Arch Ophthalmol* 1936;16:322–8.

349. SHAHIN J, GULLANE PJ, DAYAL VS. Orbital complications of acute sinusitis. *J Otolaryngology* 1986;16(1):23–7.

350. CHANDLER JR, LANGENBRUNNER DJ, STEVENS ER. The pathogenosis of orbital complications in acute sinusitis. *Laryngoscope* 1970; 80:1414–28.

351. WILLIAMS BJ, HARRISON HC. Subperiosteal abscess of the orbit due to sinusitis in childhood. *Austr NZ J Ophthal* 1991; 19(1):29–36.

352. WILLIAMS SR, CARRUTH JA. Orbital infections secondary to sinusitis in children: diagnosis and management. *Clin Otolaryngol* 1992; 17(6):550–7.

353. TARAZI AE, SHIKANI AH. Irreversible unilateral visual loss due to acute sinusitis. *Arch Otolaryngol Head Neck Surg* 1991; 117(12):1400–1.

354. SOPARKAR LN, PATRINELY JR, CUAYCONG MJ *et al.* The silent sinus syndrome: a cause of spontaneous enophthalmos. *Ophthalmology* 1994; 101(4):772–8.

355. ROTHSTEIN J, MAUSEL RH, BERLINGER NT. Relationship of optic neuritis to disease of

the paranasal sinuses. *Laryngoscope* 1984; 94(11 Pt 1):1501–8.

356. PATTERSON AW, BARNARD NA, IRVINE GH. Nasoorbital fracture leading to orbital cellulitis and visual loss as a complication of chronic sinusitis. *Br J Oral Maxillofacial Surg* 1994; 32(3):187–9.

357. JAYAMANN DG, BELL RW, ALLEN ED. Orbital cellulitis – an unusual presentation and late complication of severe facial trauma. *Br J Oral Maxillofacial Surg* 1994; 32(3):187–9.

358. PENNE RB, FLANAGEN JC, STEFANYSZYN MA *et al.* Ocular motility disorders secondary to sinus surgery. *Ophth Plastic Reconstruc Surg* 1993; 9(1):53–61.

359. BOLGER WE, PARSONS DS, MAU EA *et al.* Lacrimal drainage system injury in functional endoscopic surgery. Incidence, analysis and prevention. *Arch Otolaryngol Head Neck Surg* 1992;118(11):1179–84.

360. COREY JP, BUMSTEAD R, PANJE W *et al.* Orbital complications of functional endoscopic sinus surgery. *Otolaryngol Head Neck Surg* 1991; 117(12):1400–1.

361. CHOI S, LAWSON W, URKEN ML. Subperiosteal orbital haematoma. An unusual complication of sinusitis. *Arch Otolaryngol Head Neck Surg* 1988; 114(12):1464–6.

362. ICINO Y, NAGATA M, ISHIKAWA T. Subperiosteal orbital haemorrhage associated with chronic sinusitis: a case report and review of the literature. *Auris, Nasus, Larynx* 1985; 12(1):27–30.

363. CLUREY RA, CUNNINGHAM MJ, EAVEY RD. Orbital complications of acute sinusitis: comparison of computed tomography scan and surgical findings. *Ann Otol Rhinol Laryngol* 1992; 101(7):598–600.

364. YOUSEM DM, GALELLA SL, GUSNARD DA *et al.* MR findings in rhinocerebral mucormycosis. *J Comp Ass Tomogr* 1989; 13(5):878–82.

365. WAGENMAMM M, NACLERIO RM. Complications of sinusitis. *J Allergy Clin Immunol* 1992; 90(3 Pt 2):552–54.

366. DAVIS JP, STEARNS MP. Orbital complications of sinusitis: avoid delays in diagnosis. *Postgrad Med J* 1994; 70(820):108–10.

367. FAIRBANKS DNF, VANDERVEEN TS, BRADLEY JE. Intracranial complications of sinusitis, In English GM, ed. *Otolaryngology*, Vol 2. Philadelphia: Harper and Row: 1987.

368. RODGERS GK, TABOR E, ROAD SR *et al.* Complication of acute and chronic sinus disease. AAO-HNS SI PAC 1990.

369. POTT P. Observation of the nature and consequences of those injuries to which the head is liable from external violence. In Enbe, ed. *The Chirurgical Works of Percival Pott*, FRS. Vol 1 Philadelphia: James Webster: 1819:29–171.

370. FAIRBANKS DNF, VANDERVEEN TS, BRADLEY JE. Intracranial complications of sinusitis. In English GM, ed. *Otolaryngology*, Vol 2. Philadelphia: Harper and Row: 1987, Chap 38:1–28.

371. STANKIEWICZ MD, NEWELL DJ, PARK AH. Complications of inflammatory diseases of the sinuses. *Otolaryngol Clin N Am* 1993;26(4):639–55.

372. MANIGLIA A, VANBUREN J, BRUCE WB. Intracranial abscesses secondary to ear and paranasal sinus infections. *Otol Head Neck Surg* 1978;7:289–96.

373. MORGAN PR, MORRISON MV. Complications of frontal and ethmoid sinusitis. *Laryngoscope* 1980;90:661–6.

374. ROSENBLUM ML, HOFF JT, NORMAN O. Decreased mortality from brain abscess since advent of computerized tomography. *J Neurosurg* 1978;49:658–68.

375. CLAYMAAN GL, ADAMS GL, PAUGH DR, KOOPMANN CF. Intracranial complications of paranasal sinusitis: a combined institutional review. *Laryngoscope* 1991;101:234–39.

376. GRANT A, VON SCHOENBERG M, GRANT HR, MILLER RF. Paranasal sinus disease in HIV antibody positive patients. *Genitourin Med* 1993;69(3):208–12

377. MEITELES LZ, LUCENTE FE Sinus and nasal manifestations of the acquired immune deficiency syndrome. *Ear Nose Throat J* 1990;69:460–3.

378. BINCHALL MA, HORNER PD, STAFFORD ND. Changing patterns of HIV infection in Otolaryngology. *Clin Otolaryng* 1994;19(6):473–7.

379. SMALL CB, KAUFMAN A, ARMENEKE M, POSENSTREICH DC. Sinusitis and atopy in human immune deficiency virus infection. *J Infect Dis* 1993;167(2):283–90.

380. MEITELES LZ, LUCENTE FE. Sinus and nasal manifestations of the acquired immune deficiency syndrome. *Ear Nose Throat J* 1990;69:460–3.

381. METCALF TW, DORAN RM, ROWLANDS PC, ANY A. Microsporideal kerato-conjunctivitis in a patient with AIDS. *Brit J Ophthalmol* 1992; 76(3):177–78.

382. LI CX, SZUBA MJ, SCHUMAN P, CRANE L. *Myobacterium kansasii* sinusitis in a patient with AIDS. *Clin Infect Dis*, Oct 1994;19(4):792–3.

383. ROSENTHAL J, KATZ R, DUBOIS DB, MORRISSEY A. Chronic maxillary sinusitis associated with the mushroom *Schizophyllum commune* in a patient with AIDS. *Clin Infect Dis* 1992;14(1):46–8.

384. SCHLANGER G, LUTWICKE LI, KURZMAN M, HOCH B. Sinusitis caused by *Legionella pneumophilia* in a patient with the acquired immune deficiency syndrome. *Am J Med* 1984;77(5):957–60.

385. COLMERINO L, MONUX A, VALENCIA E, CASTRO A. Successfully treated *Candida* sinusitis in an AIDS patient. *J Cranio-Maxillo-Facial Surg* 1990;18(4):175–8.

386. BRILLHART T, CATHE J JR, PIOT D, STOOL E. Symptomatic cytomegaloviral rhinosinusitis in patients with AIDS. *International Conference on AIDS*, 16–21 June 1991;7(1):227 (Abstract No, MB 2182).

387. DAAR ES, MEYER RD. Bacterial and fungal infections. *Med Clin North Am* 1992; 76:173–203.

388. MEYER RD, GAULTIER CR, YAASHIT2A JT, BABAPOUR R, PITCHON HE. Fungal sinusitis in patients with AIDS: report of 4 cases and review of the literature. *Medicine* 1994;73(2):69–78.

389. BLUESTONE CD. State of the art: definitions and classifications. In Lim DJ, Bluestone CD, Klein JO, Nelson JD, eds *Recent Advances in Otitis Media with Effusion*. Toronto: BC Decker: 1984;1–4.

390. BLUESTONE CD, KLEIN JO. Definitions, terminology and classification. In *Otitis Media in Infants and Children*. Philadelphia: WB Saunders: 1988;1–21.

391. STOOL SE, FIELD MJ. The impact of otitis media. *Pediatr Infect Dis J* (Suppl 1): 1989;11–14.

392. NEWACHECK PW, TAYLOR WR. Childhood chronic illness: prevalence, severity and impact. *Am J Public Health* 1992;82:364.

393. WRIGHT PF, MCCONNELL KB, THOMPSON JM, VAUGHN WK. A longitudinal study of the detection of otitis media in the first two years of life. *Int J Pediatr Otorhinolaryngol* 1985;10:245–52.

394. BLUESTONE CD, KLIM JO. Epidemiology. *In Otitis Media in Infants and Children*, Philadelphia: WB Saunders: 1988;31–43.

395. RUDIN R, WELIN L, SVARDSUDD K, TIBBLIN G. Middle ear disease in samples from the general population. II. History of otitis and atorrhea in relation to tympanic membrane pathology, the study of men born in 1913 and 1923. *Acta Otolaryngol (Stockh)* 1985;99:53–9.

396. PELTON SI, SHURIN PA, KLEIN JO. Persistence of middle ear effusion after otitis media. *Pediatr Res* 1977;11:504.

397. TEELE DW, KLEIN JO, ROSNER B. Epidemiology of otitis media in children. *Ann Otol Rhinol Laryngol* 1980;89:5.

398. BLUESTONE CD, KLEIN JO. Physiology, pathophysiology and pathogenesis. In *Otitis Media in Infants and Children*. Philadelphia: WB Saunders: 1988:15–29.

399. SADLER-KIMES D, SIEGEL MI, TODHUNTER JS. Relationship between eustachian tube cartilage length and otitis media. In Sadi J, ed. *Basic Aspects of the Eustachian Tube and Middle Ear Disease*. Amsterdam: Kugler and Ghedini; 1991:353–6.

400. TAKAHASHI H, HAYESHI M, SATO H, HONJO I. Primary deficits in eustachian tube dysfunction in patients with otitis media with effusion. *Arch Otolaryngol Head Neck Surg* 1989;115:581–4.

401. SOLOMON NE, HARRIS LJ. Otitis media in children. Assessing the quality of medical care using short-term outcome measures. *Quality of Medical Care Assessment using Outcome Measures: Eight Disease-specific Applications*. Santa Monica: Rand Corp.; 1976.

402. ZONIS RD. Chronic otitis media in the Southwestern American Indian. *Arch Otolaryngol* 1968;88:360–5.

403. DUGDALE AE, LEWIS AN, CANTY AA. The natural history of otitis media. *N Engl J Med* 1982;307:1459–60.

404. PUKHANDU J, SIPILA M, KARMA P. Occurrence of and risk factors in acute otitis media. In Lim DJ, Bluestone CD, Klein JO, Nelson JD (eds.). *Recent Advances in Otitis Media with Effusion*. Burlington, Ontario: BC Decker; 1984:9–13.

405. THAELAR SB, ADDISS DG, GOODMAN RA *et al.* Infections, diseases and injuries in child day care. *JAMA* 1992;268:1720–6.

406. TULE DW, KLEIN JO, ROSNER BA. Epidemiology of otitis media in children. *Ann Otol Rhinol Laryngol* 1980;89(68):5–6.

407. DUNCAN B, EY J, HOLBERG CJ *et al.* Exclusive breast feeding for at least 4 months protects against otitis media. *Pediatrics* 1993;91:867–872.

408. TEELE DW, KLEIN JO, ROSNER B. Otitis media with effusion during the first three years of life and development of speech and language. *Paediatrics* 1984;74:282–7.

409. HENDERSON FW, COLLIER AM, SANYAL MA, WATKINS JM. A longitudinal study of respiratory viruses and bacteria in the etiology of acute otitis media with effusion. *N Engl J Med* 1982;306:1377–83.

410. ELZEL RA, PATTISHALL EN, HALEY NJ *et al.* Passive smoking and middle ear effusion among children in day care. *Pediatrics* 1992;90:228–32.

411. AROLA M, RUUSKONEN O, ZIEGLER T *et al.* Clinical role of respiratory virus infection in acute otitis media. *Pediatrics* 1990;86:848–55.

412. AROLA M, ZIEGLER T, RUUSKONEN O *et al.* Rhinovirus in acute otitis media. *J Pediatr* 1988;113:693–5.

413. CHONMAITREE T, OWEN MJ, HOWIE VM. Respiratory viruses interfere with bacteriologic response to antibiotic in children with acute otits media. *J Infect Dis* 1990;162:546–9.

414. KLEIN JO, TEELE DW. Isolation of viruses and mycoplasms from middle ear effusions: a review. *Ann Otol Rhinol Laryngol* 1976;85:140–4.

415. BLUESTONE CD, KLEIN JO. Microbiology. In *Otitis Media in Infants and Children*. Philadelphia: WB Saunders: 1988; 45–58.

416. HARRISON CJ, MARKS MI, WELCH DF. Microbiology of recently treated acute otitis media compared with previously contracted acute otitis media. *Pediatr Infect Dis* 1985;4:641–46.

417. MURPHY TF, BERSTEIN JM, DRYJA DM, CONPAGNARI AA *et al.* Outer membrane protein and lipooligosaccharide analysis of paired nasopharyngeal and middle ear isolates in otitis media due to nontypeable *Haemophilus* influenza: pathogenic and epidemiological observations. *J Infect Dis* 1987;156:723–31.

418. BERMAN SA, BALKANY TJ, SIMMONS MA. Otitis media in the neonatal intensive care unit. *Pediatrics* 1978;62:198–201.

419. ROBERTS DB. The etiology of bullous myringitis and the role of mycoplasmas in ear disease: a review. *Pediatrics* 1980;65:761–6.

420. SCHACHTER J, GROSSMAN M, HOLT J *et al.* Prospective study of chlamydial infections in neonates. *Lancet* 1979;ii:377–9.

421. LEE PYC, DRYSDALE AJ. Tuberculous otitis media: a difficult diagnosis. J Laryngology and *Otology, April* 1993;107:339–41.

422. PLESTER D, PUSALKAR A, STEINBACH E. Middle ear tuberculosis. *J Laryngol Otol* 1980;90:1415–21.

423. YANIV E. Tuberculous otitis media, a clinical record. *Laryngoscope* 1987;97:1303–6.

424. MA KH, TONG PSO, CHAN CW. Aural tuberculosis. *Am J Otol* 1990;11:174–77.

425. YANIV E, TRAUF P, CONRADIE R. Middle ear tuberculosis – a series of 24 patients. *Int J Pedia Otorhinolaryng*, Nov 1986;12(1):5–63.

426. SKOLNIK PR, NADOL JB, BAKER AS. Tuberculosis of the middle ear: review of the literature with an instructive case report. *Rev Infect Dis* 1986;8(3):403–10.

427. KALEIDA PH, STOOL SE. Assessment of otoscopists' accuracy regarding middle ear effusion: otoscopic validation. *Am J Dis Child* 1992;146:433.

428. KARMA PH, SIPILA MM, KATAJA MJ. Pneumatic otoscopy and otitis media. Value of different tympanic membrane findings and their combinations. In Lim DJ, Bluestone CD, Klein JO, Nelson JD, Ogra PL, eds. *Recent Advances in Otitis Media. Proceedings of the Fifth International Symposium*. Hamilton, Canada: Decker Periodicals 1993;41–5.

429. FINITZO T, FRIEL-PATTI S, CHINN K *et al.* Tympanometry and otoscopy prior to myringotomy: Issues in diagnosis of otitis media. *Int J Paediatr Otolaryngol* 1992; 24:101.

430. VAUGHAN-JONES R, MILLS RP. The Welch Allyn audioscope and micro-tymp: their accuracy and that of pneumatic otoscopy, tympanometry and pure tone audiometry as predictors of otitis media with effusion. *J Laryngol Otol* 1992; 106:600.

431. MCMILLAN PM, BENNETT MJ, MARCHANT CD, SHURIN PA. Ipsilateral and contralateral acoustic reflexes in neonates. *Ear Hear* 1985;6:320–4.

432. ROSENFELD RM, VERTREES J, CARR J *et al.* Clinical efficacy of antimicrobials for acute otitis media: meta-analysis of 4,700 children from 33 randomized trials. *J Pediatr* 1994;124:355–67.

433. CANAFAX DM, GIEBINK GS. Antimicrobial treatment of acute otitis media. *Ann Otol Rhinol Laryngol* 1994;103:11–14.

434. CARLIN SA, MARCHANT CD, SHURIN PA, JOHNSON CE *et al.* Early recurrences of otitis media: reinfection or relapse. *J Pediatr* 1987;110:20–5.

435. DALY K, GIEBINK GS, BATALDEN PB, ANDERSON RS *et al.* Resolution of otitis media with effusion with the use of a stepped treatment regimen of trisulthoprim-sulfamethoxazole and prednisone. *Pediatr Infect Dis J* 1991;10:500–6.

436. ROSENFELD RM. New concepts for steroid use in otitis media with effusion. *Clin Pediatr* 1992;31:615.

437. NEIL HB, KEATING LW, MCDONALD TJ. Ventilation in secretory otitis media: Effects on middle ear volume and eustachian tube function. *Arch Otolaryngol* 1977;103:228.

438. GATES GA, MUNTZ HR, GAYLIS B. Adenoidectomy and otitis media. *Ann Otol Rhinol Laryngol* 1992;101:24–31.

439. PARADISE JL, BLUESTONE CD, ROGERS KD *et al.* Efficacy of adenoidectomy for recurrent otitis media in children previously treated with tympanostomy-tube placement: results of parallel randomized and nonrandomized trials. *JAMA* 1990;263:2066–73.

440. PILLSBURY HC, KVENTON JR, SASAKI CT, FRAZIER W. Quantitative bacteriology in adenoid tissue. *Otolaryngol Head Neck Surg* 1981;89:355–63.

441. MAW AR. Chronic otitis media with effusion (glue ear) and adenotonsillectomy: prospective randomized controlled study. *Br Med J* 1983;287:1586–8.

442. CASSELBRONT ML, KALEIDA PA, ROCKETTE HE *et al.* Efficacy of antimicrobial prophylaxis and of tympanostomy tube

insertion for prevention of recurrent acute otitis media: results of a randomized clinical trial. *Pediatr Infect Dis J* 1992;11:278–86.

443. SCHULLER DE. Prophylaxis in otitis media in asthmatic children. *Pediatr Infect Dis J* 1983;2:280–3.

444. KARMA P *et al.* Finnish approach to the treatment of acute otitis media. Report of the Finnish Consensus Conference. *Ann Otol Rhinol Laryngol* 1987;96(suppl 129).

445. CANTEKIN EI, MANDEL EM, BLUESTONE CD *et al.* Lack of efficacy of a decongestant-antihistamine combination for otitis media with effusion in children. *N Engl J Med* 1983;308:297.

446. DRAPER WL. Secretory otitis media in children. *Laryngoscope* 1967;67:636–53.

447. GIEBINK GS. Epidemiology of otitis media with effusion. In Bess FH, ed. *Hearing Impairment in Children* Parikton, MD: York Press; 1988;75–90.

448. SCHACHEM PA, PAPARELLA MM, SANO J, LAMEY S. A histopathological study of the relationship between otitis media and mastoiditis. *Laryngoscope* 1991;101:1050–5.

449. PAPARELLA MM, SCHACHERN PA, SONO S. Clinical and pathological correlates of silent (subclinical) otitis media: new data. In Lim DJ, Bluestone CD, Klein JO, Nelson JD, *et al.*, eds. *Recent Advances in Otitis Media. Proceedings of the Fifth International Symposium*. Hamilton: Decker Periodicals; Canada 1993:319–22.

450. DJERIC D. Neuropathy of the facial nerve in COM without associated facial paralysis. *Eur Arch Otorhinolaryngol* 1990;247:232–6.

451. ABDELHAMID MM, PAPARELLA MM, SCHACHERN PA *et al.* Histopathology of the tensor tympani muscle in otitis media. *Eur Arch Otorhinolaryngol* 1990;248:71–8.

452. SPANDOW O, ANNIKO M, HELLSTROM S. Inner ear disturbance following inoculation of endotoxin into the middle ear. *Acta Otolaryngol (Stockh)* 1989;107:90–6.

453. IKEDA K, MORIZONO T. Changes of the permeability of the round window membrane in otitis media. *Arch Otolaryngol Head Neck Surg* 1988;114:895–7.

454. RAHKO T, KARMA P, SIPILA M. Sensorineural hearing loss and acute otitis media in children. *Acta Otolaryngol (Stockh)* 1989;108:107–12.

455. MORIZONO T, GIEBINK G, PAPARELLA MM *et al.* Sensorineural hearing loss in experimental purulent otitis media due to *Streptococcus pneumoniae Arch Otolaryngol* III 1985;794–8.

456. GRUNDFAST KM, BLUESTONE CD. Sudden or fluctuating hearing loss and vertigo in children due to *Streptococcus pneumoniae. Arch Otolaryngol* III 1985;794–8.

457. BLUESTONE CD, KLEIN JO. Complications and sequelae: intratemporal. In *Otitis Media in Infants and Children* chapter 9. Philadelphia: WB Saunders; 1988;203–47.

458. PODOSHIN L, FRADIS M, DAVID JB. Ototoxicity of ear drops in patients suffering from chronic otitis media. *J Laryngol Otol* 1989;103:46–50.

459. BROWNING GG, GATEHOUSE S, CALDER IT. Medical management of active chronic otitis media: a controlled study. *J Laryngol Otol* 1988;102:491–5.

460. TURNER AL, REYNOLDS EE. *Intracranial Pyogenic Diseases* Edinburgh: Oliver and Boyd; 1931.

461. FEIGIN RD. Bacterial meningitis beyond the neonatal period. In Feigin RD, Cherry JD, eds. *Textbook of Pediatric Infectious Diseases*. Philadelphia: WB Saunders; 1981;(I):293–308.

462. KESSLER L, DIETZMANN K, KRISH A. Beitrag zur otogenen Meningitis. *Z Laryn Rhinol-Otol* 1970;49:93–100.

463. WILLIAMS MA. Head and neck findings in paediatric acquired immune deficiency syndrome. *Laryngoscope* 97(6):713–16.

464. DESAI SD. Seropositivity, adenoid hypertrophy and secretory otitis media in adults – a recognized clinical entity. *Otolaryngol Head Neck Surg* 1992;107 (6 pt 1):755–7.

465. BARNETT ED, KLEIN JO, PELTON SI, LUGINBUHL LM. Otitis media in children born to human immunodeficiency virus-infected mothers. *Pediatr Inf Dis J* 1992;11:360–4.

466. PARK S, WUNDERLICH H, GOLDENBERG RA, MARSHALL M. *Pneumocystis carinii* infection in the middle ear. *Arch Otolaryngol Head Neck Surg* 1992;118(3):269–70.

467. GHERMAN CR, WARD PR, BASSIS ML. *Pneumocystis carinii* otitis media and mastoiditis as the initial manifestation of the acquired immune deficiency syndrome. *Am J Med* 1988;85(2):250–7.

468. MORRIS MS, PRASAD S. Otologic disease in the acquired immune deficiency syndrome. *ENT J* 1990;69:451–3.

469. SMITH ME, CANALIS RF. Otologic manifestations of AIDS: the otocyphitis connection. *Laryngoscope* 1989;99:365–72.

470. CHANDRASEKHAR SS, SIVEAL V, SEKHAR HK. Histopathologic and ultrastructural change in the temporal bone of HIV-infected adults. *Am J Otol* 13(8):207–14, 1992.

471. POOLE MD, POSTMA D, COHEN MS. Pyogenic otorhinologic infections in acquired immune deficiency syndrome. *Arch Otolaryngol* 1984;110(2):130–1.

26 Respiratory infections associated with foreign travel

C. M. PARRY* and A. D. HARRIES†

*Wellcome Trust Clinical Research Unit, Centre for Tropical Diseases, Cho Quan Hospital, Ho Chi Minh City, Vietnam, and John Radcliffe Hospital, Oxford, UK †Queen Elizabeth Central Hospital, Blantyre, Malawi, Central Africa

Introduction

International travel has become an established feature of modern life. Tourists from developed countries sunbathe on tropical beaches and trek on adventurous expeditions. Businessmen search for new trade opportunities and aid workers visit remote corners of the globe. Visitors to such tropical locations may expose themselves to unusual pathogens, including pathogens with long incubation periods whose symptoms can appear after the traveller returns home.

The wide availability of intercontinental travel has also encouraged immigrants from all parts of the world to come to developed countries, searching for political and economic security. They, in turn, may bring with them illnesses rarely if ever seen by physicians practising in temperate areas.

The purpose of this chapter is to highlight the important bacterial, parasitic and fungal infections which should be considered in the differential diagnosis of respiratory infections in the returning traveller and incoming immigrant.

Bacterial infections

Melioidosis

Melioidosis was first described in 1911 in Rangoon, Burma[1]. The post-mortem of a 10-year-old 'morphia' addict who died of pneumonia showed a 'cheesy' consolidation of the lung and subcutaneous abscesses on the legs. *Burkholderia pseudomallei* (formerly *Pseudomonas pseudomallei*) was cultured from the lung tissue. Since this first report, melioidosis has been recognised to be highly prevalent in Southeast Asia and Northern Australia[2] with additional sporadic cases in the Indian sub-continent, Africa, the West Indies and South and Central America. A few individuals appear to have acquired their infection in the Western Hemisphere in Georgia, California and Mexico[2,3].

B. pseudomallei is an aerobic, motile, free-living, Gram-negative bacillus found widely in soil and surface water in endemic areas. Infection in humans is acquired by contact with contaminated soil and water through skin abrasions or by inhalation of infectious dust particles. The infection occurs in endemic areas throughout the year but particularly during the rainy season[4,5]. The organism can infect animals, such as rats, sheep, goats and horses, but animal to human transmission has not been documented. Transmission of the organism can occur in the laboratory and in hospital[6–8]. Nosocomial spread via urinary catheters and endoscopes has been described. A case of human to human transmission has occurred by venereal transmission[9].

Serological surveys using indirect haemagglutination indicate that the infection is widespread in endemic areas but usually asymptomatic[4,10]. Between the ages of 1 and 4 exposure may occur at a rate of 25% per year[11]. The organism can also remain dormant in infected individuals, reactivating at a later date. The incubation period of clinical melioidosis can therefore vary from a few days to as long as 25 years. Soldiers, travellers and immigrants, for example, have developed the disease many years after returning from endemic areas[12–14]. Immune status appears to be a factor influencing reactivation. Melioidosis is associated with conditions in which immunity is depressed particularly diabetes mellitus and chronic renal failure but also cirrhosis, pregnancy, splenectomy, corticosteroid administration and intercurrent illness[5,15].

The clinical presentation of melioidosis is varied. An acute, subacute or chronic localised infection may progress sometimes to septicaemia. The patient may have a pyrexia of unknown origin with no localising signs. Alteratively an acute overwhelming septicaemia may be the primary event, usually with a high mortality. Localised infection is the presentation in about 40% of cases, either as an acute suppurative or chronic granulomatous process, and the respiratory tract is frequently involved. Symptoms are of fever, chest pain, weight loss and the sputum may be bloodstained. Nodular or patchy upper lobe shadowing with cavitation can be seen on the chest X-ray with, less commonly, pleural effusions or an empyema[16–22]. In the septicaemic illness, high fever and widespread subcutaneous abscesses are associated with a miliary pattern or multiple nodular lesions on the chest X-ray and abscesses in liver and spleen[5].

The pulmonary form of the disease must be distinguished from pulmonary tuberculosis, fungal infections, other pyogenic causes of lung abscess and non-infectious causes of pulmonary cavitation such as Wegener's granulomatosis and malignancy.

Physicians and microbiologists need to be alert to this condition as it is easily misdiagnosed[13,14,22]. *Pseudomonas* species or non-fermentative Gram-negative bacilli may be reported when *Burkholderia pseudomallei* is actually present in clinical specimens. The organism can be isolated from blood, sputum, skin pustules, abscess material and urine. Bone marrow cultures are useful if blood cultures are negative[23]. A careful search of Gram's-stained pus may reveal scanty numbers of small Gram-negative rods with bipolar 'safety-pin' staining (Fig. 26.1). The paucity of organisms in smears of melioidosis lesions contrasts with the large number of organisms from cavities due to *Staphylococcus aureus*, enterobacteriaceae or anaerobes. This may provide a clue to the diagnosis in a patient from an endemic area. The organism grows well on most media forming colonies which become dry and wrinkled with a distinctive earthy smell after several days incubation. A selective medium is available to aid isolation from contaminated specimens[24]. The organism is oxidase positive, gentamicin and colistin resistant and identified by its biochemical reactions and by agglutination with specific antiserum. Rapid diagnosis of melioidosis by immunofluorescence microscopy of clinical specimens and antigen detection in urine by ELISA or latex agglutination appear promising[25–27]. Histopathology of lung biopsy or other biopsy specimens will show focal necrotising suppuration or granuloma formation not specific for melioidosis. A Gram's stain of a touch preparation of the biopsy may give the diagnosis[28].

Indirect haemagglutination (IHA) is the most widely used serological test for diagnosis. An antibody titre >1:40 is generally considered to indicate infection. In endemic areas, however, titres from 1:40 to 1:160 are frequently found in healthy people or patients with other illnesses, and different serological criteria are required for diagnosis and management[29]. Titres of <1:80 are unlikely to signify infection in the absence of other evidence. Titres of 1:80 to 1:320 are suggestive of infection and should prompt a search for intra-abdominal abscesses or deep seated lesions. Infection is likely and empirical antibiotic therapy should be given for titres greater than 1:320. A fourfold or greater rise of titre in paired sera is diagnostic. IgG and IgM may be measured by ELISA or indirect immunofluorescence. IgG persists for long periods even after inapparent disease. IgM levels may reflect disease activity initially but not with relapse[30].

B. pseudomallei is resistant to penicillin, ampicillin, second generation cephalosporins, and some aminoglycosides. It is sensitive *in vitro* to co-trimoxazole, chloramphenicol, tetracycline and kanamycin. Conventional treatment in Southeast Asia usually involves a combination of one or more of these antibiotics. The septicaemic form of melioidosis, however, fails to respond to such chemotherapy. Newer antibiotics, such as ceftazidime, piperacillin and amoxycillin-clavulanic acid show reasonable *in vitro* activity against the organism although fluoroquinolones are insufficiently active at achievable serum levels[31–33]. A study in patients with septicaemia showed that parenteral ceftazidime (120 mg/kg/day in three divided doses) for a minimum of seven days followed by oral amoxycillin–clavulanic acid reduced mortality in comparison with conventional treatment by 50%[34,35]. The combination of co-trimoxazole and parenteral ceftazidime is probably as effective as ceftazidime alone but may reduce the possibility of resistance emerging during treatment[36,37]. In patients with the disease in developed countries, either of these may well prove to be the current recommended regimen. Other regimens used for the antimicrobial therapy of melioidosis are in Table 26.1. The carbapenems such as imipenem–cilastatin are very promising *in vitro*, but the results of clinical studies are awaited. Relapse may occur after treatment with conventional regimens so that treatment for 2 to 4 months is often necessary. Surgical drainage or resection of cavities is occasionally required.

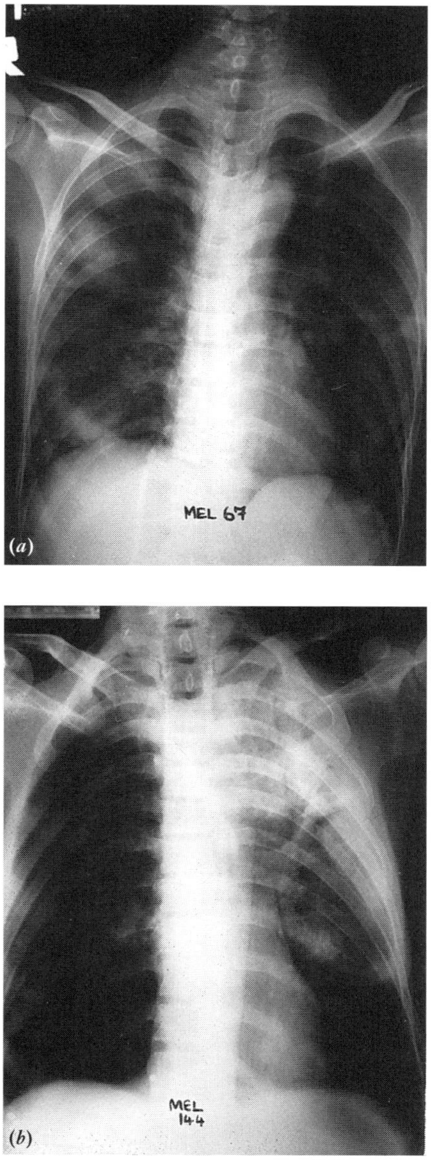

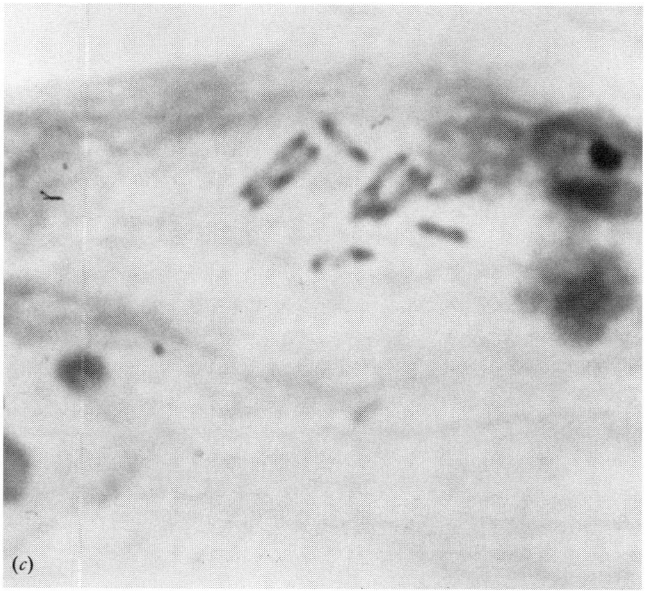

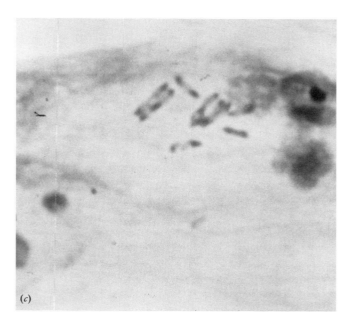

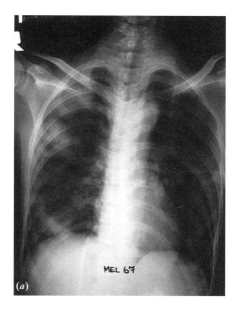

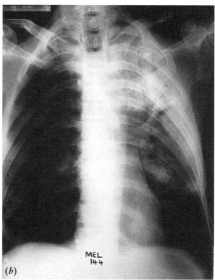

FIGURE 26.1 Gram's stain of *Burkholderia pseudomallei* showing bipolar staining. Chest X-ray of melioidosis. (Courtesy of Professor N.J. White.)

Table 26.1. *Regimens used for antimicrobial treatment of melioidosis*[b]

	Dose in mg/kg/day	(Max dose)
Agent	Septicaemic[a]	Non-septicaemic[b]
Conventional		
Chloramphenicol	100–150 (12 g/day)	50–100
Doxycycline	4–6 (400 mg/day)	4–6
Tetracycline	50 (4–6 g/day)	50
Kanamycin	20–30 (4 g/day)	–
Trimethoprim-sulphamethoxazole[c]	8–12 (800 mg/day)	4–8
Novobiocin	40–60 (6 g/day)	–
New		
Ceftazidime	150 (6–8 g/day)	–
Piperacillin	200 (16 g/day)	–
Amoxycillin–clavulanic acid	150 (7.2 g/day)	–
Imipenem-cilastatin[d]	50 (3 g/day)	–

[a]Two or three agents are combined during the septicaemic period, and treatment is rapidly tapered with clinical improvement. New agents are used singly or combined with trimethoprim-sulphamethoxazole.

[b]For the non-septicaemic period, an oral agent is used singly for a minimum of two months.

[c]Trimethoprim dose is shown.

[d]Imipenem dose is shown.

The long incubation period of the disease means that melioidosis can be easily imported to Western countries. Among healthy US army personnel who had resided for 6–12 months in endemic areas in Vietnam, 1–2% had significant antibody titres to *B. pseudomallei* and could therefore be at risk of developing overt disease[38]. Melioidosis should be considered in patients with pulmonary infection and an appropriate travel history. No vaccine or suitable antibiotic prophylaxis is currently availlable.

Brucellosis

Brucellosis is a worldwide disease of domestic animals. Four of the six species of *Brucella* may also infect man. These are *Brucella melitensis* which usually infects goats and sheep, *Brucella abortus* which infect cattle, *Brucella suis* usually in pigs and *Brucella canis* which normally infect dogs but only rarely man. Humans at highest risk of infection are those exposed to animal products such as butchers, slaughtermen, meat packers and meat inspectors. Transmission occurs by inhalation or by contamination of abraded skin or conjunctiva. In endemic areas such as the Mediterranean basin, the Arabian peninsula, the Indian subcontinent and parts of central and south America, farmers, vetinarians, agricultural engineers, laboratory technicians and anyone ingesting unpasteurised milk or milk products including soft cheeses are at risk. Other routes of transmission include accidental self-inoculation with live *Brucella* vaccines and possible human to human transmission by sexual contact[39].

Brucellosis may be acute, subacute or chronic in presentation. Acute brucellosis follows an incubation period of one week to several months and is characterised by fever, chills, headache, myalgia, back pain, arthralgia and generalised malaise. The subacute form often presents as a fever of unkown origin with non specific symptoms and signs. Chronic brucellosis also presents in a non-specific manner with lassitude and symptoms suggestive of a chronic fatigue syndrome. Localised involvement can occur in both acute and chronic disease and may involve the lung[40–49]. Bronchitis, lobar pneumonia, pleural effusions, hilar lymphadenopathy and pulmonary nodules have all been described. In two large studies of patients in Kuwait, respiratory symptoms were present in 17–23% of patients[50,51]. Dry cough, dyspnoea, pleuritic chest pains and a 'flu like' illness occurred usually in the first 2 weeks of the illness. Among the patients with respiratory symptoms, 38% had an abnormal chest X-ray in one of the studies but only 6% in the other. Abnormalities included consolidation, generalised and localised haziness, pleural effusions and in one patient a solitary granuloma.

The diagnosis is difficult, particularly in pneumonic illness. *Brucella* is a small, aerobic, non-motile, Gram-negative coccobacillus, slow growing and fastidious, requiring enriched media to grow. Blood cultures may be successful if the infection is due to *B. melitensis* or *B. suis* but are unlikely to be positive with *B. abortus*. Bone marrow culture may be superior to blood cultures, particularly in partially antibiotic treated patients[52]. Occasionally culture of pleural fluid, a liver or lymph node biopsy or pus from another site is positive although sputum is rarely so. If brucellosis is suspected, cultures should be kept for at least six weeks and are unlikely to become positive in the first 10 days. Castaneda's technique utilising a biphasic medium has been used to isolate *Brucella* from blood[53]. Alternative newer methods include the radiometric BACTEC blood culture system[54], the lysis-centrifugation technique[55] and the BACT/ALERT system[56].

Serological tests for *Brucella* are invaluable for diagnosis, given the difficulties with culture[57,58]. The principal tests available include the standard tube agglutination test (STA), a microagglutination test, the complement fixation test and enzyme linked immunoassays (ELISA). The STA test is often used as a screening test. In acute brucellosis the titres are almost always positive early in the course of the illness. A fourfold rise in the STA test titre or a single titre of 1:160 or greater is suggestive of past or present infection with *Brucella*[57,58]. False-negatives in the STA may be due to the prozone effect and sera must be diluted to 1:640 before it can be declared negative. Rarely false-negatives are due to blocking antibodies. False-positive results may be due to cross-reactions with *Francisella tularensis*, *Yersinia entercolitica* or *Vibrio cholerae*.

In chronic brucellosis the STA test may give low or negative results. When it is positive, the addition of 2-mercaptoethanol to the standard agglutination test inactivates the IgM antibodies allowing the detection of IgG antibodies. A titre in this test of greater than 1:160 more than a year after the onset of the disease is said to suggest persistent infection with *Brucella*, whereas if the titre is below 1:160, chronic brucellosis is unlikely[59]. High levels of IgG and IgA in the more sensitive ELISA tests after 1 year may reflect chronic or relapsed disease, particularly if the inital titres were low[60,61]. Skin tests give no additional information which cannot be obtained from serology.

Streptomycin in combination with tetracycline has been the treatment of choice, although rifampicin and tetracycline is just as effective. In acute brucellosis, oral rifampicin 600–900 mg/day plus oral doxycycline 200 mg/day for 6 weeks or oral doxycycline 200 mg/day for 6 weeks plus I/M streptomycin 1 g/day for 14 days gives cure rates of 95%[62,63]. Co-trimoxazole alone is unsatisfactory because of the high relapse rate but it may be used in combination with rifampicin, tetracycline or streptomycin. When used it should be given as three tablets twice daily for two weeks, followed by two tablets twice daily for 6 weeks. Oral doxycycline (5 mg/kg/day) or tetracycline (30 mg/kg/day) for 3 weeks combined with intramuscular gentamicin for the initial 5 days was effective in children over 8 years of age[64]. For those under 8, co-trimoxazole for three weeks combined with an initial 5 days of gentamicin was as effective. Co-trimoxazole in combination with rifampicin or gentamicin has been recommended for pregnant women[65]. Despite good *in vitro* activity, monotherapy with quinolones is unsatisfactory because of high relapse rates[66], although combination treatment with rifampicin appears promising[67]. Patients must be encouraged to complete a minimum course of six weeks therapy to prevent relapse, although in complicated brucellosis therapy may be required for several months depending on the response.

A vaccine is availlable for animal but not human use. Immunisation of herds, destruction of diseased animals, caution in working with animal products and correct ventilation in abbatoirs are important preventative measures. *Brucella* is a significant laboratory hazard and should be handled in a biological safety cabinet.

Typhoid fever

Typhoid or enteric fever is a common cause of fever worldwide. In the tropics, where sanitary conditions are poor, it is said to be the second commonest cause of fever lasting more than a few days[68]. It is caused by *Salmonella typhi*, *Salmonella paratyphi A*, *Salmonella schottmuelleri* (formerly *Salmonella paratyphi B*) and *Salmonella hirschfeldii* (formerly *Salmonella paratyphi C*). In developed countries the incidence of typhoid fever has generally remained at a low and stable level. In the USA, although domestic cases have dropped, those resulting from foreign travel have risen[69]. Between 1975 and 1984, 69% of typhoid cases in the USA were imported. The major sources were Mexico (39%) and India (14%). In England and Wales between 1981 and 1990, there were 1686 cases of typhoid fever, 70% of which were contracted in the Indian subcontinent, with 19% in Mediterranean, Middle East, Africa and the Far East[70].

Following an incubation period of 2 to 3 weeks, typhoid fever commonly presents with fever and headache. Many patients also complain of cough or upper respiratory symptoms. The presence of wheezes and crackles on auscultation may lead to a mistaken diagnosis of acute bronchitis. In three large series of cases, cough was found in 28–86% of patients, and sore throat in 6–84%[71–73]. Pneumonia in typhoid is an uncommon but serious complication, especially in children in whom it is usually bronchopneumonic in pattern. Lobar pneumonia has a reported incidence of 1–2%[74]. Other underlying diseases, such as diabetes mellitus or malignancy, may predispose to such complications. Lung abscess formation or empyema may complicate pneumonia[75–79].

The white cell count in typhoid fever is variable. Leukopenia is not a reliable finding and leukocytosis $>10 \times 10^9/l$ is found in 5–10% of African patients[80,81]. The definitive diagnostic method is blood culture, which is positive in up to 80% of cases. Organisms may also be isolated from clot culture, bone marrow culture, duodenal aspirate using enterotest capsules[82] and in the second or third week of illness from faeces and urine. Serological tests are of limited value in diagnosis The Widal test has been used for a long time, but false-negatives are common and false-positives occur in patients who have been vaccinated, who have previous exposure to other *Salmonella* infections or who have chronic liver disease.

The introduction of chloramphenicol in 1948 heralded effective treatment of typhoid fever and is still considered by some the drug of choice. Following reports of plasmid-mediated resistance to chloramphenicol in Mexico, India and South East Asia in the 1970s[83–85] amoxycillin and co-trimoxazole were introduced into areas with a high prevalence of chloramphenicol-resistant strains. They proved equal to chloramphenicol in terms of clinical efficacy and relapse[86]. Resistance patterns began to reflect the choice of agent used in an area. Where co-trimoxazole became the drug of choice, resistance to chloramphenicol fell dramatically[87]. Recent reports of multiresistant *S. typhi* strains resistant to chloramphenicol, ampicillin, trimethoprim and co-trimoxazole in Eastern India, Pakistan, South Africa and Vietnam[88–92] have cast uncertainty on the optimal antibiotic management. The newer quinolones (ciprofloxacin, ofloxacin, fleroxacin, perfloxacin) with their excellent penetration of biological fluids and tissues have proved very effective in typhoid fever[92,93]. For typhoid contracted in South and Southeast Asia a quinolone, such as ciprofloxacin 500 mg orally twice a day for 14 days, would probably be the treatment of choice[93] although in mild to moderate disease shorter courses are effective. A parenteral third-generation cephalosporin such as ceftriaxone is an alternative. The emergence of ciprofloxacin resistance in an isolate of *S. typhi* is of concern[94]. The choice of an oral antibiotic in children with multidrug-resistant typhoid is complicated by concerns about the saftey of quinolones. Quinolones can induce joint damage in experimental animals although use in children on a compassionate basis does not as yet appear to have resulted in similar problems[95]. A parenteral third-generation cephalosporin such as ceftriaxone would therefore be the first choice treatment although use of a quinolone may be justified if there is no other available alternative[95].

A live attenuated oral vaccine and injectable purified surface antigen vaccine are available for those travelling to endemic areas.

Plague

Plague is a zoonotic infection caused by the Gram-negative bacillus *Yersinia pestis*. It is endemic in Asia, Africa and the Americas as an enzootic in wild rodents. Human cases in the last decade have been reported from Tanzania, Vietnam, Brazil, Madagascar, Peru, Uganda, Bolivia, Burma, Kenya, Botswanna, India and the United States[96]. Pneumonic plague has occurred in epidemics in marmot trappers in Manchuria, and has also been recorded from Nigeria, Ghana, Ecuador and New Orleans[97]. A recent outbreak of bubonic and pneumonic plague in India received worldwide attention although doubts have been expressed about the accuracy of the diagnosis[98–100].

A wide variety of urban and sylvatic rodents form the natural animal reservoir for *Y.pestis*. Transmission between rodents occurs by flea bites or ingestion of contaminated animal tissue. The domestic black rat (*Rattus rattus*) and the brown sewer rat (*Rattus norvegicus*) are the most important reservoirs for plague transmission to humans in Africa, Asia and South America, although other rodents maintain transmission in the field. In the USA sylvatic rodents such as ground and rock squirrels and prairie dogs are important. Occasionally, transmission of infected fleas occurs between rodents and domestic cats or dogs who in turn may transmit infection to man. Normally low grade infection occurs in the wild with occasional animal deaths. At times, however, epizootic or epidemic spread erupts wiping out large numbers of animals. A sudden 'die-off' of urban rodents with dead rodents falling from the rafters of houses and warehouses may be followed by a large number of infected fleas looking for a blood meal. In this situation humans bitten by the rodent fleas become the accidental hosts and plague cases follow.

Plague is transmitted from rodents to man by the bite of fleas. The oriental rat flea *Xenopsylla cheopsis* is the commonest vector. Bubonic plague or septicaemic plague follows after an incubation period of 2–7 days. Bubonic plague is the commonest presentation of plague accounting for about three-quarters of the total number of cases. Secondary pneumonia may complicate bubonic or septicaemic plague.

Primary pneumonic plague is transmitted not by flea bite, but by inhalation of aerosol from a patient with either bubonic or septicaemic plague, secondary pneumonia and a productive cough. It usually occurs in the context of plague epidemics and overcrowding and is now less common than secondary plague pneumonia. Occasionally the plague bacillus may be inhaled directly into the lungs from dust contaminated with rodent faeces. Haemorrhage can occur into the intestinal canal in rodent plague, allowing the bacillus to be passed out in faeces contaminating the soil. Aerosol spread may also occur from plague-infected domestic cats[101].

Following an incubation period of 2 to 3 days, the onset of primary pneumonic plague is abrupt with rigors, headache and prostration. There is little to suggest the diagnosis in the early stages except for the marked discrepancy between the almost negligible physical signs and the gravity of the patients condition. Cough and dyspnoea rapidly follow with highly infectious watery blood stained sputum. In secondary pneumonic plague the respiratory symptoms are preceded by a several days of fever and often the presence of a bubo. In both, the clinical features may suggest pulmonary oedema with pleural effusions. Signs of consolidation are uncommon although the chest X-ray may show patchy bronchopneumonia, cavities or consolidation[102–106]. This is the most dangerous as well as the most directly infectious form of plague. Without treatment death usually occurs on the fourth or fifth day. Systemic disease may be complicated by shock and sub-clinical disseminated intravascular coagulation[107]. Necrotic purpuric lesions may also occur resulting in gangrene of distal extremities. Pathologically blood vessels show evidence of vasculitis, occlusion by fibrin thrombi leading to haemorrhage and necrosis[96].

In patients with extreme prostration, respiratory symptoms and watery blood stained sputum who have been in a known endemic area, pneumonic plague should be considered. Sputum microscopy using Giemsa or Wayson's stain reveal the characteristic bipolar bacilli (Fig. 26.2). A fluorescent antibody test is a rapid and specific means of making a presumptive diagnosis from clinical specimens. Isolation of the organism from blood, lymph node aspirate or sputum should only be attempted in laboratories with the appropriate containment facilities[108]. Serological tests help in making a final diagnosis and, although the result may be too late to help the patient, is useful for epidemiological confirmation.

The mortality of untreated pneumonic plague is high. An effective regimen for treating pneumonic plague is streptomycin 30 mg/kg of body weight im daily in two divided doses for 10 days. Alternatives include oral tetracycline 500 mg four times daily or chloramphenicol (particularly if there is associated plague meningitis) in an initial loading dose of 25 mg/kg iv, followed by 100 mg/kg daily in four divided doses for 10 days. It does not respond to penicillin. Although the fluoroquinolones appear effective *in vitro* and in a murine model of plague[109], there is currently no information concerning use in humans.

Health attendants and close contacts of patients with pneumonic plague need to take precautions. Patients should be kept in strict isolation. Attendants should wear masks and goggles, and should take chemoprophylaxis during the period of the patient's illness. Tetracycline 500 mg 6 hourly for 7–10 days is often recommended.

Preventive measures include surveillance of rodent populations and removal of habitats for urban and domestic rats and flea control, advising the public to avoid epizootic areas. A formalin-killed vaccine is available to those who are likely to become exposed in an endemic area or laboratory personnel working with *Y. pestis*. It gives some, but not complete, protection.

Anthrax

Anthrax is a disease of herbivores which may also cause infection in man. It has a worldwide distribution. Epizootic and enzootic anthrax has long been a problem in Iran, Turkey, Pakistan and the Sudan[110]. Animals are infected via the intestinal tract from food. Man is infected directly by contact with infected hides, wool or contaminated animal products, by the inhalation of spores into the lungs,

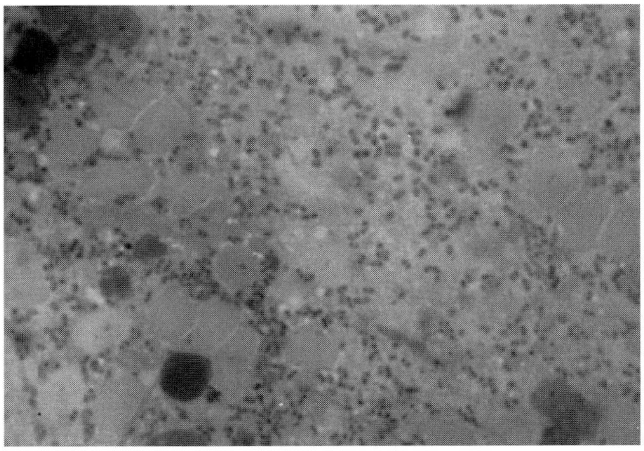

FIGURE 26.2 Methylene blue stain of *Yersinia pestis* in a bubo aspirate showing bipolar staining.

or by the ingestion of infected meat. Pulmonary anthrax was once common among workers in the textile industries of towns such as Bradford, England[111]. It is now rare in the developed world, although there have been occasional outbreaks[112,113]. Subclinical cases can occur.

Bacillus anthracis is a large, square ended, Gram-positive bacillus that sporulates under adverse condition. Virulence is related to the poly-D-glutamic acid anti-phagocytic capsule and production of a potent exotoxin which causes local oedema and necrosis[110]. In pulmonary anthrax, inhaled spores of less than 5 microns in diameter are carried to the alveoli from where they pass along the lymphatics to the mediastinal lymph nodes. In the lymph nodes the organisms multiply producing an exotoxin resulting in haemorrhagic necrosis of the thoracic lymph nodes and a haemorrhagic mediastinitis. Bacteraemia follows with secondary spread to other organs including the lungs and central nervous system[114]. Occasionally a focal haemorrhagic necrotising pneumonia occurs at the portal of entry[115].

After an incubation period of 1–5 days the illness starts with vague symptoms suggesting influenza or bronchitis. A few days later there is sudden deterioration with stridor, cyanosis, sweating, severe dyspnoea, oedema of the chest wall and neck and circulatory collapse[110,112–116]. The chest radiograph shows mediastinal widening, patchy alveolar shadowing and pleural effusions. The illness is difficult to diagnose early and may be confused with cardiac failure. Once sputum is produced, anthrax bacilli may be found by microscopy. The organism may be grown from an eschar, sputum or blood on simple or selective media. A history of inhalation exposure to animal hide products should give a clue to the diagnosis. An ELISA has been developed measuring antibodies against exotoxin components[117]. A fourfold rise in titre over a 4-week period or a single titre of greater than 1:32 is diagnostic.

Penicillin is the antibiotic of choice in a dose of one to two million units every 4 hours. The dose should be doubled if there is an associated meningitis. Chloramphenicol 1 g every 4 to 6 hours may be used in the penicillin allergic or the rare instances of penicillin resistance. Intensive care is important, although once the patient has entered the second phase of pneumonic illness, death is likely even with treatment.

Control of anthrax in animals is aided by a live, toxigenic, unencapsulated avirulent vaccine. This vaccine has not been used in humans because of concerns about its safety. A killed human anthrax vaccine derived from an exotoxin component is available and effective although requires three initial doses and recurrent booster doses. Third generation anthrax vaccines await clinical trials[110].

Tularaemia

Francisella tularensis, the bacterium that causes tularaemia, is found endemically between 30° and 70° north latitude. Cases have been reported from the USA, Scandinavian countries, Russia and Japan[118]. It is associated with wild animals, particularly squirrels and rabbits, but can also survive in water and mud for long periods. The organism is spread among animals by deerflies and ticks, or by bites. Spread to humans occurs from tick or deerfly exposure, contact with infected animals, such as during skinning or dressing and eating contaminated meat and also by inhalation. Occupations at risk include farmers, vetinarians, hunters, meat handlers and laboratory workers. Occasional minor epidemics have occurred[119,120], although human to human spread does not occur.

The organism is a tiny Gram-negative, pleomorphic coccobacillus. It grows poorly on routine media unless enriched with serum, glucose and cystine. There is a considerable risk of laboratory-acquired infection so that isolation should be restricted to reference laboratories. The organism is an facultative intracellular pathogen.

The incubation period varies between 1 and 21 days, usually 3 to 5 days. Clinical manifestations vary from asymptomatic to severe disease and death. Local growth of the organism, following a bite or contamination of skin or mucous membrane defect, leads to an ulcerated eschar and lymph node involvement. This ulceroglandular form may be complicated by bacteraemia[121]. Ingestion of the organsim can lead to pharyngitis or a 'typhoidal' form of the disease also complicated by bacteraemia. Respiratory involvement may complicate bacteraemia but may also follow inhalation[119–121]. Symptoms usually start abruptly with fever, chills, headache and a poorly productive cough with chest pain and dyspnoea. There may be radiological evidence of a bronchopneumonia, subsegmental or lobar infiltrates, apical and miliary infiltrates and hilar adenopathy. Pleural effusions are not uncommon and adult respiratory distress syndrome may be a complication. Pneumonia due to bacteraemic spread more commnly affects the lower lobes[119–122].

The diagnosis should be considered in patients with pneumonia who have had exposure to animals or arthropods in an endemic region. The presence of ulceroglandular or glandular disease may provide the clue but is not always present. Routine laboratory investigations are non-specific. Cultures of blood and lymph node pus on appropriate media may be positive but sputum is rarely so. The organism is a significant hazard to laboratory workers. A rising titre of antibodies in paired sera may be measured by agglutination, haemagglutination or ELISA and is the usual way of establishing the diagnosis[123]. A single acute titre of 1:160 or more may suggest the diagnosis but may also reflect distant infection. Antibody cross-reactions with *Brucella* spp., *Yersinia* spp. and *Proteus* OX19 may occur.

The current optimum treatment is intramuscular streptomycin 15 mg/kg twice daily for 3 days followed by 7.5 mg/kg twice daily a total of 7–14 days[118]. In children, streptomycin can be given at 40 mg/kg per day in two divided doses for 3 days followed by 20 mg/kg per day in two divided doses for the remaining 4 days. Rarely a Jarisch–Herxheimer reaction may accompany treatment. Gentamicin 3–5 mg/kg day in divided doses for 7–14 days is also effective. Tetracyclines in adults can be given as 2 g/day in divided doses for at least 14 days but may lead to higher relapse rates. Chloramphenicol can be added to streptomycin when treating meningitis. Third generation cephalosporins and fluoroquinolones are effective *in vitro* but clinical experience is currently limited. Treatment outcome is worse if treatment is delayed and in the presence of serious underlying medical disorders[124].

Avoiding exposure by wearing gloves when handling animal carcasses and cooking wild animal meat thoroughly are important methods of prevention. A live vaccine is available for those at particular risk such as laboratory workers.

Rickettsia

Louse borne typhus

This is endemic in parts of Africa, Central and South America, and Asia. The illness is caused by *Rickettsia prowazekii* acquired from the faeces of the infected body louse *Pediculus humanis corporis*. Following an incubation period of 1 week the illness develops with fever, prostration and a rash. Like typhoid fever, cough and wheeze may be part of the illness, and may on occasions lead to a mistaken diagnosis of bronchitis. Pneumonia, pleural effusion and pleurisy have been reported[125].

Scrub typhus

This has been increasingly recognised as a cause of pneumonia. It is endemic in an area that stretches from Pakistan to the Pacific Islands and Japan to North Australia. Rodents are the animal reservoir for the causative agent, *Orientia tsutsugamushi*. It is transmitted to man by the bite of a Tromboculid mite. Classically the illness commences with an eschar followed by fever, cough, rash, severe headache, myalgia and generalised lymphadenopathy. Severely ill patients may have circulatory collapse, and in untreated patients death may be associated with post-mortem changes of haemorrhagic pneumonitis and superadded bronchopneumonia[126]. In endemic areas, scrub typhus accounts for up to 20% of febrile patients admitted to hospital[127,128]. Many present with fever and non-specific symptoms. As many as 10% of scrub typhus patients have predominately chest symptoms and signs including lobar pneumonia, pleural effusion and bilateral interstitial pneumonitis[129,130].

In both louse borne and scrub typhus the peripheral leukocyte count may vary between 8 and 20×10^9/l with a neutrophilia. The diagnosis is confirmed by high or rising Weil–Felix OX-K agglutination titres and in scrub typhus, *O.tsutsugamushi* immunofluorescence antibody titres.

Typhus does not respond to penicillin, tends to relapse with erythromycin, but responds well to tetracyclines or chloramphenicol. Tetracycline is given as 25 mg/kg body weight in four divided doses, doxycycline 100 mg bd or chloramphenicol 50 mg/kg body weight for at least 7 days.

Louse borne relapsing fever

This illness, due to the spirochaete *Borrelia recurrentis*, is endemic in Ethiopia, and recent outbreaks have occurred in the Sudan, West Africa and Vietnam. The main manifestations are fever, prostration, myocarditis and liver failure. Cough and chest pain are seen in up to 50% of patients[131], although signs in the chest are rare. Pneumonia, reported in up to 5% of patients, is believed to be secondary rather than an integral part of the illness. The diagnosis is made with thick and thin blood films stained with Giemsa or Wright's stain (Fig. 26.3). Treatment is with tetracycline in a single oral dose of 0.5 g. In pregnant women and children less than 8 years old a single oral dose of 0.5 g of erythromycin should be used. A Jarisch–Herxheimer reaction may occur after the first dose of treatment.

Imported tuberculosis and drug resistance

Tuberculosis is common in developing countries. It causes substantial morbidity and mortality in Africa, Asia and parts of South America particularly in the adult working population. Globally there are estimated to be eight million new cases of tuberculosis each year. There are 2.9 million tuberculosis related deaths, more than 99% of which occur in the developing world[132]. The ease of world travel and the influx of immigrants into more affluent countries has led to an increase in imported tuberculosis.

Soon after the introduction of anti-tuberculous chemotherapy in the 1950s, the development of bacterial drug resistance was realised to be a potentially serious problem. Mutant drug-resistant bacilli, always present as a small proportion of a large bacterial population, may overgrow sensitive organisms during treatment, particularly if only one antituberculous drug is given[133]. This observation resulted in the development and use of multiple drugs to prevent the growth of resistant strains. The efficiency with which a drug prevents resistance from emerging depends on whether it can inhibit the growth of all the bacilli in the lesions all of the time. Although rifampicin and pyrazinamide are very useful in this respect, their expense often precludes their widespread use in developing countries.

Drug resistance is divided into initial drug resistance (IDR) and acquired drug resistance (ADR). ADR occurs as a result of non-compliance with a previous course of chemotherapy. IDR is, in theory, synonymous with primary drug resistance, although it may also include undisclosed acquired resistance in patients who have concealed a history of previous chemotherapy.

A world atlas of initial drug resistance was published in 1980 by the International Union against Tuberculosis[134]. Despite uncertainties concerning the reliability of data (susceptibility testing of *Mycobacterium tuberculosis* requires a high degree of laboratory skill), it was clear that high rates of initial drug resistance to isoniazid occurred in many parts of the developing world. In Thailand the levels were 52%, Egypt 34%, India 26% and Korea 24%. Much lower resistance rates were found in developed countries. In 1980 an average figure of 7% was recorded from 19 city and state laboratories in the USA; an average figure was 5% for Scotland and 3% for England and Wales[135].

An effective TB control programme will lead to a decrease in both initial and acquired drug resistance. This is well demonstrated in Birmingham, UK where a drug resistance register has been in operation since 1956[136]. Drug-resistant bacilli declined in the native born

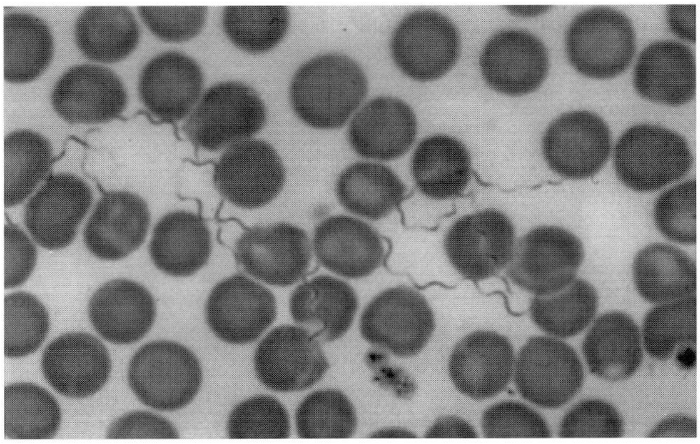

FIGURE 26.3 Blood film showing *Borrelia recurrentis*. (Courtesy of Liverpool School of Tropical Medicine.)

by 1976–1983 to 1% in males and 0.6% in females. During this period in the immigrant population the proportion of drug resistant bacilli was 5.1% for males and 6.5% for females, particularly to streptomycin and isoniazid. In Korea the introduction of improved tuberculosis control led to a fall in initial drug resistance to one or more drugs from 26% in 1965 to 15% in 1990 and acquired drug resistance from 75% in 1980 to 47% in 1990[137]. It should be noted that the reverse has occurred in some areas of the developed world in recent years. Very high levels of drug resistance have emerged particularly in areas with high rates of HIV infection, social deprivation and poor TB control programmes[138] (see Chapter 15).

The reduction in drug resistance in most of the industrialised world contrasts with an unchanged or deteriorating situation in most of the Tropics. Table 26.2 shows initial drug resistance data from selected countries. Many countries have shown an increase in IDR. Total drug resistance rose in Sierra Leone from 2.5% in 1973–77 to 11.3% in 1978–84[153]. In China, high rates of resistance to all first-line drugs have been seen in the last 30 years[154]. Initial drug resistance reflects the consequences of chemotherapy on a community. Increasing rates suggest the failure of TB control programmes. The finding of primary resistance to rifampicin in some countries, particularly in the Near East and Middle East, is worrying. It is probably related to the use of rifampicin to treat brucellosis and other conditions occurring in these areas.

Table 26.2. *Initial drug resistance to M.tuberculosis*

		Initial Drug Resistance %					
Country	Year	Total	H	S	R	E	T
Botswana [139]	77–78	11.8	7.8	0	–	–	3.9
Ghana [140]	85–87	52.6	37.0	30.0	0	0	16.0
Kenya [141]	90	14.4	10.2	1.8	0	–	–
Cote d'Ivcire [142]	89	19.9	17.0	2.0	0	0	–
India [143]	83–86	20.0	13.9	7.4	–	4.0	1.5
India [144]	88–91	19.9	10.1	7.6	3.0	2.6	–
Pakistan [145]	90s	17.0	11.0	9.0	3.0	2.0	–
Saudi Arabia [146]	86–88	11.5	9.8	1.5	3.0	0.9	–
Iran [147]	88	–	11.4	12.1	6.9	1.4	–
Turkey [148]	92	26.6	5.1	20.6	10.8	4.2	–
Indonesia [149]	84–88	13.3	9.3	8.9	0.2	0.2	–
Haiti [150]	88–89	20.0	19.0	5.0	1.0	2.0	2.0
Puerto Rico [151]	87–90	15.9	8.2	7.7	1.8	0.9	–
Latin America [152]	85–90s	16.8	6.6	11.6	1.1	0.4	2.8

H = isoniazid, S = streptomycin, R = rifampicin, E = ethambutol, T = thiacetazone.

Acquired drug resistance reflects the adequacy of antituberculous chemotherapy in individual patients. Table 26.3 shows ADR data from different areas of the world. The emergence of acquired resistance to rifampicin and the speed with which it may develop[146,155] are a cause for concern.

The reasons for high levels of drug resistance in the tropics are multifactorial (Table 26.4)[156] and the solutions difficult. Strict prescribing, improved patient compliance, well-trained health staff and improved government infrastructure should lead to a reduction in the incidence of drug resistance but are often difficult to apply in the field. The use of directly observed therapy can reduce the incidence of drug resistance in a community but is expensive. The burden of tuberculosis in developing countries will continue to strain the capacity of TB control programmes, resulting in drug-resistant tuberculosis, which may be imported into developed countries.

Parasitic infections

Paragonimiasis

Many species of *Paragonimus* occur throughout the world but only a few infect man. The three main foci of disease are: (i) the Far East, mainly China, Korea, Thailand, Taiwan, the Philippines and Japan, (ii) Africa, including Nigeria, the Cameroons, Gambia and the Congo and (iii) South America. The most important species is *Paragonimus westermani* which is found in the Far East. Paragonimiasis due to *Paragonimus kellicotti*[157] has been reported in the United States.

The life cycle is shown in Fig. 26.4. The adult fluke lives in cystic cavities in the lung where it can survive for up to 20 years. It produces ova which are released in the sputum or, if swallowed, in the patient's stool. In water the eggs hatch and release miracidia which invade certain species of snails. After about 3 months, free-swimming cercariae are released from the snail. These penetrate crustaceans where they encyst and form metacercariae. When inadequately cooked infected crustaceans or crabs are eaten, the encysted metacercariae are released in the small bowel. The young flukes penetrate the intestinal wall entering the peritoneal cavity. They undergo a long migration, eventually penetrating the diaphragm entering the pleural cavity. They cross the visceral pleura and mature in the lungs within cystic lesions.

Man is infected by eating the flesh or juices of uncooked crabs or crayfish. In Japan, raw crabs may be used in the preparation of crab soup, in Korea, the juice of raw crayfish is used as medicine for diarrhoea and in China, the stone crab is eaten alive after being immersed in wine as 'drunken crab'. The hands of cooks may become contaminated during food preparation.

The early phase of larval migration may lead to malaise, pleurisy, chest pain, an irritating cough with blood-streaked sputum and a low grade fever[158]. Eosinophilia, transient migratory soft pulmonary infiltrates, pleural effusions and pneumothoraces may be seen.

Table 26.3. *Acquired drug resistance M. tuberculosis*

		Acquired drug resistance %					
Country	Year	Total	H	S	R	E	T
Botswana[139]	77–78	70.5	70.5	27.2	–	–	25.0
Nigeria[154]	81–86	56.0	38.0	29.0	2.0	3.0	–
India[143]	86	–	55.8	26.9	37.3	–	–
Pakistan[145]	90s	36.0	30.0	12.0	15.0	9.0	–
Saudi Arabia[146]	86–88	57.6	53.7	17.9	33.7	13.7	–
Turkey[148]	92	53.4	30.0	31.9	36.2	11.2	–
Indonesia[149]	84–88	38.8	31.9	18.6	9.5	0	–
Haiti[150]	88–89	41.0	41.0	–	–	–	–
Puerto Rico[151]	87–90	33.9	22.0	18.6	13.6	6.8	–

H = isoniazid, S = streptomycin, R = rifampicin, E = ethambutol, T = thiacetazone.

Table 26.4. *Problems of drug resistance in tuberculosis*

Government	Inappropriate chemotherapy regimens
	Inadequate infrastructure for TB programmes
Pharmaceutical industry	Cost of antituberculous drugs
	Inappropriate drug combinations
Health professionals	Inappropriate prescribing habits
Patients	Poor compliance
	Self-medication

The flukes mature during the following 6 months and then begin to lay eggs. Both the adult flukes and eggs are responsible for the second phase of infection. Adult flukes found inside the bronchial lumen form 'worm cysts' or 'burrows'. The eggs excite a granulomatous response histologically resembling tuberculosis.

The onset of symptoms in this second phase is gradual with cough and haemoptysis. The sputum may be a chocolate coloured mixture of blood, inflammatory cells and *Paragonimus* eggs. Finger clubbing may develop. Complications include bronchopneumonia, lung abscesses and fibrosis[158,159]. The radiographic abnormalities are similar to those seen in pulmonary tuberculosis[158,160,161]. Ring shadows (caused by the characteristic cystic lesions), nodular lesions, diffuse or segmental infiltrates can occur. Lesions may disappear spontaneously only for new ones to appear several months later. Rarely, an empyema or bronchopleural fistula is seen. In some patients a pleural effusion is the only manifestation of infection[162,163].

In addition to the pulmonary features, flukes can migrate to ectopic sites in the skin, subcutaneous tissue, intestinal wall and peritoneum. Eggs may also enter the circulation and be carried to brain, liver and kidneys.

Eggs can be found on direct microscopy of sputum or stool and occasionally pleural fluid (Fig. 26.5). In one series of cases egg counts in sputum varied from 10^3–10^5 per day. In light infections a 24-hour collection of sputum or formol ether concentration of stool may be needed to find eggs. There is usually a mild to moderate eosinophilia.

Serological tests are useful. The ELISA is the test of choice, being highly sensitive and specific, although cross-reactions at low titre occur with hydatid disease, cysticercosis and tuberculosis.

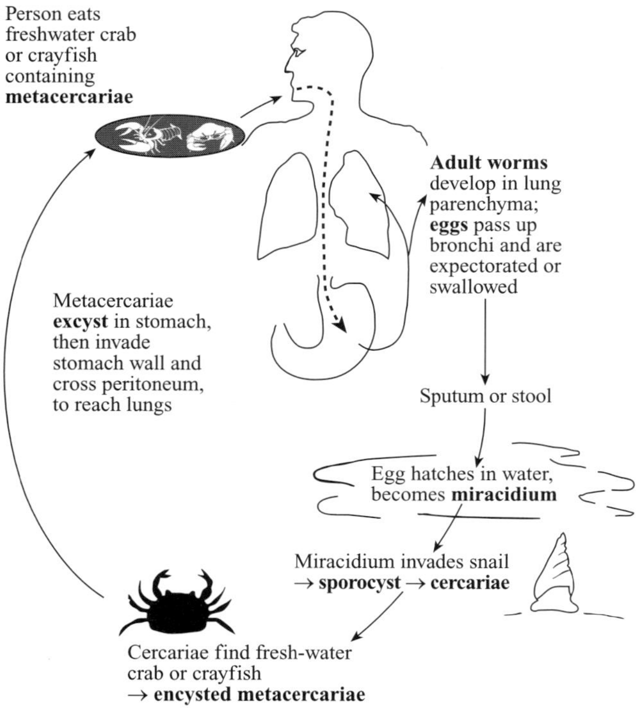

FIGURE 26.4 Schematic representation of life cycle of *Paragonimus westermani*.

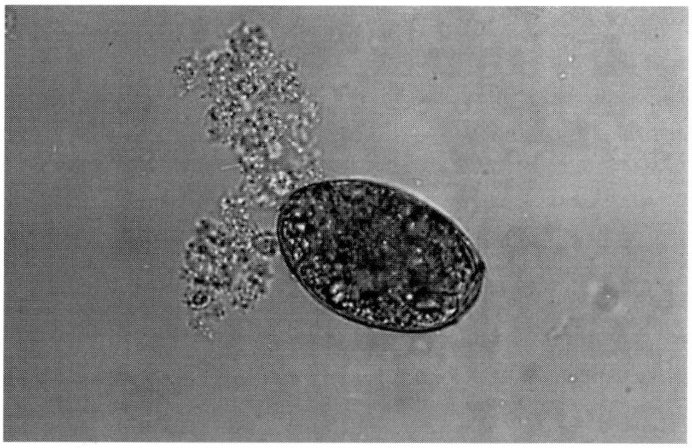

FIGURE 26.5 Egg of *Paragonimus westermani*. (Courtesy of Liverpool School of Tropical Medicine.)

The main differential diagnosis is pulmonary tuberculosis, although other conditions such as bronchiectasis, lung abscess, hydatid cyst and fungal infections should be considered.

Praziquantel is the drug of choice. A dose of 25 mg/kg taken three times a day for two days is reported to give 100% cure rate[164]. Eggs disappear 2–3 weeks after treatment with resolution of symptoms and signs. Radiographic abnormalities take several months to resolve.

Hydatid disease

Hydatid disease is a zoonosis, common in sheep-rearing countries such as Australia, New Zealand, parts of North, East and South Africa, Argentina and Southern Brazil. It also occurs sporadically in Europe, the Middle East and Asia. *Echinococcus granulosus* is maintained in dogs, sheep, goats, horses or cattle in close association with man. In Central Europe, Japan, China and Central Asia *Echinococcus multilocularis* occurs in wild canines and rodents. *Echinococcus vogelii* may be responsible for most human hydatid disease in South America[165].

The life cycle is shown in Fig. 26.6. Dogs harbour the adult *E.granulosus* in the small intestine and the worm passes eggs into the faeces. Sheep and other herbivores become infected by ingesting the taenia-like eggs on contaminated grass. After ingestion the onchospheres liberated in the gut enter the circulation and are trapped in the capillaries of certain viscera where they develop into cysts. A cyst consists of a sphere of germinal epithelium containing brood capsules and fluid. Protoscolices develop from the inner surface of the brood capsules and these can develop into daughter cysts. The daughter cysts grow within the cavity and each one may produce new brood capsules.

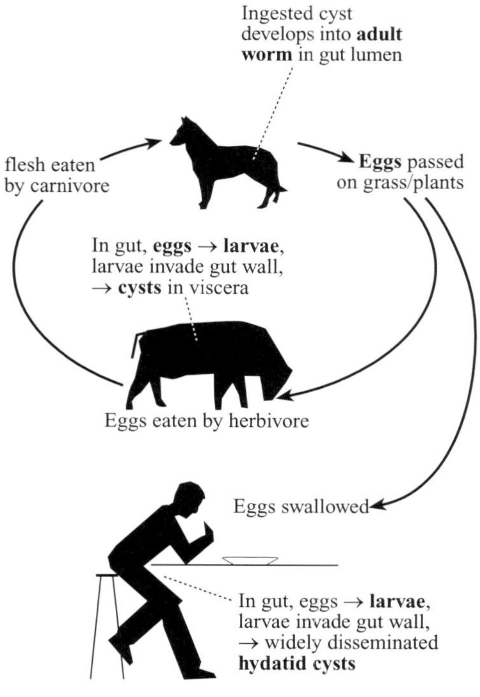

FIGURE 26.6 Schematic representation of life cycle of *Echinococcus granulosus.*

The whole structure, the 'hydatid cyst', becomes surrounded by a fibrous capsule derived of host tissue. The cyst continues to grow for years, taking on average 3 months to reach 5 mm in diameter and 6 months to reach 20 mm in diameter. Dogs, in turn, become infected by eating the contents of hydatid cysts in infected carcasses.

Man is an incidental host, infected by swallowing eggs in dog faeces. The prevalence of the disease in man is determined to a great extent by his behaviour. The highest incidence of hydatidosis in the world is found among the Turkana people living in Kenya[166]. Slaughtering of the intermediate hosts is done at home and any hydatid cysts found are fed to the dogs. This has encouraged a very high prevalence of *Echinococcus granulosus* in the large dog population. The dogs spend a lot of time in the huts, scavenging from cooking utensils left on the ground, defecating near the houses and they are allowed to clean the children of vomitus and faeces. This has resulted in an extremely high rate of infection.

The life cycle of *E. multilocularis* is similar except that the cyst produces daughter cysts by external rather than internal budding and in this way behaves like a malignant tumour. Infected foxes, other wild species of dog and wild rodents contaminate wild fruits such as strawberries, bilberries or cloudberries. Man becomes infected by eating contaminated fruit.

About 70% of cysts develop in the liver, 20% in the lungs and the remainder in other sites. The majority of cysts are found coincidentally because of radiographic investigation for unrelated symptoms. Clinical manifestations may result from the mechanical effects of the growing cyst, allergic processes due to escape of allergenic hydatid cyst fluid into the circulation, secondary bacterial infection of the cyst or cyst rupture leading to anaphylaxis. In a study from Turkey[167], one-third of patients with pulmonary hydatid were symptom-free. Their disease was diagnosed by a routine chest X-ray. In the remaining patients, cough was present in one-third, chest pain in 10% and haemoptysis in 4%. About 20% of patients may complain of coughing up pieces of ruptured membrane with a salty taste in the mouth. Lesions are bilateral in 20% of patients and multiple in 40%. The right lung is more commonly affected than the left, the lower lobe more often than the upper. Occasionally mediastinal disease occurs. Pulmonary disease due to *E. multilocularis* is less common but more aggressive than *E. granulosus*. Bronchial obstruction or bronchopulmonary fistulae are commoner complications.

In endemic areas hydatid cysts are the commonest cause of solid pulmonary shadows. They may be visualised by radiography as spherical lesions with a well defined edge and uniform density. If the cyst has ruptured a membrane may be seen floating on a fluid level, the 'water-lily' sign. Ultrasound, computed tomography or MRI scanning may also be useful[168–171] (Fig. 26.7). Direct diagnosis is only really possible if the cyst is removed at surgery. Aspiration of contents of a cyst should *not* be attempted because of the risk of leakage and anaphylaxis. The Casoni test (the injection of 0.1 ml of Seitz filtered hydatid fluid intradermally, and observation of a weal) is sensitive but not very specific and not now commonly used. Serological tests include complement fixation, haemagglutination, latex agglutination, a double diffusion test and countercurrent immuno-electrophoresis (CIE) for Arc 5 and ELISA[172–174]. The double diffusion test or CIE for Arc 5 are specific but not very sensitive and may cross-react with cystercicosis. The ELISA is more sensitive but less specific and again may cross-react with sera from patients with other cestode infections. Eosinophilia is present in less than half of patients.

Albendazole is a promising treatment for hydatid cysts. Courses of several months have been followed by disappearance of the cysts in up to 40% of cases[175–179]. A regimen of 400 mg twice a day for 4 weeks is repeated for two or three cycles, with 2-week breaks in-between. Reversible increases in liver transaminases can occur with high dose, prolonged albendazole treatment and this was the reason for the rest periods in the course of treatment. It is not clear if the rest periods are really necessary[180]. Liver function should, however, be monitored. Praziquantel is an alternative, best used peri-operatively because, although it kills the protoscolices, it does not kill the germinal epithelium of the cyst. A combination of praziquantel and albendazole may prove to be superior to either of these two agents used alone[181]. Medical treatment may be used alone, or to kill the cysts prior to surgery. Killing the cyst makes it easier to remove and also minimises the risk of spilling viable protoscolices capable of developing into new hydatids. Surgery is still probably the treatment of choice for pulmonary hydatid disease and a conservative (Cystotomy or cystectomy) or radical (lobectomy or pneumonectomy) surgical approach may be used[167,182–185].

Schistosomiasis

Human schistosomiasis is caused by flukes of the genus *Schistosoma* which live in the blood vessels of the vesical plexus around the urogenital system (*Schistosoma haematobium*), or the hepatic portal system around the gastrointestinal tract (*Schistosoma mansoni*, *Schistosoma japonicum*). Pulmonary manifestations occur as a result of the developing, migrating flukes or following chronic infection. *S. haematobium* is endemic in Africa, parts of Arabia, the Near East, Madagascar, Mauritius and a small focus in Maharashtra state, India. *S. mansoni* is widespread in Africa and Madagascar, and was exported by the slave trade to parts of South America, the Caribbean and

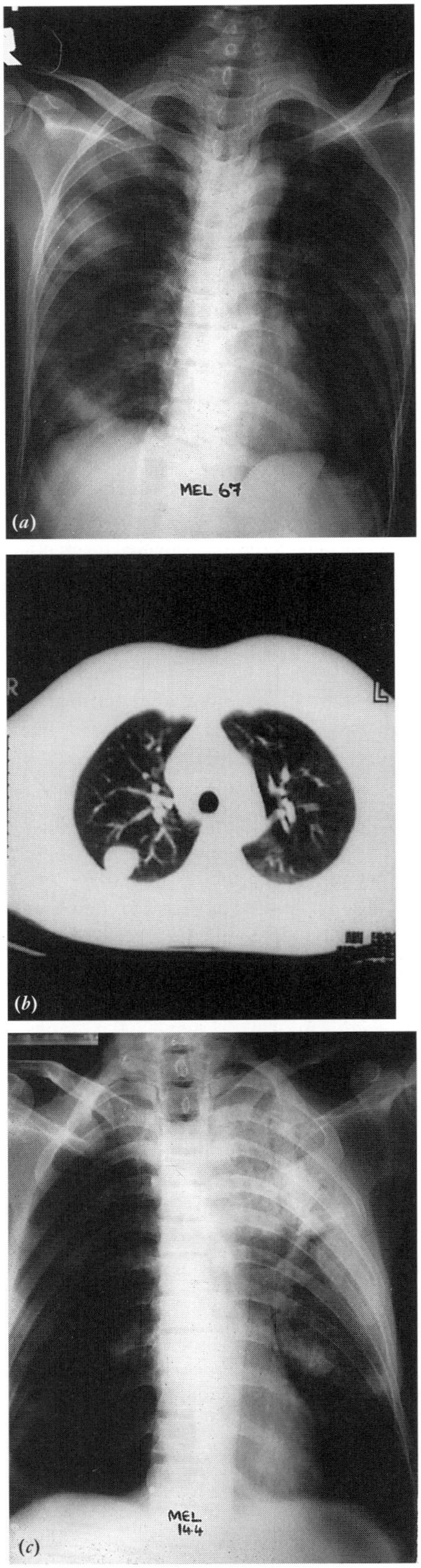

FIGURE 26.7 Chest X-ray (*a*) and CT scans (*b*) and (*c*) of a patient with pulmonary and hepatic hydatid disease.

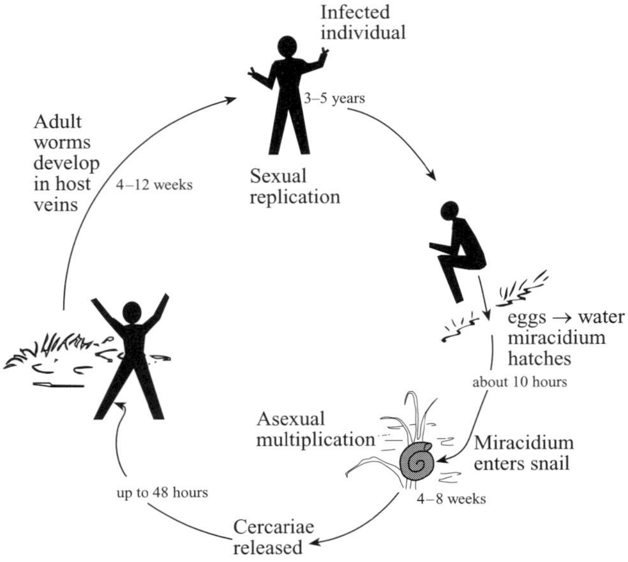

FIGURE 26.8 Schematic representation of life cycle of *Schistosome* spp.

Arabia. *S. japonicum* is the species occurring in the Orient, in China, Japan, Taiwan, the Philippines and the Celebes.

The life cycle is shown in Fig. 26.8. Fertilised female worms lay eggs in the terminal venules of the preferred host tissues. A few eggs get trapped in the tissues, where they are responsible for pathology, but most escape to the outside world via urine or faeces. In fresh water the eggs hatch to release a ciliated miracidium which penetrates the body of a suitable snail host (genus *Bulinus* for *S. haematobium*; genus *Biomphalaria* for *S. mansoni*; and genus *Oncomelania* for *S. japonicum*). Several weeks later small, fork-tailed cercariae are released from the snail and these are the infective form of the parasite. On contact with human skin, the cercaria penetrate, lose body and tail and enter the circulation as a 'schistosomule'. The shistosomule travels via the lungs to the liver, and in 4–12 weeks develops into a mature fluke in an intrahepatic portal vein. The mature females and males unite, and migrate together to reach their final habitat.

The time between infection with cercariae and the passage of eggs, the prepatent period, varies from 4–12 weeks. It tends to be shorter with *S. mansoni*, intermediate with *S. japonicum*, and longer with *S. haematobium*. The adult flukes live on average 5–8 years, although there have been instances of worms living 30 years or more.

The initial illness is an allergic larval pneumonitis occurring in non-immunes as the schistosomules migrate through the lungs. Symptoms include cough, wheeze and a peripheral eosinophilia. The diagnosis is difficult and usually only retrospective. No ova are present because the flukes have not reached maturity, and serological tests are negative. A history of water exposure in an endemic area, skin itching after bathing (cercarial dermatitis) may provide a clue. The illness is transient and treatment at this stage is ineffective.

The next phase of the illness usually starts 4 or more weeks after the initial infection. It is sometimes called Katayama fever, after the prefecture in Japan where it used to be common. The syndrome is most common with *S. japonicum*, occurs with *S. mansoni* but is extremely rarely seen with *S. haematobium*. The illness usually follows first exposure to the flukes, particularly in persons from non-endemic areas encountering the infection in endemic areas. It is rarely seen in persons, including children, from endemic areas. The reasons for this are not entirely clear, but may be because children are primed *in utero* with 'schistosomal antigen' from mothers infected during pregnancy[186].

Acute schistosomiasis, Katayama fever, is usually seen in immigrants, travellers or visitors to endemic areas. In the last decade there have been a number of reports of acute schistosomiasis in visitors, predominately to sub-Saharan Africa[187–9], and in indigenous people exposed for the first time to infected water[190]. Many patients had fever, diarrhoea, cough and urticaria in association with eosinophilia. The cough is often dry, persistent and associated with expiratory wheezing. In a study from Puerto Rico of 26 patients with acute schistosomiasis[191], 65% of subjects suffered from cough and this symptom was most often seen in patients with more severe illness.

There is strong evidence to suggest that the illness is a generalised immune complex disease occurring as the female worm starts to lay eggs which allows soluble antigen to leak out of the eggs into the circulation[191,192]. The duration of illness varies and in severe cases can be 2–3 months. Spontaneous recovery often occurs which may be related to a restoration of antigen/antibody balance as the infection matures and antibody production increases. Heavy primary infection can be fatal as it was in the Second World War in West Africa and still is in immigrant labour on large irrigation schemes in the Sudan. How common Katayama fever is in non-immune visitors to the Tropics is not established. In one study, cough and associated symptoms such as arthralgia and fever were found in about 5% of infected persons[192].

Almost all patients with Katayama fever will, at some stage of the illness, have a peripheral blood eosinophilia and also an elevated serum alkaline phosphatase as a result of granulomatous deposits around schistosomal eggs laid in the liver. Eggs of *S. mansoni* and *S. japonicum* (depending on the geographical exposure) may be found in stool specimens or from rectal snips (Fig. 26.9). In the initial phase of the illness eggs may be absent and a repeated search is necessary. Serology is very useful, and an ELISA using soluble egg antigen is both sensitive and specific.

Praziquantel in a dose 40 mg/kg as a single dose, possibly repeated after one month, is the treatment of choice for *S. mansoni* and *S. haematobium* and 20 mg/kg in three doses for 1 day for *S. japonicum* and *Schistosoma mekongi*. There is some evidence that the drug has reduced activity against immature flukes, and for this reason it is better to wait until eggs have been found before commencing treatment. The clinical state of patients may significantly deteriorate after chemotherapy. They can become more febrile and generally

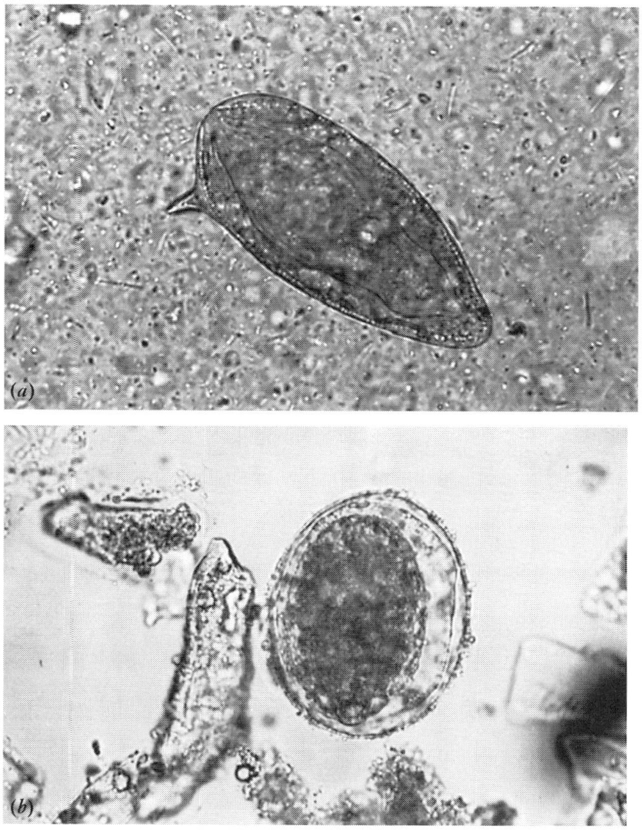

FIGURE 26.9 Eggs of *Schistosoma mansoni* (*a*) and *Schistosoma japonicum* (*b*).

unwell[193], possibly the result of a massive release of antigen from killed flukes. The administration of corticosteroids in this situation or prior administration of corticosteroids in very toxic patients may be beneficial and life saving[193,194].

Schistosomal cor pulmonale is confined to indigenous inhabitants of endemic regions who have had prolonged and heavy infection. It is seen in all three schistosome infections but is more common with *S. mansoni* and *S. japonicum*. Ova or adult worms bypass the portal system in established hepatosplenic schistosomiasis and reach the systemic circulation. As they pass through the lungs they become trapped in the small pulmonary arterioles. A granulomatous reaction follows leading to obliterative endarteritis, pulmonary hypertension and cor pulmonale. Eggs may also penetrate the wall of pulmonary arterioles, and cause a parenchymatous foreign body reaction. The clinical manifestations include chronic bronchitis, bronchiectasis and emphysema[195]. Eggs are occasionally coughed up in the sputum. The diagnosis depends on finding characteristic eggs in sputum, bronchial washings, transbronchial biopsy, stool or rectal snips. A liver biopsy will usually show characteristic Symmer's pipestem fibrosis. Treatment is with conventional anti-schistosomal drugs, but the response is variable depending on how much reversible fibrosis is present in pulmonary arterioles and lung parenchyma.

Migration phase of intestinal helminthiasis

A number of intestinal helminths may cause transient pulmonary symptoms, often with associated eosinophilia, as a result of the passage of larvae through the lungs during their developement.

Ascaris lumbricoides

Ascaris lumbricoides (roundworm) is widespread in Asia, Central and South America, Africa, and also parts of Europe and North America. Infection is acquired from the ingestion of eggs from contaminated soil or vegetables. The rhabditiform larvae hatch in the small intestine, penetrate the mucosa entering the bloodstream, reaching the lungs via the right heart. In the lungs they escape through the alveolar wall, migrate up the trachea and are swallowed down the oesophagus. The worms reach maturity in the small intestine. The first passage of ova in the stool occurs about 60–70 days after infection. *Ascaris suum*, acquired from pigs, can also invade man and give rise to pulmonary manifestations[196].

The passage of the larvae through the lungs results both in local damage and effects secondary to the non-specific and specific host response. In general, the intensity of the host pulmonary reaction is proportional to the number of *Ascaris* larvae passing through the lungs. Inflammatory infiltrates, granulomas, alveolar exudates or peribronchial infiltration can occur. Pathologically focal areas of fibrinous and eosinophilic exudative pneumonia have been documented. Seasonal attacks of *Ascaris* pneumonia have occurred in Saudi Arabia following the onset of the spring rains and the restarting of transmission[146,147].

About 1 to 2 weeks after infection patients develop clinical symptoms. The illness is usually brief, lasting less than 5 days with cough, dyspnoea and substernal discomfort being the main symptoms. There may be a mild elevation of temperature, wheezes and crackles on auscultation and radiographic signs of discrete, soft, bilateral densities. Both restrictive and obstructive abnormalities of pulmonary function have been found. *Ascaris* larvae and eosinophils may be found in sputum or gastric washings[196,197]. There is a marked eosinophilia, elevated levels of IgE and detectable antibodies to *Ascaris*. No ova are found in the stool in the acute pulmonary illness.

The pulmonary illness is self-limiting and usually needs no treatment. If symptoms are severe, however, there will be a dramatic response to corticosteroids[197]. Antihelminthics (mebendazole 100 mg bd for 3 days or albendazole 400 mg daily for 1 or 2 days or invermectin 200 μg/kg for one or two doses) may be usefully given when ova are produced in the stool 2 to 3 months later. Occasionally an adult worm migrates up the oesophagus. The worm may be vomited or aspirated leading to a secondary pneumonia[198].

Hookworm

There are two main species of hookworm. *Necator americanus* predominates in West, Central and Southern Africa, Southern USA, Central and South America and the West Indies. *Ancyclostoma duodenale* is prevalent in Southern Europe, North Africa, Northern India, China and Japan.

Infection is normally acquired when infective filariform larvae in faecally contaminated soil penetrate the skin, migrate to the lungs passing up the trachea and down the oesophagus in order to settle in the small intestine.

At the time of lung migration, a few patients complain of a cough, occasionally with blood-stained sputum, and wheezing associated with a peripheral blood eosinophilia and transient pulmonary infiltrates[199,200]. The pulmonary manifestations are mild compared with those caused by *Ascaris*. Diagnosis and treatment are as for *Ascaris*.

Strongyloides stercoralis

Although traditionally considered a tropical disease, strongyloidiasis is now reported from almost every country in Europe and North America. It is highly prevalent in parts of Brazil, Colombia and South-East Asia. Infection usually results from skin contact with soil contaminated with infective larvae. The life cycle is very similar to hookworm infection and is shown in Fig. 26.10.

In immunocompetent individuals passage of the larvae through the lungs may cause a transient cough, wheeze and peripheral eosinophilia with transient lung infiltrates.

Immunocompromised individuals may develop a hyperinfection syndrome which, if not recognised, is frequently fatal. Patients particularly at risk include those receiving cortocosteroid or cytotoxic drugs, organ transplant recipients, patients with lymphoma, leukaemia or other underlying malignancy, those with AIDs and the malnourished. In the hyperinfection syndrome auto-infection occurs as more and more rhabditiform larvae transform into filariform larvae in the large intestine, penetrate the mucosa and migrate to the lungs. Mechanical damage of the pulmonary vessels can result in extensive intra-alveolar haemorrhages[201]. Patchy changes appear on the chest X-ray and patients may die from pulmonary haemorrhage. The commonest cause of death is bacterial septicaemia, possibly because migrating filariform larvae carry enteric bacteria from the colon into the circulation.

The diagnosis of strongyloidiaisis in immunocompetent individuals requires a high index of suspicion. Stools and samples of duodenal juice, using enterotest capsules, should be examined for rhabditiform larvae[202]. Repeated stool examination and cultures may be required. Eosinophilia is commonly found. Serology, in particular the ELISA test, is useful in screening individuals at risk of *Strongyloides* infection such as candidates for immunosuppression with a history of residence in an endemic area[203, 204]. Positive serology should be an indication for a thorough parasitological investigation aimed at the demonstration of *Strongyloides stercoralis*.

In immunocompromised patients with features suggestive of disseminated strongyloidiasis a positive ELISA or indirect immunofluorescence test may be sufficient indication for immediate treatment even if parasites cannot be found. Eosinophil counts may be low or even absent. Larvae can usually be found in abundance from sputum, urine or other specimens such as CSF, ascites and skin (Fig. 26.11).

Thiabendazole 25 mg/kg bd for 3 days , or albendazole 400 mg bd for 3–5 days are the current usual treatment options. In disseminated infection these drugs should be given for 15 days[181]. Invermectin 200 μg/kg in one or two doses is emerging as an alternative[205]. It has been effective when given in up to four doses in patients with AIDS and strongyloides[206]. Careful follow-up is of all patients is required because treatment failure and subsequent relapse may occur[207].

Other helminthic infections with pulmonary manifestations

Visceral larva migrans

Toxocariasis in man results from infection with the dog ascarid *Toxocara canis* or occasionally the cat ascarid *Toxocara catis*. The worm does not undergo normal development in man but is arrested at the larval stage. Visceral larva migrans or ocular toxocariasis may result. Puppies are the main source of infection and children are usually infected if they swallow eggs when playing in contaminated soil[208,209].

In heavy infections, miliary eosinophilic granulomas form around arrested larvae. These are most prominent in the liver, but also are found in the lung, kidneys, heart, striated muscle, brain and eye. The child becomes unwell with fever, hepatomegaly, pruritic cutaneous lesions, asthma and a chronic non-productive cough. There is usually a high peripheral eosinophilia of over 30%, hypergammaglobulinaemia and bilateral peribronchial infiltrates on the chest X-ray[209–211]. In a study from Ireland[212] in patients with moderate or high antibody titres, cough was present respectively in 57% and 83%, wheeze in 43% and 61% and pneumonia in 14% and 39%. Persistent opacities on chest X-ray were seen in a small number of patients.

The condition requires differentiation from other migrating helminthiasis. Larvae are virtually never found, and diagnosis depends on a positive ELISA[213]. Treatment with diethyl-carbamazine (2–3 mg/kg three times a day for 21 days) or thiabendazole (25 mg/kg twice daily for at least 5 days) are currently recommended.

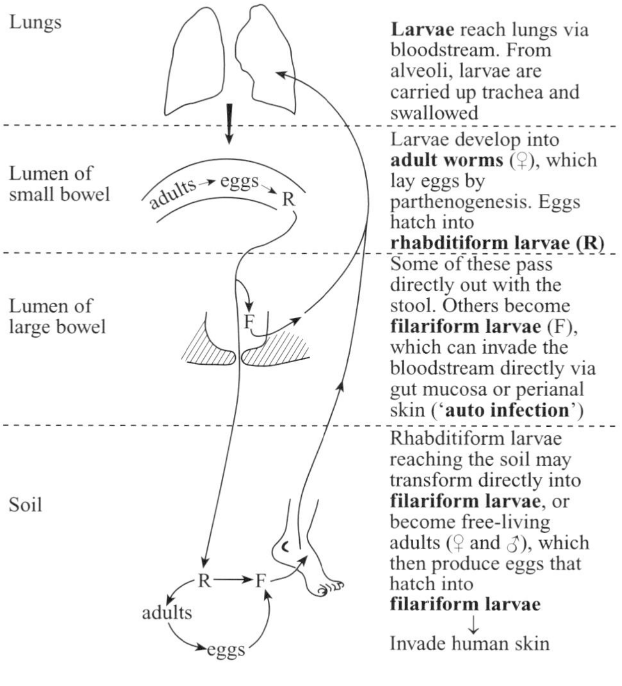

Lungs
Larvae reach lungs via bloodstream. From alveoli, larvae are carried up trachea and swallowed
Lumen of small bowel
adults
eggs
R
Larvae develop into **adult worms** (♀), which lay eggs by parthenogenesis. Eggs hatch into **rhabditiform larvae (R)**
Lumen of large bowel
F
Some of these pass directly out with the stool. Others become **filariform larvae** (F), which can invade the bloodstream directly via gut mucosa or perianal skin (‘**auto infection**’)
Soil
R
F
adults
eggs
Rhabditiform larvae reaching the soil may transform directly into **filariform larvae**, or become free-living adults (♀ and ♂), which then produce eggs that hatch into **filariform larvae**
Invade human skin

FIGURE 26.10 Schematic representation of life cycle of *Strongyloides stercoralis*.

Cutaneous larva migrans

This condition is caused by the dog or cat hookworm *Ancyclostoma brasiliense*. As it penetrates and migrates through human skin, the inflammatory reaction results in elevated, serpiginous, pruritic reddish lesions. Occasionally larvae are carried haematogenously to the lungs. A dry cough and transient migratory chest X-ray infiltrates may develop which last for 1 to 2 weeks, occasionally longer[214,215]. Blood eosinophilia is common and the syndrome is diagnosed by finding larvae, often with eosinophils in sputum. Stool examination and serology are unhelpful. The condition is usually self-limiting

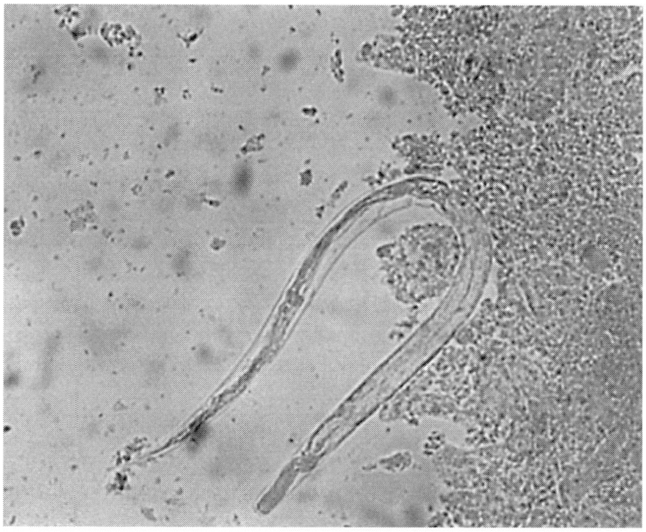

FIGURE 26.11 Unstained preparation showing a filariform larvae of *Strongyloides stercoralis* in the sputum of an African man with *Strongyloides* hyperinfection syndrome and AIDS.

and only occasionally needs treatment. Albendazole or invermectin are effective[205].

Acute fascioliasis

Fasciola hepatica is found worldwide, particularly in sheep-rearing communities. Man acquires the infection as a result of eating infected raw watercress or sucking grass on which metacercariae have encysted from contamination of water by sheep. After being swallowed, the metacercariae excyst in the small intestine, migrate through the intestinal mucosa and directly penetrate the liver. They traverse the liver parenchyma to reach the biliary system.

The acute phase of the illness, characterised by fever, tender liver and eosinophilia, resembles 'Katayama Fever'. Cough may be present and accompanied by radiographic infiltrates[216]. Eggs will not be found in the acute stage, and so the diagnosis depends on serology using an ELISA. Treatment can be tried with praziquantel (25 mg/kg three times a day for 5 days), but this is not as effective as with other fluke infections, possibly because the drug cannot penetrate the thick tegument. Bithionol (40 mg/kg on alternate days for 30 days) or emetine hydrochloride (30 mg im daily for 18 days) have been used successfully[217]. Bithionol has been regarded as the treatment of choice. Triclabendazole in a single dose of 10 mg/kg may prove to be an alternative although more experience of its use in humans is required[218].

Tropical pulmonary eosinophilia

Tropical pulmonary eosinophilia (TPE), found most commonly in South-east Asia, has also been reported from other areas where filariasis occurs such as East Africa and Brazil. The principal features of the illness are wheezing and a high peripheral eosinophilia. The disease was first described in 1939 in Indonesia[218], and its filarial origin was clarified 20–30 years later[219,220]. It is caused by occult infection with *Wuchereria bancrofti* or *Brugia* spp. which are transmitted to man by the bite of mosquitoes. TPE is the result of an immunological hypersensitivity to the microfilariae and has a genetic component as most cases are found in persons of Indian extraction. In the acute phase microfilariae are destroyed with the production of typical eosinophilic lesions (Meyer–Kouwenaar bodies) in the lung, lymph nodes and also liver and spleen. In the chronic phase lung fibrosis occurs.

Children and young adults are the most frequently affected and males more often than females[221]. The onset is gradual with fever, cough, lassitude, dyspnoea on exertion and wheezing, particularly at night. Initially there is an obstructive pulmonary picture, but this is replaced later by a more restrictive defect. In some patients, particularly in *Brugia* areas, lymphadenopathy and splenomegaly occur. Chest X-ray abnormalities, which occur in 20% of cases and may be transitory, include disseminated mottling, coarse interstitial shadowing, interstitial nodules and slight hilar lymphadenopathy.

The diagnosis of TPE should be considered in anyone with pulmonary symptoms of gradual onset from Asia and Southeast Asia. There is a high persistent eosinophilia, often $>20 \times 10^9/l$, associated with a raised ESR and elevated IgE levels. Microfilariae are absent from the peripheral blood (although are almost certainly present in the lungs). All serological tests show high antibody titres to microfilariae, and the *Dirofilaria imitis* complement fixation test is always strongly positive.

Treatment is with diethylcarbamazine (DEC). Providing irreversible fibrosis has not occurred, there is usually a rapid and complete response to DEC at a dose of 6 mg/kg per day in three divided doses given for 2–3 weeks. Radiographic changes and pulmonary function return to normal within 1–3 weeks. Bronchodilators are of value while response to treatment is awaited. About 20% of cases relapse and require repeated courses of treatment. Some have a persistent low grade alveolitis after treatment although the significance of this is not yet clear[222]. Invermectin is a possible alternative treatment currently being studied[205].

Amoebic lung infections

Entamoeba histolytica, primarily a parasite of the gastrointestinal tract, is also a rare but important cause of lung disease[223]. It has a worldwide distribution and is endemic in parts of Central and South America, South Africa, parts of North Africa, the Middle East, India and South East Asia. Amoebiasis also occurs in industrialised countries, particularly in association with institutionalised individuals, people from slum areas, immigrants from endemic areas and sexually active homosexuals. It is estimated that about one-tenth of the world's population are infected with the parasite and that there are 35–50 million symptomatic cases per year and 40–100 000 deaths[224]. Invasive disease is more prevalent and severe in crowded poor urban communities of tropical areas where there is poor sanitation and lack of hygiene.

This protozoan parasite has a life cycle with three distinct stages: trophozoite, precyst and cyst[225]. The cyst stage is the infective stage and cysts may remain viable in water for up to 4 weks. The cyst is usually ingested via faecally contaminated food, water or fingers. Occasionally transmission occurs through anal intercourse and rarely via shared colonic irrigation equipment. It passes through the stomach and excysts in the lower small bowel. Four trophozoites emerge from the cyst which then divide into eight. The trophozoites multiply and move along the intestinal canal until conditions favourable for colonisation are found, usually in the large bowel and caecal area. Once in the colon the parasite may remain a commensal, revert to the cyst form or become pathogenic with invasion of the bowel wall. The infection is usually self-limiting lasting up to 1 or 2 years although sometimes longer. Symptomless or convalescent cyst excretors are the main source of infection to others.

Both organism and host factors appear to determine invasiveness. Invasive and fulminant disease may be associated with alcoholism, malnutrition, pregnancy and immunosuppressive or cytotoxic drugs but not with HIV infection. Invasive disease may also be encouraged by concurrent helminth infection, colitis and other colonic diseases. It has been recognised for many years from epidemiological studies that *E. histolytica* may have pathogenic and non-pathogenic strains although they are morphologically indistinguishable. Investigations utilising isoenzyme analysis have shown distinct zymodemes (patterns of electrophoretic mobility of particular parasitic isoenzymes) that correlate with invasive and non-invasive infection[226,227]. DNA and antigenic analysis[225] have confirmed these clear differences between strains. It has been suggested that the non-pathogenic strains be renamed *Entamoeba dispar* and the pathogenic strains *E. histolytica*[228]. Although DNA based methods are being developed to distinguished between the two strains, they are currently only available in research laboratories[225].

The organism typically causes an ulcerative and inflammatory disease in the large bowel. When extra-intestinal invasion occurs, it is usually to the liver occasionally to the lung or peritoneum and rarely to the pericardium, brain or genitourinary system. Pleural effusions and atelectasis frequently accompany liver abscesses and do not indicate actual extension of the disease to the lung. The incidence of pleuropulmonary complications of hepatic amoebiasis has varied between 4 and 16% in different series[229]. Invasive amoebiasis is more common in men, with a male to female ratio varying between 9:1 and 15:1. People aged between 20 and 50 are most commonly affected.

Pleuropulmonary infection is almost always secondary to intestinal infection, although there have been a few isolated case reports suggesting that the organism may have been inhaled. The trophozoites migrate from intestine to lung by one of two routes. Trophozoites may invade the portal circulation and travel to the liver via the portal vein. The hepatic abscesses that can result may involve the surface of the liver, lead to the formation of adhesions between the liver and diaphragm and spread of the infection into the pleural space and lung. A perforation in the pleural space leads to an amoebic empyema and rupture into the lung can produce an abscess, consolidation or hepatobronchial fistula. Although most pleuropulmonary infection follows direct extension from an amoebic liver abscess, haemotogenous or lymphatic spread can occur rarely[231].

Amoebic liver abscesses may present acutely with a short history of malaise, fever, night sweats, anorexia, abdominal discomfort and/or pain in the right hypochondrium. Alternatively the symptoms may be more insidious with several months of ill health, weight loss or just fever. Only about 20% have a past history of dysentery and 10% will have diarrhoea at presentation. Symptoms suggesting pleuropulmonary involvement include pleuritic chest pain, right shoulder pain, hiccups or non-productive cough[230,231,234]. If the amoebic liver abscess suddenly ruptures into the chest, a tearing sensation in the chest may be followed by dyspnoea, cough or collapse. Patients who cough up chocolate-coloured 'anchovy paste', or the creamy contents of an amoebic liver abscess have a hepatobronchial fistula. Tender hepatomegaly is usual, often with a point of maximal tenderness over an intercostal space or the enlarged liver. The base of the right lung is usually dull to percussion with diminished air entry due to a raised hemi-diaphragm or accumulation of pleural fluid.

A normochromic anaemia is common. About 75% will have a leukocytosis, sometimes with band forms but generally with no eosinophilia. Liver enzymes may be elevated but can also be normal. Of patients with an amoebic liver abscess, 85–95% will have positive anti-amoeba antibodies[225]. An early negative result usually becomes positive when repeated after 7 to 10 days. The serological tests available include complement fixation, immunodiffusion, indirect fluorescent antibody (IFA), indirect haemagglutination (IHA), counter-immuno electrophoresis (CIE), enzyme-linked immunosorbent assay (ELISA) and latex agglutination. The IHA test is very sensitive, a titre of 512 is suggestive, but not diagnostic of invasive disease. Antibodies may persist after successful treatment. CIE and gel diffusion tests are usually positive for 6 to 12 months although the IHA and ELISA may remain positive for many years. A positive result from a patient in an endemic area should therefore be interpreted with caution.

Chest X-ray abnormalities are usually limited to the right side of the chest but are not diagnostic for the disease. Elevation of the right hemi-diaphragm occurs in 30–86% of cases[232]. Consolidation may be present, sometimes with cavitation in the consolidated area and pleural effusions can be variable in size. An air-containing cavity may be present under the diaphragm in the presence of a hepatobronchial fistula. Occasionally an amoebic pulmonary abscess caused by haematogenous spread may be distant from the liver. Ultrasound of the abdomen is a useful investigation and there may be various characteristic changes of a liver abscess. Usually the abscess is round or oval, has no significant wall echoes, is less echogenic than the surrounding liver parenchyma and is located peripherally. On a computed tomographic (CT) scan the liver abscess appears as a well defined rounded low density lesion with a tendency to extend beyond the surface of the liver. Isotopic liver scans, if available, show a cold abscess with a bright rim, allowing distinction from a pyogenic liver abscess, and can be positive very early in the liver disease.

Pleuropulmonary amoebiasis should therefore be considered in any patient with an unexplained right pleural effusion or consolidation in association with hepatic symptoms or signs, particularly if they have been living in an endemic area. Although the organism may be demonstrated in sputum, broncheoalveolar fluid or pleural fluid it is only found in 10% of cases and the organism is usually not found in the faeces. An US or CT scan may confirm the presence of a liver abscess and pleural effusion. Serology may be crucial for establishing the diagnosis.

Two classes of drugs are required for the treatment of invasive amoebiasis. Tissue amoebicides such as metronidazole, tinidazole, emetine, dehydroemetine and chloroquine treat the invasive parasite but luminal amoebicides such as diloxanide furoate or paromycin are required to clear the organisms from the intestinal lumen[229,235]. Metronidazole is currently considered the drug of choice for treating invasive amoebiasis. A dose of 750 mg to 800 mg three times a day, or 35–50 mg/kg/day in three divided doses in children, for 10 to 14 days is recommended. Nausea, anorexia, metallic taste and a disulfram reaction with alcohol are the common side-effects. Longer-term use may cause vertigo, ataxia and a peripheral neuropathy and an occasional transient leukopenia. Tinidazole 2 g/day in adults, 50–60 mg/kg/day in children, for 3 to 5 days is also effective. Less satisfactory and second line alternatives are emetine, dehydroemetine and chloroquine. The dose of emetine is 1 mg/kg/day to a maximum of 60 mg/day for 5 to 10 days by intramuscular or subcutaneous injection. Therapy can be repeated after 1 month. Pain and necrosis may occur at the site of injection and nausea, vomiting, diarrhoea, renal impairment, muscle aching, weakness, tenderness and stiffness have also been reported. The most important side-effects are cardiovascular with hypotension, chest pain, changes on the electrocardiogram (prolonged Q–T interval, T-wave inversion and S–T depression) and cardiac arrhythmias. These side-effects limit its use and patients should be carefully monitored if this drug is used. Dihydroemetine is a synthetic derivative of emetine which is less cardiotoxic. The dose of dehydroemetine is 1.25 mg/kg/day up to a maximum of 90 mg/day by intramuscular or subcutaneous injection.

Chloroquine has also been used, sometimes after emetine, in a dose of 600 mg base/day for 2 days followed by 300 mg base/day for 20 days. Nausea, abdominal discomfort and pruritis may occur, although the duration of treatment is usually too short for the uncommon complication of retinopathy.

Treatment with a tissue amoebicide should be followed by a luminal drug to eliminate the intestinal organism. Diloxanide furoate 500 mg three times a day or 20 mg/kg/day in three divided doses for 10 days or paromycin 25–30 mg/kg in three divided doses daily for 7 days are effective.

Large pleural effusions may require therapeutic thoracocentesis. Bronchopleural fistulae may be complicated by bacterial superinfection. An amoebic empyema is associated with a high mortality. It may be treated with anti-amoebic drugs and repeated needle aspirations, although, if the pus is thick or fails to diminish, a large bore chest tube may be required[229]. The need to resort to surgical decortication has varied in different studies.

Infection with pathogenic *E. histolytica* usually results in protective immunity and recurrent infection is rare provided the organism is eradicated from the colon. Prevention of infection requires improvements of sanitation and hygiene in endemic areas. There is currently no vaccine.

Tropical fungal infections

Although these will be covered in the section on fungal diseases, it is important to realise that fungal infections may be acquired from tropical exposure and may lead to pulmonary pathology. It is particularly important to consider these in the differential diagnosis of lung disease in immunocompromised patients who have travelled to endemic areas in the distant as well as recent past. A brief summary follows.

Sporotrichosis
This occurs in the Americas, South Africa, and China. Although usually causing cutaneous lesions, pulmonary disease (hilar lymphadenopathy, nodules, cavities) may occur.

Coccidioidomycosis
This is found in Central and South America and parts of North America. Pulmonary infiltrates and cavitation are the usual pulmonary manifestation.

Paracoccidioidomycosis
This is prevalent in Central and South America. Pulmonary manifestations include interstitial infiltrates, cavitation and hilar/mediastinal lymphadenopathy.

Blastomycosis
This is found in Central and South America and Africa with isolated reports from Israel, Saudi Arabia and India. The pulmonary features are those of an acute pneumonic illness with a small proportion going on to develop chronic pulmonary disease with infiltration and cavitation.

Table 26.5. *Problem-orientated approach*

Infections to be considered in the following circumstances
Pulmonary infiltrates with eosinophilia
Tropical pulmonary eosinophilia
Ascariasis
Toxocariasis
Hookworm
Strongyloidiasis
Schistosomiasis
Fascioliasis
Pneumonia
Anthrax
Melioidosis
Plague
Brucellosis
Typhus
Fungal infections
Acute severe respiratory illness with collapse
Anthrax
Plague
Chronic cavitating lung disease
Tuberculosis
Fungal infections
Melioidosis
Hydatid disease
Paragonimiasis
Solitary pulmonary nodule
Hydatid disease
Paragonimus
Tuberculosis
Fungal infections

Histoplasmosis
Histoplasma capsulatum is reported from more than 50 countries in temperate and tropical zones of the world; South America, Central America, the USA, Africa, India and the Far East. The pulmonary disease may be acute or chronic and similar to blastomycosis. African histoplasmosis, due to *Histoplasma dubosii*, rarely gives rise to pulmonary disease. Chronic, progressive, infiltrative and cavitatory lesions may occur with multiple abscesses usually by direct spread from clinically obvious chest lesions.

Conclusion

The diagnosis and treatment of pulmonary infections in the returning traveller or immigrant starting a new life can be challenging. A problem-orientated approach to diagnosis in such patients is provided in Table 26.5. Tables 26.6 and 26.7 summarise useful microbiological investigations which may be required. It should not be forgotten that respiratory infections in this group of patients are not solely due to

Table 26.6. *Laboratory investigations: bacterial infections*

Burkholderia pseudomallei	Microscopy	Gram's stain of sputum, pus
		Bipolar bacilli
	Culture	Sputum, blood, pus
		Non-selective and selective media
	Serology	Indirect haemagglutination
Brucella	Culture	Blood, bone marrow
		Enriched media
		Prolonged incubation
	Serology	Agglutination, CFT, ELISA
Salmonella	Culture	Blood, clot, bone marrow
		Faeces and urine in second or third week.
Yersinia pestis	Microscopy	Sputum, bubo pus
		Wayson's stain
		Bipolar bacilli
	Culture	Sputum, bubo pus
		Fluorescent antibody test
Bacillus anthracis	Microscopy	Gram's stain of sputum
	Culture	Sputum
Francisella tularensis	Serology	Agglutination, ELISA
Rickettsia prowazeckii	Serology	Weil–Felix OX-K agglutination
Rickettsia tsutsugamushi	Serology	Weil–Felix OX-K agglutination
		Immunofluorescent antibodies
Borrelia recurrentis	Microscopy	Thick and thin blood film Geimsa

Table 26.7. *Laboratory investigations: parasites*

Paragonimus	Microscopy	Sputum, stool for ova
	Serology	ELISA
Echinococcus	Microscopy	Cyst contents
	Serology	Countercurrent immune electrophoresis, complement fixation tests, ELISA
Schistosomiasis	Microscopy	Stool, rectal snips, urine, sputum for ova
	Serology	ELISA
Ascaris	Microscopy	Sputum, gastric washings for larvae
Hookworm	Microscopy	Stool for ova
Strongyloides stercoralis	Microscopy	Stool, duodenal juice (enterotest) for rhabtidiform larvae
		Repeated examination
	Culture	Stool
	Serology	ELISA
Hyperinfection syndrome	Microscopy	Stool, sputum, urine, CSF, ascites and skin for rhabtidiform larvae
Visceral larva migrans	Serology	ELISA
Cutaneous larva migrans	Sputum	Larvae
Fasciola	Serology	ELISA
Tropical pulmonary eosinophilia	Serology	Indirect haemagglutination

exotic organisms. The commonest cause of acute pneumonia in most of the tropics is *Streptococcus pneumoniae* which may be penicillin resistant. *Haemophilus influenzae* 'atypical' pneumonias and Legionnaire's disease should not be forgotten and tuberculosis remains the commonest cause of chronic pulmonary infections.

Acknowledgements

We thank Dr Malcolm Molyneux for his diagrams of the parasitic life cycles. Dr Parry is supported by the Wellcome Trust of Great Britain.

References

1. WHITMORE A, KRISHNSWAMI CS. An account of the discovery of a hitherto undescribed infectious disease occurring among the population of Rangoon. *Ind Med Gaz* 1912;47:262–7.
2. LEELARASAMEE A, BOVORNKITTI S. Melioidosis: review and update. *Rev Infect Dis* 1989;11:413–25.
3. DANCE DAB. Melioidosis: the tip of the iceberg? *Clin Microbiol Rev* 1991;4:52–60.
4. ASHDOWN LR, GAURD RW. The prevalence of human melioidosis in northern Queensland. *Am J Top Med Hyg* 1984;33:474–8.
5. CHAOGWAGUL W, WHITE NJ, DANCE DAB *et al.* Melioidosis: a major cause of community-acquired septicaemia in Northern Thailand. *J Infect Dis* 1989;159:890–9.
6. GREEN RN, TUFFNELL PG. Laboratory acquired melioidosis. *Am J Med* 1968;44:599–605.
7. ASHDOWN LR. Nosocomial infection due to *Pseudomonas pseudomallei*: two cases and an epidemiological study. *Rev Infect Dis* 1979;1:891–4.

8. SCHLECH WF III, TURCHIK JB, WESTLAKE RE JR, KLEIN GC, BAND JD, WEAVER RE. Laboratory acquired infection with *Pseudomonas pseudomallei* (melioidosis) *N Engl J Med* 1981;305:1133–5.
9. MCCORMICK JB, SEXTON DJ, MCMURRAY JG, CAREY E, HAYES P, FELDMAN RA. Human to human transmission of *Pseudomonas pseudomallei*. *Ann Intern Med* 1975;83:512–3.
10. NIGG C. Serological studies on subclinical melioidosis. *J Immunol* 1963;91:18–28.
11. KANAPHUN P, THIRAWATTASUK N, SUPUTTAMONGKOL Y *et al.* Serology and carriage of *Pseudomonas pseudomallei*: a prospective study in 1000 hospitalized children in Northeastern Thailand. *J Infect Dis* 1993;176:230–3.
12. MAYS EE, RICKETS EA. Melioidosis: recrudescence associated with bronchogenic carcinoma twenty-six years following initial geographic exposure. *Chest* 1975;68:261–3.
13. MORRISON RE, LAMB AS, CRAIG DB, JOHNSON WM. Melioidosis: a reminder. *Am J Med* 1988;84:965–7.
14. KIBBLER CC, ROBERTS CM, RIDGWAY GL, SPIRO SG. Melioidosis in a patient from Bangladesh. *Postgrad Med J* 1991;67:764–66.
15. MACKOWIAK PA, SMITH JW. Septicaemic melioidosis. Occurrence following acute influenza A six years after exposure in Vietnam. *JAMA* 1978;240:764
16. THIN RMT, BROWN M, STEWART JB, GARRETT CJ. Melioidosis: a report of ten cases. *Quart J Med* 1970;39:115–26.
17. SPOTNITZ M, RUDNITZKY J, RAMBAUD JJ. Melioidosis pneumonitis. *JAMA* 1967;202:126–30.
18. WEBER DR, DOUGLASS LE, BRUNDAGE WG, STALLKAMP TC. Acute varieties of melioidosis occurring in US soldiers in Vietnam. *Am J Med* 1969;46:234–44
19. EVERETT ED, NELSON RA. Pulmonary melioidosis: observations in thirty-nine cases. *Am Rev Resp Dis* 1975;112:331–40.
20. BATESON EM, WEBLING DD. The radiological appearances of pulmonary melioidosis. *Aust Radiol* 1981;25:239–45.
21. DHIENSIRI T, PUAPAIROJ S, SUSAENGRAT W. Roentgenonographic findings of pulmonary melioidosis: an analysis of one hundred and sixty cases. In *Abstracts of the National Workshop on Melioidosis organised by the Infectious Disease Society of Thailand and held at the Ambassador Hotel, Bangkok, 23–24 November 1985*. Bangkok: Infectious Disease Association of Thailand, 1985:61–4.
22. PUTHUCHEARY SD, PARASAKTHI N, LEE MK. Septicaemic melioidosis: a review of 50 cases from Malaysia. *Trans Roy Soc Trop Med Hyg* 1992;86:683–5.
23. DANCE DAB, WHITE NJ, SUPPUTTAMONGKOL Y, WATTANAGOON Y, WUTHIEKANUN V, CHAOWAGUL W. The use of bone marrow culture for the diagnosis of melioidosis. *Trans Roy Soc Trop Med Hyg* 1990;84:585–7.
24. ASHDOWN LR. An improved screening technique for isolation of *Pseudomonas pseudomallei* from clinical specimens. *Pathology* 1979;11:293–7.
25. SMITH MD, WUTHIEKANUM V, WALSH AL *et al.* Latex agglutination for rapid detection of *Pseudomonas pseudomallei* antigen in urine of patients with melioidosis. *J Clin Path* 1995;48:174–6.
26. DESAKORN V, SMITH MD, WUTHIEKANUM V *et al.* Detection of *Pseudomonas pseudomallei* antigen in urine for the diagnosis of melioidosis. *Am J Trop Med Hyg* 1994;51:627–33.
27. WALSH AL, SMITH MD, WUTHIEKANUM V *et al.* Immunofluorescence microscopy for the rapid diagnosis of melioidosis. *J Clin Path* 1994;47:377–9.
28. WEINBERG AN, HELLER HM. Unusual bacterial pneumonias caused by human commensal, environmental and animal associated pathogens. In Pennington JE, ed. *Respiratory Infections: Diagnosis and Management*. New York: Raven Press;1994:485–513.
29. LEELARASAMEE A. Diagnostic value of indirect haemagglutination for melioidosis in Thailand. *J Infect Dis Antimicrob Agents (Thailand)* 1985;2:213–5.
30. ASHDOWN LR, JOHNSON RW, KOEHLER JM, COONEY CA. Enzyme-linked immunosorbent assayfor the diagnosis of clinical and sub-clinical melioidosis. *J Infect Dis* 1989;160:253–60.
31. DANCE DAB, WUTHIEKANUM V, CHAOWAGUL W *et al.* The antimicrobial susceptibility of *Pseudomonas pseudomallei* emergence of resistance *in vitro* and during treatment. *J Antimicrob Chemother* 1989;24:295–309.
32. SOOKPRANEE T, SOOKPRANEE M, MELLENCAMP MA, PREHEIM LC. *Pseudomonas pseudomallei*, a common pathogen in Thailand that is resistant to the bacteriacidal effects of many antibiotics. Antimicrob Agents Chemother 1991;35:484–9.
33. SMITH MD, WUTHIEKANUM V, WALSH AL, WHITE NJ. Susceptibility of *Pseudomonas pseudomallei* to some newer beta- lactam antibiotics and antibiotic combinations using time-kill studies. *J Antimicrob Chemother* 1994;33:145–9.
34. WHITE NJ, DANCE DAB, CHAOWAGUL W, WATTANAGOON Y, WUTHIEKANUN V. PITAKWATCHARA. Halving of mortality of severe melioidosis by ceftazidime. *Lancet* 1989;ii:697–701.
35. SUPSUTTAMONGKOL Y, DANCE DAB, CHAOWAGUL W *et al.* Amoxycillin–clavulanic acid treatment of melioidosis. *Trans Roy Soc Trop Med Hyg* 1991;85:672–75.
36. SOOKRAPANEE M, BOONMA P, SUSAENGRAT W, BHURIPANYO K, PUNYAGUPTA S. Multicenter prospective randomised trial comparing ceftazidime plus co-trimoxazole with chloramphenicol plus doxycycline and co-trimoxazole for treatment of severe melioidosis. *Antimicrob Agents Chemother* 1992;36:158–62.
37. DANCE DAB, WUTHIEKANUM V, CHAOWAGUL W, SUPUTTAMONGKOL Y, WHITE NJ. Development of resistance to ceftazidime and co-amoxyclav in *Pseudomonas pseudomallei*. *J Antimicrob Chemother* 1991;28:321–4.
38. SANFORD JP, MOORE WL JR. Recrudescent melioidosis: a Southeast Asian legacy. *Am Rev Resp Dis* 1971;104:452–3.
39. RUBEN B, BAND JD, WONG P, COLVILLE J. Person-to-person transmission of *Brucella melitensis Lancet* 1991;337:14–15.
40. JOHNSON RM. Pneumonia in undulant fever: A report of three cases. *Am J Med* Sci 1935;189:483–6.
41. LAFFERTY RH, PHILLIPS CC. Pulmonary changes in patients suffering from Malta fever. *South Med J* 1937;30:595–600.
42. GREER AE. Pulmonary brucellosis. *Dis Chest* 1956;29:508–10.
43. HARVEY WA. Pulmonary brucellosis. *Ann Intern Med* 1948;28:768–81.
44. WEED LA, SLOSS PT, CLAGETT OT. Chronic localised pulmonary brucellosis. *JAMA* 1956;161:1044–7.
45. BUCHANAN TM, FABER LC, FELDMAN RA. Brucellosis in the United States, 1960–1972: an abattoir- associated disease. Part I: Clinical features and therapy. *Medicine* 1974;53:403–13.
46. CHAVEZ CA, VEACH GE. Brucellosis: localised pulmonary lesions due to *Brucella suis J Kans Med Soc* 1976;77:434–7.
47. PATEL PJ, AL-SUHAIBANI H, AL-ASKA AK, KOLAWOLE TM, AL-KASSIMI FA. The chest radiograph in brucellosis. *Clin Radiol* 1988;39:39–41.
48. GELFAND MS, KAISER AB, DALE WA. Localised brucellosis: popliteal artery aneurysm, mediastinitis, dementia and pneumonia. *Rev Infect Dis* 1989;11:783–8.
49. LUBANI MM, LULU AR, ARAJ GF, KHATEEB MI, QURTOM MAF, DUDIN KI. Pulmonary brucellosis. *Quart J Med* 1989;264:319–24.

50. MOUSA ARM. ELHAG KM, KHOGALI M, MARAFIE AA. The nature of human brucellosis in Kuwait: a study of 379 cases. *Rev Infect Dis* 1988;10:211–17.

51. LULU AR, ARAJ GF, KHATEEB MI, MUSTAFA MY, YUSUF AR, FENECH FF. Human brucellosis in Kuwait: a prospective study of 400 cases. *Quart J Med* 1988;249:39–54.

52. GOTUZZO E, CARILLO C, GUER J, LLOSA L. An evaluation of diagnostic methods for brucellosis – the value of bone marrow culture. *J Infect Dis* 1986;153:122–5.

53. CASTANEDA MR. Laboratory diagnosis of brucellosis in man. *Bull WHO* 1961;24:73–84.

54. ARNOW PM, SMARON M, ORMISTE V. Brucellosis in a group of travellers to Spain. *JAMA* 1984;251:505–7.

55. ETEMADI H, RAISSADAT A, PICKET MJ, ZAFARI Y, VAHEDIFAR P. Isolation of *Brucella* spp.from clinical specimens. *J Clin Microbiol* 1984;20:586.

56. SOLOMON HM, JACKSON D. Rapid diagnosis of *Brucella militensis* in blood: some operational characteristics of the BACT/ALERT. *J Clin Micro* 1992;30:222–4.

57. BUCHANAN TM, SULZER CR, FRIX MK, FELDMAN RA. Brucellosis in the United States, 1960–1972. An abattoir- associated disease. Part II. Diagnostic aspects. *Medicine* 1974;53:415–25.

58. YOUNG EJ. Serological diagnosis of human brucellosis: analysis of 214 cases by agglutination tests and review of the literature. *Rev Infect Dis* 1991;13:359–72.

59. BUCHANAN TM, FABER LC. 2-Mercaptoethanol *Brucella* agglutination test: usefulness for predicting recovery from brucellosis. *J Clin Microbiol* 1980;11:691–3.

60. ARAJ GF, LULU AR, MUSTAFA MY, KHATEEB MI. Evaluation of ELISA in the diagnosis of acute and chronic brucellosis in human beings. *J Hyg Camb* 1986;97:457–69.

61. ARIZA J, PELLICER T, PALLERES R, FOZ A, GUDIOL F. Specific antibody profile in human brucellosis. *Clin Infect Dis* 1992;14:131–4.

62. *Joint FAO/WHO Expert Committee on Brucellosis*. Geneva: World Health Organisation; 1986.

63. ARIZA J, GUDIOL F, PALLARES R *et al.* Treatment of human brucellosis with doxycycline plus rifampin or doxycycline plus streptomycin. A randomised double-blind study. *Ann Intern Med* 1992;117:25–30.

64. LUBANI MM, DUDKIN KI, SHARDA DC *et al.* A multi-center therepeutic study of 1100 children with brucellosis. *Paediatr Infect Dis* 1989;8:75–8.

65. YOUNG EJ. *Brucella* species. In Mandell GL, Bennett JE, Dolin R, eds. *Principles and Practice of Infectious Diseases* 4th Ed. New York, Edinburgh, London, Madrid, Melbourne, Milan, Tokyo: Churchill Livingstone; 1995:2053–60.

66. LANG R, RUBINSTEIN E. Quinolones for the treatment of brucellosis. *J Antimicrob Chemother* 1992;29:357–60.

67. AKOVA M, UZUN O, AKALIN E, HAYRAN M, UNAL S, GUR D. Quinolones in treatment of human brucellosis: comparative trial of ofloxacin–rifampin versus doxycyline–rifampin. *Antimicrob Agents Chemother* 1993;37:1831–4.

68. TYPHOID FEVER (enteric fever) In Manson-Bahr PEC, Bell DR. eds. Balliere Tindall *Mansons Tropical Diseases*. 19th Ed 1987:194–206.

69. RYAN C, HARGRETT-BEAN N, BLAKE PA. *Salmonella typhi* infections in the United States. *Rev Infect Dis* 1989;11:1–8.

70. ANON. Enteric fever in England and Wales 1981–90. *Commun Dis Rep* 1991;1:71.

71. STUART BM, PULLEN RL. Typhoid: clinical analysis of three hundred and sixty cases. *Arch Intern Med* 1946;78:629–61.

72. WALKER W. The Aberdeen typhoid outbreak of 1964. *Scot Med J* 1965;10:466–79.

73. HOFFMAN TA, RUIZ CJ, COUNTS CW *et al.* Waterborne typhoid fever in Dade County, Florida: clinical and therapeutic evaluation in 105 bacteraemic patients. *Am J Med* 1975;59:481–7

74. HUCKSTEP RL. *Typhoid Fever and other Salmonella Infections*. Edinburgh: E & S Livingstone; 1962.

75. SAPHRA I, WINTER JW. Clinical manifestations of Salmonellosis in man: an evaluation of 7779 human infections identified at the New York *Salmonella* center. *N Engl J Med* 1957;256:1128–34.

76. WEISS W, EISENBERG GM, FLIPPIN HF. *Salmonella* pleuropulmonary disease. *Am J Med* Sci 1957;233:487–96.

77. BLACK PH, KUNZ LJ, SWATZ MN. Salmonellosis – a review of some unusual aspects. *N Engl J Med* 1960;262:811–7, 864–70, 921–27.

78. ANNAMALAI A, SHREEKUMAR S, MUTHUKUMARON R. Empyema in enteric fever due to *Salmonella paratyphi B*. *Dis Chest* 1969;55:73–4.

79. MARTINEZ-VAZQUEZ JM, PAHISSA A, TORNOS A, GEMAR E, BACARDI R. Empyema due to splenic abscess in typhoid fever. *Br Med J* 1977;1:1323.

80. CHALMERS IM. Typhoid fever in an endemic area: a 'great imitator'. *S Afr Med J* 1971;45:470–2.

81. WICKS ACB, HOLMES GS, DAVIDSON L. Endemic typhoid fever: a diagnostic pitfall. *Quart J Med* 1971;40:341–54.

82. HOFFMAN SL, PUNJABI NH, ROCKHILL RC, SUTOMO A, RIVAI AR, PULUNGSIH SP. Duodenal string-capsule compared with bone-marrow, blood and rectal swab cultures for diagnosing typhoid and paratyphoid fever. *J Infect Dis* 1984;149:157–61.

83. PANIKER CK, VIMALA KN. Transferrable chloramphenicol resistance in *Salmonella typhi*. *Nature* 1972;239:109–10.

84. BUTLER T, LINH NN, ARNOLD K, POLLOCK M. Chloramphenicol-resistant typhoid fever in Vietnam associated with R factors. *Lancet* 1973;ii:983–5.

85. LAMPE PM, MANSUWAN P, DUANGMAIN C. Chloramphenicol-resistant typhoid. *Lancet* 1974;i:623–4.

86. PILLAY N, ADAMS EB, NORTH-COOMBES D. Comparative trial of amoxycillin and chloramphenicol in treatment of typhoid fever in adults. *Lancet* 1975;ii:332–4.

87. HERZOG C. Chemotherapy of typhoid fever – a review of the literature. *Infection* 1976;4:166–73.

88. THISYAKOM V, MANSUWAN P, TAYLOR D. Typhoid fever and paratyphoid fever in 192 hospitalised children in Thailand. *Am J Dis Child* 1987;141:862–5.

89. ANAND AC, KATARIA UK, SINGH W, CHATTERJEE SK. Epidemic multiresistant typhoid fever in Eastern India. *Lancet* 1990;i:352.

90. ROWE B, WARD LR, THREFALL EJ. Treatment of multiresistant typhoid fever. *Lancet* 1991;337:1422.

91. COOVADIA YM, GATHIRAM V, BHAMJEE A *et al.* An outbreak of multiresistant *Salmonella typhi* in South Africa. *Quart J Med* 1992;298:91–100.

92. HIEN TT, BETHELL DB, HOA NTT *et al.* Short course of ofloxacin for treatment of multi-drug resistant typhoid. *Clin Infect Dis* 1995;20:917–23.

93. MANDAL BK. Modern treatment of typhoid fever. *J Infect* 1991;22:1–4.

94. UMASANKAR S, WALL RA, BERGER J. A case of ciprofloxacin-resistant typhoid fever. *Commun Dis Rep* 1992;2:R139–40.

95. SCHAAD UB, WEDGWOOD J. Lack of quinolone-induced arthropathy in children. *J Antimicrob Chemother* 1992;30:414–16

96. BUTLER T. *Yersinia* species (including plague). In Mandell GR, Bennet JE, Dolin R., eds. *Principles and Practices of Infectious Diseases* Churchill Livingstone 4th Ed. 1995;2070 –8

97. PLAGUE AND MELIOIDOSIS. In Manson-Bahr PEC, Bell DR., eds. *Mansons Tropical Diseases*. Ballière Tindall 19th Ed. 1987;586–606.

98. DENNIS DT. Plague in India. *Br Med J* 1994;306:893–4

99. DAR L, THAKUR R, DAR VS. India: is it plague? *Lancet* 1994;344:1359.

100. JOHN TJ. India: is it plague? *Lancet* 1994;344:1359–60.

101. CENTERS FOR DISEASE CONTROL AND PREVENTION. Pneumonic plague – Arizona. *MMWR* 1992;268:2146–7.

102. MEYER KF. Pneumonic plague. *Bact Rev* 1961;25:249–61.

103. CONRAD FG, LECOCQ FR, KRAIN R. A recent epidemic of plague in Vietnam. *Arch Intern Med* 1968;122:193–8.

104. ALSOFROM DJ, METTLER FA JR, MANN JM. Radiographic manifestations of plague in New Mexico, 1975–1980. *Radiology* 1981;139:561–5.

105. FLORMAN AL, SPENCER RR, SHEWARD S. Multiple lung cavities in a 12-year old girl with bubonic plague, sepsis and secondary pneumonia. *Am J Med* 1986;80:1191–3.

106. CROOK LD, TEMPEST B. Plague. A clinical review of 27 cases. *Arch Intern Med* 1992;152:1253–6.

107. BUTLER T, LEVIN J, LINH NN *et al.* *Yersinia pestis* in Vietnam II. Quantitative blood cultures and detection of endotoxin in the cerebrospinal fluid of patients with meningitis. *J Infect Dis* 1976;133:493–9.

108. CHEASTY T, ROWE B. Plague: bacteriology and laboratory aspects. *PHLS Microbiol Dig* 1994;11:220–3.

109. BONACORSI SP, SCAVIZZI MR, GUIYOULE A, AMOUROUX JH, CARNIEL E. Assessment of a fluoroquinolone, three beta-lactams, two aminoglycosides, and a cycline in treatment of murine *Yersinia pestis* infection. *Antimicrob Agents Chemother* 1994;38:481–6.

110. LEW D. *Bacillus anthracis* (Anthrax). In Mandell GL, Bennett JE, Dolin R., eds. *Principles and Practice of Infectious Diseases.* Churchill Livingstone 4th Ed. 1995:1885–9.

111. LAFORCE FM. Woolsorters' disease in England. *Bull NY Acad Med* 1978;54:956–63.

112. PLOTKIN SA, BRACHMAN PS, UTELL M, BUMFORD FH, ATCHISON MM. An epidemic of inhalational anthrax, the first in the twentieth century. *Am J Med* 1960;29:992–1001.

113. SUFFIN SC, CARNES WH, KAUFMAN AF. Inhalational anthrax in a home craftsman. *Hum Pathol* 1978;9:594–7.

114. VESSAL K, YEGANEHDOUST J, DUTZ W, KOHOUT E. Radiological changes in inhalational anthrax. A report of radiological and pathological correlation in two cases. *Clin Radiol* 1975;26:471–4.

115. ABRAMOVA FA, GRINBERG LM, YAMPOLSKAYA OV, WALKER DH. Pathology of inhalational anthrax in 42 cases from the Sverdlovsk of 1979. *Proc Natl Acad Sci USA* 1993;90:2291–4.

116. BRACHMANN PS. Inhalational anthrax. *Ann NY Acad Sci*; 1980:83–93.

117. TURNBULL PC, DOGANAY M, LINDEQUE PM *et al.* Serology and anthrax in humans, livestock and Etoshosha National park Wildlife. *Epidemiol Infect* 1992;108:299–313.

118. PENN RL *Francisella tularensis* (Tularaemia) In Mandell GL, Bennett JE, Dolin R., eds. *Principles and Practice of Infectious Diseases.* Churchill Livingstone 4th Ed. 1995:2060–2068.

119. YOUNG LS, BICKNELL DS, ARCHER BG *et al.* Tularaemia epidemic: Vermont, 1968. Forty-seven cases linked to contact with muskrats. *N Engl J Med* 1969;280:1253–1260.

120. TEUTSCH SM, MARTONE WJ, BRINK EW *et al.* Pneumonic tularaemia on Martha's Vineyard. *N Engl J Med* 1979;301:826–8.

121. EVANS ME, GREGORY DW, SCHAFFNER W, MCGEE ZA. Tularaemia: a 30 year experience with 88 cases. *Medicine* 1985;64:251–69.

122. MILLER RP, BATES JH. Pleuropulmonary tularaemia. A reveiw of 29 patients. *Am Rev Resp Dis* 1969;99:31–41.

123. SATO T, FUJITA H, OHARA Y *et al.* Microagglutination test for early and specific diagnosis of tularaemia. *J Clin Microbiol* 1990;28:2372–4.

124. PENN RL, KINASEWITZ GT. Factors associated with a poor outcome in tularaemia. *Arch Intern Med* 1987;147:265–8.

125. DIAB SM, ARAJ GF, FENECH FF. Cardiovascular and pulmonary complications of epidemic typhus. *Trop Geog Med* 1989;41:76–9.

126. WIN K. Scrub typhus fever and sennetsu rickettsioses. In Weatherall DJ, Ledingham JGG, Warrell DA, eds. *Oxford Textbook of Medicine.* Oxford Medical Publications, 2nd Ed. 1987;5:353–5.

127. BROWN GW, SHIRAI A, JEGATHESEN M *et al.* Febrile illness in Malaysia – analysis of 1629 hospitalized patients. *J Trop Med Hyg* 1984;33:311–5.

128. BROWN GW, ROBINSON DM, HUXSOLL DL, NG TS, LIM KJ, SARMASEY G. Scrub typhus: a common cause of illness in indigenous populations. *Trans Roy Soc Trop Med Hyg* 1976;70:444–8.

129. EDITORIAL. Scrub typhus pneumonia. *Lancet* 1988;ii:1062.

130. CHAYKUL P, PANICH V, SILPAPOJAKUL K. Scrub typhus pneumonitis: an entity which is frequently missed. *Quart J Med* 1988;256:595–602.

131. BRYCESON ADM, PARRY EHO, PERINE PL, WARRELL DA, VUKOVICH D, LEITHEAD CS. Louse borne relapsing fever. A clinical and laboratory study of 62 cases in Ethiopia and a reconsideration of the literature. *Quart J Med* 1970;153:130–66.

132. KOCHI A. The global tuberculosis situation and the new control strategy of the World Health Organisation. *Tubercule* 1991;72:1–6.

133. MITCHESON DA. Basic mechanisms of chemotherapy. *Chest* 1979;76, suppl:771–81.

134. KLEEBERG HH, BOSHOFF MS. *A World Atlas of Initial Drug Resistance* Paris: Scientific Committee on Bacteriology and Immunology of the International Union Against Tuberculosis, 1980.

135. Editorial. Drug-resistant tuberculosis. *Br Med J* 1981;283:336–7.

136. THOMAS HE, AYRES JG. Birmingham tuberculous drug resistance register. *Tubercule* 1986, 67, 179–88.

137. KIM S, HONG Y. Drug resistance of *Mycobacterium tuberculosis* in Korea. *Tubercle Lung Dis* 1992;73:219–24.

138. FRIEDEN TR, STERLING T, PABLOS-MENDEZ, KILBURN JO, CAUTHEN GM, DOOLEY SW. The emergence of drug-resistant tuberculosis in New York City. *N Engl J Med* 1993;328:521–6.

139. NIELSEN NJ. Primary and secondary resistance of *Mycobacterium tuberculosis* Eastern Botswana. *Tubercule* 1979;60:239–43.

140. VAN DER WERF TS, GROOTHUIS DG, VAN KLINGEREN B. High initial drug resistance in pulmonary tuberculosis in Ghana. *Tubercule* 1989;70:249–55.

141. GITHUI WA, KWAMANGA D, CHAKAYA JM, KARIMI FG, WAIYAKI PG. Anti-tuberculous initial drug resistance of *Mycobacterium tuberculosis* in Kenya: a ten-year review. *E Afr Med J* 1993;70:609–12.

142. BRAUN MM, KILBURN JO, SMITHWICK RW *et al.* HIV infection and primary drug resistance to antituberculous drugs in Abidjan, Cote d'Ivoire. *AIDS* 1992;6:1327–30.

143. TRIVEDI SS, DESAI SG. Primary antituberculosis drug resistance and acquired rifampicin resistance in Gujarat, India. *Tubercule* 1988;69:37–42.

144. GUPTA PR, SINGHAL B, SHARMA TN, GUPTA RB. Prevalence of initial drug resistance in tuberculosis patients attending a chest hospital. *Ind J Med Res* 1993;97:102–3.

145. KHAN J, ISLAM N, AJANEE N, JAFRI W. Drug resistance of *Mycobacterium tuberculosis* in Karachi, Pakistan. *Trop Doct* 1993;23:13–14.

146. AL-ORAINEY IO, SAEED ES, EL-KASSIMI FA, AL-SHAREEF N. Resistance to antituberculous drugs in Riyadh, Saudi Arabia. *Tubercule* 1989;70:202–10.

147. MOHAMMADI M, MOAVEN Z, NIROUMAND-RAD I. Drug-resistant *Mycobacterium tuberculosis* in Iran. *Am Rev Resp Dis* 1990;141:A450.

148. TAHAOGLU K, KIZKIN O, TOR M, PARTAL M, SADOGLU T. High initial and acquired drug resistance in pulmonary tuberculosis in Turkey. *Tubercle Lung Dis* 1994;75:324–8.

149. HARUN M, HERAWAN Z, MARIONO A. Doctor's rush, drug resistance and treatment failure. *Am Rev Resp Dis* 1990;141:A459.

150. SCALCINI M, CARRE G, JEAN-BAPTISTE M *et al.* Antituberculous drug resistance in Central Haiti. *Am Rev Resp Dis* 1990;142:508–11.

151. GRANDES G, LOPEZ-DE-MUNAIN J, DIAZ T, RULLAN JV. Drug-resistant tuberculosis in Puerto Rico, 1987–1990. *Am Rev Resp Dis* 1993;148:6–9.

152. LASZLO A, DE KANTOR IN. A random sample survey of initial drug resistance among tuberculosis cases in Latin America. *Bull WHO* 1994;72:603–10.

153. GIBSON J. Drug resistant tuberculosis in Sierra Leone. *Tubercule* 1986;67:119–24.

154. SONG L. A review of the resistance to antituberculous drugs and the related problems during the past 30 years in China. *Am Rev Resp Dis* 1990;141:A447.

155. IDIGBE EO, DUQUE JP, JOHN EK, ANNAM O. Resistance to antituberculosis drugs in treated patients in Lagos, Nigeria. *J Trop Med Hyg* 1992;95:186–91.

156. HERSHFIELD ES. Drug resistance–response to Dr Shimao. *Tubercule* 1987;68:17–18.

157. MARIANO EG, BORJA SR, VRUNO MJ. A human infection with *Paragonimus kelicotti* (lung fluke) in the United States. Am *J Clin Path* 1986;86:204–5.

158. YANG SP, HUANG CT, CHENG CS, CHIANG LC. The clinical and roentgenologic courses of pulmonary paragonomiasis. *Dis Chest* 1959;36:494–508.

159. NWOKOLO C. Endemic paragonimus in Eastern Nigeria. *Trop Geog Med* 1972;24:138–47.

160. OGAKWU M, NWOKOLO C. Radiological findings in pulmonary paragonimiasis as seen in Nigeria: a review based on 100 cases. *Br J Radiol* 1973;46:699–705.

161. SUWANIK R, HARINSUTA C. Pulmonary paragonimiasis. An evaluation of roentgen finding in 38 positive sputum patients in an endemic area in Thailand. *Am J Roentgenol* 1959;81:236–44.

162. JOHNSON RJ, JOHNSON JR. Paragonomiasis in Indochinese refugees. Roentgonographic findings with clinical correlations. *Am Rev Resp Dis* 1983;128:534–8.

163. MINH VD, ENGLE P, GREENWOOD JR, PRENDERGAST TJ, SALNESS K, ST CLAIR R. Pleural Paragonimus in a Southeast Asian Refugee. *Am Rev Resp Dis* 1981;124:186–8.

164. JOHNSON RJ, JONG EC, DUNNING SB, CARBERRY WL, MINSHEW BH. Paragonomiasis: diagnosis and the use of praziquantel in treatment. *Rev Infect Dis* 1985;7:200–6.

165. D'ALESSANDRO A, RAUSCH RL, CUELLO C *et al. Echinococcus vogeli* in man with a review of polycystic hydatid disease in Columbia and neighbouring countries. *Am J Trop Med Hyg* 1979;28:303–17.

166. EDITORIAL. Man, dogs and hydatid disease. *Lancet* 1987;i:21–2.

167. DOGAN R, YUKSEL M, CETIN G *et al.* Surgical treatment of hydatid cysts of the lung: report on 1055 patients. Thorax 1989;44:192–9.

168. BALAKIAN JP, MUDARRIS FF. Hydatid disease of the lungs. Am J Roentgonol 1974;122:692–707.

169. BEGGS I. The radiology of hydatid disease. *Am J Roentgonol* 1985;145:639–48.

170. GOULIAMOS AD, KALIVODOURIS A, PAPAILIOU J, VLAHOS L, PAPAVASILOU. CT appearance of pulmonary hydatid disease. *Chest* 1991;100;1578–81.

171. VON-SINNER W, TE-STRAKE L, CLARK D, SHARIF H. MR imaging in hydatid disease. *Am J Roengonol* 1991;157:741–5.

172. COLTORTI EA, VARELA-DIAZ VM. Detection of antibodies against *Echinococcus granulosus* arc 5 antigens by double diffusion test. *Trans Roy Soc Trop Med Hyg* 1978;72:226–9.

173. COLTORTI EA. Standardisation and evaluation of an enzyme immunoassay as a screening test for the seroepidemiology of human hydatidosis. *Am J Trop Med Hyg* 1986;35:1000–5

174. CRAIG PS, ZEHYLE E, ROMIG T. Hydatid disease: research and control of Turkana II. The role of immunological techniques for the diagnosis of hydatid disease. *Trans Roy Soc Trop Med Hyg* 1986;80:183–92.

175. MORRIS DL, DYKES PW, DICKSON B, MARRINER SE, BOGAN JA, BURROWS FGO. Albendazole in hydatid disease. *Br Med J* 1983;286:103–4.

176. MORRIS DL, DYKES PW, MARINNER S *et al.* Albendazole – objective evidence of response in human hydatid disease. *JAMA* 1985;253:2053–7.

177. OKELO GB. A Hydatid disease: research and control in Turkana III. Albendazole in the treatment of inoperable hepatic hydatid disease in Kenya – a report of 12 cases. *Trans Roy Soc Trop Med* 1986;80:193–7.

178. HORTON RJ. Chemotherapy of *Echinococcus* infection in man with albendazole. *Trans Roy Soc Trop Med* Hyg 1989;83:97–102.

179. NAHMIAS J, GOLDSMITH R, SOIBELMAN M, EL-ON J. Three to 7 year follow-up after albendazole treatment of 68 patients with cystic echinococcus (hydatid disease). *Ann Trop Med Parasitol* 1994;88:295–304.

180. GIL-GRANDE L, RODRIQUEZ-CAABEIRO F, PRIETO JG *et al.* Randomised controlled trial of efficacy of albendazole in intra-abdominal hydatid disease. *Lancet* 1993;342:1269–72.

181. COOK GC. Review article. Antihelminthic agents: some recent developments and their clinical application. *Post Grad Med* J 1991;67:16–22.

182. XANTHAKIS D, EFTHIMIADIS M, PAPADAKIS G *et al.* Hydatid disease of the chest. Report of 91 patients surgically treated. *Thorax* 1972;27:517–28.

183. AYTAC A, YURDAKUL Y, IKZER C, OLGA R, SAYLAM A. Pulmonary hydatid disease. Report of 100 patients. *Ann Thorac Surg* 1977;23:145–51.

184. AL-OMERI M, WASIF SA. Surgical management of hydatid disease of the lung. *J Roy Coll Surg Edin* 1984;29:218–20.

185. BURGOS L, BAQUERIZO A, MUNOZ W, DE-ARETXBALA X, SOLAR C, FONSECA L. Experience in the surgical treatment of 331 patients with pulmonary hydatidosis. *J Thorac Cardiovasc Surg* 1991;102:427–30.

186. COLLEY DG. Dynamics of the human immune response to schistosomes. In *Balliere's Clinical Tropical Medicine and Communicable Diseases*. Schistosomiasis. 1987:315–32.

187. ZUIDEMA PJ. The Katayama syndrome; an outbreak in Dutch tourists to the Omo National Park, Ethiopia. *Trop Geog Med* 1981;33:30–5.

188. CHAPMAN PJC, WILKINSON PR, DAVIDSON RN. Acute schistosomiasis (Katayama fever) among British air crew. *Br Med J* 1988;297:1101.

189. FARID Z, TRABOLSI B, HAFEZ A. Acute *Schistosoma mansoni* (Katayama fever) *Am Trop Med Parasitol* 1986;80:563–4.

190. HIATT RA, SOTOMAYOR ZR, SANCHEZ G, ZAMBRANA M, KNIGHT WB. Factors in the pathogenesis of acute *Schistosoma mansoni*. *J Infect Dis* 1979;139:659–66.

191. HIATT RA, OTTESON EA, SOTOMAYOR ZR, LAWLEY TJ. Serial observations of circulating immune complexes in patients with acute schistosomiasis. *J Infect Dis* 1980;142:665–70.

192. HARRIES AD, FRYATT R, WALKER J, CHIODINI PL, BRYCESON ADM. Schistosomiasis in ex-patriots returning to Britain from the tropics: a controlled study. *Lancet* 1986;i:86–8.

193. HARRIES AD, COOK GC. Acute schistosomiasis (Katayama fever): clinical

deterioration after chemotherapy. *J Infect* 1987;14:159–61.

194. GELFAND M, CLARKE V DE V, BERNBERG H. The use of steroids in the early hypersensitivity stage of schistosomiasis. *Centr Afr J Med* 1981;27:219–21.

195. OLVEDA RM, DOMINGO EO. *Schistosoma japonicum*. In *Ballière's Clinical Tropical Medicine and Communicable Diseases.* Schistosomiasis 1987:397–417.

196. PHILLS JA, HARROLD AJ, WHITEMAN GV, PERELMUTTER L. Pulmonary infiltrates, asthma and eosinophilia due to *Ascaris suum* infestations in man. *N Engl J Med* 1972;286:965–70.

197. GELPI AP, MUSTAFA A. Seasonal pneumonitis with eosinophilia. A study of larval ascariasis in Saudi Arabia. *Am J Trop Med Hyg* 1967;16:646–57. 198.

198. GELPI AP, MUSTAFA A. *Ascaris* pneumonia. *Am J Med* 1968;44:377–89.

199. BANWELL JG, SCHAD GA. Hookworm. *Clin Gastroenterol* 1978;7:129–56.

200. NAWALINSKI TA, SCHAD GA. Arrested development in *Ancyclostoma duodenale*: course of a self induced infection in man. *Am J Trop Med Hyg* 1974;23:895–98.

201. IGRA-SIEGMAN Y, KAPILA R, SEN P, KAMINSKI ZC, LOURIA B. Syndrome of hyperinfection with *Strongyloides stercoralis*. *Rev Infect Dis* 1981;3:397–407.

202. BEAL CB, VIENS P, GRANT RG, HUGHES JM. A new technique for sampling duodenal contents. Demonstration of upper small bowel pathogens. *Am J Trop Med Hyg* 1970;19:349–52.

203. GENTA RM. Strongyloidiasis. In *Ballière's Clinical Tropical Medicine and Communicable Diseases*. Intestinal helminth infections. 1987:645–65.

204. BAILEY JW. A serological test for the diagnosis of Strongyloides antibodies in ex Far East prisoners of war. *Ann Trop Med Parasitol* 1989;83:241–7.

205. OTTESEN EA, CAMBELL WC. Invermectin in human medicine. *J Antimicrob Chemother* 1994;34:195–203.

206. TORRES JR, ISTURIZ R, MURILLO J, GUZMAN M, CONTRERAS R. Efficacy of Invermectin in the treatment of strongyloidiasis complicating AIDS. *Clin Infect Dis* 1993;17:900–2.

207. SCOWDEN EB, SCHFFNER W, STONE WJ. Overwhelming Strongyloidiasis: an unappreciated opportunistic infection. *Medicine* 1978;57:527–44.

208. HUNTLEY CC, COSTAS MC, LYERLY BS. Visceral larva migrans syndrome: Clinical characteristics and immunological studies in 51 patients. *Paediatrics* 1965;36:523–36.

209. MOK CH. Visceral larva migrans. A discussion based on review of the literature. *Clin Paediatr* 1968;7:565–73.

210. SHRAND H. Visceral larva migrans. *Toxocara canis* infection. *Lancet* 1964;i:1357–59.

211. SNYDER C. Visceral larva migrans–ten years experience. Paediatrics 1961;28:85–91.

212. TAYLOR MRH, KEANE CT, O'CONNOR P, MULVIHILL E, HOLLAND C. The expanded spectrum of Toxocaral diseases. *Lancet* 1988;i:692–4.

213. GLICKMAN L, SCHANTZ P, DOMBROSKE R *et al.* Evaluation of serodiagnostic tests for visceral larva migrans. *Am J Trop Med Hyg* 1978;27:492–8.

214. WRIGHT DO, GOLD EM. Loeffler's syndrome associated with creeping eruption (cutaneous helminthiasis): report of 26 cases. *Arch Intern Med* 1946;78:303.

215. BUTLAND RJA, COULSON IH. Pulmonary eosinophilia associated with cutaneous larva migrans. *Thorax* 1985;40:76–7

216. FLORES M, MERINO-ANGULO J, AGUIRRE ERASTI C. Pulmonary infiltrates as first sign of infection by *Fasciola hepatica*. *Eur J Resp Dis* 1982;63:231–3.

217. FARID Z, KAMAL M, WOODY J. Treatment of acute toxaemic Fascioliasis. *Trans Roy Soc Trop Med Hyg* 1988;82:299.

218. PICOT S, QUERREC M, GHEZ JL, GOULLIER–FLEURET A, GRILLOT R, AMBROISE–THOMAS P. A new report of trichlorbendazole efficacy during invading phase of fasciolasis. *Eur J Clin Microbiol Infect Dis* 1992;11:269–70.

219. MEYERS FM, KOUWENAAR W. Over hypereeosinophilie en over een merkwaardigen vorm van filiariasis. *Geneesk Tijdschr Ned-Ind* 1939;79:853–73.

220. JOE LK. Occult filiariasis: its relationship with tropical pulmonary eosinophilia. *Am J Trop Med Hyg* 1962;11:646–52.

221. BEAVER PC. Filiariasis without microfiliaraemia. *Am J Trop Med Hyg* 1970;19:181.

222. NEVA FA, OTTESEN EA. Current concepts in parasitology. Tropical (Filarial) eosinophilia. *N Engl J Med* 1978;298:1129–31.

223. OTTESEN EA, NUTMAN TB. Tropical pulmonary eosinophilia. *Annu Rev Med* 192;43:417–24.

224. WALSH JA. Problems in the recognition and diagnosis of amebiasis: estimation of the global magnitude of morbidity and mortality. *Rev Infect Dis* 1986;8:228–38.

225. RAVDIN JI. State-of-the-art clinical article. Amebiasis. *Clin Infect Dis* 1995;20:1453–66.

226. SARGEUNT PG, WILLIAMS JE, GREENE JD. The differentiation of invasive and non-invasive *Entamoeba histolytica* by isoenzyme electrophoresis. *Trans Roy Soc Trop Med Hyg* 1978;72:519–21.

227. SARGEUNT PG, WILLIAMS JD. Electrophoretic isoenzyme patterns of the pathogenic and non-pathogenic intestinal amoeba of man. *Trans Roy Soc Trop Med Hyg* 1979;73:225–7.

228. DIAMOND LS AND CLARKE CG. A redescription of *Entamoeba histolytica* Schaudinn 1903 (Emended Walker, 1911) separating it from *Entamoeba dispar* Brumpt, 1925. *J Eukaryot Microbiol* 1993;40:340–4.

229. SHARMA OP, MAHESHWARI A. Lung diseases in the tropics. Part 2: Common tropical lung diseases: diagnosis and management. *Tubercle Lung Dis* 1993;74:359–70.

230. ADAMS EB, MACLEOD IN. Invasive amoebiasis. II Amoebic liver abscess and its complications. *Medicine (Baltimore)* 1977;56:325–34.

231. RHODE FC, PRIETO O, RIVEROS O. Thoracic complications of amoebic liver abscess. *Br J Dis Chest* 1979;73:302.

232. ADEYEMO AO, ADEROUNMU A. Intrathoracic complications of amoebic liver abscess. *J Roy Sov Med* 1984;77:17–20.

234. KUBITSCHEK KR, PETERS J, NICKESON D *et al.* Amoebiasis presenting as pleuropulmonary disease. *West J Med* 1985;142:203–7.

235. RAVDIN JI, PETRI WA. *Entamoeba histolytica* (Amebiasis). In Mandell GL, Bennett JE, Dolin R, ed. *Principles and Practice of Infectious Diseases.* 4th Ed. New York, Edinburgh, London, Madrid, Melbourne, Milan, Tokyo: Churchill Livingstone; 1995;395–408.

27 Intensive care management of the critically ill patient with pneumonia

GARY MILLER

King Faisal Specialist Hospital and Research Centre, Riyadh, Saudi Arabia

Introduction

Despite the great advances in medicine this century, pneumonia remains one of the leading causes of death in industrialised countries. It currently ranks fifth among overall causes of mortality and one of the first among infectious causes[1–3]. Moreover, pneumonia is a major cause of respiratory failure in patients requiring intensive care unit admission and is one of the leading nosocomial infections in the critically ill[4–10]. In this chapter we will highlight the major categories of pneumonia syndromes managed in the intensive care unit, their pathophysiological consequences, diagnostic work-up, antimicrobial therapy, ventilatory strategies, and recent advances in the care of these patients.

Community-acquired pheumonia

Recent studies continue to provide evidence that community-acquired pneumonia remains an important cause of morbidity and mortality accounting for 3% of all hospital admissions and a mortality rate ranging from 10–25%[4–10]. Of those patients admitted to hospital with community-acquired pneumonia, 10–20% will require intensive care unit admission, among whom the mortality rate is high, ranging from 20–50% in most series. Although many of these patients who succumb from severe pneumonia have established underlying diseases, previously healthy people may also be susceptible. Factors associated with a poor prognosis include co-existent illnesses such as chronic obstructive lung disease, alcoholism, diabetes mellitus, the presence of shock, severe hypoxaemic respiratory failure, and inappropriate initial antibiotic therapy[4–10] (Table 27.1). Severe community-acquired pneumonia can be defined as 'life-threatening pneumonia acquired in a non immunosuppressed patient in the community who requires ICU admission'[11]. The proportion of patients with nosocomial pneumonia admitted to the ICU is about 20%, although the mortality rate is similar to that encountered in patients with severe community-acquired pneumonia. A recent consensus conference suggested that at least one of the following conditions justifies the definition of severe pneumonia[12].

(i) Respiratory frequency > 30 breath/min at admission.
(ii) Severe respiratory failure defined by a P_aO_2/F_iO_2 ratio of < 250.
(iii) Requirement for mechanical ventilation.
(iv) Radiological involvement of both lungs or multiple lobes or a greater than 50% increase in lung opacities within 48 hours of admission.
(v) Severe hypotension (blood pressure < 90/60 mmHg)
(vi) Vasopressor requirement for more than 4 hours.
(vii) Oliguria or acute renal failure requiring dialysis.

Criteria for ICU admission include hypoxaemic or hypercapnic respiratory failure, shock related either to sepsis or hypovolaemia, or a depressed level of consciousness. Although supportive ventilatory and haemodynamic management is similar for other causes of pneumonia, the diagnostic approach and empiric antimicrobial therapy may differ significantly.

Approximately 60% of community-acquired pneumonias are caused by common bacterial pathogens such as *Streptococcus pneumoniae*, *Staphylococcus aureus*, *Haemophilus influenzae* and Gram-negative enteric bacteria[4–12]. Atypical pneumonia especially secondary to *Legionella pneumophila* has been implicated in some series as a frequent cause of severe community-acquired pneumonia ranking second only to *S. pneumoniae*, although this has not been a universal finding and is dependent on geographical variability. In addition, other agents responsible for atypical pneumonia include *Mycoplasma pneumoniae, Chlamydia psittaci, Coxiella burnetii,* and viral agents which collectively comprise of 15–20% of severe cases of pneumonia requiring ICU admission. Aspiration pneumonia and chronic pneumonia syndromes from such agents as *Mycobacterium tuberculosis*, endemic fungi, contribute to 10% and 5% of ICU cases, respectively (Table 27.2). Most studies have only been able to isolate a specific agent in 50–70% of cases and mixed infections were reported in up to 10% of these with a positive diagnosis[4–12].

Recent studies, most of which were prospective, have all demonstrated similar findings regarding mortality rates, aetiologic agents responsible, and those factors which led to a worse outcome[7–12]. Again, mortality rates ranged from 22–42.5%, and the most common agents in all studies were *S. pneumoniae*, *L. pneumophila*, and *Staphylococcus* spp., with Gram-negative bacilli the next most common organisms. Of note, was that *M. tuberculosis* and *Pneumocystis carinii* were seen in one of the studies[7] in 11.4% and 8.5% of the cases.

Multivariate analysis identified several factors associated with a poor prognosis[7–10]. These included bacteraemia, shock, hypoxia requiring mechanical ventilation, non-pneumonia related complications, bilateral pulmonary involvement and inappropriate initial antibiotic therapy (Table 27.1).

The long term prognosis of ICU-treated community-acquired pneumonia has a favourable outlook, whereby half of those who survived the acute illness were fully recovered 1.5 to 3 years after their episode of severe pneumonia[5,13]. Clearly, intensive care therapy is a life-saving intervention in a significant number of patients who might have died from respiratory failure.

Co-morbidity

There are a number of co-morbid illnesses which have been identified as having an independent association with morbidity in patients presenting with pneumonia. These include neoplastic disease, neurological disease, immunosuppression and alcohol abuse. In patients with cancer, mortality was fivefold higher, compared to those without, and immunosuppressed patients were at least ten times more likely to have a complicated course from their pneumonia[14,15].

Pathogenesis

The major routes of microbial agents into the lung are the aspiration of oropharyngeal or gastric contents, inhalation of infected aerosols, haematogenesis spread from distant sites of infection, direct extension from adjacent tissues, or traumatic implantation.

The major pathophysiological sequelae of pneumonia is a suppurative exudate which fills the bronchi, bronchioles and adjacent alveoli resulting in maldistribution of ventilation, reduction in lung compliance and intrapulmonary shunting. Diffuse alveolar damage is usually associated with viral pneumonitis but can be seen with any type of severe pneumonia. Microscopically, hyaline membranes line alveolar walls and alveoli may be filled with proteinaceous material, sloughed alveolar lining cells, and fibrin. In other areas Type II pneumocytes indicate regenerative repair[16].

Release of proinflammatory mediators such as tumour necrosis factor, interleukin-1, interleukin-6, and other cytokines results in a myriad of systemic symptoms ranging from fever and tachycardia to septic shock and multisystem organ failure.

Physical findings

In the past, clinicians attempted to predict a 'microbiological' diagnosis on the basis of the presenting clinical data of whether the pneumonia was typical or atypical, and hence prescribe specific antimicrobial therapy. Although in some instances, clinical features can be useful in establishing a specific aetiological diagnosis, this is not possible for the majority of cases. Several studies have confirmed the unreliability of either clinical data or radiologic evaluation in providing sufficient diagnostic discrimination to permit therapeutic intervention based on this information. The presence of coexisting illnesses, and variations in virulence factors of certain pathogens may result in considerable overlap of clinical symptoms and signs.

Table 27.1. *Prognostic factors of severe community-acquired pneumonia admitted to ICU*

Anticipated demise within 5 days
Shock
Bacteraemia
Radiographical spread of pneumonia
Inappropriate initial antibiotic therapy
Non-pulmonary organ failure

Table 27.2. *Severe hospitalised community-acquired pneumonia*

Organisms
Streptococcus pneumoniae
Legionella sp.
Gram-negative bacilli
Mycoplasma pneumoniae
Respiratory viruses
Influenza A, B
Adenovirus
Varicella
RSV
Pneumocystis carinii
Mycobacterium tuberculosis
Endemic fungi

Acute bacterial pneumonia

The most common presentation of acute bacterial pneumonia is with the acute onset of fever, rigors, productive cough, dyspnoea and pleurisy. Often there is a co-morbid condition such as chronic obstructive lung disease, malignancy, alcoholism or other chronic illness. Debilitated or elderly patients may present with few notable changes including hypothermia, tachypnoea, or confusion. Physical findings compatible with consolidation are usually present with accompanying systemic signs of tachypnoea, tachycardia and fever. Radiographical features with airspace disease and air bronchograms may be seen in a lobar or diffuse pattern, although there are no specific radiological features which can differentiate between the different organisms responsible (Fig. 27.1). A PA and lateral chest X-ray is usually helpful in evaluating the severity of the process and may bring to light complicating features such as a pleural effusion or a lung abscess. An elevated leukocyte count may be present depending on the ability of the host's immune system to mount a response.

Despite extensive diagnostic testing, the pathogens responsible may only be uncovered in 50–70% of cases[3,8,17]. Routine Gram's stain and culture of sputum have shown poor sensitivity and specificity towards isolation of the pathogen responsible.

Invasive studies to obtain specimens uncontaminated by upper airway flora such as bronchoscopy with a protected specimen brush, bronchoalveolar lavage, and direct needle aspiration of the lung are not indicated in most patients but may be useful in critically ill patients, as they have a good sensitivity and specificity for identifying the aetiological agent if the patients have not been previously treated with antibiotics and if performed properly in a facility where the laboratory is experienced in processing such specimens.

In critically ill patients, routine laboratory assessment should include a CBC, renal, hepatic, and coagulation studies, as well as arterial blood gas analysis. This is important to determine if more than one system is involved, which has prognostic implications and may lead to earlier intubation and ventilation if deemed appropriate.

Blood cultures should be collected and patients with pleural effusions should have a diagnostic thoracentesis. Serological analysis for antibodies to *Legionella*, *Mycoplasma*, *Chlamydia*, and viruses, and subsequent complement fixation antibody titres to look for a fourfold rise should be taken if clinically indicated. Urine antigen detection for *Legionella* and *S. pneumonia* are easy to perform and may provide useful information (Table 27.3).

S. pneumonia and *L. pneumophila* are the most common pathogens causing pneumonia in patients requiring ICU admission. Gram-negative bacilli are usually seen only in those patients with comorbid conditions such as diabetes mellitus, COPD and alcoholism. In most ICU studies, *H. influenzae*, *S. aureus* and Gram-negative enteric bacteria were more commonly found than in ordinary hospital wards. Patients suffering from cystic fibrosis or bronchiectasis have a predilection for *Pseudomonas aeruginosa* infecting their lungs. Sporadic cases of viral, fungal, protozoal, rickettsial, tuberculosis and mixed infections have also been recognised.

It is impossible to cover all pathogens responsible for severe pneumonia and hence the choice of antimicrobial therapy should be based

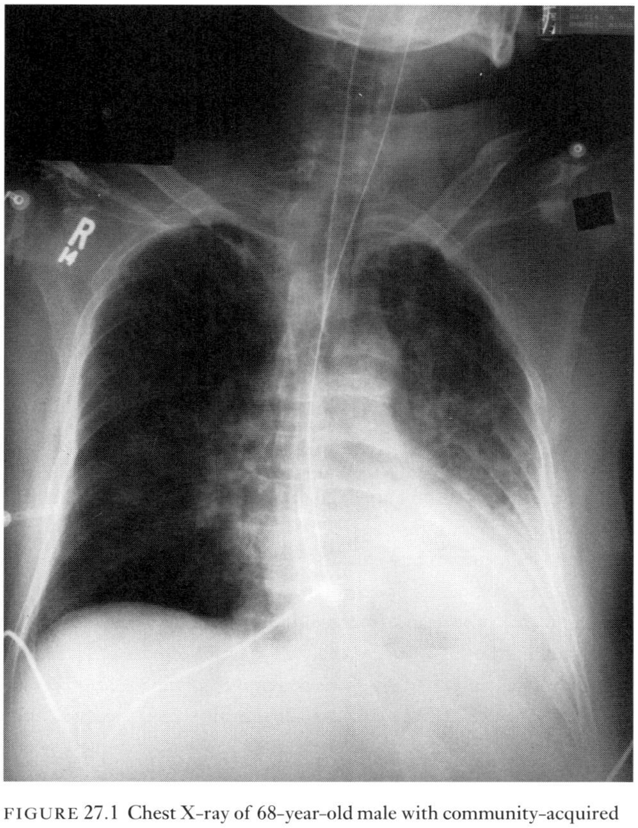

FIGURE 27.1 Chest X-ray of 68-year-old male with community-acquired pneumococcal pneumonia.

Table 27.3. *Initial diagnostic studies in patients with severe pneumonia requiring ICU admission*

Chest X-ray	
Arterial blood gas	
Blood cultures	
Serologic analysis: *Legionella*, *Mycoplasma*, *Chlamydia*	
Pleural fluid (if present): pH, cell count, glucose, protein, LDH, Gram's stain, culture, AFB culture	
Urine antigen: pneumococcus, *Legionella*	
Bronchoscopy with PSB, BAL (if available)	
Gram's stain, culture	
fungal culture	
AFB, TB culture	
viral culture	
immunofluorescence for *Legionella*	
Legionella culture	
cytology	*Pneumocystis*
	fungal stain
	virus

on the patient's premorbid status, clinical findings and epidemiological pattern most likely associated with the clinical presentation.

A recent consensus statement by the American Thoracic Society[12] recommended initiating therapy in severe hospitalised community-acquired pneumonia with a macrolide such as erythromycin plus a third-generation cephalosporin with antipseudomonal activity or another antipseudomonal agent such as imipenem or ciprofloxacin. In fulminant disease or when *Pseudomonas* is strongly suspected, the addition of an aminoglycoside should be considered. In patients with a suspicion of *P. carinii* pneumonia, trimethoprim–sulfamethoxasole should be added to the regimen. Empirical therapy with antiviral or antifungal agents are rarely indicated except for the immunocompromised patients and in transplant recipients (Table 27.4).

With effective therapy, a clinical improvement is usually seen within 48–72 hours and, unless significant clinical deterioration occurs, therapy should not be altered within the initial 3 days. It may take several days for fever to defervesce and radiographical features may lag behind clinical improvement. A number of factors may contribute to the lack of response or further deterioration, and include inappropriate antimicrobial coverage, development of organism resistance to the antibiotic or presence of an, as yet, identified atypical organism, be it viral, fungal, TB, parasitic or rickettsial. Mixed infections, metastatic infections, empyema, lung abscess or non-infectious pulmonary complications may also be a consideration. Acute respiratory distress syndrome with multisystem organ failure may be on the horizon as well as other non-infectious but inflammatory conditions such as Goodpasture's disease, Wegener's granulomatosis or bronchiolitis obliterans organising pneumonia.

Repeating diagnostic studies including bronchoscopy with protected specimen brushing and bronchoalveolar lavage in addition to obtaining a chest CT examination and possibly open lung biopsy may be necessary where the patient continues to deteriorate despite comprehensive therapy. Therefore on-going clinical assessment is of paramount importance in managing these patients.

Atypical pneumonia

A group of non-bacterial agents may produce an illness characterised by a prodromal upper respiratory tract infection, fever, dry cough and non-pulmonary complaints such as arthralgias and diarrhoea. These usually occur in younger adults and extra-pulmonary findings such as a rash, electrolyte disturbance, raised liver enzymes, haemolytic anaemia, bullous myringitis, encephalitis, rhabdomyolysis or myocarditis may accompany the variable pulmonary findings of patchy or widespread infiltrates.

The main infectious agents responsible include *M. pneumoniae, L. pneumophila* (Fig. 27.2), *C. psittaci, C. burnetti, P. carinii, Francisella tularensis* and viral agents especially influenza, respiratory syncytial virus, Epstein–Barr virus and adenovirus. *Legionella* is by far the most frequent agent responsible for atypical pneumonia severe enough to warrant ICU admission. Its incidence in community-acquired pneumonia ranges up to 27% in some series, but is most consistently reported around 6% and in the nosocomial setting ranges from 1–40%[18]. The outcome is contingent upon the early administration of appropriate antimicrobials and on the degree of immunocompetence of the patient. Fatality rates may range up to 80% in the immunocompromised patient or in those where the proper treatment has been delayed or lacking, which contrasts to a 6% mortality rate in a previously healthy patient receiving early administration of appropriate antibiotics[18].

Diagnostic studies include culturing the organism from sputum or lower airway secretions obtained from bronchoalveolar lavage or serologic assays using direct fluorescent antibody of respiratory secretions, or assessment for the presence of urinary antigen, or a fourfold rise in serum antibody titre. Recently, DNA probes have been studied but the sensitivity is much less than that of culture.

Erythromycin 1 g every 6 hours has been the standard therapy to date. In immunosuppressed patients or in those with a severe protracted illness and a confirmed diagnosis of *Legionella*, combined treatment with rifampicin 600 mg every 12 hours is recommended.

Other effective antimicrobials include doxycycline 100 mg every 12 hours and ciprofloxacin 200 mg every 6 hours. Recent studies have confirmed the effectiveness of the newer microlides such as clarithromycin 500 mg every 12 hours[19]: however, one drawback thus far is its limited availability in parenteral form.

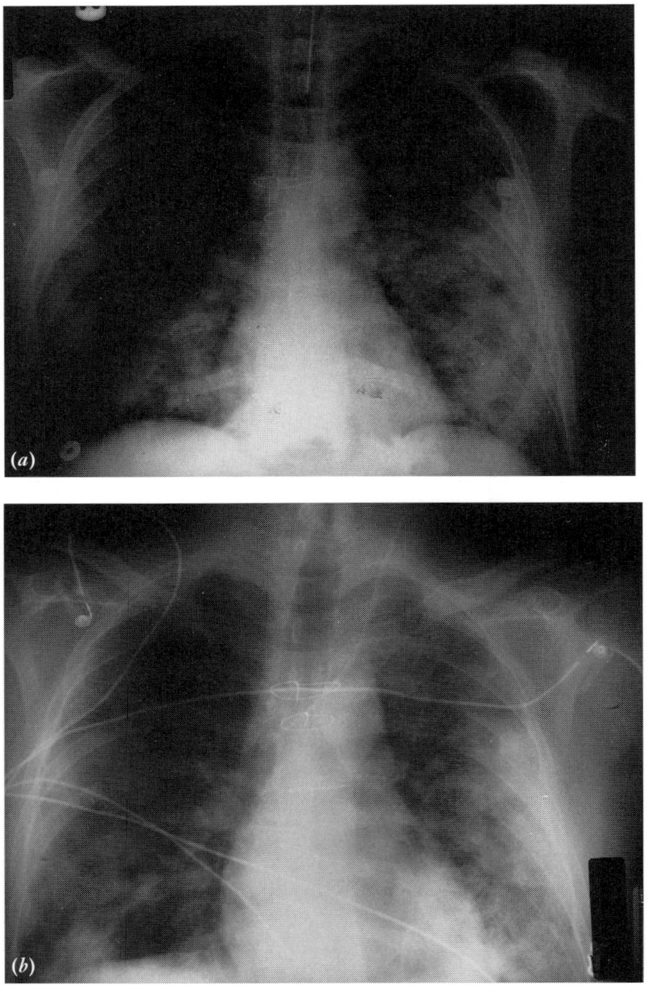

FIGURE 27.2 Chest X-ray of 42-year-old male with Legionnaire's disease.

Aspiration

The fact that occult aspiration of oropharyngeal or gastric contents is common yet clinical illness is not, demonstrates that development of lung injury is dependent on several factors including the frequency, quantity, size and composition of the material aspirated and on underlying host factors. The quality of the aspirate, namely the pH, volume, presence of food, foreign bodies, bile, mucous, tube feeding formula, faecal contamination, and bacterial concentration are all important determinants of lung injury following aspiration. Host factors such as nutritional status, comorbid lung disease, alveolar macrophage function, and ability to cough are also important. A number of varied clinical presentations include tracheal or large airway obstruction, atelectasis, pneumonia, lung abscess, chemical pneumonitis with or without acute lung injury and hypoxaemic respiratory failure (Fig. 27.3).

In most cases of witnessed pulmonary aspiration, infection plays little role in the early phase of chemical pneumonitis as the number and pathogenicity of aspirated bacteria is low, since the acid pH of normal gastric contents renders it sterile.

In this setting there is no evidence that early administration of antibiotics results in a reduced risk of infective pneumonitis, which usually only appears after 3–7 days post aspiration, and may, in fact, contribute to antimicrobial resistant organisms in those patients who do subsequently develop pneumonia. The normal bacterial density of the mouth and oropharynx is about 10^8 cfu/ml and conditions which impair host defences may increase this to more than 10^{20} cfu/ml. These include prolonged hospitalisation, malnutrition, prior antibiotic use, upper GI bleeding, bowel obstruction, ileus, enteral tube feeding, gingivitis, and increased gastric pH from histamine blockers. Aspiration of heavily contaminated gastric contents with mixed enteric aerobic and anaerobic organisms may result in fulminant necrotising pneumonia. In these instances, prompt broad spectrum coverage for Gram-negative and anaerobic bacteria is mandatory. Acceptable regimens include piperacillin 3 g IV q 4 h plus gentamicin 1.5 mg/kg q 8 h, clindamycin 900 mg IV q 8 h plus ceftazidime, or imipenem 500 mg IV q 6 h plus gentamicin 1.5 mg/kg q 8 h (Table 27.4).

Ventilation

Patients presenting with severe pneumonia require supportive care with special attention to their cardiovascular and respiratory systems. Clinical assessment of airway patency, respiratory rate and effort (work of breathing) and auscultation, provide valuable information as to whether the patient's respiratory system is able to handle the increased workload of an intercurrent infection. Level of consciousness, heart rate, blood pressure, pulse volume and urine output provides essential data on the integrity of the patient's cardiovascular system to cope with the added stress. Often patients may be intravascular volume depleted and require fluid resuscitation. If hypotension and clinical indicators of shock remain despite fluid resuscitation, inotropic agents may be required in addition to early intubation and ventilation.

For the most part, hypoxic respiratory failure is the main indication for ICU admission in patients with pneumonia. This is likely due to the presence of interstitial oedema, alveolar collapse, consolidation and atelectasis which leads to increased venous admixture, impaired oxygenation, and reduced lung compliance. Recent studies have demonstrated an inhomogenous regional distribution which are under gravitational influence of the fluid filled lung tissue with alveoli being compressed in the dependent zones, whereas aerated alveoli are found in the non-dependent regions[20].

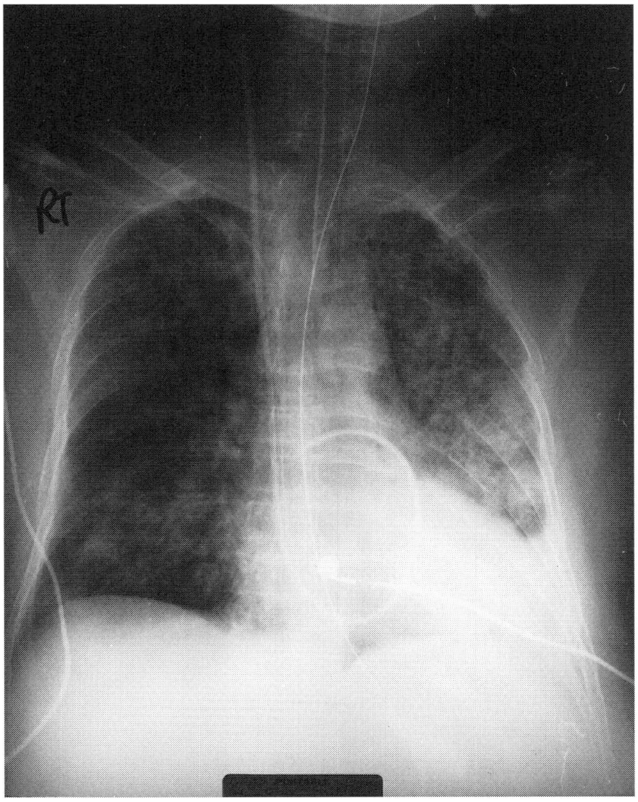

FIGURE 27.3 Chest X-ray of 75-year-old male with acute aspiration pneumonia.

Acute respiratory failure involves abnormal gas exchange with impaired oxygenation or hypoventilation. Hypoxaemia is the most life-threatening condition due to the body's minimal usable stores of oxygen. Progressive hypercapnia and acidosis are important harbingers of impending CNS depression which can lead to apnoea and hypoxaemia. Work of breathing usually requires less than 3% of the body's normal oxygen consumption, however, this may increase by 20-fold during acute respiratory failure. Tachycardia, diaphoresis, tachypnoea greater than 35/min, accessory muscle use, paradoxical breathing are signs of respiratory muscle fatigue and impending respiratory arrest. Patients with pneumonia are likely to have significant airway secretions which must be cleared to prevent aspiration, and the presence of a gag and cough reflex should be intact. The decision to intubate and begin ventilatory assistance should be based on clinical assessment with arterial blood gases or pulse oximetry being utilised only as a guide. Reasons to initiate ventilatory assistance are often multifactorial and should include implications for patient comfort and potential support of other organ systems (Table 27.5).

The benefits of intubation and mechanical ventilation include improved gas exchange, reduced work of breathing and airway protection. Patients unable to protect their airway or who have a depressed level of consciousness, are hypoxaemic despite oxygen administration, have progressively worsening hypercarbia or are in shock without adequate response to a fluid challenge, require immediate intervention with endotracheal intubation and mechanical ventilation.

Patients with severe pneumonia requiring ICU admission may present with a variety of clinical syndromes ranging from systemic inflammatory response syndrome (SIRS) to acute lung injury (ALI), acute respiratory distress syndrome (ARDS) and multisystem organ failure (MSOF). In an attempt to better understand the varied forms of clinical presentation and subsequent outcome, specific definitions to accurately stratify patients have been proposed.

In 1992 The American College of Chest Physicians and the Society of Critical Care Medicine Consensus Conference proposed a formal definition for SIRS which was to include more than one of the following clinical manifestations[21].

(i) Temperature > 38 °C or < 36 °C
(ii) Elevated heart rate > 90 beats per minute
(iii) Tachypnoea, manifested by a respiratory rate > 20 breaths per minute or hyperventilation as indicated by a P_aCO_2 < 32 mmHg (4.3 kPa)
(iv) White blood cell count > 12 000 × 10^6/l or < 4000 × 10^6/l or presence of more than 10% immature neutrophils

These changes should represent an acute alteration from baseline in the absence of other known causes for such abnormalities. When SIRS was the result of a confirmed infectious process, the term sepsis was to be used.

Table 27.4. *Empirical therapy of community-acquired pneumonia requiring ICU admission*

Patient category	Recommended regimens	Alternative regimens	Additional drugs
Immunocompetent	Second/third generation cephalosporin plus macrolide	Benzyl penicillin plus quinolone or Clindamycin plus quinolone or Clindamycin plus aztreonam	Aminoglycoside (*Pseudomonas*) Rifampicin (*Legionella*) Trimethoprim-sulfamethoxasole (*P. carinii*) Cloxacillin (*S. aureus*) Vancomycin (penicillin-resistant *Staphylococcus*)
Immunocompromised	Imipenem plus macrolide	Cephalosporin with anti-pseudomonal activity plus macrolide	Aminoglycoside Rifampicin Trimethoprim-sulfamethoxasole Cloxacillin Vancomycin
Aspiration pneumonia	Clindamycin plus third generation cephalosporin	Imipenem or Clindamycin plus quinolone or Piperacillin plus aminoglycoside	Aminoglycoside

Table 27.5. *Indications for intubation and ventilation*

Severe hypoxaemia despite maximal O_2 administration
Progressive, worsening hypercarbia
Shock
Depressed level of consciousness
Severe uncompensated acidosis

In the same year, a proposed definition for ALI and ARDS was put forth by the American Thoracic Society and European Society of Intensive Care[22]. ALI was defined as 'a syndrome of inflammation and increased lung permeability associated with a constellation of clinical radiological and physiological changes which cannot be explained although may coexist with left atrial or pulmonary capillary hypertension. ALI and ARDS are notably acute in onset and persistent (days to weeks) and are associated with one or more known risk factors, and characterised by arterial hypoxaemia resistant to oxygen therapy alone, and diffuse bilateral radiological infiltrates consistent with pulmonary oedema'. The term ARDS is reserved for the most severe end of the spectrum with a worse P_aO_2/F_iO_2 ratio of $\leq$ 200 mmHg as opposed to a P_aO_2/F_iO_2 ratio of $\leq$ 300 mmHg for ALI (Table 27.6).

The main clinical risks (Table 27.7) for development of ALI and ARDS are sepsis syndrome, multiple emergency transfusions, aspiration, diffuse pulmonary infection, near drowning, toxic inhalation, lung contusion, pancreatitis and other miscellaneous conditions by direct or indirect injury to the alveolar capillary surface[22,23]. The incidence of ARDS with these definitions ranges from 10–42% and is increased when sustained hypotension is present as part of the syndrome. Death is often caused by failure of extra-thoracic organs in response to ongoing infection and inflammation or progressive severe respiratory failure.

A recent study identified sub-populations with substantial risks for developing ARDS, including those with sepsis syndrome (43%), multiple transfusions for emergency resuscitation (40%), a combination of drug overdose and aspiration (33%) and multiple trauma (up to 40%) incidence[23]. The data collected were based on the lung injury score proposed by Murray and colleagues[24] in which four parameters (X-ray infiltrates, hypoxemia, PEEP, respiratory compliance) were graded on a point system according to severity with severe lung injury or ARDS equated with a score of > 2.5. Once a diagnosis of sepsis syndrome was made, onset of ARDS was rapid and usually within 24–48 h. Mortality was substantially higher in all patients with sepsis (57.7%) and particularly in those septic patients who developed ARDS (69%)[23]. Death is often caused by failure of other organ systems in response to ongoing infection, inflammation or progressive severe respiratory failure[25,26].

Early pathological changes in ARDS include pulmonary neutrophil sequestration and intravascular fibrin platelet aggregation[27]. Subsequent injury to the alveolar capillary interface leads to increased pulmonary vascular permeability, progressive lung inflammation and pulmonary oedema[28]. Neutrophils marginate along the endothelial surface and migrate into the interstitium and alveolae[29]. Progressive ARDS is then characterised by increasing shunt fraction, declining lung compliance and increased dead space ventilation.

Table 27.6. *Definitions*

	Temperature	Heart rate	P_aCO_2	WBC
SIRS	>38 °C <36 °C	>90 (b/min)	<32 mmHg <4.3 kPa	>12 000 × 10⁶/l < 4000 × 10⁶/l
	Oxygenation		CXR	PAWP
ALI	$P_aCO_2/F_iO_2 < 300$ mmHg		Bilateral infiltrates	≤ 18 mmHg
ARDS	$P_aCO_2/F_iO_2 \leq 200$ mmHg		Bilateral infiltrates	≤ 18 mmHg

Inflammatory cell and fibroblast infiltration, Type II pneumocyte proliferation and progressive obliteration of pulmonary microvasculature evolve. Continued fibrosis punctuated by superimposed infectious sequelae, hyperoxic induced injury and barotrauma may result in irreversible lung dysfunction. Right to left shunting of blood through non-ventilated lungs and ventilation–perfusion mismatch leads to severe hypoxaemia. Alveoli collapse secondary to inflammatory infiltrates, blood and oedema fluid, and small airways collapse due to interstitial infiltration and bronchial obstruction. Surfactant pools are also reduced in animal and human models of diffuse lung injury, secondary to alveolar epithelial cell injury[30]. Due to microvascular thrombosis with platelet and leukocyte aggregates, the number of patent capillaries decrease markedly, impairing pulmonary microvasculature[31]. This contributes to increased pulmonary vascular resistance, pulmonary hypertension, and increased dead space ventilation as lung regions are ventilated but poorly perfused leading to a marked increase in minute ventilation.

Although the disease appears to be diffuse and symmetrical, chest CT scans have demonstrated considerable heterogenicity of alveolar injury with a predilection for the dependent lung regions[20]. A number of mediators have been implicated in the process particularly activated neutrophils, which release cytokines such as TNF and interleukins that participate in the inflammatory response[32]. These processes lead to coagulopathy, platelet aggregation, induction of nitric oxide synthase and enhanced cellular oxidant production. Expression of adhesion molecules for leukocytes is increased leading to neutrophil migration and alteration in tissues, which ultimately damages cell structural components leading to oedema formation.

Patients with a localised pneumonia and focal radiographic changes may develop secondary ALI with progressive diffuse alveolar infiltrates. This may develop in the setting of community or hospital-acquired pneumonia from a variety of organisms including bacteria, viruses, mycobacteria, fungi and parasites. Patients with pneumonia requiring intensive care resulted in severe ALI in 12% of patients in one study[33]. Despite the incidence of pneumococcal pneumonia being highest in older patients, those who developed ALI from pneumococcus are younger with a mean age of 33 years[34].

Although there are some recent encouraging results regarding improved outcome from severe ALI, the overall mortality remains 50–70%. Patients who ultimately die usually develop sepsis syndrome and/or multiple system organ failure or irreversible respiratory insufficiency. A number of investigators have reported that sepsis, cardiac dysfunction and irreversible respiratory failure were the most common direct causes of death. Of interest was that deaths occurring during the first few days of lung injury resulted from the underlying injury or illness, whereas deaths occurring later in the course were associated with sepsis syndrome and multi-organ system failure. Multisystem organ failure (MSOF) has been defined as 'a clinical constellation of severe physiologic dysfunction occurring sequentially or concomitantly in multiple organs usually in the setting of sepsis or widespread perfusion deficits, after severe infection or trauma'[35]. The principal organ systems impaired include hepatic, renal, gastrointestinal, cardiovascular, haematological and central nervous system. One study[36] reported that MSOF occurred in 93% of infected patients vs 47% in those without sepsis. A second study[25] found sepsis associated with MSOF was implicated as the most common cause of late deaths. Hepatic function seems to be a major determinant of survival in patients with acute lung injury possibly through its role in clearing systemic inflammatory mediators such as bacteria and endotoxin translocated in the intestinal lumen[37,38]. Inability to clear TNF and IL-1 may perpetuate the systemic inflammatory response. Milder forms of non-pulmonary organ dysfunction are often seen in the course of ALI but resolve without progressing to frank organ failure. This may reflect an early panendothelial cell dysfunction in patients with ALI which may lead to systemic capillary leak and may be more common than appreciated.

Management in ICU

The management of patients requiring ICU admission for severe pneumonia include (i) cardiopulmonary resuscitation and stabilisation; (ii) identification and treatment of underlying conditions precipitating or perpetuating a systemic inflammatory response and ongoing ALI; (iii) achievement of adequate tissue oxygen delivery with the appropriate use of ventilatory, fluid, and haemodynamic supportive strategies and (iv) prevention, recognition and timely intervention of any complications which may result (i.e. barotrauma, nosocomial pneumonia, line sepsis, GI bleeding secondary to stress ulceration, sinusitis, and oxygen toxicity).

To date, there are no convincing prospective randomised controlled trials documenting any particular supportive modality as superior in preventing complications or improving survival in ARDS nor preventing ARDS from occurring in patients with clinical predisposition. Published clinical trials have been plagued by variable definitions, unclear comparability of treatment groups, variability in timing of interventions, differences in number and severity of non-pulmonary organ dysfunction, and lack of validated prognostic factors.

Following initial cardiopulmonary stabilisation, prompt identification and appropriate therapeutic intervention is critical for survival. Pneumonia from a diverse array of organisms has been associated with development of ALI. In the immunocompetent host bacteria, viruses, mycobacteria and fungi are among the primary infective agents while in immunocompromised patients, the clinician must have a much higher index of suspicion for *M. tuberculosis, P. carinii, Aspergillus, Legionella* and cytomegalovirus.

Table 27.7. *Most common causes of ALI/ARDS*

Sepsis syndrome	Multiple fractures
Multiple transfusions	Drug overdose
Near drowning	Diffuse pulmonary infection
Lung contusion	Toxic inhalation
Aspiration	

Bronchoscopy with protected specimen brush (PSB) and bronchoalveolar lavage (BAL) is recommended in patients with ALI from presumed community-acquired pneumonia who are not improving after initial empiric therapy[39]. Thoracoscopic or open lung biopsies may be diagnostic on selected patients presenting with idiopathic ALI and a non-diagnostic bronchoscopic BAL, either to identify the presence of an unusual infection, or diagnose an alternative non-infectious process. A comprehensive review of diagnostic strategies is discussed in Chapter 19 and in Chapter 1.

Ventilatory support

Non-invasive positive pressure mask ventilation may be utilised in patients with milder forms of ALI[40]. Prerequisites include that the patients be both alert and co-operative. Because of the tight fitting masks for positive pressure ventilation, aerophagia, emesis, and secondary aspiration are potential complications not to mention the extreme discomfort from the mask itself. Maintaining an empty stomach with a nasogastric tube and an upright posture is advisable. Patients with severe respiratory distress are usually unable to tolerate this mode of ventilation, and early elective intubation is recommended for all patients who show deterioration in gas exchange or mental status.

Mechanical ventilation

The first and highest priority is effective oxygenation (Table 27.8). After successful intubation, 100% O_2 should always be used until adequate oxygenation has been documented. For conventional ventilation tidal volumes of 10–12 ml/kg were previously suggested to achieve normal or near normal P_aCO_2 levels. However, recent data[41] suggests significant lung damage can occur with only moderate transalveolar pressures during mechanical ventilation, and therefore currently recommended tidal volume will vary from 6–8 ml/kg depending on the extent of underlying lung injury (which can be reflected by high minute ventilatory requirements and markedly elevated peak and plateau airway pressures). The relatively low tidal volume is selected to maintain low ventilating pressures in the face of the restrictive mechanical defect induced by alveolar filling and collapse. There is also recent evidence that the small tidal volume may limit further lung injury and intrapulmonary shunt[41].

The initial rate is usually set at 20–25 breaths/minute in order to achieve adequate ventilation as most patients exhibit severe tachypnoea. Controlled mechanical ventilation is the preferred mode initially as respiratory muscles can be completely rested; however, assist control (AC) or synchronised intermittent mandatory ventilation (SIMV) may be substituted once the patient is stabilised.

Human volunteer data[42] suggests that lung injury is likely to occur in patients receiving F_iO_2 in excess of 0.6 for greater than 72 hours, and after 24 hours on 100% oxygen increased levels of proinflammatory molecules can be seen in BAL fluid. In animal studies, high concentrations of oxygen can induce diffuse alveolar damage similar to ALI. Whether patients with ALI are more susceptible to hyperoxic injury remains to be determined. Hence the F_iO_2 should be reduced (≤ 0.6) as soon as possible to achieve an adequate arterial oxygen saturation of > 85–90%.

Positive end expiratory pressure (PEEP) has been the cornerstone of all ventilatory support strategies for ALI. In the lungs of patients with acute respiratory failure, the ventilated volume is considerably reduced and by increasing functional residual capacity, collapsed alveolar units can be presented for participation in gas exchange. Extravascular lung water is redistributed from the alveolar space to the interstitium and extra-alveolar space. PEEP significantly reduces parenchymal right-to-left shunt of pulmonary capillary blood thus improving arterial and tissue oxygenation, while allowing adequate oxygenation at less toxic levels of F_iO_2[43]. There is a linear relationship between increasing PEEP levels, lung volume and arterial oxygenation, however, increasing PEEP beyond a certain point may impede venous return, and hence cardiac output and tissue oxygen delivery by the mechanism of increased intrathoracic pressure[44,45]. The positive effect of resuscitating collapsed alveoli may result in over-inflation of other more distensible lung units and by compressing and obliterating those adjacent alveolar capillaries, oxygenation may be worsened, pulmonary vascular resistance may increase, and increased dead space ventilation may occur. Pulmonary hypertension, right ventricular dysfunction and a higher minute ventilation to compensate for increased dead space ventilation can lead to impaired oxygen transport.

The optimal level of external PEEP in conventional controlled ventilation is still disputed. Because of gravitational effects in the oedematous lung and the inhomogenous distribution of lung injury, there are often considerable regional differences in respiratory mechanics with accompanying local differences in compliance. Since the regional volume effects of externally applied PEEP depends on the regional compliance, this may already cause alveolar hyperinflation in the non-dependent lung zones. This conflicting distribution of external PEEP is inevitable and therefore no specific level of PEEP will be optimal for the whole lung. Therefore, application of external PEEP must be adapted to actual lung conditions in an attempt to keep less compliant alveoli open without over distension of the more compliant areas.

Therapeutic levels of PEEP range from 7–15 cm H_2O in contrast to physiologic levels of PEEP (3–5 cm H_2O) which are used to normalise lung volumes in the supine position and correct for loss of glottic function following endotracheal intubation. To assess what the optimal PEEP level is for a given patient with ALI, one approach is to systematically increase PEEP levels by 2–5 cm H_2O and assess the physiological effects after 10–20 minutes by measuring arterial blood gases, static lung compliance, blood pressure, cardiac output and pulmonary capillary wedge pressure. Incremental increases in PEEP while monitoring static compliance, blood pressure and pulse oximetry, can be rapidly performed at the bedside. When further increments in PEEP do not alter lung compliance or cause it to fall, it is likely that hyperexpansion has occurred and adverse consequences on venous return with tachycardia and hypotension may be observed. The goal is to achieve a significant increase in arterial oxygenation with little or no haemodynamic deterioration. In addition, one must be cognizant to limit airway pressures to ≤ 35 cm H_2O (plateau pressure) to avoid further perpetuation of lung injury. Thus the least PEEP necessary to reduce F_iO_2 to a less toxic range (≤ 0.6) and not impair haemodynamic function is the current practice.

Adverse cardiovascular effects of positive pressure ventilation and PEEP[44,45] may occur at any point following its institution, particularly if the patient is hypovolaemic or receives drugs which may impair reflex alterations in venous pressure and accordingly, hypotension must be urgently treated with volume expansion and/or vasoactive drugs. Once the most appropriate PEEP level has been applied, airway disconnections should be kept to a minimum as rapid alveolar flooding and oxygen desaturation may occur.

Patients with focal lung disease (lobar pneumonia) may warrant a cautious trial of PEEP as often more diffuse lung oedema and atelectasis may be present than can be appreciated on a chest radiograph. PEEP therapy may worsen gas exchange and should be abandoned if no improvement in shunt fraction or oxygenation is noted. Positioning the patient with the 'good lung down' may improve ventilation perfusion matching and hence oxygenation.

Ancillary methods to reduce oxygen consumption in patients with pneumonia include adequate sedation and muscle relaxation, correction of hyperthermia and avoidance of shivering.

Alternative ventilatory strategies

Until recently a number of adverse effects complicating mechanical ventilation were well known including oxygen toxicity and barotrauma, and major efforts have been made to prevent, minimise and treat these complications. Three strategies aimed at limiting airway pressure and tidal volume have recently been utilised in managing these patients suffering from ALI, namely permissive hypercapnia, pressure-controlled ventilation and pressure-limited volume-cycled ventilation.

Permissive hypercapnia

Use of permissive hypercapnia for ALI was predicated on the improved survival and minimal side effects where the strategy was used for ventilating patients with severe status asthmaticus. Hickling and co-workers[46–48] first demonstrated that in patients with acute respiratory failure, moderate elevation of P_aCO_2 (62 mmHg) (8.3 kPa) is generally well tolerated, and the reduction of peak airway pressure reduced mortality considerably. In patients with adequate oxygenation but persistently elevated plateau pressure, reduction in tidal volume and minute ventilation reduces airway pressures at the expense of an elevated P_aCO_2. In the absence of raised intracranial pressure, P_aCO_2 is allowed to increase as long as a pH of 3 7.2 can be maintained. Buffering of acidosis with bicarbonate under these circumstances is not generally recommended as additional CO_2 is generated.

Pressure-limited ventilation

Pressure-controlled (limited) ventilation (PCV) utilises a fixed or preset pressure applied to the airways for a specified time or percentage of the respiratory cycle. Thus the delivered tidal volume is not fixed (as in volume-controlled ventilation) but varies with the actual lung mechanics, namely airway resistance and lung compliance. Ventilation may be further influenced by spontaneous respiratory activity which, by interaction, may reduce tidal volume or minute ventilation mandating the need for careful monitoring[49–51].

Pressure-controlled inverse ratio ventilation (PC-IRV) is an alternate form of ventilation where inspiratory time is prolonged to 50% or greater of the respiratory cycle (I:E> 1). Prolongation of the inspiratory time sustains elevated mean airway pressure and as a consequence, reduction in peak and plateau airway pressures and possibly PEEP requirements. Inspiratory pressures remain constant throughout the entire period of inspiration and by recruitment and maintaining patency of alveoli, gas exchange and lung compliance may improve. Thus the principal advantage of PC-IRV is to limit peak airway pressure to a preset level. In addition, the more rapid inspiratory flow and pressure rise provides time for gas redistribution to slow filling alveoli and is especially useful for patients with non-homogenous lung injury[50,51].

Complications of PC-IRV are similar to those of conventional ventilation, namely barotrauma and haemodynamic compromise. The development of air trapping (intrinsic or auto PEEP) is a distinctive possibility as the inspiratory time is prolonged with insufficient time for exhalation. Monitoring for adequacy of tidal volume and for auto PEEP is crucial if employing this ventilatory strategy. Deep sedation and/or neuromuscular blockade are usually required to maintain patient ventilator synchrony.

Recent studies have failed to convincingly demonstrate the superiority of any specific ventilatory mode regarding the outcome of patients with ALI[52]. However, guidelines published in the consensus conference on mechanical ventilation of 1993[53], recommends that:

(i) a ventilator mode should be chosen which has been shown to support oxygenation and ventilation in patients with ARDS.
(ii) plateau pressure ≥ 35 cm H_2O be avoided.
(iii) $S_aO_2 \geq 90\%$ be targeted.
(iv) The level of F_iO_2 should be minimal.
(v) a PEEP trial be initiated at the lowest level which improves oxygenation and minimises deleterious side-effects.
(vi) a trial of permissive hypercapnia be employed if plateau pressures exceed 35 cm H_2O and no contraindication to a raised P_aCO_2 (e.g. raised ICP) is noted.
(vii) When oxygenation is inadequate, sedation, paralysis and position change may be useful therapeutic manoeuvres.

There is some evidence demonstrating improved gas exchange by placing the patient in the prone position[54].

Adjunctive measures

Other adjunctive measures at enhancing tissue oxygen delivery include increasing intracaval (IVOX) gas exchange[55], tracheal insufflation[56], high frequency ventilation[57,58] and perfluorocarbon liquid ventilation[59]. These modalities have been tried to decrease exposure of the lung to high pressures (and volumes) and enable better gas exchange than is otherwise possible. At present their utility for general medical practice is considered unproven.

Table 27.8. *Mechanical ventilation for acute lung injury*

	Conventional	Pressure limited
Settings		
Mode	Assist control, SIMV	Pressure control
Tidal volume	6–8 ml/kg	P plat $\leq$ 35 cm H_2O
Rate	18–24 breath/min	18–24 breath/min
F_iO_2	1.0 $\rightarrow$ taper to $\leq$ 0.6	1.0 $\rightarrow$ taper to $\leq$ 0.6
PEEP	5–15 cm H_2O	5–15 cm H_2O
I:E ratio	1:2 – 1:4	1:2 – 4:1
Goals		
S_aO_2	$\geq$ 90%	$\geq$ 90%
F_iO_2	$\leq$ 0.6	$\leq$ 0.6
P_aCO_2	38–45 mmHg (5.1–6.0 kPa)	
pH	7.36 – 7.44	$\geq$ 7.20
DO_2	$\geq$ 500 ml/min/m^2	$\geq$ 500 ml/min/m^2

Haemodynamic management

The optimal fluid and haemodynamic management of patients with ARDS is currently hotly debated. Some investigators advocate improved outcome in patients kept euvolemic with fluid restriction and pulmonary artery occlusion pressure reduction[60–62]. Others have argued for aggressive volume support and inotropic management to achieve supranormal physiologic values for oxygen delivery and oxygen consumption[63,64]. The relationship between oxygen delivery and oxygen consumption in patients with ARDS is controversial and beyond the scope of this review. Other topical issues include the use of colloids to support patients with leaky pulmonary capillaries, the need for placement of Swan-Ganz catheters in all patients with ARDS, and whether augmentation of tissue oxygen delivery bears any relationship to development of multisystem organ failure and/or improved outcome.

To answer the first question, thus far, animal and retrospective human studies support the concept that lower pulmonary capillary wedge pressures and extravascular lung water may lead to improved outcome from severe lung injury. Overall, decreased intravenous fluid repletion and judicious use of diuretics are well tolerated. Aiming for a normal PAWP of 8–12 mmHg seems reasonable as long as this does not lead to severe haemodynamic compromise and taking into account the effect of PEEP (usually $\geq$ 10 cm H_2O) on interfering with interpretation of haemodynamic measurements.

Patients with ALI have increased permeability for large molecular weight proteins including albumin, which diffuse into the alveolar spaces. Thus administration of colloids in the early stages of lung injury are also likely to leak from the capillaries to the pulmonary interstitium perhaps leading to worsening of the process and has been observed in several animal models of ALI[65]. There is no clinical data whether colloids may be beneficial in the later stages when endothelial permeability barriers are restored.

To date, the use of haemodynamic monitoring has failed to demonstrate improved clinical outcome; however, it by itself is not a therapeutic intervention and is merely a monitoring device. Especially in the early stages of severe lung injury, swan ganz catheterisation is useful in distinguishing cardiogenic vs non-cardiogenic pulmonary oedema and provides a basis and assessment for therapeutic strategies involving fluids, inotropic agents, and ventilatory support modalities. Patients with underlying cardiac disease and diminished cardiac reserve will also probably be easier to manage with haemodynamic monitoring. Recognising the many potential side-effects, these catheters should be removed once the patient has been stabilised.

Whether or not to augment tissue oxygen delivery by use of fluids or inotropic agents (dobutamine) to supra-physiologic ranges, has until now not demonstrated any significant improval in outcome in patients with ARDS and moreover, in one recent study, the group randomised to receive inotropic support had a greater mortality[66]. That is not to say one should ignore tissue oxygen delivery; however, a simplified approach based on an individual patient's requirement seems justified with optimal fluid replacement and a haematocrit of $\geq$ 30% being the initial step, following which the addition of an inotropic agent may be added if clinically indicated to maintain adequate end organ perfusion.

To date, specific treatment in patients with ARDS secondary to pneumonia includes appropriate antimicrobials, maintenance of cardiovascular stability, adequate oxygenation, sedation and/or neuromuscular blocking agents, prophylaxis for deep vein thrombosis, and upper GI haemorrhage, nutritional support and ongoing monitoring and timely intervention of any potential complications. The diagnosis of nosocomial pneumonia in ventilated patients is difficult and invasive techniques with quantitative microbiological cultures may improve diagnostic sensitivity and specificity and decrease inappropriate use of antibiotics.

Novel therapeutic interventions

A number of novel therapeutic interventions have been the subject of recent studies and for the sake of completeness will be only briefly mentioned. Extracorporeal membrane oxygenation (ECMO) for patient with severe ALI was not found to improve outcome. Subsequent trials with veno–veno bypass and extracorporeal CO_2 removal ($ECCO_2$-R), partial oxygenation across the artificial membrane and apnoeic oxygenation with non toxic oxygen concentrations resulted in improved survival in ARDS patients compared with historical controls[67].

A recent study where extracorporeal CO_2 removal in patients who failed pressure control inverse ratio ventilation (PC-IRV) compared to patients with tightly controlled routine support, showed lower mortality in both groups compared to historical controls but no survival advantage with the extracorporeal technique[51].

Surfactant replacement therapy has been successful in improving morbidity and mortality in premature newborns with respiratory distress syndrome. Surfactant is known to be deficient in animal models and patients with ALI and if exogenously administered could potentially maintain alveolar stability, improve recruitment of alveoli, and decrease the driving force for oedema formation[68,69]. Although initial reports from a clinical trial of synthetic surfactant in ARDS were promising, recent analysis of the multi-centred randomised placebo-controlled trial showed no significant survival benefit for the surfactant treated group[70].

Clinical trials to evaluate compounds which neutralise proinflammatory cytokines, namely TNFα and 1L-1B, thus far have not shown any overall survival advantage[32].

Monoclonal antibodies directed against the lipid A component of endotoxin showed improved survival in certain subsets of patients with Gram-negative infections[71]. However a subsequent trial of anti-endotoxin HA-IA was prematurely halted because of excess deaths in patients without Gram-negative infections. Additional trials of murine anti-endotoxin E5 similarly showed no benefit in patients with Gram-negative infections, however ongoing studies are still being conducted to evaluate the possibility of improvement in end organ dysfunction and multi-system organ failure.

Cyclo-oxygenase inhibitors have been shown to improve survival in animal models of sepsis and in an early pilot trial of humans[72]. Currently a multicentre randomised double-blind trial is being carried out investigating the effects of intravenous ibuprofen.

Antioxidant therapy has potential impact in patients with severe infections and ALI. A number of agents including vitamin E, superoxide dismutase and *N*-acetyl cysteine has shown some improved survival in animal models[73] but the effect has been inconsistent.

A number of studies have focused on treatment of pulmonary hypertension which can be severe and progressive in ARDS leading to right ventricular dysfunction. Vasodilators such as prostaglandin E1 (PGE1) were examined as a 7-day infusion in patients who developed severe ARDS following sepsis, trauma, or surgery. Despite reduction in pulmonary and systemic vascular resistance, increased cardiac output and oxygen consumption, no survival advantage was found in a well-controlled multicentre study[74].

Inhaled nitric oxide (NO) is a new investigational drug used for selective vasodilation of the pulmonary vasculature, by mimicking the effects of endogenously produced endothelium-derived relaxing factor. In addition to selective pulmonary vasodilation, nitric oxide can improve hypoxaemia by improving ventilation perfusion relationships within the lung. Inhaled nitric oxide is inactivated following its rapid binding to haemoglobin thereby limiting its effect on the pulmonary vasculature. Unfortunately nitric oxide has the potential to generate increased amounts of highly reactive oxidant peroxynitrate.

A number of recent trials[75,76] have indicated that, although some patients with severe ARDS have an excellent response with improved P_aO_2/F_iO_2 ratios, reduction of pulmonary artery pressure and shunt fraction, no improvement in survival has yet been observed.

The role of corticosteroids in ARDS has been closely evaluated with prospective randomised trials which have failed to show any benefit either in the prevention of ARDS in septic patients, or in the outcome of those with established lung injury treated early in their course[77,78]. Recently anecdotal reports have described improved gas exchange after corticosteroid treatment in patients during the late or fibro-proliferative phase of their illness[79]. However, prospective randomised studies are necessary to confirm these observations.

Withdrawal of ventilatory support

Once the patient has improved from the underlying illness for which mechanical ventilation was instituted, an attempt at withdrawing ventilatory support is justified. Several modes of partial ventilatory support have been proposed with the aim of gradually decreasing the level of mechanical assistance to eventually liberate the patient from the ventilator. The complications associated with mechanical ventilation are many and are best avoided or minimised by active efforts to shorten the duration of its use. Patients with acute hypoxaemic respiratory failure from pneumonia may respond to therapeutic interventions within several days to a level such that supplemented oxygen delivered by mask would be sufficient to maintain arterial haemoglobin saturation above 90%. Most patients can be weaned from the ventilator if the following conditions are met:

(i) Stable cardiovascular system and absence of sepsis, myocardial ischaemia and uncontrolled acidosis.
(ii) Adequate respiratory drive.
(iii) Adequate pulmonary gas exchange as evidenced by arterial oxygenation saturation of > 90% with an $F_iO_2 < 0.5$ and PEEP < 7.5 cm H_2O.
(iv) Adequate spontaneous ventilation (tidal volume > 5 ml/kg, negative inspiratory force > 25 cm H_2O and respiratory rate < 36/min, respiratory rate/tidal volume < 100).
(v) Absence of excessive respiratory workload.

Extubation requires sufficient level of consciousness, co-operation and strength to ensure maintenance of a patient airway, presence of airway reflexes to prevent aspiration, and adequate cough to clear secretions.

Ventilator dependence is usually due to respiratory muscle overload as a result of lung stiffness, excessive work of breathing, or muscle strength (60–80%) as opposed to problems of oxygenation or ventilatory drive (10–20%). Other important factors to consider are cardiac dysfunction, subjective dyspnoea, pain, or psychological problems.

Once the underlying process is resolving, oxygenation is adequate and ventilatory drive present, one of the partial ventilatory support modes can be chosen to gradually wean the patient, if spontaneous breathing without mechanical support is not tolerated.

Two recent studies have examined strategies to progressively reduce the contribution of the ventilator for respiratory support[80,81]. These include T-piece trials or periods of spontaneous breathing followed by full support, intermittent mandatory ventilation (whereby gradual reduction in the number of support breaths is delivered) and pressure support ventilation (where the patient is given a pressure boost with each spontaneous breath). The main goals are to maintain adequate oxygenation without overloading or fatiguing respiratory muscles and gradually reduce the support as the patient is able to assume greater workloads.

Of the current partial support modes either gradual reduction with intermittent mandatory ventilation with pressure support, or stand alone pressure support may be better tolerated by patients as opposed to acute withdrawal of total support. In the latter method, patients who do not tolerate breathing without assistance may deteriorate rapidly. Pressure support has been shown to reduce the pressure volume characteristics of work of breathing and seems better tolerated on subjective enquiry. Whichever modality is chosen, careful monitoring of potentially reversible factors which can adversely affect outcome is necessary which includes electrolyte imbalance, anaemia, infection, cardiac failure, acid-base disturbances and adverse effects of medications (Table 27.9).

Table 27.9. *Ventilator complications*

Ventilation hazards	
Endotracheal tube	Dislodgement, aspiration, imposed work of breathing
Dys-synchrony	Timing, flow
Barotrauma	Plateau pressure > 35 cm H_2O
Oxygen	$F_iO_2 > 0.6$
Cardiac	Hypotension
Infection	Nosocomial pneumonia, sinusitis

Line infections

Vascular catheters are the most frequently used indwelling medical devices and are widely utilised in the treatment of critically ill patients in the ICU. Central venous access is typically used for administration of fluids, blood products, medications and TPN for haemodynamic monitoring or for procedures such as haemodialysis and plasmapharesis. Although useful, they also pose a hazard for significant infections and mechanical complications. Bloodstream infection is a serious catheter related complication with more than 50 000 cases occurring annually in the US with an estimated case facility rate of 10–20%[82]. Major mechanical complications occur in approximately 4% of line insertions including pneumothorax, haemothorax, phlebitis, and cardiac arrhythmias.

Numerous factors are associated with the development of catheter related infections involving both host and environmental variables. These include catheter composition and lumen number, insertion site, improper aseptic technique, prolonged catheterisation, frequent manipulations, dressing type and severity of underlying illness. In prospective studies that have used semi-quantitative cultures, the most common organisms responsible for catheter infections are coagulase negative staphylococci, *S. aureus* and *Candida* species. *Corynebacterium*, especially JK strains and *Bacillus* species can also cause catheter-related infections and may be introduced from the skin or catheter hub. Gram-negative bacilli acquired from the hospital environment such as *Pseudomonas* spp., *Acinetobacter* spp. and *Xanthomonas maltophilia* have also been reported to cause catheter related sepsis. Finally, enteric organisms like *E. coli*, *Klebsiella* and enterococci rarely are responsible for catheter related infections.

Some centres routinely replace catheters after 72 hours or 7 days by guidewire exchange or *de novo*, but this has not been found to reduce the infectious complications and may lead to increased mechanical complications[83]. Currently, there is no evidence to support routine central line removal or replacement despite the documented association between duration of catheterisation and infection, as long as the site appears clean and the patient is stable. However, the need for central venous access should be reviewed daily and the catheter removed at the earliest possible time. Should the site appear infected with pus, heat, erythema or tenderness, the line should be removed and cultured and simultaneous blood cultures should be drawn. A new site can then be chosen for central line placement if it is still deemed necessary.

In those patients with clinical signs of sepsis, without other known cause and a central vein catheter in place for more than 72 hours, empirical removal with either guidewire exchange with culture of the original catheter or replacement at a different site are reasonable options given the paucity of prospective data to guide the clinician.

Most catheter-related septicaemias are uncomplicated bloodstream infections that respond well to intravenous antibiotic therapy. Should bacteraemia persist for more than 48 hours after catheter removal and initiation of appropriate antimicrobial therapy, a complicated intravascular focus such as endocarditis or septic thrombophlebitis bears consideration. Echocardiography and Doppler ultrasound or distal venography of the limb are warranted. Infective endocarditis or central vein thrombophlebitis should be treated with parenteral antibiotics for at least 4 weeks.

Since the most common bacterial infections are coagulase negative *Staphylococcus* and *S. aureus* and given that most coagulase-negative staphylococci are sensitive only to vancomycin, this antibiotic is the initial agent of choice pending culture results. Although the optimal duration of therapy is unknown, a 7–10 day course is usually adequate unless complicated by deep-seated infections or septic thrombophlebitis, where at least 4 weeks of therapy is recommended.

Catheter-related candidaemia can be treated with a short course of amphotericin B 5–7 mg/kg (0.5 mg/kg/d) for 7–10 days or alternately fluconazole 400 mg/d if the organism is sensitive. Fundoscopic examination is helpful to rule out retinitis. Similarly, ongoing candidaemia after catheter removal while on anti-fungal therapy should alert the clinician to endocarditis and septic thrombophlebitis.

Recent studies with the use of chlorhexidine/silver sulfadiazine bonded catheters have reduced catheter related bacteraemias and further investigations are ongoing[84].

Nutritional support

Nutritional support is essential in the management of critically ill patients. It has been estimated that 30–50% of hospitalised patients have clinical evidence of malnutrition and preliminary evidence indicates a relationship between initial nutritional status and in-hospital mortality[85]. Physiologic stress is associated with elevated catecholamines and other counter regulatory hormone levels while septicaemia, common in critically ill patients, is associated with elevated levels of cytokines in the blood including TNF, interleukin-1 and interleukin-6. Although cytokines may have beneficial properties such as stimulation of antimicrobial function, mobilisation of substrate stores and promotion of wound healing, excessive or prolonged release may lead to an exaggerated inflammatory response, a depletion of protein and energy stores and a development of a nutritionally depleted state[86]. Undernutrition is associated with loss of body proteins leading to respiratory muscle weakness with associated ventilator dependency, in addition to impaired cellular immune function, wound healing and increased susceptibility for infection. On the other hand, overfeeding critically ill patients has been associated with increased CO_2 production and respiratory insufficiency, hyperglycaemia, hypertriglyceridaemia, abnormal hepatic function and azotaemia.

Nutritional assessment of the critically ill patient is often difficult as the effect of malnutrition on body weight may be masked by fluid retention. A history of decreased food intake, presence of chronic illness and physical features on examination of muscle weakness, loss of subcutaneous fat stores, features of chronic liver disease or signs of specific nutritional depletion is quite useful in ascertaining nutritional status.

Although there are no specific laboratory indicators specific for nutritional status, adequacy of body stores of magnesium, calcium, phosphate, in addition to liver and renal function, blood count, pre-albumin levels are useful. Bioelectric impedance is a new non-invasive method, allowing bedside quantitation of lean body mass.

Caloric requirements in critically ill patients remain the focus of much controversy and range from routine use of indirect calorimetry to linear regression equations using height, weight, age and estimates based on weight multiplied by standard references. For the most part, energy requirements range between 25 and 35 kcal/kg/day[87,88]. The exceptions to this requirement are burn and trauma patients whose requirements may increase to 40–45 kcal/kg/day or individuals who are severely calorie depleted and will need increased calories over a longer period of time to increase body fat mass.

Studies of protein requirements in critically ill patients ranges from 1.2–1.8 g/kg/day above which utilisation of exogenously provided protein for synthetic purposes plateaus off. Nitrogen balance may remain consistently negative in this patient population and positive nitrogen balance should not be the ultimate goal. More importantly is the improved muscle function with nutritional support, which is seen before any increase in body protein or muscle mass is observed[89].

In the stressed critically ill patient carbohydrate improves nitrogen retention and calorie to protein ratios of 150 calories per gram of nitrogen are generally accepted as standard. Carbohydrate should be provided at a rate no greater than 4–5 mg/kg/min for optimal metabolic benefit and minimal adverse complications. Excess glucose infusion rates may lead to fatty liver infiltration, cholestasis, steatosis and possible hypercarbia.

Based on current information, it appears optimal to provide non-protein calories as a mixture of carbohydrate and fat in a ratio of 70:30. Infusion of lipid emulsion of 0.5–1 mg/kg/day may add a nutrient dense caloric source as well as providing a preferred substrate for mechanically ventilated patients. Excess fat intake may lead to increased triglyceride levels, cholestasis and decreased immune function. Addition of omega-3 fatty acids has been shown to improve immune responses and creation of new triglyceride moieties incorporating different ratios of medium chain triglycerides, essential fatty acids and omega-3 and omega-6 fatty acids may prove useful for treating specific disease states.

The addition of vitamins and minerals to the nutritional recipe is extremely important with additional supplements as clinically necessary to meet the specific requirements of individual patients.

Current practice supports the use of early enteral feeding over parenteral nutrition in critically ill patients. This can usually be accomplished by nasogastric silastic feeding tubes although percutaneous gastrostomy tubes can also be placed. Enteral feeding is preferred because of lower cost, fewer serious complications and promotion of gut integrity and immune function, thereby reducing the risk of translocation of bacteria. Early initiation of enteral feeding (within 6–12 hours of insult) has been shown to have a significant effect on septic complications in critically ill patients fed a formula enriched with arginine, RNA and omega 3 fatty acids[90]. It may also modify hormonal response to stress and improve wound healing. One of the major drawbacks of enteral feeding is the limitation on calorie intake and the discrepancy between prescribed and delivered feeds whereby patients may only receive 50–85% of their requirements. This is usually due to large gastric residual volumes, diarrhoea, clogging of the tube, etc.

Some patients cannot maintain adequate calorie intake by enteral feeding alone or may not be able to tolerate any enteral nutrition and parenteral nutrition may be essential. Newer information has suggested that although some patients (post-op not severely malnourished) may have some functional deficiency of selected electrolytes, vitamins and minerals within 24 to 48 hours of an acute catabolic event, energy substrate stores are not depleted for several days.

When a patient who is critically ill is started on total parenteral nutrition, careful monitoring for complications involving the central line, fluid balance, electrolyte, acid–base status and organ function is essential.

Recent studies utilising growth factors to stimulate anabolic activity to enhance the maintenance of lean body mass during hypocaloric feeding and to stimulate expansion of body protein during refeeding, have shown promise[91]. Further trials are ongoing to study the effects of growth hormone administration on outcome, length of stay, weaning time and immunological function in critically ill patients.

Disseminated intravascular coagulation

DIC is a dynamic pathological syndrome characterised by activation of the coagulation and fibrinolytic systems resulting in diffuse thrombus formation and clinically presents with bleeding. Unlike most disease states, DIC is not a primary entity but is secondary to a variety of underlying severe systemic illnesses such as septicaemia, major tissue injury, malignancy, obstetrical complications, and intravascular haemolysis. The clinical presentation of DIC is quite variable depending primarily on the underlying disease and degree of haemostasis activation. Most features of DIC are attributable to the generation of thrombin or a thromboplastic substance and plasmin from a variety of inciting events. Clinical manifestations range from microvascular thrombosis (particularly of the kidneys, lungs, and brain) resulting in minor organ dysfunction to severe bleeding and multi-organ system failure.

Early symptoms include mild cerebral dysfunction, hypoxaemia and respiratory distress, petechial and mucocutaneous bleeding, and renal impairment. As the process progresses, the symptoms may become quite severe leading to ARDS, renal failure, multifocal spontaneous bleeding, hepatic dysfunction, shock, seizures and thromboembolic events. Organ failure results from vascular deposition of fibrin and is aggravated by consumption of coagulation inhibitors. Bleeding is induced by concurrent consumption of coagulation factors, fibrinolysis activation, and by appearance of fibrinogen or fibrin degradation products that compromises platelet aggregation and inhibits fibrin polymerisation.

It has been observed that levels of protein C, antithrombin III, fibrinogen, platelets, and factors V, VIII, and IX are significantly reduced in DIC; however as the clinical manifestations are varied, so are the laboratory investigations necessary to secure the diagnosis at an early stage.

To date, there is no one diagnostic study useful on its own and complete clinical and laboratory evaluation is needed. In addition to the above noted findings, D-dimer levels are elevated, PT, PTT prolonged, and a microangiopathic haemolytic anaemia may be present (schistocytes on blood film).

The key to management is treatment of the underlying disease. Transfusion of blood products with packed red blood cells, platelets and fresh frozen plasma, and if required cryoprecipitate for correction of hypofibrinogenaemia, may protect the patient from haemorrhagic complications while the mechanism triggering the DIC is corrected.

Heparin therapy remains controversial and is usually only recommended for cases of purpura fulminans, severe obstetric DIC, and Trousseau syndrome with massive thromboembolism. Antifibrinolytic agents such as epsilon aminocaproic acid or tranexamic acid are contraindicated because of the risk of extensive thrombotic complications. Clinical trials are currently ongoing, utilising Protein C and antithrombin III for treatment of DIC.

Renal failure

Acute renal failure may be seen in up to 25% of critically ill patients requiring intensive care unit admission and despite technological advances, the mortality still exceeds 50% in those who develop renal failure as part of multi-system organ failure. In fact, the mortality of patients who require some form of dialysis is 65–80%, or more than twofold higher than of patients not requiring such support. Isolated renal failure has a mortality of less than 10%; however, the addition of one other organ system failure increases mortality to 60%. Factors associated with reduced survival include hypotension, requirement of inotropic support, sepsis, pancreatitis, immunosuppression, and heart failure. Oliguric renal failure (< 15 ml/h) carries double the mortality than non-oliguric renal failure which is probably due to associated shock and other severe underlying conditions.

The pathophysiologic mechanism of acute renal failure as part of multi-system organ dysfunction has recently focused on a systemic or uncontrolled inflammatory response resulting in the release and activation of a myriad of cytokines such as endotoxin, tumour necrosis factor, interleukin-1 and vasoconstrictor mediators as endothelin, thromboxane, and leukoteines. These substances may lead to organ failure by direct or indirect effects on organ function. Increased circulating concentrations of these cytokines has been correlated with a poor outcome in human and animal models of sepsis.

Renal function is critically dependent on adequate perfusion and hence on an adequate circulatory status. Impaired renal perfusion may result from circulatory failure, hypotension, vascular obstruction, hypovolaemia, or maldistribution of cardiac output. Certain forms of renal insufficiency (hepatorenal syndrome) mimic pre-renal physiology by re-distributing blood flow away from the glomerulus. Prolonged renal ischaemia (mean arterial pressure below 60–70 mmHg) for longer than 30 minutes risks renal injury and glomerular filtration stops at a mean arterial pressure of about 50 mmHg. At an early or moderate stage of impaired renal perfusion (secondary to ECF volume contraction) early recovery occurs if the circulation is restored. If the process is more severe, acute renal failure supervenes and recovery may be delayed weeks or months and thus prompt restoration of renal perfusion before onset of tubular necrosis is critical.

Once pre-renal causes have been excluded, post-renal (obstructive) causes should be considered. These include urinary calculi, tumour, prostatic hypertrophy, blood clot and retro-peritoneal haemorrhage. Although post-renal disease accounts for only a small proportion of acute renal failure, this should not be overlooked and is easily assessed by ultrasonography and can be appropriately treated.

Intra-renal abnormalities include tubular disorders, interstitial nephritis, glomerulonephritis and small vessel vasculitis. After pre-renal azotaemia, nephrotoxic drugs are the most common cause of acute renal failure. Aminoglycosides, contrast agents, non-steroidal anti-inflammatory drugs are the worst offenders and the adverse effect of these nephrotoxins are potentiated by pre-existing renal insufficiency and volume contraction. Myoglobin and haemoglobin may cause acute renal failure when released into the serum from haemolysis or rhabdomyolysis. Appropriate therapy for rhabdomyolysis includes volume loading, osmotic diuretics, and alkalinising agents in order to keep these compounds in solution and prevent precipitation and obstruction in the renal tubules.

Interstitial nephritis is a common but frequently unrecognised allergic reaction in the renal interstitium usually in response to a specific drug such as penicillin, rifampin or frusemide. Urine eosinophils is the most useful diagnostic study and removal of the offending agent plus corticosteroids are accepted modalities of treatment.

Glomerulonephritis and vasculitis are uncommon causes of abrupt renal failure in the ICU but may be seen in conjunction with other systemic illnesses as endocarditis, systemic lupus erythematosus or polyarteritis nodosa.

Insults to the kidneys are virtually inevitable in the acutely ill patients but their impact can be minimised by optimising circulatory volume, judicious use of inotropic agents only after volume expansion, minimising potential septic insults by removing intravascular devices as soon as possible, avoidance of nephrotoxic antibiotics if possible, monitoring of nephrotoxic drug concentrations, minimising contrast studies, and use of appropriate volume loading regimens for optimal hydration prior to contrast media and nephrotoxins such as amphotericin B.

Currently there is little support for the use of low dose dopamine for prophylaxis against renal failure.

A number of compounding problems may result from acute renal failure, namely electrolyte imbalances, fluid overload, hypertension, anaemia, coagulopathy, GI bleeding, seizures, infections, severe catabolism, and drug toxicity.

Currently, the main indications for dialysis or haemofiltration include fluid overload, refractory hyperkalaemia, life threatening acidosis, symptomatic uraemia and persistent bleeding caused by platelet dysfunction.

Currently dialysis can be provided by intermittent or continuous renal replacement therapies both of which have advantages and disadvantages and can be selected on the basis of individual patient's requirements and equipment availability.

In summary, in the patient with relatively uncomplicated renal failure, a good outcome may be expected; however, when it supervenes in a patient with multi-system disease, it is an important marker of severity of illness in addition to increasing the complexity of management.

Psychological care of ICU patients

Patients on mechanical ventilation experience distress related to a variety of factors, namely their underlying illness, the critical care environment and most often the endotracheal tube. In addition to the discomfort of suctioning, the frustration of being unable to speak and the overall fear and anxiety most intensive care patients experience, a number of other factors such as sleeplessness, pain, restraints, noise, immobility and confusion may also be experienced. Although pharmacological therapy is often required, sedating medications will never replace the concern, competence and communication skills of the health care providers. It has been demonstrated that the degree to which staff effectively interact with patients, families and each other, has an impact on patient recovery. Increased patient agitation may easily result from misunderstood verbal or non-verbal communication and hence effective communication is extremely important for successful weaning of ventilated patients.

It is important for all members of the health care team to communicate with patients and provide continual reassurance, be it for a specified procedure, prior to suctioning, or just for repositioning of the patient in bed.

A number of cognitive behavioural strategies to limit patient distress ranges from relaxation therapy, distraction and music therapy, relaxed visiting policies and minimal use of physical restraints.

References

1. MARRIE TW, DURANT H, YATES L. Community-acquired pneumonia requiring hospitalization: 5 year prospective study. *Rev Infect Dis* 1989; 11: 586–99.
2. FARR B M, SLOMAN A J, FISCH M J. Predicting death in patients hospitalized for community-acquired pneumonia. *Ann Intern Med* 1991; 115: 428–36.
3. TORRES A, SERRA BATLLES J, FERRER A *et al.* Severe community-acquired pneumonia: epidemiology and prognostic factors. *Am Rev Resp Dis* 1991; 144: 312–18.
4. POTGIETER PD, HAMMOND JMJ. Etiology and diagnosis of pneumonia requiring ICU admission. *Chest* 1992; 101: 199–203.
5. ORTQUIST A, STERNER G, NILSSON JA. Severe community-acquired pneumonia requiring hospitalization: factors influencing need of intensive care treatment and prognosis. *Scand J Infect Dis* 1985; 17: 377–86.
6. SORENSON J, CEDERHOLM I, CARLSSON C. Pneumonia: a deadly disease despite intensive care treatment. *Scand J Infect Dis* 1986; 18: 329–35.
7. RELLO J, QUINTANA E, AUSSINA V, NET A, PRATS G. A three year study of severe community-acquired pneumonia with emphasis on outcome. *Chest* 1993; 103: 232–5.
8. MOINE P, VERCKEN JB, CHEVRET S, CHASTANG C, GAJDOS P and the French study group for community-acquired pneumonia in the Intensive Care Unit. Severe community-acquired pneumonia. *Chest* 1994; 105: 1487–95.
9. ALMIRALL J, MESALLES E, KLAMBURG J, PARRA O, AGUDA A. Prognostic factors of pneumonia requiring admission to the Intensive Care Unit. *Chest* 1995; 107: 511–16.
10. LEROY O, SANTRE C, BEUSCART C *et al.* A five year study of severe community-acquired pneumonia with emphasis on prognosis in patients admitted to an Intensive Care Unit. *Intens Care Med* 1995; 21: 24–31.
11. TORRES A, EL-EBIARY M, RODRIGUEZ-ROISIN R. Severe community-acquired pneumonia; a New clinical entity. In J L Vincent, ed. *Yearbook of Intensive Care and Emergency Medicine* 1994: 600–16.
12. THE AMERICAN THORACIC SOCIETY. Guidelines for the initial management of adults with community-acquired pneumonia: diagnosis, assessment of severity, and initial antimicrobial therapy. *Am Rev Resp Dis* 1993; 148: 1418–26.
13. THE BRITISH THORACIC SOCIETY. The aetiology, management and outcome of severe community-acquired pneumonia on the Intensive Care Unit. *Resp Med* 1992; 86: 7–13.
14. FINE M J, ORLOFF J J, ARISUMI D *et al.* Prognosis of patients hospitalized with community-acquired pneumonia. *Am J Med* 1990; 88: 1N–8N.
15. FINE M J, SMITH D N, SINGER D E Z. Hospitalization decision in patients with community-acquired pneumonia: a prospective cohort study. *Am J Med* 1990; 89: 713–21.
16. BARNES P. The pathology of community-acquired pneumonia. *Semin Resp Infect* 1994; 9: 130–9.
17. PACHON J, PRADOS M D, CAPOTE F, CUELLO J A, GURNACHO J, VERANO A. Severe community-acquired pneumonia. *Am Rev Resp Dis* 1990; 142: 369–73.
18. ROIG J, DOMINGO C, MORERA J. Legionnaires disease. *Chest* 1994; 105: 1817–25.
19. HAMEDANI P, ALI J, HAFEEZ S *et al.* The Safety and efficacy of Clarithromycin in patients with *Legionella* pneumonia. *Chest* 1991; 100: 1503–6.
20. GATTINONI L, PELOSI P, VITALE G *et al.* Body position changes redistribute lung computed-tomographic density in patients with acute respiratory failure. *Anesthesiology* 1991; 74: 15–23.
21. BONE R C, BALK RA, CERRA FB *et al.* Definitions for sepsis and organ failure and guidelines for the use of innovative therapies in sepsis. *Chest* 1992; 101: 1644–55.
22. BERNARD GR, ARTIGAS A, BRIGHAM K *et al.* The American–European Consensus Conference on ARDS. *Am J Resp Crit Care Med* 1994; 149: 818–24.
23. HUDSON L, MILBERG J, ANARDI D, MAUNDER R. Clinical risks for development of the Acute Respiratory Distress Syndrome. *Am Rev Resp Crit Care Med* 1995; 151: 293–301.
24. MURRAY JF, MATTHAY MA, LUCE JM, FLICK MR. An expanded definition of the Adult Respiratory Distress Syndrome. *Am Rev Resp Dis* 1988; 138: 720–3.
25. MONTGOMERY A, STAGER M, CARRICO C, HUDSON L. Causes of mortality in patients with Adult Respiratory Distress Syndrome. *Am Rev Resp Dis* 1985; 132: 485–9.
26. SUCHYTA M, CLEMMER T, ELLIOTT C, ORME J, WEAVER L. The Adult Respiratory Distress Syndrome. A report of survival and modifying factors. *Chest* 1992; 101: 1074–9.
27. LAMY M, FALLAT R, KOENIGER *et al.* Pathologic features and mechanisms of hypoxemia in Adult Respiratory Distress Syndrome. *Am Rev Resp Dis* 1976; 114: 267–84.

28. BACHOFEN M, WEIBEL E. Alterations of the gas exchange apparatus in adult respiratory insufficiency associated with septicemia. *Am Rev Resp Dis* 1977; 116: 589–615.
29. PRATT PC. Pathology of the Adult Respiratory Distress Syndrome. In Thorlbeck W M, Abel MR, eds. *The Lung: Structure, Function and Disease*. Baltimore Md: Williams and Wilkins Co.; 1978: 43–57.
30. PISON V, SEEGER W, BUCHHORN R *et al.* Surfactant abnormalities in patients with respiratory failure after multiple trauma. *Am Rev Resp Dis* 1989; 140: 1033–9.
31. ZAPOL W M, KOBAYASHI K, SNIDER MT *et al.* Vascular obstruction causes pulmonary hypertension in severe acute respiratory failure. *Chest* 1977; 7: 306–7.
32. DINARELLO CA, GELTAND J A, WOLFF SM. Anticytokine strategies in the treatment of the systemic inflammatory response syndrome. *JAMA* 1993; 269: 1829–35.
33. FOWLER AA, HAMMON RF, GOOD JT *et al.* Adult Respiratory Distress Syndrome: risk with common predispositions. *Ann Intern Med* 1983; 98: 593–7.
34. FRUCHTMAN SM, GOMBERT ME, LYONS HA. Adult Respiratory Distress Syndrome as a cause of death in pneumococcal pneumonia. *Chest* 1983; 83: 598–601.
35. MATUSCHAK GM. Multiple system organ failure: clinical expression, pathogenesis, and therapy. In Hall J B, Schmidt G A, Wood LDH, eds. *Principles of Critical Care* New York: McGraw-Hill, 1992: 613–36.
36. BELL RC, COALSON JJ, SMITH JD *et al.* Multiple organ system failure in Adult Respiratory Distress Syndrome. *Ann Intern Med* 1983; 99: 293–8.
37. MATUSCHAK GM, RINALDO JE. Organ interactions in the Adult Respiratory Distress Syndrome during sepsis: role of the liver in host defense. *Chest* 1988; 94: 400–6.
38. SCHWARTZ DB, BONE RC, BALK RA *et al.* Hepatic dysfunction in the Adult Respiratory Distress Syndrome. *Chest* 1989; 95: 871–5.
39. ORTQVIST A, KALIN M, LEJDEBORN L, LUNDBERG B. Diagnostic fibreoptic bronchoscopy and protected specimen brush in patients with community-acquired pneumonia. *Chest* 1990; 97: 576–82.
40. MEDURI GU, CONOSCENTI CC, MENASHE PH *et al.* Non-invasive face mask, ventilation in patients with acute respiratory failure. *Chest* 1989; 95: 865–70.
41. KIISKI R, TAKALA J, KARI A, MILIC-EMILI J. Effect of tidal volume on gas exchange and oxygen transport in the Adult Respiratory Distress Syndrome. *Am Rev Resp Dis* 1992; 148: 1131–5.
42. LODATO RF. Oxygen toxicity. *Crit Care Clin* 1990; 6: 749–65.
43. PETTY TL. The use, abuse, and mystique of positive end expiratory pressure. *Am Rev Resp Dis* 1988; 138: 475–8.
44. LUCE JM. The cardiovascular effects of mechanical ventilation and positive end expiratory pressure. *JAMA* 1984; 252: 807–11.
45. VAN HOOK CJ, CARILLI AD, HAPONIK EF. Hemodynamic effects of positive end expiratory pressure. *Am J Med* 1986; 81: 307–10.
46. HICKLING KG, HENDERSON SJ, JACKSON R. Low mortality associated with low volume pressure-limited ventilation with permissive hypercapnia in severe Adult Respiratory Distress Syndrome. *Intens Care Med* 1990; 16: 372–7.
47. HICKLING KG, WALSH J, HENDERSON S, JACKSON R. Low mortality rate in Adult Respiratory Distress Syndrome using low-volume, pressure limited ventilation with permissive hypercapnia: a prospective study. *Crit Care Med* 1994; 22: 1568–78.
48. TUXEN D. Permissive hypercapnic ventilation. *Am J Resp Crit Care Med* 1994; 150: 870–4.
49. MACINTYRE N. Clinically available new strategies for mechanical ventilatory support. *Chest* 1993; 104: 560–5.
50. MARCY TW, MARINI JJ. Inverse ratio ventilation in ARDS. *Chest* 1991; 100: 494–504.
51. MORRIS AH, WALLACE CJ, MENLOVE RL *et al.* Randomized clinical trial of pressure-controlled inverse ratio ventilation and extracorporeal CO_2 removal for Adult Respiratory Distress Syndrome. *Am J Resp Crit Care Med* 1994; 149: 295–305.
52. SHANHOLTZ C, BROWER R. Should inverse ratio ventilation be used in Adult Respiratory Distress Syndrome? *Am J Resp Crit Care Med* 1994; 149: 1354–8.
53. SLUTSKY AS. Concensus Conference on Mechanical Ventilation Part I. *Intens Care Med* 1994; 20: 64–79. Part II 1994; 20: 150–62.
54. LANGER M, MASCHERONI D, MARCOLIN R *et al.* The prone position in ARDS patients. *Chest* 1988; 94: 103–7.
55. MORTENSON JD. Augmentation of blood gas transfer by means of an intravascular blood gas exchanger (IVOX). In Marini J J, Roussos C, eds. *Ventilatory Failure*. London: Springer-Verlag; 1991: 318–46.
56. RAVENSCRAFT S, BURKE W, NAHUM A, ADAMS A, NAKOS G, MARINI J. Tracheal gas insufflation augments CO_2 clearance during mechanical ventilation. *Am Rev Resp Dis* 1993; 148: 345–51.
57. FROESE AB, BRYAN AC. High frequency ventilation. *Am Rev Resp Dis* 1987; 135: 1363–74.
58. GLUCK E, HEARD S, PATEL C *et al.* Use of ultrahigh frequency ventilation in patients with ARDS. *Chest* 1993; 103: 1413–20.
59. TUTUNCU AS, FAITHFULL NS, LACHMANN B. Comparison of ventilatory support with intratracheal perfluorocarbon administration and conventional mechanical ventilation in animals with acute respiratory failure. *Am Rev Resp Dis* 1993; 148: 785–92.
60. SIMMONS RS, BERNDINE GG, SEIDENFIELD JJ *et al.* Fluid balance and the Adult Respiratory Distress Syndrome. *Am Rev Resp Dis* 1987; 135: 924–9.
61. HUMPHREY H, HALL J, SZAJDER I, SILVERSTEIN M, WOOD L. Improved survival in ARDS patients associated with a reduction in Pulmonary Capillary Wedge Pressure. *Chest* 1990; 97: 1176–80.
62. HUDSON L. Fluid management strategy in Acute Lung Injury. *Am Rev Resp Dis* 1992; 145: 988–9.
63. TUCHSHMIDT J, FRIED J, ASTIZ M *et al.* Elevation of cardiac output and oxygen delivery improves outcome in septic shock. *Chest* 1992; 102: 216–20.
64. SHOEMAKER WC, APPEL PL, KRAM HB *et al.* Prospective trial of supranormal values of survivors as therapeutic goals in high risk surgical patients. *Chest* 1988; 94: 1176–86.
65. NANJO S, BHATTACHARYA J, STAUB NC. Concentrated albumin does not affect lung edema formation after acid instillation in the dog. *Am Rev Resp Dis* 1983; 128: 884–9.
66. HAYES MA, TIMMINS AC, YAU EHS, PALAZZO M, HINDS C, WATSON D. Elevation of systemic oxygen delivery in the treatment of critically ill patients. *N Engl J Med* 1994; 330: 1717–22.
67. GATTINONI L, PRESENTI A, MASCHERONI D *et al.* Low frequency positive pressure ventilation with extracorporeal CO_2 removal in severe acute respiratory failure. *JAMA* 1986; 256: 881–6.
68. JOBE AH. Pulmonary surfactant therapy. *N Engl J Med* 1993; 328: 861–8.
69. LEWIS JF, JOBE AH. Surfactant and the Adult Respiratory Distress Syndrome. *Am Rev Resp Dis* 1993; 147: 218–33.
70. WIEDEMAN H, BAUGHMAN R, DEBRISBLANC B. Multicenter trial in human sepsis-induced ARDS of an aerosolized synthetic surfactant (Exosurf). *Am Rev Resp Dis (Abstract)* 1992; 145: A184.
71. ZIEGLER E, FISCHER C, SPRUNG C *et al.* Treatment of Gram-negative bacteremia and septic shock with HA-IA human monoclonal antibody against endotoxin. A randomized double-blind, placebo controlled trial. *N Engl J Med* 1991; 324: 429–36.

72. BERNARD GR, REINES HD, HALUSHKA P *et al.* Prostacyclin and Thromboxane A_2 formation is increased in human sepsis syndrome. *Am Rev Resp Dis* 1991; 144: 1095–101.

73. POWELL R, MACHIEDO G, RUSH B *et al.* Effect of oxygen free radical scavengers on survival in sepsis. *Am Surg* 1991; 57: 86–8.

74. BONE RC, SLOTMAN G, MAUNDER R *et al.* Randomized double-blind multicenter study of prostaglandin E1 in patients with the Adult Respiratory Distress Syndrome. *Chest* 1989; 96: 114–19.

75. ROISSAINT R, FALKE KJ, LOPEZ F, SLAMA K, PISON V, ZAPOL W M. Inhaled nitric oxide for the Adult Respiratory Distress Syndrome. *N Engl J Med* 1993; 328: 399–405.

76. BIGATELLO LM, HURFORD WE, KACMAREK RM, ROBERTS JD JR, ZAPOL W M. Prolonged inhalation of low concentrations of nitric oxide in patients with severe Adult Respiratory Distress Syndrome; effects on pulmonary hemodynamics and oxygenation. *Anesthesiology* 1994; 80: 761–70.

77. BERNARD GR, LUCE JM, SPRUNG CL *et al.* High dose corticosteroids in patients with the Adult Respiratory Distress Syndrome. *N Engl J Med* 1987; 317: 1565–70.

78. BONE RC, FISCHER CJ, CLEMMER TP *et al.* Early methylprednisolone treatment for septic syndrome and the Adult Respiratory Distress Syndrome. *Chest* 1987; 92: 1032–6.

79. MEDURI GU, CHINN AJ, LEEPER KV *et al.* Corticosteroid rescue treatment of progressive fibroproliferation in late ARDS: Patterns of response and predictors of outcome. *Chest* 1994; 105: 1516–27.

80. BROCHARD L, RAUSS A, BENITO S *et al.* Comparison of three methods of gradual withdrawal from ventilatory support during weaning from mechanical ventilation. *Am J Resp Crit Care Med* 1994; 150: 896–903.

81. ESTEBAN A, FRUTOS F, TOBIN MJ *et al.* A comparison of four methods of weaning patients from mechanical ventilation. *N Engl J Med* 1995; 332: 345–50.

82. HAMPTON AA, SHERETZ RJ. Vascular access infections in hospitalized patients. *Surg Clin N Am* 1988; 68: 57–71.

83. COBB DK, HIGH KP, SAWYER RG. A controlled trial of scheduled replacement of central venous and pulmonary artery catheters. *N Engl J Med* 1992: 327: 1062–8.

84. MAKI DG, WHEELER SJ, STOLZ SM, MERMEL LA. Clinical trial of a novel antiseptic central venous catheter. *The 31st Interscience Conference on Antimicrobial Agents and Chemotherapy*, Chicago, September 1991, Abstract 176.

85. MURRAY MJ, MARSH HM, WOCHOS DN, MOXNESS KE, OFFORD KP, CALLAWAY CW. Nutritional assessment of Intensive Care Unit patients. *Mayo Clin Proc* 1988; 63: 1106–15.

86. SHAW JHF, KOEA JB. Metabolic basis for management of the septic surgical patient. *World J Surg* 1993; 17: 154–64.

87. MCMAHON MM, FARNELL MB, MURRAY MJ. Nutritional support of critically ill patients. *Mayo Clin Proc* 1993; 68: 911–20.

88. DE BIASSE MA, WILMORE DW. What is optimal nutritional support? *New Horizons* 1994; 2: 122–30.

89. JEEJEEBHOY KN. How should we monitor nutritional support: structure or function? *New Horizons* 1994; 2: 131–8.

90. BOWER RH, CERRA FB, BERSHADSKY B *et al.* Early enteral administration of a formula (Impact) supplemented with arginine, nucleotides and fish oil in Intensive Care Unit patients: results of a multicenter, prospective, randomized, clinical trial. *Crit Care Med* 1995; 23: 436–49.

91. ROSS RJM, RODRIGUEZ-ARNAO J, BENTHAM J, COAKLEY JH. The role of insulin, growth hormone and IGF-1 as anabolic agents in the critically ill. *Intens Care Med* 1993; 19: S54–7.

28 Diseases associated with persistent or recurrent pulmonary infiltrates

MICHAEL E. ELLIS

King Faisal Specialist Hospital and Research Centre, Riyadh, Saudi Arabia

Introduction

Some patients with pulmonary infiltrates and a supposed infectious pneumonia may not respond in a seemingly appropriate fashion to antimicrobial therapy. Their progress may be unduly prolonged, the pneumonic process may recur or may not resolve on antibiotics. There are four possibilities viz: (a) a truly infectious pneumonia of common aetiology, e.g. caused by *Streptococcus pneumoniae*, *Haemophilus* or *Legionella* spp, which is resolving at a perceived slow but a normal expected rate; (b) an infectious pneumonia of either an uncommon aetiology, for example, *Mycobacterium tuberculosis*, or of a common aetiology but in which the organism is resistant, the mode of antimicrobial treatment is not appropriate (e.g. low dosages) or there are suppurative or indirect complications arising from the pneumonia, but which, once recognised and treated appropriately, will respond accordingly; (c) an infectious pneumonia which is resolving slowly or which recurs as a result of an underlying host mechanical defect, or immunocompromisation, including aged and pregnant patients; (d) an apparent infectious pneumonia which does not resolve or recurs and is in reality non-microbial in origin. This chapter will address each of these categories, highlighting some of the more major examples (Fig. 28.1). The special setting of nosocomial pneumonia is addressed in Chapter 19.

Definitions: slowly resolving, chronic and recurrent pneumonia

These terms are, to some extent, arbitrary and variable. Some reports focus on radiographical abnormalities, others on the accompanying acute/chronic pulmonary and systemic features such as cough, malaise and fatigue. Definitions of a *slowly resolving pneumonia* include: less than complete clearing of radiological infiltrates at 4 weeks,[1] less than 50% clearing of radiographical infiltrates at 4 weeks in the patient who has defervesced and improved symptomatically[2], non-resolution of a radiographical infiltrate in an expected period of time based on a presumptive diagnosis and at least 10 days of antibiotic therapy[3], failure to resolve an apparent routine infection within 30 days[4], signs and symptoms slow to resolve following optimal therapy[5], persistence of radiographical infiltrates, cough, temperature > 38.1 °C/leukocytosis/sputum, for ≥ 10 days having received antibiotics ≥ 1 week[6].

A slowly resolving pneumonia merges into a *chronic pneumonia* syndrome if substantial radiographical changes and symptoms persist for more than 4–6 weeks, though such a clear distinction is not always possible. *Recurrent pneumonia*, on the other hand, is defined as the occurrence of at least two or three distinct clinical and radiological episodes of pneumonia[7,8].

Truly infectious pneumonias resolving normally but 'slowly'

It is clear that the course of pneumonia will be influenced by microbial aetiology, age, antimicrobial therapy and underlying co-morbid or host defence factors. The pneumonia may be evolving 'slowly' in an absolute sense, but as expected relative to the presence of these factors. A number of studies provide information relating to the influence of the microbial organism on the temporal progression of the pneumonia. The most frequently implicated microorganisms in community-acquired pneumonia are *S. pneumoniae*, *Mycoplasma pneumoniae*, *Legionella* species and *Chlamydia psittaci* or *Chlamydia pneumoniae* (see Chapters 5, 13 and 14). Some of these studies provide a reference time to decide when a pneumonia is resolving slowly or is chronic.

There is very little disagreement that the use of antibiotics has a substantial impact in accelerating the rate of resolution and reducing the mortality associated with pneumococcal pneumonia. With this antibiotic variable 'fixed', early reports suggested that some individuals still appeared to respond slowly[9], but it was the classic paper of van Metre[10] who described the expected clinical and radiographical course of pneumococcal pneumonia in 358 patients. Of these patients, 71% defervesced by day 5 and 94% by day 15. In addition, 83% had cleared their chest radiograph of lung parenchymal infiltrates by day 30. Persistence of fever beyond 10 days and consolidation beyond 30 days occurred in a greater proportion of patients who were aged > 50 years, had multilobar rather than lobar disease, presence of bacteremia, a peripheral white cell count of $< 5 \times 10^9$/l, type I/type II pneumococcus, chronic alcoholism and antibiotic treatment initiated after the first day of disease. These features tended to be present also in patients with suppurative complications such as lung abscess, empyema and atelectasis. At least two of these different features were present in patients who subsequently died. Of some interest is that 'concomitant diseases' (chronic pulmonary disease, ischaemic heart disease, cardiac failure, diabetes mellitus, thyrotoxicosis, hemiplegia, hepatic cirrhosis, uraemia, leukaemia and lymphosarcoma) did not appear to prolong time to defervescence but were associated with prolonged consolidation.

By comparison, Jay found that only approximately 60% of patients had cleared their consolidation by 4 weeks, but 97% had done so by 8 weeks, although at that time 30% still had residual non-consolidation abnormalities such as volume loss, pleural disease and stranding. By 18 weeks, chest radiographs were normal in all patients[11]. However, in all of the 72 patients in Jay's series compared to only 63 of the 358 patients in van Metre's series – bacteraemia had already been identified as a factor associated with a slower resolution of pneumonia. Alcoholism, age > 50 years, chronic obstructive pulmonary disease and extensive initial pneumonia were confirmed as factors associated with those patients whose resolution was delayed beyond 6 weeks (Fig. 28.2).

A more recent study from the UK indicated that 30% of patients with non-bacteraemic pneumococcal pneumonia but only 15% with bacteraemic/antigenemic pneumococcal pneumonia had achieved a normal chest radiograph at 4 weeks[12]. By 24 weeks, the majority of patients had a normal chest radiograph (Fig. 28.3). In this study, no attempt was made to differentiate radiographical consolidation from other radiographical abnormalities such as pleural fluid, volume loss, cavitation and hilar lymphadenopathy. Of some interest was that radiographical *deterioration* occurred in 52% of bacteraemic (and 26% of non-bacteraemic) pneumococcal pneumonic patients following admission prior to the start of resolution. Secondary adult respiratory distress syndrome may be one explanation[12].

Generally in pneumococcal pneumonia, substantial defervescence, sputum volume reduction and bacterial conversion settle within a few days and the radiographical improvement consistently lags behind this clinical and microbiological improvement[10,13]. Chronic fatigue has been poorly studied in patients with community-acquired pneumonia but may be the last symptom to disappear and only then after many weeks or even months. Cough and auscultatory lung findings disappear in most patients by the second week[14]. Feinsilver *et al.*[6] used persistence of *symptoms* for at least 10 days as part of their working definition of non-resolving pneumonia. It is important to manage the patient's symptoms and not 'treat' the chest radiological abnormalities.

The crude non-concordance of these various studies may reflect different microbial diagnostic techniques, incidences of bacteraemia, definitions and interpretations of radiological abnormalities, antimicrobial choices, dosages and duration, and variations in background population demographics. A synthesis of these reports would be that, in a heterogenous population of patients admitted to hospital with community-acquired pneumococcal pneumonia, initial radiological deterioration might occur in up to a quarter of patients in the first week, but in the second week, substantial clearing of infiltrates should take place. A completely normal chest radiograph would be returned by 4 months in the vast majority of patients and in all patients by 6 months. Fever and sputum volume would be expected to substantially improve by the end of the first week. Dissection of this group further suggests that for patients aged < 50 years with no chronic obstructive pulmonary disease or history of alcoholism and who have limited pulmonary involvement on presentation, radiological and clinical resolution should be more rapid and a completely normal chest radiograph would be expected by 4–6 weeks. In contrast, a patient aged > 50 years who has identified co-morbid conditions would 'normally' result in the time course of resolution at the right of this spectrum.

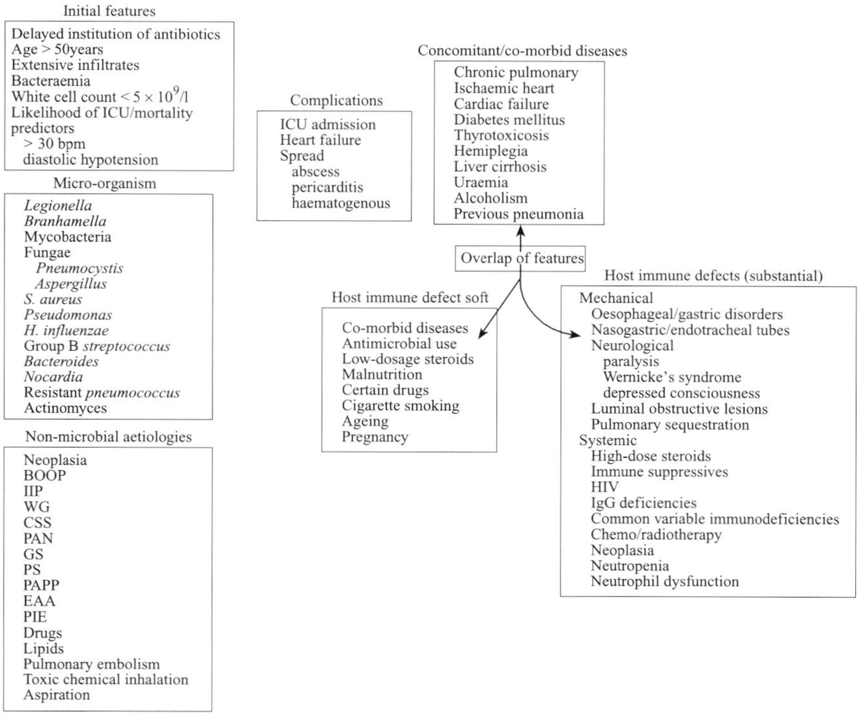

FIGURE 28.1 Factors associated with/responsible for prolonged resolution of, or recurrent, pneumonia/pulmonary infiltrates.

In contrast to the situation with pneumococcal pneumonia, 50% of patients with uncomplicated *M. pneumoniae* clear their radiographical abnormalities by 4 weeks in 90% by 12 weeks[12]. This was similar to Finnegan's series[15] (40% at 4 weeks, 96% at 8 weeks). Initial radiological deterioration similar to that observed in pneumococcal pneumonia was again described for 25% of patients in the Macfarlane study, a feature supported by others[16,17] but was relatively uncommon in Finnegan's report[15]. Residual cough and fatigue may be found in some patients for several weeks or months. In a minority, permanent lung sequelae such as fibrosis and bronchiolitis obliterans may occur.

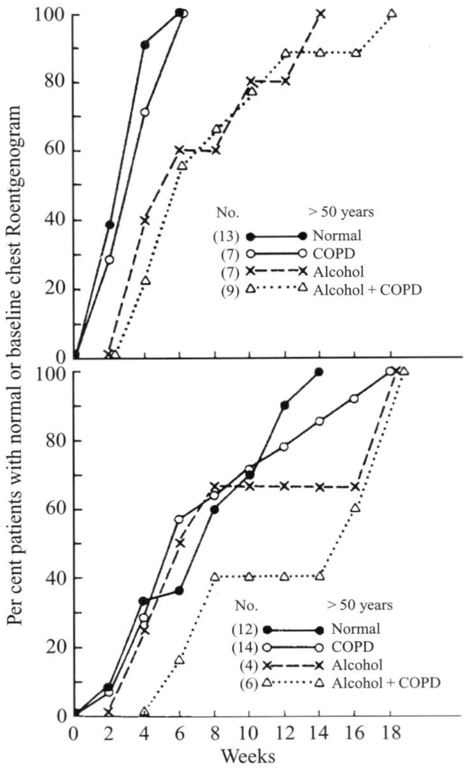

FIGURE 28.2 [from Jay, Ref. 11, with permission]. Effects of age, absence of underlying disease (normal), chronic obstructive pulmonary disease (COPD), acute alcoholism (alcohol) and both (COPD + alcohol) on radiographical resolution of *Streptococcus pneumoniae* pneumonia.

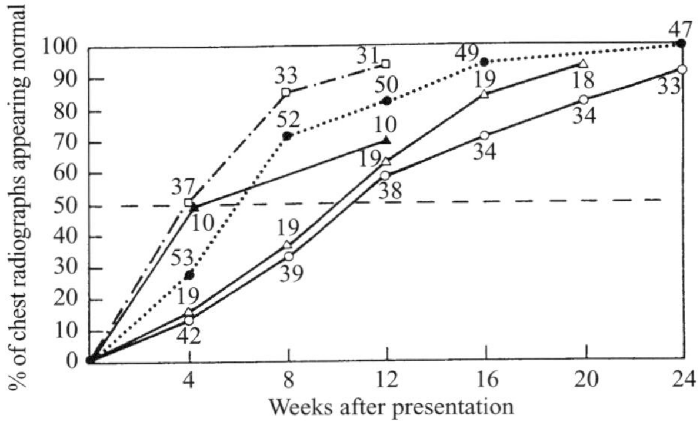

FIGURE 28.3 [from Macfarlane, Ref. 12, with permission]. Percentages of surviving patients showing radiographical clearance at four weekly intervals after admission to hospital.
o—o Legionnaires' disease ($n=42$); △—△ bacteraemic or antigenaemic pneumococcal pneumonia ($n=19$); •·····• other pneumococcal pneumonias ($n=53$); □-·-□ mycoplasma pneumonia ($n=37$); ▲—▲ psittacosis pneumonia ($n=10$).

Legionnaire's disease is associated with a relatively longer period of resolution; it is also common to witness initial substantial radiological deterioration in as many as 65% of patients[12]. It is thought that the organism *per se* rather than underlying co-morbid disease is directly responsible for this, since for example only 29% have pre-existing chronic diseases[18]. Thus, only 15% of patients at 4 weeks show a normal chest radiograph; the figure improving to 55% at 12 weeks and 80% at 20 weeks. At 24 weeks, 15% of patients still exhibit radiographical abnormalities[12]. Some series describe an even slower rate of resolution: 75% of patients surviving Legionnaire's disease had radiographical abnormalities at 3 months[19]. The fact that up to one-quarter of cases of Legionnaire's disease in some centres require ventilation (often prolonged) reflects the inherent chronicity of this illness[18]. These findings are similar to those reported by others[20] although some are at variance, for example, a higher rate of resolution with only 30% having X-ray abnormalities at 8 weeks is seen by Kirby[21]. In summary, substantial clearing in Legionnaire's disease would be expected by the second and third week in most patients. Several patients may be ventilated and have a much longer course. A working leeway of 6–7 months to complete radiological clearance is therefore an acceptable time before concern is generated over the possible existence of a significant/sinister underlying disease, other than that known to be present. Furthermore, many patients recovering from Legionnaire's disease may be expected to have residual dyspnoea associated with objective pulmonary function abnormalities one year later[22].

C. psittaci and *C. pneumoniae* generally show a rate of resolution intermediate between that described for bacteraemic/antigenemic pneumococcal pneumonia and non-bacteraemic/antigenemic pneumococcal pneumonia, so that 50% will have a normal radiograph by 4 weeks and 60–80% by 8 weeks[12,23]. *Moraxella catarrhalis* is being increasingly implicated as a cause of pneumonia in the debilitated and elderly. Many patients have severe lung disease and mortality is high. Resolution is often prolonged[24]. For most patients with community-acquired pneumonia, therefore, a substantial XR/clinical improvement should occur by 2 weeks.

Infectious pneumonia with complications or due to uncommon organisms

A slowly resolving pneumonic situation may also arise as a result of the complications which may, for example, result in ICU admission, or if certain predictors for mortality are present. Multilobar involvement, tachypnoea > 30 breaths per minute, diastolic hypotension < 60 mmHg, age > 65 years, other underlying diseases and hypoxaemia are among these predictors[25–29]. Furthermore, abscess formation, pericarditis, heart failure, extrapulmonary haematogenous dissemination may also result in a protracted course of the pneumonia itself or prolongation of certain symptoms, e.g. fever. The mere presence of an unusual pathogen might also account for slow resolution. However, the presence of certain pathogens *per se* should in some cases heighten the suspicion of a more serious underlying problem. For example, *Pneumocystis carinii* is highly suggestive of an advanced immunosuppressive state such as HIV infection; *Aspergillus* could reflect neutrophil dysfunction or chronic necrotising pulmonary aspergillosis. Travel to, or residence in, endemic areas such as the Mississippi River Valley necessitates exclusion of histoplasmosis, or coccidioidomycosis for Arizona. A careful travel history is needed in all patients presenting with pulmonary symptomatology (see Chapter 26). *Mycobacterium tuberculosis* commonly produces a chronic pulmonary illness and should always be ruled out particularly in patients with risks determined by social class, exposure to intravenous drug abuse, exposure in a highly endemic area and in HIV-positive patients. Other agents that may be associated with a prolonged course include the pneumonic destructive organisms such as *Staphylococcus aureus*, *Pseudomonas*, and other enteric Gram-negative organisms, *H. influenzae*, group B *streptococcus*, anaerobic organisms such as *bacteroides*, non-tuberculous mycobacteria, fungi, *Actinomyces*, exotic or tropical worms and protozoa, viruses such as influenza and RSV, and *Nocardia* (see relevant chapters). Finally, resistance to antimicrobial agents, for example, as reflected by the rising MICs of pneumococci to penicillin[30], failure to select appropriate antibiotics or deliver a therapeutic dose may also determine the course of the pneumonia (See Chapter 4).

Infectious pneumonia in patients with underlying host defence defects

The host immunity is the other major factor which determines response rate and outcome. Patients with no overt co-morbid conditions would be expected to resolve most of their presenting symptoms and radiological abnormalities relatively rapidly, i.e. they would comprise the left of the resolution time spectrum for the given microorganism. Patients with chronic preexisting diseases would exhibit a longer but still 'normal' period of resolution. The vast majority of these conditions produce depressed host response to infection[10,11]. They include cardiac failure (impaired pulmonary clearance of bacteria, reduced surfactant, enhanced bacterial multiplication), diabetes mellitus (dysfunctional polymorphs), alcohol use (dysfunctional polymorphs, dysfunctional alveolar macrophages including defective toxic oxygen radical formation, chemotaxis, mucociliary function and diminished cytokine responsiveness), cigarette smoking (mucus changes, mucociliary escalator impediment, alveolar macrophage dysfunction, airway immunoglobulin changes, bacterial colonisation of the lower respiratory tract and chronic obstructive pulmonary disease), malnutrition (reduced immunoglobulins, polymorph and alveolar macrophage dysfunction), the elderly (see later this chapter), possibly prior sepsis itself (via a delicate serum/pulmonary imbalance of the TNF-mediated inflammatory response and reduced complement levels)[31], drug administration (theophylines, antimicrobials such as the macrolides, e.g. erythromycin, anaesthetics, and corticosteroids, which reduce bacterial clearance) and mechanical breaches of the upper airways defences, e.g. endotracheal tubes (see Chapter 3).

These somewhat 'soft' features of a defective host response are relatively common in patients with community-acquired pneumonia admitted to hospital. For example, alcoholism was present in 28% and other chronic illnesses in 20% of all hospitalised pneumococcal pneumonia patients in van Metre's series[10]. These confounding illnesses are usually documented at the initial patient assessment. In the past, it has been suggested that provided such a feature has been identified further detailed investigations are deemed unnecessary since the chance of diagnosing a new predisposing factor, particularly malignancy, is remote. This has been supported by the work of Jay[11] who found no incidence of lung cancer in 7 of 72 bacteraemic patients who had slowly resolving pneumococcal pneumonia despite their chest radiographs suggesting the presence of an underlying cancer. However, among the remaining patients, who cleared their pneumonia without delay, 6 (8%) did have sinister immunocompromisation – all malignancies of the lung, blood or reticulo-endothelial system. Thus, lung cancer was not responsible for the delayed resolution of pneumonia. Van Metre's report on 358 patients did not mention lung cancer or other malignancies as a contributory factor in slowly resolving pneumonia[10]. Obviously, the presence of an unsuspected abnormality on routine haematology, biochemistry or chest radiography should be fully investigated since lung abscess, pericarditis, tumour, etc. may occur in *any* patient with pneumonia. More recent publications have also suggested that the incidence of serious/sinister underlying lung disease or of other alternative diagnoses or immunodeficiency in patients admitted with pneumonia may be more common than previously suspected or increasing in incidence. This may be as a result of more detailed investigations being undertaken on patients, access to more sophisticated diagnostic techniques, and a changing general population which is characterised by increased longevity and a greater incidence of iatrogenic and indigenous immunosuppressive illnesses. Thus, in a study by Fang *et al.*[32] in 359 patients with community-acquired pneumonia, whereas the frequency of chronic obstructive pulmonary disease (31%), alcohol abuse (33%), diabetes (13%), congestive cardiac failure (13%) was not surprising, 36% of patients had in addition haematological malignancy, solid organ malignancy, neutropenia or chronic steroid administration, and 2.5% had AIDS. Feinsilver[6] investigated 35 patients with non-resolving presumed infectious community-acquired pneumonia, by fibreoptic bronchoscopy/open lung biopsy. Patients with *known* HIV or lung cancer were excluded. Of these patients 14 (40%) had new specific diagnoses established – mainly by fibreoptic bronchoscopy. They included bronchoalveolar carcinoma and adenocarcinoma in four. A further seven patients had unusual respiratory infections which were unsuspected at admission which mimicked regular community-acquired pneumonia. These included tuberculosis, cytomegalovirus disease, *Pneumocystis* and actinomycosis. One other patient had Wegener's granulomatosis and 1 had bronchiolitis obliterans with organising pneumonia (BOOP). However, a new diagnosis was most likely to be found in younger (< 55 years) non-smokers with multi-lobar findings on chest radiography and who had symptoms persisting > 4–6 weeks. Patients without these features who have slow resolution do not normally have unsuspected serious underlying disease, and the appropriate management is clinical observation, provided no obvious radiological, clinical or laboratory abnormalities are apparent. These recent observations suggest that the traditional approach of monitoring patients with slowly resolving pneumonia for several weeks without investigating – particularly young individuals with no 'soft' host defects – may require re-evaluation. The finding of malignancy in several patients with a normal rate of radiological resolution[11] supports this. More contemporary data is needed to clarify the issue.

Recurrent pneumonia

Data reflecting the incidence of recurrent pneumonia is sparse and limited to patients admitted to hospital with community-acquired pneumonia. Ekdahl reported 90/2542 (3%) patients with community-acquired pneumonia who had at least three episodes[8] and Fang 12/359 (3.3%) for patients with at least two episodes[32].

It has already been mentioned that some patients with pneumonia may have predisposing or underlying chronic disease. It is, therefore, not surprising that patients with recurrent pneumonia will have similar pre-morbid conditions. However, it is not clear whether the frequency and/or severity of these is enhanced in patients with recurrent pneumonia. For example, in a large Finnish *community-based* study of community-acquired pneumonia performed in 1982[33] 546 of 46,979 inhabitants had community-acquired pneumonia (of which 42% were admitted to hospital) and for most patients this was presumably the first episode. However, only 104/546 (19%) had pre-defined chronic conditions, among which cancer and immunosuppressive therapy accounted for the minority (14/104, 13%), severe chronic lung disease/severe chronic heart disease and diabetes accounting for the majority (90/104: 86%). By contrast, a prospective study of 359 patients admitted to hospital in Pittsburgh, USA in 1987 (of whom only 12 patients had recurrent pneumonia) indicated underlying disease was present in 70% of *all* patients. Although chronic obstructive pulmonary disease, alcoholism, diabetes mellitus and congestive cardiac failure were the most frequently described underlying diseases severe immune deficiency as represented by haematologic and solid organ cancer was present in 28.4% of patients[32]. The difference in underlying disease frequency and spectrum between these two studies may reflect differences in patient demography, frequency of use of antibiotics in the community, variation in microbial diagnostic techniques or an increasing percentage of some populations which are more immunocompromised. Indeed, the high incidence of unusual infections such as TB, *P. carinii* and fungi in some recent series, e.g. 20%[6] is witness to these factors. Nevertheless, in patients with documented recurrent pneumonia, the incidence of co-morbid illness appears to be high. All patients in Ekdahl's series[8] had predisposing illnesses of whom 18/90 (20%) had solid organ cancer, 7/90 (8%) had haematological malignancy, 11/90 (12%) had hypogammaglobulinaemia and one patient had AIDS – that is severe/sinister predisposing diseases occurred in 37/90 (41%) of cases. The spectrum of underlying disease is similar to that described in an earlier report[7] although hypogammaglobulinaemia was not as common (but neither was it looked for as carefully as in Ekdahl's series and may be therefore rather more common than realised). The available evidence does therefore suggest that in recurrent pneumonia, underlying conditions *are* found more frequently and are probably more serious than in patients who have only one episode of community-acquired pneumonia.

The same factors predisposing to pneumonia and to its slow resolution or chronicity may also play a role in recurrence, namely, cardiac failure, diabetes mellitus, alcohol abuse, cigarette smoking, malnutrition, the elderly, prior sepsis, certain drug administrations and mechanical breaches of the respiratory tract defence systems. In addition, there are other well-recognised risks and these are described as follows. It is of some interest that pneumonia *per se* is a risk factor for subsequent pneumonia. In a study of 241 patients previously admitted to hospital with pneumonia, the overall incidence rate for subsequent pneumonia was 5.45 times significantly greater (even more so in patients aged > 65 years) over a 3-year follow-up period, compared to a group of 332 patients admitted with non-pulmonary infections. The patients with recurrent pneumonia also had a higher mortality due to pneumonia[34].

HIV-associated immune deficiency

HIV-infected individuals are at increased risk from capsulated bacterial pneumonia. Thus, the incidence of pneumococcal pneumonia in such patients is some sevenfold increased compared to those who are HIV negative[35]. Recurrent bacterial pneumonia due to *S. pneumoniae* and *H. influenzae* is also well described in patients with HIV infection[36]. This has led to the inclusion of recurrent bacterial pneumonia as an AIDS defining condition[37], the risk of recurrence rising as the CD4 count falls. These features appear to be, in part, related to B-cell abnormalities resulting in non-specific polyclonal gammopathic associated dysfunction and reduction in specific protective antibodies against capsulated organisms. Other factors include selective serum and mucosal encapsulated bacterial protective IgA2 deficiency[38], heightened complement activation and defective neutrophil and macrophage functions. HIV-positive intravenous drug abusers who smoke illicit drugs and patients with limited access to health care services are additional risk features which may increase their susceptibility to bacterial pneumonia[35]. Pneumococcal pneumonia is now the most common cause of HIV-associated lower respiratory tract infection, and responsible for nearly one half of first HIV-related manifestations in some areas[39] and may supersede by almost 50% the incidence of *Pneumocystis* pneumonia among intravenous drug abusers[40]. Pneumococcal pneumonia in these patients is usually twofold more likely to be bacteraemic compared to HIV-negative patients. Of some interest is that response to antimicrobial therapy is usually prompt and satisfactory – prolongation of each pneumococcal pneumonic episode is not usually a feature with no increased pneumonia-associated mortality[39,40]. *H. influenzae*, *S. aureus*, *M. catarrhalis*, legionellosis, and *M. pneumoniae* infections are also seen (albeit less commonly than streptococcal pneumonia) but the data relating to recurrence with them is somewhat sparse[35]. Recurrence has, however, been documented in the somewhat uncommon situation of HIV *Pseudomonas* pneumonia which is often associated with neutropenia, indwelling catheters and prolonged steroid use[41]. *Nocardia* pneumonia is also a cause of protracted pneumonia in some 0.25% cases of AIDS patients, is likely to relapse and recur[42], despite appropriate chemoprophylaxis. *Rhodococcus equi* has been described in HIV-positive and other immunosuppressed patients and produces a cavitary pneumonia. Its acid fast staining and radiological features mimic TB or occasionally tumour. Bacteraemic-seeded subcutaneous cerebral abscesses may also occur. Lung fibrosis may result and relapse appears to be particularly common[43,44]. Recurrent bacterial and other pneumonias should always raise the suspicion of HIV infection and a careful, social, sexual and past history together with an HIV antibody test should be performed in suspected cases. Other aspects of HIV-associated respiratory tract disease including *P. carinii* particularly are described in detail in Chapter 22.

Non-HIV-associated immunodeficiency states

Several other causes of humoral and cellular immune deficiency predispose to recurrent bacterial pneumonias. These include selective IgG2 and IgG4 deficiency[45], agammaglobulinaemia, and common variable hypogammaglobulinaemia[46]. Ekdahl's study[8] highlighted that immunoglobulin deficiencies may be underdiagnosed in many patients with recurrent pneumonias – 11/38 patients investigated (29%) had total hypoimmunoglobulinaemia. Isolated IgA deficiency does not usually produce recurrent infections but hypoimmunoglobulinaemia A *with* hypoimmunoglobulinaemia G2 does[47]. Screening for IgG and IgA deficiency in all patients with recurrent pneumonias is therefore suggested.

Common variable immunodeficiency (CVI) is a multifaceted syndrome affecting males and females equally in their 20s and 30s. A key manifestation is an increased incidence of recurrent bacterial infections due to encapsulated bacteria such as *S. pneumoniae* and *H. influenzae*, particularly of the upper respiratory tract (sinusitis, otitis media) and lower respiratory tract (pneumonia and bronchitis) which ultimately lead to chronic lung disease. The heterogenous nature of CVI is reflected by the finding that recurrent mycobacterial, fungal, viral (particularly CMV and enteroviral) and protozoal (*P. carinii*) infection also occur, as do multiple gastrointestinal, lymphoproliferative and autoimmune diseases. Diarrhoea due to *Salmonella*, *Campylobacter* and *Giardia* characterise the infective gastrointestinal disorders whilst gastric adenocarcinoma, intestinal lymphoma[48], inflammatory bowel disease and a pseudo-gluten sensitive enteropathy are also found. A wide range of benign lymphoreticuloses occur including splenomegaly and lymphadenopathy due to lymphoid hyperplasia, but malignant lymphoma can occur. Haemolytic anaemia, granulocyte antibody-associated neutropenia, immune thrombocytopenic purpura and pernicious anaemia are common. A major underlying defect in all patients is the variable inability of B-cells to secrete normal immunoglobulin[49]. There also appears to be CD4 T-cell deficiency production of IL2[50]. Some patients have abnormally high numbers of CD8 cytotoxic/suppressive (on B-cell immunoglobulin production) T-cells[51]. These combined B and T disorders provide a basis for understanding the wide range of illnesses in this complex disease. The current status of therapy involves appropriate prolonged antimicrobial therapy, treatment and prophylaxis-directed intravenous immunoglobulin replacement and immunomodulatory therapy with such modalities as recombinant interleukin-2[52].

Iatrogenic immunosuppression is a well-established cause of sepsis in general and recurrent pulmonary infections particularly. Organ transplantation is a major contributor and this has been covered in detail in Chapter 21. Bone marrow transplantation, chemo/radiotherapy and immunosuppressive drugs lower the host's mechanical, mucosal and systemic defences to critical levels. The gastrointestinal, upper and lower respiratory tracts and skin are major sources for a variety of bacterial, viral and protozoal pulmonary infections which, unconstrained by poor antibody responses, hypogammaglobulinaemia, functional hyposplenism, mucositis, graft vs. host disease, associated airways damage, severe and prolonged neutropenia, abnormal T-cell population, etc. manifest a variety of severe pneumonias which may recur until immunoreconstitution has taken place. Occult and overt pneumonias due to *S. pneumoniae*, *Staphylococcus*, *Pseudomonas* and other Gram-negatives, *Aspergillus* and other fungi, cytomegalovirus and other viruses are particularly common. They require a high degree of diagnostic suspicion and prompt institution of broad spectrum empiric, or definitive therapy. Invasive investigative techniques are in some cases limited by the patient's poor general condition. Prophylactic antimicrobial regimes often result in the emergence of resistant organisms. For further details, refer to Chapter 21.

Defects of the gastrointestinal and upper respiratory tracts

Breaches in the anatomical and functional boundaries in these systems or their associated dysfunction result in the recurrent transfer of oropharyngeal/oesophageal contents into the sterile lower airways with subsequent risk for recurrent pneumonia. For instance, oesophageal lesions and oesophageal–gastric/sphincter incompetency, oesophageal diverticulosis, hiatus hernia, scleroderma, ascites, tracheal-oesophageal fistula and diabetic associated gastroparesis can produce recurrent pneumonia secondary to recurrent aspiration. Placement of endotracheal tubes and naso-gastric feeding tubes will result in bypassing normal protective mechanisms. Patients with kyphoscoliosis or partial diaphragmatic paralysis secondary to poliomyelitis (for example), patients with phrenic nerve paralysis secondary to tumour or laryngeal paralysis may have suboptimal protective cough mechanisms and be prone to reduced upper airways clearance. Similarly, alcoholics, as a result of a diminished level of consciousness, repeated vomiting episodes or Wernicke's encephalopathy are highly prone to recurrent aspiration. Other at risk situations due to depressed consciousness include meningitis/encephalitis, intracranial oedema (trauma, CVA) and drug overdosage. Chronic neurological disease provides alternative risks for recurrent pulmonary aspiration. Most commonly these are seizure disorders, bulbar and suprabulbar palsies, amyotrophic lateral sclerosis, Guillain–Barré syndrome, Parkinsonism and botulism. Finally, pregnancy and head down positions will present aspiration risks. Chronic pulmonary diseases including bronchiectasis, cystic fibrosis and chronic bronchitis provide a bacterial milieu and recurrent local aspiration facilitates recurrent pneumonia (see Chapters 29 and 24).

Mechanical abnormalities of the more distal airways may provide the means for circumventing normal host defences. These include luminal airways obstruction by tumour such as bronchial carcinoma, carcinoid, inhaled foreign body, endobronchial Kaposi's sarcoma and lymphoma, rhinoscleroma and amyloidosis. Bronchopulmonary sequestration or accessory lung tissue, particularly of the extra-lobar type (which is associated with foregut communications), can present with regurgitation of food or cough and recurrent pneumonia, chest pain and haemoptysis[53].

Special problems in the aged

The elderly are particularly prone to pneumonia and its complications such as extrapulmonary manifestations, for example, meningitis. A severe or protracted course may occur more frequently in this group of individuals. Age may be the single most important factor producing delay in the resolution of pneumonia. The reasons for this include an increased propensity for heart failure, chronic obstructive airways disease, diabetes, malnutrition, neoplasia, neurological disorders, renal dysfunction, etc., all of which have been described in detail elsewhere in this chapter. The increased use of hypnotics in this age-group also predisposes to increased aspiration risk. In addition, the ageing immune system with a diminished inflammatory response may lead to delayed resolution of many pneumonias. As an indication of this, as many as a half of all patients over the age of 65 years with community-acquired pneumonia have no febrile response[54], and bacteraemic pneumococcal pneumonia tends to occur mainly in the elderly[12]. Specific age-related suboptimal immune function includes a diminished IgM level, diminished cell-mediated immune responsiveness and neutrophil reserve. There is also mechanical dysfunction as part of the ageing process – reduced lung elasticity, cough reflexes and reduction in mucociliary function, all of which will negatively impact in the response to pneumonia. Lack of 'classical' features of pneumonia itself in this age-group such as fever and a relative inability of an elderly person to provide a clear history may lead to delayed diagnosis and treatment. The elderly are also vulnerable to several non-infectious mimicks – including an increased risk for malignancy, drug reactions, thromboembolic disease and aspiration (including lipoid) pneumonia. Certain pathogens tend to be more common in the elderly age group including *M. catarrhalis*, RSV, group B *Streptococcus*, enteric Gram-negative organisms and tuberculosis. These pathogens tend to have an association with a longer course. Being elderly will also influence the physician's decision in favour of admitting the patient with community-acquired pneumonia to hospital rather than managing at home despite disagreement on age being an independent predictor of mortality[55]. Nevertheless, the presence of associated factors (which are more common in the elderly) such as altered mentation, neoplasia, Gram-negative rod aetiology/aspiration pneumonia and poor cardiovascular reserve as indicated by hypotension are predictors of increased mortality and should weigh heavily in favour of hospitalisation[55,56]. The elderly may have social performance disabilities including difficulties in coping with personal body care, shopping and eating, and in the absence of community social services or relative support are additional features that result in hospitalisation and may well impact on the speed of recovery.

Special problems in pregnancy

Although uncommon, affecting between 0.1 and 0.3% of all deliveries[57,58], pneumonia of pregnancy and the peripartum period is special since it poses important problems for both mother and child.

Maternal problems

Physiological (reduced ventilatory reserve, increased likelihood of aspiration and increase in lung water content) and immunological (reduced cell-mediated immune protection) changes place a pregnant woman at high risk for more severe pneumonic infections and diminished tolerance to hypoxaemia. The microbial aetiological spectrum is not different from community-acquired pneumonia (apart from septic pulmonary embolism secondary to suppurative thrombophlebitis). However, the course of pneumonia is often complicated by, for example, empyema, more frequent ventilatory support, in up to a half of all patients[58]. This may possibly be due to an element of misdiagnosis in that some presenting signs may be mistaken as normal physiological pregnancy changes, for example, dyspnoea. However, mortality from pregnancy-associated pneumonia has declined from almost 10% in the 1960s[59] to well below 5%[58,60].

Pregnancy is one known risk factor for the development of third trimester associated varicella pneumonia. The course is often complicated with many patients requiring assisted ventilation. The mortality can be between 11% and 35%[61,62]. However, acyclovir appears to have substantially reduced the need for assisted ventilation and mortality. There is also an increased mortality due to viral pneumonias caused by influenza, measles and Epstein–Barr virus.

Pregnancy poses a risk for the deterioration of health in HIV-infected women which includes the development of fulminant *P. carinii* pneumonia with an associated high mortality[63].

Pregnant women are particularly vulnerable to oropharyngeal gastric aspiration and subsequent aspiration pneumonia due to a progesterone related lax eosophageal gastric sphincter coupled with an increase in intragastric pressure.

Foetal problems

Foetal morbidity including low birth weight and prematurity, and mortality are increased as a result of maternal pneumonia[58]. Although congenital malformations in general are not increased, the congenital zoster syndrome can occur as a result of maternal viraemia. Trans-uterine spread of HIV can also occur, resulting in asymptomatic HIV infection or the foetal AIDS syndrome.

Certain antimicrobials can cross the placental barrier and place the foetus at risk from drug toxicity. Included among these are tetracyclines (bone and teeth malformation), aminoglycosides and vancomycin (ototoxicity and renal dysfunction), sulphonamides (kernicterus) and chloramphenicol (grey baby syndrome). The current data suggests that acyclovir is safe[64].

Management of pneumonia in pregnancy involves prophylaxis against aspiration (use of regional rather than general anaesthesia, together with antacids or H2 blockers during caesarian section), a high index of diagnostic suspicion and hence earlier diagnosis, appropriate management of the pneumonia with antimicrobials as well as its complications with supportive treatment, delay of preterm delivery for a no risk foetus using uterine relaxants, and foetal monitoring during delivery if foetal distress occurs.

Non-microbial pseudo-infectious pneumonias

Several non-infectious conditions not only mimic an infectious pneumonia, but can predispose to infectious pneumonia.

Pulmonary neoplasia

Primary bronchial carcinoma can be mistakened for a slowly resolving pneumonia (though the converse is more likely). It can also be causative of a slowly or resolving recurrent pneumonia, either directly via mechanical airways obstruction or indirectly via mechanical derangement of the cough and other airways' protective mechanisms (for example, recurrent laryngeal nerve or phrenic nerve paralysis), or secondary via depressed systemic immunity. Radiography most often presents a distinctive radiological picture which is unlikely to be confused or missed in the setting of pneumonia (Fig. 28.4). Rarely pneumonia of infectious aetiology can masquerade radiographicalally as a tumour, e.g. 'round' pneumonia (see Fig. 10.4, CMV chapter). Its frequency of occurrence in non-resolving pneumonias appears to be small but not negligible[6,10,11]. A particularly aggressive form has been recognised in young male HIV smokers.

Bronchoalveolar carcinoma, on the other hand, is more likely to be confused with pneumonia, particularly in those patients who present with fever, productive cough and diffuse alveolar densities mimicking lobar consolidation. Nevertheless, the presentation most often is in a patient with chronic lung disease who has an afebrile presentation, a chronic non-productive cough (excessive bronchorrhea is uncommon), weight loss and with focal mass lesions or multiple nodules on chest radiography.

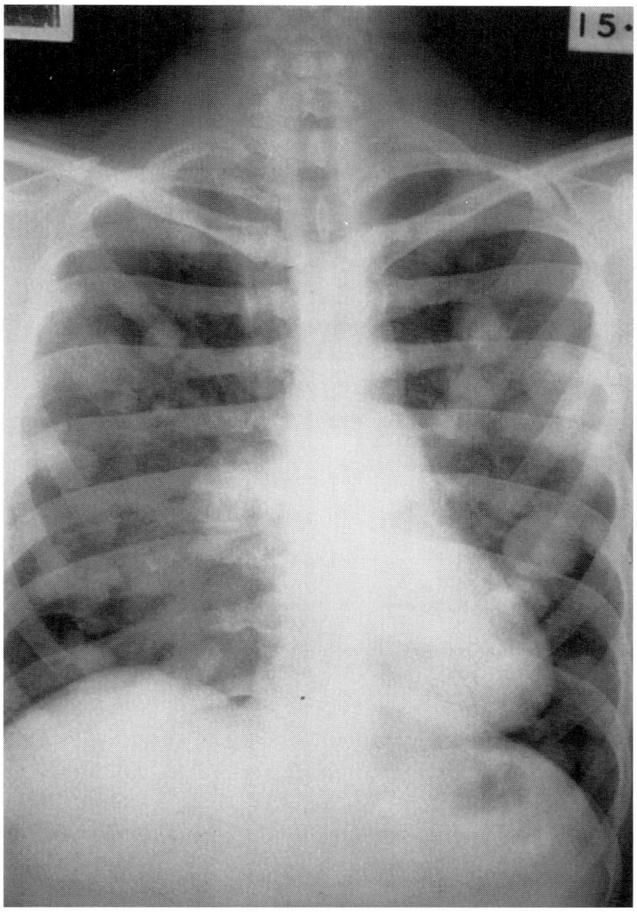

FIGURE 28.4 Metastatic cancer with well circumscribed nodular lesions and interspersed with bilateral pulmonary infiltrates.

Thoracic lymphoma (and pseudolymphoma) usually presents as part of disseminated and nodal disease. However, primary pulmonary lymphoma does occur, but less commonly. Hodgkin's lymphoma affects the pulmonary system more often than non-Hodgkin's lymphoma. Absence of hilar/mediastinal lymphadenopathy is more in favour of non-Hodgkin's or primary pulmonary rather than Hodgkin's lymphoma in patients with lymphomatous parenchymal involvement. Most cases present subacutely with increasing dyspnoea, fever and systemic disturbance. Chest radiography may show focal infiltrates with air bronchograms, nodules, pleural involvement or lymphadenopathy. Definitive diagnosis is made by lung biopsy, though initial histological findings may prove difficult to differentiate from a non-specific inflammatory response. Presence of cellular atypia, positive specific monoclonal antibody stains for surface markers or abnormal cytological analysis are confirmatory.

Secondary pulmonary tumours can present either as well-demarcated nodules due to haematogenous spread, or less well demarcated reticular densities/perihilar thickening, or with Kerley A or B lines which represent lymphangitic carcinomatosis. It is the latter particularly which may be confused with an infectious pneumonia, especially when accompanied by tumour related fever and cough. In some cases, the presentation is as abrupt as community-acquired pneumonia. The most common tumours with propensity for secondary lung spread include lung, breast, colon, kidney and testicle, with lung and breast being largely responsible for lymphangitis carcinomatosis.

HIV-associated Kaposi's sarcoma may produce interstitial or endobronchial lung disease.

Bronchiolitis obliterans and organising pneumonia (BOOP)

In 1981, two patients with several years' history of recurrent pneumonia were described[65]. Their most recent hospital admissions were characterised by a few weeks of cough, fever, sputum, progressive dyspnoea and bilateral infiltrates which were unresponsive to antibiotics but responded well to systemic corticosteroids. One patient in addition had subacute thyroiditis. Initially, it was perceived that the patients had chronic interstitial pneumonia probably of the desquamative type. However, lung biopsy showed thickening of alveolar walls with a lymphocytic infiltrate and the alveolar spaces were filled with large nodules of loose connective tissue. There was no evidence for bronchiectasis, carcinoma, granulomatous disease or pulmonary microbial infection. This apparent newly recognised entity was called 'an organising pneumonia-like process'. Two years later, eight further patients were reported from the Brompton Hospital London, with similar clinical, radiological and histological features, with no evidence of an infective agent or other aetiologies and the term 'cryptogenic organising pneumonitis' was coined[66]. In 1985, 50 of 94 patients with bronchiolitis obliterans (BO) were found to have associated patchy organising pneumonia and the term bronchiolitis obliterans with organising pneumonia (BOOP) was used to describe this association[67]. It is now generally considered that BOOP is probably not a new disease but has been previously described under various synonyms at several instances in the literature.

BOOP is distinct from BO and the two terms have produced some confusion. BO is an irreversible, destructive fibrotic scarred state of small airways following their plugging by an inflammatory process; the alveoli are spared. A hypertranslucent chest radiograph without infiltrates is normally found, although nodules, linear and diffuse infiltrates may later supervene. A predominantly obstructive defect (a greater reduction in FEV1 greater than in DLCO) is found on pulmonary function testing. The disease is unresponsive to steroids and in general carries a worse prognosis than BOOP. In contrast BOOP involves mainly the alveolar lumen and walls with some variable extension to the alveolar ducts and distal/respiratory bronchioles. All patients have chest radiological infiltrates. The FEV1 is normal but the DLCO is substantially reduced. The main features[68] include a flu-like illness (fever, fatigue and malaise) or cough or mild dyspnoea starting abruptly but progressing over 1–2 months despite antibiotic therapy. Crackles on auscultation is the most common physical abnormality, bilateral inhomogenous infiltrates are present on plain chest radiography, whereas a CT scan reveals patchy airspace consolidation or interstitial shadows. The lung infiltrates may be fleeting and mimic pulmonary eosinophilia. Infiltrates may also be localised, and present as focal lesions (e.g. an isolated pulmonary nodule) often in asymptomatic patients. A reticulonodular pattern or merely hyperinflation in the absence of infiltrates is sometimes seen. Rarely cavitation and pleural effusions occur. Pulmonary function tests show a substantially low DLCO, reduced vital capacity and total lung volume but no airways obstruction, apart from smokers. Bronchoalveolar lavage often reveals increased lymphocytes although in some patients eosinophils may predominate – this produces confusion with pulmonary eosinophilia. Polymorphs may also be present. It is quite possible that the clinical spectrum is wider than realised, with milder cases resolving spontaneously and with some overlap with other syndromes. Lung tissue shows the histological changes characterised by granulation tissue plugs or buds, with foam cells within the alveolar ducts and alveoli (Fig. 28.5 (*a*) and (*b*)). A largely monocytic and fibroblastic chronic infiltration of the alveolar walls in the absence of honey-combing or extensive interstitial fibrosis is found. Interstitial involvement is minor. If no underlying trigger is identifiable, the disease is called idiopathic BOOP or cryptogenic organising pneumonia (COP). The use of the term COP avoids the confusion surrounding the term BOOP. There are, however, a number of *associated* illnesses or factors which accompany COP – these include connective tissue disorders[67] such as SLE and polymyositis[69], drugs including cocaine and amiodorone[68] thyroiditis[65], bone marrow transplant with CMV infection[66], HIV infection[67], radiotherapy[70] and viruses including adenovirus[71]. Some of these processes, however, have BOOP pattern *histology* and the *clinical and radiological features* may not always be characteristic of BOOP. Of some importance are recent reports that BOOP may complicate bone marrow transplantation[72,73] – although BO has been widely recognised in bone marrow transplantation, BOOP previously had not been reported. It is quite possible that previous cases diagnosed as BO may in fact have been BOOP and the issue requires clarification because of the implication for steroid therapy in these patients.

In some patients, BOOP may settle spontaneously whilst in others there is a dramatic response to one or more courses of high tapering dosage prednisolone, given for 3 to 12 months or even longer, the regimen individualised. Patients with associated underlying diseases such as SLE appear to do less well and deteriorate despite therapy. Overall, between 60% and 80% of patients respond to steroids. For severe cases, cytotoxic drugs can be used. The mortality rate is approximately 5%; pulmonary fibrosis occurs in up to 20%.

BOOP has to be distinguished from BO (as above), and from a number of other infiltrative lung diseases. A tissue biopsy is therefore necessary for definitive differentiation from infectious pulmonary diseases, usual interstitial pneumonia, diffuse alveolar damage, unclassified interstitial pneumonia, chronic eosinophilic pneumonia, hypersensitivity pneumonitis, Wegener's granulomatosis, collagen vascular diseases, pulmonary drug toxicity, pulmonary lymphoproliferative disorders, etc.[74]. BOOP or COP and other idiopathic pulmonary interstitial/alveolar inflammatory reactions such as pulmonary eosinophilia may represent different responses in different patients to the same as yet unidentified inhaled or ingested antigens, and this may explain the overlap seen in some cases. The importance of differentiation pivots around the generally favourable impact of steroids[75]. Recently thoracoscopic video-aided lung biopsy has proved useful[76]. However, CT-guided transbronchial biopsy may return a low diagnostic yield because of its patchy nature. Open lung biopsy

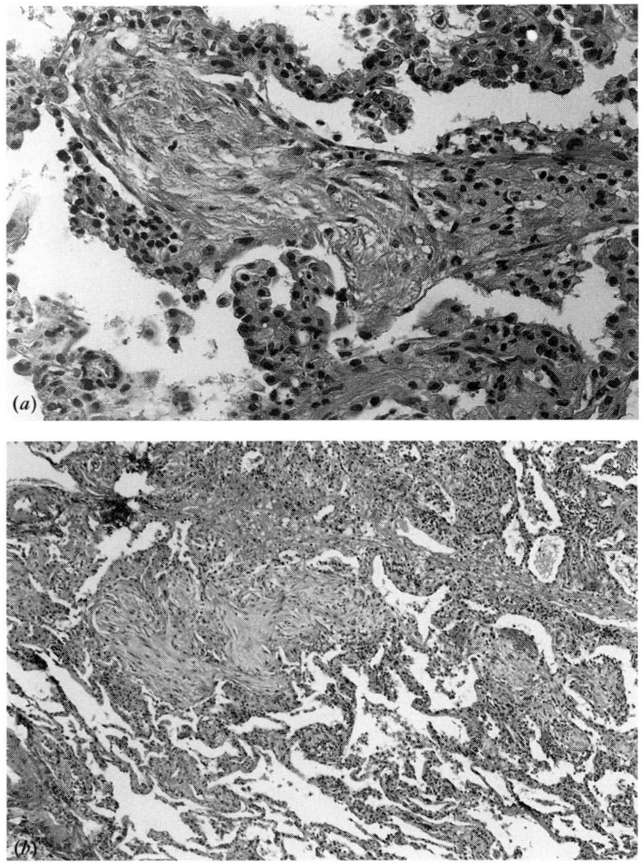

FIGURE 28.5 (*a*) COP: fibroblasts in myxoid matrix with macrophages filling the alveolar duct. (*b*) COP: low power view illustrating patchy area of involvement. (Courtesy of Dr F. Al Dayed.)

may not always be feasible. There may have to be reliance on collating clues obtained through less invasive means for diagnosing BOOP e.g. a pneumonia unresponsive to antibiotics, absence of microorganisms, lymphocytic BAL and absent autoantibodies. A trial of steroid therapy would be justifiable in such patients.

The causation of BOOP remains unclear and only 7/57 cases reported by Eppler[67] had a specific cause or associated disorder of connective tissue. Furthermore, the finding of a histological BOOP pattern in relation to infections, drugs, etc. clouds the relationship further. One contender for pathogenesis is an initial temporary infection which triggers a subsequent response, leading to BOOP. Evidence in support of a microbial aetiology for BO or BOOP is found in the case of nocardial infections[77] adenoviral infections[78] HIV disease[67]. Viral infections may enhance MHC-2 antigens in bronchiolar respiratory cells and may be the trigger for subsequent T-cell disease immune cytopathy.

Idiopathic interstitial pneumonia following bone marrow transplantation (IIP)

Approximately 40% of allografts and 10% of autologous/syngeneic bone marrow grafts develop interstitial pneumonitis of whom one-third to one-half have idiopathic interstitial pneumonitis (IIP)[79–82]. Onset is typically during the fifth transplant week but can vary considerably. Symptoms typically include dyspnoea, unproductive cough, hypoxaemia, and pulmonary infiltrates which are usually diffuse but which may be focal[83,84]. In many respects, the presentation has characteristics not dissimilar to cytomegalovirus or *P. carinii* interstitial pneumonia, but a careful search in the peripheral blood and in open lung biopsies reveals no pathogens. Histological features of non-specific interstitial pneumonitis or diffuse alveolar damage with bronchiolitis, vascular alterations and cellular atypia are found.

The clinical course is downhill, with approximately 30% of patients dying with progressive respiratory failure, and 30% from other causes (mainly infective but also some with fatal coagulopathy and organ failure)[83]. The majority of survivors have minimal (usually subclinical pulmonary function) abnormalities at follow-up a year later (reduced DLCO, reduced total lung capacity), but a few may go on to develop pulmonary fibrosis. Of some interest is that a major pulmonary infection, usually fungal or viral, which may be disseminated, appears to supervene later in the course of IIP in approximately one-third of patients[83]. However, only a minority of these were apparently missed on the first lung biopsy specimen. Curiously, patients who had previously received high dose total body irradiation and also those with acute graft vs. host disease, although they have a higher incidence of IIP, paradoxically have a better survival[83]. The reason for this is unclear; one explanation is that distinct aetiologies for IIP exist among patients who develop acute GVHD or receive high dose TBI.

The precise aetiology of IIP is unknown. Microbiologically it does not fit with missed or cryptic CMV disease or indeed other commonly known infectious processes such as polyomavirus, Epstein–Barr virus, *Mycoplasma* and *Legionella*[20,85]. Although low levels of CMV may be detected in patients with IIP, their clinical features are quite distinct from those with definite CMV lung disease. The possibility remains, however, that CMV could activate the host immune response and produce lung damage[85]. Furthermore, there is an equal frequency of occurrence of IIP in allogeneic and syngeneic transplants and it is not related to GVHD. Moreover, the lower incidence in patients transplanted for aplastic anaemia suggests that TBI or chemotherapy *per se* appears to be a major risk factor[86]. The risk for IIP as well as for infectious interstitial pneumonitis appears to be related to the absolute dosage of TBI[87]. Further evidence in support of TBI comes from patients who have a lower incidence of IIP if they receive fractionated rather than single exposure TBI[87]. If fractionated TBI is combined with lung shielding, the incidence of IIP is substantially lowered from some 26% to 0%[88].

Following its discovery in 1986, the human herpes virus 6 (HHV6) has contended for a pathogenic role in the supposed IIP of bone marrow transplant patients. Most of the general population has been infected with this virus by the age of 4 years. It is a cause of exanthem subitum in children and may contribute towards reticulo-endothelial disorders and the chronic fatigue syndrome. In 1991, Carrigan[89] showed that HHV6 infected intraalveolar macrophages and lymphocytes in patients with BMT-associated IIP. Cone in 1993[90] showed that the lung tissue of all 15 patients with bone marrow transplantation (of whom eight had interstitial pneumonitis or diffuse alveolar damage or bronchiolitis and seven had concomitant cytomegalovirus, *P. carinii* pneumonia or Hodgkin's disease) contained HHV6-DNA. The levels of HHV6-DNA were up to 500 times those compared to controls or those with concomitant infections. Their work suggested an association between HHV6 and bone marrow transplant interstitial pneumonitis. Higher levels of lung tissue HHV6 DNA were found in association with supposed IIP compared to those patients who had other pathogens such as CMV. The survival was better in those patients who had higher HHV6 DNA levels (two of eight with HHV6 died compared with five of seven who had concomitant CMV or other processes), and this suggested that HHV6 associated interstitial pneumonitis may be less severe than CMV pneumonitis. It is not clear from this report how prophylaxis or treatment with acyclovir or ganciclovir influences the findings – an issue of some importance given the apparent *in vitro* susceptibility pattern of HHV6 to these drugs. The recent identification of HHV7 may further confuse the issue[91] and more data is needed to clarify the exact incidence and influence of antiviral therapy.

Recently, BOOP has been described in association with bone marrow transplantation[72,73] and should be excluded in cases of bone marrow transplantation associated idiopathic pneumonia.

Most cases of IIP following bone marrow transplantation occur early. However, *late IIP* is a recognised but rare condition which appears between 120 and 445 days following bone marrow transplantation[92,93]. Non-infectious aetiologies such as lymphocytic alveolitis syndrome contribute towards these. The cardinal features include dyspnoea, dry cough, absence of fever, local or diffuse interstitial opacities on plain chest radiology or alveolar airspace consolidation on high resolution CT scan, chronic graft versus host disease and predominantly CD8 BAL lymphocytosis[94]. The clinical pulmonary function and radiological course in contrast to early onset IIP is good with apparent response to immunosuppressive drugs including prednisolone. One possible aetiology is that this syndrome represents a pulmonary manifestation of chronic graft versus host disease due to an interaction of allogeneic lymphocytes with bronchiolar epithelial cells which express MHLC antigens, induced by previous (? cryptic) cytomegalovirus infection.

The management of those patients who present with an idiopathic interstitial pneumonitis after bone marrow transplantation involves an assiduous and appropriate diagnostic work-up to exclude an infectious cause such as cytomegalovirus or PCP. Open lung biopsy may be diagnostically more sensitive compared to BAL[95] and may influence treatment decisions, although it is not as yet been shown to impact on outcome. Empirical therapy directed towards *P. carinii* or cytomegalovirus is justified whilst awaiting results of investigations. However, antiviral, antiprotozoal, immunomodulatory and corticosteroid therapies have had no impact on the outcome of IIP.

Pulmonary vasculitides

Systemic vasculitides which involve the lung may masquerade or predispose to infectious pneumonia. The more important of these are Wegener's granulomatosis, Churg–Strauss syndrome and polyarteritis nodosa (and its variants). They may be suspected from extra-pulmonary manifestations, non-response to antibiotics, tissue biopsy and in some instances serology.

Wegener's granulomatosis (WG)

This is an idiopathic necrotising granulomatous vasculopathy in which the lungs and/or upper airways are involved in all patients without exception. Lung disease is found in 85%, renal disease in 85%, and there is a variable incidence of multi-organ disease[96]. WG affects men and women aged between 14 and 75 years, (mean age 41 years). A respiratory presentation predominates in 90% of patients who may have severe/persistent rhinorrhoea and otitis media (often mistaken as infection or allergy) sinusitis, nasal deformity, subglottic stenosis, fever, dyspnoea, cough, haemoptysis (due to alveolar haemorrhage) or pleural pain as the most common presentations[96,97]. Onset can be sudden with extensive pulmonary haemorrhage or renal failure. It is the febrile pulmonary presentation with fever that leads to the initial mistakened diagnosis of an infectious pneumonia. Furthermore, overlap between WG and infection occurs and is reflected by recurrent post-obstructive infectious pneumonia secondary to endobronchial WG lesions, depressed mucosal immunity or immunosuppressive therapy. The responsible organisms include *P. aeruginosa*, fungae (*Aspergillus*, *Candida*), *P. carinii*, *S. pneumoniae*, *H. influenzae*, *M. tuberculosis* and non-tuberculous mycobacteria[97]. Sight-threatening retro-orbital pseudotumours which produce proptosis and dysconjugate gaze, pseudo-rheumatoid arthritis (symmetrical small joint involvement and false positive rheumatoid serology), skin disease (ulcers, nodules, etc.), and mononeuritis multiplex cranial nerve abnormalities commonly occur. Many of these emerge during the follow-up period. Initial symptoms may be mild or even absent in up to one-half of all patients who are proven to have radiographical and pulmonary histological abnormalities. This could substantially delay the diagnosis and is partly responsible for the mean time of 8–15 months from onset of symptoms to diagnosis.

Radiographically in 50–60% of patients, multiple bilateral nodular infiltrates (which may cavitate) or diffuse parenchymal/alveolar infiltrates (which may fleet) are seen equally commonly. Focal segmental or lobar densities occur and pleural effusions are present in 20%; mediastinal lymphadenopathy is distinctly unusual. Histological abnormalities from open lung biopsy (which produces a better yield than transbronchial biopsy) include small vessel vasculopathy consisting of granulomas, fibrinoid necrosis and cicatricial stenosis together with parenchymal changes of geographic necrosis, poorly formed granulomas, scattered giant cells and micro-abscesses. Alveolar haemorrhage may also be present. These changes are of course not pathognomonic for WG and a fungal or bacterial aaetiology should be ruled out[97]. Focal, segmental glomerulonephritis or rapidly progressive crescentic glomerulonephritis is present in patients with renal disease. Circulating and pulmonary (BAL) IgG antineutrophil cytoplasmic and antimonocyte lysosomal antibodies are present in most patients with WG, and have generated considerable interest and controversy in recent years. ANCA, although first described and thought specific for WG, can be found in other vasculitides. By contrast, ANCA with diffuse granular cytoplasmic distribution of staining (c-ANCA) appears to be more specific than ANCA with perinuclear staining distribution (p-ANCA) for WG[98], though this is not absolute and c-ANCA like p-ANCA have also been found in other systemic vasculitides. ANCA is therefore useful as a supportive diagnostic tool; it can also be used to monitor and predict the course of WG.

Without treatment the disease is almost universally fatal but prolonged combination treatment with cyclophosphamide (given for at least 1 year) and steroids (tapered over several months) induces and maintains remission in most patients. However, permanent respiratory and pulmonary sequelae, such as bronchostenosis, chronic obstructive airways disease and restrictive lung disease may occur in approximately one-fifth of patients. Chronic sinus dysfunction occurs in approximately half of all patients. Other non-pulmonary long term sequelae include chronic renal insufficiency, hearing loss, nasal dysfunction and visual loss. Treatment related morbidity, for example, steroid side-effects and cyclophosphamide cystitis is frequent but alternative treatments, for example, pulse cyclophosphamide, methotrexate, azathioprine or chlorambucil are as yet unproven. Following a surprise observation that patients with WG improved after cotrimoxazole was given for intercurrent bacterial infections[99], the antibiotic has been claimed to be at least as successful as standard therapy[100], an experience not shared by others[97] and clearly requires further study.

Churg–Strauss syndrome (CSS)

Compared to WG this is rare[101,102]. Clinical pointers which differentiate CSS include a background long standing history of atopy or asthma, a pseudo-community-acquired pneumonic presentation (cough, fever, constitutional disturbance) combined with features of atopy – particularly nasal polyposis and sinusitis. Extrapulmonary and systemic vasculopathic manifestations are common and include multi-organ involvement such as sinusitis, polyps, skin nodules, mononeuritis multiplex and abdominal pain. These are also found in WG, but severe renal failure is less common (although microscopic haematuria on presentation is present in up to one-third) whilst hypertension (often treatment resistant) occurs in up to 50% of patients. Cardiac associated mortality is high[103]. The onset of vasculopathy coincides with improvement of the patient's asthma.

Radiographically, the infiltrates are usually patchy, transient, peripheral, focal and alveolar. There is usually substantial blood and tissue eosinophilia. Serum IgE is elevated. Angiography may demonstrate aneurysms in the liver. p-ANCA and c-ANCA may be positive in approximately a half of patients. The combined eosinophilic-granulomatous histology of necrotising vasculopathy in small/medium blood vessels and pulmonary tissues, and spread extravascularly are other differentiating features. However, overreliance on the pathological rather than the clinical features for diagnosis may result in underdiagnosis of several cases of CSS[104]. Usually symptoms respond to steroids with/without immunosupportive treatment such as azathioprine or cyclophosphamide, but long-term maintenance therapy is essential. Mortality without steroid treatment is of the order of 50%.

Polyarteritis nodosa (PAN) and the overlap syndrome (OS)

In one-third of cases of PAN a predominantly respiratory presentation is found, with fever, cough and minor haemoptysis, although fleeting chest radiographical infiltrates are less common[105]. Pulmonary symptoms may be overshadowed by the effect of aneurysmal formations in other organs, which can produce hypertension, muscular pain and coronary ischaemia. A syndrome composed of features of WG, CSS and PAN and characterised by alveolar haemorrhage, macroscopic aneurysms, positive ANCA, nodular eosinophilic and pulmonary alveolar infiltrates has been termed the OS[101].

Goodpasture's syndrome (GS)

Pulmonary haemorrhage found in association with glomerulonephritis is termed Goodpasture's Syndrome. For diagnosis some authorities require the presence of antibodies to the capillary basement membrane of the glomerulus but more than 50% of patients do not have this antibody[106]. Some of these patients may have WG, SLE, etc. or may be called idiopathic GS[106]. Confusion in terminology therefore exists and probably considerable overlap of clinical pathology occurs in different presentations.

In smokers or other situations which trigger increased lung capillary permeability, circulating antibodies to the capillary basement membrane of the glomerulus may cross-react with alveolar antigens and produce alveolar haemorrhage. The clinical spectrum of GS varies from the isolated incidental pseudoinfective alveolar infiltrates, to frank haemoptysis (in up to 75%) which may be fulminant. Anaemia and renal failure are also found. Usually, it is the pulmonary presentation with haemoptysis and respiratory failure which heralds in this disease, although renal involvement is invariable and rapidly progressive glomerulonephritis follows. It is, therefore, important to diagnose GS early since prognosis clearly relates to the speed with which treatment is instituted[106]. Diagnosis is made on renal biopsy (lung biopsy is not specific for GS) by demonstrating the characteristic linear deposits of complement with IgG/IgM, against a background of diffuse proliferative, crescentic glomerulonephritis. Crescent formation is found in all IgM antibody-positive patients, whereas other histological patterns are found in IgM negative (idiopathic GS) patients. A similar syndrome of idiopathic, rapidly progressive glomerulonephritis but with a milder and less frequent pulmonary component, absence of antibodies to glomerular membrane but with circulating immune complexes and ANCA, has also been described[107].

Overall, the prognosis of GS is guarded. A presenting creatinine > 600 μmoles/l, oliguria, and > 50% crescents on renal biopsy bode a poor outcome[106]. Aggressive treatment with plasmapheresis, pulse methylprednisolone and cytotoxic therapy is standard practice[106,108].

Alveolar haemorrhage can also occur rarely in other vasculitides including WG, SLE, idiopathic pulmonary haemosiderosis (confined to the lung) and secondary to certain drugs such as penicillamine.

Pulmonary sarcoidosis (PS)

Sarcoidosis is a disease of uncertain aetiology characterised histologically by multisystem involvement with granulomas, clinically most often by hilar lymphadenopathy and pulmonary infiltrates (although the CXR in a minority may be normal) and less frequently by constitutional disease, skin and eye lesions, biochemically by hypercalcaemia/hypercalcuria and immunologically by depressed cell-mediated immunity and hyperimmunoglobulinaemia. Its incidence and severity varies with race and country, genetic predisposition, age and sex. Variation in diagnostic techniques and disease presentation may contribute towards the varying incidence. Overall, the highest incidence appears to be in black males in their 30s to 40s. The incidence per a hundred thousand population is approximately 20 in the UK, 60 in Norway and less than 1 in Brazil[109]. A number of families have been documented with more than one case and a high incidence of HLA-B8, CW7 and DR3 has been found indicating genetic disposition.

The immunopathology of pulmonary sarcoid is complex[110] but it is thought that an initial unknown antigenic stimulus in the lungs activates alveolar macrophages and T-cells to release IL-1 and IL-2/γIFN/macrophage inhibitory factors respectively. Peripheral blood T-lymphocytes are sequestered to the lung (resulting in lymphopenia, particularly CD4 penia which is responsible for impaired delayed type hypersensitivity) together with monocytes, under the influence of IL-1/IL-2. This produces an alveolitis. Cytokines, including interferon and macrophage migration inhibitory factor, interact to produce localised granulomas, their evolution regulated by T lymphocytes (CD4 lymphocytes being found in active disease, suppressor lymphocytes being found in quiescent or inactive disease) and by IL-1 and IL-2 induced release of PGE2. Subsequently, the inflammatory/granulomatous response may resolve or may produce lung parenchymal disease or fibrosis. Evidence exist that fibrosis is promoted by IL-1/immune interferon/fibronectin stimulation of human lung fibroblasts which is inhibited by PGE2. In addition to these local pulmonary effects, hyperimmunoglobulinaemia arises from T-cell production of immunoglobulins; hypercalcaemia from increased 1:25 dihydroxy-vitamin D activity from activated mononuclear phagocytes in the granulomas, and constitutional features such as fever and myasthenia from IL-1 directly or via PGE2.

Active sarcoid granulomas histologically consist of nodules of epitheliod cells containing Schaumann doubly refractile crystalline or asteroid inclusion bodies usually with minimal necrosis. However, necrotising sarcoid granulomatosis is described and may be a separate clinical pathological entity[111]. Multinucleated giant cells occur at the periphery and centrally. Evolution of the lesions results in collagenous change, hyalinosis and sclerosis or resolution. However, the lesions are not pathognomonic for sarcoid. TB, brucellosis, fungal disease, all have to be excluded.

Pine pollen, beryllium and various microbial agents have been suggested as providing the antigenic stimulus. Partial evidence for transmissible agents has been provided from mice experiments where sarcoid lesions were induced from human sarcoid homogenates[112], from epidemiological studies, e.g. a much higher incidence of prior contact with other cases compared to controls, and time-space clustering of cases[113]. The evidence that TB might be incriminated includes: the finding of AFB on histology, *M. tuberculosis* on culture and *M. tuberculosis* DNA from sarcoid tissues[114]. The relative difficulty of identifying *M. tuberculosis* in some instances may be related to the ability of the organism to exist without a cell wall.

There is a plethora of presenting symptoms[115–117]. A respiratory presentation, however, is the most frequent manifestation of sarcoid. Symptoms include acute or insidious onset of unproductive cough, ill-defined chest pain or the patient may be asymptomatic with incidental chest radiographical abnormalities. Dyspnoea in general indicates advanced disease. Constitutional symptoms include fever, myasthenia, weight loss and fatigue. Other symptoms are large joint effusion-free polyarthralgia, peripheral neuropathy, cranial nerve palsies, transverse myelitis, uveitis, conjunctivitis, Sjörgren-like syndrome, hepatosplenomegaly, skin plaques, erythema nodosum, cardiomyopathy and conduction defects, upper airways granulomatosis and renal dysfunction. Chest radiographical lesions include most commonly reticulo-nodular or small nodular shadows (Fig. 28.6). Pneumonic-like lesions, diffuse patchy infiltrates, miliary shadows, perihilar linear infiltrates, cavitation, fibrosis and upper lobe infiltrates mimicking pulmonary tuberculosis can also be found. Lesions may be apparent on CT scanning (Fig. 28.7) despite a normal plain chest radiograph. In addition, pleural effusions (uncommon), endobronchial sarcoid (more common than suspected) and hilar lymphadenopathy (usually symmetrical) can occur. Differentiation is from pulmonary tuberculosis, fungal lung disease, drug-induced lung disease, neoplasia, extrinsic allergic alveolitis and other pulmonary granulomatosis. Thoracic sarcoid is staged: I : hilar lymphadenopathy (50% of patients); II : hilar lymphadenopathy + pulmonary opacities (25% of patients); III : pulmonary opacities alone (15% of patients); IV : pulmonary fibrosis (10% of patients) – and this staging provides a basis for prognosis.

Pulmonary function tests are variable and not always related to chest X-ray abnormalities but include reduced DLCO (even in patients with a normal chest radiograph), reduced pulmonary compliance and evidence of airways obstruction.

Spontaneous resolution occurs in 65% of patients in Stage I, 50% of patients in Stage II and 20% of patients in Stage III. Acute presentation, constitutional symptoms, erythema nodosum and Stage I disease are good prognostic indicators for spontaneous resolution. Chronic disease, Stage III, nephrolithiasis, increased age, ethnic Blacks and associated dyspnoea, all carry a poor prognosis for progression to progressive pulmonary fibrosis and cor pulmonale. The overall mortality rate for patients with pulmonary opacities is approximately 8% with up to 20% developing pulmonary fibrosis.

The presence of bilateral hilar lymphadenopathy in a young person is highly suspicious of sarcoid but the diagnosis in most cases pivots on the demonstration of non-caseating granulomas from accessible lymph nodes (peripheral or via mediastinoscopy) or from pulmonary tissue via transbronchial biopsy (an excellent yield) or from other tissue in an appropriate clinical presentation. The diagnosis is strengthened if other compatible extra-thoracic manifestations are present. The Kveim test using correctly prepared Kveim substance is highly specific (98%) and 75% sensitive in patients with active disease[118]. The serum angiotensin converting enzyme (SACE) has low specificity

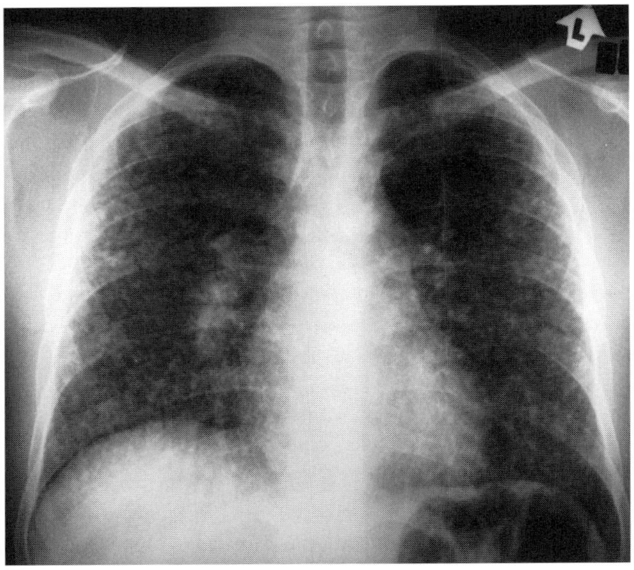

FIGURE 28.6 Sarcoidosis. Diffuse micronodular infiltrates in both lungs associated with bilateral hilar lymphadenopathy. (Courtesy of Dr M. Bazarbashi.)

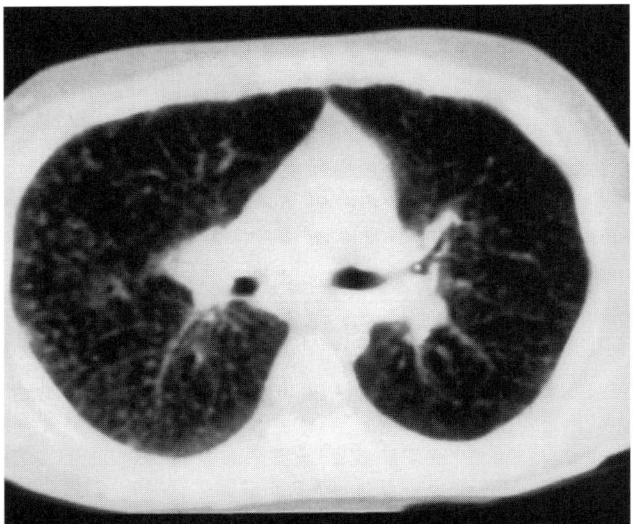

FIGURE 28.7 Sarcoidosis. CT Chest demonstrating peripheral pruning of bronchovascular bundles and thickened interlobular septae. (Courtesy of Dr M. Bazarbashi.)

(about 80%) and is 75% sensitive[118] – it may reflect extent of the disease. Gallium-67 scanning (Fig. 28.8) is rather non-specific, being positive in any pulmonary inflammatory disease; however, a positive parotid gland uptake is highly suggestive of sarcoid. BAL may show an increase in CD4 lymphocytes but this is non-specific and suffers from an intra-technique variability[119]. These ancillary diagnostic techniques are not routinely used but may be helpful in difficult cases. SACE and gallium scanning may delineate disease; SACE may be useful for monitoring progress as may serum neopterin[120] and positron emission tomographic measurement of fluorine 18 deoxyglucose uptake[121].

Although steroids are effective in sarcoid, controversy exists regarding their specific indications, dosage and duration[118,122]. Eye involvement, hypercalcaemia, neurological manifestations (though often resistant), severe constitutional features and other symptomatic organ involvements are generally accepted indications[122]. The major areas of controversy centre over thoracic sarcoid. Most Stage I patients are asymptomatic and undergo spontaneous resolution and steroids are not indicated. Most Stage II/III patients show benefit but in most this is only temporary, and trials have not proven an end survival benefit[123]. However, patient selection bias probably occurred in some trials (those with relatively good prognosis were recruited) and has made interpretation difficult. Most authorities therefore treat patients who have troublesome pulmonary disability[118]. Other indications might be significant radiographical or pulmonary function test deterioration from presentation[122]. Commonly used dosages are between 20 and 40 mg of prednisolone on alternate days or daily for 6–12 months and tapering according to the individual response. Relapse is of the order of 20% but much higher in Blacks. In an attempt to minimise systemic steroid side-effects, inhaled high dose steroids have been used. The current evidence is conflicting –

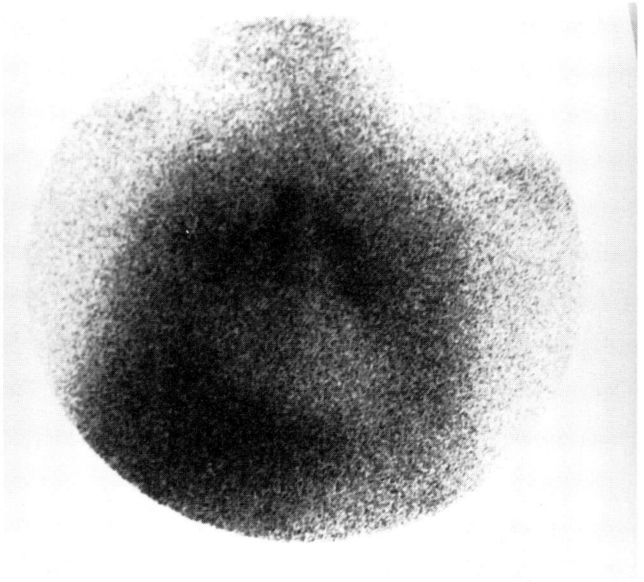

FIGURE 28.8 Sarcoidosis. Gallium scan demonstrating multiple areas of increased uptake in the mediastinum, and bilateral hilar pulmonary regions (lymphadenopathy). The diffuse abnormal uptake in both lungs is only slightly less than the liver. (Courtesy of Dr M. Bazarbashi.)

some have shown no recognisable therapeutic effect[124] and others indicate that, for maintenance purposes of early disease, inhaled budesonide is as effective as oral steroids[125]. Adjunctive therapies include cyclosporin, methetrexate and chloroquine with some anecdotal successes. Lung transplantation is potentially curative for end-stage pulmonary sarcoid but recipients are prone to recurrent disease in the allograft accompanied by more severe early rejection episodes[126]. In the future, anticytokines and immunocytotoxics may prove to have a role.

Pulmonary alveolar phospholipoproteinosis (PAPP)

PAPP is a life-threatening, yet eminently treatable condition, characterised by the accumulation of viscid lipid rich proteinaceous material in alveolar and terminal bronchioles, which stains with periodic acid Schiff[127]. Many cases are idiopathic but some series have reported that a half of all patients have exposure to pneumoconiotic dusts in an industrial setting, or to busulfan, chlorambucil, aluminum, asbestos, aerosolised chemical cleaners, etc. Animal models and quantitative elemental analysis of BAL fluid lend some support that these agents can trigger PAPP[127]. An association with haematological malignancies has been described. Infections including non-tuberculous mycobacteria, *Pseudomonas*, *Nocardia*, fungi, *P. carinii*, bacteria and viruses have been also incriminated. Since these have been documented mainly in patients not having access to therapeutic bronchoalveolar lavage[128], they may have occurred secondary to prolonged antibiotic/steroid administration and to the microbial growth promoting nature of the phospholipids. Reduced clearance of microorganisms by defective alveolar macrophages may also be responsible. PAPP is therefore generally considered to be a particular non-specific noninfectious, possibly genetically determined alveolar response to injury from both unknown and specifically known factors. In the case of drug-induced PAPP stimulation of phospholipid (mainly dipalmitoyl lecithin of lung surfactant) production by type II pneumocysts is an important mechanism.

Clinically, the major complaints are of dyspnoea, cough, fever, and chest pain. There may be haemoptysis and clubbing. Chest radiography shows ground glass bilateral perihilar alveolar densities (Figs. 28.9, 28.10); reticulo-nodular densities, unilateral shadows and interstitial infiltrates are less commonly observed. Profound hypoxaemia is the most frequent abnormal pulmonary function but reduced transfer factor for carbon monoxide and lung volumes are also found. Raised serum lactate dehydrogenase is common. Untreated, the course is relapsing and leads to progressive deterioration in respiratory function due to pulmonary fibrosis in many patients – spontaneous resolution occurs in approximately 20%[129]. The mortality rate in the pretherapeutic BAL era was approximately 30%; currently it is 10%. However, mortality may have been overestimated as cases have included mistaken diagnoses, or death from associated problems[129,130]. Death directly due to PAPP is rare, provided patients receive therapeutic BAL, apart from the occasional unfortunate complication of BAL associated iatrogenic aspiration. Treatment is with controlled large volume (10 litres or more) therapeutic BAL to remove the intraalveolar phospholipids (Figs. 28.11, 28.12). The success rate is of the order of 75% of whom 60–80% will have no recurrence within 5 years[129,130].

Extrinsic allergic alveolitis (EAA)

Exposure, often intense and prolonged, to inhaled appropriately sized organic antigens in some individuals produces an intense cell mediated immune reaction and results in recurrent episodes of dyspnoea, non-productive cough, fever, chills, fatigue and weight loss[131]. Onset may be acute depending on antigen concentration – if antigen concentration is low, then symptoms are less striking – normally little fever/chills. An occupational exposure history with a clear temporal relationship (onset of symptoms 4–6 hours – occasionally more – after exposure and relief within 1–2 days following removal from the antigen source) provides a solid diagnosis in most patients. The presence of diffuse or basal bilateral fine crepitations accompanied by disseminated interstitial/alveolar infiltrates on chest radiography or CT scanning is typical though lobar, segmental and other patterns are described. Reticulo-nodular and cystic appearances may occur in chronic EAA. However, many cases are initially misdiagnosed as atypical pneumonias. Untreated or unrecognised the mortality rate is some 30% at 5 years[132]. Classical EAA diseases include Farmer's lung, Bagassosis and Humidifier lung due to thermophilic *Actinomyces*

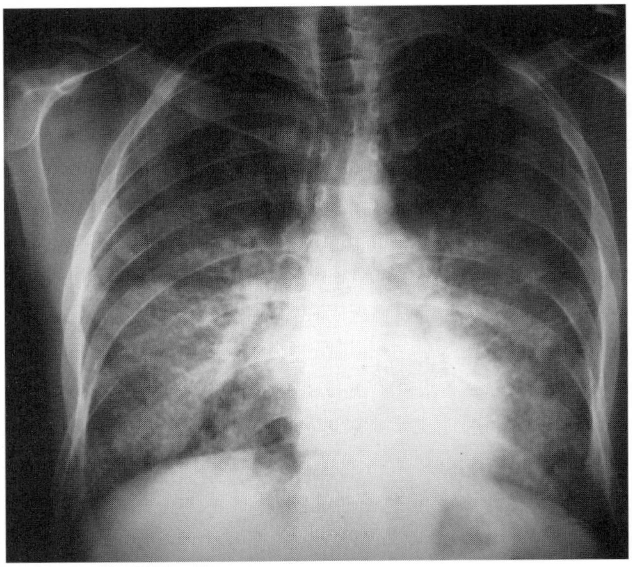

FIGURE 28.9 PAPP. Bilateral diffuse airspace consolidation. (Courtesy of Dr M. Bazarbashi.)

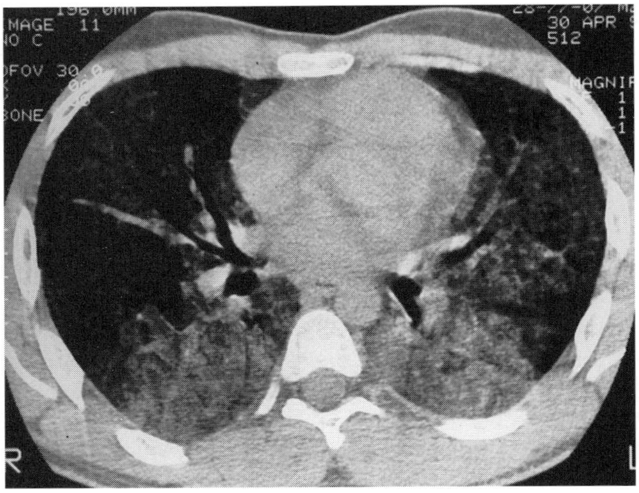

FIGURE 28.10 PAPP. CT chest showing severe patchy air space obliteration and striking air bronchograms. (Courtesy of Dr M. Bazarbashi.)

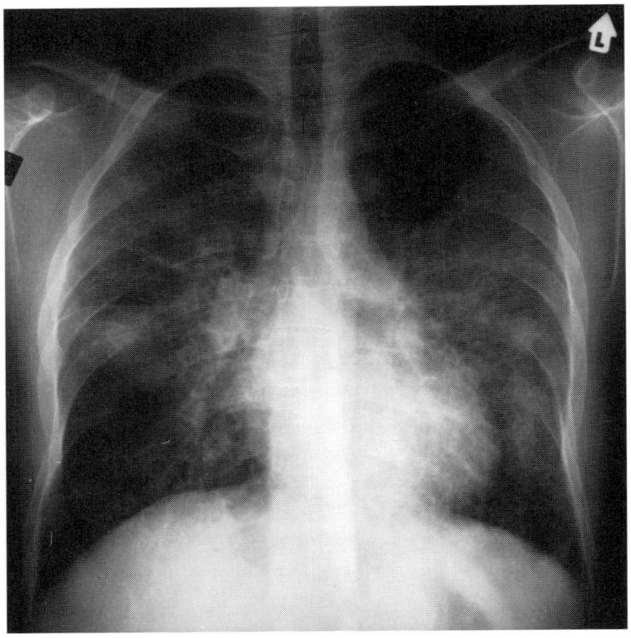

FIGURE 28.11 PAPP. (Courtesy of Dr M. Bazarbashi.)

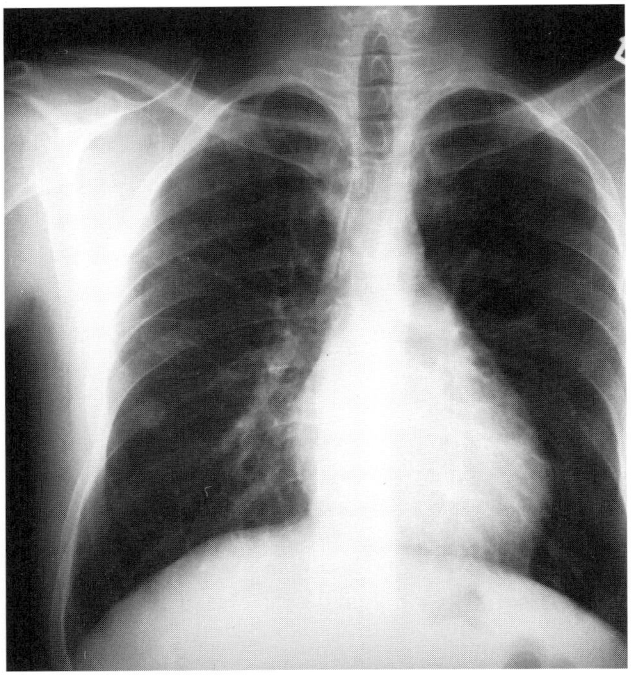

FIGURE 28.12 PAPP. Follow up films after large volume therapeutic lavage. (Courtesy of Dr M. Bazarbashi.)

present in mouldy hay, sugarcane and contaminated humidifiers respectively, Maltworker's lung due to *Aspergillus clavatus* contaminating barley, and thatched roof disease due to *Saccharomonospora* in dried grasses. However, the list is extensive and includes EAA caused by animal products, insect products and chemicals such as diisocyanates[133].

Restrictive dysfunction is the key finding on pulmonary function testing. Long-term follow-up indicates evolution into a mixed obstructive: restrictive pattern in the setting of predominant pulmonary fibrosis and respiratory failure[133]. A striking peripheral leukocytosis (occasionally $> 15 \times 10^9/l$) without eosinophilia accompanies the clinical picture. The WCC response may be blunted in chronic EAA. Skin tests are crude and unhelpful in diagnosis. Specific precipitating antibodies merely indicate exposure and are not pathognomonic of disease. Occasionally, no precipitins can be identified and in these cases, ELISA, RIA, and other more sensitive tests may be positive but again only indicate previous exposure. Serum and bronchial IgG antibodies are increased. The IgE is normal. Thus, there is no specific test for *disease*. The diagnosis hinges firmly on a carefully elicited occupational history, monitored biological real-life challenge to the patient's environment and occasionally, laboratory based broncho-provocation to the suspected antigen. BAL usually shows predominantly increased lymphocytes (up to 80%) of which usually more than a half are suppressor (CD8) or cytotoxic cells, the remainder being helper cells (CD4)[131]. In some forms of EAA, CD4 cells predominate – and is associated with a worse prognosis. This cellular ratio of less than 1 serves to distinguish EAA from pulmonary sarcoid which has a ratio in excess of 5. Histopathologically, the alveoli are filled with mononuclear cells, accompanied by T-lymphocytes or foamy macrophages and non-caseating granulomas resembling sarcoidosis. There may also be an element of bronchiolitis obliterans and fibrosis, particularly in chronic EAA.

The mainstay of management of these patients involves avoidance, of or reduction in, antigen exposure by suitable filter-masks or ventilation. Although systemic steroids are used, evidence for a long term benefit is not available[134] and indeed might be associated with an increased recurrence rate. Removal from the source results in alleviation of symptoms and improvement of lung function with a generally good prognosis. Chronic low level exposure to the antigen may result in pulmonary fibrosis and respiratory failure.

Pulmonary infiltrates associated with peripheral blood or pulmonary eosinophilia (PIE)

Several idiopathic and secondary disorders contribute towards this syndrome complex with a variable degree of overlap in which the common key mediator of disease is the eosinophil. A 100-fold pulmonary tissue to blood sequestration of the wandering eosinophil is a normal phenomenon and explains why some patients with PIE syndromes may have no *blood* eosinophilia. Stimulated eosinophilic granules release a number of lung toxigenic products, among which are major basic protein, neurotoxin, cationic protein and reactive oxygen species. Triggers for eosinophil activation are varied and not always understood. Eosinophils are cytotoxic and anti-inflammatory – they may be stimulated in a number of ways, for example, surface cell receptors (for complement immunoglobulin, etc.), and may combine with helminth derived antibodies. β-adrenergic blockade, menstrual factors, cytokine derived prolongation of eosinophil survival, GMCSF stimulated eosinophilic products and activation, tumour related eosinophil stimulating factors, are among some of the other triggers. Löffler described mildly symptomatic patients who had transient pulmonary infiltrates and peripheral blood eosinophilia (Löffler's syndrome)[135]. Later, Crofton recognised five groups of patients which were variants of this description[136]. However, there have been further variants and the final clear classification of PIE is not yet complete. Most of the diseases can mimic pneumonia and it is important to distinguish these at an early stage to effect appropriate treatment and management.

Löffler's syndrome – simple pulmonary eosinophilia

In the original account, many of the patients may have had *Ascaris* infection from garden fertiliser and other parasites including *Toxicara*, *Ancylostoma*, *Necator*, *Strongyloides* may be causative. Drugs, microbial agents and other factors may be involved in Löffler's syndrome but approximately one-third of patients do not have underlying disease. Cough, dyspnoea, fever, wheeze are commonly found. Löffler's syndrome is the most benign of the PIE syndrome and prognosis for full recovery is excellent without therapy.

Chronic eosinophilic pneumonia (CEP)

CEP is characterised by at least 2 weeks of pulmonary infiltrates – usually situated in the central lung fields, peripheral eosinophilia in excess of 6%, and lung biopsy which shows eosinophilic and histiocytic infiltration of alveolar/interstitial/bronchiolar compartments[137,138]. Eosinophilic abscesses may be found. Alveolar macrophages may contain Charcot-Leyden crystal protein. There is no vasculitis/necrosis. The typical presentation is of a middle-aged person (predominantly female) who has pre-existing asthma, (although this may occur later) sinusitis or nasal polyposis, and presents with protracted (6–7 months), progressive or relapsing cough, fever, dyspnoea and weight loss[137]. Less frequent symptoms include sputum production, wheeze, fatigue and chills. Extra-pulmonary manifestations are not found. An initial diagnosis of infectious pneumonia such as TB or atypical pneumonia is frequently entertained in these patients. Classically, plain chest radiography shows specific findings of patchy alveolar infiltrates in the outer two-thirds (particularly upper lobes) of the lung fields appearing as 'photographic negative pulmonary oedema'. However, a recent review suggested that such infiltrates are actually uncommon on plain radiography, and CT scanning is much more sensitive in demonstrating this pattern which is then recognised in the majority of patients[139]. This radiographical pattern, however, is not pathognomonic for CEP and can occur in BOOP and sarcoid. Lobar, nodular, pleural effusions, lymphadenopathy and cavitations are also found[139]. High peripheral (> 60% of the total white count), sputum and BAL (> 20%) eosinophilia is common. Lysis and degranulation of alveolar eosinophils may preclude their easy identification on standard light microscopy. The total serum IgE is often raised; thrombocytosis may occur. Pulmonary function abnormalities include hypoxaemia, an increased alveolar–arterial gradient, reduction in carbon monoxide transfer factor, and a restrictive defect (which however may be mixed with obstructive elements if concurrent asthma is present). Biopsy is not usually necessary to make the diagnosis. Clinical, radiological and laboratory variations from the above occur including overriding constitutional features, an acute presentation with rapidly progressive respiratory failure[140], non-peripheral infiltrates or lobar consolidation, and the presence of eosinophilic abscesses or multi-nucleate giant cells forming non-caseating granulomas. The clinical and radiological response to high dose (60 mg prednisolone equivalent) systemic steroids is often dramatic and rapid – non-responsiveness after 2 days or at latest a week should lead to re-evaluation of the diagnosis. Laboratory markers which may prove a useful ancillary guide in assessing response include urinary neurotoxin[141] and BAL PGE2[142] although chest radiographical response is usually sufficient. Relapse after discontinuation of treatment is common (80% of patients) and a one and a half year of course of steroids (50 mg of prednisolone on alternate day and tapered) is often necessary. The occasional patient requires maintenance steroids indefinitely but most patients will eventually not be steroid dependent. The role of inhaled steroids remains to be determined. Significant residual pulmonary function abnormalities and pulmonary fibrosis are uncommon. The underlying asthma rather than CEP is thought to be responsible for this. The mortality rate is extremely low.

Acute eosinophilic pneumonia (AEP)

This is a relatively recently recognised syndrome of unknown cause and of acute life threatening onset[143]. It was first described separately by Badesch[144] and Allen[140]. Following an acute highly febrile illness of a few days duration, hypoxic respiratory failure, often requiring IPPV, rapidly supervenes. There may be a prior history of allergic rhinitis although this was absent in earlier reports[140]. Chest radiography shows pan-lobar, mixed alveolar/interstitial infiltrates in a non-peripheral distribution (unlike CEP) and without lymphadenopathy. There may be pleural effusions and Kerley B-lines. Peripheral blood eosinophilia may be mild or absent but BAL shows an impressively high eosinophil percentage (it may approach 50%). Pulmonary function testing shows reduced transfer factor for carbon monoxide and a pure restrictive defect. Lung biopsy does not show vasculitis but rather eosinophilic infiltration of alveolar walls, bronchial walls and interstitium. Part of the diagnostic criteria demands the absence of microbial or other aetiological agents. Despite this, an association with inhaled cocaine has been described[145] and a hypersensitivity type response to inhaled antigens has been proposed as causative. Although some cases apparently resolve spontaneously, the response to high dose steroids is dramatic and apparently life saving. There is no relapse subsequently. The nature of the acute onset makes it one of the more difficult non-infectious pneumonias to differentiate from infection. The presence of the high BAL eosinophilia is a strong pointer away from bacterial or viral pneumonia[146], although fungal and protozoal pneumonias can be associated with BAL eosinophilia. A low diagnostic threshold is essential in this condition since fatalities could possibly be prevented by early intervention with steroids.

Pulmonary eosinophilia due to parasites (PEP)

Ascaris lumbricoides was the incriminating agent in Loeffler's original description of simple pulmonary eosinophilia. This and other parasites (either mature worms, larvae, microfilariae, eggs or unknown antigens) enjoy a migratory pulmonary journey which is associated with eosinophilia. *Strongyloides*, *Ascaris*, *Toxocara*, *Ankylostoma*, *Wucheria* and *Schistosoma* have been discussed in detail in Chapter 26.

Drug-induced pulmonary eosinophilia

This will be discussed under drug-induced toxicity. See pages 543–546.

The hyper-eosinophilic syndrome (HES)

HES is characterised by symptoms of at least 6 months duration due to multisystem failure as a result of widespread infiltration by eosinophils, and associated with a peripheral blood eosinophil count of $> 1{,}5 \times 10^9/l$. Although recognised for decades, it has eluded aetiological determination[147,148]. Eosinophilic leukaemia is a rare association; presence of the Philadelphia chromosome, increased B12, polycythemia rubra-vera, and abnormal leukocyte alkaline phosphatase scores are pointers to this particular diagnosis. Hypereosinophilia can, however, precede cutaneous T-cell lymphoma[149]. Other more common clinical features include eosinophilic cardiac involvement[150] in approximately 60% of patients, as a result of direct endo-myocardial damage from the release of eosinophil granule substances. Restrictive or obliterative cardiomyopathy, Löffler's eosinophilic endocarditis and mural thrombosis occur. Diffuse central nervous system damage resulting from either released neurotoxins or secondary to cerebral arterial thrombo-emboli is manifest by intellectual dysfunction. More focal involvement gives rise to stroke or cranial nerve paralysis. Pulmonary involvement is found in about 50% of patients with HES. An asthma-like presentation is common, characterised by episodic nocturnal cough, fever, and sweats but without airways resistance on pulmonary function testing[148]. Associated focal or diffuse interstitial infiltrates or sometimes pleural effusions are found. Occasionally, angio-oedema with a raised IgE is encountered. Pulmonary hypertension with vessel thrombosis, lung infarction and hilar lymphadenopathy has also been described. Recently, the adult respiratory distress syndrome in association with HES has been documented[151]. In patients with HES, the presence of a high BAL eosinophil count suggests HES pulmonary involvement[152]. Other manifestations of HES include disseminated thromboembolic disease to the skin, kidneys and bowel, thrombocytopenia, anaemia, generalised myalgia and myopathy. Clonal proliferation of type II T-helper cells with associated high levels of interleukin-4 and 5 but diminished levels of interleukin-2 and gamma interferon may produce the features of HES[153]. Soluble interleukin-2 receptors have been found to be increased in HES, the highest levels being associated with T-cell lymphoma. Measurement of levels may prove useful for monitoring the progress of patients[149]. Response to corticosteroids in about a half of patients is good, particularly in those with a raised IgE or without neurological disease. Other treatment approaches include suppression of eosinophil production or actions by hydroxyurea, interferon, vincristine, cyclosporin A and azathioprine.

Miscellaneous conditions associated with pulmonary eosinophilia

Several pulmonary and extrapulmonary diseases unusually have a variable, mild pulmonary eosinophilic component. These include non-infective conditions such as sarcoidosis (but usually causes a lymphocytic alveolitis), bronchial carcinoma, lymphomas and lymphocytic leukaemia (particularly in association with GMCSF)[154], pulmonary infections such as tuberculosis and atypical mycobacterial infections[155] (suggesting a hypersensitivity response to acid fast bacilli) fungal diseases particularly *Aspergillus*, coccidioidomycosis and *P. carinii*, and BOOP (see page 533), pulmonary fibrosis both idiopathic and secondary to connective tissue disorders in which the tissue fibrosis is directly linked to eosinophil degranulation[156] and respiratory syncytial virus infection. Histiocytosis X typified by pneumothorax, lung cysts or nodules, with deposits of immunoglobulin G or complement in alveolar walls and vessels and cytoplasmic x-bodies can also be associated with PIE[157]. Inflammatory bowel disease (particularly ulcerative colitis) can also be found in association with PIE. The association with CSS has already been described (page 33) and allergic bronco-pulmonary aspergillosis in Chapter 16.

Drug-induced pulmonary disease

Virtually any medicament or drug can produce lung disease through direct toxic, hypersensitivity or miscellaneous mechanisms. Occasionally, the presentation can mimic an infectious pneumonia but a drug causation is suggested by non-response to antibiotics, resolution if the drug is stopped, rapid reappearance of symptoms if the patient is rechallenged, absence of a respiratory pathogen, and in some cases presence of peripheral or lung eosinophilia or compatible lung histology. Classification is complex and difficult and therefore some of the more important or common drugs known to produce pulmonary disease will be discussed individually. A detailed account of pulmonary drug toxicity including mechanisms is provided in some excellent reviews[158,159].

Drug-induced pulmonary disease associated with pronounced pulmonary eosinophilia

Anecdotal reports suggest that most drugs are capable of inducing a degree of eosinophilic associated pulmonary toxicity. However, sulphonamides and nitrofurantoin are among those studied in detail.

Sulphasalazine and other sulpha-drugs

It is generally believed that the sulphapyridine moiety triggers a hypersensitivity reaction. Symptoms usually manifest within 3 months of starting the treatment, but delay for as long as 6 years has been reported[160]. Progressive dyspnoea, cough, chest pain, is common and associated pulmonary infiltrates and accompanying blood eosinophilia occur in approximately a half of all cases[161]. The chest radiograph shows bilateral peripheral infiltrates (Fig. 28.13) but these are sometimes better visualised on CT scanning (Fig. 28.14). Bronchiolitis obliterans and fibrosing alveolitis can occur unusually as a result of exposure. Other sulpha drugs which have been implicated include sulphamethoxypyridazine (alveolitis)[162] and cotrimoxazole[163]. The sulphonamide moiety of Fansidar (sulphadoxine–pyrimethamine) was implicated using lymphocyte transformation testing[164]. Histological examination confirms a marked eosinophilic/monocytitic infiltration of alveolar spaces and walls, with epithelioid and multinucleated giant cell granulomas surrounding eosinophilic necrotic areas, but without vasculitis. Once the drug is withdrawn, the outcome is usually good but steroids may hasten recovery. Reexposure to the drug may produce recurrent symptoms and continued exposure may lead to death[165].

Nitrofurantoin

In contrast to sulpha drugs which have been studied infrequently and rarely cause pneumonitis, this drug has been studied in more detail and may cause pneumonitis in as many as 1% of patients taking the drug. The decline in its use in recent years has seen a substantial drop of reported cases[166]. Oxidant production and hypersensitivity (presence

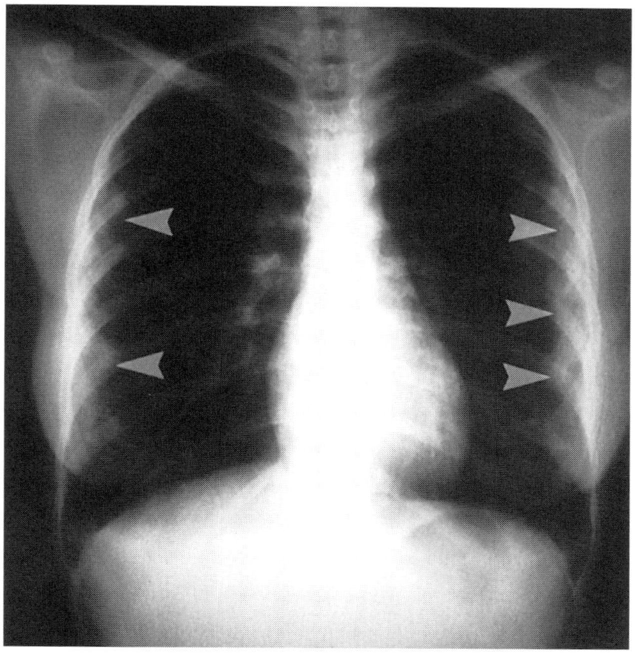

FIGURE 28.13 16-year-old female received co-trimoxazole; developed cough, dyspnea, fever, myalgia at 1 week. Blood eosinophils 1.1. $\times 10^9$/l ($n < 0.4$). Chest radiograph shows diffuse peripheral/sub-pleural infiltrates. Lung parenchyma clear.

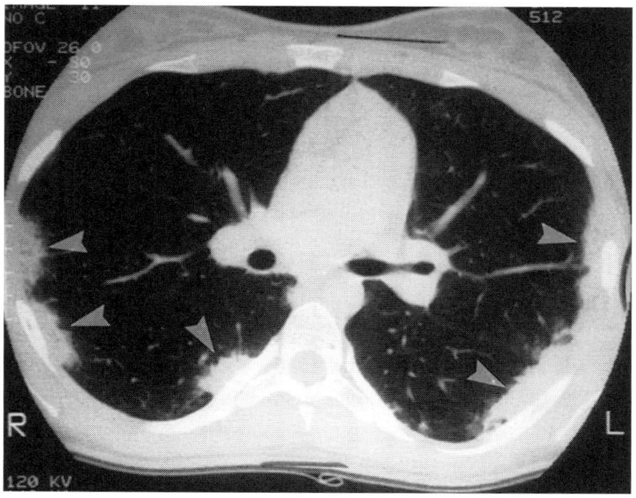

FIGURE 28.14 CT scan of PIE.

of albumin antibodies and albumin immune complexes) are pathogenesis contenders. The more common acute presentation (occurring within one month of taking the drug but even more rapidly if rechallenged) is characterised by fever, dyspnoea, dry cough, chest pain, rash, malaise, myalgia and arthralgia[167]. There is peripheral eosinophilia in 75% of the patients. Some patients develop respiratory failure. In the chronic (2 months' to 5 years' duration) presentation, dyspnoea and cough are the only features usually found, which may not become apparent for months or years after the start of the drug therapy. Radiographically, there are bibasilar or alveolar and interstitial infiltrates. The transfer factor for carbon monoxide is reduced and there is a restrictive pattern on pulmonary function testing. Histologically, vasculitis may be present with monocyte/polymorph/eosinophil infiltration of alveoli and the interstitium. Removal of the drug is associated with an excellent immediate response (resolution of symptoms and infiltrates within a few days) and a good long term outcome for the acute form. Patients with a more chronic presentation carry a 10% mortality risk and risk of irreversible pulmonary fibrosis. Steroids do not help but are often administered.

Other drugs producing pulmonary eosinophilia

These include antimicrobials such as penicillin, ampicillin, minocycline, PAS and tetracycline.

Notable among other drugs is oleoanilide which was responsible for contaminating Spanish rapeseed oil and produced disease in 19 828 persons of whom 315 died[168]. The presentation was characterised by an early phase (first week) illness dominated by pulmonary, lymphoreticular and dermatological symptoms, an intermediate phase (second–eighth week) characterised by gastroenteritis and haematological abnormalities, and a late phase (after the second month) in which neuromuscular and rheumatological findings were found. *Mycoplasma* pneumonia was often misdiagnosed. Late permanent sequelae included fibrosis, pulmonary hypertension and neuromuscular disability such as jaw contractures.

L-Tryptophan ingestion is thought to be responsible for the eosinophilia-myalgic syndrome[169,170], characterised by respiratory failure due to interstitial/alveolar infiltration by lymphocytes and eosinophils, vasculopathy and respiratory muscle weakness (which may be severe), myalgias and pulmonary hypertension. Steroids may be effective[170].

Drug-induced pulmonary disease with a lesser eosinophilic contribution or without eosinophilia

Chemotherapeutic drugs

Carmustine

Used mainly for brain neoplasias, this has been associated with a 25% incidence of pulmonary toxicity, the onset usually paralleling the cumulative dose. Interstitial fibrosis causes basal lung changes[158]. However, an atypical presentation is of delayed (by several years) upper zonal pulmonary fibrosis. Improved survival from the underlying disease in some patients has probably permitted the recognition of this new presentation[171].

Busulfan

This can also produce alveolar proteinosis (see pages 539–40). Occurring in patients with leukaemia, this entity may be resistant to lavage therapy.

Bleomycin

This is an important antitumour antibiotic commonly used in the treatment of a number of solid tumours and lymphomas. Pulmonary damage is reported in approximately 4% of patients but can be as high as 40%[158, 172]. Interstitial fibrosis, hypersensitivity pneumonitis and chest pain syndrome are the three major manifestations. Several mechanisms have been proposed. These include generation of reactive oxygen metabolites, concentration of the drug in those lung cells which are defective in hydrolase inactivating enzymes – these include the type II pneumocytes – stimulation of polymorphs and lymphocytes and increase in lung hydroxyproline. Bleomycin toxicity is enhanced in the older person, by a cumulative dose in excess of 500 units, a continuous infusion route (possibly), diminished creatinine clearance (possibly), concomitant radiotherapy, concomitant use of an F_iO_2 in excess of an average of 0.39, and other chemotherapeutics such as cyclophosphamide (possibly). Histologically, there are no pathognomonic changes but dysplastic alveolar type II pneumocysts are found together with type I pneumocyte necrosis and intraalveolar lamellar body accumulation. BAL may reveal increased cholesterol and an alteration of the proportions of phospholipids which possibly affects surfactant function. There may be an increase in both polymorphonuclear neutrophils and eosinophils. A predominance of mononuclear or polymorphonuclear cellular infiltrate is found, which may progress to collagenous nodular formation and interstitial/intraalveolar fibrosis. Patients who have a predominantly hypersensitivity presentation have eosinophilic infiltration but only mild interstitial fibrosis. Those with the chest pain syndrome do not develop pulmonary fibrosis.

Clinically, low grade fever, dyspnoea, and dry cough are common. However, sputum collection may reveal dysplastic cells. Bi-basilar or lower zone crepitations can be auscultated in most patients. Some, however, may have a normal physical examination and no symptoms despite histological evidence of lung damage. A fulminant course with cyanosis and respiratory failure has also been described. The chest radiograph usually shows bilateral basal reticular shadowing though small nodules can be seen which can be confused with metastases which can also occur in such patients receiving tumour therapy[173]. Alveolar airspace filling can be seen. CT scanning is much more sensitive and will show changes even in the presence of a normal routine plain chest radiograph[174]. A reduced transfer factor for carbon monoxide, decreased lung volumes and vital capacity are often present even when the chest radiograph is normal. However, their interpretation may be difficult in the presence of confounding factors such as lung metastases, opportunistic infections, and technical problems due to patient's poor compliance secondary to poor performance status. In patients with a predominantly hypersensitivity presentation, physical examination is usually normal. They may also have normal X-ray findings.

Acute severe chest pain without cough or dyspnoea and mimicking myocardial ischaemia or pulmonary embolism occurs in approximately

3% of patients receiving intravenous infusions of bleomycin[175] – acute chest pain syndrome. However, no long-term sequelae occurs in these patients and this syndrome is not a contraindication to receiving further bleomycin.

The outcome for patients with acute hypersensitivity pneumonitis or the acute chest pain syndrome is generally excellent. For other patients who have early mild disease, discontinuation of drug is associated with reversal of symptoms and signs. Patients with more advanced or progressive disease require steroids – they often respond but residual pulmonary dysfunction may occur. Some have a fulminant course despite steroids. The mortality rate for bleomycin lung toxicity is approximately 20%.

As cytokines become available in a therapeutic mode, increasing reports of their pulmonary toxicity are emerging. Thus, 50% of patients on interleukin-2 experience pulmonary oedema[176] and many patients receiving tumour necrosis factor experience respiratory distress or alteration in pulmonary function tests[177].

Amioradone and other cardiovascular drugs

Patients with resistant arrhythmias may be treated with amioradone but this drug accumulates in lung tissue and causes pulmonary damage in about 8% of patients, of whom up to one-fifth will die as a result[178]. Toxicity appears in part to be dose related (more than 400 mg daily), possibly synergistic with high F_iO_2 and increased in patients with chronic lung disease. The pathogenesis may be related to hypersensitivity or triggering of uncontrolled intrapulmonary collagen synthesis with subsequent widespread pulmonary fibrosis, possibly mediated by cystosolic calcium[179] or the iodide moiety, oxygen radicals or phospholipids.

Symptoms commence during amioradone treatment or occasionally following discontinuation of the drug. The presentation is usually subacute with breathlessness and productive cough, fever, weight loss, and malaise. However, an acute onset rapidly progressive course sometimes occurs mimicking acute infection. Post-surgical adult respiratory distress syndrome in some patients has been linked to the use of pre-operative and post-operative amioradone[180,181]. Heart failure, trauma and infection are possible triggers. In one study, the practice of giving prophylactic postoperative amioradone was discontinued because of the high rate (9.3%) of amioradone associated adult respiratory distress syndrome[181]. Plain chest radiography demonstrates a bilateral, patchy, mixed consolidation/interstitial pattern although mass-like lesions can occur. Recently, CT scanning has demonstrated increased densities of lung tissue due to lipophilic accumulated amioradone[182]. Reduced DLCO occurs and reflects severity. Reduced lung volumes and hypoxaemia occur later. Leucocytosis is common. BAL shows increased polymorphs and an increase in CD8 cells. Lung tissue indicates diffuse alveolar damage, features of a chronic interstitial pneumonia or BOOP. Collections of foamy macrophages are present and although non-specific for amioradone toxicity, their absence is a strong pointer away from the diagnosis. The management is withdrawal of the drug if at all possible which, however, may not stop the progression of the disease partly due to its extremely long half-life, and supportive measures and corticosteroids are also indicated.

Other cardiovascular drugs having a rare propensity for pulmonary injury include tocainide (pulmonary fibrosis) and captopril (alveolitis).

Non-steroidal anti-inflammatory drug-associated lung disease

Although toxic doses of aspirin, usually in the setting of attempted suicide can induce non-cardiogenic pulmonary oedema[183], it appears that chronic salicylate medication induces an underdiagnosed pseudosepsis syndrome[184]. Key points include fever, leucocytosis with bands, hypotension, low systemic vascular resistance and multiorgan failure which includes the adult respiratory distress syndrome. Two of five patients died in one series.

Gold pneumonitis occurs in about 1% of patients and is mediated by a hypersensitivity mechanism and is associated with eosinophilia and BAL lymphocytosis[185].

Methotrexate produces pulmonary toxicity in 5% of patients and is usually associated with subacute onset of constitutional symptoms, fever and rash[186]. The chest radiograph may demonstrate bilateral diffuse mixed alveolar/interstitial infiltrates, and hilar lymphadenopathy; there may be pulmonary eosinophilia. BAL may show a predominance of CD8 lymphocytes. Tissue may reveal non-caseating granulomas. Some patients have a history of receiving other antirheumatic drugs such as gold, some patients progress despite stopping the drug. Steroids are given for severe symptomatology.

D-Penicillamine is a relatively unusual and less clear-cut cause of pulmonary toxicity and produces a variety of syndromes including pulmonary haemorrhage and bronchiolitis obliterans[158].

Miscellaneous drugs/toxic substances/other causes

Drug abuse either intravenously or by inhalation is frequently associated with pulmonary toxicity. 'Crack' lung due to *cocaine* smoking[187] may produce acute onset dyspnoea associated with alveolar haemorrhage and eosinophilic infiltration, and may progress to respiratory failure and BOOP quite distinct from the secondary pulmonary effects arising from the cardio-toxic effects of the drug.

Contamination of heroin and other opiate drugs with talc may result in intravenous talcosis – slowly progressive respiratory failure associated with upper lobe nodular fibrosis[188]. Alternatively an acute reaction may occur – manifest by rapid onset dyspnoea, cough, and bilateral interstitial/alveolar infiltrates due to mainly non-cardiogenic and to a lesser extent cardiac pulmonary oedema[158].

The presence of *lipids* within the airways lumen is known to stimulate a tissue reaction, the severity of which relates to the source and particular composition of the lipid. This is known as lipoid pneumonia. If an airway becomes obstructed, for example, secondary to carcinoma, then endogenous lipids are released producing a foamy macrophage response. Exogenous lipoid pneumonia, on the other hand, results when inhalation of foreign lipoid substances such as 'ghee' instilled into infant's nostrils[189] or the use of paraffin[190]. The resultant tissue reaction is severe if animal lipids are implicated whereas vegetable oils are relatively benign. The setting is usually of an elderly person who habitually uses oils or an infant given 'ghee' who may or may not have a reason for recurrent aspiration and has chronic cough possibly accompanied by fevers and sweats[191]. Chest radiography may show ill-defined opacities; bronchial carcinoma may be simulated. The presence of fat globules in respiratory secretion is diagnostic. Tissue histology will show lipid deposits and alveolar foamy macrophages. Multinucleated giant cells may be found. The lesions may become fibrotic. An association with non-tuberculous mycobacteria has been described[192, 193]. Hypercalcaemia may result from dihydroxy vitamin D production from the lung granulomas[194]. The outcome is variable. Some patients show regression, others remain static and some may progress to lung fibrosis.

Non-cardiogenic pulmonary oedema can also be induced by low molecular weight dextran[195], thiazide diuretics[158], tocolytic therapy (uterine-inhibitor)[196] and tricyclic and phenothiazine drug overdosage[158].

Pulmonary embolism is well known to be overlooked or mistakenly diagnosed as pneumonia. A high index of suspicion is required in patients at risk. Ventilation/perfusion lung scans, pelvic and peripheral venography and pulmonary angiography should be considered. Treatment is with anticoagulation, thrombolysis or vena caval filters according to the severity or recurrency of the clinical situation.

Inhalation of toxic chemicals

A number of gaseous chemicals if inhaled, usually in an industrial setting damage the lower respiratory tract and result in acute non-cardiogenic pulmonary oedema, pulmonary haemorrhage and long term sequelae. These can simulate pneumonic illnesses. True secondary bacterial pneumonia is also a consequence. The mechanism is thought to be direct mucosal damage in the case of irritant gases such as ammonia, chlorine, hydrochloric acid, nitrogen oxides, phosgene, sulphadioxide and ozone. Usually there is a clear exposure history with pulmonary symptoms developing within minutes or hours and the presence of clear physical features of pulmonary oedema namely chest tightness, cough productive of frothy, clear or blood stained sputum leaves no doubt as to the diagnosis. Bronchospasm due to bronchial hyperreactivity – sometimes prolonged – is often present. In some instances of irritant gas exposure there is a second phase in which respiratory failure and pulmonary infiltrates develop a few weeks after initial exposure and this may lead to BOOP, for example, with nitrogen dioxide, sulphadioxide and ammonia[67]. The other major mechanism of injury is via tissue hypoxia, for example, with carbon monoxide or cyanide poisoning. Polymer-fume fever due to fluorocarbon exposure is thought to have an immune-mediated basis[197]. In the situation of smoke inhalation, injury is caused by the toxic inhalants, thermal burns and inhaled carbonaceous particles. Histological changes include pulmonary oedema, alveolar proteinaceous fluid or haemorrhage, interstitial haemorrhage, hyaline membrane formation, vascular thrombosis, sloughing or mucosal epithelium and submucosal necrosis.

Treatment of chemical inhalation injury is supportive with ventilation as necessary. Specific measures are sometimes indicated, for example, methylene blue for nitrogen dioxide-associated methemoglobulinaemia, hyperbaric oxygen for carbon monoxide poisoning and sodium nitrite/thiosulphate/hydrocobalamin/hyperbaric oxygen for cyanide poisoning. Corticosteroids are sometimes used in the acute situation despite a clear benefit on the epithelial and parenchymal damage but may be useful in controlling the associated airways obstruction and in managing BOOP. Prophylactic antibiotics should be deferred in favour of their early appropriate institution for established secondary microbial pneumonia. In individuals who recover, long-term sequelae[198] include bronchiectasis and obstructive airways disease in addition to BOOP.

Non-infectious aspiration pneumonia

The consequences of aspiration depend on the nature of the aspirated material. Inhalation of solid objects can produce sudden death – the café coronary syndrome[199] or lead to recurrent pneumonia or may be missed. Although the concept of recurrent/persistent pneumonia in the context of the presence of a foreign body is well recognised, recurrent or slowly resolving pneumonia as a chronic irritant/inflammatory post-extraction procedure phenomenon[200] (in addition to acute post-extraction pulmonary oedema) is not always appreciated.

Pulmonary manifestations from aspiration of sea water are due to acute pulmonary oedema from its hypertonicity. Co-aspiration of particulate matter, e.g. sand or microbes, development of ARDS and trauma secondary to resuscitation measures may complicate the presentation. In contrast fresh water aspiration being hypotonic does not produce pulmonary oedema but directly damages lung surfactant, alveolar capillaries and interstitial tissue.

Aspiration of acid ($pH < 2.5$), gastric contents results in extensive tissue damage including alveolar wall disintegration, haemorrhage and larger airways desquamation. This produces severe hypoxemia, pulmonary oedema and pulmonary hypertension with an associated mortality of up to 70% in cases of massive gastric acid aspiration. Concomitant particulate aspiration compounds this morbidity and mortality. Particulate aspiration not only includes food stuffs but antacids (which, although elevating the gastric pH, can produce *per se* an intense tissue reaction including pulmonary haemorrhage)[201]. Chronic lung disease may occur in long-term survivors. Should the pH of the gastric contents be above 2.5, provided there is no particulate matter, severe and persistent histological or clinical changes are unusual[202]. Lipoid aspiration has been discussed previously.

In addition to chemical pneumonia, aspiration carries with it the risk of bacterial pneumonia from the accompanying oropharyngeal gastric flora. Anaerobes are most often implicated particularly *Bacteroides, Fusobacterium*, and *Peptostreptococcus* spp. although aerobic streptococci are sometimes found. In the hospitalised or chronically ill patients, Gram-negative rods and *S. aureus* often feature.

Clinically, patients with aspiration may present with wheezing, stridor, aphonia, or cough if there is foreign body airways obstruction. Gastric contents aspiration leads to cyanosis, fever, wheeze and cough which rapidly progresses to respiratory failure in the case of acidic aspiration. However, this usually quickly clears within 24 hours if the contents have a pH of > 2.5[202]. Features of pulmonary oedema are characterised by frothy or blood stained sputum and may be mistaken for acute bronchitis. Continuation of the fever or leukocytosis, often present initially in chemical aspiration, which if accompanied by purulent sputum production suggests a secondary bacterial pneumonia.

Radiologically, in the case of foreign body aspiration, there may be hyperlucency and mediastinal shift due to air trapping with reduced diaphragmatic excursion. Patchy diffuse alveolar consolidation, with irregular or discrete infiltrates, predominantly in dependent zones (upper lobe posterior segment; lower lobe apical segments) is com-

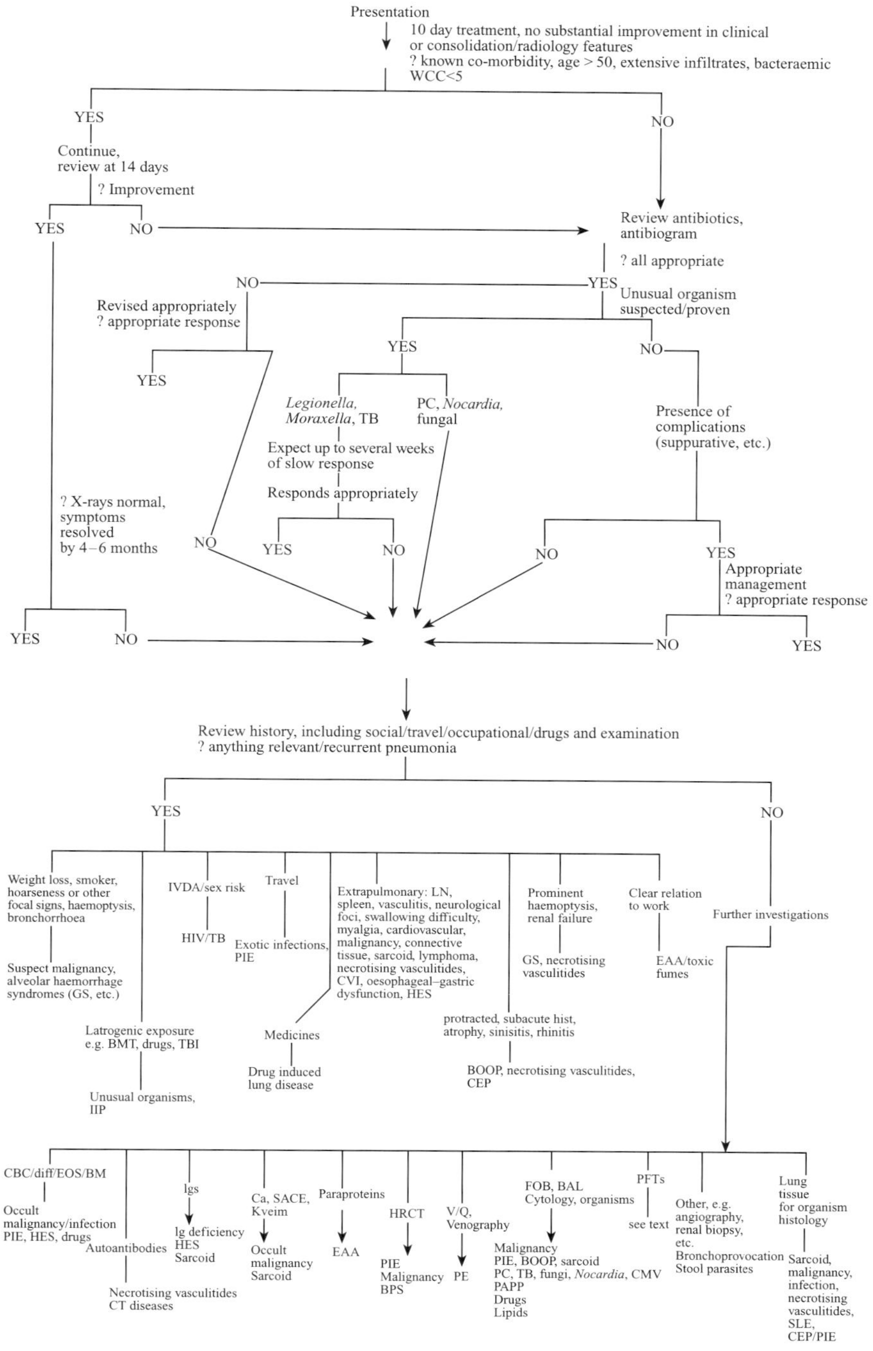

BAL	Bronchoalveolar lavage	Igdef	Immunoglobulin deficiency
BM	Bone marrow examination	Igs	Immunoglobulins
BMT	Bone marrow transplantation	IIP	Idiopathic interstitial pneumonitis
BOOP	Bronchiolitis obliterans/organising pneumonia	IVDA	Intra-venous drug abuse
BPS	Bronchopulmonary sequestration	LN	Lymphadenopathy
Ca	Calcium	Malig	Malignancy
CDC/diff	Complete blood count + differential + blood film	PAPP	Pulmonary alveolar phospholipoproteinosis
CEP	Chronic eosinophilic pneumonia	PC	*Pneumocystis*
CMV	Cytomegalovirus	PE	Pulmonary embolism
CVI	Common variable immunodeficiency	PFTs	Pulmonary function tests
EAA	Extrinsic allergic alveolitis	PIE	Pulmonary infiltration with eosinophilia
EOS	Eosinophils	Pptns	Precipitins
FOB	Fibreoptic bronchoscopy	SACE	Serum angiotensin converting enzyme
GS	Goodpasture's syndrome	SLE	Systemic eosinophilic pneumonia
HRCT	High resolution CT scan chest	TBI	Total body irradiation
HES	Hypereosinophilic syndrome		

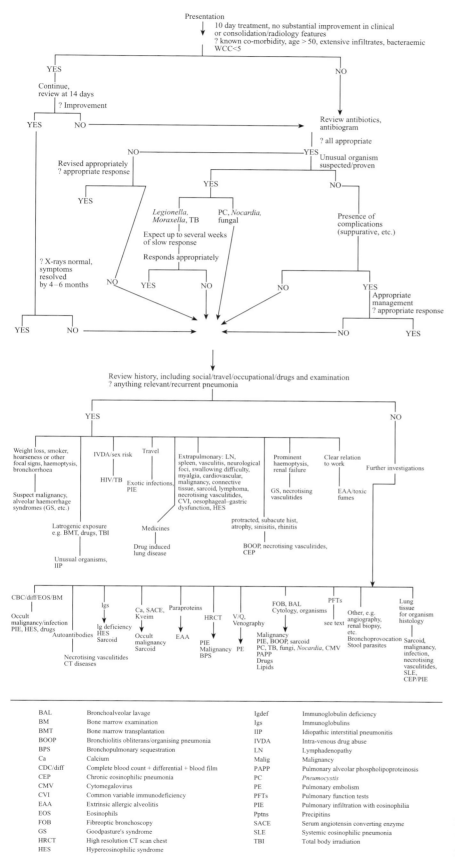

FIGURE 28.15 Clinical approach to the patient with protracted pulmonary infiltrates/pneumonia.

mon. Widespread diffuse radiographical involvement, on the other hand, is found in massive aspiration, particularly of gastric contents and in subsequent bacterial pneumonia.

Management pivots around (i) removal or bypassing the foreign body by Heimlich's manoeuvre, or cricothyroidectomy in the life threatening situation, or bronchoscopy possibly through a formal thoracotomy for subacute presentations; (ii) supportive measures with oxygen, inotropes and ventilation; and (iii) use of appropriate antibiotics in a therapeutic mode if secondary bacterial pneumonia is suspected. Metronidazole alone for aspiration pneumonia is relatively ineffective whereas clindamycin is highly effective for most cases. Gram-negative cover with for example, ceftriaxone, ceftazidime or imipenem should be added in selected circumstances, for example, the prolonged hospitalised chronically ill or immunocompromised patient. An aminoglycoside is often added in patients with septic shock or who are neutropenic. Prophylactic antibiotics and corticosteroids are currently thought to have no impact in the management of these patients. Experimental treatment modalities include surfactant replacement[203] and nitric oxide. Awareness of the risk for aspiration coupled with appropriate preventative strategies, are probably the most important measures, and include the use of antacids, expert induction/general anaesthetic techniques, care over nasogastric tube feeding and nursing at risk patients in a semi-erect position.

Finally, it is important to remember that many drugs with pulmonary toxicity may not only produce a syndrome mimicking infectious pneumonia but may cause pneumothorax (e.g. bleomycin), bronchospasm (e.g. aspirin, cocaine, β-blockers, cytokines and nitrofurantoin) and pleural effusion (e.g. chemotherapeutics, tryptophan, amioradone, and sclerotherapy agents).

Summary

In a patient with community-acquired pneumonia the time course for resolution will depend on the aetiological organism, initial clinical features, co-morbid diseases and integrity of the host immune defence system. For most patients, substantial symptomatic improvement is expected by 10–14 days with a lag in radiological improvement and sometimes initial temporary deterioration. Substantial clearing of infective infiltrates for consolidation should occur by 2–3 weeks and a return to the baseline pre-pneumonic or normal X-ray by approximately 6 months. In general, younger and otherwise healthy patients would experience a more rapid resolution than this whilst patients > 50 years with chronic pulmonary and other diseases might not achieve clinical and radiological cure until the more conservative time limit had expired. Certain organisms, although themselves sometimes associated with co-morbid factors, would be associated with a long time course. For patients whose time course appears to be unduly prolonged both at the time of initial presentation and for those who by 4–6 months have still not totally resolved symptoms and radiological features and as well as those whose pneumonia is recurrent, further assessment is indicated. A proposed scheme is shown in Fig. 28.15 and is directed primarily to the patient with a protracted pneumonia – aspects of these are also relevant to the patient with recurrent pneumonia or suspected pneumonia. It is important to keep in mind that patients with an apparent normal rate of pneumonia resolution may also have underlying diseases.

References

1. ISRAEL HL, WEISS W, EISENBERG GM *et al.* Delayed resolution of pneumonias. *Med Clin N Am* 1956;40:1291–303.
2. KIRKLAND SH, WINTERBAUER RH. Slowly resolving, chronic and recurrent pneumonia. *Clin Chest Med* 1991;12:303–18.
3. FEIN AM, FEINSILVER SH, NIEDERMAN MS. Non resolving and slowly resolving pneumonia. *Clin Chest Med* 1993;14:555–69.
4. GLEICHMAN TK, LEDER M, ZAHN D. Major etiologic factors producing delayed resolution in pneumonia. *Am J Med Sci* 1949;218:309–20.
5. FEIN AM, FEINSILVER SH, NIEDERMAN MS, FIEL S, PAI PB. When the pneumonia doesn't get better. *Clin Chest Med* 1987;8:529–41.
6. FEINSILVER SH, FEIN AM, NEIDERMAN MS, SCHULTZ DE, FAEGENBURG DH. Utility of fiberoptic bronchoscopy in non-resolving pneumonia. *Chest* 1990;98:1322–6.
7. WINTERBAUER RH, BEDON GA, BALL WC, JR. Recurrent pneumonia. Predisposing illness and clinical patters in 158 patients. *Ann Intern Med* 1969;70: 689–700.
8. EKDAHL K, BRACONIER JH, ROLLOF J. Recurrent pneumonia: a review of 90 adult patients. *Scand J Infect Dis* 1992;24:71–6.
9. Conference on therapy: treatment of pneumonia. *Am J Med* 1948;4423–35.
10. VAN METRE TE JR. Pneumococcal pneumonia treated with antibiotics. *N Engl J Med* 1954;251:1048–52.
11. JAY SJ, JOHANSON WG, PIERCE AK. The radiographical resolution of *Streptococcus pneumoniae* pneumonia. *N Engl J Med* 1975;293:798–801.
12. MACFARLANE JT, MILLER AC, RODERICK SMITH WH, MORRIS AH, ROSE DH. Comparative radiographical features of community-acquired legionnaires' disease, pneumococcal pneumonia, mycoplasma pneumonia, and psittacosis. *Thorax* 1984;39:28–33.
13. GRAHAM WGB, BRADLEY DA. Efficacy of chest physiotherapy and intermittent positive-pressure breathing in the resolution of pneumonia. *N Engl J Med* 978;299:624–7.
14. LEHTOMAKI K. Clinical diagnosis of pneumococcal, adenoviral, mycoplasmal and mixed pneumonias in young men. *Eur J Resp Dis* 1988;1:324–9.
15. FINNEGAN OC, FOWLES SJ, WHITE RJ. Radiographic appearances of mycoplasma pneumonia. *Thorax* 1981;36:469–72.
16. BORTHWICK RC, CAMERON DC, PHILIP T. Radiographic patterns of pulmonary involvement in acute mycoplasmal infection. *Scand J Resp Dis* 1978;59:190–3.
17. HEBERT DH. The roentgen features of Eaton agent pneumonia. Am J Roentgenol 1966;98:300–4.
18. WOODHEAD MA, MACFARLANE JT. Legionnaires' disease: a review of 79 community-acquired cases in Nottingham. *Thorax* 1986;41:635–40.
19. MILLER AC. Early clinical differentiation between legionnaires' disease and other sporadic pneumonias. *Ann Intern Med* 1979;90:526–8.
20. FAIRBANK JT, MAMOURIAN AC, DIETRICH PA AND GIROD JC. The chest radiograph in legionnaires' disease. *Radiology* 1983;147:33–4.

21. KIRBY BD, PECK H, MEYER RD. Radiographic features of legionnaires' disease. *Chest* 1979;76:562–5.

22. LO CD, MACKEEN AD, CAMPBELL DR *et al.* Radiographic analysis of the course of Legionella pneumonia. *J Can Assoc Radiol* 1983;34:116–19.

23. STRENGSTROM P, JANSSON E, WAGER O *et al.* Pneumonia with special reference to roentgenological lung findings. *Acta Med Scand* 1962;171:349–56.

24. WRIGHT P, WALLACE R JR, SHEPPERD J. A descriptive study of 42 cases of *Branhamella catarrhalis* pneumonia. *Am J Med* 1990;88:2–8.

25. MARRIE TJ, DURANT H, YATES L. Community-acquired pneumonia requiring hospitalisation: 5-year prospective study. *Rev Infect Dis* 1989;11:586–99.

26. RESEARCH COMMITTEE OF THE BRITISH THORACIC SOCIETY AND THE PUBLIC HEALTH LABORATORY SERVICE. Community acquired pneumonia in adults in British Hospitals in 1982–1983: a survey of aetiology, mortality, prognostic factors and outcome. *Quart J Med* 1987;62:195–200.

27. FINE MJ, SMITH DN, SINGER DE. Hospitalisation decision in patients with community-acquired pneumonia: a prospective cohort study. *Am J Med* 1990;89:713–21.

28. BRITISH THORACIC SOCIETY RESEARCH COMMITTEE. The aetiology, management and outcome of severe community-acquired pneumonia on the intensive care unit. *Resp Med* 1992;86:7–13.

29. VAN EEDEN SF, COETZEE AR, JOUBERT JR. Community acquired pneumonia – factors influencing intensive care admission. *South Afr Med J* 1988;73:77–81.

30. AL ZAMIL F, SHIBL A, QADRI SMH. Detection of pneumococci with increased resistance to penicillin and their clinical significance. *Ann Saudi Med* 1992;12(3):279–82.

31. NELSON S, CHIDIAC C, BAGBY G, SUMMER WR. Endotoxin induced suppression of lung host defences. *J Med* 1990;21:85–103.

32. FANG G-D, FINE M, ORLOFF J, ARISUMI D *et al.* New and emerging etiologies for comunity-acquired pneumonia with implications for therapy. A prospective multicenter study of 359 cases. *Medicine* 1990;69:307–16.

33. JOKINEN C, HEISKANEN L, JUVONEN H *et al.* Incidence of community-acquired pneumonia in the population of four municipalities in Eastern Finland. *Am J Epidemiol* 1993;137:977–88.

34. HEDLUND JU, ÖRTQVIST ÅB, KALIN M, SCALIA-TOMBA G, GIESECKE J. Risk of pneumonia in patients previously treated in hospital for pneumonia. *Lancet* 1992;340:396–7.

35. CAIAFFA WT, GRAHAM NMH, VLAHOV D. Bacterial pneumonia in adult populations with human immunodeficiency virus (HIV) infection. *Am J Epidemiol* 1993;138:909–22.

36. POLSKY B, GOLD JWM, WHIMBEY YE *et al.* Bacterial pneumonia in patients with the acquired immunodeficiency syndrome. *Ann Intern Med* 1986;104:38–41.

37. CENTERS FOR DISEASE CONTROL. 1993 revised classification system for HIV infection and expanded surveillance case definition for AIDS among adolescents and adults. *MMWR* 1992;41:1–19.

38. MULLER F, FROLAND SS, BRANDTZAEG P. Altered IgG subclass distribution in lymph node cells and serum of adults infected with human immunodeficiency virus (HIV). *Clin Exp Immunol* 1989;78:153–8.

39. GARCIA-LEONI ME, MORENO S, RODENO P. Pneumococcal pneumonia in adult hospitalised patients infected with the human immunodeficiency virus. *Arch Intern Med* 1992;152:1808–12.

40. MAGNENAT JL, NICOD LP, AUCKENTHALER R, JUNOD AF. Mode of presentation and diagnosis of bacterial pneumonia in human immunodeficiency virus infected patients. *Am Rev Resp Dis* 1991;144:917–22.

41. KIELHOFNER M, ATMAR RL, HAMILL RJ *et al.* Life threatening *Pseudomonas aeruginosa* infections in patients with human immunodeficiency virus infection. *Clin Infect Dis* 1990;14:403–11.

42. JAVALY K, HOROWITZ HW, WORMSFR GP. Nocardiosis in patients with human immunodeficiency virus infection. *Medicine* 1992;71:128–38.

43. VESTBO J, LUNDGREN JB, GAUB J *et al.* Severe *Rhodococcus equi* pneumonia : case report and literature review. *Eur J Clin Microbiol Infect Dis* 1991;10:762–8.

44. FRAME C, PETKUS AF. *Rhodococcus equi* pneumonia : case report and literature review. Ann Pharmacother 1993;27:1340–2.

45. MATTER L, WILHELM JA, ANGEHM W, SKVARIL F, SCHOPFER K. Selective antibody deficiency and recurrent pneumococcal bacteremia in a patient with Sjorgren's syndrome, hyperimmunoglobulinemia G and deficiencies of IgG2 and IgG4. *NEJM* 1985;312(16):1039–42.

46. WATTS WJ, WATTS MB, DAI W *et al.* Respiratory dysfunction in patients with common variable hypoglobulinemia. *Ann Intern Med* 1986;104:38–41.

47. OXELIUS V-A, LAURELL A-B, LINDQUIST B *et al.* IgG subclasses in selective IgA deficiency. Importance of AgG-IgA deficiency. *N Engl J Med* 1981;304:1476–7.

48. KINLIN LJ, WEBSTER ABD, BIRD AG *et al.* Prospective study of cancer in patients with hypogammaglobulinemia. *Lancet* 1985;1:263–6.

49. BRYANT A, CALVER NC, TOUBI E, WEBSTER ADB, FARRANT J. Classification of patients with common variable immunodeficiency by B cell secretion of IgM and IgG in response to anti-IgM and interleukin-2. *Clin Immunol Immunopathol* 1990;56:239–48.

50. KRUGER G, WELTE K, CIOBANU N *et al.* Interleukin-2 correction of defective in vitro T-cell mitogenesis in patients with common varied immunodeficiency. *J Clin Immunol* 1984;4:295–303.

51. JAFFE J, STROBER W, SNELLER MC. Functional abnormalities of CD8 T cells define a unique subset of patients with common variable immunodeficiency. *FASEB* 1992;6:A1120.

52. CUNNINGHAM-RUNDELS C, MAYER L, SAPIRA E, MENDELSOHN L. Restoration of immunoglobulin secretion in vitro in common variable immunodeficiency by *in vivo* treatment with polyethylene glycolconjugated human recombinant interleukin-2. *Clin Immunol Immunopathol* 1992;64:46–56.

53. JAVAID A, AAMIR AUH. Pulmonary sequestration: a case report and review. *Resp Med* 1994;88:65–6.

54. MARRIE T, HALDANE V, FAULKNER R *et al.* Community acquired pneumonia requiring hospitalisation : is it different in the elderly? *J Am Geriatr Soc* 1985;33:671–80.

55. FINE MJ, ARENA VC, HANUSA BH *et al.* Prognosis of patients hospitalised with community-acquired pneumonia. *Am J Med* 1990;88:(5N)IN–8N.

56. FINE MJ, SINGER DE, SMITH D. Hospitalisation decision in patients with community-acquired pneumonia : a prospective cohort study. *Am J Med* 1990:89;713–21.

57. BERKOWITZ K, LASALA A. Risk factors associated with the increasing prevalence of pneumonia during pregnancy. *Am J Obstet Gynecol* 1990;163:981–5.

58. MADINGER NE, GREENSPOON JS, ELLRODT AG. Pneumonia during pregnancy: has modern technology improved maternal and fetal outcome. *Am J Obstet Gynecol* 1989;161:657–62.

59. HOPWOOD HG. Pneumonia in pregnancy. *Obstet Gynecol* 1965;25:875–9.

60. BENEDETTI TJ, VALLE R, LEDGER WJ. Antepartum pneumonia in pregnancy. *Am J Obstet Gynecol* 1982;144:413–17.

61. ESMONDE TF, HERDMAN G, ANDERSON G. Chicken pox pneumonia: an association with pregnancy. *Thorax* 1989;44:812–15.

62. HAAKE DA, ZAKOWSKI PC, HAAKE DL AND BRYSON YJ. Early treatment with acyclovir for varicella pneumonia in otherwise healthy adults : retrospective controlled study and review. *Rev Infect Dis* 1990;12:788–98.

63. KOONIN LM, ELLERBROCK TV, ALTRASH HK. Pregnancy-associated death due to AIDS in the United States. *J Am Med Assoc* 1989;261:1306–9.

64. ANDREWS EB, YANKASKAS BC, CORDERO JF, SCHOEFFLER K, HAMPP S AND THE ACYCLOVIR IN PREGNANCY REGISTRY ADVISORY COMMITTEE. Acyclovir in pregnancy registry : six years experience. *Obstet Gynecol* 1992;79:7–13.

65. GRINBLAT J, MECHLIS S, LEWITUS Z. Organizing pneumonia-like process. An unusual observation in steroid responsive cases with features of chronic interstitial pneumonia. *Chest* 1981;80:259–63.

66. DAVISON AG, HEARD BE, MCALLISTER WAC, TURNER-WARWICK MEH. Cryptogenic organizing pneumonitis. *Quart J Med* 1983;207:382–94.

67. EPLER GR, COLBY TV, MCLOUD TC, CARRINGTON CB, GAENSLER EA. Bronchiolitis obliterans organizing pneumonia. *N Engl J Med* 1985;312:152–8.

68. COSTABEL U, TESCHLER H, SCHOENFELD B, HARTUNG W, NUSCH A, GUZMAN J, GRESCHUCHNA D, KONIETZKO N. BOOP in Europe. *Chest* 1992;102:14S–20S.

69. HSUE Y-T, PAULUS HE, COULSON WF. Bronchiolitis obliterans organizing pneumonia in polymyositis. A case report with longterm survival. *J Rheumatol* 1993;20:877–9.

70. KAUFMAN J, KOMOROWSKI R. Bronchiolitis obliterans : a new clinical-pathological complication of irradiation pneumonitis. *Chest* 1990;97:1243–4.

71. KUWANOK K, HAYASHI S, MACKENZIE A, HOGG JC. Detection of adenovirus DNA in paraffin-embedded lung tissues from patients with bronchiolitis obliterans and organizing pneumonia (BOOP) using *in situ* hybridisation. *Am Rev Resp Dis* 1990;141:A319.

72. THIRMAN MJ, DEVINE SM, O'TOOLE K, CIZEK G, JESSURUN J, HERTZ M, GELLER RB. Bronchiolitis obliterans organizing pneumonia as a complication of allogeneic bone marrow transplantation. *Bone Marrow Transpl* 1992;10:307–11.

73. PRZEPIOKA D, ABU-ELMAGD K, HUARINGA A *et al.* Bronchiolitis obliterans organizing pneumonia in a BMT patient receiving FK506 (letter). *Bone Marrow Transpl* 1993;11:502.

74. KITAICHI M. Differential diagnosis of bronchiolitis obliterans organizing pneumonia. *Chest* 1992;102:44S–9S.

75. KING JR, TE, MORTENSON RL. Cryptogenic organizing pneumonitis. The North American experience. *Chest* 1992;102:8S–13S.

76. BENSARD DD, MCINTYRE RC JR, WARING BJ *et al.* Comparison of video thorascopic lung biopsy to open lung biopsy in the diagnosis of interstitial lung disease. *Chest* 1993;103:765–70.

77. CAMP M, MEHTA JB, WHITSON M. *Bronchiolitis obliterans* and *Norcardia asteroides* infection of the lung. *Chest* 1987;92:1107–8.

78. KUWANO K, HAYASHI S, MACKENZIE A, HOGG JC. Detection of adenovirus DNA in paraffin-embedded lung tissues from patients with *Bronchiolitis obliterans* and organising pneumonia (BOOP) using *in situ* hybridisation. *Am Rev Resp Dis* 1990;141:A319.

79. CORDONNIER C, BERNAUDIN JF, BIERLING P, HUET Y, VERNANAT JP. Pulmonary complications occurring after allogeneic bone marrow transplantation: a study of 130 consecutive transplanted patients. *Cancer* 1986;58:1047–54.

80. MEYERS JD, FLOURNOY N, THOMAS ED. Nonbacterial pneumonia after allogeneic marrow transplantation: a review of ten year's experience. *Rev Infect Dis* 1982;4:1119–32.

81. APPELBAUM FR, MEYERS JD, FEFER A *et al.* Nonbacterial nonfungal pneumonia following bone marrow transplantation in 100 identical twins. *Transplantation* 1983;33:265–8.

82. PEREGO R, HILL R, APPELBAUM FR *et al.* Interstitial pneumonitis following autologous bone marrow transplantation. *Transplantation* 1986;42:515–17.

83. CRAWFORD SW, HACKMAN RC. Clinical course of idiopathic pneumonia after bone marrow transplantation. *Am Rev Resp Dis* 1993;147:1393–400.

84. KAPLAN EB, PIETRA GG, AUGUST CS. Interstitial pneumonitis, pulmonary fibrosis and chronic graft versus host disease. *Bone Marrow Transpl* 1992;9:71–5.

85. GRUNDY JE, SHANLEY JD, GRIFFITH PD. Is cytomegalovirus interstitial pneumonitis in transplant recipients an immunopathological condition? *Lancet* 1987;ii:996–9.

86. MEYERS JD, FLOURNOY N, WADE JC *et al.* Biology of interstitial pneumonia after marrow transplantation. Proceedings of the UCLA Symposia Conference. *Rec Adv Bone Marrow Transpl* 1983;405–23.

87. LATINI P, ARISTEI C, AVERSA F *et al.* Interstitial pneumonitis after hyperfractionate/total body irradiation in HLA-matched T-depleted bone marow transplantation. *Int J Radiat Oncol Biol Phy* 1992;23:401–5.

88. WESHLER Z, BREURER R, OR .R Interstitial pneumonias after total body irradiation: effect of partial lung shielding. *Br J Haematol* 1990;74:61–4.

89. CARRIGAN DR, DROBYSKI WR, RUSSLER SK, TAPPER MA, KNOWX KK, ASH RC. Interstitial pneumonitis associated with human herpesvirus-6 infection after marrow transplantation. *Lancet* 1991;338:147–9.

90. CONE RW, HACKMAN RC, HUANG M-L *et al.* Human herpesvirus 6 in lung tissue from patients with pneumonitis after bone marrow transplantation. *N Engl J Med* 1993;329:156–61.

91. FRENKEL N, SCHIRMER EC, WYATT LS. Isolation of a new herpesvirus from human CD4+ T cells. *Proc Nat Acad Sci USA* 1990;87:748–52.

92. WINGARD JR, SANTOS GW, SARAL R. Late-onset interstitial pneumonia following allogeneic bone marrow transplantation. *Transplantation* 1985;39:21–3.

93. PERREAULT C, COUSINEAU S, D'ANGELO G *et al.* Lymphoid interstitial pneumonia after allogeneic bone marrow transplantation. A possible manifestation of chronic graft-versus-host disease. *Cancer* 1985;55:1–9.

94. LEBLOND V, ZOUABI H, SUTTON L *et al.* Late CD8+ lymphocytic alveolitis after allogeneic bone marrow transplantation and chronic graft-versus-host disease. *Am J Resp Crit Care Med* 1994;150:1056–61.

95. ELLIS ME, SPENCE D, BOUCHAMA A *et al.* Open lung biopsy provides a higher and more specific diagnostic yield compared to broncho-alveolar lavage in immunocompromised patients. *Scand J Infect Dis* 1995: 157–62.

96. FAUCI AS, HAYNES BF, KATZ P, WOLFF SM. Wegener's granulomatosis: prospective clinical and therapeutic experience with 85 patients for 21 years. *Ann Intern Med* 1983;98:76–85.

97. HOFFMAN GS, KERR GS, LEAVITT RY *et al.* Wegener's granulomatosis: an analysis of 158 patients. *Ann Intern Med* 1992;116:488–98.

98. FALK RJ, HOGAN S, CAREY TS, JENNETTE JC. Clinical course of antineutrophil cytoplasmic autoantibody-associated glomerulonephritis and systemic vasculitis. *Ann Intern Med* 1990;113:656–63.

99. DEREMEE RA. The treatment of Wegener's granulomatosis with trimethoprim/sulfamethoxazole: illusion or vision? *Arthr Rheumatol* 1988;31: 1068–72.

100. ISRAEL HL. Sulfamethoxazole-trimethoprim therapy for Wegener's granulomatosis. *Arch Intern Med* 1988;148:2293–5.

101. LEAVITT RY, FAUCI AS. Pulmonary vasculitis. *Am Rev Resp Dis* 1986;134:140–66.

102. CHURG J, STRAUSS L. Allergic granulomatosis, allergic angiitis and periarteritis nodosa. *Am J Pathol* 1951;27:277–301.

103. CHUMBLEY LC, HARRISONE G, DEREMEE RA. Allergic granulomatosis and angiitis (Churg–Strauss Syndrome): report and analysis of 30 cases. *Mayo Clin Proc* 1977;52:477–84.

104. LANHAM JG, ELKON KB, PUSEY CD, HUGHES GR. Systemic vasculitis with asthma and eosinophilia: a clinical approach to the Churg–Strauss syndrome. *Medicine* 1984;63:65–81.

105. FROHNETT PP, SHEPS SG. Long term follow up study of periarteritis nodosa. *Am J Med* 1967;43:8–14.

106. HOLDSWORTH S, BOYCE N, THOMSON NM, ATKINS RC. The clinical spectrum of acute glomerulonephritis and lung haemorrhage (Goodpasture's syndrome). *Quart J Med New Series* 55 1985;216;75–86.

107. COUSER WG. Rapidly progressive glomerulonephritis: classification, pathogenetic mechanisms and therapy. *Am J Kidney Dis* 1988;6:448–64.

108. JOHNSON JP, MOORE J, AUSTIN HA, BALOW JE, ANTONOYCH TT, WILSON CB. Therapy of anti-glomerular basement membrane antibody disease: analysis of prognostic significance of clinical, pathologic and treatment factors. *Medicine* (*Baltimore*) 1985:219–27.

109. Proceedings of the Third International Conference on Sarcoidosis. *Acta Med Scand* Suppl 1962:425–32

110. THOMAS PD AND HUNNINGHAKE GW. Current concepts of the pathogenesis of sarcoidosis. *Am Rev Resp Dis* 1987;135:747–60.

111. CHITTOCK DR, JOSEPH MG, PATERSON NA, MCFADDEN RG. Necrotizing sarcoid granulomatosis with pleural involvement. Clinical and radiographical features. *Chest* 1994;106:672–6.

112. MITCHELL DN, REES RJW. The nature and physical characteristics of a transmissible agent from human sarcoid tissue. *Ann NY Acad Sci* 1976;278:233–48.

113. KERN DG, NEILL MA, WRENN DS, VARONE, JC. Investigation of a unique time-space cluster of sarcoidosis in firefighters. *Am Rev Resp Dis* 1993;148:974–80.

114. FIDLER HM, ROOK GA, MCIJOHNSON N, MCFADDEN J. *Mycobacterium* tuberculosis DNA in tissue affected by sarcoidosis. *Br Med J* 1993;306:546–9.

115. SILTZBACK LE, JAMES DG, NEVILLE E *et al.* Course and prognosis of sarcoidosis around the world. *Am J Med* 1974;57:847–52.

116. MAYCOCK RL, BERTRAND P, MORRISON CE, SCOTT JH. Manifestations of sarcoidosis. Analysis of 145 patients with a review of nine series selected from the literature. *Am J Med* 1963;35:67–9.

117. MITCHELL DN, SCADDING JG. Sarcoidosis. *Am Rev Resp Dis* 1974;110:774–802.

118. SEATON A, SEATON D, LEITCH AG. Sarcoidosis. In *Crofton and Douglas's Respiratory Diseases*, Oxford: Blackwell Scientific Publications: 4th Ed 1989: 630–59.

119. CRYSTAL RB, ROBERTS WE, HUNNINGHAKE GW *et al.* Pulmonary sarcoidosis : a disease characterised and perpetuated by activated lung T-lymphocytes. *Ann Intern Med* 1981;94:73–94.

120. MULLER-QUERNHEIM J. Monitoring sarcoidosis therapy with immunopathologic parameters. *Pneumologie* 1994;48:47–9.

121. BRUDIN LH, VALIND SO, RHODES CG *et al.* Fluorine-18 deoxyglucose uptake in sarcoidosis measured with positron emission tomography. *Eur J Nucl Med* 1994;21:297–305.

122. HUNNINGHARE GW, GILBERT S, PUERINGER R *et al.* Outcome of the treatment for sarcoidosis. *Am J Resp Crit Case Med* 1994;149:893–8.

123. STONE DJ, SCHWARTZ A. A long-term study of sarcoid and its modification by steroid therapy. *Am J Med* 1966:41: 528–40.

124. MILMAN N, GRAUDAL N, GRODE G, MUNCH E. No effect of high-dose inhaled steroids in pulmonary sarcoidosis: a double-blind, placebo-controlled study. *J Int Med* 1994;236:285–90.

125. ZYCH D, PAWLICKA L, ZIELINSKI J. Inhaled budesonide vs prednisone in the maintenance treatment of pulmonary sarcoidosis. *Sarcoidosis* 1993;10:56–61.

126. JOHNSON BA, DUNCAN SR, OHORI NP *et al.* Recurrence of sarcoidosis in pulmonary allograft recipients. *Am Rev Resp Dis* 1993;148:1373–7.

127. ROSEN SH, CASTLEMAN B, LIEBOW AA. Pulmonary alveolar proteinosis. *N Engl J Med* 1958;258:1123–42.

128. BEDROSSIAN CWM, LUNA MA, CONKLIN RH, MILLER WC. Alveolar proteinosis as a consequence of immunosuppression: a hypothesis based on clinical and pathologic observations. *Hum Pathol* 1980;11:527–35.

129. CLAYPOOL WD, ROGERS RM, MATUSCHAK GM. Update on the clinical diagnosis, management and pathogenesis of pulmonary alveolar proteinosis (phospholipidosis). *Chest* 1984;85:550–8.

130. PRAKASH UBS, BARHAM SS, CARPENTER HA, DINES DE, MARSH HM. Pulmonary alveolar phospholipoproteinosis: experience with 34 cases and a review. *Mayo Clin Proc* 1987;62:499–518.

131. COSTABEL U. The alveolitis of hypersensitivity pneumonitis. *Eur Resp J* 1988;1:5–9.

132. BRAUN SR, DO PICO G, TSIATIS A, HORRATH E, DICKIE HA, RANKIN J. Farmer's lung disease: long term clinical and physiological outcome. *Am Rev Resp Dis* 1797;119:185–91.

133. SALVAGGIO JE. Hypersensitivity pneumonitis. *J Allerg Clin Immunol* 1986;79:558–71.

134. KOKKARINEN JI, TUKIAINEN HO, TERHO EO. Effect of corticosteroid treatment on the recovery of pulmonary function in Farmer's lung.' *Am Rev Resp Dis* 1992;145:3–5.

135. LÖFFLER, W. Zur differential-diagnose der lungen-infiltrierungen, II: über flüchtige Succedan-infiltrate (mit Eosinophilie). *Beitrage Klini Tuberkul* 1932;79:368–92.

136. CROFTON JW, LIVINGSTONE JL, OSWALD NC, ROBERTS ATM. Pulmonary eosinophilia. *Thorax* 1952;7:1–35.

137. JEDERLINC PJ, SICILLIAN L, GAENSLER EA. Chronic eosinophilic pneumonia. A report of 19 cases and a review of the literature. *Medicine* 1988;67:154–62.

138. CARRINGTON CB, ADDINGTON WW, GOFF AM *et al.* Chronic eosinophilic pneumonia. *N Engl J Med* 1969;280:787–98.

139. MAYO JR, MÜLLER NL, ROAD J, SISLER J, LILLINGTON G. Chronic eosinophilic pneumonia. CT findings in six cases. *Am J Roentgenol* 1989;727–30.

140. ALLEN JN, PACHT ER, GADEK JE, DAVIS WB. Acute eosinophilic pneumonia as a reversible cause of noninfectious respiratory failure. *N Engl J Med* 1989;321:569–73.

141. DEVILLER P, GRUART V, PRIN L *et al.* Detection of an eosinophil derived neurotoxin in the urine of a patient with idiopathic chronic eosinophilic pneumonia. *Clin Chim Acta* 1991;20:105–12.

142. OGUSHI F, OZAKI T, KAWANO T, YASUOKA S. PGE_2 and $PGF^2\alpha$ content in bronchoalveolar lavage fluid obtained from patients with eosinophilic pneumonia. *Chest* 1987;91:204–6.

143. BUCHHEIT J, NEMR E, RODGERS JR G, FEGER T, YAKOUB O. Acute eosinophilic pneumonia with respiratory failure: a new syndrome? *Am Rev Resp Dis* 1992;145:716–18.

144. BADESCH DB, KING TE, SCHWARTZ MI. Acute eosinophilic pneumonia: a hypersensitivity phenomenon? *Am Rev Resp Dis* 1989;139:249–52.

145. CLINICOPATHOLOGIC CONFERENCE.

Respiratory Failure and eosinophilia in a young man. *Am J Med* 1993;94:533–42.

146. RICKER DH, TAYLOR SR, GARTNER JR JC, KURLAND G. Fatal pulmonary aspergillosis presenting as acute eosinophilic pneumonia in a previously healthy child. *Chest* 1991;100:875–7.

147. CHUSID MJ, DALE DC, WEST BC, WOLFF SM. The hypereosinophilic syndrome. Analysis of fourteen cases with review of the literature. *Medicine* 1975;54:1–27.

148. SPRY CJF, DAVIES J, TAI PC *et al.* Clinical features of fifteen patients with the hypereosinophilic syndrome. *Quart J Med* 1983;205:1–22.

149. PRIN L, PLUMAS J, GRUART V *et al.* Elevated serum levels of soluble interleukin-2 receptor: a marker of disease activity in the hypereosinophilic syndrome. *Blood* 1991;78:2626–32.

150. DAVIES J, SPRY CJF, SAPSFORD R *et al.* Cardiovascular features of 11 patients with eosinophilic endomyocardial disease. *Quart J Med* 1983;52:23–9.

151. WINN RE, KOLLEF MH, MEYER JI. Pulmonary involvement in the hypereosinophilic syndrome. *Chest* 1994;105:656–60.

152. SLABBYNCK H, IMPENS N, NAEGELS S, DEWALE M, SCHANDEVYL W. Idiopathic hypereosinophilic syndrome-related pulmonary involvement diagnosed by bronchoalveolar lavage. *Chest* 1992;101:1178–80.

153. COGAN E, SCHANDENÉ L, CRUSIAUX A, COCHAUX P, VELU T, GOLDMAN M. Clonal proliferation of type 2 helper T cells in a man with the hypereosinophilic syndrome. *N Engl J Med* 1994;330:535–8.

154. SAWYERS CL, GOLDE DW, QUAN S, NIMER SD. Production of granulocyte-macrophage colony-stimulating factor in two patients with lung cancer, leukocytosis and eosinophilia. *Cancer* 1992;69:1342–6.

155. VIJAYAN V-K, REETHA A-M, JAWAHAR MS, SANKARAN K, PRABHAKAR R. Pulmonary eosinophilia in pulmonary tuberculosis. Chest 1992;101:1708–9.

156. NOGUCHI H, KEPHART GM, COLBY TV, GLEICH GJ. Tissue eosinophil degranulation in syndromes associated with fibrosis. *Am J Pathol* 1992;140:521–8.

157. TRAVIS WD, BOROK Z, ROUM JH *et al.* Pulmonary Langerhans' cell granulomatosis (Histiocytosis X). A clinico-pathological study of 48 cases. *Am J Surg Pathol* 1993;17:971–86.

158. COOPER JA, WHITE DA, MATTHAY RA. Drug induced pulmonary disease. Part I: cytotoxic drugs. *Am Rev Resp Dis* 1986;133:321–40.

159. COOPER JAD, WHITE DA, MATTHAY RA. Drug-induced pulmonary disease. *Am Rev Resp Dis* 1986;133:488–505.

160. JORDAN A, COWAN RE. Reversible pulmonary disease and eosinophilia associated with sulphasalazine. *J Roy Soc Med* 1988;81:233–5.

161. WANG KK, BOWYER BA, FLEMING CR, SCHROEDER KW. Pulmonary infiltrates and eosinophilia associated with sulfasalazine. *Mayo Clin Proc* 1984;59:343–6.

162. STEINFORT CL, WIGGINS J, SHEFFIELD EA, KEAL EE. Alveolitis associated with sulphamethoxypyridazine. *Thorax* 1989;44:310–11.

163. FIEGENBERG DS, WEISS H, KIRSHMAN H. Migratory pneuomnia with eosinophilia. *Arch Int Med* 1967;120:85–9.

164. DANIEL PT, HOLZSCHUH J, BERG PA. Sulfadoxine specific lymphocyte transformation in a patient with eosinophilic pneumonia induced by sulfadoxine-pyrimethamine (Fansidar). *Thorax* 1989;44:307–9.

165. DAVIES D, MCFARLANE A. Fibrosing alveolitis and treatment with sulphasalazine. *Gut* 1974;15:185–8.

166. SOVIJARVI ARA, LEMOLA M, STENMS B *et al.* Nitrofurantoin-induced acute, subacute and chronic pulmonary reactions : a report of 66 cases. *Sci J Resp Dis* 1977;58:41.

167. HOLMBERG L, BOMAN G. Pulmonary reactions to nitrofurantoin. 447 cases reported to the Swedish Adverse Drug Reaction Committee 1966–1976. *Eur J Resp Dis* 1981;62:180–9.

168. KILBOURNE EM, RIGAU-PEREZ JG, HEATH JR CW *et al.* Clinical epidemiology of toxic-oil syndrome. Manifestations of a new illness. *N Engl J Med* 1983;309:1408–14.

169. PHILEN RM, HILL JR RH, FLANDERS WD *et al.* and the Eosinophilia-Myalgia Studies of Oregon, New York, and New Mexico. Tryptophan contaminants associated with eosinophlia-myalgia syndrome. *Am J Epidemiol* 1993;138: 154–9.

170. BANNER AS, BOROCHOVITZ D. Acute respiratory failure caused by pulmonary vasculitis after L-Tryptohan infection. *Am Rev Resp Dis* 1991;143:661–4.

171. O'DRISCOLL BR, HASLETON PS, TAYLOR PM, POULTER LW, GATTAMANENIN HR, WOODCOCK AA. Active lung fibrosis up to 17 years after chemotherapy with carmustine (BCNU) in childhood. *N Engl J Med* 1990;323:378–82.

172. JULES-ELYSEE K, WHITE DA. Bleomycin-induced pulmonary toxicity. *Clin Chest Med* 1990;11:1–20.

173. SANTRACH PJ, ASKIN FB, WELLS RJ, AZIZKHAN RG, MERTEN DF. Nodular form of bleomycin-related pulmonary injury in patients with osteogenic sarcoma. *Cancer* 1989;15:806–11.

174. BELLAMY EA, HUSBAND JE, BLAQUIERE RM, LAW MR. Bleomycin-related lung damage : CT evidence. *Radiology* 1985;156:155–8.

175. WHITE DA, SCHWARTZBERG LS, KRIS MG, BOSL GJ. Acute chest pain syndrome during bleomycin infusions. *Cancer* 1987;59:1582–5.

176. SAXON RR, KLEIN JS, BAR MH, BLANC P, GAMSU G, WEBB WR *et al.* Pathogenesis of pulmonary edema during interleukin-2 therapy: correlation of chest radiographical and clinical findings in 54 patients. *Am J Roentgenol* 1991;156:281–5.

177. KUEI JH, TASHKIN DP, FIGLIN RA. Pulmonary toxicity of recombinant human tumor neurosis factor. *Chest* 1989;96:334–8.

178. MARTIN WJ II, ROSENOW EC III. Amiodarone pulmonary toxicity. Recognition and pathogenesis. *Chest* 1988;93:1067–75.

179. MARTIN WJ II, KACHEL DL, STANDING JE, OLSEN R, POWES GW. Amidarone-toxicity of human pulmonary endothelial cells is mediated by an increase in cystosolic calcium. Abstract. *Clin Res* 1989;37:49A.

180. GREENSPON AJ, KIDWEU GA, HURLEY W, MANNION J. Amiodarone-related postoperative adult respiratory distress syndrome. *Circulation* 1991;84:407–15.

181. VAN MIEGHEM W, COOLEN L, MALYSSE I, LACQUET LM, DENEFFE GJD, DEMEDTS MGP. Amiodarone and the development of ARDS after lung surgery. *Chest* 1994;105:1642–5.

182. REN H, KUHLMAN JE, KRUBAN RH, FISHMAN EK, WHEELER PS, HUTCHINS GM. CT-pathology correlation of amiodarone lung. *J Comp Assist Tomogr* 1990;14: 760–5.

183. HEFFNER JE, SAHN SA. Salicylate-induced pulmonary edema. *Ann Intern Med* 1981;95:405–9.

184. LEATHERMAN JW, SCHMITZ PG. Fever, hyperdynamic shock, and multiple-system organ failure. A pseudo-sepsis syndrome associated with chronic salicylate intoxication. *Chest* 1991;100:1391–6.

185. EVANS RB, ETTENSOHN DB, FAWAZ-ESTRUP F, CALLY EV, KAPLAN SR. Gold lung: recent development in pathogenesis, diagnosis and therapy. *Semin Arthr Rheum* 1987;16:196–205.

186. CARSON CW, CANNON GW, EGGER MJ, WARD JR, CLEGS DO. Pulmonary disease during the treatment of rheumatoid arthritis with low dose pulse methotrexate. *Semin Arthr Rheum* 1987;16:186–95.

187. FORRESTER JM, STEELE AW, WALDRON

JA, PARSONS PE. Crack lung : an acute pulmonary syndrome with a spectrum of clinical and histopathological findings. *Am Rev Resp Dis* 1990;142:462–7.

188. PARE JP, COTE G, FRASER RS. Long-term follow-up of drug abusers with intravenous talcosis. *Am Rev Resp Dis* 1989;139:233–41.

189. ANNOBIL SH, BENJAMIN B, KAMESWARAN M, KHAN AR. Lipod pneumonia in children following aspiration of animal fat (ghee). *Ann Trop Paediat* 1991;11:87–94.

190. WAGNER JC, ADLER DI, FULLER DN. Foreign body granulomatosis of the lungs due to liquid paraffin. *Thorax* 1955;10:157–70.

191. LIPINSKI JK, WEISBROD GL, SANDERS GE. Exogenous lipoid pneumonitis. *J Can Assoc Radiol* 1980;31:92–8.

192. HUTCHINS GM, BOITNOTT JK. A typical mycobacterial infection complicating mineral oil pneumonia. *J Am Med Assoc* 1978;240:539–41.

193. ELLIS ME, QADRI SMH. *Mycobacteria* other than tuberculosis producing disease in a tertiary referral hospital. *Ann Saudi Med* 1993;13:505–15.

194. GREENAWAY TM, CATERSON ID. Hypercalcemia and lipoid pneumonia. *Aust NZ J Med* 1989;19:713–15.

195. KITZIGER KJ, SANDERS WE, ANDREWS CP. Acute pulmonary edema associated with use of low-molecular weight dextrose for prevention of microvascular thrombosis. *J Hand Surg* 1990;15A:902–5.

196. PISANI RJ, ROSENOW III EC. Pulmonary edema associated with tocolytic therapy. *Ann Intern Med* 1989;110:714–18.

197. HARRIS KD. Polymer-fume fever. *Lancet* 1951;ii:1008–10.

198. LEDUC D, GRIS P, LHEUREUX P, GENENVOIS PA, DE VUYST P, YERNAULT JC. Acute and long term respiratory damage following inhalation of ammonia. *Thorax* 1992;47:755–7.

199. HAUGEN RK. The cafe coronary : sudden deaths in restaurants. *J Am Med Assoc* 1963;186:142–6.

200. MCGUIRT WF, HOLMES KD, FEEHS R, BROWNE JD. Tracheobronchial foreign bodies. Laryngoscope 1988;98:615–18.

201. SHEPHERD KE, FAULKNER CS, LEITER JC. Acute histologic effects of simulated large volume aspiration of sucralfate into the lungs of rats. *Crit Care Med* 1990;18:524–8.

202. SCHWARTZ DJ, WYNNE JW, GIBBS CP *et al.* The pulmonary consequences of aspiration of gastric contents at pH values greater than 2.5. *Am Rev Resp Dis* 1980;121:119–26.

203. ENHORNING G. Surfactant replacement in adult respiratory distress syndrome. *Am Rev Resp Dis* 1989;140:281–3.

29 Chronic air flow obstruction, acute and chronic bronchitis, and bronchiectasis

HAROLD H. REA* and ATHOL U. WELLS†
*King Faisal Specialist Hospital and Research Centre, Riyadh, Saudi Arabia; †Department of Respiratory Medicine, Green Lane Hospital, Auckland, New Zealand

Introduction

A complex inter-relationship exists between respiratory tract infection and bronchitis, asthma, emphysema and bronchiectasis. This chapter will address the role of infection within the context of the current knowledge of the overall respiratory pathology of these conditions.

Acute bronchitis

The authors agree with Pennington's[1] view that 'acute bronchitis in the normal host simply represents a less extensive version of community-acquired pneumonia. In the absence of chronic bronchopulmonary disease the aetiological agents are virtually identical.' Cough is the only consistent symptom but is typically associated with sputum production at some stage of the illness. The discomfort of tracheitis and a preceding cold or influenza-like illness are common. Unless there is co-existent bronchopulmonary disease there are usually no physical signs or auscultatory changes and physiologically there may be no change in pulmonary function although airway reactivity may increase.

Depending on the age of the patient, severity of the illness and the possibility of co-morbidity, a chest X-ray and sputum and serological testing may be indicated, but usually symptomatic treatment and observation or empirical antibiotic therapy is started without other investigation. Antibiotic selection should be based on the same rationale as for community-acquired pneumonia[2]. See also Chapter 17.

Differentiating between viral, mycoplasma, bacterial, allergic and toxic gas aetiologies may be very difficult. An occupational history may be important and with recurrent episodes of so-called 'bronchitis' one must bear in mind the possibility of asthma or a non-infectious aetiology. The inter-relationship between recurrent 'acute bronchitis' and asthma is very complex and of course depends on the definition of asthma. Suffice to say that viral respiratory tract infections can undoubtedly increase bronchial reactivity and this effect may persist for a long time. There is some evidence that *Chlamydia* and *Mycoplasma* infection can initiate asthma[3,4] and asthmatics may, of course, develop acute bronchitis. Asthmatics may be predisposed to bronchial infection and certainly in children viral infections are a common cause of exacerbations of asthma.

Thus with symptoms of recurrent or prolonged 'acute bronchitis' if there is any supporting evidence for a diagnosis of asthma (atopy, family history, variable pulmonary function) or with post viral bronchial hyperresponsiveness 'anti-asthma' treatment may be indicated, i.e. inhaled bronchodilators and inhaled steroids.

In adults, acute bronchitis or upper respiratory infection may initiate a series of self-perpetuating problems which cause chronic cough (see below). Treatment may need to be directed to more than one of the elements to break this cycle.

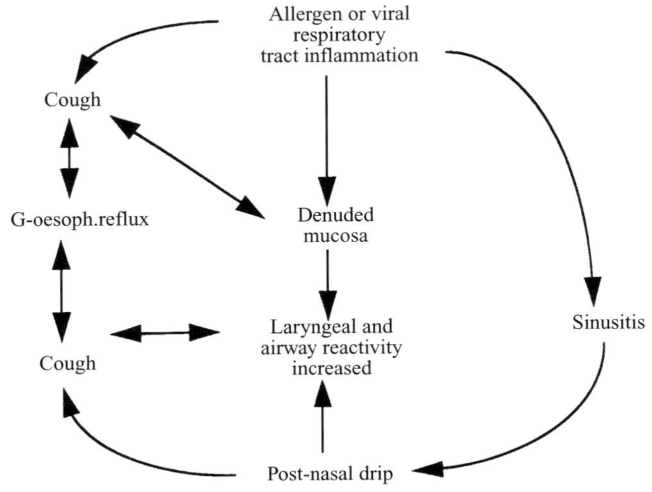

Chronic air flow obstruction and chronic bronchitis

Introduction and definitions

Substantial contributions to this section have come from the outstanding reviews by Drs Benjamin Burrows[5], Sonia Buist[6] and Murphy and Sethi[7]. This chapter will deal with a variety of intrapulmonary airway diseases in adults, whose definition and pathogenesis remain unclear. Discussion will apply to:

(i) Chronic bronchitis – epidemiological studies in the United States suggest that up to 25% of adults have symptoms of chronic bronchitis[8].
(ii) Emphysema
(iii) Other diseases causing airway and air flow obstruction with little variability and incomplete reversibility. Small airways disease (chronic obstructive bronchiolitis) will be discussed excluding that due to drugs, collagen vascular diseases, transplantation and associated with organising pneumonia.

Bronchiectasis is covered in the second part of this chapter and cystic fibrosis is dealt within Chapter 24.

A variety of pathogenetic pathways can lead to chronic air flow obstruction (CAO), e.g. smoking or chronic asthma. Mostly this section will deal with chronic airway disease related to smoking but there is no doubt that asthma can progress to severe, little variable and largely irreversible air flow obstruction even in non-smokers. In the absence of a thorough history, clinical testing or histological examination, this entity may be indistinguishable from smoking-related chronic air flow obstruction. As about 30% of asthmatics will be smokers and that some smokers may develop late or adult onset asthma, much overlap is to be expected. Asthma and smoking induced CAO are quite different diseases but current routine clinical testing and management means that they are often indistinguishable if they present with severe shortness of breath and late in adult life. The risk factors for ventilatory defect in these two aetiologies may be quite different. It is reasonable to combine chronic bronchitis (excess bronchial mucus producing sputum for at least 3 months of the year for at least two consecutive years and not due to other disease) and CAO which varies little and is incompletely reversible under the heading 'chronic obstructive pulmonary disease' (COPD), especially if the origin of the disease is unclear. However, nowadays more information should be available, and diagnostic labels applied to patients with CAO should be descriptive where possible with regard to aetiology and physiology, for example: (i) Chronic air flow obstruction due to asthma now with little variability and best FEV_1 50% predicted.(ii) Smoking-related air flow obstruction with no variability and best FEV_1 30% of predicted.

Thus, the term COPD should be used as little as possible, but has a use due to familiarity and as rubric to include chronic bronchitis and CAO of uncertain cause.

Although cigarette smoking is the most common aetiological factor in the diseases to be discussed in this chapter, other ways of arriving at the same airway problems are possible. It is clear that pulmonary disease caused by cigarette smoking is multifaceted and that chronic bronchitis, emphysema and small airways disease on their own or in any combination can occur. This chapter discusses the microbiology and treatment of diseases producing chronic bronchitis and irreversible air flow obstruction in adults irrespective of aetiology. CAO may be caused by either emphysema or irreversible obstructive changes in peripheral airways or both. Large airway, inflammation and collapsibility may contribute too. These may, or may not, be pathogenetically related processes.

Morphology

Smoking cigarettes almost invariably produces chronic bronchitis and the histology associated with this, i.e. inflammation on mucosal surfaces of bronchi greater than 2 mm and around glands and gland ducts in bronchi greater than 4 mm in diameter. The study of Mullen *et al.*[9] shows that the term chronic bronchitis is justified as patients with mucous hypersecretion do have inflammation of cartilaginous airways. However, only 15–20% of smokers develop significant obstruction of air flow and the site of the air flow obstruction is thought to be airways less than 2 mm internal diameter. Obstruction in these airways may be due to small airways inflammation or emphysema or a mixture of these. In the latter, air flow obstruction is thought to be contributed to by loss of the airway elastic support. Several studies have shown the importance of the relationship between inflammation and fibrosis of the membranous and respiratory bronchioles and goblet cell metaplasia of the membranous bronchioles, to limitation of air flow[10–16]. The data of Mullen *et al.* support the hypothesis that chronic bronchitis, chronic limitation of air flow, emphysema and disease of small airways are separate though interrelated entities.

Aguayo reviews the morphological correlates of CAO[17]. In addition to emphysematous changes, peribronchiolar inflammation and airway wall thickening (i.e. airway wall remodelling) are other morphological features found in smokers with chronic air flow obstruction. Morphometric analysis of small airway dimensions in smokers with and without CAO have shown that in those with obstruction the small airways are narrowed and thickened[18]. In addition to causing airway narrowing these changes can cause airway hyperresponsiveness[19].

Risk factors, pathogenesis and natural history

The reader is referred to the superb chapters by Burrows and Dosman and others in the Medical Clinics of North America, May 1990[5].

The authors of this chapter share the views of Burrows that controversy persists with regard to the question of susceptibility to cigarette smoke – clearly not just due to protease/antiprotease imbalance, the interrelationship of small airway inflammation to emphysema (do inflammatory changes in peripheral airways precede the mechanical changes in the alveoli and the development of emphysema?), the role of bronchial hyperresponsiveness (inherited aetiological factor or merely a marker of airway inflammation and narrowing?) and the great difficulty in most epidemiological studies of separating those whose chronic air flow obstruction has developed as a result of asthma as opposed to those whose aetiological pathway is different.

Although, as already stated, these questions are important in terms of future preventative strategies they actually have little effect currently on management. No matter what the aetiological pathway, current pharmaceutical treatment of severe CAO is largely determined by the degree of variability of air flow obstruction, the extent to which air flow obstruction is reversible and the frequency and severity of infections.

Bronchial responsiveness and allergy as a risk factor

In 1961 the Dutch investigator Orie observed that many patients with chronic bronchitis had an allergic background and displayed increased airway response to histamine[20]. The idea that bronchial hyperresponsiveness (BHR) is a risk factor for CAO has become known as the 'Dutch hypothesis' but it remains unclear whether BHR is a cause or result of the disease. In a recent study[21] responsiveness was not increased in young smokers with normal lung function but was significantly related to baseline lung function. Even if BHR is not a direct causal factor it could well be an intermediate part of a causal pathway and could be a marker for high risk.

Orie and co-workers felt that asthma and chronic bronchitis were different manifestations of the same underlying 'basic disturbance', the specific clinical pattern depending on age, gender, environmental exposure and the relative severity of atopy and BHR.

Atopy is associated with asthma, BHR and reduced pulmonary function but there is no clear evidence that it is a risk factor for irreversible air flow obstruction in non-asthmatics. Reports vary as to whether the relationship of eosinophil count to level of pulmonary function remains after excluding asthmatics. Among smokers BHR appears to be associated with accelerated longitudinal decline of pulmonary function although most studies showing this are limited by retrospective design or lack of adjustment for pre-challenge level of pulmonary function. It is unclear whether BHR is a risk factor that precedes and predisposes to chronic air flow obstruction or is a manifestation of airway inflammation and narrowing and reduced tractional support for the airways. Additional questions that wait to be answered are – does treatment of bronchial hyperresponsiveness with β-2 agonist or inhaled steroid offer protection against deterioration of pulmonary function? Do allergy and BHR have significant impact on lung growth and if so, does this influence the risk of CAO in adult life?

Burrows and coworkers[5] suggest that two forms of chronic air flow obstruction in adults should be differentiated on the basis of whether or not there are asthmatic features. Patients whom Burrows labels chronic asthmatic bronchitis appear to have a better prognosis, smaller exposure to tobacco and greater prevalence of allergic features as compared to patients with chronic air flow obstruction who lack an asthmatic background and suffer primarily from emphysema. Burrows suggests that the Dutch hypothesis is relevant to the syndrome he calls chronic asthmatic bronchitis, but not to other patients with chronic air flow obstruction. He feels that if asthmatic patients are excluded from studies of CAO then the correlation of ventilatory defect with atopy, BHR, eosinophilia, etc. may disappear. It may also be that lower respiratory tract infection plays a lesser role in the progress of chronic air flow obstruction due to asthma than it does in chronic air flow obstruction due to smoking.

The two pathogenetic pathways for chronic air flow obstruction hypothesised by Burrows[5] are represented in Fig. 29.1 and 29.2. Added to Fig. 29.1 could be a potential contribution from air pollution, occupational exposures to dust, fumes and gases, passive smoking, socioeconomic status and living conditions (such as cooking indoors), and airway hyperresponsiveness as already mentioned.

It should be noted that lower respiratory tract infections in infancy are prominent in both hypothetical pathways. In the Tuscon[22] studies even in non-asthmatics a history of childhood respiratory trouble identified smokers and ex-smokers with severe ventilatory impairment. It seems the history of non-asthmatic childhood respiratory trouble could increase susceptibility to damage due to smoking later in life. Non-asthmatic childhood respiratory trouble may mean recurrent and frequent respiratory tract infections.

It also may be that some of the most susceptible smokers have been born with less than ideal pulmonary function. Perhaps severe asthma, or severe and recurrent lower respiratory tract infections and/or bronchopulmonary dysplasia lead to a situation in which the lungs do not grow properly and capacity achieved at the end of growth is sub-optimal. If rapid decline in pulmonary function is then added to this then clearly such a person will become symptomatic at an early age.

Natural history of chronic air flow obstruction

Fig. 29.3 and 29.4 show hypothetical courses for the development of severe chronic air flow obstruction[5]. In Fig. 29.3, course A represents a person with childhood respiratory trouble who enters adulthood with poor pulmonary function, and then despite not having a very rapid decline in pulmonary function becomes symptomatic at 55 or 60 years of age.

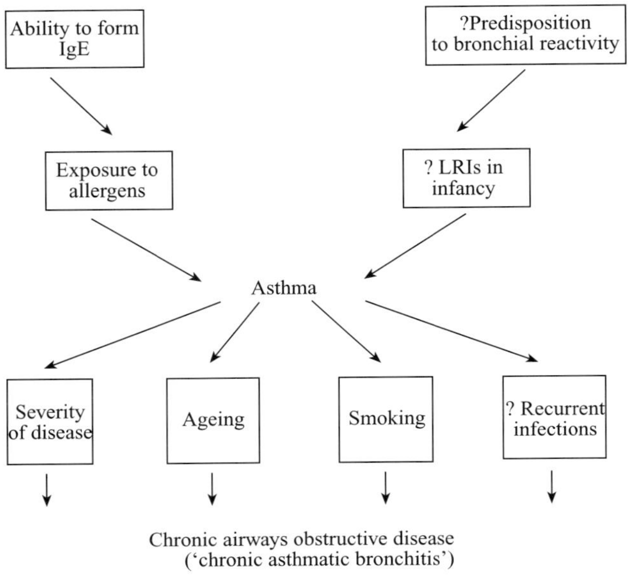

FIGURE 29.1 Hypothetical pathways for the development of persistent forms of asthma, called chronic asthmatic bronchitis in this chapter. This diagram conforms reasonably well with the original hypothesis.

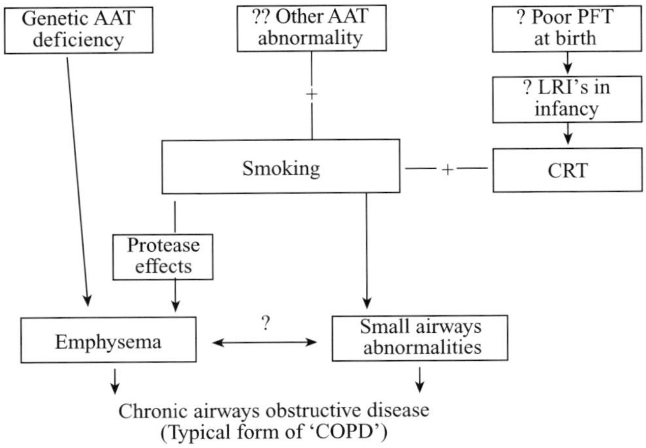

FIGURE 29.2 Hypothetical pathways for the development of the typical form of COPD that is characteristic of smokers showing no evidence of asthma.

Course B shows attainment of normal lung function but very rapid decline in middle age in a susceptible smoker. Also shown on this diagram is the course of decline of pulmonary function in a normal nonsmoker and in a smoker who is not predisposed to chronic air flow obstruction.

Burrows has the impression that asthmatics with chronic air flow obstruction have a much less rapid decline in pulmonary function and diffusion capacity is usually well maintained. He wonders if this less rapid decline is due to the effect of treatment with inhaled β_2-agonist and/or steroids.

Cigarette smoking as a risk factor

Undoubtedly, cigarette smoking is the most important risk factor for chronic air flow obstruction. Cigarette smokers have a higher than average rate of decline of pulmonary function and the decline is to some extent dose related[23–27]. The fact that only 20% develop clinically significant air flow obstruction[28,29] suggests that host factors are important in determining which smokers get disease. Although chronic bronchitis and emphysema have causal relationships with cigarette smoking they do not necessarily share the same risk factors. Chronic bronchitis is an airway disease and emphysema a parenchymal disease. Small airway inflammation or disease is usually the earliest detectable structural change in smokers. It is unclear whether small airways disease is causally related to emphysema. Buist[30] feels that it is more likely that both are due to cigarette smoking but are independent processes. Some smokers with small airway disease do not go on to develop severe air flow obstruction and emphysema. It is generally accepted now that chronic bronchitis is not always associated with air flow obstruction or severe loss of pulmonary function. Buist[6] feels that this was not true as recently as the mid 1960s in the United Kingdom when complex bronchitis with repeated chest infections and progressive shortness of breath was common. This more severe form of chronic bronchitis is still common in developing countries. Severe fixed air flow obstruction is seen in nonsmoking women in the Kingdom of Saudi Arabia[31]. In the developing world the high incidence of chronic bronchitis in never smoking women may be contributed to by infections, domestic smoke exposure and incense burning[31,32]. Perhaps aggressive treatment of airway infection and use of inhaled bronchodilators or steroids and/or reductions of indoor and outdoor air pollution have changed this destructive ongoing airway effect of chronic bronchitis.

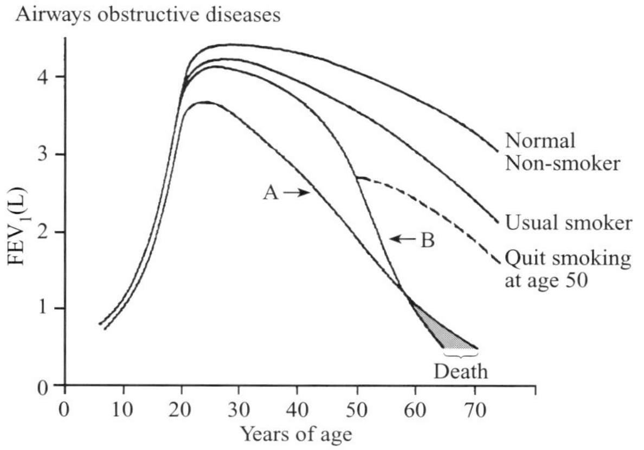

FIGURE 29.3 Hypothetical preclinical courses for the development of the typical COPD characteristic of smokers showing no evidence of asthma. (See text for explanation of curves A and B.)

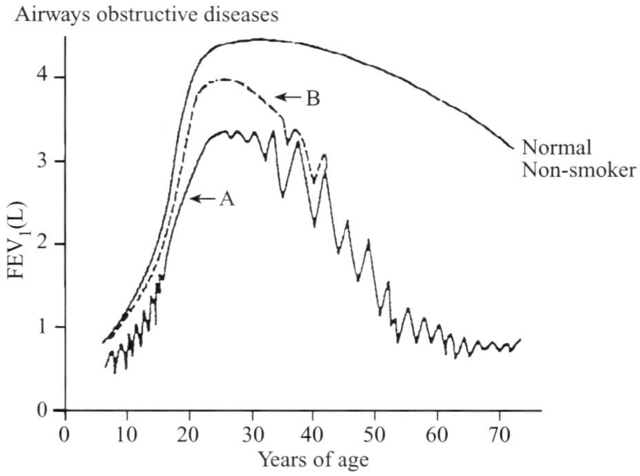

FIGURE 29.4 Hypothetical courses for the development of severe 'chronic asthmatic bronchitis' in adulthood. The course of this disorder is probably extremely variable. Curve A is intended to depict early childhood asthma, which remits during adolescence, but recurs later in adulthood. Curve B is meant to represent late onset asthma with a progressive course. (From Burrows B[5], reproduced with permission.)

Smoking cessation has been shown to produce a small improvement in lung function (not normalisation) and an immediate decrease in cough and sputum[33,34].

The role of infection in aetiology and natural history

In general, studies report an association between symptoms of recurrent respiratory infection and lower pulmonary function[35–40]. The association of respiratory syncytial virus bronchiolitis in the first year of life with continued wheezing and pulmonary function test abnormalities is well known[41]. Barker and Osman[42] demonstrated a strong geographical relationship in England and Wales between death rates from chronic bronchitis and emphysema in 1959 to 1978 and infant mortality from bronchitis and pneumonia during 1921 to 1925. They concluded that this provided strong evidence for a direct causal link between acute lower respiratory tract infections in early childhood and chronic bronchitis in adult life.

It appears that respiratory infections in childhood may cause permanent airway damage and predispose the sufferer to chronic disease especially if the individual is subsequently exposed to other risk factors. As Leeder points out in a review of the role of infection[43], during the first six years of life 50 000 000 new alveoli are budding annually and it is surprising that so many respiratory infections occur without permanent consequence! Longitudinal studies which examine the relationship between respiratory infections and rate of decline of pulmonary function are bedeviled by the need to rely on questionnaire data to define infections.

The 8-year follow-up study of London Transport Workers[28,29] showed no significant association between decline in pulmonary function and recurrent respiratory infections. In the Tuscon study[44], however, more adults with a history of 'childhood respiratory trouble' had impaired lung function compared to those who did not. The contributions of respiratory infection to CAO may be less in the United States and Western Europe than in developing countries where very high rates of recurrent respiratory infections still occur. This author's impression is that the high prevalence of chronic air flow obstruction seen in non-smoking middle-aged women in Saudi Arabia may be due in part to high frequency of respiratory infections.

In general, longitudinal studies show little effect of acute exacerbations on the rate of decline of pulmonary function in adults but studies using sophisticated measures of pulmonary function and better definition of infective exacerbations might show different results. Also, it may be that some infectious agents or some subgroups of patients are at particular risk from infective exacerbations.

Whatever the long-term consequences there is no doubt that infection can cause acute decompensation in people with poor ventilatory reserve. Acute infection was by far the most common observable cause of death in a prospective study[45].

Murphy and Sethi[7] elaborate on the hypothesis of Cole[46] that chronic colonisation/infection of the lower respiratory tract can contribute to progressive lung damage ('vicious circle hypothesis') – see Fig. 29.5. Although originally proposed in the pathogenesis of bronchiectasis similar mechanisms may be operative in COPD. The presence of bacteria in the lower respiratory tract alters host defences, predisposing to further infection. Bacterial products and proteases from inflammatory cells inhibit ciliary activity and damage the respiratory epithelium producing continuing respiratory tract damage. Thus, as Cole says, 'noninvasive organisms have damaging properties and should be considered pathogenic.' This concept has proved contentious for some microbiologists/physicians who believe that antimicrobial treatment should be directed only towards organisms displaying clinical features of invasiveness.

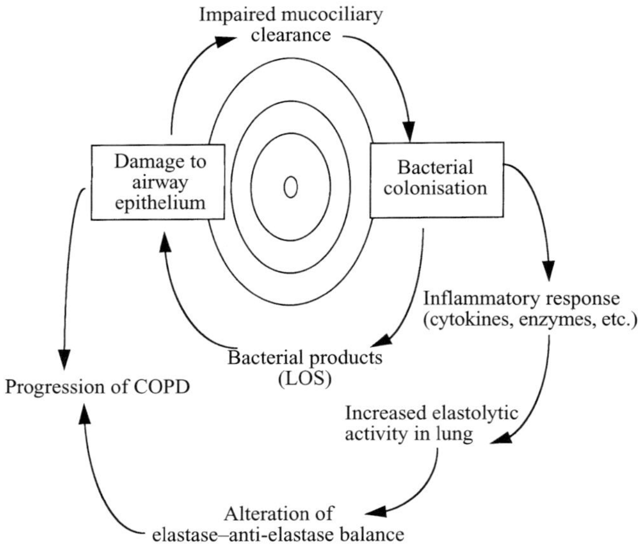

FIGURE 29.5 Schematic diagram of the vicious circle hypothesis of the role of bacterial infection in COPD. LOS = lipoligosaccharide. Initiating factors, e.g. smoking, childhood respiratory disease.

Protease/antiprotease imbalance as a risk factor

There is familial aggregation of chronic air flow obstruction and the discovery that some patients with emphysema had very low levels of α_1-protease inhibitors (α_1Pi) supports the possibility of a genetic component. However, α_1Pi deficiency accounts for less than 10% of chronic air flow obstruction so presumably there are other genetic factors not yet understood.

Individuals with severe α_1Pi deficiency are at considerable risk of developing emphysema[47–49]. There is no firm evidence yet, but individuals with intermediate levels may also have an increased risk. It seems probable that they are and that the elastase imbalance can be worsened by cigarette smoking and possibly by lower respiratory tract infection – producing increased numbers of neutrophils and alveolar macrophages.

Buist[6] classifies risk factors for chronic air flow obstruction into known and possible (Table 29.1). This author would add atopy and asthma to this list as already discussed. Buist discusses a list of 'agents' which may play a part in the development of chronic air flow obstruction but which may not by themselves be sufficient to cause it.

Air pollution

Buist summarises this debate by stating 'air pollution can result in mucus hypersecretion and a small reduction in pulmonary function. The role of air pollution in emphysema is not known. One could argue that the particulates and oxidants are likely to contribute to both sides of the protease/antiprotease balance: the particulates by causing an influx of neutrophils and macrophages and therefore an increase in elastase, and the oxidants by inactivating α_1Pi.'
Indoor air pollution may include oxides of nitrogen, formaldehyde, sidestream cigarette smoke, etc. and with tight sealing of buildings to conserve energy in developing countries this may reach toxic levels.

Occupational dust, fumes and gases

There is no doubt that these exposures can cause chronic bronchitis and can contribute to an increase in the rate of decline of FEV_1[50].

Passive smoking

Small but significant differences can be detected in both children and adults between those who are and those who are not regularly exposed to other people's smoke – respiratory symptoms and prevalence are increased[51–53] and pulmonary function slightly lower[54,55]. Respiratory infections are more common in infants with smoking parents[56–58]. If, as has been proposed, respiratory illness in childhood has a carryover effect in adult life, it may place the adult at greater risk of CAO – either by inducing BHR or failure to achieve maximum lung growth. A longitudinal study in East Boston showed that maternal smoking was found to be associated with a reduced rate of annual increase in FEV_1 in children – 3–5% decrease in expected lung growth[59].

Socioeconomic status and living conditions

Studies in the UK have shown a very clear social class gradient for CAO and chronic bronchitis[35]. This may have lessened with improved living conditions. This gradient may be related to occupation, air pollution and a higher rate of respiratory infection.

Table 29.1. *Risk factors for COPD*

	Known	Possible/probable
Age	Cigarette smoke	Air pollution
		Occupational dusts, fumes, gases
		Passive (involuntary) smoking
		Respiratory viruses
		Socioeconomic factors; living conditions
		Alcohol
Host	α_1Pi deficiency	Age
		Gender
		Familial/genetic
		Airway hyperresponsiveness
		Atopy and asthma

From Buist S[6]. Reproduced (with some modification) with permission.

Micrology of chronic air flow obstruction

The reader is referred to the review by Murphy and Sethi[7].

In contrast to normal people, the lower respiratory tract of patients with chronic bronchitis and CAO is not sterile. Bacteria are recovered from the sputum of patients with chronic bronchitis in the absence of signs and symptoms of infection; the condition referred to as colonisation. Several epidemiological studies show that patients with chronic bronchitis are more susceptible to respiratory infection and have a higher rate of acute respiratory illness than normals[60].

Defining an exacerbation is difficult (various combinations of increased sputum, shortness of breath, cough and sputum purulence and temperature). Exacerbations may be caused by viruses, mycoplasma, bacteria and non-infectious factors. No reliable method of differentiating those caused by bacteria from exacerbations caused by other agents currently exists. Gram's stain of a sputum sample may be helpful if it shows abundant neutrophils and a single predominant morphological type of organism. Sputum culture does not distinguish colonisation and infection. Acute exacerbations are predominantly mucosal infections and may resolve without antibiotic. Often exacerbations are not associated with bacteraemia, but of course some may progress to this and/or bronchopneumonia[7].

Non-typable *Haemophilus influenzae*, *Streptococcus pneumoniae* and *Moraxella catarrhalis* are common in the normal upper respiratory tract, commonly present in the lower respiratory tract in stable patients with chronic bronchitis and CAO (presumably colonisation) and common causes of exacerbations. The determination of the cause of an exacerbation is complicated by the difficulty in isolating and culturing viruses, and by the fact that serological data are hard to interpret – it is conceivable that bacteria may cause an exacerbation without changing serum markers.

The pathological and physiological abnormalities in chronic bronchitis which predispose to bacterial infection probably include impaired mucociliary clearance, obstruction of bronchi and the chronic presence of bacteria in the bronchial epithelium.

The association of acute exacerbations with viral agents is clearer than with bacteria. Isolation of virus from the respiratory tract is uncommon in humans except during acute illness; thus virus isolated during acute flare-ups probably do represent primary infection. Eadie *et al.*[61] drew attention to the role of rhinovirus, Carilli *et al.*[62] and Sommerville[63] to the respiratory syncytial virus, influenzae A and adenovirus in COPD.

Gump *et al.*[64] reported 116 exacerbations in 25 patients. A third were related to viral infection or mycoplasma. The discovery of *H. influenzae* and *S. pneumoniae* was similar in viral and non-viral exacerbations, thus bacteria may be the primary cause of exacerbations or secondary invaders following viral infection. Some serologically diagnosed viral infections did not result in worsening of the chronic bronchitis. There are very discrepant reports on the incidence of *Mycoplasma pneumoniae* in acute exacerbations of COPD. Between 30 and 50% of exacerbations remain unexplained.

Sputum culture is unable to distinguish colonisation from infection unless used quantitatively or with cytological or biopsy evidence. The same may also be true for protected specimen brushing via a bronchoscope. However, in using the latter *H. influenzae* and *S. pneumoniae* are almost always isolated. Although many patients with CAO are chronically colonised, there is some evidence that there is a quantitative increase during acute exacerbations[65]. Documenting a serological response to an organism has been considered a valid method to demonstrate infection and several studies have used this approach in COPD[7]. These studies give conflicting results but as Murphy and Sethi point out this may be due to the fact that most of these studies use a single isolate of, e.g. non-typable *H. influenzae* as the source of the antigen for the immunoassay and recent work has established that marked antigenic heterogeneity exists in surface antigens amongst strains.

In the last several years increasing reports link *M. catarrhalis* with exacerbations of COPD[66,67]. It is also postulated that *M. catarrhalis* may act as an indirect pathogen protecting other pathogens by producing a β-lactamase.

Fagon *et al.*[68] obtained protected brush specimens via a flexible bronchoscope from 54 patients admitted to hospital with an exacerbation of chronic bronchitis and CAO who required mechanical ventilation. Patients were excluded if they had received antibiotics. A total of 44 microorganisms were cultured from 27 patients. Patients with chest X-ray evidence of pneumonia were also excluded. Only 50% had demonstrable bacterial infection and the organisms isolated are illustrated in Table 29.2. The role of *Chlamydia pneumoniae* in exacerbations of chronic bronchitis is unclear, but may be important and in Fagon's study it seemed that *Haemophilus parainfluenzae* was important also. Special culture media are required for the isolation of *M. pneumoniae* and *C. pneumoniae* and neither are visible on Gram's stain so they may account for some culture negative flares of bronchitis.

Pulmonary defence and immunological response in chronic bronchitis and CAO

The morphological features of chronic bronchitis predispose the patients to infection. Independent of the structural changes, tobacco smoke inhibits ciliary motility, and impairs neutrophil phagocytosis and bactericidal function. Some investigators have noted defective

Table 29.2. *Frequency of organisms recovered from protected brush specimens in 27 patients during acute exacerbation of chronic bronchitis*

	Total		Concentrations (cfu/ml)					
Organisms	n	%	10^2	10^3	10^4	10^5	10^6	10^7
Gram-negative bacteria	28	64	7	5	7	7		2
Haemophilus parainfluenzae	11	25		2	3	4		2
Haemophilus influenzae	6	14	1	1	2	2		
Moraxella catarrhalis	3	7		2	1			
Pseudomonas aeruginosa	3	7	3					
Proteus mirabilis	3	7	2		1			
Escherichia coli	2	4	1			1		
Gram-positive bacteria	16	36	4	4	1	5	1	1
Streptococcus pneumoniae	7	16		2	1	2	1	1
Other streptococci	4	9	2			2		
Staphylococcus spp.	4	9	2	2				
Corynebacterium spp.	1	2				1		
Total	44		11	9	8	12	1	3

From Fagon J[68]. Reprinted with permission.

local production of IgA[69–71] and abnormal levels of IgA in bronchial secretions have been seen in the presence of normal serum IgA[72]. It is unclear whether abnormal immunity can be a cause rather than just a consequence of COPD. A primary site of microbial persistence and multiplication in COPD is respiratory mucus within airways. The most important bacterial organisms are not particularly virulent but should be considered pathogenic, because they produce chronic inflammation which causes disease (Cole's 'vicious circle' where the microbes become parasitic – second line humoral and cellular immunological defences damage the lung increasing bacterial colonisation)[46].

Saetta *et al.*[73] examined the nature of leukocyte infiltration in ten chronic bronchitics by comparing their bronchoscopic biopsies with six normal non-smoking controls. Lobar bronchial biopsy showed that the bronchitics had an increased total number of leukocytes both in the epithelium and lamina propria whereas the number of neutrophils, eosinophils, and mast cells were similar in the two groups. Airway macrophages and T-lymphocytes were increased and the subjects with chronic bronchitis also had increased expression of markers of lymphocyte activation. This specific description of the type of inflammation in airway walls in chronic bronchitis is important as it is the airway inflammation that correlates with destruction of alveolar attachments[74] and is found to be a characteristic of those who developed centrilobular emphysema[75].

That Saetta *et al.* did not demonstrate differences in the number of neutrophils infiltrating the bronchial mucosa is of interest but may be due to selection of subjects, small numbers or the fact that they used biopsies and not bronchoalveolar lavage. Saetta concludes that mononuclear cell infiltration and T-cell activation suggest their involvement in the pathogenesis of chronic bronchitis.

Thompsom and Rennard review the assessment of airways inflammation in chronic bronchitis[76]. Bronchoalveolar lavage (BAL) can be performed in a manner which includes airway contents. BAL in young smokers has increased macrophages and neutrophils[77]. Chronic bronchitics have increased neutrophils and goblet cells. Airway neutrophilia is correlated with airways obstruction, sputum production and smoking history and goblet cell numbers with ventilatory defect (FEV_1)[78–80]. Therapeutic interventions – smoking reduction, theophylline and inhaled steroids have been shown to reduce these indices of inflammation[81–83].

In this editorial[76] Thompson and Rennard go on to discuss the exciting future role of bronchial brushing (associated with molecular biology techniques) and bronchial biopsy in exploring inflammation of airways and hence, pathogenetic mechanisms and therapies in COPD; showing that a therapy reduces airway inflammation may provide rationale for longitudinal clinical studies.

Murphy and Sethi[7] include a fascinating update of recent advances in cell biology and molecular mechanisms in a superb review of 'Bacterial Infection in COPD'. They list four potential contributions of infection to the clinical course of COPD:

(i) Recurrent acute infectious exacerbations accelerate lung damage and decline in pulmonary function.
(ii) Bacteria cause acute exacerbations which themselves cause morbidity and mortality[45].
(iii) Chronic colonization/infection of the lower respiratory tract contributes to progressive lung damage (the vicious circle hypothesis).
(iv) Childhood respiratory tract infection predisposes to COPD in later life.

Murphy and Sethi review the responses to *H. influenzae*, *S. pneumoniae* and *M. catarrhalis* in the respiratory tract.

H. influenzae

Virtually all strains of *H. influenzae* recovered from the respiratory tract of patients with chronic bronchitis are non-encapsulated and termed 'non-typable'. Outer membrane protein analysis indicates that this is a diverse group of bacteria[84]. The molecular basis by which these organisms adhere to epithelial cells is not fully elucidated but when it is it may provide a basis for preventative action such as vaccines[85,86]. *H. influenzae* express pili on their surface and those may have a role in adherence to respiratory tract epithelium. Bacteria adhere to mucus before they adhere to damaged epithelial cells – they do not adhere to normal epithelium. Epithelium is damaged by lipo-oligosaccharide or other soluble bacterial toxins thus, microbial factors promote further colonisation[87].

P_2 is the major protein in the outer membrane of *H. influenzae* and it expresses an immunodominant and highly strain-specific epitope on the bacterial surface[88]. Murphy suggests that the induction of a strain-specific immune response stops induction of antibodies that would protect from infection by other strains. Longitudinal changes in the P_2 protein further enable the organism to evade host defences. The P_6 outer membrane protein seems to have potential as a vaccine antigen[89]. Lipo-oligosaccharide is another outer membrane constituent. It is a biologically active molecule and potent mediator of inflammation[90].

Respiratory tract infection in patients with COPD represents a spectrum from clinically mild mucosal infection to more invasive forms including pneumonia. Thus it is important to study both the mucosal and systemic immune responses. The serum and sputum of patients with COPD contain abundant antibodies to most outer membrane proteins of the patient's own isolates of Non-typable *H. influenzae*[91]. Patients are infected and colonised despite these antibodies. Molecular biological techniques will allow elucidation of this problem and may help in development of vaccines. Clancy *et al.*[92] have trialled a formalin-killed strain of Non-typable *H. influenzae* vaccine in patients with COPD. Oral administered vaccine induced a tenfold reduction in the incidence of purulent exacerbations compared with placebo. Protection was observed through one winter season only, i.e. no protection was observed the following year.

S. pneumoniae

A reliable method to distinguish colonisation, which is common in patients with COPD from infection does not exist. Most infections in COPD are not associated with bacteraemia. *S. pneumoniae* attaches to human pharyngeal cells through the specific interaction of bacterial surface adhesins and a carbohydrate receptor on the host cell[93]. Cell wall antigens stimulate peripheral blood monocytes to secrete interleukin (IL-1), a cytokine which is a central mediator of inflammation[94]. Phagocytosis is essential for protection from infection by *S. pneumoniae* and the capsular polysaccharide has antiphagocytic properties. The role of anti-capsular antibody in protection is well defined thus, its role in chronic bronchitis requires further definition.

Pneumococcal vaccine is of uncertain efficacy in COPD; however, the potential benefit seems to outweigh the risk and it is recommended by the American Thoracic Society and the Immunization Practices Advisory Committee of the Centers for Disease Control[95].

Moraxella catarrhalis

Murphy and Sethi[7] discuss three problems which have made it difficult to assess the role of this organism as a lower respiratory tract pathogen:

(i) It is part of the normal upper respiratory tract flora.
(ii) It is morphologically indistinguishable on Gram's stain and colonies are indistinguishable on culture plates from commensal *Neisseria* spp.
(iii) The disease it produces is non-invasive in nature.

Strong evidence now implicates *M. catarrhalis* as a pathogen in purulent exacerbations and in pneumonic illnesses in patients with COPD[96–100].

The predominance of Gram-negative diplococci extracellularly and especially intracellularly is highly predictive of growth of *M. catarrhalis* in culture[97]. Up to 75% of *M. catarrhalis* strains are β-lactamase producers[100]. Bacterial infections in COPD are predominantly mucosal infections. Studies of mucosal antibody responses are needed to understand colonisation and infection.

Clinical features and complications of chronic air flow obstruction

Significant symptoms usually do not occur until middle age. Mild abnormalities of pulmonary function may be discernible before the onset of clinical symptoms. This has led to recommendations for spirometric screening of smokers to detect those most at risk. A mild 'smoker's cough' is often present many years before onset of dyspnea.

Progressive exertional dyspnoea is the most common presenting complaint. Patients may date the onset of dyspnoea to an acute respiratory illness; the acute infection may reduce an already limited respiratory reserve giving the false impression that the onset was acute. Cough, wheezing and recurrent respiratory infections, may also be initial manifestations. Rarely, initial complaints are related to cor pulmonale, because some patients apparently ignore cough and dyspnoea.

Cough and sputum production are extremely variable. Sputum varies from a few ml of clear viscid mucus to large quantities of purulent material. Wheezing also varies in character and intensity. Asthma-like episodes may occur with acute infections, but many patients deny having any wheeze. A history of marked fluctuation in disease severity or childhood wheezing should make one suspect chronic asthma.

Physical findings in COPD are notoriously variable, especially in the early stages. A consistent abnormality is obstruction to expiratory air flow. Some wheeze is often noted toward the end of a forced expiration. Gross pulmonary hyperinflation, prolonged expiration, depressed diaphragm, pursed-lip breathing, stooped posture, and use of accessory muscles of respiration are seen only in later stages of COPD. Other findings, including wheeze, diminished vesicular breath sounds, tachycardia, and decreased diaphragmatic motion are not consistently present. The chest may be 'quiet' in advanced stages of emphysema. Late in the disease, there may be hypoxaemia, secondary polycythaemia and cor pulmonale.

Chest X-ray findings are also variable. In early stages of the disease, the X-ray is often normal. Changes indicative of hyperinflation (e.g. depressed diaphragm, generalised radiolucency of the lung fields, increase retrosternal air space) are common and suggestive of emphysematous disease, but are not diagnostic and tend to appear only with advanced COPD. They may also be found in patients with asthma and occasionally in healthy persons. Localised radiolucency with attenuation of vascular markings or bullae is a more reliable indicator of emphysema. In patients with recurrent chest infections, a variety of post-inflammatory abnormalities may be noted on the plain chest film, e.g. localised fibrotic changes, honeycombing, or contraction atelectasis of a segment or lobe.

Bullae are seen occasionally with COPD. Large bullae are generally well seen on ordinary X-rays, but small ones are more reliably detected with CT scans. Bronchitis itself does not have a characteristic appearance on ordinary chest X-ray nor on CT scan. Sometimes small airway disease can be seen on CT Fig. 29.6 (*a*) and (*b*).

COPD should be suspected in any patient with chronic productive cough or exertional dyspnea of uncertain aetiology, or whose physical examination reveals evidence of air flow obstruction. Definite diagnosis depends on a compatible history and demonstration of physiological evidence of airways obstruction that is incompletely reversible and varies little despite intensive and maximal medical management and for which no other specific cause can be found.

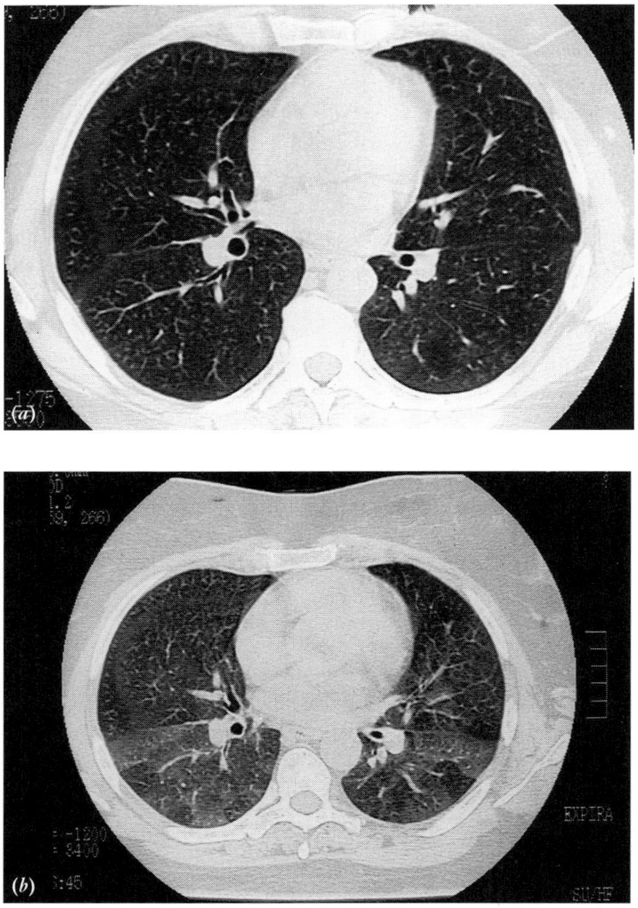

FIGURE 29.6 Inspiratory (*a*) and expiratory (*b*) CT scans of a patient with exertional dyspnoea and non-productive cough. The inspiratory image is normal. At end expiration the CT scan shows widespread areas of decreased attenuation (blackness), indicative of regional hypovascularity, in keeping with the patchy gas trapping seen in obliterative bronchiolitis. The diagnosis was confirmed histologically.

Spirometric testing reveals characteristic obstruction of expiratory flow with a reduced FEV_1 and a low maximum mid-expiratory flow. Slowing of forced expiration is also evident on flow–volume curves. The vital capacity (VC) and forced vital capacity (FVC) are somewhat impaired in patients with severe disease, but are better maintained than flow rates. The FEV_1 is well below predicted and the FEV_1/VC ratio is regularly reduced to < 60% with clinically significant COPD (see Fig. 29.7).

Maldistribution of ventilation and perfusion occurs in COPD and produces an increased physiologic dead-space (i.e. areas of the lung in which ventilation is high relative to blood flow), resulting in 'wasted' ventilation. Venous admixture is also increased by the presence of alveoli with reduced ventilation in relation to blood flow (a low V/Q ratio), resulting in hypoxemia.

Diffusing capacity is regularly reduced in patients with severe emphysema, but is more variable in those with airways obstruction associated with predominant intrinsic airways disease and is generally normal in stable chronic asthma. In patients with severe emphysema and a well-maintained ventilatory drive, resting hypoxaemia is usually mild and hypercapnia does not occur until terminal stages. In these patients, sometimes called 'pink puffers', the P_aCO_2 may even be reduced and frank pulmonary hypertension and cor pulmonale usually develop late. In other patients with airways obstruction, hypoxaemia and hypercapnia may be noted relatively early. Such patients, sometimes called 'blue bloaters', tend to develop hypoxaemia with pulmonary hypertension and chronic cor pulmonale. A reduced ventilatory drive, obesity or sleep apnoea appear to contribute to the early development of cor pulmonale. Polysomnography may be indicated in patients with severe blood gas abnormalities or cor pulmonale who have only a moderate reduction in FEV_1.

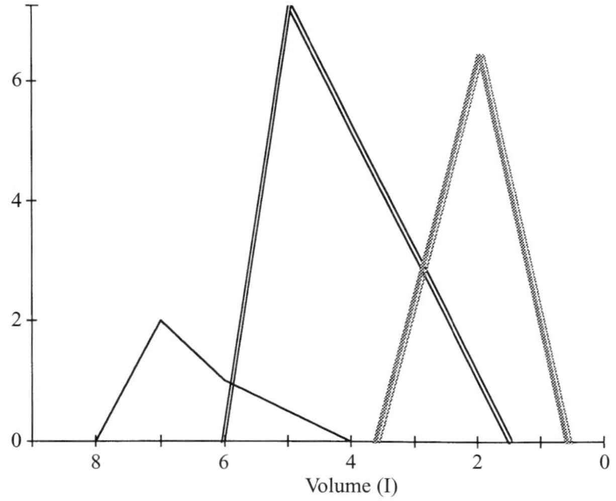

FIGURE 29.7 Forced expiratory flow as a function of total lung volume is shown for normal subjects and for subjects with COPD and pulmonary fibrosis. Note that for COPD, the total lung volume is high, whereas expiratory flow is decreased. In fibrotic disease, flows are near normal, but total lung volume is much smaller.

The residual volume (RV) and total lung capacity (TLC) are markedly elevated in emphysematous patients, while pulmonary hyperinflation may be relatively slight in the bronchial type of COPD, but the ratio of RV/TLC tends to be elevated in both types of disease.

Treatment of chronic bronchitis and chronic air flow obstruction

Antibiotics

As discussed by Murphy and Sethi[7] there are four hypothetical objectives in the use of antibiotics in diseases producing chronic bronchitis or chronic air flow obstruction:

(i) To treat acute infective exacerbations to reduce symptoms, time lost from work and possibly deterioration in pulmonary function.
(ii) To treat acute exacerbations to reduce mortality or respiratory failure.
(iii) To treat chronic colonisation/infection in the hope of reducing progressive lung damage and to interrupt the vicious circle or to reduce frequency of acute exacerbations.
(iv) To treat childhood respiratory tract infection in the hope that this will reduce the risk of COPD in adulthood.

Controversy exists regarding the role of antibiotics in managing exacerbations of COPD[65,101–103].

The reader is referred to the excellent papers debating pro: antibiotics[65] and con: antibiotics[102] for the treatment of exacerbations in *Seminars in Respiratory Infections*. This author believes this controversy is academic. There is little doubt that antibiotics should be used since they make the patient feel better more quickly, reduce time lost from work, may avoid life-threatening complications in those with poor respiratory reserve, have a low cost and high benefit to risk ratio and theoretically, at least, may slow decline in pulmonary function. It seems intuitively that having 'bacteria and pus' in the lower airways is not a good idea! Having said this, it seems true that some exacerbations are not due to bacteria that there is no reliable method for determining the aetiology of exacerbations.

The benefits of antibiotics are most often to be seen in patients with severe exacerbations and with severe underlying lung disease[96,104]. These authors support the approach of Murphy and Sethi (see Fig. 29.8).

Prophylactic antibiotics have been used in an attempt to reduce the frequency of exacerbations. This may be of value in patients having four or more exacerbations per year[105,106]. Table 29.3 summarises antimicrobial susceptibility for the three major bacterial pathogens – local patterns may differ from this.

The use of antibiotics to break the putative vicious circle and clear colonisation cannot be recommended because airway penetration is poor, large concentrations are required for long periods to reduce the number of micro-organisms and since muco-ciliary clearance and epithelial damage will not be restored to normal, the microorganism will quickly recolonise. In the future the vicious circle may be broken by anti-inflammatory therapy, e.g. vaccines or immunosuppressants.

Treatment of COPD (other than with antibiotics)

Kolbe[107] has produced an algorithm for management of COPD (Fig. 29.9). Smoking cessation is the most important modality. The role of *H. influenzae* vaccines awaits clearer definition.

Bronchodilators undoubtedly improve symptoms but whether they alter the natural history of the diseases is unclear. A recent publication from 'The Lung Health Study'[108] reports the effects of smoking intervention and use of an inhaled anticholinergic bronchodilator on the rate of decline of FEV_1 in smokers aged 35–60 years with mild COPD.

This large randomised trial examined pulmonary function change over 5 years and concluded that a smoking intervention programme had significantly beneficial effects; that regular use of an anticholinergic bronchodilator had acute benefits, but did not influence the long-term decline of FEV_1. A two-week trial of oral corticosteroids is often valuable in defining the degree of reversibility of air flow obstruction and may predict those who will benefit from inhaled steroids. As has been pointed out big responders to oral steroids, may be those who have asthma as a contributor to their chronic air flow obstruction.

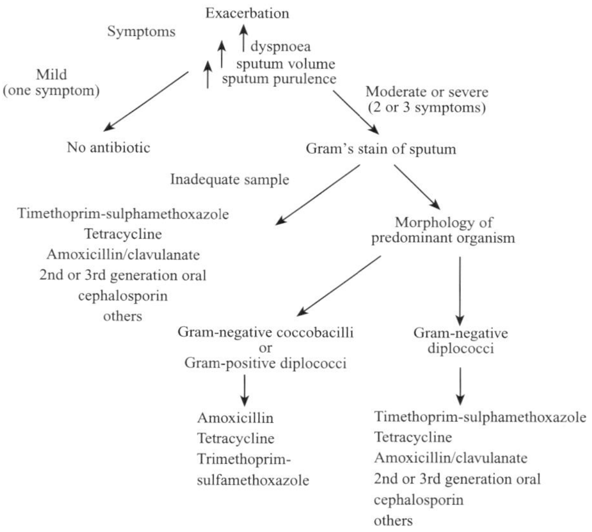

FIGURE 29.8 Algorithm of the authors' approach to evaluation of antimicrobial therapy of exacerbations of chronic obstructive pulmonary disease. Because no single antibiotic is appropriate for all patients, these recommendations are intended as general guidelines. A history of an adverse event to an antibiotic should be sought before administration of the agent.

1. If the symptom is clinically severe, the exacerbation should be evaluated as moderate or severe.
2. Inadequate sputum sample defined by presence of squamous epithelial cells or no predominant morphological type of bacterium.
3. Some strains of *Streptococcus pneumoniae* are resistant to trimethoprim-sulfamethoxazole.
4. Some strains of non-typable *Haemophilus influenzae* and *Streptococcus pneumoniae* are resistant to tetracyline.
5. Up to 25% of strains of non-typable *Haemophilus influenzae* are resistant to amoxicillin.
6. Clarithromycin, azithromycin, ofloxacin, and ciprofloxacin are broad spectrum agents which are also effective.

Table 29.3 *(a) Antimicrobial susceptibility to eight oral antimicrobial agents of bacterial isolates recovered from 15 US Medical Centers*[a]

Organism	Percentage of strains susceptible to (%) Ampicillin	Amoxicillin plus clavulanate	Amoxicillin plus Cefaclor	Cefurozime
Haemophilus influenzae[b]	83[e]	100	100	100
Streptococcus pneumoniae	100[d]	100	100	100
Moraxella catarrhalis[c]	16	100	100	100

[a]From a national surveillance study: Jorgensen *et al. Antimicrob Agents Chemother* 1990; 34: 2075.
[b]90% of *H. influenzae* isolates were non-typable.
[c]No specific guidelines for correlation of minimal inhibitory concentrations with susceptibility have been established for *M. carrhalis*; however, with the exception of ampicillin, isolates were susceptible to levels of antibiotics attainable in serum following usual doses.
[d]One isolate of *S. pneumoniae* was resistant to penicillin, and 3.8% were relatively resistant (MIC 0.12 to 1 mg/ml).
[e]Numbers represent percentage of isolates susceptible based on NCCLS guidelines[102].

Table 29.3 *(b). Antimicrobial susceptibility to eight oral antimicrobial agents of bacterial isolates recovered from 15 US Medical Centers*[a]

Organism	Percentage of strains susceptible to (%) Erythromycin	Tetracycline	Trimethoprim sulfamethoxazole
Haemophilus influenzae	–[b]	98	99
Streptococcus pneumoniae	100	98[c]	95
Branhamella catarrhalis	100	100	100

[a]From a national surveillance study: Jorgensen *et al. Antimicrob Agents Chemother* 1990; 34: 2075.
[b]No reliable *in vitro* data or methods for susceptibility exist.
[c]Other studies have shown more resistance of *S. pneumoniae* to tetracycline.
From Murphy, T. and Sethi, S. [7] Reprinted with permission.

The response to inhaled β_2-agonists may be a predictor of response to oral steroids but the bottom line is that predicting response in an individual patient is impossible so a therapeutic trial is required. A significant minority of patients with CAO will respond to oral steroids; therefore in all patients, if symptom control is unacceptable with bronchodilators, inhaled steroids and the other measures outlined in the algorithm, a trial of oral steroids is indicated[109].

In judging response one must be aware that within-subject variability of peak expiratory flow or FEV_1 may be large so detecting treatment effect may be difficult. A large placebo effect is described and the definition of FEV_1 response is contentious. Should FEV_1 response be expressed as percentage change from baseline or increase of FEV_1 as percentage of the predicted FEV_1?

Substantial benefit may occur from reduction of 'gas trapping' and/or better gas exchange. These effects are only measurable by more sophisticated tests of pulmonary function, i.e. body box, arterial blood gas or exercise testing. Thus tests like the 12 minute walking test and quality of life assessments should be part of the methods used to judge response.

The role of inhaled steroids in smoking related CAO is unclear. To some extent the response to an oral steroid trial will predict response to inhaled steroids, but Shim *et al.*[110] concluded that only 4 of 12 respondents to oral prednisone maintained the response with inhaled steroids.

Theoretically, inhaled steroids might reduce airway inflammation and could slow or interrupt the vicious circle. This might have an effect on the natural history of the disease or rate of decline of ventilatory function. Thomson *et al.*[83] showed a 10% improvement in FEV_1 and reduction in bronchoalveolar lavage cellularity and other parameters of inflammation when patients with chronic bronchitis were given inhaled beclomethasone, five puffs four times per day.

Bronchiectasis

The authors would like to acknowledge the strong influence of Professor Peter Cole, both in his personal guidance, and through his definitive chapter on bronchiectasis[111].

Definition

The term 'bronchiectasis', signifying chronic dilatation of one or more bronchi, was first applied in a translation of Hasse's textbook in

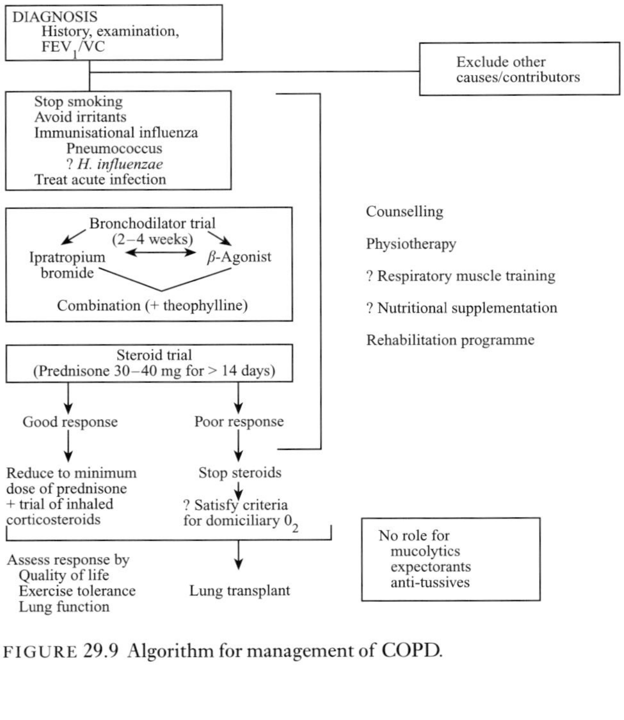

FIGURE 29.9 Algorithm for management of COPD.

1846[112], nearly 30 years after the original description of bronchial dilatation by Laennec[113]. The definition of bronchiectasis is purely morphological and is not, in itself, a statement of disease pathogenesis. Bronchiectasis should not be viewed as a final diagnosis but as the final common outcome of a number of mechanisms and primary causes[111].

Morphology of bronchiectasis

Airway abnormalities in bronchiectasis may be categorized histologically or bronchographically. No modern investigator has surpassed the definitive histological characterisation of Whitwell in 1952, a description of 200 resected bronchiectatic specimens, including neoprene casts of the bronchial tree in 20 instances[114]. Whitwell identified the three histological subcategories recognized today: follicular, saccular and atelectatic bronchiectasis. Follicular bronchiectasis, the most common appearance in the modern era, is characterised by the formation of lymphoid follicles within bronchial and bronchiolar walls, in association with prominent mural inflammation and interstitial pneumonia within the adjacent parenchyma. Enlarged follicles may completely occlude the bronchiolar lumen; in mild disease, subepithelial follicle formation may be the only obvious abnormality but elastin stains generally demonstrate loss of elastic tissue within the bronchial wall. By contrast, follicle formation is not prominent in saccular bronchiectasis and interstitial pneumonia is not observed in the lung parenchyma adjacent to the characteristic grossly dilated bronchial saccules.

In the third subgroup, 'atelectatic bronchiectasis', the defining feature is loss of alveolar volume, probably as a result of obstruction of lobar bronchi[114]; however, this group is heterogenous in other regards. Bronchial compression by enlarged lymph nodes is found in many cases; atelectatic bronchiectasis most frequently affects the right middle lobe bronchus, in keeping with its vulnerability to compression by nodal tissue[115].

In early histological studies, distal obstruction of small airways was a striking feature, especially in severe disease[114,116,117]. Reid showed that the reduction in the number of normal subdivisions of bronchi seen on bronchography corresponded microscopically to obliterative bronchiolitis[118]; recently, a high prevalence of small airways disease has been demonstrated on high resolution CT scans in bronchiectasis[119]. Other structural derangements at a pathological level include localized emphysema in regions of severe bronchiectasis[117] and parenchymal distortion by fibrotic bands, a particularly frequent finding in advanced disease[114].

The microscopic findings are well summarised by Cole[111]. Chronic inflammation of the bronchial wall by mononuclear cells is common to all types of bronchiectasis; recent immunohistological studies have demonstrated the presence of an active cell-mediated immune response, with marked increases in suppressor (cytotoxic) CD8-positive activated T-lymphocytes, as well as antigen-processing cells and mature effector macrophages[120]. Excess mucus and large numbers of polymorphonuclear cells are seen in the airway lumen; recently, elevated levels of interleukin-8, a potent neutrophil chemoattractant, have been measured in the sputum of patients with bronchiectasis[121]. In severe disease, degeneration of ciliated epithelium is usual, with replacement by squamous or columnar epithelium, loss of the bronchial wall elastin layer and destruction of bronchial muscle and cartilage. The bronchial arteries hypertrophy and anastomose with pulmonary arteries[122], leading, in extreme cases, to shunting from systemic to pulmonary arteries[123].

Some confusion has arisen from the use of separate bronchographic classifications of bronchiectasis into cylindrical, cystic/saccular and varicose appearances. Cylindrical bronchiectasis (Fig. 29.10 and 29.11), consisting of symmetrical dilatation of airways along a longitudinal axis, is synonymous with follicular bronchiectasis; cystic bronchiectasis (Fig. 29.12 and 29.13) corresponds to the saccular histological subtype. Varicose bronchiectasis (Fig. 29.14) can belong to either histological category, shares bronchographic features with both other subtypes, and can be regarded as an intermediate form of disease. In the modern era, cylindrical bronchiectasis is much the most common appearance in idiopathic disease[124].

The pathogenesis of bronchiectasis

Many theories of pathogenesis have been debated during recent decades only to be discarded, with the notable exception of the 'vicious circle' hypothesis, proposed by Cole in 1984. It is now clear that idiopathic bronchiectasis cannot be ascribed to traction from parenchymal fibrosis, the effect of mechanical stress upon normal bronchi, or developmental deficiencies within the bronchial wall[111,114]. In animal studies, bronchiectasis develops only if obstruction and active infection coexist[125,126]. However, the extrapolation of

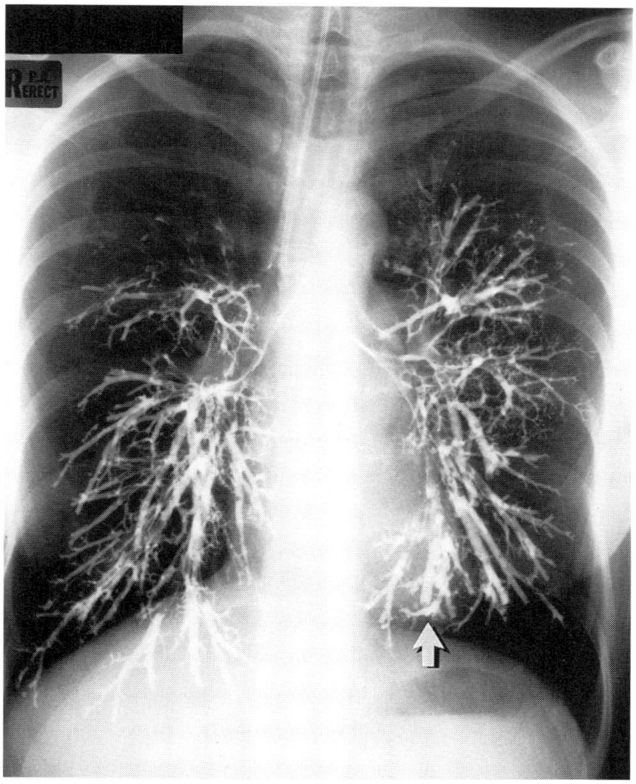

FIGURE 29.10 Bronchogram showing early cylindrical bronchiectasis in the left lower lobe (arrowed). Distal filling by contrast is poor despite 5 minutes in the erect posture.

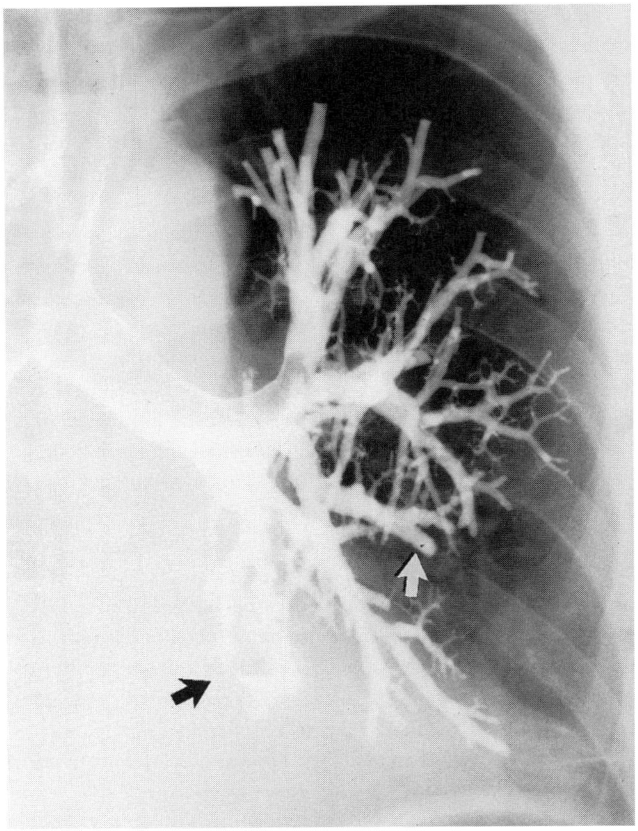

FIGURE 29.11 Bronchogram showing cylindrical bronchiectasis in the lingula (white arrow): note the absence of distal filling and symmetrical bronchial dilatation along the longitudinal axis. There is cystic bronchiectasis within the left lower lobe (black arrow).

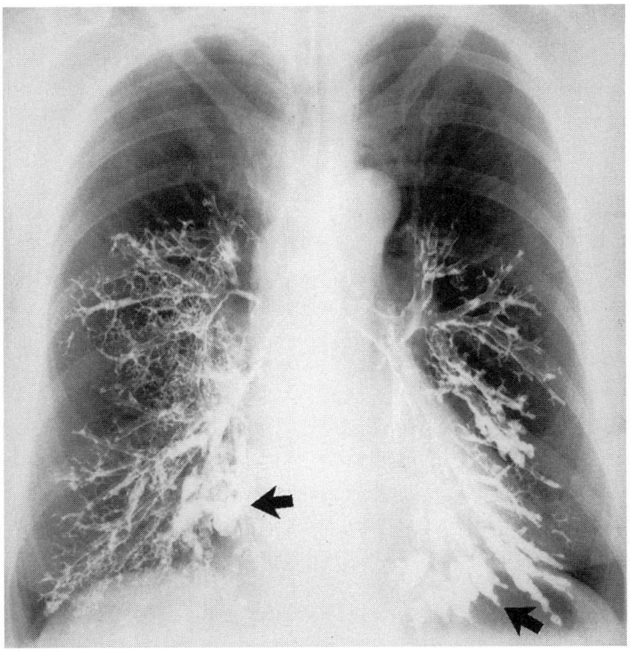

FIGURE 29.12 Bronchogram showing gross cystic bronchiectasis within the right middle and left lower lobes (arrowed).

animal data to human disease is problematic. In the animal model, bronchiectasis is induced by bronchial occlusion whereas in most patients, there is no antecedent evidence of endobronchial obstruction involving the large airways; atelectatic histological appearances

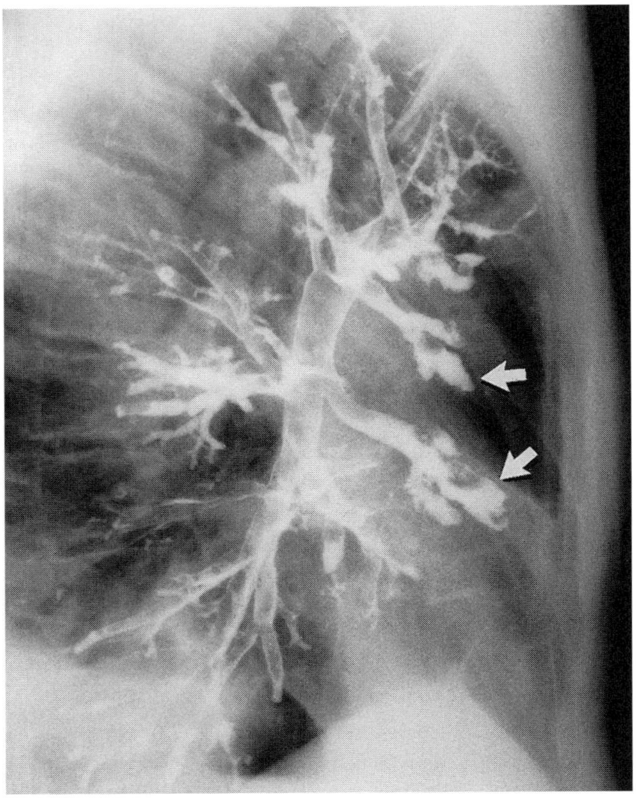

FIGURE 29.13 Bronchogram showing cystic bronchiectasis in the right middle lobe and anterior segment of the right upper lobe (arrowed), seen on lateral projection.

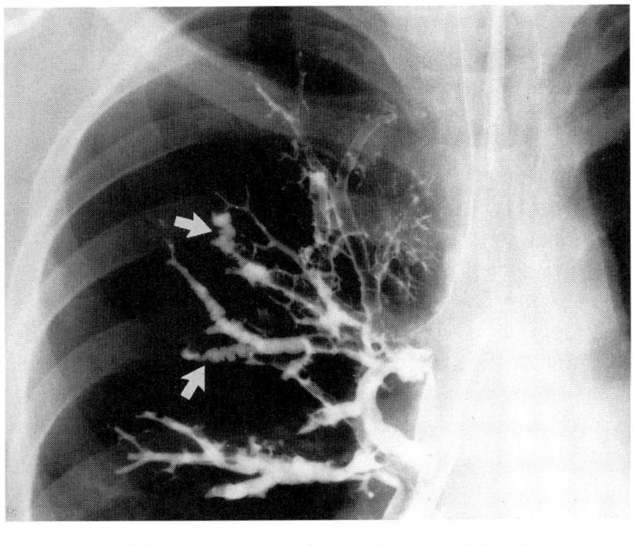

FIGURE 29.14 Bronchogram showing the characteristic beading appearances of varicose bronchiectasis, seen in the right upper lobe (arrowed).

were seen in only 10% of specimens in the series of Whitwell[114]. Thus, the fundamental question of the exact anatomic sequence of events, including the site of initial airflow obstruction, remains uncertain; the airflow obstruction seen in advanced disease has been variously ascribed to obliterative bronchiolitis, asthma, the collapse of large airways during expiration and the retention of secretions.

Obliterative bronchiolitis is part and parcel of severe bronchiectasis[114,116,117] and is likely to be an integral part of pathogenesis, judging from recent CT work, which demonstrates a close relationship between the severity of bronchiectasis and the extent of small airways disease within the same lobe[119]. Physiological evidence of small airways disease is common in bronchiectasis, even in mild disease[127]. However, the temporal relationship between small airways involvement and the genesis of bronchiectasis has never been definitively studied. It is possible that chronic infection begins in the large airways and spreads peripherally, leading to secondary bronchiolar obliteration[118] or that initiating insults, such as viral infection, induce simultaneous damage to the bronchi and bronchioles[128]. However an intriguing alternative hypothesis is that bronchiolitis is the initial event in idiopathic bronchiectasis, preceding and leading to overt large airways involvement. The susceptibility of the small airways to damage is well documented in studies of smokers[129] and childhood bronchiolitis is known to precede chronic lung disease in adulthood in some instances[130]. It is possible that the scarring and atelectasis associated with infective bronchiolitis obliterans leads to bronchial dilatation[131]. Alternatively, the mechanical consequences of persistent bronchiolar obstruction may play a crucial indirect pathogenetic role; in severe bronchiolitis, the markedly increased resistance to expiratory airflow in the small airways may impair the efficacy of cough and reduce the clearance of large airway secretions, leading to recurrent or prolonged bacterial infection and thus to progressive bronchiectasis. Circumstantial evidence in support of this contention includes the presence of small airways disease on CT in bronchiectatic patients in a number of lobes in which bronchiectasis has yet to develop[119]. Similarly, regional ventilation studies have shown that reduced ventilation in bronchiectasis is not confined to bronchiectatic lobes[132]. In cystic fibrosis, an obliterative bronchiolitis is believed to be the earliest lung lesion[133]. Finally, Becroft has reported the development of bronchiectasis in a cohort of children during the 13 years following episodes of severe adenovirus bronchiolitis[128].

The importance of asthma in pathogenesis is contentious. A recent study has suggested that the prevalence of asthma is not increased in bronchiectasis[134]; however, increases in bronchial hyperreactivity have been widely reported in bronchiectasis[135–137], leading many to argue that bronchospasm makes a major contribution to disease progression, by retarding the clearance of secretions. This debate remains unresolved. Severe narrowing of the airway lumen in inflammatory airways disease may be enough to give the clinical picture of asthma, without the need to invoke smooth muscle hyperresponsiveness of the airways or eosinophilic bronchiolitis[138]. Thus, variable airflow obstruction may be inseparable from the bronchiolitis of bronchiectasis; the indiscriminate use of the term 'asthma' does little to advance our understanding of pathogenesis and may be a source of considerable semantic confusion.

Emphysema has been described histologically in severe bronchiectasis[117,139] but has not been widely described radiologically and is unlikely to play an important role in the early evolution of disease. The combination of emphysema and bronchiectasis has been described in alpha-l-antitrypsin deficiency[140]. However, relative preservation of the total gas transfer (DLCO) is usual in bronchiectasis[119], a finding known to be indicative of intrinsic small airways disease rather than emphysema in the context of airflow obstruction[141].

The 'vicious circle' hypothesis

Irrespective of the anatomic sequence of events, pathogenetic hypothesis must explain a number of observations of the host–microbe interaction. Patients with chronic suppurative lung disease usually have hypergammaglobulinemia[142] and are plainly able to mount an exuberant immune response to colonising organisms; the organisms themselves are not virulent, have little propensity to invade systemically, and are seldom associated with rapidly progressive lung disease in the modern era[143]. The prevalence of immune deficiency is low in bronchiectasis, except when recurrent acute infection is a prominent feature[142]. The paradoxical persistence of infection in the absence of immune deficiency, despite an active immune response, led to the formulation by Cole of the 'vicious circle' hypothesis in 1984[144].

The 'vicious circle' hypothesis proposes that colonizing microbes subvert normal host clearance mechanisms, thereby modulating the respiratory environment and facilitating further microbial proliferation. As a result, clearance of infection by the host immune response is predestined to fail; paradoxically, the immune system succeeds only in amplifying damage to mucociliary clearance, resulting in a 'vicious circle' of host damage and increasing microbial colonisation. In part, bronchiectasis can be viewed as an autoimmune disease.

In advancing his hypothesis, Cole presupposes an initial insult resulting in impairment of mucociliary clearance, leading to retention of secretions and allowing the selection of colonising bacteria. Organisms such as *Pseudomonas aeruginosa*, *S. pneumoniae*, and *H. influenzae* then secrete compounds that inhibit mucus transport by inducing ciliary dyskinesia[145], and possibly by a direct toxic effect upon ciliated epithelium. Cole also speculates that increases in the viscosity and volume of mucus, shown to be stimulated by infection in animal studies[146,147], might uncouple ciliary beating from mucus, resulting in stasis of a thicker outer layer of secretions[111]; however, recent studies of sputum viscoelasticity and its relationship to regional lung clearance have cast doubt upon the importance of this mechanism in human disease[148].

The continued stimulation of the host immune system is an integral part of the 'vicious circle' hypothesis. The contribution of activated T-cells and local antibody production to damage of the bronchial wall is unclear. The non-specific component of the inflammatory response is likely to play an important role. The chemoattractant properties of microbial products for neutrophils are well recognised[149]; it is likely that a wide variety of microbial and host factors, including interleukin-8 and changes in expression of adhesion protein receptors on endothelial cells, sustain and amplify the influx of immune cells. Studies of ^{111}indium-labelled granulocytes reveal that in bronchiectasis approximately 50% of circulating granulocytes leave the body via the bronchial lumen[150]; the traffic of such large numbers of cells is likely to have major damaging consequences, even if the amount of enzymatic release by each cell is small. Both neutrophil elastase and purulent sputum damage ciliated cells and slow ciliary beating[151,152].

Thus, the host response may play a major role in amplifying the 'vicious circle' of tissue damage. The primary deficiency in idiopathic bronchiectasis, leading to this putative cascade of events, remains undefined; possible factors include genetic predisposition, the severity of the initial insult, the stage of lung development at the time of the initial insult, underlying immune responses to specific antigens and the overall function of the immune system, modulated by diet and general health. Essentially, the 'vicious circle' hypothesis argues for 'uncoupling' of the normal microbe–host interaction, whether primarily due to intrinsic host factors, environmental considerations or fortuity in the timing and severity of the initial episode.

Prevalence

Although responsible for severe morbidity and mortality before the advent of antimicrobial agents[153], bronchiectasis has not been widely studied in the modern era, due in part to a perceived decline in the prevalence and severity of disease in developed countries, ascribed to improved socioeconomic status, immunisation against pertussis and measles, and the widespread availability of antimicrobial agents[154]. Evidence supporting a recent fall in prevalence include a reduction in hospital admission[155] and deaths from bronchiectasis[156,157] in recent decades. However, hospital admissions and mortality are markers of severe disease and may not reflect the prevalence of milder disease. The prevalence of bronchiectasis approximated 0.1% in the 1950s, judging from chest radiographic appearances[116,158] but has not been defined in the modern era. Cole emphasises his perception, based upon a very large clinical experience of the investigation of patients with chronic purulent sputum production, that bronchiectasis is now widely under-diagnosed, even by respiratory physicians[111].

The relative importance of race and low socioeconomic status in increasing the prevalence of chronic pulmonary suppuration has not been formally quantified. Unemployment, malnutrition and barriers to medical care are all likely to influence the prevalence and natural history of bronchiectasis adversely; poor and uneducated patients with chronic illness are unlikely to present early or to receive regular primary medical care[159]. These factors and the lack of ready availability of antimicrobial agents may explain the high prevalence of bronchiectasis reported anecdotally in the third world. The importance of racial susceptibility to bronchiectasis remains unclear. A markedly higher prevalence and/or mortality of bronchiectasis has been reported in a number of ethnic groups, including North American Indians[160], New Zealand Maori[161] and Western Samoans[162]. These racial groups have, in common, a change to a European style of life after centuries of geographic isolation. In general, social or ethnic minorities contribute disproportionately to the mortality and morbidity of respiratory disease[163]; to date, no definitive attempt has been made to distinguish between a genetic predilection for bronchiectasis in these races and environmental considerations, including changes in diet, housing and the introduction by Europeans of microbes to which indigenous populations had not been exposed. However, it appears unlikely that a genetic predilection for chronic lung suppuration is the sole explanation for the marked racial disparities detailed above. Early historical accounts stress the health and vigour of both North American Indians and New Zealand Maori prior to European colonisation. The introduction of microbial organisms such as measles, tuberculosis and pertussis, amongst others, to a population with no acquired immunity, had a devastating effect; the Maori population fell from 100 000 to 42 000 in the course of only two decades, largely as a result of disease[164].

The aetiology of bronchiectasis: characteristic features

The recognition of an underlying cause is important as it may profoundly influence management (e.g. oral corticosteriod therapy for allergic bronchopulmonary aspergillosis, immunoglobulin infusions in hypogammaglobulinaemia). The diagnosis of bronchiectasis represents the final common outcome of a wide variety of pathogenetic mechanisms, most of which have in common an element of airway obstruction and the presence of bacterial infection within the bronchial tree. Attempts to define the morphological characteristics of secondary bronchiectasis have centred upon bronchographic and/or CT descriptions of the site and nature of disease but have taken little account of the problem of selection bias. Descriptive studies tend to exaggerate perceived 'characteristic' features and their use as diagnostic discriminators. A recent CT study of a large unselected population of bronchiectatic patients has demonstrated that no single morphological feature is diagnostic of any particular aetiology of bronchiectasis[124].

The diagnosis of *idiopathic* bronchiectasis is one of exclusion. Idiopathic disease remains the most common form of bronchiectasis in the modern era and is characterised by cylindrical appearances, follicular histological findings, and a predilection for involvement of the lower lobes. The proportion of cases that can be attributed to a discrete infective episode is contentious; in many retrospective series, a high prevalence of an antecedent history of severe lower respiratory infection has been documented[165–167]. Microorganisms reported to predispose to bronchiectasis include *Bordetella pertussis*, measles virus, adenovirus and *M. pneumoniae*[168,169]. However, isolated infective episodes in childhood often appear significant to the patient because of their dramatic nature; the causal significance of such episodes in the pathogenesis of bronchiectasis remains speculative, with the notable exception of tuberculosis which is known to result in upper lobe fibrosis and bronchiectasis.

Mucociliary clearance defects

These are the commonest genetic disorders associated with suppurative lung disease. In cystic fibrosis, the development of bronchiectasis is likely to reflect the reduction of mucus transport[170] which results from the abnormal viscidity of secretions. Bronchiectasis in cystic fibrosis (Fig. 29.15) has been reported as predominantly central[171] and to involve the upper lobes early in disease[172] and all lobes in advanced disease[173]. Bronchographic appearances have been variously described as predominantly cylindrical[172] and predominantly varicose[174], perhaps reflecting variations in the severity of disease.

Primary ciliary dyskinesia

This is an autosomal recessive condition with a frequency of approximately 1:20 000[175]. Ciliary beating is slow and poorly coordinated;

ciliary ultrastructure is disordered throughout the respiratory tract and in the uterine tract. In many cases, spermatozoal ciliary abnormalities give rise to male infertility. Ciliary dyskinesia is accompanied by dextrocardia or situs inversus in about 50% of instances. This combination may be associated with sinusitis (Kartagener's syndrome); the radiographic features are similar to those of idiopathic bronchiectasis[124,176], apart from a reported predilection for middle lobe involvement[177].

Other congenital forms of bronchiectasis are rare and often associated with other anomalies such as congenital heart disease, Klippel–Feil syndrome and pulmonary sequestration[178]. Deficiencies of bronchial cartilage may manifest as bronchiectasis early in life, as in the Williams–Campbell syndrome[179], or in adulthood, as in tracheobronchomegaly[180].

A number of *acquired mucociliary defects* have been described. In 'secondary ciliary dyskinesia', seen in severe asthma[181], viral or bacterial infection[182,183] and chronic bronchitis due to smoking[184], ciliary structures are normal but ciliary beating is impaired. *Young's syndrome* consists of bronchiectasis, sinusitis and obstructive azoospermia[185]; this often manifests in adult life and has been linked to mercury poisoning in infancy (pink disease)[186]. Sperm production is normal on testicular biopsy[187] but spermatozoal accumulation does not occur, due to a functional obstruction of the vas deferens. The abnormally viscid nature of secretions is likely to be responsible; similarly viscid respiratory secretions result in prolongation of mucociliary transport[188] and secondary bacterial infection.

Hypogammaglobulinaemia

This is the most frequent immune deficiency associated with adult bronchiectasis. This may take the form of acquired panhypogammaglobulinaemia, selective deficiencies of IgG and IgM, or IgG subclass deficiency: IgG subclass 2 deficiency is associated with recurrent infection by *S. pneumoniae* or *H. influenzae*[189]. Complete absence of humoral immune function (X-linked hypogammaglobulinaemia) is relatively infrequent. All these conditions are treatable by immunoglobulin replacement, unlike the rare deficiencies of phagocytic or cellular immune function, which are generally fatal in childhood. The bronchiectasis of hypogammaglobulinemia (Fig. 29.16) is generally cylindrical[190,191], with relatively more bronchial wall thickening than bronchial dilatation[124,191], and may have a predilection for the middle lobes[191].

Bronchiectasis is a prominent feature of severe *allergic bronchopulmonary aspergillosis (ABPA)*. Early in the course of disease, bronchospasm is often the predominant clinical abnormality, but in advanced ABPA, chronic secondary lung suppuration may supervene, giving rise to very extensive airway destruction[124] and a clinical picture similar to that of severe idiopathic disease. Lobar collapse from mucus plugging is an occasional feature. In the bronchiectasis of ABPA, involvement of the central airways in the upper and middle lobes is disproportionate[192]; central bronchiectasis has been considered virtually pathognomonic of ABPA by some authors (Fig. 29.17)[193,194] but is not an invariable finding[124,195].

Endobronchial obstruction of large airways should always be suspected when bronchiectasis coexists with regional atelectasis. Mechanical obstruction is often surgically remediable, especially when due to a benign tumour or inhaled foreign body. Bronchiectasis may arise from intense inflammatory endobronchial obstruction, especially when complicated by infection, as in aspiration of toxic chemicals[196], aspiration associated with dysphagia (Fig. 29.18) or severe gastro-esophageal regurgitation; the last may give rise to localised or generalised disease but is often under-recognised in clinical practice, due to the high prevalence of symptom of reflux in the community.

Radiological evidence of bronchiectasis may be evident in a number of diffuse interstitial lung diseases, especially sarcoidosis, in which cough and airflow obstruction may be the predominant clinical abnormalities; fibrotic distortion is generally held responsible. 'Traction bronchiectasis' is also seen in lone cryptogenic fibrosing alveolitis, but the clinical significance of this finding is unclear.

Diseases associated with bronchiectasis

Rhinosinusitis

This is probably the condition most frequently associated with bronchiectasis. Upper respiratory symptoms are reported by more

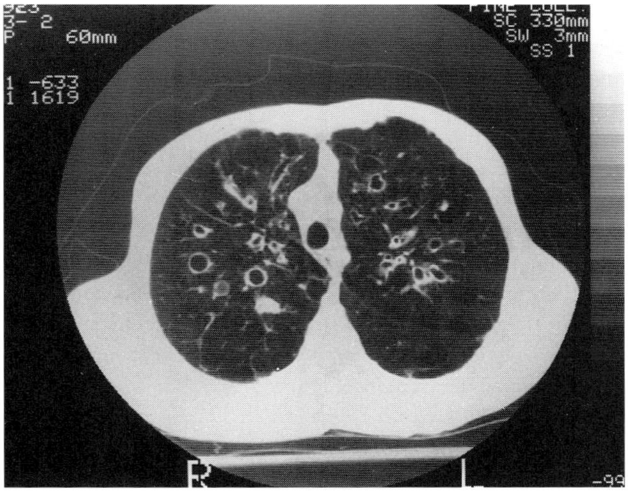

FIGURE 29.15 High resolution CT scan showing severe bilateral cystic upper lobe bronchiectasis in a patient with cystic fibrosis.

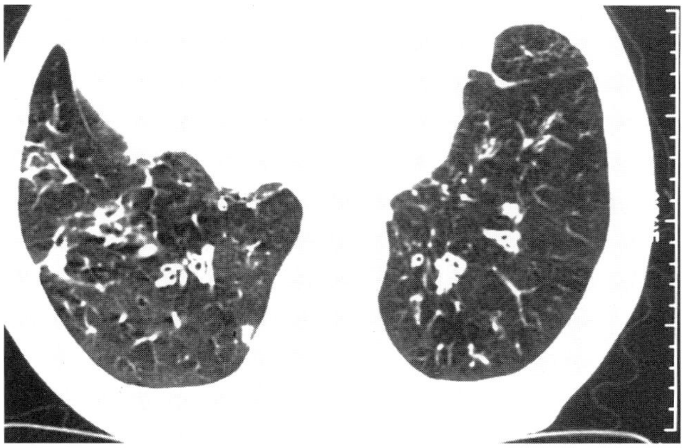

FIGURE 29.16 High resolution CT scan appearances typical of hypogammaglobulinaemia. Bronchial wall thickening is prominent in the absence of severe bronchial wall dilatation.

than 75% of patients and 30% have chronic purulent sinusitis[197] Nasal disease with post-nasal drip is believed by some to play a causative role in bronchiectasis, but this hypothesis is unproved.

Amongst the *collagen vascular diseases*, bronchiectasis most commonly complicates rheumatoid arthritis (RA)[198–201]; in RA, bronchiectasis and lung fibrosis have a similar prevalence[198]. Bronchiectasis often precedes systemic evidence of RA by a number of years[199,200], but may also be a feature of advanced RA[201]; however, it does not appear to be a marker for more rapid progression of systemic disease[200]. Bronchiectasis has also been described in Sjögren's syndrome[202] and systemic lupus erythematosus[203]. The histological similarities between the small airways' abnormalities in follicular idiopathic bronchiectasis and the follicular bronchiolitis of RA and Sjögren's syndrome[204] may indicate common pathogenetic mechanisms in these diseases.

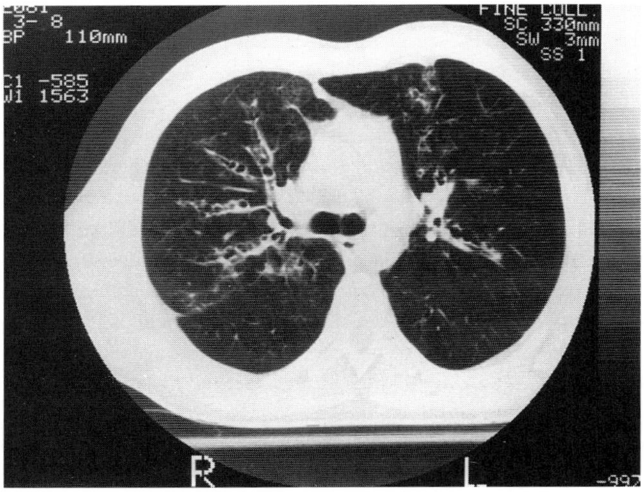

FIGURE 29.17 High resolution CT section in a patient with allergic bronchopulmonary aspergillosis. Bronchiectasis in the upper lobes is extensive and central with prominent varicosity.

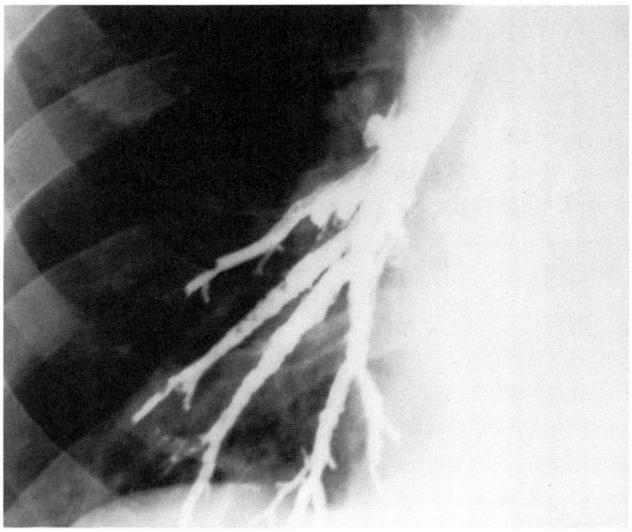

FIGURE 29.18 Plain chest radiographic appearances immediately following barium swallow in a patient with severe dysphagia, post laryngectomy. Aspirated contrast material outlines bronchiectatic airways within the right middle lobe.

The association between *ulcerative colitis* and bronchiectasis is now well recognized[205,206]; either disease may precede the other, often by many years. In a striking subgroup, purulent sputum production develops days or weeks after total colectomy for ulcerative colitis[111]. The absence of antecedent respiratory symptoms and the efficacy of steroid therapy in suppressing sputum production have given rise to a hypothesis of shared tissue epitopes between the two 'target organs'; it has been suggested that the major focus of immunological activity switches to the bronchial tree after removal of the diseased colon[111].

Mechanisms of the development of bronchiectasis in *malignancy* include localised endobronchial obstruction, especially in lung tumours, and the immunosuppression inherent in acute or chronic lymphatic leukaemia, due either to the diseases themselves or to the effects of chemotherapy[207]. Lymphoreticular malignancy and bronchiectasis may also be associated with the yellow nail syndrome, which consists of two or more of the triad of lymphoedema, recurrent or chronic pleural effusions, and the characteristic nail dystrophy from which the syndrome takes its name[208].

Bronchiectasis has been reported in a handful of patients with homozygous alpha-1-antitrypsin deficiency[209,210], lending limited support to the suggestion that a subtle antiprotease defect might contribute to the pathogenesis of bronchiectasis. The contribution of concomitant hypogammaglobulinaemia to this association has yet to be evaluated; selective IgG deficiency and/or IgG subclass deficiency has been reported in five patients with homozygous alpha-1-antitrypsin deficiency[211,212] and identified in a further six cases known to the authors. Loci for alpha-1-antitrypsin and the heavy chain of immunoglobulin are adjacent on chromosome 14[213].

The clinical features of bronchiectasis

Before the advent of antimicrobial agents, the typical picture of bronchiectasis included the persistent production of large volumes of purulent sputum, recurrent haemoptysis, frequent infective exacerbations, prominent wheeze, fatigue, weight loss, halitosis, clubbing, widespread crackles on auscultation and evidence of obvious bronchiectasis on chest radiography. In the modern era, many patients present with recurrent episodes of acute bronchitis but low-grade chronic sputum production and little other clinical or chest radiographic evidence of disease. Two other clinical profiles are occasionally encountered. Recurrent haemoptysis, often admixed with sputum, may be the only manifestation of disease. An important subgroup of patients present with recurrent fever, pleuritic pain and repeated episodes of pneumonia in a single site; this constellation is often seen in bronchial obstruction. The absence of chronic sputum production ('dry bronchiectasis') often results in under-diagnosis.

A number of historical features should give rise to suspicion of an underlying cause of bronchiectasis. A history of tuberculosis, prominent gastro-oesophageal regurgitation or foreign body inhalation are of obvious importance. Lifelong symptoms increase the likelihood of cystic fibrosis or primary ciliary dyskinesia. Prominent bronchospasm and the production of plugs of viscid sputum are usual in ABPA. Recurrent episodes of acute infection, out of proportion with the severity of underlying bronchiectasis, are often seen in immunodeficiency; in a study of 800 patients with lung infection, immunodeficiency was identified in over two thirds of patients with recurrent pneumonia but in less than 10% of those with chronic lung suppuration[142].

Sputum cultures have a sensitivity of nearly 90%, in identifying organisms colonizing the lower respiratory tract[214]. However, the clinical utility of sputum cultures is often limited by their low specificity; contamination by oropharyngeal flora is virtually inescapable, creating difficulties in determining the significance of individual isolates. In general, bacteria colonizing the lower respiratory tract in bronchiectasis are not virulent; *H. influenzae* is found in over 70%[215]. *P. aeruginosa* or *Staphylococcus aureus* are commonly found in cystic fibrosis; the former is also isolated in patients with idiopathic bronchiectasis, especially in extensive disease[216] and may also play a role in disease progression[217]. The possibility of active tuberculosis should not be overlooked; in a recent study of patients with typical bronchiectasis with little upper lobe involvement and no other features suggestive of tuberculosis, *Mycobacterium tuberculosis* was isolated in 10% on routine culture[218].

The interpretation of lung function tests in bronchiectasis is not always straightforward. Airflow obstruction, often partially reversible, is found in the majority of cases[135,219] and bronchial hyperreactivity has been widely reported[135–137]. However, analyses of the relationship between the severity of airflow obstruction and the extent of bronchiectasis have given both good[220] and poor[221] correlations. A significant minority of patients have a restrictive or mixed defect[219,221], presumably as a consequence of parenchymal fibrosis. Functional indices may also be modulated by retained secretions[222], reducing their precision as a guide to disease severity.

The investigation of known or suspected bronchiectasis is governed by three major goals: the achievement of a secure diagnosis of bronchiectasis, the accurate evaluation of disease extent and severity, and the identification of a primary underlying cause. An algorithm for the investigation of bronchiectasis is detailed in Table 29.4. In recent decades, advances in the evaluation of bronchiectasis have been largely diagnostic, centring upon the increasing use of high resolution computed tomography (CT).

The diagnosis of bronchiectasis

The diagnosis of bronchiectasis is essentially radiological. There is usually little difficulty in reaching a confident diagnosis on plain chest radiography in severe disease; the characteristic findings were well documented by Gudjberg, in the pre-antibiotic era[139] and include parallel opacities ('tramlines') denoting thickened bronchial walls, ring and curvilinear shadows representing dilated airway walls seen en face, and band shadows generated by airways filled with secretions. Optional features include fluid levels within cystic structures, generalised hyperinflation, regional volume loss, consolidation, scarring and pleural thickening. In early series, chest radiography was regarded as sensitive; Gudjberg reported that only 5% of chest radiographs were normal in bronchiectasis[139]. However, this finding was based upon the severe bronchiectasis commonly encountered 40 years ago in clinical practice; even in that era, the true percentage of patients with normal chest radiographs was almost certainly higher than 5%, as a normal radiograph would have pre-empted the demonstration of subtle bronchiectasis by invasive investigations in many instances. More recently, with the decline in prevalence of very severe bronchiectasis, the insensitivity of chest radiography in detecting bronchiectasis has been widely recognised; in the modern era, up to 50% of patients with bronchographically-proven bronchiectasis have normal chest radiographs[223]. Moreover, even when bronchiectasis is apparent on plain radiography, the extent of disease may be grossly underestimated, an important consideration if resection surgery is contemplated for apparently localized disease.

Historically, the procedure of choice, both to diagnose bronchiectasis and to stage the extent of disease, has been bronchography. The preeminence of bronchography arose largely by default; the procedure is cumbersome, unpleasant for the patient (frequently resulting in a poor quality of images) and associated with difficulties in interpretation and significant interobserver variation[223]. The test itself consists of the introduction of aqueous contrast material into the respiratory tree, either by endotracheal tube or via the bronchoscope. Despite its limitations, which include the inability to evaluate bronchial wall thickening, bronchography has been the 'gold-standard' against which other diagnostic techniques have been evaluated.

High resolution CT scanning has now supplanted bronchography in routine clinical practice. The change from thick to thin section collimation has greatly improved the sensitivity of CT, compared to bronchography. Thick section CT had a sensitivity of between 50% and 80%[224,225]; however, the use of 1.5 mm collimation has improved this figure to approximately 95%[226,227]. The recent development of low-dose radiation protocols[228], which do not appear to reduce sensitivity, can only serve to increase the routine use of CT; the radiation burden of such protocols, with the acquisition of 1.5 mm sections at 10 mm intervals, is now equivalent to that of ten plain chest radiographs or less.

The CT appearances of bronchiectasis are dependent upon the orientation of bronchi relative to the plane of CT sections. In the upper and lower lobes, airways will be depicted in transverse section and should normally have a diameter similar to that of the accompanying pulmonary artery; in bronchiectasis, the increased diameter of the airway, relative to the artery, gives rise to the characteristic 'signet ring' sign (Fig. 29.19(*a*) and (*b*). In the mid-zones, airways run horizontally to the plane of CT sections and will be imaged along their length; bronchiectatic airways do not taper distally and may flare peripherally, in severe disease. Bronchial wall thickening is often seen but is not an invariable sign.

The major difficulty in the use of CT in diagnosis is the problem of false positivity, which can be minimised by the services of experienced radiologists and an awareness of technical limitations. Cardiac pulsation commonly gives rise to movement artefact which may simulate the presence of bronchiectasis in the middle lobes, by double imaging of blood vessels. Branching of airways may simulate the 'signet-ring' sign of bronchiectasis; this difficulty can be overcome by close attention to adjacent sections. An awareness of the pretest probability of the diagnosis is indispensable; subtle bronchial dilatation may be seen in long-standing asthma and in normal individuals[229]. Similarly, in horizontal airways, there is no exact point beyond which the identification of peripheral bronchi is abnormal, although most authorities regard airways as bronchiectatic if they are visible within 3 cm of the pleural surface or over two-thirds of the distance

Table 29.4. *An algorithm for the investigation and management of suspected bronchiectasis*

1. *Diagnosis*
   Suspect underlying bronchiectasis in all patients with unexplained chronic purulent sputum production. Unless characteristic features are present on plain chest radiography, proceed to thin section CT to make the diagnosis
2. *Stage severity of bronchiectasis*
   Extent and severity of disease quantified by thin section CT and formal lung function tests. Baseline measurement of disease severity allows definitive evaluation of subsequent progression of disease.
3. *Exclude underlying causes of bronchiectasis*
   Full tuberculosis screen and measurement of serum immunoglobulins should be performed in all patients. Allergic bronchopulmonary aspergillosis, ciliary dyskinesia, and cystic fibrosis should be excluded when clinically warranted. Consider bronchoscopy to exclude endobronchial obstruction in localised disease.
4. *Identify associated disorders*
   Base the need for investigation upon historical and clinical evidence of rhinosinusitis, gastro-oesophageal regurgitation or collagen vascular disease.
   Document the presence of reversible airflow obstruction by means of peak-flow monitoring and/or bronchial provocation testing.
5. *Routine medical management*
   Daily postural drainage, except in trivial bronchiectasis. Inhaled corticosteroid therapy: the authors recommend a high initial dose (e.g. 2400–3200 μg/day) in troublesome disease, titrating against clinical response.
   Short courses (e.g. 1–2 weeks) of broad spectrum antibacterial agents, starting on the first day of an acute infective exacerbation.
   Vigorous treatment of associated rhinosinusitis and gastro-oesophageal regurgitation.
6. *Management of severe bronchiectasis*
   Consider a 1–2 week course of intravenous antibiotics accompanied by intensive physiotherapy to bring about an initial response.
   Continuous oral antibiotics may be required in relapsing disease.
   Domiciliary oxygen therapy may be required in chronic hypoxic respiratory failure.
   Bronchial artery embolisation may be life-saving in recurrent major haemoptysis.
7. *Indications for surgery*
   Bronchiectasis due to endobronchial obstruction
   Localised bronchiectasis in patients who fail medical management
   Resection of severe local disease in generalised bronchiectasis (contentious)

from the hilum to the lung periphery[230,231]. Useful ancillary signs include crowding of the bronchi associated with lobar volume loss, and mucous plugging of the small airways, giving rise to 'spottiness' of the lung periphery within a bronchiectatic lobe (Fig. 29.20)[232].

The medical management of bronchiectasis

Daily postural drainage and intermittent antibacterial therapy are widely cited as the mainstay of treatment. However, there have been few controlled therapeutic trials in patients with bronchiectasis; treatment has largely been based upon anecdotal evidence. One major difficulty, which has precluded definitive therapeutic evaluation, has been the need to distinguish between two separate goals: the treatment of infection and reversible inflammatory disease, designed to bring about an immediate reduction in morbidity, and the prevention of progression of irreversible fibrotic disease in the long term. However, not all patients have a major reversible component. Moreover, the natural history of bronchiectasis is highly variable; any attempt to evaluate the prevention of progression of disease would require the definitive staging of disease severity in large numbers of patients followed by many years of treatment. This question has never been properly addressed; thus, therapies in bronchiectasis remain symptomatic and largely empirical.

The difficulties in evaluating treatment are exemplified by the widespread use of *postural drainage*, which is regarded by most clinicians as the cornerstone of therapy. The performance of postural drainage requires specialist instruction, in order to ensure that the diseased areas are drained effectively by the correct choice of posture, and the investment of a great deal of time by the patient; compliance is often poor[233]. However, the efficacy of postural drainage has never been definitively studied in idiopathic bronchiectasis; evidence for its use is circumstantial. In cystic fibrosis, rigorous daily postural drainage and the early use of antibiotics for infective exacerbations have been associated with a major improvement in life expectancy during recent decades. Patients with idiopathic bronchiectasis frequently report that failure to perform postural drainage is associated with an immediate increase in sputum production and the prevalence of infective exacerbations. The anecdotal efficacy of postural drainage has caused many to argue that the withholding of postural drainage, a prerequisite in a controlled trial, would be unethical. It is now unlikely that the long-term efficacy of postural drainage in the prevention of progression of disease will ever be definitely studied; thus, the central role of postural drainage will remain unchallenged.

Similar analytic difficulties apply to the use of *antibacterial agents* in bronchiectasis, which has been associated with a major reduction

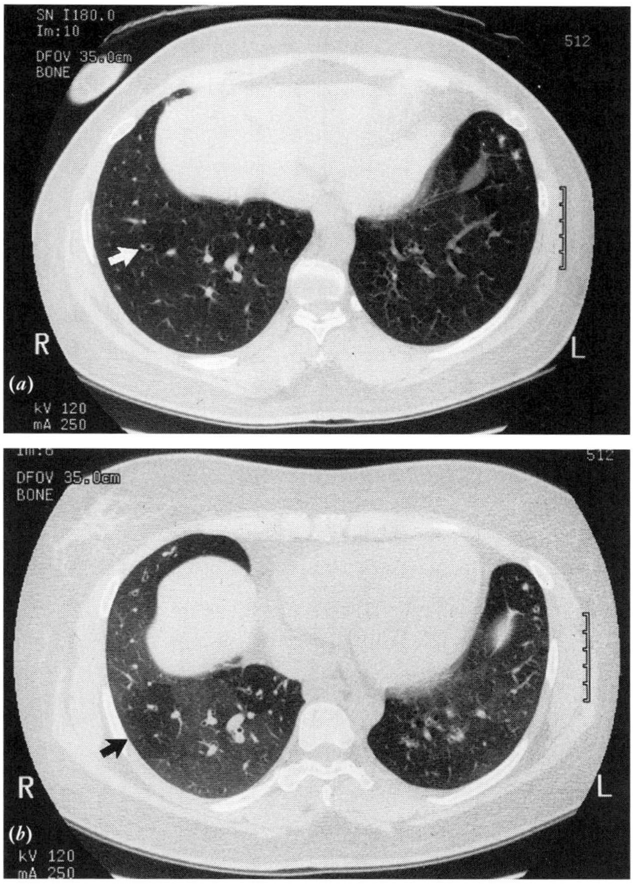

FIGURE 29.19 (*a*) High resolution CT section in a patient with chronic mucus hypersecretion. The 'signet-ring' sign (arrowed), demonstrating increased bronchial diameter (compared to the adjacent pulmonary artery), is diagnostic of bronchiectasis. (*b*) CT section acquired in expiration at the same level: the bronchiectatic airway has collapsed and is surrounded by prominent transradiancy, indicative of regional gas trapping.

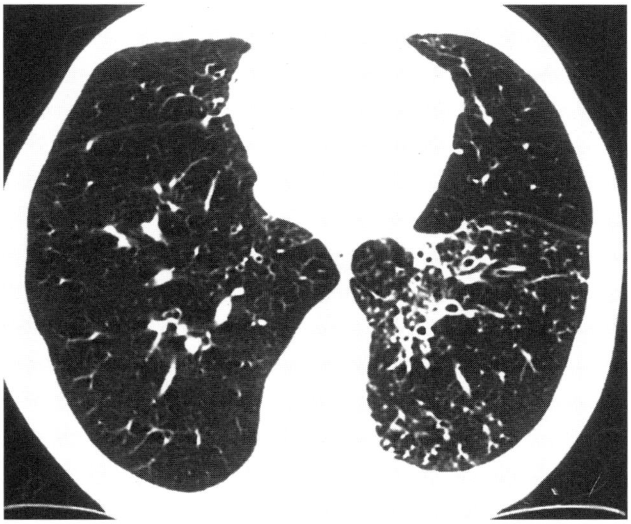

FIGURE 29.20 High resolution CT scan showing bronchiectasis in the left lower lobe with 'signet-ring' appearances and striking plugging of centrilobular bronchioles.

in mortality in the modern era. The intermittent use of short course of broad spectrum oral antibacterial agents, early in acute infective exacerbations, is accepted by all clinicians on symptomatic grounds. The improved survival in cystic fibrosis suggests that this approach almost certainly reduces tissue damage and slows the rate of progression of disease. However, the role of continuous antibacterial therapy is unclear. High dose amoxycillin (3g twice daily) has been invaluable in some patients, in reducing short-term morbidity[234]; maintenance antibacterial regimens have been associated with reductions in sputum microbial load[235], sputum purulence[236], and granulocyte traffic to the lungs[150]. However, the efficacy of treatment in improving functional lung indices is highly variable[237,238]. A number of *in vivo* and bronchial biopsy studies have focused upon the penetration of antibiotics into bronchial mucosal cells and sputum. The tissue concentrations of β-lactams (penicillins and cephalosporins) are a consistent fraction of simultaneous concentrations in serum (ratios of between 0.05 and 0.25); fluoroquinolones such as ciprofloxacin have superior penetration (ratios of between 0.80 and 2.0)[239]. However, the clinical value of measuring antimicrobial concentrations at sites of infection in the lung remains uncertain.

In the absence of definitive therapeutic evidence, many clinicians adopt an approach based on anecdotal experience and tailored to individual requirements. Patients unresponsive to intermittent oral agents may benefit from intravenous antibacterial therapy and intensive physiotherapy, which serves to reduce bacterial antigenic load and break the "vicious circle" of infection and tissue damage resulting from an over-exuberant immune response; an initial response may be maintained by continuous therapy with oral broad spectrum agents such as amoxycillin[234]. Nebulised antibiotics, especially anti-pseudomonal agents such as aminoglycosides and carbenicillin, have also been used in maintenance treatment, specially in cystic fibrosis[240], but their role in idiopathic bronchiectasis is unproven.

The indications for maintenance antibiotic regimens remain imprecise. The possibility of increasing bacterial resistance with this approach is a major concern to many, but is entirely unproven. As Cole compellingly observes, a rigidly conservative approach does not meet the needs of patients with inexorably progressive disease[111]. Thus, the best way to use antibiotic treatment in bronchiectasis remains unclear; the overall consensus amongst experienced clinicians favours the restriction of continuous therapy to patients with major chronic morbidity or extensive disease.

Anti-inflammatory or immunosuppressive therapy has the important theoretical benefit of breaking the 'vicious circle' of infection and tissue damage by quelling an over-exuberant, destructive immune response. However, the efficacy of systemic anti-inflammatory agents has not been formally evaluated, with the exception of oral corticosteroid therapy, which has resulted in a sustained functional benefit in the bronchiectasis of cystic fibrosis[241]. There has been increasing interest in the use of inhaled corticosteroids, recently shown to reduce cough and sputum production in idiopathic bronchiectasis[242]. The concentration of nitric oxide in exhaled air, a marker of airway inflammation, is markedly elevated in untreated bronchiectasis but lies within the normal range in patients treated with inhaled steroid therapy[243]. The role of corticosteroids in preventing progression of bronchiectasis merits further evaluation as there are excellent theoretical reasons for their use. It is the authors' experience that many patients with acute severe exacerbations of bronchiectasis respond to oral or high dose inhaled corticosteroids once pulmonary sepsis has been controlled.

The treatment of disorders associated with bronchiectasis may be central to effective medical treatment in many instances. Symptoms attributable to *hypogammaglobulinaemia*, including rhinosinusitis and sputum production, often respond to human immunoglobulin replacement; intravenous preparations are safer than intramuscular preparations and are efficacious and less distressing to patients[244], with the important proviso that replacement is ineffective in selective IgA deficiency and is associated with a risk of anaphylaxis. The efficacy of immunoglobulin replacement in preventing the progression of bronchiectasis is unproven. The definitive treatment of *gastro-oesophageal regurgitation* may make a major difference to morbidity in a small subgroup of patients. *Rhinosinusitis* is common in bronchiectasis[198], often very distressing to the patient and merits aggressive medical or surgical therapy. Despite the common observation that acute sinusitis often precedes acute lower respiratory infective exacerbations, the beneficial effect of suppression of rhinosinusitis in the medical treatment of bronchiectasis has not been studied.

A number of treatments have as their primary aim the *improvement of clearance of airway secretions*, in the belief that the retention of secretions contributes to pathogenesis. Bronchodilator therapy has been advocated by some and may play an important role in increasing sputum clearance in patients with bronchospasm, whether due to asthma or the bronchiolitis of bronchiectasis. Significant functional benefits, especially improvements in indices of airflow obstruction, have been reported with the use of inhaled fenoterol[135] and subcutaneous terbutaline[245]. The place of mucolytic therapy in increasing tracheobronchial clearance remains controversial, despite limited support for the use of bromhexine in bronchiectasis[246]. Humidification via nebulisation has been advocated as an adjunct to chest physiotherapy in aiding tracheobronchial clearance, based on a study of seven patients[247] but has no proven role as yet in routine management.

Two major complications of bronchiectasis may pose particular difficulties in advanced disease. Domiciliary oxygen therapy is commonly prescribed in chronic hypoxic respiratory failure; in the absence of evidence to the contrary, it is difficult to disagree with this approach. While haemoptysis is usually minor, recurrent major haemoptysis may be life threatening; recently, excellent results have been reported with therapeutic bronchial artery embolisation in over 200 patients with major relapse haemoptysis complicating bronchiectasis, tuberculosis, cystic fibrosis or aspergillosis[248].

The surgical treatment of bronchiectasis

Resection surgery was widely performed in the pre-antibiotic era and merits constant consideration as the only curative treatment in bronchiectases. The interpretation of early surgical results is difficult; whilst an apparent cure or major improvement was reported in over 50% of patients, a significant proportion had no immediate benefit or developed recurrent bronchiectasis[249–251]. These results, the absence of clearcut indications for surgery and improvements in medical management have engendered a nihilistic view of surgery among physicians. However, it should be stressed that case severity and selection differed substantially from that in the modern era. In recent years, there has been renewed interest in resection surgery in carefully selected cases, with satisfactory or excellent outcomes reported in 62% of 73 patients[252] and 67% of 48 patients[253]. Surprisingly, a good outcome was seen in four patients with hypogammaglobulinaemia, with resection of localised disease[254]. However, the indications for surgery remain extremely imprecise, except in the context of local endobronchial obstruction due to a benign tumour. Most clinicians espouse the view first expressed in the 1950s that surgery for localised disease should not be attempted without a trial of aggressive medical management and should be delayed for at least 12 months after the onset of symptoms[255].

Occasionally, resection surgery has been advocated for a 'sump' of infection in generalized bronchiectasis[111], in the belief that removal of severe localised disease might improve the efficacy of medical management, however, experience with this approach is purely anecdotal.

Lung transplantation is an important consideration in extensive progressive bronchiectasis, but experience has been strictly limited, to date. The excellent results achieved in cystic fibrosis suggest that transplantation may have an important future role in idiopathic disease.

References

1. PENNINGTON JE. *Community Acquired Pneumonia and Acute Bronchitis in Respiratory Infections: Diagnosis and Management*. 2nd Ed. New York: Raven Press;1988.
2. AMERICAN THORACIC SOCIETY, Guidelines for the initial management of adults with community-acquired pneumonia: diagnosis assessment of severity, and initial antimicrobial therapy. *Am Rev Resp Dis* 1993; 148:1418–26.
3. HAHN DL, DODGE RW, GOLABJATNIKOV R. Association of *Chlamydia pneumoniae* (TWAR) infection with wheezing, asthmatic bronchitis and adult onset of asthma. *JAMA* 1991; 266:225–30.
4. YANO H, ICHIKAWA Y, KOMATU S, ARAIS S, OIZUMI K. Association of *Mycoplasma pneumoniae* antigen with initial onset of bronchial asthma. *Am J Resp Crit Care Med* 1994; 149:1348–53.
5. BURROWS B. Obstructive lung disease. In Dosman J, and Cockcroft D, eds. *The Medical Clinics of North America*. May 1990; 74:547–61.
6. BUIST S. Smoking and other risk factors. Section I – Obstructive Diseases: 1001–1030. Murray JK, Nadel JA, eds. *Textbook of Respiratory Medicine*. Philadelphia: WB Saunders, 1988.
7. MURPHY T., SETHI S. State-of-the-art. Bacterial infection in chronic obstructive pulmonary disease. *Am Rev Resp Dis*. 1992; 146:1067–83.
8. WOOLCOCK AJ. Epidemiology of chronic airways disease. *Chest* 1989; 96(3 Suppl): 302S–6S.
9. MULLEN JB, WRIGHT JL, WIGGS BR, PARE PD, HOGG JC. Reassessment of inflammation of airways in chronic bronchitis. *BMJ* 1985; 291:1235–9.

10. COSIO M, GHEZZO H HOGG JC *et al.* The relations between structural changes in small airways and pulmonary function test. *N Engl J Med* 1978; 298: 1277–81.
11. BEREND N, WOOLCOCK AJ, MARLIN GE. Correlation between the function and structure of the lung in smokers. *Am Rev Resp Dis* 1979; 119:695–705.
12. COSIO MG, HALE KA, NIEWOEHNER DE. Morphologic and morphometric effects of prolonged ciragette smoking on the small airways. *Am Rev Resp Dis* 1980; 122:265–71.
13. PETTY TL, SILVERS W, STANDFORD RE, BAIRD D, MITCHEL RS. Small airways pathology is related to increased closing capacity and abnormal slope of phase III in excised human lungs. *Am Rev Resp Dis* 1980; 129:449–56.
14. BEREND N, WRIGHT JL, THURLBECK WM, MARLIN GE, WOOLCOCK AJ. Small airways disease: reproducibility of measurements and correlation with lung function. *Chest* 1981; 79:263–8.
15. WRIGHT JL, LAWSON LM, PARE PD, KENNEDY S, WIGGS B, HOGG JC. The detection of small airways disease. *Am Rev Resp Dis* 1984; 129:989–94.
16. WRIGHT JL, WIGGS BJ, HOGG JC. Airway disease in upper and lower lobes in lungs of patients with and without emphysema. *Thorax* 1984; 39:282–5.
17. AGUAYO SM. Determinants of susceptibility to cigarette smoke. *Am J Resp Crit Care Med* 1994; 149:1692–8.
18. BOSKEN C, WIGGS BR, PARE PD, HOGG JC. Small airway dimensions in smokers with obstruction to air flow. *Am Rev Resp Dis* 1990; 142:563–70.
19. WIGGS BR, BOSKEN C, PARE PD, HOGG JC. A model of airway narrowing in asthma and chronic obstructive pulmonary disease. *Am Rev Resp Dis* 1992; 145:1291–8.
20. ORIE NG, SLUITER HJ, DE VRIES K, TAMMALING GJ, WITKOP J. The host factor in bronchitis. In Orie NG, Sluiter JH, eds. *Bronchitis*. Assem, The Netherlands: Royal Vangorcum, 1961: 43–59.
21. TAYLOR RG, CLARKE SW. Bronchial reactivity to histamine in young male smokers. *Eur J Resp Dis* 1985; 66: 320–6.
22. BURROWS B, KNUDSON RJ, LEBOWITZ MD. The relationship of childhood respiratory illness to adult obstructive airway disease. *Am Rev Resp Dis* 1977; 119:751–60.
23. US Department of Health Education and Welfare. *The Health Consequences of Smoking. Chronic Obstructive Lung Disease*. US Department of Health and Human Services, Public Health Service, Office of Smoking, Rockville MD 20857, DHHS (PHS) 84–50205, 1984.
24. US Department of Health Education and Welfare. *Smoking and Health: A Report of the Advisory Committee to the Surgeon General of the Public Health Service*. US Department of Health Education and Welfare, Washington DC, Public Health Service, Publication No. 1103, 1964.
25. BUIST AS, DUCIC S. Smoking: evaluation of studies which have demonstrated pulmonary function changes. In Macklem PT, Permutt S, eds. *The Lung in Transition Between Health and Disease Vol. 12. Lung Biology in Health and Disease*, C. Lenfort, ed. New York: Marcel Dekken; 1979.
26. BURROWS B, KNUDSON RJ, CLINE MG, LEBOWITZ MD. Quantitative relationships between cigarette smoking and ventilatory function. *Am Rev Resp Dis* 1977; 119:195–205.
27. BECK GJ. DOYLE CA, SCHACKTER EN. Smoking and lung function. *Am Rev Resp Dis* 1981; 123:149–55.
28. FLETCHER CR, PETO R, TINKER C, SPEIZER FE. *The Natural History of Chronic Bronchitis and Emphysema*. New York, Oxford University Press, 1976.
29. FLETCHER CR, PETO R. The natural history of chronic air flow obstruction. *Br Med J* 1977; 1:1645–8.
30. BUIST AS. Current status of small airways disease. *Chest* 1984; 86:100–5.
31. DOSSING M, KHAN J, AL RABIAH F. Risk factors for chronic obstructive lung disease in Saudi Arabia. *Resp Med* 1944; 88:519–22.
32. PANDEY MR. Prevalence of chronic bronchitis in a rural community of the Hill Region of Nepal. *Thorax* 1984; 39:331–6.
33. BUIST AS, NAGY JM, SEXTON GJ. The effect of smoking cessation on lung function: a 30-month follow-up of two smoking cessation clinics. *Am Rev Resp Dis* 1979; 120:953–88.
34. CHERNIAK RM, MCCARTHY DS. Reversibility of abnormalities of pulmonary function. In Macklem PT, Permutt S, eds. *The Lung in the Transition Between Health and Disease*. New York: Marcel Dekker; 1979: 329–38.
35. HOLLAND WW, HALIL T, BENNETT AE, ELLIOTT A. Factors influencing the onset of chronic respiratory disease. *Br Med J* 1969; 2:205–8.
36. MONTO AS, ROSS HW. The Tecumseh study of respiratory illness. X. Relation of acute infections to smoking, lung function and chronic symptoms. *Am J Epidemiol* 1978; 107:57–64.
37. HOLLAND W, BAILEY P, BLAND JM. Long-term consequences of respiratory disease in infancy. *J Epidemiol Commun Health* 1978; 32:256–9.
38. COLLEY J, DOUGLAS J REID D. Respiratory disease in young adults: Influence of early childhood lower respiratory tract illness, social class, air pollution and smoking. *Br Med J* 1973; 3:195–8.
39. YARNELL J, ST. LEGER A. Respiratory infections and their influence on lung function in children: a multiple regression analysis. *Thorax* 1981; 36:847–51.
40. LEEDER S, WOOLCOCK A, BLACKBURN CR. Prevalence and natural history of lung disease in NSW school children. *Int J Epidemiol* 1974; 3:15–23.
41. PULLAN C, HEY E. Wheezing, asthma and pulmonary dysfunction 10 years after infection with *respiratory syncytial virus* in infancy. *Br Med J* 1982; 284:1665–9.
42. BARKER D, OSMOND C. Childhood respiratory infection and adult chronic bronchitis in England and Wales. *Br Med J*. 1986; 293:1271–4.
43. LEEDER SR. Role of infection in the cause and course of chronic bronchitis and emphysema. *J Infect Dis* 1975; 131:731–42.
44. BURROWS B, KNUDSON RJ, LEBOWITZ MD. The relationship of childhood respiratory illness to adult obstructive airway disease. *Am Rev Resp Dis* 1977; 119:751–60.
45. BURROWS B, EARLE RH. Course and prognosis of chronic obstructive lung disease. *N Engl J Med* 1969; 280:397–404.
46. COLE PJ. Microbial–host interactions in the airways in chronic respiratory infection. *Clin Therap* 1991; 13:194–8.
47. SNIDER GL. Pathogenesis of emphysema – twenty years of progress. *Am Rev Resp Dis* 1981; 124:321–4.
48. SNIDER GL. Pathogenesis of emphysema and chronic bronchitis. *Med Clin North Am* 1981; 65: 647–65.
49. JANOFF A. Biochemical links between cigarette smoking and pulmonary emphysema. J *Appl Physiol* 1983; 55:285–93.
50. KAUFFMANN F, DROUET D, LELLOUCH J, BRILLE D. Twelve years spirometric changes among Paris area workers. *Int J Epidemiol* 1979; 8:207.
51. COLLEY JRT. Respiratory symptoms in children and parental cigarette smoking and phlegm production. *Br Med J* 1974; 2:201–24.
52. BLAND M, BEWLEY B, POLLAND V, BANKO M. Effect of children and parents smoking on respiratory symptoms. *Arch Dis Child* 1978; 53: 100–5.
53. LEBOWITZ MD, BURROWS B. Respiratory symptoms related to smoking habits of family adults. *Chest* 1976; 69: 48–50.
54. WEISS ST, TAGER IB, SPEIZER FE, ROSNER B. Persistent wheeze. Its relation to respiratory illness, cigarette smoking, and level of pulmonary function in a population sample

of children. *Am Rev Resp Dis* 1980; 122:679–707.

55. TAGER IB, WEISS ST, ROSNER B, SPEIZER FE. Effect of parental smoking on the pulmonary function of children. *Am J Epidemiol* 1969; 110:15–26.
56. HARLAP S, DAVIES AM. Infant admissions to hospital and maternal smoking. *Lancet* 1974; i:529–32.
57. COLLEY JRT, HOLLAND WW, CORKHILL RT. Influence of passive smoking and parental phlegm on pneumonia and bronchitis in early childhood. *Lancet* 1974; ii:1031–4.
58. FERGUSSON DM, HORWOOD LJ, SHANNON FT, TAYLOR B. Parental smoking and lower respiratory illnesses in the first three years of life. *J Epidemiol Commun Health* 1981; 35:180–4.
59. TAGER IB, WEISS ST, MUNOZ A, ROSNER B, SPEIZER FE. Longitudinal study of the effects of maternal smoking on pulmonary function in children. *N Engl J Med* 1983; 309: 699–703.
60. MONTO AS, HIAGGENS MW, ROSS HW. The Tecumseh study of respiratory illness. VIII. Acute infection in chronic respiratory disease and comparison groups. *Am Rev Resp Dis* 1975; 111:27–36.
61. EADIE MB, STOTT EJ, GRIST NR. Virological studies in chronic bronchitis. *Br Med J* 1966; 2:671–3.
62. CARILLI AD, GOHD RS, GORDON W. A virologic study of chronic bronchitis. *N Engl J Med* 1964; 270:123–7.
63. SOMMERVILLE RG. *Respiratory syncytial virus* in acute exacerbations of chronic bronchitis. *Lancet* 1963; ii:1247–8.
64. GUMP DW, PHILLIPS CA, FORSYTH BR. Role of infection in chronic bronchitis. *Am Rev Resp Dis* 1976; 117:465–74.
65. ISADA CM. Pro: antibiotics for chronic bronchitis with exacerbations. *Semin Resp Infect* 1993; 8:243–53.
66. HAGEN H, VERGHESE A, ALVAREZ S, BERK SL. *Branhamella catarrhalis* respiratory infections. *Rev Infect Dis* 1987; 9:1140–9.
67. NICOTRA B, RIVERA M, LUMAN J, WALLACE RJ. *Branhamella catarrhalis* as a lower respiratory tract pathogen in patients with chronic lung disease. *Arch Int Med* 1986; 146:890–3.
68. FAGON J, CHASTRE J, TROUILLET J *et al.* Characterisation of distal bronchial micro flora during acute exacerbations of chronic bronchitis. *Am Rev Resp Dis* 1990; 142:1004–8.
69. MEDICI TC. Buergi H. The role of immunoglobulin A in endogenous bronchial defense mechanism in chronic bronchitis. *Am Rev Resp Dis* 1971; 103:784–91.
70. CLARKE CW. Aspects of serum and sputum antibody in chronic airways obstruction. *Thorax* 1976; 31:702–7.
71. SOUTAR CA. Distribution of plasma cells and other cells containing immunoglobulin in the respiratory tract in chronic bronchitis. *Thorax* 1977; 32:387–96.
72. STOCKLEY RA, AFFORD SC, BURNETT D. Assessment of 7S and 11S immunoglobulin in sputum. *Am Rev Resp Dis* 1980; 122:959–64.
73. SAETTA M, STEFANO A, MAESTRELLI P *et al.* Activated T-lymphocytes and macrophages in bronchial mucosa of subjects with chronic bronchitis. *Am Rev Resp Dis.* 1993; 147:301–6.
74. SAETTA M, GHEZZO H, KIM WD *et al.* Loss of alveolar attachments in smokers. A morphometric correlate of lung function impairment. *Am Rev Resp Dis* 1985; 132:894–900.
75. KIM WD, EIDELMAN DH, IZQUIERDO J, GHEZZO H, SAETTA MP, COSIO MG. Centrilobular and panlobular emphysema in smokers. Two distinct morphologic and functional entities. *Am Rev Resp Dis* 1991; 144:1385–90.
76. THOMPSOM AB, RENNARD SI. Assessment of airways inflammation in chronic bronchitis. *Eur Resp J* 1993; 6:461–4.
77. REYNOLDS HY, MENNIL WW. Airway changes in young smokers that may antedate chronic obstructive lung disease. *Med Clin North Am* 1981; 65:667–89.
78. MARTIN TR, RAGHU G. Maunder RJ, Springmeyer SC. The effects of chronic bronchitis and chronic air flow obstruction on lung cell populations recovery by bronchoalveolar lavage. *Am Rev Resp Dis* 1985; 132:254–60.
79. THOMPSON AB, DAUGHTON D, ROBBINS R, GHAFOURI MA, OCHLARKING M, RENNARD SI. Intraluminal airway inflammation in chronic bronchitis: characterization and correlation with clinical parameters. *Am Rev Resp Dis* 1989; 140:1527–37.
80. SPURZEM JR, THOMPSOM AB, DAUGHTON DM, MUELLER M, LINDER J, RENNARD SI. Chronic inflammation is associated with an increased proportion of goblet cells recovered by bronchial lavage. *Chest* 1991; 100:389–93.
81. RENNARD SI, DAUGHTON D, FUJITA J *et al.* Short-term smoking reduction is associated with reduction in measures of lower respiratory tract inflammation in heavy smokers. *Eur Respir J* 1990; 3:752–9.
82. RENNARD S, THOMPSON A, DAUGHTON D *et al.* Theophylline reduces neutrophil recruitment *in vitro* and lowers airway neutrophilia in chronic bronchitis. *Eur Resp J* 1990; 3:116 Abstr.
83. THOMPSON AB, MUELLER MB, HEIRES AJ *et al.* Aerobolized beclomethasone in chronic bronchitis: improved pulmonary function and diminished airway inflammation. *Am Rev Resp Dis* 1992; 146:389–95.
84. MURPHY TF, DUDAS KC, MYLOTTE JM, APICELLA MA. A subtyping system for non-typable *Haemophilus influenzae* based on outer membrane proteins. *J Infect Dis* 1983; 147:838–46.
85. READ RC, WILSON R, RUTMAN A *et al.* Interaction of non-typable *Haemophilus influenzae* with human respiratory mucosa *in vitro*. *J Infect Dis* 1991; 163:549–58.
86. LOEB MR, CONNOR E, PENNY D. A comparison of adherence of fimbriated and nonfimbriated *Haemophilus influenzae* type b to human adenoids in organ culture. *Infect Immun* 1988; 56:484–9.
87. JOHNSON AP, INZANA TJ. Loss of ciliary activity in organ cultures of rat trachea treated with lipo-oligosaccharide from *Haemophilus influenzae*. *J Med Microbiol* 1986; 22:265–8.
88. HAASE EM, CAMPAGNARI AA, SARWAR J *et al.* Strain-specific and immunodominant surface epitopes of the P_2 porin protein of non-typable *H. influenzae*. *Infect Immun* 1991; 59:1278–84.
89. GREEN BA, METCALF BJ, QUINN-DEY T, KIRKLEY DH, QUATAERT SA, DEICH RA. A recombinant non-fatty acylated form of the Hi-Pal (P_6) protein of *H. influenzae* elicits biologically active antibody against both Non-typable and type b *H. influezae*. *Infect Immun* 1990; 58:3275–8.
90. ZWAHLEN A, RUBIN LG, MOXON ER. Contribution of lipo-oligosaccharide to the pathogenicity of *H. influenzae*: comparative virulence of genetically related strains in rats. Microbiol Pathology 1986; 1:465–73.
91. HANZEN MV, MUSHEN MD, BAUGHN RE. Outer membrane proteins of Non-typable *H. influenzae* and reactivity of paired sera from infected patients with their homologous isolates. *Infect Immun* 1985; 47:843–6.
92. CLANCY R, CRIPPS A, MURREE-ALLEN K, YOUNG S, ENGEL M. Oral immunization with killed *H. influenzae* for protection against acute bronchitis in chronic obstruction lung disease. *Lancet* 1985; ii:1395–7.
93. ANDERSSON B, BEACHEY EH, TOMASZ A, TUOMANEN E, SVANBORG-EDEN C. A sandwich adhesin on *Streptococcus pneumoniae* attaching to human oropharyngeal epithelial cells *in vitro*. *Microbiol Pathogen* 1988; 4:267–8.
94. RIESENFELD-ORM I, WOLPE S, GARCIA-BUSTOS JK, HOFFMAN MK, TUOMANEN E. Production of interleukin-1 but not tumour necrosis factor by human monocytes stimulated with pneumococcal cell

surface components. *Infect Immun* 1989; 57:1890–3.

95. CENTERS FOR DISEASE CONTROL. Pneumococcal polysaccharide vaccine. *MMWR* 1989; 38:64–76.

96. SRINIVASAN G, RAFF MJ, TEMPLETON WC, GIVENS SJ, GRAVES RC, MELO JC. *Branhamella catarrhalis* pneumonia. Report of two cases and review of the literature. *Am Rev Resp Dis* 1981; 123:553–5.

97. NICOTRA B, RIVERA M, LUMAN JI, WALLACE RJ JR. *Branhamella catarrhalis* as a lower respiratory tract pathogen in patients with chronic lung disease. *Arch Intern Med* 1986; 146:890–3.

98. CHAPMAN AJ, MUSHER DM, JONSSON S, CLARRIDGE JE, WALLACE RJ JR. Development of bactericidal antibody during *Branhamella catarrhalis* infection. *J Infect Dis* 1985; 151:878–82.

99. AITKEN JM, THORNLEY PE. Isolation of *Branhamella catarrhalis* from sputum and tracheal aspirate. *J Clin Microbiol* 1983; 18:1262–3.

100. WALLACE RJ JR, STEINGRUBE VA, NASH DR *et al.* BRO β-lactamases of *Branhamella catarrhalis* and *Moraxella subgenus Moraxella*, including evidence for chromosomal β-lactamase transfer by conjugation in *B. catarrhalis*. *Antimicrob Agents Chemother* 1989; 33:1845–54.

101. American Thoracic Society. Standards for the diagnosis and care of patients with chronic obstructive pulmonary disease (COPD) and asthma. *Am Rev Resp Dis* 1987; 136:225–44.

102. NICOTRA MB, KRONENBERG RS. Con: antibiotic use in exacerbations of chronic bronchitis. *Semin Respi Infect* 1993; 8:254–8.

103. PINES A, RAAFAT H, GREENFIELD JS *et al.* Antibiotic regimens in moderately ill patients with purulent exacerbations of chronic bronchitis. *Br J Dis Chest* 19175; 66:107–19.

104. ANTHONISEN NR, MANFREDA J, WARREN CP, HERSHFIELD ES, HARDING GK, NELSON SK. Antibiotic therapy in exacerbations of chronic obstructive pulmonary disease. *Ann Intern Med* 1987; 106:196–204.

105. DAVIS AL, GROBOW EJ, TOMPSETT R *et al.* Bacterial infection and some effects of chemoprophylaxis in chronic pulmonary emphysema. I. Chemoprophylaxis with intermittent tetracycline. *Am J Med* 1961; 31:365–81.

106. PINES A. Controlled trials of a sulphonamide given weekly to prevent exacerbations of chronic bronchitis. *Br Med J* 1967; 3:202–4.

107. KOLBE J. An algorithm for the management of COPD. Auckland Medical School Grand Round. June 1991.

108. ANTHONISEN NR, CONNETT JE, KILEY JP *et al.* The Lung Health Study. Effects of smoking intervention and the use of an inhaled anticholinergic bronchodilator on the rate of decline of FEV_1. *JAMA* 1994; 2175:1497–1505.

109. POSTMA DS, RENKEMA TE, KOETER GH. Effects of corticosteroids in chronic obstructive airways disease. *Agents and Actions* Suppl. 1990; 30:41–57.

110. SHIM CS, WILLIAMS MH. Aerosol beclomethasone in patients with steroids responsive chronic obstructive pulmonary disease. *Am J Med* 1985; 78:655–8.

111. COLE P. BRONCHIECTASIS. IN GEDDES, D.M., EDS. BREWIS R.A.L.CORRIN, B.& GIBSON, G.J. *'Respiratory Medicine'*. Ballière-Tindall, 1990: 1756–9.

112. HASSE C.SWAINE WE, trans/ed. *An Original Description of the Diseases of the Organs of Circulation and Respiration*. London: London Sydenham Society; 1846.

113. LAENNEC RTH. *In A Treatise on the Diseases of the Chest and on Mediate Auscultation*, 4th ed. Forbes, J. Translat Br. New York: Wood. 1835.

114. WHITWELL F. A study of the pathology and pathogenesis of bronchiectasis. *Thorax* 1952; 7: 213–39.

115. BROCK RC. Post tuberculous bronchostenosis and bronchiectasis of the middle lobe. *Thorax* 1950; 5: 5–39.

116. CHURCHILL ED. The segmental and lobular physiology and pathology of the lung. *J Thorac Surg* 1949; 18: 279–87.

117. CULLINER MM. Obliterative bronchitis and bronchiolitis with bronchiectasis. *Dis Chest* 1963; 44: 351–61.

118. REID LM. Reduction in bronchial subdivision in bronchiectasis. *Thorax* 1950; 5:233–47.

119. HANSELL DM, WELLS AU, RUBENS MB, COLE PJ. Bronchiectasis: functional significance of areas of decreased attenuation at expiratory CT. *Radiology* 1994; 193: 369–74.

120. LAPA E SILVA JR, JONES JAH, COLE PJ, POULTER LW. The immunological component of the cellular inflammatory infiltrate in bronchiectasis. *Thorax* 1989; 44: 668–73.

121. RICHMAN-EISENSTAT JB, JORENS PG, HEBERT CA, UEKI I, NADEL JA. Interleukin-8: an important chemoattractant in sputum of patients with chronic inflammatory airways diseases. *Am J Physiol* 1993; 264: 413–18.

122. LIEBOW AA, HALES MR, LINDSBERG GE. Enlargement of the bronchial arteries and their anastomoses with pulmonary arteries in bronchiectasis. *Am J Pathol* 1949; 25:211–31.

123. VAN FRAENHOVEN L, WILMS G, VERSCHAKELEN J, PEENE P. Systemic to pulmonary artery shunting. *J Belge Radiol* 1993; 76:373–4.

124. REIFF DB, WELLS AU, CARR DH, COLE PJ, HANSELL DM. CT findings in bronchiectasis:limited value in distinguishing between idiopathic and specific types. *AJR* 1995; 165:261–7.

125. TANNENBERG J, PINNER M. Atelectasis and bronchiectasis: an experimental study concerning their relationship. *J Thorac Surg* 1942; 11:571–616.

126. LAPA E SILVA JR, GUERRIRO D, NOBLE B, POULTER LW, COLE PJ. Immunopathology of experimental bronchiectasis. *Am J Resp Cell Mol Biol* 1989; 1:297–304.

127. LANDAU LI, PHELAN PD, WILLIAMS HE. Ventilatory mechanics in patients with bronchiectasis starting in childhood. *Thorax* 1974; 29:304–12.

128. BECROFT DMO. Bronchiolitis obliterans, bronchiectasis, and other sequelae of *adenovirus* type 21 infection in young children. *J Clin Pathol* 1971; 24:175–82.

129. NIEWOEHNER DE, KLEINERMAN J, RICE DB. There is a chronic inflammatory process present in the peripheral airways of all young smokers. *N Engl J Med* 1974; 291:775–7.

130. PAGTAKHAN RD, REED MH, CHERNICK V. Is Bronchiolitis in infancy an antecedent of chronic lung disease in adolescence and adulthood? *J Thorac Imag* 1986; 1:34–40.

131. THURLBECK WM. Chronic airflow obstruction. In Thurlbeck WM, ed. *Pathology of the Lung*. New York, NY: Thieme, 1988; 519–75.

132. BASS H, HENDERSON JAM, HECKSCHER T, ORIOL A, ANTHONISEN NR. Regional structure and function in bronchiectasis. *Am Rev Resp Dis* 1968; 97:598–609.

133. MELLINS RB. The site of airway obstruction in cystic fibrosis. *Pediatrics* 1969; 44:315–18.

134. PANG J, CHAN HS, SUNG JY. Prevalence of asthma, atopy and bronchial; hyperreactivity in bronchiectasis: a controlled study. *Thorax* 1989; 44:948–51.

135. MURPHY MB, REEN DJ, FITZGERALD MX. Atopy, immunological changes, and respiratory function in bronchiectasis. *Thorax* 1984; 39:179–84.

136. VARPELA E, LAITINEN LA, KESKINEN H, KORHOLA O. Asthma, allergy and bronchial hyperreactivity to histamine in patients with bronchiectasis. *Clin Allerg* 197; 8:273–80.

137. IP MS, SO SY, LAM WK, YAM L, LIONG E. High prevalence of asthma in patients with bronchiectasis in Hong Kong. *Eur Respir J* 1992; 5:418–23.

138. HOGG JC. Bronchiolitis in asthma and chronic obstructive airways pulmonary disease. *Clin Chest Med* 1993; 14:733–40.

139. GUDBJERG CE. Roentgenologic diagnosis of bronchiectasis: an analysis of 122 cases. *Acta Radiol* 1955; 43:209–26.

140. GUEST PJ, HANSELL DM. High resolution computed tomography in emphysema associated with alpha-1-antitrypsin deficiency. *Clin Radiol* 1992; 45:260–6.

141. GELB AF, ZAMEL N. Simplified diagnosis of small-airway obstruction. *N Engl J Med* 1973; 288:395–8.

142. COLE PJ. Host-microbial interactions in chronic respiratory disease. In Reeves D and Geddes A, Eds. *Recent Advances in Infection* 3. Edinburgh: Churchill Livingstone; 1989.

143. ELLIS DA, THORNLEY PE, WIGHTMAN AJ, WALKER M, CHALMERS J, CROFTON JW. Present outlook in bronchiectasis: clinical and social study and review of factors influencing prognosis. *Thorax* 1981; 36:659–64.

144. COLE PJ, A new look at the pathogenesis and management of persistent bronchial sepsis: a vicious circle hypothesis and its logical therapeutic connotations. In Davies RJ, ed. *Strategies for the Management of Chronic Bronchial Sepsis*. Oxford: The Medicine Publishing Foundation; 1984.

145. WILSON R, ROBERTS D AND COLE PJ. Effect of bacterial products on human ciliary function *in vitro*. *Thorax* 1985; 40:129–31.

146. ADLER KB, HINDLEY DD, DAVIS GS. Bacteria associated with obstructive pulmonary disease elaborate extracellular products that stimulate secretion by explants of guinea-pig airways. *Am J Pathol* 1986; 129:501–14.

147. SOMERVILLE M, RICHARDSON PS, TAYLOR GW, WILSON RW, COLE PJ. Chloroform extract of *Pseudomonas aeruginosa* stimulates mucus output into cat trachea *in vivo*. *Am Rev Resp Dis* 1988; 137:A1175.

148. HASANI A, PAVIA D, AGNEW JE, CLARKE SW. Regional lung clearance during cough and forced expiration technique (FET): effects of flow and viscoelasticity. *Thorax* 1994; 49:557–61.

149. RAS G, WILSON R, TODD H, COLE PJ. In vitro chemotactic effect of bacterial products on neutrophils in chronic bronchial sepsis. *Am Rev Resp Dis* 1988; 137:A171.

150. CURRIE DC, SAVERYMUTTU SH, PETERS AM *et al.* Indium-111-labelled granulocyte accumulation in respiratory tract of patients with bronchiectasis. *Lancet* 1987; i:1335–9.

151. SMALLMAN LA, HILL SL, STOCKLEY RA. Reduction of ciliary beat frequency *in vitro* by sputum from patients with bronchiectasis; a serine proteinase effect. *Thorax* 1984; 39:663–7.

152. SYKES DA, WILSON R, GREENSTONE M, CURRIE DC, STEINFORT C, COLE PJ. Deleterious effects of purulent sputum sol on human ciliary function *in vitro*; at least two factors identified. *Thorax* 1987; 42:256–61.

153. PERRY KMA, KING DS. Bronchiectasis: a study of prognosis based on a follow-up of 400 patients. *Am Rev Resp Dis* 1940; 41: 531–48.

154. DAVIS AL, Bronchiectasis. In Fishman AP ed. *Pulmonary Diseases and Disorders*. New York: McGraw-Hill; 1980:1209–19.

155. FIELD CE. Bronchiectasis. Third report on a follow-up study of medical and surgical cases from childhood. *Arch Dis Child* 1969; 44:551–61.

156. KONIETZKO NFJ, CARTON RW, LEROY EP. Causes of death in patients with bronchiectasis. *Am Rev Resp Dis* 1969; 100:852–8.

157. SANDERSON JM, KENNEDY MCS, JOHNSON MF, MANLEY DCE. Bronchiectasis: results of surgical and conservative management. *Thorax* 1974; 29:407–16.

158. WYNNE-WILLIAMS N. Bronchiectasis: a study centred on Bedford and its environs. *Br Med J* 1953; i:1194–9.

159. MCCLELLAN V, GARRETT J. Appointment-keeping behaviour of Middlemore Hospital's outpatient Asthma Clinic. *NZ Med J* 1989; 102:211–13.

160. MURRAY JF, NADEL JA. *Textbook of Respiratory Medicine*. Philadelphia: WB Saunders Co; 1988:1109.

161. O'NEILL M, KOLBE J, WELLS AU. Bronchiectasis in New Zealand: a dying disease or a neglected epidemic? *Am J Resp Crit Care Med* 1995; 151:A201.

162. WAKEFIELD ST J, WAITE D. Abnormal cilia in Polynesians with bronchiectasis. *Am Rev Resp Dis* 1980; 129:1003–9.

163. GIBSON K. Respiratory disease in minorities: issues of access, race and ethnicity. *Am J Resp Crit Care Med* 1994; 149:570–1.

164. WELLS AU. Tuberculosis in New Zealand Maoris. In AJ Proust ed. '*History of Tuberculosis in Australia, New Zealand and Papua New Guinea*'. Curtin: Brolga Press; 1991: 97–102.

165. LINDSKOG GE, GUBBELL DS. An analysis of 215 cases of bronchiectasis. *Surg Gynecol Obstet* 1955; 100:643–50.

166. STRANG C. The fate of children with bronchiectasis. *Ann Intern Med* 1956; 44:630–56.

167. LEES AW. Atelectasis and bronchiectasis in pertussis. *Br Med J* 1950; 2:1178–41.

168. SIMILA S, LININA O, LANNING P, HEIKKINEN E, ALA-HOUHALA M. Chronic lung damage caused by *adenovirus* Type 7: a ten-year follow-up study. *Chest* 1981; 80:127–31.

169. WHYTE KF, WILLIAMS GR. Bronchiectasis after *mycoplasma pneumonia*. *Thorax* 1984; 39:390–1.

170. WOOD RE, WANNER A, HIRSCH J, FARRELL PM. Tracheal mucociliary transport in patients with cystic fibrosis and its stimulation by terbutaline. *Am Rev Resp Dis* 1975; 111:733–41.

171. HANSELL DM, STRICKLAND B. High resolution computed tomography in pulmonary cystic fibrosis. *Br J Radiol* 1989; 62:1–5.

172. SANTIS G. HODSON ME, STRICKLAND B. High resolution computed tomography in adult cystic fibrosis patients with mild lung disease. *Clin Radiol* 1991; 44:20–2.

173. BHALLA M, TURCIOS N, APONTE V *et al.* Cystic fibrosis: scoring system with thin-section CT. *Radiology* 1991; 179:783–8.

174. JACKSON LE, HOUSTON S, HABBICK BF, GENEREUX S, HOWIE JL. Cystic fibrosis: a comparison of computed tomography and plain chest radiographs. *J Can Assoc Radiol* 1986; 37:17–21.

175. GREENSTONE M, RUTMAN A, DEWAR A, MACKAY I, COLE PJ. Primary ciliary dyskinesia: cytological and clinical features. *Quart J Med* 1988; 67:405–523.

176. FRASER RG, PARE JAP, PARE PD, FRASER RS, GENERAUX GP. Diagnosis of diseases of the chest, 3rd ed. Philadelphia: WB Saunders Co; 1990:2186–20.

177. NADEL HR, STRINGER DA, LEVISON H, TURNER JAP, STURGESS JM. The immotile cilia syndrome: radiological manifestations. *Radiology* 1985; 154:651–5.

178. BELOVSKA A. Pulmonary sequestration: a report of an unusual case and a review of the literature. *Thorax* 1967; 22:351–7.

179. WILLIAMS H, CAMPBELL P. Generalised bronchiectasis associated with deficiency of cartilage in the bronchial tree. *Arch Dis Child* 1960; 35:182–91.

180. WOODRING JH, HOWARD RS, REHM SR. Congenital tracheobronchomegaly (Mounier–Kuhn syndrome): a report of 10 cases and review of the literature. *J Thorac Imaging* 1991; 6(2):1–10.

181. DULPHANO MJ, LUK CK. Sputum and ciliary inhibition in asthma. *Thorax* 1982; 37:646–51.

182. WILSON R, ALTON E, RUTMAN A *et al.* Upper respiratory tract viral infection and mucocilliary clearance. *Eur J Resp Dis* 1987; 70:2175–9.

183. WILSON R, COLE PJ. The effect of bacterial products on ciliary function. *Am Rev Resp Dis* 1988; 138:S49.

184. BALLENGER JJ. Experimental effect of cigarette smoke on human respiratory cilia. *N Engl J Med* 1960; 263:832–5.

185. YOUNG D. Surgical treatment of male infertility. *J Reprod Infertil* 1970; 23:541–2.

186. HENDRY WF, A'HERN RP, COLE PJ. Was Young's syndrome caused by exposure to mercy in childhood? *BMJ* 1993; 307:1579–82.

187. HENDRY WF, KNIGHT RK, WHITFIELD HN *et al.* Obstructive azoospermia: respiratory function tests, electron microscopy and results of surgery. *Br J Urol* 1978; 50:598–604.

188. HANDELSMAN DFJ, CONWAY AJ, BOYLAN LM, TURTLE JR. Young's syndrome: obstructive azoospermia and chronic sinopulmonary infections. *N Engl Med J* 1984; 310:3–9.

189. UMETSU DT, AMBROSINO DM, OUNTI I, SIBER GR, GEHA RS. Recurrent sino-pulmonary infection and impaired antibody response to bacterial capsular polysaccharide antigen in children with selective IgG-subclass deficiency. *N Engl Med J* 1985; 313: 47–1291.

190. DUKES RJ, ROSENOW EC, HERMANS PE. Pulmonary manifestations of hypogamma-globulinaemia. *Thorax* 1978; 33:603–7.

191. CURTIN JJ, WEBSTER ADB, FARRANT J, KATZ D. Bronchiectasis in hypogamma-globulinaemia – a computed tomography assessment. *Clin Radiol* 1991; 44:82–4.

192. NEELD DA, GOODMAN LR, GURNEY JW, GREENBURGER PA, FINK JN. Computed tomography in the evaluation of allergic bronchopulmonary aspergillosis. *Am Rev Resp Dis* 1990; 142:1200–5.

193. GREENBERGER PA. Allergic bronchopulmonary aspergillosis and fungoses. *Clin Chest Med* 1988; 9:599–608.

194. PANCHAL N, PANT C, BHAGAT R, SHAH A. Central bronchiectasis in allergic bronchopulmonary aspergillosis: comparative evaluation of computed tomography with bronchography. *Eur Resp J* 1994; 7:1290–3.

195. CURRIE DC, GOLDMAN JM, COLE PJ, STRICKLAND B. Comparison of narrow section computed tomography and plain chest radiography in chronic allergic bronchopulmonary aspergillosis. *Clin Radiol* 1987; 38:593–6.

196. KASS I, ZAMEL N, DOBRY CA, HOLZER M. Bronchiectasis following ammonia burns of the respiratory tract. A review of two cases. *Chest* 19175; 62:282–5.

197. MACKAY IS, COLE PJ. Rhinitis, sinusitis and associated chest disease. In Mackay IS, Bull TR, eds. R*hinology Vol 4, Scott-Brown's Otolaryngology*, 5th ed. London: Butterworths, 1987.

198. SOLANKI T, NEVILLE E. Bronchiectasis and rheumatoid disease: is there an association? *Br J Rheumatol* 1992; 31:691–3.

199. BAMJI A, COOKE N. Rheumatoid arthritis and chronic bronchial suppuration. *Scand J Rheumatol* 1985; 114:15–21.

200. MCMAHON MJ, SWINSON DR, SHETTAR S *et al.* Bronchiectasis and rheumatoid arthritis: a clinical study. *Ann Rheum Dis* 1993; 52:776–9.

201. SHADICK NA, FANTA CH, WEINBLATT ME, O'CONNELL W, COBLYN JS. Bronchiectasis: a late feature of severe rheumatoid arthritis. *Medicine (Baltimore)* 1994; 73:161–70.

202. FAIRFAX AJ, HASLAM PL, PAVIA D *et al.* Pulmonary disorders associated with Sjogren's syndrome. *Quart J Med* 1981; 50:279–95.

203. CLAUSE HP, SANGER PW, TAYLOR FH, ROBICSEK F. Systemic lupus erythematosus associated with bronchiectasis. *Dis Chest* 1964; 45:219–24.

204. FORTOUL TI, CANO-VALLE F, OLIVA E *et al.* Follicular bronchiolitis in association with connective tissue diseases. *Lung* 1985; 163:305–14.

205. BUTLAND RJA, COLE PJ, CITRON KM, TURNER-WARWICK M. Chronic bronchial suppuration and inflammatory bowel disease. *Quart J Med* 1981; 50:63–75.

206. GARG K, LYNCH DA, NEWELL JD. Inflammatory airways disease in ulcerative colitis: CT and high-resolution CT feature. *J Thorac Imaging* 1993; 8:159–63.

207. KEARNEY PJ, KERSHAW CR, STEVENSON PA, Bronchiectasis in acute leukaemia. *Br Med J* 1977; 2:857–9.

208. HILLER E, ROSENOW EC III, OLSSEN AM. Pulmonary manifestations of the yellow nail syndrome. *Chest* 1975; 61;452–8.

209. LONGSTRETCH GF, WEITZMAN SA, BROWING RJ, LIEBERMAN J. Bronchiectasis and homozygous alpha-1-antitrypsin deficiency. *Chest* 1975; 67:233–5.

210. JONES DK, GODDEN D, CAVANAGH P. Alpha-1-antitrypsin deficiency presenting as bronchiectasis. *Br J Dis Chest* 1985; 79:301–4.

211. PHUNG ND, KUBO RT, SPECTOR SL. Alpha-1-antitrypsin deficiency and common variable hypogammaglobulinaemia in a patient with asthma. *Chest* 1982; 81:116–19.

212. BARTH J, WINKLER I, SCHMIDT EW, BRAUN BE, MOLLMANN HW, SKVARII F. IgG-subklassenverteilung im serum von patienten mit homozygotem a1-antitrypsinmangel. *Pneumologie* 1990; 44:561–2.

213. COX DW, MARKOVIC VD, TESHIMA IE. Genes for immunoglobulin heavy chains and for a1-antitrypsin are localised to specific regions of chromosome 14q. *Nature* 1982; 297:428–30.

214. STEINFORT CL, TODD H, HIGGS E, COLE PJ. Bacteriology of daily purulent sputum. *Thorax* 1987; 42:235.

215. ROBERTS DE, COLE PJ. Use of selective media in bacteriological investigation of patients with chronic suppurative respiratory infection. *Lancet* 1980; i:796–7.

216. WELLS AU, DESAI S, WETTON C, WILSON R, COLE PJ. The isolation of *Pseudomonas aeruginosa* from sputum in idiopathic bronchiectasis: an association with extensive disease and severe airflow obstruction. *Am Rev Resp Dis* 1993; 147: A645.

217. NAGAKI M, SHIMURA S, TANNO Y, ISHIBASHI T, SASAKI H, TAKISHIMA T. Role of chronic *Pseudomonas aeruginosa* infection in the development of bronchiectasis. *Chest* 1992; 102:1464–9.

218. CHAN CH, HO AK, CHAN RC, CHEUNG H, CHENG AK. Mycobacteria as a cause of infective exacerbation in bronchiectasis. *Postgrad Med J* 1992; 68:896–9.

219. CHERNIACK NS, CARTON RW. Factors associated with respiratory insufficiency in bronchiectasis. *Am J Med* 1966; 41:564–71.

220. WONG-YOU-CHEONG JJ, LEAHY BC, TAYLOR PM, CHURCH SE. Airways obstruction and bronchiectasis: correlation with duration of symptoms and extent of bronchiectasis on computed tomography. *Clin Radiol* 1992; 45:256–9.

221. PANDE JN, JAIN BP, GUPTA RG, GULERIA JS. Pulmonary ventilation and gas exchange in bronchiectasis. *Thorax* 1971; 26:727–33.

222. COCHRANE M, WEBBER BA, CLARKE SW. Effects of sputum on pulmonary function. *BMJ* 1977; 2:1181–3.

223. CURRIE DC, COOKE JC, MORGAN DA *et al.* Interpretation of bronchograms and chest radiographs in patients with chronic sputum production. *Thorax* 1987; 42:278–84.

224. COOKE JC, CURRIE DC, MORGAN AD *et al.* Role of computed tomography in diagnosis of bronchiectasis. *Thorax* 1987; 42:272–7.

225. SILVERMAN PM, GODWIN JD. CT/bronchgraphic correlations in bronchiectasis. *J Comput Assist Tomogr* 1987; 11:52–6.

226. GRENIER P, MAURICE F, MUSSET D *et al.* Bronchiectasis: assessment by thin-section CT. *Radiology* 1986; 161:95–9.

227. JOHARJY JA, BASHI SA, ABDULLAH AK. Value of medium thickness CT in the diagnosis of bronchiectasis. *AJR* 1987; 149:1173–7.

228. ZWIREWICH CV, MAYO JR, MULLER NL. Low dose high resolution CT of lung parenchyma. *Radiology* 1991; 180:413–17.

229. LYNCH DA, NEWELL JD, TSCHOMPER BA, CLINK TM, NEWMAN LS, BETHEL R. Uncomplicated asthma in adults: comparison of

CT appearances of the lungs in asthmatic and healthy subjects. *Radiology* 1993; 188:829–33.

230. MURATA K, ITOH H, TODO G *et al.* Centrilobular lesions of the lung: demonstration by high resolution CT and pathologic correlation. *Radiology* 1986; 161:641–5.

231. WEBB WR, STEIN MG, FINKBEINER WE, IM JG, LYNCH D, GAMSU G. Normal and diseased isolated lungs; high resolution CT. *Radiology* 1988; 166:81–7.

232. HANSELL DM. High resolution computed tomography of the lungs. In Armstrong P, Wilson AG, Dee P, Hansell DM, eds. '*Imaging of Disease of the Chest*', 2nd ed.St Louis: Mosby; 1995:141–2.

233. CURRIE DC, MUNRO C, GASKELL D, COLE PJ. Practice, problems and compliance with postural drainage: a survey of chronic sputum producers. *Br J Dis Chest* 1986; 80:249–53.

234. CURRIE DC, GARBETT NS, CHAN KL *et al.* Double-blind randomised study of prolonged higher-dose oral amoxycillin in purulent bronchiectasis. *Quart J Med* 1990; 76:799–816.

235. CURRIE DC, HIGGS E, METCALFE S, ROBERTS DE, COLE PJ. Simple method of monitoring microbial load in chronic bronchial sepsis: pilot comparison of reduction in colonising microbial load with antibiotics given intermittently and continuously. *J Clin Pathol* 1987; 40:830–6.

236. STOCKLEY RA, HILL SL, MORRISON HM. Effect of antibiotic treatment on sputum elastase in bronchiectatic outpatients in a stable clinical state. *Thorax* 1984; 39:414–19.

237. HILL SL, STOCKLEY RA. The effect of short and long term antibiotic response on lung function in bronchiectasis. *Thorax* 1986; 41:798–800.

238. COLE PJ, ROBERTS DE, DAVIES SF, KNIGHT RK. A simple oral antimicrobial regimen effective in severe chronic bronchial suppuration associated with culturable *Haemophilus influenzae*. *J Antimicrob Chemother* 1983; 11:109–17.

239. BALDWIN DR, HONEYBOURNE D, WISE R. Pulmonary deposition of antimicrobial agents: methodological considerations. *Antimicrob Agents Chemother* 1992; 36:1171–5.

240. HODSON ME, PENKETH AR, NATTEM KC. Aerosol carbenicillin and gentamicin treatment of *Pseudomonas aeruginosa* infection in patients with cystic fibrosis. *Lancet* 1981; ii:1137–9.

241. AUERBACH HS, WILLIAMS M, KIRKPATRICK JA, COLTEN HR. Alternate-day prednisolone reduces morbidity and improves pulmonary function in cystic fibrosis. *Lancet* 1985; ii:686–7.

242. ELBORN JS, JOHNSTON B, ALLEN F, CLARKE J, MCGARRY J, VARGHESE G. Inhaled steroids in patients with bronchiectasis. *Resp Med* 1992; 86:121–4.

243. KHARITONOX S, WELLS AU, O'CONNOR B *et al.* Elevated levels of exhaled nitric oxide in bronchiectasis. *Am J Resp Crit Care Med* 1995; 151:1889–93.

244. GARBETT ND, CURRIE DC, COLE PJ. Comparison of the clinical efficacy and safety of an intramuscular and an intravenous immunoglobulin preparation for replacement therapy in idiopathic adult onset panhypogammaglobulinaemia. *Clin Exp Immunol* 1989; 76:1–7.

245. JAIN NK, GUPTA KN, SHARMA TN, GARG VK, AGNIHOTRI SP. Airway obstruction in bronchiectasis and its reversibility. *Ind J Chest Dis Allied Sci* 1992; 34:7–10.

246. OLIVIERI D, CIACCIA A, MARANGIO E, MARSICO S, TODISCO T, DEL-VITA M. Role of bromhexine in exacerbations of bronchiectasis: double-blind randomized multicenter study versus placebo. *Respiration* 1991; 58:117–29.

247. CONWAY JH, FLEMING JS, PERRING S, HOLGATE ST. Humidification as an adjunct to chest physiotherapy in aiding tracheo-bronchial clearance in patients with bronchiectasis. *Resp Med* 1992; 86:109–14.

248. CREMASCHI P, NASCIMBENE C, VITULO P *et al.* Therapeutic embolization of bronchial artery: a successful treatment in 209 cases of relapse haemoptysis. *Angiology* 1993; 44:295–9.

249. GUDBJERG CE. Radiological diagnosis of bronchiectasis and prognosis after operative treatment. *Acta Radiol* 1957; suppl 143.

250. CLARK NS. Bronchiectasis in childhood. *Br Med J* 1963; 1:80–8.

251. BORRIE J, LICHTER I. Surgical treatment of bronchiectasis: ten year survey. *Br Med J* 1965; 2:908–12.

252. ETIENNE T, SPILIOPOULOS A, MEGEVAND R. Bronchiectasis and timing for surgery. *Ann Chir* 1993; 47:729–35.

253. THEVENET F, GAMONDES JP, CORDIER JF *et al.* Surgery for bronchiectasis: operative indications and results – 48 observations. *Rev Mal Resp* 1993; 10:245–50.

254. COHEN AJ, ROIFMAN C, BRENDAN J *et al.* Localised pulmonary resection for bronchiectasis in hypogammaglobulinaemic patients. *Thorax* 1994; 49:509–10.

255. LEE-LANDER FP. Bronchiectasis. *Br Med J* 1950; 2:1486–8.

30 Miscellaneous agents of pneumonia and lower respiratory tract infections

MICHAEL E. ELLIS

King Faisal Specialist Hospital and Research Centre, Riyadh, Saudi Arabia

This chapter is devoted to the presentation of pneumonia and lower respiratory tract infections due to various unusual, newly recognised, rarely described or changing presentations of previously recognised pathogens.

STREPTOCOCCAL (OTHER THAN *Streptococcus pneumoniae*) PNEUMONIA

In excess of 30 species belong to the *Streptococcus* genus. Blood agar haemolysis patterns, biochemical reactions, growth and morphological characterisation and genetic analysis are used to classify them. Streptococci showing a β-haemolytic pattern (and some with α haemolysis and γ (non-haemolysis) patterns) can be sero grouped – mainly A, B, C, D and G. The group D streptococci are now divided and regrouped into the enterococci and non-enterococci. Viridans streptococci are a heterogenous α haemolytical group. This section deals with pneumonia produced by streptococci other than *S. pneumoniae*. Although relatively uncommon, striking epidemiological and clinical changes are having important impacts on patient management.

Group A β haemolytic streptococcal pneumonia

Much concern and attention has been focused on the resurgence of severe life-threatening group A β haemolytic *Streptococcus* infections (GAS) in recent years. Invasive GAS are not new – necrotising fasciitis, pueperal fever, scarlet fever, and pneumonia have been known for centuries. Up to 5% of all cases of pneumonia in the UK were due to GAS in the preantibiotic era. Improved socioeconomic circumstances and infection control policies were associated with dramatic falls in GAS infections in the first half of this century. The introduction of sulphonamides and penicillin had a smaller impact on the death rate. However, from the mid 1980s onwards, there has been a reversal of this state of affairs. A focal outbreak of acute rheumatic fever in Salt Lake City, Utah was one of the earliest heralded phenomena[1]. Following reports of increased occurrence of non-suppurative sequelae of GAS infections, severe suppurative invasive disease including pneumonia was described from Europe and North America. Thus the proportion of GAS in published cases of bacteraemia has increased in the last 10 years and case reports have suddenly increased[2–4]. In one study from Norway, there has been a tenfold increase in age specific GAS bacteraemia in the 4 years from 1986[3–5]. Normally less than ten reports per year of GAS necrotising fasciitis would be reported in England and Wales, but within the first 6 months of 1994, 25 cases had been notified[6,7]. GAS infections may be fulminant, many occurring in younger patients who have no predisposition.

In a recent review of severe invasive GAS in Ontario over a recent 5-year period, 9/50 cases had a respiratory tract focus of which six were lower respiratory tract infections (pneumonia, empyema, mediastinitis)[8]. Estimates of the frequency of involvement of the respiratory tract/occurrence of pneumonia in patients with GAS bacteraemia are around 0–30%[4,9–11]. However, as a cause of either community acquired or hospital acquired pneumonia in general, GAS is uncommon.

GAS are Gram-positive facultatively anaerobic paired/short-chained cocci. The somatic M protein conveys virulence – its major property is antiphagocytic and hence permits invasiveness. Absence of circulatory or mucosal antibodies to the M protein leads to local infection and risk of bacteraemia. The second most important microbe determinants are three streptococcal pyogenic exotoxins (SPE: A,B, and C), particularly SPE-A. The SPE-A gene is present in the majority of isolates of GAS in severe disease[12]. SPE results in fever, tissue destruction, destruction of alveolar capillary and blood brain barriers and multiorgan failure, mediated through cytokine recruitment which includes interleukin-1 B, interleukin-6 and TNFα. Direct stimulation of T-helper cells may occur through direct binding to class II major histocompatibility complexes of antigen presenting cells and Vβ region of the T cell receptor through a 'superantigen' effect of SPE-A or M proteins. SPE-B is cytotoxic against heart and other tissues. Bacteraemia produced by a non-SPE producing strain is proposed to be mild and self-limiting. Bacteraemia caused by an SPE producing strain may be severe – presence of pre-existing host antibodies will result in severe clinical disease with shock (rare), DIC and death in those individuals who are predisposed by their disability, immunocompromisation or extremes of age. Absence of pre-existing SPE antibody will allow more severe disease more often – with shock (common), toxic shock-like syndrome, myocardial failure, necrotising fasciitis and death in all groups and irrespective of background immune status[13].

M types 1 and 3 (and to a lesser extent 12, 18, and 28) predominate in the toxic shock-like syndrome patients and the majority of these strains contain the SPE-A gene. Production of the toxin occurs in just over one-half of these[12,14].

The recent upsurge in severe GAS infections is postulated to have arisen because of a relative increase in M types 1 and 3 particularly, from 20% of GAS bacteraemias to 80% over the last decade[13], coupled to a low level of host immunity.

Acquisition of GAS infection occurs as a result of either a mechanical breach of the skin through burns, varicella, trauma, intravenous drug abuse or surgical procedures or via the respiratory tract or the female genital tract. Person-to-person transmission is also known to occur. Such reported cases have sometimes documented the development of streptococcal toxic shock-like syndrome in the close contacts of the index case of streptococcal toxic shock-like syndrome, for example, a fire fighter who resuscitated a child[15]. Clusters of invasive GAS infection have also been documented in families, hospital and nursing homes[16]. Outbreaks of GAS pneumonia have been described in the military[17] in long-term care institutions[18] and during viral epidemics due to influenza and measles[19]. However, as a cause of either community-acquired or hospital-acquired pneumonia in general it is uncommon.

Manifestations determined by host immunity and microbial virulence factors include skin infections such as cellulitis, impetigo, erisipelas and necrotising fasciitis, scarlet fever, bacteraemia and streptococcal toxic shock syndrome.

The respiratory tract may be involved in three ways. Direct inhalation acquired pneumonia may follow a viral illness. The classical description of streptococcal pneumonia is among military recruits[17]. Direct suppurative extension to the mediastinum and parenchymal lung tissue may occur in septic scarlet fever. Finally, the lung may be involved as part of the streptococcal toxic shock-like syndrome with ARDS.

The case definition for streptococcal toxic shock-like syndrome includes hypotension (< 90 mmHg systolic blood pressure) or shock and two of: renal impairment, DIC, disordered liver function, ARDS, erythema ± desquamating rash, soft tissue necrosis, in the presence of GAS isolated from blood or normally sterile sites (= definite toxic shock-like syndrome) or from normally non-sterile sites (= probable toxic shock-like syndrome)[20]. Prodromal influenza-like features often lead to an initial erroneous diagnosis. Common clinical features include severe pain at the site of infection, often abrupt in onset, fever, confusion, together with cutaneous signs if the skin is the portal of entry. Hypocalcaemia, raised creatinine kinase, disordered liver function, hypoalbuminaemia, lymphopenia have been described in association with this syndrome[8].

Clinical features of GAS pneumonia include sudden onset of high fever and chills, pleuritic chest pain, cough, productive of sputum and dyspnoea. The rapid accumulation of pleural fluid in 80% of patients is said to be typical of GAS[21]. Non-specific features include nausea, vomiting, diarrhoea and abdominal pain[11]. Bacteraemia occurs in between 2 and 12% of cases and carries with it an increased mortality risk[22]. There may be additional complicating features including shock, rash, DIC and multiorgan failure including ARDS. An identifiable portal of entry is often absent. When it is apparent, the throat is often the source[17,23]. Alternatively, a cutaneous source may be present[24]. In the latter instance, haemorrhagic or bullous skin rash is highly suggestive (Fig. 30.1).

Empyema (40% of cases) and less commonly abscess formation (< 5%) have been described[11,22,25]. Radiographical features include bronchopneumonic changes and lobar consolidation which may be necrotising. Underlying conditions may be present including corticosteroid treatment, malignancy, immunosuppression, diabetes mellitus, alcoholism and intravenous drug abuse. However, in recent years there has been an increasing proportion of individuals with severe invasive GAS having no predisposing conditions.

The prognosis is guarded. GAS bacteraemia in general carries a mortality rate of around 20–25%[11], although some other series report mortalities of over 50%[8]. Shock, increased age, pneumonia, absence of a leukocyte response, hyperbilirubinaemia are poor prognostic indicators.

Management involves appropriate antimicrobials, intensive care, and surgical resection of accessible foci such as amputation in the case of necrotising fasciitis. Although the organism is still highly susceptible to penicillin, treatment failures have been documented. This may be due to large inoculum sizes, associated with slow growth rates, hence reducing therapeutic efficacy of cell wall acting antibiotics such as penicillins[26]. For this reason, the use of protein synthesis inhibiting antibiotics such as clindamycin or erythromycin have been preferred in cases of GAS pneumonia to reduce M protein synthesis or toxin production[27]. Failure of antimicrobial penetration into relatively avascular or oedematous infective foci is undoubtedly an additional

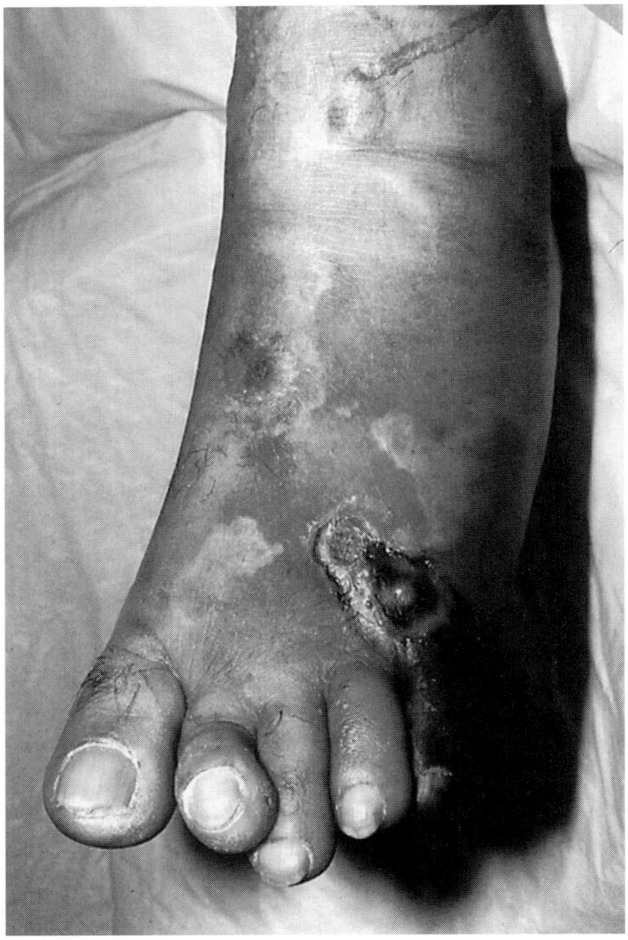

FIGURE 30.1 GAS with haemorrhagic skin changes.

factor. Thus, surgical debridement, fasciotomy or amputation as appropriate should be performed without hesitation. Hyperbaric oxygen therapy, if available, may be employed as adjunctive therapy. For patients with cutaneous foci this is advocated on the basis of its antimicrobial effect, ability to reverse critical tissue organ hypoxia and apparent good effect in other severe necrotising infections. Although it is a controversial issue with no prospective human controlled studies in this area, there is anecdotal and other literature support[28].

Case

A patient with GAS, toxic shock-like syndrome, primary focus foot (Fig.30.1) with ARDS and pneumonia. He remained febrile, toxic, despite below knee amputation and antimicrobials. Further new blisters appeared post-op. Following three dives HBO 2 atm × 2 h – patient became afebrile, need for inotropic support was curtailed and blisters resolved. Patient recovered.

Group B streptococcal respiratory infections

Group B streptococcal (GBS) infections are responsible for the majority of cases of neonatal sepsis, including meningitis, and for much of the bacterial-related disease of pregnancy. Formerly, it appeared that GBS largely targeted these groups of patients. However, evidence has emerged that GBS disease currently involves a third group of individuals – non-pregnant adults. This is reflected in a 2-year prospective bacteraemia/meningitis surveillance project in eight metropolitan Atlanta counties[29]. Although 67% of 424 patients with invasive GBS disease occurred in traditional target groups, 33% occurred in non-pregnant adults. The annual incidence of 4.4/100 000 population had doubled compared to a retrospective study 6 years previously. Although soft tissue, bacteraemias of unknown source or urinary tract infections accounted for the majority of infection, pneumonia occurred in 9%[29]. The incidence of pneumonia was, however, higher among 28 non-pregnant adults with GBS bacteraemia presenting to a large community hospital in whom 18% had pneumonia[30]. The incidence of pneumonia or tracheobronchitis was 44% in another series[31]. However, as an overall cause of pneumonia it appears to be rare with only 13 well-identified cases being reported up to 1982[32]. Between 17% and 90% of cases appear to be nosocomial acquired[29,30,32].

GBS are Gram-positive β haemolytic facultative diplococci. Although absence of or low levels of pre-existing capsular type specific antibodies appear to predispose to neonatal/maternal sepsis, this has not been addressed in non-pregnant adults. GBS have a propensity for causing extensive necrotising parenchymal lung destruction[32].

The vast majority of patients with GBS pneumonia have at least one serious underlying disease. Diabetes, dementia, cerebral vascular disease, paralysis, renal failure, malignancy (both solid tumour and haematological), liver disease, alcoholism and steroid treatment account for the majority[29,30,31]. Patients with HIV, diabetes mellitus or carcinoma present a 30-fold increased risk for invasive GBS[29]. Many patients with GBS pneumonia are also elderly and debilitated. In one series the average age was 73 years[32]. However, the age range is wide 18–99 years[29]. Concomitant urinary tract infection/wound infection are not usually found, suggesting that the portal entry is the oropharynx[32].

GBS infections, in general, are often part of a polymicrobial picture in 15% to 70% of patients[29,30,32], *Staphylococcus aureus*, *Staphylococcus epidermidis*, and a variety of Gram-negative rods being particularly common[29].

The clinical setting for GBS pneumonia, therefore, usually involves an elderly individual with significant underlying disease or risk for aspiration. Fever, tachypnoea, tachycardia, hypotension, hypoxia, leukocytosis and anaemia are common[32]. Chest radiology usually shows bilateral infiltrates. The mortality rate, in general, is high but varies between 30% and 85%[30,32] and in some patients, for example, those with advanced carcinoma GBS pneumonia is a contributory rather than primary cause of death.

The treatment of choice is usually high dose (12 Mu/day) intravenous benzyl penicillin. Alternatives include ceftriaxone. Resistance to erythromycin or clindamycin may be encountered. Antimicrobial treatment may need to be modified in the light of response or presence of other pathogens.

Group C streptococcal respiratory tract infections

Group C streptocci (GCS) include four species and commonly cause a wide range of domestic animal disease including pneumonia, mastitis, septicaemia and arthritis. *Streptococcus equisimilis* and *Streptococcus zooepidemicus* causes pneumonia. In horses, *S. equisimilis* is responsible for the respiratory infection ‘strangles’. Although GCS can be found in the human pharynx, gastrointestinal, and genitourinary tracts where it is regarded as part of the normal flora, at least 88 cases of human disease have been described[33]. *S. equisimilis* and *S. zooepidemicus* are the commonest identifiable but two-thirds are not speciated[33]. Endocarditis, bacteraemia and meningitis account for 60% of cases. Pneumonia, sinusitis, pharyngitis or epiglottitis are found in 9%. Association of GCS pneumonia with *Eikenella corrodens* has been described[34,35]. An underlying condition is present in 74% of patients and includes cardiovascular disease, haematological/solid organ malignancy, immunosuppression and substance abuse in two-thirds of patients. The pharynx is the portal of entry for one-fifth of cases and a history of exposure to animals or animal products may be found in a quarter of patients.

Only relatively few of the infections have been pneumonic in presentation and in some cases where is an association with *E. corrodens*[33–37] a concise clinical description is not possible. Acquisition seems to be community acquired. The onset of pneumonia appears to be sudden and the course protacted or severe[36,37]. Mortality for GCS infections in general is high (25%) particularly in older patients with significant underlying illnesses[33]. Antimicrobial susceptibility includes penicillins, cephalosporins and vancomycin. It is not clear whether *in vitro* penicillin tolerance exists.

Group G streptococcal respiratory infections

The group G streptococci (GGS) account for 8% of all blood culture isolates of β haemolytic and group D streptococci[38] and this quantitative contribution appears to have remained constant for two decades. Underlying disease, particularly solid tumour or haematological malignancy is found in most patients[38,39]. However, it is a moot point whether it is depressed host immunity or anatomical barrier breach which leads to infection, by providing a portal of entry from the skin, vagina, gastrointestinal or upper respiratory tract reservoirs. Community-acquired cutaneous infections and skin focal infection account for approximately two-thirds of all clinical presentations[38]. Other reports have emphasised endovascular infections, particularly endocarditis and septic arthritis[39].

In some reports patients usually older than 50 years are implicated[38,40], whilst others indicate that most patients are less than 50 years[39]. However, this difference probably reflects the different population groups being studied.

Pneumonia accounts for up to 11% of associated GGS bacteraemias[38]. Septic thrombophlebitis with septic pulmonary embolism has been described in the puerperal period[41]. There is little information to comment specifically on the clinical features of pneumonia.

A single drug regimen, which is usually a β-lactam antibiotic, appears to be effective. In general, the immediate outcome for GGS bacteraemia disease is good except for patients with severe focal disease, impaired host resistance, or in some cases of endocarditis[38,40]. In these cases, the persistent septic focus or impaired killing of GGS[38,39] may be the explanation.

Lower respiratory tract infections due to viridans group streptococci

Viridans streptococci (VS) are a heterogenous group that usually inhabit the oro-pharynx and proximal gastrointestinal tract. Precise taxonomonic classification is difficult. This produces confusion when comparing literature published at different times. Currently 13 species are recognized as belonging to this group[41]. VS produce α haemolysis on blood agar, fail to conform to specific sero-groups, and can be distinguished from *S. pneumoniae* by optochin resistance and lack of bile solubility[41]. Infective endocarditis and bacteraemia in general are the commonest clinical manifestations[42,43] although certain species preferentially target different organs and tissues.

The role of VS in the pathogenesis and occurrence of pneumonia is not clear but is currently accepted as probably uncommon. However, pneumonia may well be underdiagnosed due to dismissing VS as contaminants in clinical specimens. Their presence as normal commensals and hence interpretation in positive cultures as contaminants, their sensitivity to antibiotics commonly used for treating respiratory tract infections and the lack of a pathonomonic clinical picture may be responsible for underdiagnosis. VS are frequently found in association with other respiratory tract organisms in cases of aspiration pneumonia. Nevertheless, there are a number of reports which do support a pathogenic pulmonary role for VS[43–48]. Repeated positive blood cultures, culture from material obtained by protected methods or from closed spaces such as the pleural cavity and absence of other organisms, together with an appropriate clinical radiological setting provide strong evidence for this. In addition, the emergence of penicillin-resistant strains (see later) should be regarded as an additional factor promoting consideration of their pathogenic potential. There are few estimates of their contribution to pneumonia. One report suggested that 7% of bacterial pneumonias may be due to VS[49]. Another more recent study of over 1000 patients with community-acquired pneumonia indicated that 9.2% of the bacteremic cases were due to VS (*Streptococcus mitis*, *Streptococcus sanguis 1 and 2*, *Streptococcus intermedius*)[50]. Some other reports suggest that primary VS pneumonia is not so rare as has been previously reported[45,47].

In 71 children with VS bacteraemia, 13 were judged to have a relevant clinical illness of which 3 (23%) had pneumonia[43]. *S. mitis* and *S. sanguis* were the responsible VS species. In an additional 22 patients, VS may have contributed to the patients' lower respiratory tract and upper respiratory tract illnesses. Among 20 patients with an isolate of *S. mitis*, five (25%) were thought to be clinically relevant, of which two caused serious pulmonary infections (empyema, tracheo-oesophageal fistula with mediastinitis)[46]. Among 153 clinical isolates of the *Streptococcus milleri* group, 12 strains originated from patients with respiratory tract infections (*Streptococcus constellatis*, *Streptococcus anginosis*, and *S. intermedius*), although no information was given as to the clinical significance[51]. *S. milleri* pneumonia may occur as a result of spread from the primary pathological focus within the gastrointestinal tract, for example, liver abscess[52]. It appears that VS can cause lower respiratory tract infections in both children and adults with males being affected more than females. In adults several cases are described in patients less than 50 years[44,45,47,48]. Patients are not usually significantly immunocompromised although certain risk factors may be present[43,44]. However, in recent studies of neutropenic patients, VS appears to play an important role in the development of ARDS[53,54]. VS have also been described in association with ARDS. In a review of five studies of neutropenic patients up to 39% of bacteraemias in 2000 episodes of neutropenia were due to VS[54]. *S. mitis* and *S. sanguis II* were found most frequently. ARDS occurred in up to 33% of these patients probably as a result of the combined action of chemotherapy-related pulmonary toxicity and the subsequent VS infection producing increased capillary permeability. Heavy colonisation by VS, severe neutropenia, prophylactic quinolones or cotrimoxazole and mucositis were among the risk factors. Another study has indicated that VS was the most common cause of streptococcal bacteraemia in neutropenic patients undergoing intensive chemotherapy particulary with cytarabine[53]. One-third of these had diffuse pneumopathy with frequent isolation of streptococci from BAL. Alcoholism and chronic airways disease may also be present. Most cases are community acquired. In patients with chronic destructive pneumonia, VS with *Bacteroides* spp. are often found, but again the exact role of VS has not been determined in this setting[55].

Purulent productive cough, pleuritic chest pain, fever, and chills of abrupt onset (over 24 hours) are common presenting symptoms. Shock may also be present[47]. The chest radiograph usually shows non-specific infiltrates. Segmented alveolar opacities may be commonly seen[50]. Empyema, lung abscess, mediastinitis from tracheo-oesophageal fistula are not uncommon complications[44,46,48].

In general, response to a β-lactam antibiotic including penicillin is good with most patients recovering. However, penicillin-resistant VS strains have emerged recently. Most of these show intermediate resistance (MICs 0.25–2 μg/ml) but some are highly resistant (MICs 3–4 μg/ml). Thus, in Europe up to 46% of bacteraemias due to VS are penicillin resistant in contrast to the USA where only 1% are penicillin resistant[56]. The mechanisms appear to be alterations in the penicillin-binding proteins. Often these strains are also resistant to macrolides. Infections with such strains should be treated with imipenem, vancomycin or fourth generation cephalosporins.

Enterococcal pneumonia

The enterococci were recently reclassified from streptococci (Group D) into their own genus. Facultatively anaerobic these Gram-positive singlet/paired/short chained gram positive cocci grow at temperature extremes, in high saline concentrations and in 40% bile salts. *Enterococcus faecalis* accounts for 85% of clinical isolates and *Enterococus faecium* 7.5%. Commensal in the mouth and the gastrointestinal tract, most infections are urinary tract infections, bacteraemias, endocarditis, and intra-abdominal. Respiratory tract infections are exceedingly rare. Ammiotic fluid aspiration pneumonia in a neonate has been described[57,59]. The use of broad spectrum antibiotics appears to lead to enterococcal superinfection including pneumonia[58,59]. This has occurred after moxalactam therapy[58], cephalosporins/aminoglycosides in conjunction with enteral feeding[59] and prophylactic non-absorbable antibiotics (tobramycin and colistin) given to mechanically ventilated patients on the ICU[60]. In the last instance, six of the eight patients with clinically significant enterococcal infections had pneumonia. It is postulated that antimicrobial pressure selects out resistant enterococci, leading to tracheal and oropharynx colonisation, usually with *E. faecalis*, and subsequent aspiration pneumonia.

The enterococci are intrinsically resistant to β lactams and aminoglycosides. A combination of these two classes of antibiotics is, however, in general effective and synergistic and is the treatment of choice for enterococcal pneumonia. Dosages should be with penicillin up to 20 mu/day and gentamicin 3–5 mg/kg/day. However, the organisms can acquire resistance by novel mechanisms. In addition to at least four mechanisms for intrinsic resistance, acquired resistance mechanisms include diminished affinity of penicillin binding proteins, β-lactamase production, ribosomal mutations, production of aminoglycoside modifying enzymes and enzymic resistance to combination synergisms. It is the emergence of vancomycin resistance since the late 1980s which was previously felt to be highly unlikely which has caused great concern. The mechanism of resistance to this glycopeptide is an alteration of preterminal peptide amino acids dALA-d-ALA to dALA-dLAC resulting in inhibition of vancomycin binding to the bacterial cell wall. Furthermore, the emergence of multiply resistant enterococci to all approved classes of antimicrobial agents has made it impossible to offer any form of antimicrobial treatment to some individuals, who usually die of uncontrolled sepsis[61]. In order to detect these rather unusual resistant patterns, specialised testing techniques are necessary, for example, for high level aminoglycoside resistance or combination studies with time-kill methods. Alternative antimicrobial strategies for these patients include amoxicillin plus vancomycin or imipenem plus vancomycin, fluoroquinolones and tetracycline analogues.

Stomatococcus mucilaginosus

This seemingly harmless commensal of the oral cavity poses a threat for immunocompromised adults and children. It was previously known as *Staphylococcus salivarius* or *Micrococcus mucilaginosus*. It can be misidentified as *Staphylococcus, Micrococcus* or *Streptococcus* spp. However, its strong adherence to agar, weakly positive or negative catalase production, intolerance to sodium chloride and other biochemical reactions enable specific identification. Only recently has it been implicated in serious disease particularly septicaemia, endocarditis and catheter-related sepsis[62,63]. Pneumonia was found in 50% and ARDS in 13% in a small series[64]. Most patients have serious underlying disease, particularly conditions which produce severe neutropenia or in patients with cancer. The organism is often resistant to penicillin and methicillin. Resistance may also be seen to tetracycline, cotrimoxazole, quinolones and other antibiotics. Antibiotic pressure may lead to clinical disease with the organism. *S. mucilaginosus* appears to be susceptible to vancomycin which is the antibiotic of choice but the mortality remains high particularly in patients with associated central nervous system infection[63,64].

Listeria lower respiratory tract infections

Listeria monocytogenes is a Gram-positive intracellular motile bacillus. It is found in a wide variety of animals, plants and the soil and is asymptomatically present in the stools of humans in one-sixth of cases. Sixteen sero-types have been identified of which 4b, 1/2b and 1/2a cause most human disease. Foodstuffs such as certain cheese products and milk are sources for human infections which are mainly targeted to the central nervous system. Most susceptible people are the new-born, pregnant adults, the elderly and the immunocompromised. Pleuropulmonary infections are uncommon with less than a dozen cases reported in the literature.

In a review of eight cases[65] all but one had predisposing underlying conditions: Hodgkin's, carcinoma, alcoholism, diabetes mellitus and HIV. Although HIV-positive persons have an approximately 100 times increased risk for acquiring listeriosis compared to the general population[66], listerial pneumonia is a distinctly rare event, perhaps as a result of the widespread use of cotrimoxazole prophylaxis in that population. Nine cases of pleural fluid infection secondary to *L. monocytogenes* have been documented[67]. As with the pneumonic cases, all but one had serious concomitant conditions mainly, Hodgkin's, or non-Hodgkin's lymphoma and leukaemia. *Listeria* pneumonia does occur in the immunocompetent host[68]. Although infection in pregnancy poses a significant risk for serious congenital listeriosis because most infections are uterine, the illness in the mother is generally mild. Only two cases of maternal listeriosis with pulmonary complications due to ARDS have been described[69].

The clinical manifestations of listerial pneumonia include fever, cough and chills. Onset is variably acute or chronic. Features of empyema may be present. The pneumonia can be severe with progression to lung necrosis[70]. Diagnosis usually depends on positive cultures from blood, pleural fluid or from tracheo-bronchial secretions[65,67,68,70].

Antimicrobial management involves ampicillin or penicillin in combination with an aminoglycoside, since β-lactam antibiotics are bacterostatic against *Listeria*. The required duration of treatment for pneumonia is unclear though up to 6 weeks for non-pneumonic infections is generally recommended. Alternative effective antibiotics include trimethoprim-sulphamethoxazole, rifampicin and possibly vancomycin/ erythromycin/piperacillin and tetracycline[67]. Since there is poor penetration of aminoglycosides into the pleural fluid, intercostal tube drainage is indicated for empyema. Occasional open drainage may be needed[67]. Mortality is between 12 and 40% for treated cases[65,67]. In cases of severe respiratory failure secondary to listerial sepsis including necrotising pneumonia, extra-corporeal membrane oxygenation (ECMO) may be life-saving[70].

Bacillus infections (apart from those due to *Bacillus anthracis*)

Bacillus spp. are Gram-positive aerobic spore forming rods. Infections due to *B. anthracis* are undoubtedly pathogenic whilst many other *Bacillus* spp. are generally considered to be of low virulence and often play a commensal/non-pathogenic role. Ubiquitous in soil, dust and water, their isolation from clinical specimens has always been regarded as of dubious significance and often taken to be due to contamination. It is now recognised, however, that *Bacillus* spp. other than *B. anthracis* can produce disease in both immunocompetent and immunocompromised patients. These include *Bacillus cereus* food poisoning, *Bacillus subtilis* deep tissue infections including panopthalmitis, osteomyelitis, endocarditis, cellulitis, splenic abscess, necrotising fasciitis and pneumonia[71–73].

B. cereus pneumonia

Pneumonia due to *Bacillus* spp. including *B. cereus* is unusual[71–80]. Over a five and a quarter years' period, 38 infections caused by *Bacillus* spp. from five major Cleveland hospitals were identified[73] – only two caused pneumonia. In a literature review of cases of disseminated *Bacillus* infections from 1913 to 1978[72] 32 cases were identified of which seven had pneumonia (one with pleurisy), *B. cereus* accounted for four, *Bacillus subtilis* two, *Bacillus sphaericus* two. Recently, a *Bacillus* spp. resembling *Bacillus alvei* was thought to produce pneumonia and empyema in a 62-year-old immunocompetent man[80]. *B. cereus* pneumonia is often necrotising[76,79]. This may be related to the production of exotoxins with cytolytic enterotoxin activity including protease, haemolysin, phospholipase and lecithinase. Because of the ubiquity of these organisms, isolation from a regular sputum sample poses a dilemma for significance interpretation. Isolation from tissue, blood or closed cavities should therefore be attempted for a firm diagnosis.

The mechanism of acquisition of pulmonary disease due to non-anthrax *Bacillus* spp. is not known but may occur as a result of primary infection of the skin from trauma and inoculation with subsequent haematogenous dissemination. A primary inhalational route has also been postulated in those individuals exposed to soil dust[76] or by aspiration of oral contents. Nosocomial transmission has been mooted in the case of neonatal disease – possible sources being contaminated resuscitation devices and during intrapulmonary drug instillation[79].

Most patients with *Bacillus* pneumonia are adults and have significant associated conditions particularly haematogenous malignancy. Less frequently diabetes mellitus, chronic hepatitis, alcoholism and nephrotic syndrome are described. Occasionally patients are described with no underlying immune defect[72,76,77,80]. It has recently been reported in premature neonates[80] but otherwise seems to be less common in children[81]. Most infections occur in men.

Non-specific features include fever, cough, chest pain. Haemoptysis occurs in several patients and may be life threatening[82]. Pneumothorax has been reported[82]. Persistence of *B. cereus* spores in patients with bronchiectasis may lead to recurrent infections[77]. The chest radiographical findings include infiltrates, cavitation, pleural effusions and even pseudotumour[14,82]. The mortality rate ranges from 30% to 80%[72,82] and is mainly due to the underlying immunosuppression. *B. cereus* and non *B. cereus* strains are resistant to penicillin/cephalosporins through β-lactamase production but remain sensitive to aminoglycosides, chloramphenicol, clindamycin, vancomycin, erythromycin and ciprofloxacin. *B. alvei* may be more resistant to vancomycin and ciprofloxacin compared to the other *Bacillus* spp.[80]. In general, vancomycin is the antimicrobial of choice for non-anthracis *Bacillus* pneumonia. Surgical drainage of closed space infections and resection of necrotic tissue when indicated are important adjunctive surgical therapeutic manoeuvres[82].

Corynebacterium infections of the respiratory tract

Corynebacterium spp. also known as diphtheroids constitute part of the normal upper respiratory tract and skin flora. They are Gram-positive pleomorphic non-motile non-sporing bacilli. Some do cause human disease. *Corynebacterium ulcerans* (pharyngotonsillitis), *Corynebacterium xerosis* (skin infections), *Corynebacterium pseudodiphtheriticum* (endocarditis), *Corynebacterium haemolyticum* (skin infection pharyngitis) and *Corynebacterium JK* (skin infection) are the commonest. Of these, *C. xerosis*, *C. group JK* and also *Corynebacterium equi* are established aetiological agents of pneumonia. *C. pseudodiphtheriticum* and *Corynebacterium striatum* have also been recognised recently to produce pneumonia.

C. xerosis

A brief summary of reported cases of invasive disease was given recently[83]. Three of nine patients had pneumonia of which two had additional complications namely, empyema, pericarditis and endocarditis. Patients have underlying predispositions including haemodialysis, lung cancer, patent ductus- arteriosus and leukemia[84]. Usually the organisms are sensitive to penicillin and β- lactams, erythromycin, cotrimoxazole, chloramphenicol, aminoglycosides and vancomycin, although resistance, sometimes multiple, has been described[84].

Corynebacterium group JK

Most infections have been described in patients with haematological malignancy particularly bone marrow transplant recipients. Prolonged neutropenia, broad spectrum antibiotics and skin abrasion predispose to infection. Skin infections at intravenous insertion sites, bacteraemia and pneumonia are all described. Resistance to penicillin, cephaloporins and aminoglycosides is common and vancomycin is the antimicrobial of choice.

C. striaticum

This has been associated with exacerbation of COAD[85], with respiratory tract infection in patients mechanically ventilated[86], as well as other infections including bacteraemias and peritonitis.

C. pseudodiphtheriticum

Cases of pneumonia, lung abscess, tracheitis, and tracheobronchitis due to this organism have been occasionally described in the past, and usually in the immunocompromised host and then only since 1983[87–89]. Recent evidence has emerged, however, suggesting that this organism may be implicated in pneumonia more commonly than formally appreciated. Bronchitis, pneumonia, bronchiectasis and chronic pulmonary disease have been described in 33 patients in recent years[87,88]. SLE, immunosuppressive therapy, chronic lung disease, HIV, diabetes, mechanical ventilation, congestive heart failure, malignancy, adult T cell lymphotropic virus infection, VSD and pulmonary hypertension have been mentioned as underlying conditions. In general, however, recent reports[87,88] suggest that most patients did not have severe immunodeficiency. Isolation of the organism in pure growth, phagocytised intracellular diphtheroids particularly as demonstrated by electron microscopy[87] organisms within tissue, plentiful polymorphs in sputum, and $\geq 10^7$ cfu/ml of organisms in sputum together with clinical and microbiological response[87,88] provide strong evidence for their pathogenic role rather than mere contaminants or commensals. Isolates are usually sensitive to β-lactams, tetracycline, vancomycin and cotrimoxazole but resistant to clindamycin and erythromycin. Sensitivity to ciprofloxacin is variable[88].

Concomitantly isolated organisms are found in approximately 15–30% of patients particularly those with underlying COPD – their role as co-pathogens cannot be ruled out.

Patients are usually male with underlying conditions and with a mean age around 70 years. Onset is acute, fever is relatively uncommon. There is usually purulent sputum and cough. The white cell count is elevated in most cases. Treatment is usually satisfactory when penicillin, ampicillin or cefazoline are used and the mortality rate is around 10%. Deaths are apparently only indirectly related to the infection.

Rhodococcus respiratory infections

Rhodococcus equi has long been recognised as producing pneumonia and extrapulmonary infections in fowls, older horses, cattle, sheep and pigs. It was first recognized as a human pathogen in 1967, in a patient with a lung abscess[89] and since that time many cases have been described in the literature. Some 77 published cases had accrued by 1995[90]. The global increase in the immunocompromised host population and awareness that several microbiological and clinical characteristics of this organism overlap with other more common organisms may be responsible for the recent increase in reported cases.

R. equi is a facultatively intracellular aerobic, pleomorphic Gram-positive non-sporing cocco-bacillus (coccal forms more plentiful than bacillary forms), weakly acid fast and producing dry orange colonies on mycobacterial media. It has been confused with other organisms which include diphtheroids, *M. tuberculosis*, non- tuberculous mycobacteria, *L. monocytogenes* and *Nocardia* spp. Capsular serotypes I and II account for 90% of clinical isolates.

It is usually acquired through inhalation, less commonly orally, from reservoir sources which include infected animals, manure of animal runs, soils, or soiled vegetables. Characteristically, T-lymphocyte cell dysfunction aided by humoral dysfunction is present in the majority of patients. Defective histiocytic type processing of *R. equi* occurs. Lung lesions are characterised by polymorph and histiocytic infiltrates forming microabscesses. Macrophage/giant cell necrotising granulomas are also found. Malakoplakia has been described[91].

Predisposing clinical conditions for *R. equi* infections include HIV infection, renal or heart transplantation, reticulo-endothelial and haematological malignancies with/without chemotherapy, prednisolone treatment of connective tissue diseases and alcoholism[92–94].

Most patients are in some way immunocompromised. A few are immunocompetent[93–95]. Prior exposure to animals has been documented in between 18% and 45%[94]. HIV positive patients are less likely to give such a history. Although the clinical spectrum is wide and encompasses extrapulmonary target sites such as skin abscesses, central nervous system abscesses, osteomyelitis, cervical lymphadenopathy, joints and endometrium, pneumonia has been the most frequent disease manifestation occurring in over 75% of cases[94,96].

Most cases occur in young/middle-aged adults with a male predominance. Paediatric cases have, however, been described[94]. Symptoms include an insidious onset characterised by high grade fever, cough which may be productive, fatigue and dyspnoea[94,95,96]. There may also be pleuritic chest pain and haemoptysis[93,97]. Chest radiology initially reveals infiltrates in an upper lobe; the lower lobes can also be affected. Cavitation occurs in more than 50% of patients. Pleural effusion/empyema is not uncommon. Endobronchial masses and lung abscesses may occur[97]. Although the presentation is not dissimilar in HIV-positive/HIV-negative patients[94] HIV positive patients tend to be coinfected with other pulmonary organisms including *Pneumocystis*, non-tuberculous mycobacteria, histoplasmosis and *Toxoplasma*[94,98]. Occasionally, concomitant extrapulmonary sites of infection are present. The disease therefore commonly mimicks tuberculosis clinically and microbiologically[99]. The white cell response is often normal.

The organism can be cultured most often from blood, sputum, bronchoscopical specimens, pleural fluid and lung tissue.

Mortality is substantial – 20% in HIV negative and 55% in HIV-positive patients[94].

Treatment is difficult and optimal antimicrobial therapy has not been defined. Unlike animal strains, *R. equi* isolated from human clinical specimens are resistant to penicillin and first-generation cephalosporins. Less than 5% are resistant to erythromycin, rifampicin, tetracycline or septrin[100]. The most active agents *in vitro* are penicillin, doxycycline, erythromycin, lincomycin, vancomycin, chloramphenicol and aminoglycosides[93,96]. Most individuals would be treated with two antimicrobials (utilising some agents which concentrate into polymorphs) usually vancomycin + erythromycin or rifampicin + erythromycin or imipenem + vancomycin[93,101]. Some authors advocate initial treatment with drugs exhibiting high bacteriocidal activity but poor intracellular penetration (e.g. imipenem) since bacterial load is substantial in neutropenic patients, followed by maintenance therapy with intracellularly active agents[102]. Duration of treatment should be at least 2 months – perhaps up to 6 months – since relapse is high[93] and the organism persists within alveolar macrophages even on treatment[103]. For abscesses and empyema which fail to resolve on antibiotics, appropriate surgical intervention including drainage or resection should be undertaken.

Rochalimaea respiratory infections

Rochalimaea spp. are small Gram-negative bacilli producing a variety of diseases including cat-scratch disease, trench fever, bacillary angiomatosis, bacteraemia, peliosis hepatitis and disseminated infection[104]. *Rochalimaea* spp. are now considered in the *Bartonella* genus. Extracutaneous bacillary angiomatosis is manifest by multisystem visceral involvement including the mucosal surfaces of the respiratory tract. Bacillary angiomatosis is thought to be acquired from a cat-scratch or bite, the soil or other vectors. Lung infiltrates, pleural effusions and polypoid endobronchial lesions can occur[105]. Definitive diagnosis is made on the clinical features, histological appearances of angiomatous changes with oedema and inflammatory cells consisting of eosinophilic aggregates with neutropenic debris, cavitary masses of bacillary structures on Warthin Starry stains[104], culture, blood and serology. Treatment is with several weeks of doxycycline/minocycline/tetracycline/chloramphenicol/cotrimoxazole/azithromycin/ciprofloxacin, together with surgical excision as appropriate.

Ehrlichia respiratory infections

Ehrlichia spp., usually *Ehrlichia canis* or *Ehrlichia chaffeensis* are obligate intracellular Gram-negative cocci, probably tick-borne. Different species parasitise monocytes, granulocytes or platelets. Cases have been described in Japan and the USA, particularly the South Central and Southeastern states since 1986.

Fever, skin rash, chills and headaches are the most common among a myriad of non-specific symptoms[106,107]. Leukopenia is a hallmark of the disease. Lymphopenia, thrombocytopenia, hepatic dysfunction are other laboratory markers. Aseptic meningoencephalitis can also occur. Respiratory distress is present in between 6% and 10% of adult cases[106]. Acute pulmonary infiltrates have also been noted[107]. The illness is sometimes fatal particularly in delayed diagnosis cases, with an overall mortality of about 20%. Confirmatory diagnosis is by immunofluorescence antibody staining, PCR and histological search for the characteristic morulae (Wright's purple staining aggregates in blood cells). However, diagnosis is most often empirical and requires a high degree of suspicion since microbiological tests are rather insensitive or experimental. Thus, *Ehrlichia* pneumonia should be suspected in patients with an appropriate travel history, history of tick exposure together with acute fever with leukopenia and thrombocytopenia. Treatment is with tetracycline or chloramphenicol.

Respiratory infection due to *Neisseria* spp.

Most cases of pulmonary infection due to *Neisseria* spp. are caused by *Neisseria meningitidis*. *Neisseria catarrhalis* now called *Branhamella* or *Moraxella catarrhalis* is considered separately (see Chapter 7). *N. meningitidis* is a Gram-negative diplococcus. The capsular polysaccharide enables serogrouping, groups A,B,C,X,Y,W-135 and L commonly causing human disease. Meningococci attach via pili to nasopharyngeal cells producing a carrier state. Earlier theories that outbreaks of meningocococcal diseases are preceded by an increase in the carriage rate in the population have generated considerable controversy.

Occult bacteraemia in association with an upper respiratory infection, acute meningococcaemia with skin rash and hypotension, meningitis with and without meningococcaemia, meningoencephalitis, chronic meningococcaemia and complement deficiency-associated recurrent meningococcaemia are the most frequently described manifestations of meningococcal disease. Some of these particularly acute meningococcaemia with or without meningitis carry a poor prognosis.

Respiratory disease due to meningococci is long recognised. However, the asymptomatic, chronic, intermittent or transient oropharyngeal carriage state may lead to problems in precisely defining cases. Nevertheless, meningococcal pharyngitis has been described. Meningococcal pneumonia due to *N. meningitidis* group B or C occurs in about 10% of meningococcal disease occurring with these sero groups[108]. Although the clinical spectrum of disease due to *N. meningitidis* group Y has been said to be similar to that caused by groups B and C[109], other studies suggest that group Y disease produces primary pneumonia which predominates 4 : 1 over meningococcaemia/meningitic presentations[108]. Thus, 68/78 Air Force recruits with group Y disease had primary pneumonia[108].

A prior history of upper respiratory infection is common in patients with meningococcal pneumonia – for example, influenza may enhance the acquisition of meningococci after exposure to these bacteria[110].

The features of group Y meningococcal pneumonia are non-pathognomonic but include cough, fever and rales in 96–100% and commonly sore throat, chest pain, chills, a history of upper respiratory infection, fatigue and pharyngitis[108]. The patients do not usually have a predisposing severe illness although pre-existing leukopenia or mechanical respiratory support have been described as possible predisposing factors. Chest radiology usually shows patchy alveolar infiltrates and small pleural effusions are found in 22% of patients. Lower unilobar involvement is the most frequent radiographical presentation. A firm microbiological diagnosis depends on collecting respiratory samples uncontaminated by upper respiratory tract secretions. Only 1 of 44 patients from a Dutch district general hospital with *N. meningitidis* on culture actually had pneumonia[111]. A positive blood culture is found in 15% of primary group Y meningococcal pneumonia[108]. The peripheral white cell count is elevated, but occasionally leukopenia is described in patients with more severe disease. The serum adenosine deaminase activity seems to be significantly lower in patients with meningococcal pneumonia compared to patients with pneumonia due to *S. pneumoniae*, *Haemophilus influenzae*, *Mycoplasma* or viral aetiologies[112]. Response to antibiotics (usually penicillin) is brisk and virtually all patients with primary pneumonia due to group Y meningococci recover. This compares to a mortality rate of > 5% in patients with group B or C meningococcal disease. However, in patients with group Y meningococcal disease who have meningococcaemia and/or meningitis, the course and outcome is less favourable than those with primary pneumonia only.

Rarely other *Neisseria* spp. have been incriminated in pneumonia. These include *Neisseria sicca*, part of the normal flora of the oropharynx. This has produced pneumonia in patients with predisposing conditions including pregnancy, bullous pemphigoid and steroid therapy, and arteriosclerotic heart disease[113]. *Neisseria mucosa*, another normal inhabitant of the oropharynx, has also been described in the pathogenesis of the empyema, following pneumonectomy[114]. *N. sicca* and *Neisseria perflava* have been isolated from patients with HIV infection, including patients with pulmonary and disseminated infection in association with positive blood cultures[115].

Pneumocystis carinii pneumonia

P. carinii is reviewed in this chapter because of its controversial classification (see below). Emphasis will be on *P. carinii* pneumonia

(PCP) in the patient without HIV (see Chapter 22 for details of HIV associated PCP).

Although Chagas was the first to identify the organism in 1909 and Delano and Delano described it in Parisian sewer rats in 1912[116], it was initially implicated in human pulmonary disease only in 1942[117]. Since that time it has been recognised as producing subclinical and limiting infection in the first few years of life and clinical disease in the immunocompetent host but its major impact is to produce severe pneumonia in patients immunocompromised through iatrogenic congenital or acquired modes.

Originally believed to be a protozoan, recent molecular biological techniques have revealed properties more consistent with fungi. The precise classification, however, still remains elusive. Features favouring a protozoan taxonomy include: response to antimicrobials used to treat other protozoa, lack of ergosterol in the plasma membrane, no response to antifungals, existence of cysts containing sporozoites and absence of growth on fungal media. Fungal characteristics include: ability of the cell wall to take up fungal stains, dihydrofolate reductase and thymidylate synthase enzymes encoded on different chromosomes, 'fungal-like' ribosomal RNA sequences[118], e.g. PCR products with sequences very similar to those of ustomycetous red yeast fungi[119], and the fungal-like protein products e.g. β tubulin, β 1–3 glucan components of cell wall and response to β glucan inhibitors, evidence of aerosol transmissibility, and presence of elongation factor 3 (found only in fungi).

The life cycle of *P. carinii* involves (i) trophozoites - tiny (approximately 2–5 μ) thin-walled (Geimsa staining), pleomorphic forms which leads to (ii) precysts: an intermediate slightly larger stage which leads to (iii) cysts (approximately 4–8 μ) – containing up to eight internal daughter thick-walled cysts (methenamine silver staining). *P. carinii* exists extracellularly within alveoli (Fig.30.2*a*, *b*). It undergoes both sexual (cysts) and asexual (trophozoites) reproduction. β glucan inhibitors block cyst development, whilst folate antagonists target the trophozoites. No *in vitro* culture system exists for propagating *P. carinii*; with rat derived *P. carinii* strains short-term (10 days) culture can be achieved.

P. carinii is found in a variety of animals but different species have different host specificity[120]. However, for rats, more than one species can infect at the same/different times; there is controversial evidence for this in the human.

Histopathogenesis

Although the natural reservoir for *P. carinii* is unknown, contenders include animals or soil environments. The organism is acquired by man by the aerosol route. Following inhalation, attachment of trophozoites to type I alveolar cells occurs, followed by its extracellular prolonged survival, perhaps as a constituent of the flora, in alveolar fluid. Serological evidence suggests that 75% of healthy children worldwide have had subclinical infection by their fourth year of life[121]. An intact immune system prevents infection developing into clinical apparent disease. Conversely, severely malnourished children with hypoimmunoglobulinaemia and hypoalbuminaemia have been prone to interstitial plasma cell pneumonitis due to *P. carinii*. It appears that CD4 lymphocytes play a major role in host defence – hence, the high probability of PCP occurring in HIV-positive individuals when the CD4 count is much less than $200/mm^3$. To a lesser extent, β lymphocyte function is also important (hence passive immunisation is sometimes helpful). Among the cytokines, γ interferon and interleukin-1 play contributory roles. Once the host immune defence is jeopardised, uncontrolled intra-alveolar proliferation of *P. carinii* occurs.

Characteristically, an eosinophilic intra-alveolar foamy exudate occurs which contains trophozoites. There is only a mild interstitial inflammatory reaction. Alveolar capillary membrane integrity is threatened. Surfactant phospholipid secretion may be diminished. Hyaline membrane formation and fibrosis may result. The inflammatory responses are responsible for the characteristic increase in the alveolar arterial oxygen gradient, leading to hypoxaemia, and for the

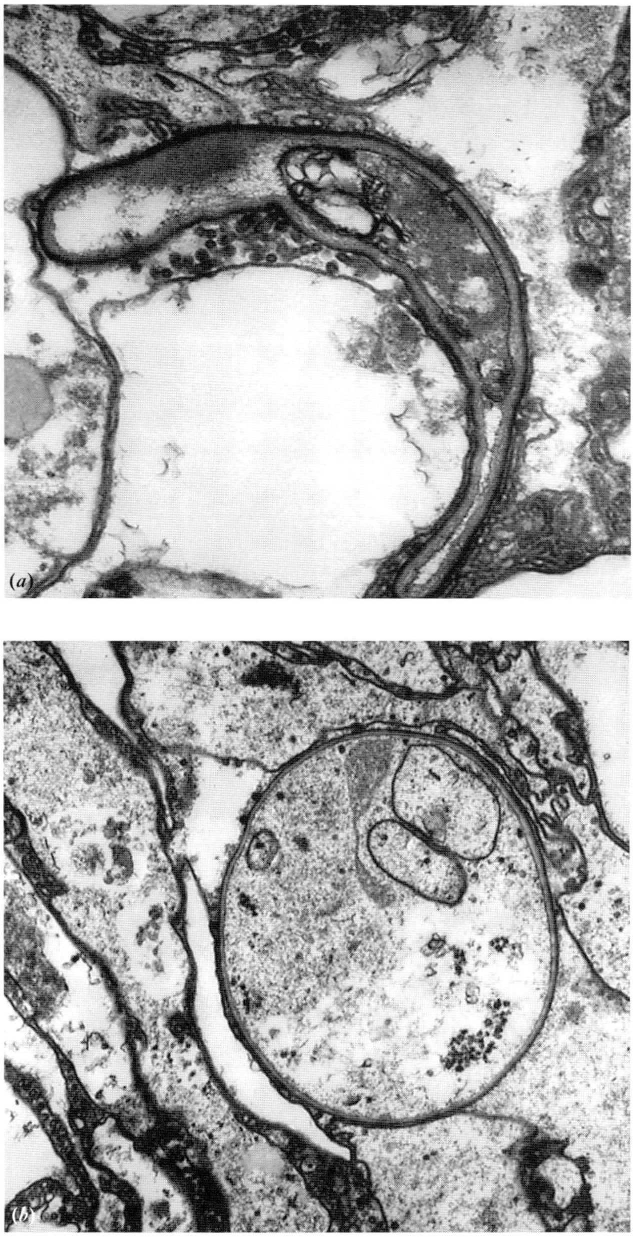

FIGURE 30.2 (*a*), (*b*) Electron microscopic appearances of *P. carinii*.

reduction in TLCO. These can be reversed by the early administration of corticosteroids.

Atypical histological changes as derived from autopsy, open lung biopsy or routine transbronchial biopsy studies may also be found. These include absence of the alveolar exudate, granulomatous inflammation, interstitial/intraluminal fibrosis, honeycombing cavities and pneumocystoma *(Pneumocystis* within a collection of fibroblasts and eosinophils) formation, diffuse alveolar damage, patchy calcification, and BOOP. Some cases also show extrapulmonary pneumocystosis e.g. in hilar lymph nodes[122,123]. Coexistence of cytomegalovirus occurs in about 10% of patients with PCP and may increase the severity of the illness. In patients with HIV, other concomitant diagnoses may be present, for example, Kaposi's sarcoma.

Susceptible individuals include persons with HIV infection (Chapter 22), solid organ transplants, chemotherapy, steroid therapy and severe combined immunodeficiency syndrome (SCID), haematological malignancies and solid organ malignancies, autoimmune deficiencies and patients with the nephrotic syndrome. The degree of risk varies with the particular background immunocompromised profile, type of transplant and other factors. Thus, heart transplant recipients carry a risk of clinically apparent PCP of around 5% compared to 40% for lung or heart–lung transplants[124–126], whereas in HIV patients on no prophylaxis whose CD4 count is 0.1×10^9/l the risk is over 60%/person/year[127]. Another factor is perhaps the geographical location. Thus, PCP in the same risk groups in Africa is rare compared to North America. However, this may be due to the striking disparity of diagnostic facilities. The incidence of asymptomatic infection in transplant recipients may be substantially higher, reaching almost 8% in some. An interesting observation from the renal transplant population is that of an outbreak of PCP and other pneumonias in association with CD4 counts less than 0.2×10^9/l[128]. This was similar to that found in liver transplants, and of course in AIDS patients.

Although it is generally believed that reactivation of dormant infection previously acquired in childhood is the principal mechanism, the occurrence of clusters of cases provides evidence of *de novo* acquisition and possible person-to-person transmission in several instances[128–131].

Although unusual PCP is well recognised to occur in otherwise healthy individuals[130,132]. Recent reports have ruled out known immunosuppressive conditions at presentation and during prolonged follow-up after recovery[132]. None of five patients described recently had CD4 or CD8 abnormalities or other risk factors. One had documented *Mycoplasma pneumoniae* infection and it was postulated that temporary cutaneous anergy might have been induced by polyclonal activation of B cells and suppression of T-cells by the *M. pneumoniae*, leading to subsequent PCP[132].

Clinical

The clinical manifestations of PCP vary with the particular risk setting. Even within the risk setting, the onset, of course, can vary considerably between patients[133]. In malnourished or premature infants feeding difficulties may be the first manifestation prior to established respiratory distress. In all groups of patients other than those with HIV, onset is generally sudden and progression rapid. In patients with organ transplantation onset occurs around 8 weeks post-transplant or during periods of heightened immunosuppressive therapy. Cough, fever, dyspnoea are usual features. Sputum is unusual. Chest pain and myalgias can occur. Physical examination reveals features of respiratory distress with crepitations heard in most but not all patients.

Certain patients may be largely asymptomatic. For example, in heart–lung transplant recipients, more than 80% are infected but only half of these have overt disease[124]. Furthermore, immunosuppressive therapy, steroids, cyclosporin may all modify the clinical feature.

Clinical features of extrapulmonary pneumocystosis may be apparent, for example, lymphadenopathy, retinal cotton wool lesions but are rarely observed clinically (in less than 5%) compared to autopsy evidence where histological involvement of other organs can be found in nearly 50% of cases[134].

Complications include pneumothorax and pneumomediastinum possibly related to the use of aerosol pentamidine.

Hypoxaemia due to a wide alveolar arterial gradient is common. Leukocytosis occurs in immunocompetent patients but not in other groups. The serum lactate dehydrogenase (LDH) and serum angiotensin-converting enzyme (SACE) may be elevated and reflect the degree of non-specific lung injury.

The chest radiograph usually shows perihilar, bilateral infiltrates with sparing of the lung bases and apices (except in those patients receiving inhaled pentamidine prophylaxis when infiltrates tend to be apical or basal). The chest radiograph initially may be normal. Unusual radiological manifestations of PCP include cavitation, pneumothorax, unilateral infiltrates, nodules and pleural effusions. In immunosuppressed patients, chemotherapy, coexistent pathogens such as CMV and rejection phenomena may supervene and complicate the radiological features. A number of other radiological imaging techniques may provide additional information or clarify that. CT scanning is more sensitive than plain radiology and is useful therefore when the plain radiograph is normal. MRI is not so helpful.

Although a presumptive diagnosis of PCP can be made in HIV-positive patients on clinical grounds alone[135] (see Chapter 22) and a diagnostic empirical trial instigated, in other patients in whom the differential diagnosis is wider, it is preferable to make a specific diagnosis prior to starting therapy. Multilobe BAL is the sampling technique of choice[136], although the yield is less in non-AIDS patients compared to over 95% in AIDS patients. This probably reflects the greater load of *P. carinii* in AIDS patients. Tissue sampling by transbronchial biopsy or open lung biopsy may provide a higher yield (90–95%) compared to BAL (approximately 70%) in non-AIDS patients[137]. Open lung biopsy has the added advantage of providing the highest 'catch-all' diagnosis. Induced sputum[138] has only a sensitivity of around 40% but some centres have claimed up to 90% (see Chapter 22).

A number of stains can be used to visualise *P. carinii*. This includes methenamine silver (for cyst wall), Diff-Quick version of Wright–Giemsa (for intracystic components and developmental stages), immunofluorescence monoclonal antibodies and immunohistochemicals. PCR appears to be the most sensitive diagnostic test – offering a threefold increased sensitivity diagnostic rate compared with silver staining techniques on induced sputum, and an 80% sensitivity rate from oropharyngeal mouthwash samples[139,140,144]. It can also be positive on blood samples[141]. Its high sensitivity raises concern in distinguishing clinical disease/infection/artefacts. Positive PCRs become negative a few days after commencing treatment.

Several other non-invasive diagnostic techniques are available but are rather non-specific in general or at the research stage only. Radiolabelled isotope scans, including gallium-67, technicium-99 labelled *P. carinii* monoclonal antibodies, technicium-99 M. diethylentriamine penta-acetate scans for alveolar capillary membrane permeability indicators may provide evidence of abnormalities in the presence of a normal chest radiograph but are rather non-specific. Indium-111 human polyclonal immunoglobulin has been found to be capable of identifying *P. carinii* with 80% sensitivity[142] but is also positive in some patients without PCP but who have other infections. Of some importance is that this scan appears to differentiate infections from lymphoma and Kaposi's sarcoma giving an advantage over gallium scanning. Immunoscintigraphy using specific *P. carinii* monoclonal antibodies may provide a basis for further investigations.

LDH activity in the serum though non-specific may indicate immediate relapse of PCP as well as indicating prognosis. Exercise-induced desaturation of the arterial blood oxygen in an appropriate clinical and radiological setting has been proved useful for predicting PCP[143]. A reduced DLCO may be found even in the presence of a normal chest radiograph.

Treatment and outcome

Specific antimicrobials, corticosteroids, supportive ventilation and treatment of concomitant infections are the four mainstays in the management of PCP. The two major equi-effective antimicrobials are high dose cotrimoxazole and parenteral pentamidine. However, the folic acid antagonist cotrimoxazole is preferred. Dosage is 20 mg/kg/day of trimethoprim and 100 mg/kg/day of sulphamethoxazole, given for 14 days (21 days is preferred for AIDS related PCP and for severely immunocompromised non-HIV patients). Mild PCP can sometimes be managed successfully with oral treatment and on an outpatient basis. Serum levels are rarely performed in practice; however, a trimethoprim peak level of 5–50 μg/ml (sulphamethoxazole 100–150 μg/ml) is said to render the best balance of efficacy/ toxicity. Side-effects in non-HIV patients are infrequent and mild but in HIV-positive patients are frequent and may be severe. These include skin rash which may occasionally progress to life-threatening Stevens–Johnson syndrome, fever, bone marrow suppression, anaphylaxis and hepatotoxicity. The mechanism is unclear – hypersensitivity or a direct toxic effect due to slow acetylator status or glutathione deficiencies are possibilities. Bone marrow suppression can be additive in patients with haematological disease. Supplemental folinic acid protection as used in HIV positive patients is controversial in leukaemic patients. A mild skin rash in HIV patients is not an indication to discontinue cotrimoxazole as it often disappears spontaneously. Desensitisation can be attempted if cotrimoxazole needs to be given again but this subject is controversial[144].

Pentamidine is an alternative treatment for patients who cannot tolerate cotrimoxazole or fail to respond to it. However, definite evidence of heightened efficacy in those patients who switch treatment because of therapeutic failure is lacking. Combination treatment of cotrimoxazole and pentamidine offers no advantage. The dosage is 4 mg/kg/day. Pentamidine's toxic profile is formidable in both HIV-positive and HIV-negative patients with cardiac dysrhythmias, hypotension, hypo/hypercalcaemia, hypomagnesaemia, hypo/hyperglycaemia, uraemia, pancreatitis, neutropenia and injection site abscesses. Some of these may be ameliorated by administering only 3 mg/kg/day. Inhaled pentamidine cannot be recommended for definitive treatment though it has been given when all other modalities fail.

Response to cotrimoxazole or pentamidine occurs by the third/fourth day in non-HIV patients and by about a week in HIV positive patients. There may be an initial worsening of the patient's condition shortly after starting treatment presumably due to the host's inflammatory reaction. The use of steroids within the first 72 hours of antimicrobial therapy for moderate to severe HIV-associated PCP ($p_aO_2 \leq 9.3$ kPa or alveolar/arterial gradient ≥ 4.7 kPa) has been associated with a better outcome. The dose of prednisolone is 80 mg daily tapering to 20 mg at days 11 to 20 then discontinuation. Other immunomodifiers showing some benefit in animal models but yet to be tested in humans include γ interferon, replacement of surfactant and aerosolised heat-killed *Escherichia coli*.

Alternative drugs (and their efficacy) include dapsone (poor), dapsone and trimethoprim (good), trimetrexate (good as salvage treatment but increased PCP recurrence), clindamycin and primaquine (? good), atovaquone (fair), the purine scavenger eflornithine (no longer in use), nebulized pentamidine (fair, but upper lobe relapse and extrapulmonary disseminated pneumocystosis) and a variety of experimental drugs which include piratrexim, β glucan synthesis inhibitors, purine nucleoside analogues, combinations of clarithromycin and sulphamethoxazole, quinolones and echinocandins. However, extensive and/or comparative trials vs cotrimoxazole or pentamidine have not been performed. In addition, specific problems or side-effects have been encountered with some of these treatments, for example, haemolysis in G6PDH deficient patients with dapsone or primaquine, skin and liver toxicity with trimetrexate, rash and diarrhoea with clindamycin + primaquine, GI tract disturbances, fever and rash with atovaquone.

Intensive care for patients with PCP appears currently to be in vogue again following the experience in the 1980s when the survival rate for patients with PCP admitted to an intensive care unit was less than 15%. Now survival rates in excess of 35% are reported[145]. This may be due to the use of steroids, prophylactic cotrimoxazole, earlier and empirical therapy, earlier and more rapid diagnosis and better standards of care.

Although there is no concrete evidence of person-to-person transmission as supported by epidemiological – molecular studies, in view of the animal evidence of transmissibility of *P. carinii* and reported clusters of cases, it is desirable that patients with PCP should be managed in single rooms and separated from other immunocompromised hosts, with airborne control of infection precautions.

Response to treatment overall for PCP is generally good – survival rates of in excess of 80% are attainable. HIV-positive patients, however, usually do less well compared to HIV-negative patients. Poor prognostic factors include initial hypoxaemia, extensive chest radiographical changes, presence of BAL neutrophilia, raised serum LDH levels, coexistent fungal/bacterial/viral disease, malnutrition, and lack of management expertise. Recurrence is a definite possibility and the frequency of this is higher in HIV-positive patients (50%/year) – but recurrent disease is generally milder.

Prophylaxis

Primary and secondary prophylaxis should be offered to all patients at high risk for *P. carinii* infection. For discussion of this issue in HIV-positive patients refer to Chapter 22. The risk for PCP in other immunosuppressed populations varies with the risk group and the geographical centre. As a general rule : SCID, acute lymphatic leukaemia, human T-cell lymphotropic leukaemia and lymphoma, lung, heart–lung transplants, brain tumours and all immunocompromised patients with a previous episode of PCP provide the greatest risk and should receive long-term prophylaxis.

Cotrimoxazole has been the favourite chemoprophylaxis for 20 years[146] at a dose of 5 mg of trimethoprim equivalent/kg/day given in two divided doses. Alternatively, it may be given three times a week. This has been proved effective in haematological malignancies/patients receiving chemotherapy, bone marrow transplantation, renal transplantation, cardiac transplantation and lung transplantation[126,146–149]. Side-effects are generally quite mild. The issue of whether prophylaxis with cotrimoxazole in patients with cardiac allografts is warranted is controversial – on the basis of a very low incidence of PCP in some programmes and also of particularly potentially serious drug interactions with immunosuppressive regimes particularly azathioprine which produce life threatening rejection. This was addressed in a recent prospective randomised three-arm study (twice daily cotrimoxazole vs three times a week cotrimoxazole vs no treatment) given for 14 days post-transplant for 4 months[126]. A significant reduction in PCP was documented with either cotrimoxazole arm; there was no excess rejection. Although both active arms were equally effective, those in the intermittent group tended to develop PCP following discontinuation of prophylaxis.

Pentamidine administered by aerosol (see Chapter 22) is an alternative prophylactic mode for patients who cannot tolerate cotrimoxazole. Although avoiding the systemic side-effects associated with parenteral pentamidine, it is far more expensive than cotrimoxazole, equipment has to be standardised to optimise particle size delivery, bronchospasm may be problematic, potential risk of chemical toxicity and other respiratory pathogens such as TB transmissible to attendees, a higher incidence of apical pulmonary and extrapulmonary pneumocystosis, and pneumothorax are disadvantages. In HIV-positive patients, comparative studies suggest that inhaled pentamidine is not as efficacious as cotrimoxazole. However, it has been used successfully in some other risk groups who have a contraindication to cotrimoxazole. Aerosolised pentamidine (300 mg monthly by Respigard II nebuliser) was administered to nine patients post-lung transplant for a mean of 10 months[150]. It was safe and no patient developed PCP compared with an expected incidence of up to 43%. The theoretical risk that pentamidine by upregulating class II MHC antigens in bronchial epithelium might produce rejection was not seen.

Alternative prophylaxis include dapsone ± pyrimethamine and sulfadoxine with pyrimethamine, whislt clindamycin with privaquine and atovaquone are investigational in this regard.

References

1. VEASY LG, WIEDMEIER SE ORSMOND GS *et al.* Resurgence of acute rheumatic fever in the intermountain area of the United States. *N Engl J Med* 1987;316:421–7.
2. STRÖMBERG A, ROMANUS V, BURMAN LG. Outbreak of group A streptococcal bacteraemia in Sweden: An epidemiologic and clinical study. *J Infect Dis* 1991;164:595–8.
3. LENTNEK AL, GIGER O, O'ROURKE E. Group A β-hemolytic streptococcal bacteraemia in intravenous substance abuse. A growing clinical problem? *Arch Intern Med* 1990;150:89–93.
4. ISPAHANI P, DONALD FE, AVELINE AJD. *Streptococcus pyogenes* bacteraemia in Cambridge – a review of 67 episodes. *Quart J Med* 1988;68:603–13.
5. MARTIN PR, HOIBY EA. Streptococcal serogroup A epidemic in Norway 1987–1988. *Scand J Infect Dis* 1990;22:421–9.
6. NECROTISING FASCIITIS. *Weekly Epidemiol Rec* 1994;22:165–6.
7. STREPTOCOCCAL INFECTIONS. *Weekly Epidemiol Rec* 1995;22:146–7.
8. DEMERS B, SIMOR AE, VELLEND PM *et al.* Severe invasive group A streptococcal infections in Ontario, Canada: 1987–1991. *Clin Infect Dis* 1993;16:792–800.
9. HENKEL JS, ARMSTRONG D, BLEVINS A, MOODY MD. Group A β-hemolytic *Streptococcus* bacteraemia in a cancer hospital. *JAMA* 1970;21:983–6.
10. BARNHAM M. Invasive streptococcal infections in the era before the acquired immune deficiency syndrome: a 10 years' compilation of patients with streptococcal bacteraemia in North Yorkshire. *J Infect* 1989;18:231–48.
11. BURKERT T, WATANAKUNAKORN C. Group A streptococcal bacteraemia in a community teaching hospital – 1980–1989. *Clin Infect Dis* 1992;14:29–37.
12. CLEARY PP, KAPLAN EL, HANDLEY JP *et al.* Clonal basis for resurgence of serious *Streptococcus pyogenes* disease in the 1980s. *Lancet* 1992;339:518–21.
13. SPENCER RC. Invasive streptococci. *Eur J Clin Microbiol Infect Dis* 1995;S1:26–32.
14. HAUSER AR, STEVENS DL, KAPLAN EL, SCHLIEVERT PM. Molecular analysis of pyrogenic exotoxins from *Streptococcus pyogenes* isolates associated with toxic shock-like syndrome. *J Clin Microbiol* 1991;29:1562–7.
15. VALENZUELA TD, HOOTON TM, KAPLAN EL, SCHLIEVERT P. Transmission of 'toxic strep' syndrome from an infected child to a firefighter during CPR. *Ann Emerg Med* 1991;20:123–5.
16. SCHWARTZ B, ELLIOTT JA, BUTLER JC *et al.* Clusters of invasive group A streptococcal infections in family, hospital, and nursing home settings. *Clin Infect Dis* 1992; 15:277–84.
17. BRASILIER JL, BISTRONG HW, SPENCE WF. Streptococcal pneumonia in recent outbreaks in military recruitment populations. *Am J Med* 1968;44:580–99.
18. BARNHAM M, KERBY J. *Streptococcus pyogenes* pneumonia in residential homes: probability of spread of infection from the staff. *J Hosp Infect* 1981;2:255–7.
19. KEVY GW, LOWE BA. Streptococcal pneumonia and empyema in childhood. *N Engl J Med* 1961;205:738–43.
20. BREIMAN R, DAVIS J, FACKLAM R *et al.* Defining the group A streptococcal toxic shock syndrome: rationale and consensus definition. *JAMA* 1993;269:390–1.

21. BURMEISTER RW, OVERHOLT EL. Pneumonia caused by haemolytic *Streptococcus*. *Arch Int Med* 1968;III:367–75.

22. MCINTYRE HD, ARMSTRONG JG, MITCHELL CA. *Streptococcus pyogenes* pneumonia with abscess formation. *Aust NZ J Med* 1989;19:248–9.

23. CHAPNICK EK, GRADON JD, LUTWICK LI *et al.* Streptococcal toxic shock syndrome due to noninvasive pharyngitis. *Clin Infect Dis* 1992;14:1074–7.

24. COWAN MR, PRIMM PA, SCOTT SM, ABRAMO TJ, WIEBE RA. Serious group A β-hemolytic streptococcal infections complicating varicella. *Ann Emerg Med* 1994;23:818–22.

25. FRIEDEN TR, BIEBUYCK J, HIERHOLZER WJ JR. Lung abscess with group A β-hemolytic *Streptococcus*. *Arch Intern Med* 1991;151:1655–7.

26. STEVENS DL, GIBBONS AE, BERGSTROM R, WINN V. The Eagle effect revisited: efficacy of clindamycin, erythromycin, and penicillin in the treatment of streptococcal myositis. *J Infect Dis* 1988;158:23–8.

27. GEMMELL CG, PETERSON PK, SCHMELING D *et al.* Potentiation of opsonisation and phagocytosis of *Streptococcus pyogenes* following growth in the presence of clindamycin. *J Clin Invest* 1981;67:1249–56.

28. ROSS BROWN D, DAVIS NL, LEPAWSKY M, CUNNINGHAM J, KORTBEEK J. A multicenter review of the treatment of major truncal necrotizing infections with and without hyperbaric oxygen therapy. *Am J Surg* 1994;167:485–9.

29. FARLEY MM, CHRISTOPHER HARVEY R, STULL T *et al.* A population- based assessment of invasive disease due to group B *Streptococcus* in nonpregnant adults. *N Engl J Med* 1993;328:1807–11.

30. GALLAGHER PG, WATANAKUNAKRN C. Group B streptococcal bacteraemia in a community teaching hospital. *Am J Med* 1985;78:795–800.

31. BAYER A, CHOW A, ANTHONY B, GUZE L. Serious infections in adults due to group B streptococci. *Am J Med* 1976;61:498–503.

32. VERGHESE A, BERK SL, BOELEN LJ, KELLY SMITH J. Group B streptococcal pneumonia in the elderly. *Arch Intern Med* 1982;142:1642–5.

33. BRADLEY SF, GORDON JJ, BAUMGARTNER DD, MARASO WA, KAUFFMAN CA. Group C streptococcal bacteraemia: analysis of 88 cases. *Rev Infect Dis* 1991;13:270–80.

34. STONE DR. *Eikenella corrodens* and group C streptococci. *Clin Infect Dis* 1992;14:789.

35. JOSHI N, O'BRYAN T, APPELBAUM PC. Pleuropulmonary infections caused by *Eikenella corrodens*. *Rev Infect Dis* 1991;13:1207–12.

36. VARTIAN CV. Bacteremic pneumonia due to group C streptococci. *Rev Infect Dis* 1991;13:1029–30.

37. MIGUEL DE J, COLLAZOS J, ECHEVERRIA J *et al.* Group C streptococcal pneumonia and aneurysm infection. *Chest* 1993;104:1644.

38. WATSKY KL, KOLLISCH N, DENSEN P. Group G streptococcal bacteraemia. The clinical experience at Boston University Medical Center and a critical review of the literature. *Arch Intern Med* 1995;145:58–61.

39. LAM K, BAYER AS. Serious infections due to group G streptococci. Report of 15 cases with *in vitro–in vivo* correlations. *Am J Med* 1983;75:561–70.

40. PACKE GE, SMITH DF, REID TM, SMITH CC. Group G streptococcal bacteraemia – a review of thirteen cases in Grampian. *Scot Med J* 1991;36(2):42–4.

41. JOHNSON CC, TUNKEL AR. Viridans streptococci and groups C and G streptococci. In Bannett JE, Dolin R, eds. Mandell GL, *Principles and Practice of Infectious Disease.* 4th Ed; Churchill Livingstone 1995:1845–61.

42. WATANAKUNAKORN C, PANTELAKIS J. Alpha-hemolytic streptococcal bacteraemia: a review of 203 episodes during 1980–1981. *Scand J Infect Dis* 1993;25:403–8.

43. GAUDREAU C, DELAGE G, ROUSSEAU D, CANTOR ED. Bacteraemia caused by *viridans* streptococci in 71 children. *CMA J* 1981;125:1246–9.

44. PRATTER MR, IRWIN RS. Viridans streptococcal pulmonary parenchymal infections. *JAMA* 1980;243:2515–17.

45. MAHOMED GOOLAM A, FELDMAN C, SMITH C, PROMNITZ DA, KAKA S. Does primary *Streptococcus viridans* pneumonia exist? *S Afr Med J* 1992;82:432–4.

46. CATTO BA, JACOBS MR, SHLAES DM. *Streptococcus mitis*. A cause of serious infection in adults. *Arch Intern Med* 1987;147:885–8.

47. SARKAR TK, MURARKA RS, GILARDI GL. Primary *Streptococcus viridans* pneumonia. *Chest* 1989;96:831–4.

48. CARRASCOSA M, PEREZ-CASTRILLON JL, SAMPEDRO I, VALLE R, CILLERO L, MENDEZ MA. Lung abscess due to *Streptococcus mitis*: case report and review. *Clin Infect Dis* 1994;19:781–3.

49. BARTLETT JG. Diagnostic accuracy of transtracheal aspiration bacteriologic studies. *Am Rev Resp Dis* 1977;115:777–82.

50. MARRIE TJ. Bacteremic community-acquired pneumonia due to *viridans* group streptococci. *Clin Invest Med* 1993;16:38–44.

51. WHILEY RA, BEIGHTON D, WINSTANLEY TG, FRASER HY, HARDIE JM. *Streptococcus intermedius*, *Streptococcus constrellatus*, and *Streptococcus anginosus* (the *Streptococcus milleri* group): association with different body sites and clinical infections. *J Clin Microbiol* 1992:30:243–4.

52. HENDERSON A, WALL D. *Streptococcus milleri* liver abscess presenting as fulminant pneumonia. *Aust NZ J Surg* 1993;63:237–40.

53. DEVAUX Y, ARCHIMBAUD E, GUYOTAT D *et al.* Streptococcal bacteraemia in neutropenic adult patients. *Nouv Rev Franc Hematol* 1992;34:191–5.

54. BOCHUD P, CALANDRA T, FRANCIOLI P. Bacteraemia due to *viridans* streptococci in neutropenic patients: a review. *Am J Med* 1994;97:256–64.

55. CAMERON EWJ, APPELBAUM PC, PUDIFIN D, HUTTON WS, CHATTERTON SA, DUURSMA J. Characteristics and management of chronic destructive pneumonia. *Thorax* 1980;35:340–6.

56. CARRATALÁ J, GUDIOL F. Life-threatening infections due to penicillin-resistant *viridans* streptococci. *Curr Opin Infect Dis* 1995;8:123–6.

57. SHLAES DM, LEVY J, WOLINSKY E. Enterococcal bacteraemia without endocarditis. *Arch Intern Med* 1981;141:578.

58. YU VL. Enterococcal superinfection and colonization after therapy with Moxalactam a new broad-spectrum antibiotic. *Ann Intern Med* 1981;94:784–5.

59. BERK SL, VERGHESE A, HOLTSCLAW SA, KELLY SMITH J. Enterococcal pneumonia. Occurrence in patients receiving broad-spectrum antibiotic regimens and enteral feeding. *Am J Med* 1983;74:153–4.

60. BONTEN MJM, VAN TIEL FH, VAN DER GEEST S, STOBBERINGH EE, GAILLARD CA. *Enterococcus faecalis* pneumonia complicating topical antimicrobial prophylaxis. *N Engl J Med* 1993;328:209–10.

61. MONTECALVO MA, HOROWITZ H, GEDRIS C *et al.* Outbreak of Vancomycin-, Ampicillin- , and Aminoglycoside- resistant *Enterococcus faecium* bacteraemia in an adult oncology unit. *Antimicrob Agents Chemother* 1994;38:1363–7.

62. ASCHER DP, ZBICK C, WHITE C, FISHER GW. Infection due to *Stomatococcus mucilaginosus*: 10 cases and review. *Rev Infect Dis* 1991;13:1048–52.

63. AL FIAR F, ELLIS M, QADRI SMH, ERNST P. *Stomatococcus mucilaginosus* meningitis in a patient with acute lymphoblastic leukemia. *Ann Sandi Med* 1995;15:393–5

64. HENWICK S, KOEHLER M, PATRICK CC. Complications of bacteraemia due to

Stomatococcus mucilaginosus in neutropenic children. *Clin Infect Dis* 1993;17:667–71.

65. DOMINGO P, SERRA J, SAMBEAT MA, AUSINA V. Pneumonia due to *Listeria monocytogenes*. *Clin Infect Dis* 1992;14:787–9.

66. JURADO RL, FARLEY MM, PEREIRA E, HARVEY RC, SCHUCHAT A, WENGER JD, STEPHENS DS. Increased risk of meningitis and bacteraemia due to *Listeria monocytogenes* in patients with human immunodeficiency virus infection. *Clin Infect Dis* 1993;17:224–7.

67. MAZZULLI T, SALIT IE. Pleural fluid infection caused by *Listeria monocytogenes:* case report and review. *Rev Infect Dis* 1991;13:564–70.

68. WHITELOCK-JONES L, CARSWELL J, RASMUSSEN KC. *Listeria* pneumonia. *S Afr Med J* 1989;75:188–9.

69. BOUCHER M, YONEKURA ML, WALLACE RJ, PHELAN JP. Adult respiratory distress syndrome: a rare manifestation of *Listeria monocytogenes* infection in pregnancy. *Am J Obstet Gynecol* 1984;149:686–8.

70. HIRSCHL RB, BUTLER M, COBURN CE, BARTLETT RH, BAUMGART S. Listeria monocytogenes and severe newborn respiratory failure supported with extracorporeal membrane oxygenation. *Arch Pediatr Adolesc Med* 1994;148:513–17.

71. PEARSON HE. Human infections caused by organisms of the *Bacillus* species. *Am J Clin Pathol* 1970;53:506–15.

72. TUAZON CU, MURRAY HW, LEVY C, SOLNY MN, CURTIN JA, SHEAGREN JN. Serious infections from *Bacillus* spp. *JAMA* 1979;241:1137–40.

73. SLIMAN R, REHM S, SHLAES DM. Serious infections caused by *Bacillus* species. *Medicine* 1987;66:218–23.

74. ISAACSON P, JACOBS PH, MACKENZIE AMR, MATHEWS AW. Pseudotumour of the lung caused by infection with *Bacillus sphaericus*. *J Clin Pathol* 1976;29:806–11.

75. COONROD JD, LEADLEY PJ, EICKHOFF TC. Bacillus cereus pneumonia and bacteraemia. *Am Rev Resp Dis* 1971;103:711–14.

76. JONSSON S, CLARRIDGE J, YOUNG EJ. Necrotizing pneumonia and empyema caused by *Bacillus cereus* and *Clostridium bifermentans*. *Am Rev Resp Dis* 1983;127:357–9.

77. GASCOIGNE AD, RICHARDS J, GOULD K, GIBSON GJ. Successful treatment of *Bacillus cereus* infection with ciprofloxacin. *Thorax* 1991;46:220–221.

78. LEFF A, JACOBS R, GOODING V, HAUCH J, CONTE J, STULBARG M. *Bacillus cereus* pneumonia. Survival in a patient with cavitary disease treated with gentamicin. *Am J Rev Resp Dis* 1977;115:151–4.

79. JEVON GP, MICHAEL DUNNE JR W, JOHN HICKS M, LANGSTON C. *Bacillus cereus* pneumonia in premature neonates: a report of two cases. *Pediatr Infect Dis J* 1993; 12:251–3.

80. COUDRON PE, PAYNE JM, MARKOWITZ SM. Pneumonia and empyema infection associated with a *Bacillus* species that resembles *B. alvei J Clin Microbiol* 1991;29:1777–9.

81. FELDMAN S, PEARSON TA. Fatal *Bacillus cereus* pneumonia and sepsis in a child with cancer. *Clin Pediatr* 1974;13:649–55.

82. BEKEMEYER WB, ZIMMERMAN GA. Life-threatening complications associated with *Bacillus cereus* pneumonia. *Am Rev Resp Dis* 1985;131:466–9.

83. MALIK AS, JOHARI MR. Pneumonia, pericarditis, and endocarditis in a child with *Corynebacterium xerosis* septicemia. *Clin Infect Dis* 1995;20:191–2.

84. WALLET F, MARQUETTE CH, COURCOL RJ. Multiresistant *Corynebacterium xerosis* as a cause of pneumonia in a patient with acute leukemia. *Clin Infect Dis* 1994;18:845–6.

85. COWLING P, HALL L. *Corynebacterium striatum*: a clinically significant isolate from sputum in chronic obstructive airways disease. *J Infect* 1993;20:335–6.

86. MARTINEZ-MARTINEZ L, SUAREZ AI, DEL CARMEN ORTEGA M, RODRIGUEZ-JIMENEZ R. Fatal pulmonary infection caused by *Corynebacterium striatum*. *Clin Infect Dis* 1994;19:806–7.

87. AHMED K, KAWAKAMI K, WATANABE K, MITSUSHIMA H, NAGATAKE T, MATSUMOTO K. *Corynebacterium pseudodiphtheriticum*: a respiratory tract pathogen. *Clin Infect Dis* 1995;20:41–6.

88. MANZELLA JP, KELLOGG JA, PARSEY KS. *Corynebacterium pseudodiphtheriticum*: a respiratory tract pathogen in adults. *Clin Infect Dis* 1995;20:37–40.

89. GOLUB B, FALK G, SPINK WW. Lung abscess due to *Corynebacterium equi*. Report of first human infection. *Ann Intern Med* 1967;66:1174–7.

90. SCOTT MA, GRAHAM BS, VERRALL R, DIXON R, SCHAFFNER W, THAM KT. *Rhodococcus equi* – an increasingly recognized opportunistic pathogen. Report of 12 cases and review of 65 cases in the literature. *Am J Clin Pathol* 1995;103:649–55.

91. KWON KY, COLBY TV. *Rhodococcus equi* pneumonia and pulmonary malakoplakia in acquired immunodeficiency syndrome. Pathologic features. *Arch Pathol Lab Med* 1994;118:744–8.

92. SEGOVIA J, PULPON LA, CRESPO MG *et al*. Rhodococcus equi: first case in a heart transplant recipient. *J Heart Lung Transpl* 1994;13:332–5.

93. LASKY JA, PULKINGHAM N, POWERS MA, DURACK DT. *Rhodococcus equi* causing human pulmonary infection: review of 29 cases. *South Med J* 1991;84:1217–20.

94. HARVEY RL, SUNSTRUM JC. *Rhodococcus equi* infection in patients with and without human immunodeficiency virus infection. *Rev Infect Dis* 1991;13:139–45.

95. SPARK RP, MCNEIL MM, BROWN JM, LASKER BA, MONTANO MA, GARFIELD MD. *Rhodococcus* species fatal infection in an immunocompetent host. *Arch Pathol Lab Med* 1993;117:515–20.

96. EMMONS W, REICHWEIN B, WINSLOW DL. *Rhodococcus equi* infection in the patient with AIDS: literature review and report of an unusual case. *Rev Infect Dis* 1991;13:91–6.

97. SHAPIRO JM, ROMNEY BM, WEIDEN MD, WHITE CS, O'TOOLE KM. *Rhodococcus equi* endobronchial mass with lung abscess in a patient with AIDS. *Thorax* 1992;47:62–3.

98. GILLET-JUVIN K, STERN M, ISRAEL-BIET D, PENAUD D, CARNOT F. A highly unusual combination of pulmonary pathogens in an HIV infected patient. *Scand J Infect Dis* 1994;26:215–17.

99. MAGNANI G, ELIA GF, MCNEIL MM *et al*.. Rhodococcus equi cavitary pneumonia in HIV-infected patients: an unsuspected opportunistic pathogen. *J Acquir Immune Defic Syndr* 1992;5:1059–64.

100. MCNEIL MM, BROWN JM. Distribution and antimicrobial susceptibility of *Rhodococcus equi* from clinical specimens. *Eur J Epidemiol* 1992;8:437–43.

101. NORDMANN P, ROUVEX E, GUENOUNOU M, NICOLAS MH. Pulmonary abscess due to a rifampin and fluoroquinolone resistant *Rhodococcus equi* strain in HIV infected patient. *Eur J Clin Microbiol Infect Dis* 1992;11:557–8.

102. CHAVANET P, BONNOTTE B, CAILLOT D, PORTIER H. Imipenem/teicoplanin for *Rhodococcus equi* pulmonary infection in AIDS patient. *Lancet* 1991;337:794–5.

103. VAN ETTA LL, FILICE GA, FERGUSON RM, GERDING DN. *Corynebacterium equi*: a review of 12 cases of human infection. *Rev Infect Dis* 1983:5:1012–18.

104. COCKERELL CJ. Rochalimaea infections. Curr Opin Infect Dis 1995;8:130–6.

105. SLATER LN, Min K-W. Polypoid endobronchial lesions. A manifestation of bacillary angiomatosis. *Chest* 1992;102:972–4.

106. DALE EVERETT E, EVANS KA, BETH HENRY R, MCDONALD G. Human ehrlichiosis in adults after tick exposure. *Ann Intern Med* 1994;120:730–5.

107. FISHBEIN DB, DAWSON JE, ROBINSON

LE. Human ehrlichiosis in the United States, 1985–1990. *Ann Intern Med* 1994;120:736–43.

108. KOPPES GM, ELLENBOGEN C, GEBHART RJ. Group Y meningococcal disease in United States Air Force Recruits. *Am J Med* 1977;62:661–6.

109. SMILACK JD. Group Y meningococcal disease. Twelve cases at an Army training center. *Ann Intern Med* 1974;81:740.

110. YOUNG LS, MARC LAFORCE F, JAMES HEAD J, FEELY JC, BENNETT JV. A simultaneous outbreak of meningococcal and influenza infections. *N Engl J Med* 1987;287:5–9.

111. DAVIES BI, SPANJAARD L, DANKERT J. Meningococcal chest infections in a general hospital. *Eur J Clin Microbiol Infect Dis* 1991;10:399–404.

112. KLOCKARS M, KLEEMOLA M, LEINONEN M, KOSKELA M. Serum adenosine deaminase in viral and bacterial pneumonia. *Chest* 1991;99:623–6.

113. GILRANE T, TRACY JD, GREENLEE RM, SCHELPERT III JW, BRANDSTETTER RD. Neisseria sicca pneumonia. *Am J Med* 1985;78:1038–40.

114. THORSTEINSSON SB, MINUTH JN, MUSHER DM. Postpneumonectomy empyema due to *Neisseria mucosa*. *Am J Clin Path* 1975;64:534–6.

115. MORLA N, GUIBOURDENCHE M, RIOU J-Y. *Neisseria* spp and AIDS. *J Clin Microbiol* 1992;30:2290–4.

116. DELANO P, DELANO M. Sur les rapports des kystes de *carinii* du poumon des rats avec le *Trypanosoma lewisii*. *CR Acad Sci* 1912;155:658–60.

117. VAN DER MEER G, BRUG SL. Infection par *Pneumocystis* chez l'home et chez les animaux. *Ann Soc Belg Med Trop* 1942;22:301–9.

118. EDMAN JC, KOVACS JA, MASUR H, SANTI DV, ELWOOD HJ, SOGUN MI. Ribosomal RNA sequences show *Pneumocystis carinii* to be a member of the fungi. *Nature* 1988;334:519–22.

119. WAKEFIELD AE, PETERS SE, BANERJI S *et al. Pneumocystis carinii* shows DNA homology with the ustomycetous red yeast fungi. *Mol Microbiol* 1992;6:1903–11.

120. BAUER NL, PARULSRUD JR, BARTLETT MS, SMITH JW, WILDE CE. *Pneumocystis carinii* organisms obtained from rats, ferrets and mice are antigenically different. *Infect Immunol* 1993;61:1315–9.

121. PIFER LL, HUGHES WT, STAGNO S, WOODS D. *Pneumocystis carinii* infection; evidence for high prevalence in normal and immunosuppressed children. *Pediatrics* 1978;61:35–41.

122. TRAVIS WD, PITTALUGA S, LIPSCHIK GY *et al.* Atypical pathologic manifestations of *Pneumocystis carinii* pneumonia in the acquired immune deficiency syndrome. *Am J Surg Pathol* 1990;14:615–25.

123. FOLEY NM, GRIFFITHS MH, MILELR RF. Histologically atypical *Pneumocystis carinii* pneumonia. *Thorax* 1993; 48:996–1001.

124. GRYZAN S, PARADIS IL, ZEEVI A *et al.* Unexpectedly high incidence of *Pneumocystis carinii* infection after lung–heart transplantation. *Am Rev Resp Dis* 1988;137:1268–74.

125. DUMMER JS, MONTER CG, GRIFFITH BP, HARDESTY RL, PARADIS IL, HO M. Infections in heart–lung recipients. *Transplantation* 1986;41:725–9.

126. OLSEN SL, RENLUND DG, O'CONNELL JB *et al.* Prevention of *Pneumocystis carinii* pneumonia in cardiac transplant recipients by trimethoprim sulfamethoxazole. *Transplantation* 1993;56:359–62.

127. MUNOZ A. Trends in the incidence of outcomes defining acquired immunodeficiency syndrome (AIDS) in the Multicenter AIDS Cohort Study: 1985–1991. *Am J Epidemiol* 1993;137:423–38.

128. BOURBIGOT B, BENSOUSSAN T, GARO B *et al.* CD4 T-lymphocyte counts as predictors of pneumonia after kidney transplantation. *Transpl Proc* 1993;25:1491–2.

129. CHAVE J, DAVID S, WAUTERS J *et al.* Transmission of Pneumocystis carinii from AIDS patients to other immunosuppressed patients: a cluster of *Pneumocystis carinii* pneumonia in renal transplant patients. *AIDS* 1991;5:927–32.

130. JACOBS JL, LIBBY DM, WINTERS RA, GELMONT DM, HARTMAN BJ, LAURENCE J. A cluster of *Pneumocystis carinii* pneumonia in adults without predisposing illnesses. *N Engl J Med* 1991;324:246–50.

131. SINGER C, ARMSTRONG D, ROSEN PP, SCHOTTENFELD D. *Pneumocystis carinii* pneumonia: a cluster of eleven cases. *Ann Intern Med* 1975;82:772–7.

132. CANO S, CAPOTE F, PEREIRA A, CALDERON E, CASTILLO J. *Pneumocystis carinii* pneumonia in patients without predisposing illnesses. Acute episode and follow-up of five cases. *Chest* 1993;104:376–81.

133. KOVACS JA, HIEMENZ JW, MACHER AM *et al. Pneumocystis carinii* pneumonia: a comparison between patients with the acquired immunodeficiency syndrome and patients with other immunodeficiencies. *Ann Intern Med* 1984;100:663–71.

134. RAVIGLIONE MC. Extrapulmonary pneumocytosis: The first 50 cases. *Rev Infect Dis* 1990;12:1127–38.

135. CENTRES FOR DISEASE CONTROL. Revision o the CDC Surveillance case definition for acquired immunodeficiency syndrome. *MMWR* 1987;36(Suppl):35–155.

136. LEVINE SJ, MASUR H, GILL VJ *et al.* Effect of aerosolised pentamidine prophylaxis on the diagnosis of *Pneumocystis carinii* pneumonia by induced sputum examination in patients infected with the human immunodeficiency virus. *Am Rev Resp Dis* 1991;144:760–4.

137. ELLIS ME, SPENCE D, BOUCHAMA A *et al.* Open lung biopsy provides a higher and more specific diagnostic yield compared to broncho-alveolar lavage in immunocompromised patients. *Scand J Infect Dis* 1995;27:157–62.

138. KIRSCH CM, JENSEN WA, KAGAWA FT *et al.* Analysis of induced sputum for the diagnosis of recurrent *Pneumocystis carinii* pneumonia. *Chest* 1992;102:1152–4.

139. WAKEFIELD AE, GUIVER L, MILLER RF, HOPKIN JM. DNA amplification on induced sputum samples for diagnosis of *Pneumocystis carinii* pneumonia. *Lancet* 1991;337:1378–9.

140. WAKEFIELD AE, MILLER RF, GUIVER LA, HOPKIN JM. Oropharyngeal samples for detection of *Pneumocystis carinii* by DNA amplifications. *Quart J Med* 1993;86:401–6.

141. LIPSCHIK GY, GILL VJ, LUNDGREN JD *et al.* Improved diagnosis of *Pneumocystis carinii* infection by polymerase chain reaction on induced sputum and blood. *Lancet* 1992;340:203–6.

142. BUSCOMBE JR, OYEN WJG, GRANT A *et al.* ^{111}Indium labelled polyclonal human immunoglobulin: identifying focal infection in patients positive for human immunodeficiency virus. *J Nucl Med* 1993;34:1621–5.

143. SMITH DE, FORBES A, DAVIES S, BARTON SE, GAZZARD BG. Diagnosis of *Pneumocystis carinii* pneumonia in HIV antibody positive patients by simple outpatient assessment. *Thorax* 1992;47:1005–9.

144. SMITH RM, IWAMOTO GK, RICHERSON HB *et al.* Trimethoprim – sulfamethoxazole desensitisation in the acquired immunodeficiency syndrome. *Ann Intern Med* 1987;106:335.

145. JEFFREY AA, BULLEN C, MILLER RF. Intensive care management of *Pneumocystis carinii* pneumonia. *Care Crit III* 1993;9:258–60.

146. HUGHES WT, KUHN S, FELDMAN S *et al.* Successful chemoprophylaxis for *Pneumocystis carinii* pneumonitis. *N Engl J Med* 1977;297:1419–26.

147. WINSTON DJ, HO WG, GALE RP, CHAMPLIN RE. Prophylaxis of infection in bone marrow transplants. *Eur J Cancer Clin Oncol* 1988;24(Suppl):S15.

148. HIGGINS RM, BLOOM SL, HOPKIN JM,

MORRIS PJ. The risks and benefits of low-dose co-trimoxazole prophylaxis for *Pneumocystis* pneumonia in renal transplantation. *Transplantation* 1989;47:558.

149. KRAMER KR, STOEHR C, LEWISTON NJ, STARNES V, THEODORE J. Trimethoprim-sulfamethoxazole prophylaxis for *Pneumocystis carinii* infections in heart–lung and lung transplantation: how effective and for how long? *Transplantation* 1992;53:586–9.

150. NATHAN SD, ROSS DJ, ZAKOWSKI P, KASS RM, KOERNER SK. Utility of inhaled pentamidine prophylaxis in lung transplant recipients. *Chest* 1994;105:417–20.

Index

Note: main discussions of drugs are in bold typeface